**The Maudsley®
Prescribing Guidelines
in Psychiatry**

The Maudsley Guidelines

Other books in the *Maudsley Prescribing Guidelines* series include:

The Maudsley Practice Guidelines for Physical Health Conditions in Psychiatry
David Taylor, Fiona Gaughran, Toby Pillinger

The Maudsley Guidelines on Advanced Prescribing in Psychosis
Paul Morrison, David Taylor, Phillip McGuire

The Maudsley Prescribing Guidelines for Mental Health Conditions in Physical Illness
Siobhan Gee, David M. Taylor

The Maudsley Deprescribing Guidelines: Antidepressants, Benzodiazepines, Gabapentinoids and Z-drugs
Mark Horowitz, David M. Taylor

The Maudsley® Prescribing Guidelines in Psychiatry

15th Edition

David M. Taylor, BSc, MSc, PhD, FFRPS, FRPharmS, FRCPEdin, FRCPsychHon

Director of Pharmacy and Pathology, Maudsley Hospital and
Professor of Psychopharmacology, King's College, London, UK

Thomas R. E. Barnes, MBBS, MD, FRCPsych, DSc

Emeritus Professor of Clinical Psychiatry at Imperial College London and joint head of the Prescribing
Observatory for Mental Health at the Royal College of Psychiatrists' Centre for Quality Improvement, London, UK

Allan H. Young, MB, ChB, MPhil, PhD, FRCP, FRCPsych

Chair of Mood Disorders and Director of the Centre for Affective Disorders in the Department of Psychological Medicine
in the Institute of Psychiatry, Psychology and Neuroscience at King's College, London, UK

WILEY Blackwell

This edition first published 2025
© 2025 David M. Taylor

The right of David M. Taylor, Thomas R. E. Barnes and Allan H. Young to be identified as the authors of this has been asserted in accordance with law.

Registered Office(s)
John Wiley & Sons, Inc., 111 River Street, Hoboken, NJ 07030, USA
John Wiley & Sons Ltd, New Era House, 8 Oldlands Way, Bognor Regis, West Sussex, PO22 8NQ, UK

For details of our global editorial offices, customer services, and more information about Wiley products visit us at www.wiley.com.

The manufacturer's authorized representative according to the EU General Product Safety Regulation is Wiley-VCH GmbH, Boschstr. 12, 69469 Weinheim, Germany, e-mail: Product_Safety@wiley.com.

Wiley also publishes its books in a variety of electronic formats and by print-on-demand. Some content that appears in standard print versions of this book may not be available in other formats.

Library of Congress Cataloging-in-Publication Data Applied for:

Paperback: 9781394238767

Cover Design: Wiley

Set in 10/12pt Sabon by Straive, Pondicherry, India

Printed and bound in Great Britain by Bell and Bain Ltd, Glasgow
B127854_110325

Contents

Preface

The *Maudsley® Prescribing Guidelines in Psychiatry* is now just one of several books in the Maudsley® *Guidelines* series. Since the publication of the 14th edition of the 'big' *MPG*, it has been joined by the *Maudsley® Deprescribing Guidelines: Antidepressants, Benzodiazepines, Gabapentinoids and Z-drugs* and by the *Maudsley® Prescribing Guidelines for Mental Health Conditions in Physical Illness*. These books cover some of the ground usually tackled in the main *MPG* but in much greater detail. In an effort to reduce repetition we have, in this 15th edition, left out (or let out) sections on such subjects as delirium, psychotropics in surgery and alternative routes of antidepressant administration and considerably reduced the size of sections on stopping psychotropics. What space has been made available by these changes has been filled by new sections on, for example, premenstrual syndrome, menopause, gambling disorder, ADHD in adults and relational aspects of prescribing practice.

This 15th edition of the *MPG* appears at a time when there is a growing antipathy towards the use of psychotropic drugs in mental illness. The prescribing advice given here assumes a decision to prescribe has already been made and so, to a large extent, we skirt the issue of whether or not prescribing is necessarily the right thing to do. Nonetheless, we do acknowledge that drug treatment is not always the best treatment for everyone in every situation. There are of course a range of effective non-drug treatments for mental health problems. The advice and guidance given in this and previous editions is aimed at optimising prescribing practice rather than promoting prescribing *per se*.

As ever, I and my fellow authors are indebted to a large number of expert contributors who have enabled us to provide information and guidance on such a wide range of topics; a feature that is possibly unique to the *Maudsley® Prescribing Guidelines in Psychiatry*. Sincere thanks are also due to Ivana Clark, the managing editor of this edition.

Even though some sections have been transplanted to other books in *The Guidelines* series, the scope of this edition is greater than the last and, as a consequence, it is a weightier book. It is probably worth pointing out that a special effort has been made to be economic with words and references although I suspect this is of little consolation to those lugging the book from ward to ward or home to hospital. It is the 'big' *MPG*, after all.

David M. Taylor
January 2025

Acknowledgements

The following have contributed to the 15th edition of *The Maudsley® Prescribing Guidelines in Psychiatry*.

Aditya Sharma
Alys Cawson
Andrea Danese
Anna Walder
Bruce Clark
Daniel Harwood
Daniel Hayes
David Rogalski
Delia Bishara
Derek Tracy
Dimitrios Chartonas
Ebenezer Oloyede
Emily Finch
Emmert Roberts
Eromona Whiskey
Ewa Zadeh
Faiza Hoda
Frankie Anderson
Haroula Konstantinidou
Ian Osborne
Ilaria Bonoldi
Ivana Clark
Jacob Kranowski
Justin Sauer
Kalliopi Vallianatou
Kate Organ

Livia Martucci
Mariam Mustapha
Marinos Kyriakopoulos
Mark Horowitz
Marta Di Forti
Martina Carboni
Mary Thornton
Michael Craig
Michael Newson
Michele Sie
Mike Kelleher
Nicola Funnell
Nicola Kalk
Nicoletta Adamo
Oliver Howes
Paul Gringras
Paul Moran
Petrina Douglas-Hall
Phillip Timms
Ray McGrath
Shubhra Mace
Siobhan Gee
Stephanie Lewis
Tennyson Lee
Thomas Reilly
Yuya Mizuno

Contributors' conflict of interest

Many of the contributors to *The Guidelines* have received funding from pharmaceutical manufacturers for research, consultancy or lectures. Readers should be aware that these relationships inevitably colour opinions on such matters as drug selection or preference.

We cannot therefore guarantee that guidance provided here is free of indirect influence of the pharmaceutical industry but hope to have mitigated this risk by providing copious literature support for statements made. As regards direct influence, no pharmaceutical company has been allowed to view or comment on any drafts or proofs of *The Guidelines* and none has made any request for the inclusion or omission of any topic, advice or guidance. To this extent, *The Guidelines* have been written independent of the pharmaceutical industry.

List of abbreviations

5HT3	5-hydroxytryptamine 3	AF	atrial fibrillation
22q11.2DS	22q11.2 deletion syndrome	AIDS	acquired immune deficiency syndrome
%w/v	percentage weight per volume	ALAI	aripiprazole long-acting injection
AACAP	American Academy of Child and Adolescent Psychiatry	ALP	alkaline phosphate
		ALT	alanine aminotransferase
ACE	angiotensin-converting enzyme	AMPA	alpha-amino-3-hydroxy-5-methyl-4-isoxazolepropionic acid
Ach	acetylcholine	AN	anorexia nervosa
AChE	acetylcholinesterase	ANC	absolute neutrophil count
AChE-I	acetylcholinesterase inhibitors	ANI	asymptomatic neurocognitive impairment
ACOG	American College of Obstetricians and Gynecologists	APP	amyloid precursor protein
		ARIA	amyloid-related imaging abnormality
AD	Alzheimer's disease	ART	antiretroviral therapy
ADAPT	Adolescent Depression Antidepressants and Psychotherapy Trial	ASD	autism spectrum disorder
		AST	aspartate aminotransferase
ADAS-cog	Alzheimer's Disease Assessment Scale – cognitive subscale	ATPase	adenosine triphosphatase
		AUD	alcohol use disorder
ADH	alcohol dehydrogenase	AUDIT	Alcohol Use Disorders Identification Test
ADHD	attention deficit hyperactivity disorder	Aβ	beta amyloid
		BAC	blood alcohol concentration
ADIS	Anxiety Disorders Interview Schedule	BAP	British Association for Psychopharmacology
ADL	activities of daily living		
ADR	adverse drug reactions	BBB	blood–brain barrier
AEC	Anticholinergic Effect on Cognition Scale	bd	twice a day
		BDD	body dysmorphic disorder

BDNF	brain-derived neurotrophic factor	CNS	central nervous system
BED	binge eating disorder	COCP	combined oral contraceptive pill
BEN	benign ethnic neutropenia	COMT	catechol-O-methyltransferase
BMI	body mass index		
BN	bulimia nervosa	COPD	chronic obstructive pulmonary disease
BNF	*British National Formulary*	COWS	Clinical Opiate Withdrawal Scale
BP	blood pressure		
BPD	Borderline personality disorder	CQC	Care Quality Commission
BPSD	behavioural and psychological symptoms of dementia	CrCl	creatinine clearance
		CRLTA	clozapine-related life-threatening agranulocytosis
BuChE	butyrylcholinesterase		
CAMS	Childhood Anxiety Multimodal Study	CRP	C-reactive protein
		CTO	Community Treatment Order
CATIE	Clinical Antipsychosis Trials of Intervention Effectiveness	CUtLASS	Cost Utility of the Latest Antipsychotic Drugs in Schizophrenia Study
CBT	cognitive behavioural therapy		
CDRS	Children's Depression Rating Scale	CVD	cardiovascular disease
		CY-BOCS	Children's Yale-Brown Obsessive Compulsive Scale
CDR-SB	Clinical Dementia Rating Scale – Sums of Boxes		
CDRS-R	Children's Depression Rating Scale-Revised	CYP	cytochrome P450
		DAI	Drug Attitude Inventory
CGAS	Children's Global Assessment Scale	DBM	dibenzoylmethane
		DBT	dialectical behaviour therapy
CGI	Clinical Global Impression	DEXA	dual-energy x-ray absorptiometry
CI	confidence interval		
CIBIC-plus	Clinician's Interview-Based Impression of Change plus caregiver input	DHA	docosahexaenoic acid
		DHEA	dehydroepiandrosterone
		DIVA-5	Diagnostic Interview for ADHD in Adults
CIGH	clozapine-induced GI hypomotility	DLB	dementia with Lewy bodies
CIWA-Ar	Clinical Institute Withdrawal Assessment of Alcohol Scale Revised	DMDD	disruptive mood dysregulation disorder
		DMq	dextromethorphan and low-dose quinidine
CK	creatine kinase		
CKD	chronic kidney disease	DOACs	direct-acting oral anticoagulants
CKD-EPI	Chronic Kidney Disease Epidemiology Collaboration	DoLS	Deprivation of Liberty Safeguards

DSM-5	*Diagnostic and Statistical Manual of Mental Disorders*, 5th edition	GGT	gamma-glutamyl transferase
DVLA	Driver and Vehicle Licensing Agency	GHB	gamma-hydroxybutyrate
		GHB/GBL	gamma-hydroxybutyrate/ gamma-butyrolactone
ECG	electrocardiogram	GI	gastrointestinal
ECT	electroconvulsive therapy	GLP-1	glucagon-like peptide-1
EEG	electroencephalogram	GP	general practitioner
eGFR	estimated glomerular filtration rate	GRDS	gastric reduction duodenal switch
EMDR	eye movement desensitisation and reprocessing	GSM	genitourinary symptoms of menopause
		HAD	HIV-associated dementia
EOSS	early-onset schizophrenia spectrum	HAM-D	Hamilton Depression Rating Scale
EPA	eicosapentaenoic acid	HAND	HIV-assocated neurocognitive disorders
EPS	extrapyramidal symptoms		
EPSE	extrapyramidal side effect		
ER	extended release	HbA_{1c}	glycated haemoglobin
ERK	extracellular signal-regulated kinase	HCl	hydrogen chloride
		HD	Huntington's disease
ES	effect size	HDL	high-density lipoprotein
EU	European Union	hERG	human ether-a-go-go-related gene
FBC	full blood count		
FDA	Food and Drug Administration	HIV	human immunodeficiency virus
FGA	first-generation antipsychotic	HLA	human lymphocyte antigen
FPG	fasting plasma glucose	HPA	hypothalamic–pituitary–adrenal
FRAMES principles	feedback, responsibility, advice, menu, empathy, self-efficacy		
		HR	hazard ratio
		HRT	hormone replacement therapy
FSH	follicle-stimulating hormone	IADL	instrumental activities of daily living
FTI	Fatal Toxicity Index		
GABA	gamma-aminobutyric acid	ICD-10	*International Classification of Diseases 10*
GAD	generalised anxiety disorder		
		ICH	intracranial/intracerebral haemorrhage
GASS	Glasgow Antipsychotic Side-effect Scale	IGSLI	International Study Group on Lithium
GBL	gamma-butyrolactone		
G-CSF	granulocyte colony-stimulating factor	IHD	ischaemic heart disease
		IM	intramuscular
GERD	gastro-esophageal reflux disease	INR	international normalised ratio
GFR	glomerular filtration rate	IR	immediate release

ISBD	International Society for Bipolar Disorders		MR	modified release
ISTSS	International Society for Traumatic Stress Studies		MS	mood stabilisers/multiple sclerosis
IV	intravenous		MSM	men who have sex with men
Kiddie-SADS	Kiddie-Schedule for Affective Disorders and Schizophrenia		NAPLS	North American Prodromal Longitudinal Studies
LAI	long-acting injection		NaSSA	noradrenergic and specific serotonergic antidepressant
LC-MS	liquid chromatography and mass spectrometry		NbN	neuroscience-based nomenclature
LD	learning disabilities		NEET	not in education, employment or education
LDL	low-density lipoprotein			
LFT	liver function test		NICE	National Institute for Health and Care Excellence
LGIB	lower gastrointestinal bleeding			
LMP	last menstrual period		NIMH	National Institute of Mental Health
MADRS	Montgomery–Asberg Depression Rating Scale		NMDA	N-methyl-D-aspartate
MAO	monoamine oxidase		NMDAR	N-methyl-D-aspartate receptor
MAOI	monoamine oxidase inhibitor		NMS	neuroleptic malignant syndrome
MARS	Medication Adherence Rating Scale		NNH	number needed to harm
MASC	Multidimensional Anxiety Scale for Children		NNT	number needed to treat
MCA	Mental Capacity Act		NPIS	National Poisons Information Service
MCI	mild cognitive impairment			
MDD	major depressive disorder		NPS	new psychoactive substances
MDMA	3,4-methylenedioxymethamphetamine		NPV	negative predictive value
MDRD	Modification of Diet in Renal Disease		NRT	nicotine replacement therapy
MDT	multidisciplinary team		NSAID	non-steroidal anti-inflammatory drug
MFQ	Mood and Feelings Questionnaire		OCD	obsessive compulsive disorder
MHA	Mental Health Act			
MHRA	Medicines and Healthcare products Regulatory Authority		od	once daily
			OGTT	oral glucose tolerance test
MI	myocardial infarction			
MMSE	Mini Mental State Examination		on	at night
			OOWS	Objective Opiate Withdrawal Scale
MND	mild neurocognitive disorder			
			OR	odds ratio
MoCA	Montreal Cognitive Assessment		OST	opioid substitution treatment

PAIN	Peri-operative Pain and Addiction Interdisciplinary Network	PTSD	post-traumatic stress disorder
PANDAS	paediatric autoimmune neuropsychiatric disorder associated with *Streptococcus*	PUFA	polyunsaturated fatty acid
		PWE	people with epilepsy
		RANZCP	Royal Australian and New Zealand College of Psychiatrists
PANS	paediatric acute-onset neuropsychiatric syndrome	RC	Responsible Clinician
		RCADS	Revised Children's Anxiety and Depression Scale
PANSS	Positive and Negative Syndrome Scale	RCT	randomised controlled trial
PAWS	post-acute withdrawal syndrome	REM	rapid eye movement
PBA	pseudobulbar affect	RID	relative infant dose
PD	Parkinson's disease	RIMA	reversible inhibitor of monoamine oxidase A
PDSS	post-injection delirium sedation syndrome	RLAI	risperidone long-acting injection
PE	pulmonary embolism	ROMI	Rating of Medication Influences
PET	positron emission tomography	RR	respiratory rate/risk ratio
PG	propylene glycol	RRBI	restricted repetitive behaviours and interests
P-gp	P-glycoprotein	RT	rapid tranquillisation
PHQ-9	Patient Health Questionnaire-9	RTA	road traffic accident
PLWH	people living with HIV	rTMS	repetitive transcranial magnetic stimulation
PMDD	premenstrual dysphoric disorder	RUPP	Research Units on Paediatric Psychopharmacology
PMR	postmortem redistribution	RYGB	Roux-en-Y gastric bypass
PMS	premenstrual syndrome	SADQ	Severity of Alcohol Dependence Questionnaire
po	by mouth		
POI	premature ovarian insufficiency	SAWS	Short Alcohol Withdrawal Scale
PORT	Program of Rehabilitation and Therapy	SC	subcutaneous
PP1M	paliperidone long-acting injection 1-monthly	SCARED	Screen for Child Anxiety and Related Emotional Disorders
PP3M	paliperidone long-acting injection 3-monthly	SCRA	synthetic cannabinoid receptor agonist
PPH	postpartum haemorrhage	SD	sexual dysfunction
PPI	proton pump inhibitor	SERM	selective oestrogen receptor modulators
PPV	positive predictive value		
prn	as required		
PSSD	post-SSRI sexual dysfunction		
PT	prothrombin time	SERT	serotonin receptor

SGA	second-generation antipsychotic	tMS	transcranial magnetic stimulation
SIADH	syndrome of inappropriate secretion of antidiuretic hormone	TORDIA	Treatment of Resistant Depression in Adolescents
		TRBD	treatment-resistant bipolar disorder
SIB	Severe Impairment Battery		
SJW	St John's wort	TRD	treatment-resistant depression
SNRI	serotonin–noradrenaline reuptake inhibitor	TREC	Tranquilização Rápida-Ensaio Clínico [Rapid Tranquillisation Clinical Trial]
SOAD	Second Opinion Appointed Doctor		
SPC	Summary of Product Characteristics	TRS	treatment-resistant schizophrenia
SROM	slow-release oral morphine	TS	Tourette syndrome
SSRI	selective serotonin reuptake inhibitor	U&Es	urea and electrolytes
		UDP	uridine diphosphate
STAR*D	Sequenced Treatment Alternatives to Relieve Depression	UGT	UDP-glucuronosyltransferase
		UGIB	upper gastrointestinal bleeding
STOP-PD II	Study of the Pharmacotherapy of Psychotic Depression II	UGT	UDP-glucuronosyltransferase
SUD	stimulant use disorder	UKTIS	UK Teratology Information Service
TADS	Treatment of Adolescents with Depression Study	VaD	vascular dementia
TCA	tricyclic antidepressant	VG	vegetable glycerine
TD	tardive dyskinesia	VHR	Vienna High Risk
tDCS	transcranial direct current stimulation	VMAT-2	vesicular monoamine transporter 2
TDM	therapeutic drug monitoring	VNS	vagal nerve stimulation
		VTE	venous thromboembolism
TdP	torsades de pointes	WBC	white blood cell
tds	three times a day	WCC	white cell count
TF-CBT	trauma-focused cognitive behavioural therapy	WHO	World Health Organization
TFT	thyroid function test	YMRS	Young Mania Rating Scale
TIA	transient ischaemic attack	ZA	zuclopenthixol acetate

Chapter 1

Schizophrenia and related psychoses

ANTIPSYCHOTIC DRUGS

General introduction

Classification of antipsychotics

Before the 1990s, antipsychotics (or major tranquillisers as they were then known) were classified according to their chemistry. The first antipsychotic, chlorpromazine, was a phenothiazine compound – a tricyclic structure incorporating a nitrogen and a sulphur atom. Further phenothiazines were generated and marketed, as were chemically similar thioxanthenes such as flupentixol. Later, entirely different chemical structures were developed according to pharmacological paradigms. These included butyrophenones (haloperidol), diphenylbutylpiperidines (pimozide) and substituted benzamides (sulpiride, amisulpride).

Chemical classification remains useful but is rendered somewhat redundant by the broad range of chemical entities now available and by the absence of any clear structure–activity relationships for newer drugs. The chemistry of some older drugs does relate to their propensity to cause movement disorders. Piperazine phenothiazines (e.g. fluphenazine, trifluoperazine), butyrophenones and thioxanthenes are most likely to cause extrapyramidal effects, while piperidine phenothiazines (e.g. pipotiazine) and benzamides are the least likely. Aliphatic phenothiazines (e.g. chlorpromazine) and diphenylbutylpiperidines (pimozide) are perhaps somewhere in between.

Relative liability for inducing extrapyramidal side effects (EPSEs) was originally the primary factor behind the typical/atypical classification. Clozapine had long been known as an atypical antipsychotic on the basis of its low liability to cause EPSEs and its failure in animal-based antipsychotic screening tests. Its remarketing in 1990 signalled the beginning of a series of new medications, all of which were introduced with claims (to varying degrees of accuracy) of 'atypicality'. Of these medications, perhaps only clozapine, and possibly quetiapine, is completely atypical, seemingly having a

The Maudsley® Prescribing Guidelines in Psychiatry, Fifteenth Edition. David M. Taylor, Thomas R. E. Barnes and Allan H. Young.
© 2025 David M. Taylor. Published 2025 by John Wiley & Sons Ltd.

very low or zero liability for extrapyramidal symptoms (EPS). Others show dose-related effects, although, unlike with typical drugs, therapeutic activity can usually be achieved without EPSEs. This is possibly the real distinction between typical and atypical drugs: the ease with which a dose can be chosen within the licensed dosage range that is effective but does not cause EPSEs (for example, compare haloperidol with olanzapine).

The typical/atypical dichotomy does not lend itself well to classification of antipsychotics in the middle ground of EPSE liability. Thioridazine was widely described as atypical in the 1980s but is a 'conventional' phenothiazine. Sulpiride was marketed as an atypical but is often classified as typical. Risperidone, at its maximum dose of 16mg/day, is just about as 'typical' as a drug can be. Alongside these difficulties is the fact that there is nothing either pharmacologically or chemically which clearly binds these so-called atypicals together as a group, save perhaps a general but not universal finding of preference for D2 receptors outside the striatum. Nor are atypicals characterised by improved efficacy over older drugs (clozapine and one or two others excepted) or the absence of hyperprolactinaemia (which is usually worse with risperidone, paliperidone and amisulpride than with typical drugs). Lastly, some more recently introduced agents (e.g. pimavanserin, xanomeline) have antipsychotic activity and do not cause EPS but have almost nothing in common with other atypicals in respect to chemistry, pharmacology or adverse-effect profile.

In an attempt to get round some of these problems, typicals and atypicals were reclassified as first- or second-generation antipsychotics (FGA/SGA). All drugs introduced since 1990 are classified as SGAs (i.e. all atypicals) but the new nomenclature dispenses with any connotations regarding atypicality, whatever that may mean. However, the FGA/SGA classification remains problematic because neither group is defined by anything other than time of introduction – hardly the most sophisticated pharmacological classification system. Perhaps more importantly, date of introduction is often wildly distant from date of first synthesis. Clozapine is one of the oldest antipsychotics (synthesised in 1959) while olanzapine is hardly in its first flush of youth, having first been patented in 1971. These two drugs are of course SGAs, apparently the most modern of antipsychotics.

In this edition of the *Maudsley Prescribing Guidelines*, we conserve the FGA/SGA distinction more because of convention than some scientific basis. Also, we feel that most people know which drugs belong to each group – it thus serves as a useful shorthand. However, it is clearly more sensible to consider the properties of *individual* antipsychotics when choosing drugs to prescribe or in discussions with patients and carers. With this in mind, the use of Neuroscience-based Nomenclature (NbN)[1] – a naming system that reflects pharmacological activity – is strongly recommended.

Choosing an antipsychotic

In the UK, the National Institute for Health and Care Excellence (NICE) guideline for medicines adherence[2] recommends that patients should be as involved as possible in decisions about the choice of medicines that are prescribed for them, and that clinicians should be aware that illness beliefs and beliefs about medicines influence adherence. Consistent with this general advice that covers all healthcare, the NICE guideline for schizophrenia emphasises the importance of patient choice rather than specifically recommending a class or individual antipsychotic as first-line treatment.[3]

Antipsychotics are effective in both the acute and maintenance treatment of schizophrenia and other psychotic disorders. They differ in their pharmacology, pharmacokinetics, overall efficacy/effectiveness and tolerability, and, perhaps more importantly, response and tolerability differ between patients. This variability of individual response means that there is no clear first-line antipsychotic medication that is preferable for all.

Relative efficacy

After the publication of the independent CATIE[4] and CUtLASS[5] studies, the World Psychiatric Association reviewed the evidence relating to the relative efficacy of 51 FGAs and 11 SGAs and concluded that, if differences in EPS could be minimised (by careful dosing) and anticholinergic use avoided, there was no convincing evidence to support any advantage for SGAs over FGAs.[6] As a class, SGAs may have a lower propensity for EPS and tardive dyskinesia (TD),[7] but this was somewhat offset by a higher propensity to cause metabolic adverse effects. A meta-analysis of antipsychotic medications for first-episode psychosis[8] found few differences between FGAs and SGAs as groups of drugs but minor advantages for olanzapine and amisulpride individually. A later network meta-analysis of first-episode studies found small efficacy advantages for olanzapine and amisulpride and overall poor performance for haloperidol.[9]

When individual non-clozapine SGAs are compared, summary data suggest that olanzapine is marginally more effective than aripiprazole, risperidone, quetiapine and ziprasidone, and that risperidone has a minor advantage over quetiapine and ziprasidone.[10] FGA-controlled trials also suggest an advantage for olanzapine, risperidone and amisulpride over older drugs.[11,12] A network meta-analysis[13] broadly confirmed these findings, ranking amisulpride second behind clozapine and olanzapine third. These three drugs were the only ones to show clear efficacy advantages over haloperidol. The magnitude of differences was again small (but potentially substantial enough to be clinically important)[13] and must be weighed against the very different adverse effect profiles associated with individual antipsychotics. A 2019 network meta-analysis of 32 antipsychotics[14] ranked amisulpride as the most effective drug for positive symptoms and clozapine as the best for both negative symptoms and overall symptom improvement. Olanzapine and risperidone were also highly ranked for positive symptom response. The greatest (beneficial) effect on depressive symptoms was seen with sulpiride, clozapine, amisulpride, olanzapine and the dopamine partial agonists, perhaps reflecting the relative absence of neuroleptic-induced dysphoria common to most FGAs.[15] In the longer term, olanzapine may have advantages over some other antipsychotics.[16] There was a tendency for more recently introduced drugs to have a lower estimated efficacy – a phenomenon that derives from the substantial increase in placebo response since 1970.[17]

Clozapine is clearly the drug of choice in refractory schizophrenia,[18] although bizarrely, this is not a universal finding,[19] probably because of the biased nature and quality of many active–comparator trials.[20,21]

Both FGAs and SGAs are associated with a number of adverse effects. These include weight gain, dyslipidaemia, increases in plasma glucose/diabetes,[22,23] hyperprolactinaemia, hip fracture,[24] sexual dysfunction, EPS including neuroleptic malignant syndrome,[25] anticholinergic effects, venous thromboembolism (VTE),[26] sedation and postural hypotension. The exact profile is drug specific (see individual sections on specific adverse effects), although comparative data are not robust[27] (see large-scale meta-analyses[13,28] for rankings of some adverse-effect risks).

Adverse effects are a common reason for treatment discontinuation,[29] particularly when efficacy is poor.[13] Patients do not always spontaneously report adverse effects, however,[30] and psychiatrists' views of the prevalence and importance of adverse effects differ markedly from patient experience.[31] Systematic enquiry, together with a physical examination and appropriate biochemical tests, is the only way accurately to assess their presence and severity or perceived severity. Patient-completed checklists such as the Glasgow Antipsychotic Side-effect Scale (GASS)[32] can be a useful first step in this process. The clinician-completed Antipsychotic Non-Neurological Side-Effects Rating Scale facilitates more detailed and comprehensive assessment.[33]

Non-adherence to antipsychotic treatment is common and here the guaranteed medication delivery associated with depot/long-acting injectable antipsychotic preparations (LAIs) is unequivocally advantageous. In comparison with oral antipsychotics, there is strong evidence that depots are associated with a reduced risk of relapse and rehospitalisation,[34–36] although randomised controlled trials (RCTs) do not always reflect this difference.[37] Any logical assessment of the benefits of LAIs and the damage caused by relapse would conclude that LAIs should be first-line treatments, rather than reserved for those who have already relapsed on oral medication. Moreover, the wider use of SGA LAIs has to some extent changed the image of depots, which were sometimes perceived as punishments for miscreant patients. Their tolerability advantage probably relates partly to the better definition of their therapeutic dose range, meaning that the optimal dose is more likely to be prescribed (compare aripiprazole, with a licensed dose 300mg or 400mg/month, with flupentixol, which has a licensed dose in the UK of 50mg every 4 weeks to 400mg/week). The optimal dose of flupentixol is around 40mg every 2 weeks[28] – just 5% of the maximum allowed.

As already mentioned, for patients whose symptoms have not responded sufficiently to adequate, sequential trials of two or more antipsychotic drugs, clozapine is the most effective treatment.[38–40] Its use in these circumstances is recommended by NICE[3] and probably every schizophrenia guideline besides. The biological basis for the superior efficacy of clozapine is uncertain.[41] Olanzapine should probably be one of the two drugs used before clozapine.[10,42] A case might also be made for a trial of amisulpride: it has a uniformly high ranking in meta-analyses and one trial found continuation with amisulpride to be as effective as switching to olanzapine.[43] This same trial also suggested clozapine might be best placed as the second drug used, given that switching provided no benefit over continuing with the first prescribed drug.

This chapter covers the treatment of schizophrenia with antipsychotic drugs, the relative adverse effect profile of these drugs and how adverse effects can be managed.

References

1. Zohar J, et al. Neuroscience-based Nomenclature (NbN): a call for action. *World J Biol Psychiatry* 2016; **17**:318–320.
2. National Institute for Health and Care Excellence. Medicines adherence: involving patients in decisions about prescribed medicines and supporting adherence. Clinical guideline [CG76]. 2009 (last updated March 2019, last checked December 2024); https://www.nice.org.uk/Guidance/CG76.
3. National Institute for Health and Care Excellence. Psychosis and schizophrenia in adults: prevention and management. Clinical guideline [CG178]. 2014 (last checked November 2024); https://www.nice.org.uk/guidance/cg178.
4. Lieberman JA, et al. Effectiveness of antipsychotic drugs in patients with chronic schizophrenia. *N Engl J Med* 2005; **353**:1209–1223.
5. Jones PB, et al. Randomized controlled trial of the effect on quality of life of second- vs first-generation antipsychotic drugs in schizophrenia: Cost Utility of the Latest Antipsychotic Drugs in Schizophrenia Study (CUtLASS 1). *Arch Gen Psychiatry* 2006; **63**:1079–1087.
6. Tandon R, et al. World Psychiatric Association Pharmacopsychiatry Section statement on comparative effectiveness of antipsychotics in the treatment of schizophrenia. *Schizophr Res* 2008; **100**:20–38.
7. Tarsy D, et al. Epidemiology of tardive dyskinesia before and during the era of modern antipsychotic drugs. *Handb Clin Neurol* 2011; **100**:601–616.
8. Zhang JP, et al. Efficacy and safety of individual second-generation vs. first-generation antipsychotics in first-episode psychosis: a systematic review and meta-analysis. *Int J Neuropsychopharmacol* 2013; **16**:1205–1218.
9. Zhu Y, et al. Antipsychotic drugs for the acute treatment of patients with a first episode of schizophrenia: a systematic review with pairwise and network meta-analyses. *Lancet Psychiatry*; **4**:694–705.
10. Leucht S, et al. A meta-analysis of head-to-head comparisons of second-generation antipsychotics in the treatment of schizophrenia. *Am J Psychiatry* 2009; **166**:152–163.
11. Davis JM, et al. A meta-analysis of the efficacy of second-generation antipsychotics. *Archives of General Psychiatry* 2003; **60**:553–564.
12. Leucht S, et al. Second-generation versus first-generation antipsychotic drugs for schizophrenia: a meta-analysis. *Lancet* 2009; **373**:31–41.
13. Leucht S, et al. Comparative efficacy and tolerability of 15 antipsychotic drugs in schizophrenia: a multiple-treatments meta-analysis. *Lancet* 2013; **382**:951–962.
14. Huhn M, et al. Comparative efficacy and tolerability of 32 oral antipsychotics for the acute treatment of adults with multi-episode schizophrenia: a systematic review and network meta-analysis. *Lancet* 2019; **394**:939–951.
15. Voruganti L, et al. Neuroleptic dysphoria: towards a new synthesis. *Psychopharmacology (Berl)* 2004; **171**:121–132.
16. Leucht S, et al. Long-term efficacy of antipsychotic drugs in initially acutely ill adults with schizophrenia: systematic review and network meta-analysis. *World Psychiatry* 2023; **22**:315–324.
17. Leucht S, et al. Sixty years of placebo-controlled antipsychotic drug trials in acute schizophrenia: systematic review, Bayesian meta-analysis, and meta-regression of efficacy predictors. *Am J Psychiatry* 2017; **174**:927–942.
18. Siskind D, et al. Clozapine v. first- and second-generation antipsychotics in treatment-refractory schizophrenia: systematic review and meta-analysis. *Br J Psychiatry* 2016; **209**:385–392.
19. Samara MT, et al. Efficacy, acceptability, and tolerability of antipsychotics in treatment-resistant schizophrenia: a network meta-analysis. *JAMA Psychiatry* 2016; **73**:199–210.
20. Taylor DM. Clozapine for treatment-resistant schizophrenia: still the gold standard? *CNS Drugs* 2017; **31**:177–180.
21. Kane JM, et al. The role of clozapine in treatment-resistant schizophrenia. *JAMA Psychiatry* 2016; **73**:187–188.
22. Manu P, et al. Prediabetes in patients treated with antipsychotic drugs. *J Clin Psychiatry* 2012; **73**:460–466.
23. Rummel-Kluge C, et al. Head-to-head comparisons of metabolic side effects of second generation antipsychotics in the treatment of schizophrenia: a systematic review and meta-analysis. *Schizophr Res* 2010; **123**:225–233.
24. Sorensen HJ, et al. Schizophrenia, antipsychotics and risk of hip fracture: a population-based analysis. *Eur Neuropsychopharmacol* 2013; **23**:872–878.
25. Trollor JN, et al. Comparison of neuroleptic malignant syndrome induced by first- and second-generation antipsychotics. *Br J Psychiatry* 2012; **201**:52–56.
26. Masopust J, et al. Risk of venous thromboembolism during treatment with antipsychotic agents. *Psychiatry Clin Neurosci* 2012; **66**:541–552.
27. Pope A, et al. Assessment of adverse effects in clinical studies of antipsychotic medication: survey of methods used. *Br J Psychiatry* 2010; **197**:67–72.
28. Bailey L, et al. Estimating the optimal dose of flupentixol decanoate in the maintenance treatment of schizophrenia: a systematic review of the literature. *Psychopharmacology (Berl)* 2019; **236**:3081–3092.
29. Falkai P. Limitations of current therapies: why do patients switch therapies? *Eur Neuropsychopharmacol* 2008; **18** Suppl 3:S135–S139.
30. Yusufi B, et al. Prevalence and nature of side effects during clozapine maintenance treatment and the relationship with clozapine dose and plasma concentration. *Int Clin Psychopharmacol* 2007; **22**:238–243.
31. Day JC, et al. A comparison of patients' and prescribers' beliefs about neuroleptic side-effects: prevalence, distress and causation. *Acta Psychiatr Scand* 1998; **97**:93–97.
32. Waddell L, et al. A new self-rating scale for detecting atypical or second-generation antipsychotic side effects. *J Psychopharmacol* 2008; **22**:238–243.
33. Ohlsen RI, et al. Interrater reliability of the Antipsychotic Non-Neurological Side-Effects Rating Scale measured in patients treated with clozapine. *J Psychopharmacol* 2008; **22**:323–329.

34. Tiihonen J, et al. Effectiveness of antipsychotic treatments in a nationwide cohort of patients in community care after first hospitalisation due to schizophrenia and schizoaffective disorder: observational follow-up study. *BMJ* 2006; 333:224.

35. Leucht C, et al. Oral versus depot antipsychotic drugs for schizophrenia—a critical systematic review and meta-analysis of randomised long-term trials. *Schizophr Res* 2011; **127**:83–92.

36. Leucht S, et al. Antipsychotic drugs versus placebo for relapse prevention in schizophrenia: a systematic review and meta-analysis. *Lancet* 2012; **379**:2063–2071.

37. Schneider-Thoma J, et al. Comparative efficacy and tolerability of 32 oral and long-acting injectable antipsychotics for the maintenance treatment of adults with schizophrenia: a systematic review and network meta-analysis. *Lancet* 2022; **399**:824–836.

38. Kane J, et al. Clozapine for the treatment-resistant schizophrenic. A double-blind comparison with chlorpromazine. *Arch Gen Psychiatry* 1988; **45**:789–796.

39. McEvoy JP, et al. Effectiveness of clozapine versus olanzapine, quetiapine, and risperidone in patients with chronic schizophrenia who did not respond to prior atypical antipsychotic treatment. *Am J Psychiatry* 2006; **163**:600–610.

40. Lewis SW, et al. Randomized controlled trial of effect of prescription of clozapine versus other second-generation antipsychotic drugs in resistant schizophrenia. *Schizophr Bull* 2006; **32**:715–723.

41. Stone JM, et al. Review: the biological basis of antipsychotic response in schizophrenia. *J Psychopharmacol* 2010; **24**:953–964.

42. Agid O, et al. An algorithm-based approach to first-episode schizophrenia: response rates over 3 prospective antipsychotic trials with a retrospective data analysis. *J Clin Psychiatry* 2011; **72**:1439–1444.

43. Kahn RS, et al. Amisulpride and olanzapine followed by open-label treatment with clozapine in first-episode schizophrenia and schizophreniform disorder (OPTiMiSE): a three-phase switching study. *Lancet Psychiatry* 2018; **5**:797–807.

General principles of prescribing

- The lowest possible dose should be used. For each patient, the dose should be titrated to the lowest known to be effective (see section on minimum effective doses in this chapter). Dose increases should then take place only after 1–2 weeks of assessment, during which the patient is clearly showing poor or no response.
- With regular dosing of LAIs, plasma levels rise for at least 6–12 weeks after initiation, even without a change in dose (see section on depot pharmacokinetics in this chapter). Dose increases during this time are therefore difficult to evaluate. The preferred method is to establish efficacy and tolerability of oral medication at a particular dose and then give the equivalent dose of the oral drug in LAI form. Where this is not possible, the target dose of LAI for an individual should be the dose established to be optimal in clinical trials (although such data are not always available for older LAIs).
- Antipsychotic LAIs provide better relapse protection than oral treatment. LAIs should be used as first-line treatment aimed at preventing relapse. They should not be reserved only for those who have already relapsed on oral treatment.
- Clozapine should be offered as soon as treatment resistance is apparent. The sooner clozapine is prescribed, the more effective it will be.
- For the large majority of patients, the use of a single antipsychotic (with or without additional mood stabiliser or sedatives) is recommended. Apart from some exceptional circumstances (e.g. clozapine augmentation or adjunctive aripiprazole for prolactin elevation) antipsychotic polypharmacy should generally be avoided because of the increased adverse-effect burden and risks associated with QT prolongation and sudden cardiac death (see section on antipsychotic polypharmacy in this chapter).
- Combinations of antipsychotics should only be used where response to a single antipsychotic (including clozapine) has been clearly demonstrated to be inadequate. In such cases, the effect of the combination against target symptoms and on adverse effects should be carefully evaluated and documented. Where there is no clear benefit, treatment should revert to single antipsychotic therapy.
- In general, antipsychotics should not be used as 'when necessary' sedatives. Time-limited prescriptions of benzodiazepines or general sedatives (e.g. promethazine) are preferred (see section on rapid tranquillisation in this chapter).
- Response to antipsychotic drug treatment should be assessed using recognised rating scales and outcomes documented in patients' records.
- Those receiving antipsychotics should undergo close monitoring of physical health (including blood pressure, pulse, ECG, plasma glucose and plasma lipids; see appropriate sections in this chapter).
- When withdrawing antipsychotics, reduce the dose slowly in a hyperbolic regimen, which minimises the risks of withdrawal symptoms and rebound psychosis.

Note – this section is not referenced. Please see relevant individual sections in this chapter for detailed and referenced guidance.

Antipsychotics – minimum effective doses

Table 1.1 suggests the minimum dose of individual antipsychotics likely to be effective in first- or multi-episode schizophrenia. Most patients will respond to the dose suggested, although others may require higher doses. Given the variation in individual response, all doses should be considered approximate. Primary references are provided where available, but some consensus opinion has also been used. Only oral treatment with commonly used drugs is covered.

Table 1.1 Minimum effective dose/day – antipsychotics

Drug	First episode	Multi-episode
First-generation		
Chlorpromazine[1]	200mg*	300mg
Haloperidol[2–6]	2mg	4mg
Sulpiride[7]	400mg*	800mg
Trifluoperazine[8,9]	10mg*	15mg
Second-generation		
Amisulpride[10,11]	300mg*	400mg*
Aripiprazole[6,12–16]	10mg	10mg
Asenapine[6,16,17]	5mg*	10mg
Blonanserin[18]	Not known	8mg
Brexpiprazole[19,20]	2mg*	4mg
Cariprazine[21,22]	1.5mg*	1.5mg
Clotiapine[23,24]	Not known	120mg
Iloperidone[6,16,25]	4mg*	8mg
Lumateperone[26]	Not known	42mg*
Lurasidone[6,27]	40mg HCl/37mg base*	40mg HCl/37mg base
Olanzapine[6,28–31]	5mg	7.5mg
Paliperidone[16]	3mg*	3mg
Pimavanserin[32–34]	Not known	34mg**
Quetiapine[35,36]	150mg* (but higher doses often used[37])	300mg IR
		500mg MR[38]
Risperidone[3,6,39–42]	2mg	4mg
Xanomeline[43,44]	200mg*	200mg*
Ziprasidone[6,15,45–47]	40mg*	80mg

* Estimate – too few data available.

** US Food and Drug Administration-approved for Parkinson's disease psychosis; dose in schizophrenia not clear.

References

1. Dudley K, et al. Chlorpromazine dose for people with schizophrenia. *Cochrane Database Syst Rev* 2017; 4(4):CD007778.
2. McGorry PD. Recommended haloperidol and risperidone doses in first-episode psychosis. *J Clin Psychiatry* 1999; 60:794–795.
3. Schooler N, et al. Risperidone and haloperidol in first-episode psychosis: a long-term randomized trial. *Am J Psychiatry* 2005; 162:947–953.
4. Donnelly L, et al. Haloperidol dose for the acute phase of schizophrenia. *Cochrane Database Syst Rev* 2013; (8):CD001951.
5. Oosthuizen P, et al. A randomized, controlled comparison of the efficacy and tolerability of low and high doses of haloperidol in the treatment of first-episode psychosis. *Int J Neuropsychopharmacol* 2004; 7:125–131.
6. Leucht S, et al. Dose equivalents for second-generation antipsychotics: the minimum effective dose method. *Schizophr Bull* 2014; 40:314–326.
7. Soares BG, et al. Sulpiride for schizophrenia. *Cochrane Database Syst Rev* 2000; (2):CD001162.
8. Armenteros JL, et al. Antipsychotics in early onset schizophrenia: systematic review and meta-analysis. *Eur Child Adolesc Psychiatry* 2006; 15:141–148.
9. Koch K, et al. Trifluoperazine versus placebo for schizophrenia. *Cochrane Database Syst Rev* 2014; (1):CD010226.
10. Sparshatt A, et al. Amisulpride - dose, plasma concentration, occupancy and response: implications for therapeutic drug monitoring. *Acta Psychiatr Scand* 2009; 120:416–428.
11. Buchanan RW, et al. The 2009 schizophrenia PORT psychopharmacological treatment recommendations and summary statements. *Schizophr Bull* 2010; 36:71–93.
12. Cutler AJ, et al. The efficacy and safety of lower doses of aripiprazole for the treatment of patients with acute exacerbation of schizophrenia. *CNS Spectr* 2006; 11:691–702.
13. Mace S, et al. Aripiprazole: dose–response relationship in schizophrenia and schizoaffective disorder. *CNS Drugs* 2008; 23:773–780.
14. Sparshatt A, et al. A systematic review of aripiprazole: dose, plasma concentration, receptor occupancy and response: implications for therapeutic drug monitoring. *J Clin Psychiatry* 2010; 71:1447–1456.
15. Liu CC, et al. Aripiprazole for drug-naive or antipsychotic-short-exposure subjects with ultra-high risk state and first-episode psychosis: an open-label study. *J Clin Psychopharmacol* 2013; 33:18–23.
16. Leucht S, et al. Dose-response meta-analysis of antipsychotic drugs for acute schizophrenia. *Am J Psychiatry* 2020; 177:342–353.
17. Citrome L. Role of sublingual asenapine in treatment of schizophrenia. *Neuropsychiatr Dis Treat* 2011; 7:325-339.
18. Tenjin T, et al. Profile of blonanserin for the treatment of schizophrenia. *Neuropsychiatr Dis Treat* 2013; 9:587–594.
19. Correll CU, et al. Efficacy of brexpiprazole in patients with acute schizophrenia: review of three randomized, double-blind, placebo-controlled studies. *Schizophr Res* 2016; 174:82–92.
20. Antoun Reyad A, et al. Efficacy and safety of brexpiprazole in acute management of psychiatric disorders: a meta-analysis of randomized controlled trials. *Int Clin Psychopharmacol* 2020; 35:119–128.
21. Garnock-Jones KP. Cariprazine: a review in schizophrenia. *CNS Drugs* 2017; 31:513–525.
22. Citrome L. Cariprazine for acute and maintenance treatment of adults with schizophrenia: an evidence-based review and place in therapy. *Neuropsychiatr Dis Treat* 2018; 14:2563–2577.
23. Lokshin P, et al. Clotiapine: an old neuroleptic with possible clozapine-like properties. *Progr Neuro Psychopharmacol Biol Psychiatry* 1998; 22:1289–1293.
24. Lyseng-Williamson K. Clotiapine in schizophrenia: a guide to its use. *Drugs Ther Perspect* 2015; 31:365–371.
25. Crabtree BL, et al. Iloperidone for the management of adults with schizophrenia. *Clin Ther* 2011; 33:330–345.
26. Peng H, et al. Efficacy and safety of lumateperone for bipolar depression and schizophrenia: a systematic review and meta-analysis. *Int J Neuropsychopharmacol* 2024; 27:pyae052.
27. Meltzer HY, et al. Lurasidone in the treatment of schizophrenia: a randomized, double-blind, placebo- and olanzapine-controlled study. *Am J Psychiatry* 2011; 168:957–967.
28. Sanger TM, et al. Olanzapine versus haloperidol treatment in first-episode psychosis. *Am J Psychiatry* 1999; 156:79–87.
29. Kasper S. Risperidone and olanzapine: optimal dosing for efficacy and tolerability in patients with schizophrenia. *Int Clin Psychopharmacol* 1998; 13:253–262.
30. Keefe RS, et al. Long-term neurocognitive effects of olanzapine or low-dose haloperidol in first-episode psychosis. *Biol Psychiatry* 2006; 59:97–105.
31. Bishara D, et al. Olanzapine: a systematic review and meta-regression of the relationships between dose, plasma concentration, receptor occupancy, and response. *J Clin Psychopharmacol* 2013; 33:329–335.
32. Mathis MV, et al. The US Food and Drug Administration's perspective on the new antipsychotic pimavanserin. *J Clin Psychiatry* 2017; 78:e668–e673.
33. Ballard C, et al. Pimavanserin in Alzheimer's disease psychosis: efficacy in patients with more pronounced psychotic symptoms. *J Prev Alzheimers Dis* 2019; 6:27–33.
34. Nasrallah HA, et al. Successful treatment of clozapine-nonresponsive refractory hallucinations and delusions with pimavanserin, a serotonin 5HT-2A receptor inverse agonist. *Schizophr Res* 2019; 208:217–220.
35. Sparshatt A, et al. Quetiapine: dose–response relationship in schizophrenia. *CNS Drugs* 2008; 22:49–68.
36. Sparshatt A, et al. Relationship between daily dose, plasma concentrations, dopamine receptor occupancy, and clinical response to quetiapine: a review. *J Clin Psychiatry* 2011; 72:1108–1123.
37. Pagsberg AK, et al. Quetiapine extended release versus aripiprazole in children and adolescents with first-episode psychosis: the multicentre, double-blind, randomised tolerability and efficacy of antipsychotics (TEA) trial. *Lancet Psychiatry* 2017; 4:605–618.

38. Terao I, et al. Comparative efficacy of quetiapine by dose and formulation for psychosis in schizophrenia: a systematic review and dose-response model-based network meta-analysis. *J Psychopharmacol* 2023; **37**:953–959.
39. Lane HY, et al. Risperidone in acutely exacerbated schizophrenia: dosing strategies and plasma levels. *J Clin Psychiatry* 2000; **61**:209–214.
40. Williams R. Optimal dosing with risperidone: updated recommendations. *J Clin Psychiatry* 2001; **62**:282–289.
41. Ezewuzie N, et al. Establishing a dose-response relationship for oral risperidone in relapsed schizophrenia. *J Psychopharmacol* 2006; **20**:86–90.
42. Li C, et al. Risperidone dose for schizophrenia. *Cochrane Database Syst Rev* 2009; (4):CD007474.
43. Kaul I, et al. Efficacy and safety of the muscarinic receptor agonist KarXT (xanomeline-trospium) in schizophrenia (EMERGENT-2) in the USA: results from a randomised, double-blind, placebo-controlled, flexible-dose phase 3 trial. *Lancet* 2024; **403**:160–170.
44. Kaul I, et al. Efficacy of xanomeline and trospium chloride in schizophrenia: pooled results from three 5-week, randomized, double-blind, placebo-controlled, EMERGENT trials. *Schizophrenia (Heidelb)* 2024; **10**:102.
45. Bagnall A, et al. Ziprasidone for schizophrenia and severe mental illness. *Cochrane Database Syst Rev* 2000; (4):CD001945.
46. Taylor D. Ziprasidone: an atypical antipsychotic. *Pharmaceutical J* 2001; **266**:396401.
47. Joyce AT, et al. Effect of initial ziprasidone dose on length of therapy in schizophrenia. *Schizophr Res* 2006; **83**:285–292.

Quick reference for licensed maximum doses

Table 1.2 lists the licensed maximum doses of antipsychotics according to the European Medicines Agency, as of January 2025.[1]

Table 1.2 Maximum doses of antipsychotics according to European Medicines Agency labelling.[1]

Drug	Maximum dose
FGAs – oral	
Chlorpromazine	1000mg/day
Flupentixol	18mg/day
Haloperidol	20mg/day
Levomepromazine	1200mg/day
Pericyazine	300mg/day
Perphenazine	24mg/day (64mg/day hospitalised patients)
Pimozide	20mg/day
Sulpiride	2400mg/day
Trifluoperazine	20mg/day (maximum dose not formally specified)
Zuclopenthixol	150mg/day
SGAs – oral	
Amisulpride	1200mg/day
Aripiprazole	30mg/day
Asenapine	20mg/day (sublingual)
Cariprazine	6mg/day
Clozapine	900mg/day
Lurasidone	160mg (HCl)/148mg (base)/day
Olanzapine	20mg/day
Paliperidone	12mg/day
Quetiapine	750mg/day schizophrenia (800mg/day MR)
	800mg/day bipolar disorder
Risperidone	16mg/day
Sertindole	24mg/day
Long-acting injections	
Aripiprazole 1-monthly	400mg/month (SPC implies 'every 4 weeks')
Aripiprazole 2-monthly	960mg/2 months (SPC states 'every 56 days')
Flupentixol decanoate	400mg/week
Haloperidol decanoate	300mg/4 weeks
Olanzapine pamoate	300mg/2 weeks
Paliperidone palmitate 1-monthly	150mg/month
Paliperidone palmitate 3-monthly	525mg/3 months

(Continued)

Table 1.2 (Continued)

Drug	Maximum dose
Paliperidone depot 6-monthly	1000mg/6 months
Risperidone (Consta®)	50mg/2 weeks
Risperidone (Okedi®)	100mg/4 weeks
Zuclopenthixol decanote	600mg/week

Table 1.3 lists the licensed maximum doses of antipsychotics available outside the EU, according to the US Food and Drug Administration, where available (as of December 2024).[2]

Table 1.3 Licensed maximum doses of antipsychotics, according to US Food and Drug Administration labelling, where available.[2]

Drug	Maximum dose
FGAs – oral	
Fluphenazine	40mg/day
Thiothixene	60mg/day
SGAs – oral	
Blonanserin*	24mg/day[3]
Brexpiprazole	4mg/day
Iloperidone	24mg/day
Lumateperone	42mg/day
Molindone	225mg/day
Perospirone**	48mg/day
Pimavanserin	34mg/day
Xanomeline and trospium chloride	250mg/60mg/day
Ziprasidone	160mg/day
Long-acting injections	
Aripiprazole lauroxil (Aristada Initio®)[†]	675mg
Aripiprazole lauroxil (Aristada®)	882mg/month or 1064mg/2 months
Fluphenazine decanoate	100mg/14 days
Risperidone (Uzedy®)	125mg/month or 250mg/2 months
Risperidone (Rykindo®)	50mg/2 weeks
Transdermal patch	
Asenapine	7.6mg/24hr
Blonanserin*	80mg/24hr patch[4]

* Available only in China, Japan and South Korea at the time of writing.
** Available only in Japan at the time of writing.
[†] Used to initiate treatment with Aristada, not for repeat dosing.

References

1. Electronic Medicines Compendium. Summaries of Product Characteristics. (Last accessed January 2025); https://www.medicines.org.uk/emc.
2. US Food and Drug Administration. Highlights of Prescribing Information. 2024; https://www.fda.gov/drugs.
3. Inoue Y, et al. Safety and effectiveness of oral blonanserin for schizophrenia: a review of Japanese post-marketing surveillances. *J Pharmacolog Sci* 2021; **145**:42–51.
4. Nishibe H, et al. Striatal dopamine D2 receptor occupancy induced by daily application of blonanserin transdermal patches: phase 2 study in Japanese patients with schizophrenia. *Int J Neuropsychopharmacol* 2021; **24**:108–117.

Equivalent doses

Knowledge of equivalent dosages is useful when switching between FGAs. Estimates of 'neuroleptic' or 'chlorpromazine' equivalence, in mg/day, between these medications are based on clinical experience, expert panel opinion (using various methods) and any dopamine binding studies available.

Table 1.4 provides approximate equivalent doses for FGAs.[1–3] The values given should be seen as a rough guide when switching from one FGA to another and are no substitute for clinical titration of the new medication dose against adverse effects and response.

Equivalent doses of SGAs may be less clinically relevant, as these medications tend to have better defined, evidence-based licensed dose ranges. There are several different ways of calculating equivalence based on, for example, defined daily dose,[4] minimum effective dose[5,6] and average dose.[7] These methods give different estimates of equivalence. A very rough guide to equivalent SGA daily dosages is given in Table 1.5.[3,6–10] There is considerable disagreement about exact equivalencies, even among the references cited here. Clozapine is not included because this has a distinct initial titration schedule and a high dose–plasma level variability and because it probably has a different mechanism of action.

Comparing potencies of FGAs with SGAs introduces yet more uncertainty in respect to dose equivalence. Very approximately, 100mg chlorpromazine is equivalent to 1.5mg risperidone.[3] An online calculator is available from the American Association of Psychiatric Pharmacists.[11]

Table 1.4 Equivalent doses of first-generation antipsychotic medications.

Drug	Equivalent dose (consensus)	Range of values in literature
FGAs – oral		
Chlorpromazine	100mg/day	Reference
Flupentixol	3mg/day	2–3mg/day
Fluphenazine	2mg/day	1–5mg/day
Haloperidol	2mg/day	1.5–5mg/day
Pericyazine	10mg/day	10mg/day
Perphenazine	10mg/day	5–10mg/day
Pimozide	2mg/day	1.33–2mg/day
Sulpiride	200mg/day	133–300mg/day
Trifluoperazine	5mg/day	2.5–5mg/day
Zuclopenthixol	25mg/day	25–60mg/day
FGAs – long-acting injections		
Flupentixol decanoate	10mg/week	10–20mg/week
Fluphenazine decanoate	5mg/week	1–12.5mg/week
Haloperidol decanoate	15mg/week	5–25mg/week
Zuclopenthixol decanoate	100mg/week	40–100mg/week

Schizophrenia and related psychoses **15**

CHAPTER 1

Table 1.5 Second-generation antipsychotics – approximate equivalent doses.[3-10]

Drug	Approximate equivalent dose
SGAs – oral	
Amisulpride	400mg
Aripiprazole	15mg
Asenapine	10mg
Blonanserin	~
Brexpiprazole	2mg
Cariprazine	1.5mg
Clotiapine	100mg
Iloperidone	12mg
Lumateperone	21mg*
Lurasidone	80mg (74mg base)
Melperone	300mg
Molindone	50mg
Olanzapine	10mg
Pimavaserin	17mg*
Quetiapine	400mg
Risperidone	4mg
Sertindole	10mg*
Xanomeline	~
Ziprasidone	80mg
SGAs – long-acting injections	
Aripiprazole 1-monthly	300mg/month
Aripiprazole lauroxil	441mg every 2 months
Olanzapine pamoate	405mg/4 weeks
Paliperidone palmitate	100mg/month
Risperidone (Consta)	50mg/2 weeks
Risperidone (Okedi)	100mg/4 weeks
Risperidone (Uzedy)	100mg/month or 200mg every 2 months
Transdermal patch	
Asenapine	5.7mg/24 hr

~ Unknown equivalence at time of writing.
* Expert consensus recommendation.

CHAPTER 1

References

1. Foster P. Neuroleptic equivalence. *Pharmaceutical J* 1989; **243**:431–432.
2. Atkins M, et al. Chlorpromazine equivalents: a consensus of opinion for both clinical and research implications. *Psychiatr Bull* 1997; **21**:224–226.
3. Patel MX, et al. How to compare doses of different antipsychotics: a systematic review of methods. *Schizophr Res* 2013; **149**:141–148.
4. Leucht S, et al. Dose equivalents for antipsychotic drugs: the DDD method. *Schizophr Bull* 2016; **42** Suppl 1:S90–S94.
5. Rothe PH, et al. Dose equivalents for second generation long-acting injectable antipsychotics: the minimum effective dose method. *Schizophr Res* 2018; **193**:23–28.
6. Leucht S, et al. Dose equivalents for second-generation antipsychotics: the minimum effective dose method. *Schizophr Bull* 2014; **40**:314–326.
7. Leucht S, et al. Dose equivalents for second-generation antipsychotic drugs: the classical mean dose method. *Schizophr Bull* 2015; **41**:1397–1402.
8. Woods SW. Chlorpromazine equivalent doses for the newer atypical antipsychotics. *J Clin Psychiatry* 2003; **64**:663–667.
9. McAdam MK, et al. Second International Consensus Study of Antipsychotic Dosing (ICSAD-2). *J Psychopharmacol* 2023; **37**:982–991.
10. Leucht S, et al. Dose–response meta-analysis of antipsychotic drugs for acute schizophrenia. *Am J Psychiatry* 2020; **177**:342–353.
11. American Association of Psychiatric Pharmacists. Antipsychotic dose conversion website (last accessed February 2025); https://aapp.org/guideline/essentials/antipsychotic-dose-equivalents.

High-dose antipsychotic medication: prescribing and monitoring

'High-dose' antipsychotic medication can result from the prescription of either a single antipsychotic medication at a dose above the recommended maximum or two or more antipsychotic medications concurrently that, when expressed as a percentage of their respective maximum recommended doses and added together, results in a cumulative dose of more than 100%.[1] In clinical practice, antipsychotic polypharmacy and prn antipsychotic medication are strongly associated with high-dose prescribing.[2,3]

Efficacy

There is no firm evidence that high doses of antipsychotic medication are any more effective than standard doses for schizophrenia. This holds true for the use of antipsychotic medication for rapid tranquillisation, relapse prevention, persistent aggression and the management of acute psychotic episodes.[1] Nevertheless, the prescription of high-dose antipsychotic medication remains relatively common in clinical practice.[4-6] In the UK, the national audit of schizophrenia in 2013, reporting on prescribing practice for over 5,000 predominantly community-based patients, found that, overall, 10% were prescribed a high dose of antipsychotic medication.[7] A 2022 audit of adult inpatients in mental health services[8] found that in over 4,000 patients on acute adult wards, just under 10% were prescribed high-dose antipsychotic medication, and for over 2,000 patients on forensic wards, the respective figure was 13%. In both settings, a high-dose prescription was predominantly a consequence of combined antipsychotic medications.

Examination of the dose–response effects of a variety of antipsychotic medications has not found any evidence of greater efficacy for doses above accepted licensed ranges.[9,10] Efficacy appears to be optimal at relatively low doses, such as 4mg/day risperidone,[11] 300mg/day quetiapine,[12] and olanzapine 10mg.[13,14] Similarly, treatment with LAI risperidone at a dose of 100mg 2-weekly offers no benefits over 50mg 2-weekly,[15] and 320mg/day ziprasidone[16] is no better than 160mg/day. All currently available antipsychotic medications (with the possible exception of clozapine) exert their antipsychotic effect primarily through antagonism (or partial agonism) at post-synaptic dopamine receptors. But there is increasing evidence that refractory symptoms in some patients with treatment-resistant schizophrenia may not be driven by dysfunction of dopamine pathways,[17-20] so prescribing a higher dosage to increase dopamine blockade in such patients would seem to be of uncertain value.

Dold and colleagues[21] conducted a meta-analysis of RCTs that compared continuation of standard-dose antipsychotic medication with dose escalation in patients whose schizophrenia had proved to be unresponsive to a prospective trial of standard-dose pharmacotherapy with the same antipsychotic medication. In this context, there was no evidence of any benefit associated with the increased dosage. In a study of patients with first-episode schizophrenia, increasing the dose of olanzapine up to 30mg/day and the dose of risperidone up to 10mg/day in those cases where the illness was non-responsive to treatment with standard doses yielded only a 4% absolute increase in overall response rate. Switching to an alternative antipsychotic, including clozapine, was considerably more successful.[22]

A small number of RCTs have examined the efficacy of high versus standard dosage in patients with treatment-resistant schizophrenia (TRS).[1] Some have demonstrated benefit[23] but the majority of these studies are old, the number of patients randomised is small and study design is poor by current standards. Some studies used daily doses equivalent to more than 10g chlorpromazine. One small (n = 12) open study of high-dose quetiapine (up to 1400mg/day) in refractory schizophrenia found modest benefits in a third of patients[24] but other, larger studies of quetiapine for such patients have shown no benefit for higher doses.[22,23] A further RCT of high-dose olanzapine (up to 45mg/day) versus clozapine for TRS found similar efficacy for the two treatments but concluded that, given the small sample size, it would be premature to conclude that they were equivalent.[25] Subsequent systematic reviews of relevant studies addressing high-dose olanzapine for TRS have similarly concluded that while such a regimen may be superior to other, non-clozapine antipsychotic medications, it may be seen as a safe and effective alternative for refractory illness only when clozapine use is not appropriate.[26,27]

Perhaps the most comprehensive systematic analysis of dose–response[28] largely confirmed the observation that the dose–response curve reaches a plateau above a certain dose for nearly all antipsychotic medications, with the possible exceptions of olanzapine and lurasidone. (With these two medications there is some evidence that doses at the upper end of the licensed range are somewhat more effective than lower doses.)[14,29] This systematic review also suggested that the doses above which no additional benefit was likely (e.g. risperidone 6.3mg/day; quetiapine 482mg/day) were somewhat higher than the doses of optimal efficacy previously determined (see above). Importantly, however, there was no evidence to support the use of doses of any antipsychotic medication above its licensed dose range.

Consensus panel recommendations are broadly in line with clinical trial outcomes. A 2023 international consensus study[30] suggested maximum effective doses exceeded licensed doses in only two cases: olanzapine (30mg/day) and quetiapine (800mg/day).

A 2023 systematic review of dose–response relationships[31] found that the effect of all antipsychotics reached a plateau within the licensed dose range, with the possible exceptions of lumateperone, olanzapine and lurasidone.

Adverse effects

The majority of adverse effects associated with antipsychotic treatment are dose-related.[32] These include EPS,[31] weight gain,[33] sedation, postural hypotension, anticholinergic effects, QTc prolongation[34] and coronary heart disease mortality.[35–38] High-dose antipsychotic treatment is clearly associated with a greater adverse-effect burden.[16,35,39–41] There is some evidence that antipsychotic dose reduction from a very high (mean 2253mg chlorpromazine equivalents per day) to a high (mean 1315mg chlorpromazine equivalents per day) dose can lead to improvements in cognition and negative symptoms.[42]

Recommendations

- The use of high-dose antipsychotic medication should be an exceptional clinical practice and only ever employed when adequate trials of such medication (including clozapine) at standard dosage have failed.
- If high-dose antipsychotic medication is prescribed, it should be standard practice to review and document the target symptoms, therapeutic response and adverse effects, ideally using validated rating scales, so that there is ongoing consideration of the risk–benefit balance for the patient. Close physical monitoring (including ECG) is essential.

Prescribing high-dose antipsychotic medication

Before using high doses, ensure that:

- Sufficient time has been allowed for response (see section on 'time to response').
- There have been adequate trials of at least two different antipsychotic medications (including, if possible, olanzapine), conducted sequentially.
- Clozapine has failed or not been tolerated because of agranulocytosis or other serious adverse effects. Most other adverse effects can be managed. A small proportion of patients may also decline to take clozapine.

The decision to prescribe high doses should:

- Be made by a senior psychiatrist.
- Involve the multidisciplinary team.
- Be done, if possible, with a patient's informed consent.

Process

- Rule out contraindications (e.g. ECG abnormalities, hepatic impairment).
- Consider and minimise any risks posed by concomitant medication (e.g. potential to cause QTc prolongation, electrolyte disturbance or pharmacokinetic interactions via CYP inhibition).
- Document the decision to prescribe high dosage in the clinical notes, together with a description of the target symptoms. The use of an appropriate rating scale is advised.
- Adequate time for response should be allowed after each dosage increment before a further increase is made.

Monitoring

- Physical monitoring should be carried out as outlined in the section on 'monitoring'.
- All patients on high doses should have regular ECGs (at baseline, when steady-state serum levels have been reached after each dosage increment, and then every 6–12 months). Additional biochemical/ECG monitoring is advised if drugs that are known to cause electrolyte disturbances or QTc prolongation are subsequently co-prescribed.
- Target symptoms should be assessed after 6 weeks and 3 months. If insufficient improvement in these symptoms has occurred, the dose should be decreased to the normal range.

References

1. Royal College of Psychiatrists. *The Risks and Benefits of High-Dose Antipsychotic Medication*. College Report CR190. London: Royal College of Psychiatrists; 2014.
2. Paton C, et al. High-dose and combination antipsychotic prescribing in acute adult wards in the UK: the challenges posed by p.r.n. prescribing. *Br J Psychiatry* 2008; 192:435–439.
3. Roh D, et al. Antipsychotic polypharmacy and high-dose prescription in schizophrenia: a 5-year comparison. *Aust N Z J Psychiatry* 2014; 48:52–60.
4. Campos Mendes J, et al. Patterns of antipsychotics' prescription in Portuguese acute psychiatric wards: a cross-sectional study. *Psychiatry Res* 2016; 246:142–148.
5. Martinho S, et al. Antipsychotic polypharmacy and high-dose antipsychotics in involuntary patients: a seven-year audit of discharge prescriptions in an acute care unit. *Psychiatr Q* 2021; 92:1–14.
6. Kaikoushi K, et al. Prescription patterns in psychiatric compulsory care: polypharmacy and high-dose antipsychotics. *BJPsych Open* 2021; 7:e149.
7. Patel MX, et al. Quality of prescribing for schizophrenia: evidence from a national audit in England and Wales. *Eur Neuropsychopharmacol* 2014; 24:499–509.
8. Royal College of Psychiatrists. Prescribing Observatory for Mental Health. Topic 1h & 3e: Prescribing of antipsychotic medication in adult mental health services, including high dose, combined, and PRN. CCQI 422. 2022 (last accessed February 2025); https://www.rcpsych.ac.uk/improving-care/ccqi/national-clinical-audits/pomh.
9. Davis JM, et al. Dose response and dose equivalence of antipsychotics. *J Clin Psychopharmacol* 2004; 24:192–208.
10. Gardner DM, et al. International consensus study of antipsychotic dosing. *Am J Psychiatry* 2010; 167:686–693.
11. Ezewuzie N, et al. Establishing a dose-response relationship for oral risperidone in relapsed schizophrenia. *J Psychopharm* 2006; 20:86–90.
12. Sparshatt A, et al. Quetiapine: dose–response relationship in schizophrenia. *CNS Drugs* 2008; 22:49–68.
13. Kinon BJ, et al. Standard and higher dose of olanzapine in patients with schizophrenia or schizoaffective disorder: a randomized, double-blind, fixed-dose study. *J Clin Psychopharmacol* 2008; 28:392–400.
14. Bishara D, et al. Olanzapine: a systematic review and meta-regression of the relationships between dose, plasma concentration, receptor occupancy, and response. *J Clin Psychopharmacol* 2013; 33:329–335.
15. Meltzer HY, et al. A six month randomized controlled trial of long acting injectable risperidone 50 and 100mg in treatment resistant schizophrenia. *Schizophr Res* 2014; 154:14–22.
16. Goff DC, et al. High-dose oral ziprasidone versus conventional dosing in schizophrenia patients with residual symptoms: the ZEBRAS study. *J Clin Psychopharmacol* 2013; 33:485–490.
17. Egerton A, et al. Dopamine and glutamate in antipsychotic-responsive compared with antipsychotic-nonresponsive psychosis: a multicenter positron emission tomography and magnetic resonance spectroscopy study (STRATA). *Schizophr Bull* 2021; 47:505–516.
18. Kapur S, et al. Relationship between dopamine D2 occupancy, clinical response, and side effects: a double-blind PET study of first-episode schizophrenia. *Am J Psychiatry* 2000; 157:514–520.
19. Demjaha A, et al. Dopamine synthesis capacity in patients with treatment-resistant schizophrenia. *Am J Psychiatry* 2012; 169:1203–1210.
20. Gillespie AL, et al. Is treatment-resistant schizophrenia categorically distinct from treatment-responsive schizophrenia? A systematic review. *BMC Psychiatry* 2017; 17:12.
21. Dold M, et al. Dose escalation of antipsychotic drugs in schizophrenia: a meta-analysis of randomized controlled trials. *Schizophr Res* 2015; 166:187–193.
22. Agid O, et al. An algorithm-based approach to first-episode schizophrenia: response rates over 3 prospective antipsychotic trials with a retrospective data analysis. *J Clin Psychiatry* 2011; 72:1439–1444.
23. Aubree JC, et al. High and very high dosage antipsychotics: a critical review. *J Clin Psychiatry* 1980; 41:341–350.
24. Boggs DL, et al. Quetiapine at high doses for the treatment of refractory schizophrenia. *Schizophr Res* 2008; 101:347–348.
25. Meltzer HY, et al. A randomized, double-blind comparison of clozapine and high-dose olanzapine in treatment-resistant patients with schizophrenia. *J Clin Psychiatry* 2008; 69:274–285.
26. Souza JS, et al. Efficacy of olanzapine in comparison with clozapine for treatment-resistant schizophrenia: evidence from a systematic review and meta-analyses. *CNS Spectr* 2013; 18:82–89.
27. Gannon L, et al. High-dose olanzapine in treatment-resistant schizophrenia: a systematic review. *Ther Adv Psychopharmacol* 2023; 13:20451253231168788.
28. Leucht S, et al. Dose-response meta-analysis of antipsychotic drugs for acute schizophrenia. *Am J Psychiatry* 2020; 177:342–353.
29. Loebel A, et al. Lurasidone dose escalation in early nonresponding patients with schizophrenia: a randomized, placebo-controlled study. *J Clin Psychiatry* 2016; 77:1672–1680.
30. McAdam MK, et al. Second International Consensus Study of Antipsychotic Dosing (ICSAD-2). *J Psychopharmacol* 2023; 37:982–991.
31. Siafis S, et al. Antipsychotic dose, dopamine D2 receptor occupancy and extrapyramidal side-effects: a systematic review and dose-response meta-analysis. *Mol Psychiatry* 2023; 28:3267–3277.
32. Yoshida K, et al. Dose-dependent effects of antipsychotics on efficacy and adverse effects in schizophrenia. *Behav Brain Res* 2021; 402:113098.
33. Wu H, et al. Antipsychotic-induced weight gain: dose-response meta-analysis of randomized controlled trials. *Schizophr Bull* 2022; 48:643–654.
34. He L, et al. A real-world study of risk factors for QTc prolongation in schizophrenia patients receiving atypical antipsychotics. *J Clin Psychopharmacol* 2022; 42:71–74.
35. Osborn DP, et al. Relative risk of cardiovascular and cancer mortality in people with severe mental illness from the United Kingdom's General Practice Research Database. *Arch Gen Psychiatry* 2007; 64:242–249.

36. Ray WA, et al. Atypical antipsychotic drugs and the risk of sudden cardiac death. *N Engl J Med* 2009; **360**:225–235.

37. Barbui C, et al. Antipsychotic dose mediates the association between polypharmacy and corrected QT interval. *PLoS One* 2016; **11**:e0148212.

38. Weinmann S, et al. Influence of antipsychotics on mortality in schizophrenia: systematic review. *Schizophr Res* 2009; **113**:1–11.

39. Honer WG, et al. A randomized, double-blind, placebo-controlled study of the safety and tolerability of high-dose quetiapine in patients with persistent symptoms of schizophrenia or schizoaffective disorder. *J Clin Psychiatry* 2012; **73**:13–20.

40. Bollini P, et al. Antipsychotic drugs: is more worse? A meta-analysis of the published randomized control trials. *Psychol Med* 1994; **24**:307–316.

41. Baldessarini RJ, et al. Significance of neuroleptic dose and plasma level in the pharmacological treatment of psychoses. *Arch Gen Psychiatry* 1988; **45**:79–90.

42. Kawai N, et al. High-dose of multiple antipsychotics and cognitive function in schizophrenia: the effect of dose-reduction. *Prog Neuropsychopharmacol Biol Psychiatry* 2006; **30**:1009–1014.

Combined antipsychotics (antipsychotic polypharmacy)

In psychiatric practice, prescriptions for combined antipsychotic medications are common[1-3] and often long term.[4] The medications combined are likely to include LAI antipsychotic preparations,[5,6] quetiapine[7] and FGAs,[8] the last of these perhaps reflecting the frequent use of haloperidol and chlorpromazine as prn medications.

Poor response to antipsychotic monotherapy

A national clinical audit conducted in the UK in 2022[9] found that by far the most common reason recorded for prescribing regular, combined antipsychotic medications was an insufficient response to antipsychotic monotherapy. The use of combined antipsychotic medications has been found to be associated with younger patient age, male gender, increased illness severity, complexity and chronicity, as well as poorer functioning, inpatient status and a diagnosis of schizophrenia.[2,7,10-12] These associations largely reinforce the notion that antipsychotic polypharmacy is used where schizophrenia has proved to be refractory to trials of antipsychotic monotherapy.[10,13-15]

Importantly, there is a lack of robust evidence that the efficacy of combined antipsychotic medications is superior to treatment with a single antipsychotic.[16,17] A meta-analysis of 16 RCTs in schizophrenia, comparing augmentation with a second antipsychotic with continued antipsychotic monotherapy, found that combining antipsychotic medications lacked double-blind/high-quality evidence of efficacy.[18] In addition, in patients with schizophrenia, the effects of a change back from antipsychotic polypharmacy to monotherapy, even when carefully conducted, are uncertain. The findings of two randomised studies suggested that the majority of patients may be successfully switched from antipsychotic polypharmacy to monotherapy without loss of symptom control,[19,20] and an open-label trial in institutionalised patients with chronic psychotic disorders found that such a switch did not increase the likelihood of relapse.[21] However, an RCT in outpatients with schizophrenia reported greater increases in symptoms 6 months after a switch from two co-prescribed antipsychotic medications to one,[22] although the expectation is that such exacerbations can be successfully managed.[19]

Long-term antipsychotic treatment

A non-interventional, population-based study in Hungary sought to compare the effectiveness of antipsychotic monotherapy with the use of combined antipsychotic medications over a 1-year observation period.

While the results provided evidence for the superiority of monotherapy over polypharmacy for SGAs in terms of all-cause treatment discontinuation in schizophrenia, polypharmacy was associated with a lower likelihood of mortality and psychiatric hospitalisations.[23] Similarly, a 20-year observational study in Finland reported on the risk of rehospitalisation in a cohort of 62,250 hospital-treated patients with schizophrenia. To minimise selection bias, the investigators used within-individual analyses, with each patient used as their own control. The main finding was that antipsychotic combinations, particularly those including clozapine and LAI antipsychotic medications, were associated with a slightly lower risk of psychiatric rehospitalisation than monotherapy.[24] Although the interpretation of such real-world findings is hindered by the issue of confounding by indication,[25] there are perhaps several plausible explanations for improved efficacy with polypharmacy. It may be that combining antipsychotic medications with different receptor profiles can be more effective and lead to better therapeutic efficacy and/or a lower adverse-effect burden and therefore better outcomes. It may be also that co-prescribing two antipsychotic medications improves medication adherence in that it increases the likelihood that a patient may use at least one of them.[24] Notably, clozapine and LAI antipsychotic preparations appear to be the most effective monotherapies for relapse prevention in schizophrenia.[26] Thus, adding a second antipsychotic medication to clozapine or an LAI antipsychotic medication in an attempt to mitigate metabolic adverse effects (e.g. by adding aripiprazole) or manage symptoms of agitation, anxiety or sleep disturbance (e.g. by adding olanzapine or quetiapine) might enhance a patient's engagement in their treatment and improve adherence to the effective antipsychotic treatment that has been augmented.

Adverse effects

Evidence for possible harm with combined antipsychotic medications is perhaps more convincing. Clinically significant adverse effects have been associated with combined antipsychotic medications, which may partly reflect that polypharmacy regimens are commonly a high-dose prescription.[8,27] There is an increased prevalence and severity of EPS,[28,29] increased metabolic adverse effects and diabetes,[22,30,31] sexual dysfunction,[32] an increased risk of hip fracture,[33] paralytic ileus,[34] grand mal seizures,[35] prolonged QTc,[36] hypertension[37] and arrhythmias.[13] Switching from antipsychotic polypharmacy to monotherapy has been shown to lead to worthwhile improvements in cognitive functioning.[20]

The evidence relating to an increased mortality with a continuing antipsychotic polypharmacy regimen is inconsistent. Two large case–control studies and a database study[38–40] found no increased mortality in patients with schizophrenia receiving antipsychotic polypharmacy compared with antipsychotic monotherapy. However, a 10-year prospective study of a cohort of 88 patients with schizophrenia found that receiving more than one antipsychotic medication concurrently was associated with substantially increased mortality.[18,41] These investigators explored the possibility that the use of combined antipsychotic medications might be a proxy for greater severity/increased refractoriness of psychiatric illness but found no association between mortality and any measured index of illness severity, although these measures focused on negative symptoms and cognitive deficits. Further, analysis of data from a large anonymised mental healthcare database (2007–2014) of 10,945 adult patients with serious mental illness who had been prescribed a single antipsychotic or polypharmacy for 6 months or more revealed a weak association between regular, long-term antipsychotic polypharmacy and all-cause mortality and natural causes of death.[42] However, the authors concluded that the evidence for the association was limited, even after controlling for the effect of dose. Another study, involving the follow-up of 99 patients with schizophrenia over a 25-year period, found that those prescribed three antipsychotics simultaneously were twice as likely to die as those who had been prescribed only one.[43] These authors also considered the possibility of indication bias influencing the findings, speculating that combined antipsychotic medication might be more likely to be prescribed for the most severe schizophrenia.

Given the association between combined antipsychotic medication and a greater adverse-effect burden,[15,44] it follows that it should be standard practice to document in the clinical records the rationale for prescribing combined antipsychotics in individual cases, together with a clear account of the benefits and adverse effects of an individual trial of the strategy. Medicolegally, this would seem to be prudent, although in practice it is not always done.[45]

The use of combined antipsychotic medications in clinical practice

There are myriad possible antipsychotic medication combinations but very limited data on their relative risk–benefit profiles in relation to overall therapeutic response or target symptom clusters. The clinical disadvantages of antipsychotic polypharmacy include an increased adverse-effect burden, higher total dosage, increased risk of drug–drug interactions, poorer medication adherence related to the complexity of the treatment and difficulties in the attribution of any response to one or more of the individual antipsychotic medications prescribed, leading to difficulty in determining the implications for an optimal longer-term regimen.[6]

Despite the limited supportive evidence base, the use of antipsychotic polypharmacy is an established custom and practice in many countries.[46–48] Further, the general consensus across treatment guidelines that the use of combined antipsychotic medication for the treatment of refractory psychotic illness should be considered only after other, evidence-based, pharmacological treatments such as clozapine have been exhausted is not consistently followed in clinical practice.[6,12,13,49–51] However, a trial of clozapine augmentation with a second antipsychotic medication to enhance efficacy is a potentially supportable practice[52–56] (see section on optimising clozapine treatment in this chapter). Other antipsychotic polypharmacy strategies with potentially valid rationales are the addition of aripiprazole to reduce body weight in patients receiving clozapine.[57,58] Adjunctive aripiprazole can also normalise prolactin levels, although, while the study findings on resolving hyperprolactinaemia are generally positive, they are not entirely consistent.[59–64] Such polypharmacy with aripiprazole may be seen as worthwhile, evidence-based practice, albeit in the absence of regulatory trials demonstrating safety. In some cases, the use of aripiprazole alone might be a more logical choice.

Conclusion

Prescribing more than one antipsychotic medication may improve efficacy and very probably increases medical morbidity.[65,66] Nevertheless, based on evidence currently available relating to efficacy and the potential for serious adverse effects, the routine use of combined, non-clozapine, antipsychotic medications is probably best avoided.

Summary

- There is a dearth of robust evidence supporting the superiority of combined, non-clozapine, antipsychotic medications over antipsychotic monotherapy.
- There is more substantial evidence supporting the potential for harm and so the use of combined antipsychotic medications, which is commonly a high-dose prescription, should generally be avoided.

- Combined antipsychotic medications are commonly prescribed and this practice seems to be relatively resistant to change.
- As a minimum requirement, all patients who are prescribed combined antipsychotic medications should be systematically monitored for adverse effects (including an ECG) and any beneficial effect on the symptoms of psychotic illness carefully documented.
- Some antipsychotic polypharmacy strategies (e.g. combinations with aripiprazole) show clear benefits for tolerability but not efficacy.

References

1. Harrington M, et al. The results of a multi-centre audit of the prescribing of antipsychotic drugs for in-patients in the UK. *Psychiatr Bull* 2002; **26**:414–418.
2. Gallego JA, et al. Prevalence and correlates of antipsychotic polypharmacy: a systematic review and meta-regression of global and regional trends from the 1970s to 2009. *Schizophr Res* 2012; **138**:18–28.
3. Sneider B, et al. Frequency and correlates of antipsychotic polypharmacy among patients with schizophrenia in Denmark: a nation-wide pharmacoepidemiological study. *Eur Neuropsychopharmacol* 2015; **25**:1669–1676.
4. Procyshyn RM, et al. Persistent antipsychotic polypharmacy and excessive dosing in the community psychiatric treatment setting: a review of medication profiles in 435 Canadian outpatients. *J Clin Psychiatry* 2010; **71**:566–573.
5. Aggarwal NK, et al. Prevalence of concomitant oral antipsychotic drug use among patients treated with long-acting, intramuscular, antipsychotic medications. *J Clin Psychopharmacol* 2012; **32**:323–328.
6. Barnes T, et al. Antipsychotic long acting injections: prescribing practice in the UK. *Br J Psychiatry Suppl* 2009; **52**:S37–S42.
7. Novick D, et al. Antipsychotic monotherapy and polypharmacy in the treatment of outpatients with schizophrenia in the European Schizophrenia Outpatient Health Outcomes Study. *J Nerv Ment Dis* 2012; **200**:637–643.
8. Paton C, et al. High-dose and combination antipsychotic prescribing in acute adult wards in the UK: the challenges posed by p.r.n. prescribing. *Br J Psychiatry* 2008; **192**:435–439.
9. Royal College of Psychiatrists. Prescribing Observatory for Mental Health. Topic 1h & 3e: Prescribing of antipsychotic medication in adult mental health services, including high dose, combined, and PRN. CCQI 442. 2022 (last accessed February 2025); https://www.rcpsych.ac.uk/improving-care/ccqi/national-clinical-audits/pomh.
10. Correll CU, et al. Antipsychotic polypharmacy: a comprehensive evaluation of relevant correlates of a long-standing clinical practice. *Psychiatr Clin North Am* 2012; **35**:661–681.
11. Baandrup L, et al. Association of antipsychotic polypharmacy with health service cost: a register-based cost analysis. *Eur J Health Econ* 2012; **13**:355–363.
12. Kadra G, et al. Predictors of long-term (≥6months) antipsychotic polypharmacy prescribing in secondary mental healthcare. *Schizophr Res* 2016; **174**:106–112.
13. Grech P, et al. Long-term antipsychotic polypharmacy: how does it start, why does it continue? *Ther Adv Psychopharmacol* 2012; **2**:5–11.
14. Malandain L, et al. Correlates and predictors of antipsychotic drug polypharmacy in real-life settings: results from a nationwide cohort study. *Schizophr Res* 2018; **192**:213–218.
15. Fleischhacker WW, et al. Critical review of antipsychotic polypharmacy in the treatment of schizophrenia. *Int J Neuropsychopharmacol* 2014; **17**:1083–1093.
16. Korkmaz Ş A, et al. Real-world evidence of antipsychotic monotherapy versus polypharmacy in the treatment of schizophrenia spectrum disorders. *J Clin Psychopharmacol* 2024; **44**:250–257.
17. Ortiz-Orendain J, et al. Antipsychotic combinations for schizophrenia. *Schizophr Bull* 2018; **44**:15–17.
18. Galling B, et al. Antipsychotic augmentation vs. monotherapy in schizophrenia: systematic review, meta-analysis and meta-regression analysis. *World Psychiatry* 2017; **16**:77–89.
19. Essock SM, et al. Effectiveness of switching from antipsychotic polypharmacy to monotherapy. *Am J Psychiatry* 2011; **168**:702–708.
20. Hori H, et al. Switching to antipsychotic monotherapy can improve attention and processing speed, and social activity in chronic schizophrenia patients. *J Psychiatr Res* 2013; **47**:1843–1848.
21. Shakir M, et al. The effect on relapse rate and psychiatric symptomatology: switching a combination of first- and second-generation antipsychotic polypharmacy to antipsychotic monotherapy in long-term inpatients with schizophrenia and related disorders: a pragmatic randomized open-label trial (SwAP trial). *Schizophr Res* 2022; **243**:187–194.
22. Constantine RJ, et al. The risks and benefits of switching patients with schizophrenia or schizoaffective disorder from two to one antipsychotic medication: a randomized controlled trial. *Schizophr Res* 2015; **166**:194–200.
23. Katona L, et al. Real-world effectiveness of antipsychotic monotherapy vs. polypharmacy in schizophrenia: to switch or to combine? A nationwide study in Hungary. *Schizophr Res* 2014; **152**:246–254.
24. Tiihonen J, et al. Association of antipsychotic polypharmacy vs monotherapy with psychiatric rehospitalization among adults with schizophrenia. *JAMA Psychiatry* 2019; **76**:499–507.
25. Goff DC. Can adjunctive pharmacotherapy reduce hospitalization in schizophrenia? Insights from administrative databases. *JAMA Psychiatry* 2019; **76**:468–470.

26. Tiihonen J, et al. Real-world effectiveness of antipsychotic treatments in a nationwide cohort of 29823 patients with schizophrenia. *JAMA Psychiatry* 2017; **74**:686–693.

27. López de Torre A, et al. Antipsychotic polypharmacy: a needle in a haystack? *Gen Hosp Psychiatry* 2012; **34**:423–432.

28. Carnahan RM, et al. Increased risk of extrapyramidal side-effect treatment associated with atypical antipsychotic polytherapy. *Acta Psychiatr Scand* 2006; **113**:135–141.

29. Gomberg RF. Interaction between olanzapine and haloperidol. *J Clin Psychopharmacol* 1999; **19**:272–273.

30. Suzuki T, et al. Effectiveness of antipsychotic polypharmacy for patients with treatment refractory schizophrenia: an open-label trial of olanzapine plus risperidone for those who failed to respond to a sequential treatment with olanzapine, quetiapine and risperidone. *Hum Psychopharmacol* 2008; **23**:455–463.

31. Gallego JA, et al. Safety and tolerability of antipsychotic polypharmacy. *Expert Opin Drug Saf* 2012; **11**:527–542.

32. Hashimoto Y, et al. Effects of antipsychotic polypharmacy on side-effects and concurrent use of medications in schizophrenic outpatients. *Psychiatry Clin Neurosci* 2012; **66**:405–410.

33. Sorensen HJ, et al. Schizophrenia, antipsychotics and risk of hip fracture: a population-based analysis. *Eur Neuropsychopharmacol* 2013; **23**:872–878.

34. Dome P, et al. Paralytic ileus associated with combined atypical antipsychotic therapy. *Prog Neuropsychopharmacol Biol Psychiatry* 2007; **31**:557–560.

35. Hedges DW, et al. New-onset seizure associated with quetiapine and olanzapine. *Ann Pharmacother* 2002; **36**:437–439.

36. Beelen AP, et al. Asymptomatic QTc prolongation associated with quetiapine fumarate overdose in a patient being treated with risperidone. *Hum Exp Toxicol* 2001; **20**:215–219.

37. Eyles E, et al. Antipsychotic medication and risk of metabolic disorders in people with schizophrenia: a longitudinal study using the UK clinical practice research datalink. *Schizophr Bull* 2024; **50**:447–459.

38. Baandrup L, et al. Antipsychotic polypharmacy and risk of death from natural causes in patients with schizophrenia: a population-based nested case–control study. *J Clin Psychiatry* 2010; **71**:103–108.

39. Chen Y, et al. Antipsychotics and risk of natural death in patients with schizophrenia. *Neuropsychiatr Dis Treat* 2019; **15**:1863–1871.

40. Tiihonen J, et al. Polypharmacy with antipsychotics, antidepressants, or benzodiazepines and mortality in schizophrenia. *Arch Gen Psychiatry* 2012; **69**:476–483.

41. Waddington JL, et al. Mortality in schizophrenia: antipsychotic polypharmacy and absence of adjunctive anticholinergics over the course of a 10-year prospective study. *Br J Psychiatry* 1998; **173**:325–329.

42. Kadra G, et al. Long-term antipsychotic polypharmacy prescribing in secondary mental health care and the risk of mortality. *Acta Psychiatr Scand* 2018; **138**:123–132.

43. Joukamaa M, et al. Schizophrenia, neuroleptic medication and mortality. *Br J Psychiatry* 2006; **188**:122–127.

44. Centorrino F, et al. Multiple versus single antipsychotic agents for hospitalized psychiatric patients: case-control study of risks versus benefits. *Am J Psychiatry* 2004; **161**:700–706.

45. Taylor D, et al. Co-prescribing of atypical and typical antipsychotics: prescribing sequence and documented outcome. *Psychiatr Bull* 2002; **26**:170–172.

46. Kreyenbuhl J, et al. Adding or switching antipsychotic medications in treatment-refractory schizophrenia. *Psychiatr Serv* 2007; **58**:983–990.

47. Nielsen J, et al. Psychiatrists' attitude towards and knowledge of clozapine treatment. *J Psychopharmacol* 2010; **24**:965–971.

48. Ascher-Svanum H, et al. Comparison of patients undergoing switching versus augmentation of antipsychotic medications during treatment for schizophrenia. *Neuropsychiatr Dis Treat* 2012; **8**:113–118.

49. Goren JL, et al. Antipsychotic prescribing pathways, polypharmacy, and clozapine use in treatment of schizophrenia. *Psychiatr Serv* 2013; **64**:527–533.

50. Howes OD, et al. Adherence to treatment guidelines in clinical practice: study of antipsychotic treatment prior to clozapine initiation. *Br J Psychiatry* 2012; **201**:481–485.

51. Thompson JV, et al. Antipsychotic polypharmacy and augmentation strategies prior to clozapine initiation: a historical cohort study of 310 adults with treatment-resistant schizophrenic disorders. *J Psychopharmacol* 2016; **30**:436–443.

52. Shiloh R, et al. Sulpiride augmentation in people with schizophrenia partially responsive to clozapine: a double-blind, placebo-controlled study. *Br J Psychiatry* 1997; **171**:569–573.

53. Josiassen RC, et al. Clozapine augmented with risperidone in the treatment of schizophrenia: a randomized, double-blind, placebo-controlled trial. *Am J Psychiatry* 2005; **162**:130–136.

54. Paton C, et al. Augmentation with a second antipsychotic in patients with schizophrenia who partially respond to clozapine: a meta-analysis. *J Clin Psychopharmacol* 2007; **27**:198–204.

55. Barbui C, et al. Does the addition of a second antipsychotic drug improve clozapine treatment? *Schizophr Bull* 2009; **35**:458–468.

56. Taylor DM, et al. Augmentation of clozapine with a second antipsychotic: a meta-analysis of randomized, placebo-controlled studies. *Acta Psychiatr Scand* 2009; **119**:419–425.

57. Fleischhacker WW, et al. Effects of adjunctive treatment with aripiprazole on body weight and clinical efficacy in schizophrenia patients treated with clozapine: a randomized, double-blind, placebo-controlled trial. *Int J Neuropsychopharmacol* 2010; **13**:1115–1125.

58. Cooper SJ, et al. BAP guidelines on the management of weight gain, metabolic disturbances and cardiovascular risk associated with psychosis and antipsychotic drug treatment. *J Psychopharmacol* 2016; **30**:717–748.

59. Byerly MJ, et al. Effects of aripiprazole on prolactin levels in subjects with schizophrenia during cross-titration with risperidone or olanzapine: analysis of a randomized, open-label study. *Schizophr Res* 2009; **107**:218–222.

60. Liu X, et al. Co-prescription of aripiprazole on prolactin levels in long-term hospitalized chronic schizophrenic patients with co-morbid type 2 diabetes: a retrospective clinical study. *Front Psychiatry* 2023; **14**:1124691.

61. Jiang Q, et al. Treatment of antipsychotic-induced hyperprolactinemia: an umbrella review of systematic reviews and meta-analyses. *Front Psychiatry* 2024; **15**:1337274.
62. Shim JC, et al. Adjunctive treatment with a dopamine partial agonist, aripiprazole, for antipsychotic-induced hyperprolactinemia: a placebo-controlled trial. *Am J Psychiatry* 2007; **164**:1404–1410.
63. Trives MZ, et al. Effect of the addition of aripiprazole on hyperprolactinemia associated with risperidone long-acting injection. *J Clin Psychopharmacol* 2013; **33**:538–541.
64. Chen CK, et al. Differential add-on effects of aripiprazole in resolving hyperprolactinemia induced by risperidone in comparison to benzamide antipsychotics. *Prog Neuropsychopharmacol Biol Psychiatry* 2010; **34**:1495–1499.
65. Lin SK. Antipsychotic polypharmacy: a dirty little secret or a fashion? *Int J Neuropsychopharmacol* 2020; **23**:125–131.
66. Guinart D, et al. Antipsychotic polypharmacy in schizophrenia: why not? *J Clin Psychiatry* 2020; **81**:19ac13118.

Antipsychotic prophylaxis

First episode of psychosis

Antipsychotics provide effective protection against relapse, at least in the short to medium term,[1] and the introduction of antipsychotics in the 1950s seems to have improved outcomes overall.[2] A meta-analysis of placebo-controlled trials found that 26% of patients with first-episode schizophrenia on maintenance antipsychotic relapsed after 6–12 months compared with 61% on placebo.[3] Although the current consensus is that antipsychotics should be prescribed for 1–2 years after a first episode of schizophrenia,[4,5] one study[6] found that withdrawing antipsychotic treatment in line with this view led to a relapse rate of almost 80% after 1 year medication-free and 98% after 2 years. A 2019 Swedish population study revealed that the longer the treatment with antipsychotics, the lower the risk of hospitalisation (e.g. those with 5 years' treatment had half the hospitalisation rate of those treated for less than 6 months).[7]

Other studies in first-episode schizophrenia confirmed that only a small minority of patients who discontinue remain well 1–2 years later[8–11] (e.g. a small study found 94% of patients with first-episode schizophrenia relapsed within 2 years of stopping risperidone long-acting injection; 97% at three years).[12] A 2018 meta-analysis of eight RCTs was rather more optimistic and found relapse rates averaged 35% (treated) and 61% (discontinued) at 18–24 months.[13]

A 5-year follow-up of a 2-year RCT, during which patients either received maintenance antipsychotic treatment or had their antipsychotic dose reduced or discontinued completely, found that while there was a clear advantage for maintenance treatment with respect to reducing short-term relapse this advantage was lost in the medium term. Further, the dose-reduction/discontinuation group were receiving lower doses of antipsychotic drugs at follow-up and had better functional outcomes.[14] There are numerous interpretations of these outcomes but the most that can be concluded is that dose reduction is a possible option in first-episode psychosis. The study has been heavily criticised[15] and there are certainly other studies showing disastrous outcomes from antipsychotic discontinuation,[16] albeit over shorter periods with fewer patients. Nonetheless, some patients with first-episode psychosis will not need long-term antipsychotics to stay well – figures as high as 18–30% have been put forward.[17]

There are no reliable patient factors linked to outcome following discontinuation of antipsychotics in patients with first-episode psychosis (other than cannabis use)[18] and there remains more evidence in favour of continuing antipsychotics than for stopping them.[19] There are indications that very prolonged discontinuation regimens using hyperbolic tapering (see section on stopping antipsychotics in this chapter) may offer the best chance of successfully withdrawing from antipsychotic treatment.[20,21]

Definitions of relapse usually focus on the severity of positive symptoms and largely ignore cognitive and negative symptoms: positive symptoms are more likely to lead to hospitalisation while cognitive and negative symptoms (which respond less well, and in some circumstances may even be exacerbated by antipsychotic treatment) have a greater overall impact on quality of life.

With respect to antipsychotic choice, in the context of an RCT, clozapine did not offer any advantage over chlorpromazine in the medium term in patients with first-episode non-refractory schizophrenia.[22] However, in a large naturalistic study of patients with a first admission for schizophrenia, clozapine and olanzapine fared better with respect to preventing readmission than other oral antipsychotics.[23] In this same study, the use of a long-acting antipsychotic injection seemed to offer advantages over oral antipsychotics, despite confounding by indication (depots will have been prescribed to those considered to be poor adherers, oral to those perceived to have good adherence).[23] Later studies show a huge advantage for long-acting risperidone over oral risperidone in the first episode[24] and a smaller but substantial benefit for paliperidone LAI over oral antipsychotics in 'recently diagnosed schizophrenia'.[25] In a later study, amisulpride was shown to give good outcomes and staying on amisulpride after not initially reaching remission was as successful as switching to olanzapine.[26]

In practice, a firm diagnosis of schizophrenia is rarely made after a first episode and the majority of prescribers and/or patients will have at least attempted to stop antipsychotic treatment within one year.[27] Ideally, patients should have their dose reduced very gradually and all relevant family members and healthcare staff should be aware of the discontinuation (such a situation is most likely to be achieved by using LAI). It is vital that patients, carers and keyworkers are aware of the early signs of relapse and how to access help. Antipsychotics should not be considered the only intervention. Evidence-based psychosocial and psychological interventions are clearly also important.[28]

Multi-episode schizophrenia

The majority of those who have one episode of schizophrenia will go on to have further episodes. Patients with residual symptoms, a greater adverse-effect burden and a less positive attitude to treatment are at greater risk of relapse.[29] With each subsequent episode, the baseline level of functioning deteriorates[30] and the majority of this decline is seen in the first decade of illness. Suicide risk (10%) is also concentrated in the first decade of illness. Antipsychotic drugs, when taken regularly, protect against relapse in the short, medium and (with less certainty) long term.[3,31] Those who receive targeted antipsychotics (i.e. only when symptoms re-emerge) seem to have a worse outcome than those who receive prophylactic antipsychotics[32,33] and the risk of TD may also be higher. Similarly, low-dose antipsychotics are less effective than standard doses.[34] The optimal dose to prevent relapse is 5mg/day risperidone equivalents.[35] Higher doses offer no benefit and ensure poorer tolerability.

Depot preparations may have an advantage over oral in maintenance treatment, most likely because of guaranteed medication delivery (or at least guaranteed awareness of medication delivery). Meta-analyses of clinical trials have shown that the relative and absolute risks of relapse with depot maintenance treatment were 30% and 10% lower, respectively, than with oral treatment.[3,36] Long-acting preparations of antipsychotics may thus be preferred by both prescribers and patients.

Summary

- Relapse rates in patients discontinuing antipsychotics are extremely high.
- Antipsychotics significantly reduce relapse, readmission and violence/aggression.
- Long-acting depot formulations provide the best protection against relapse.

A large meta-analysis concluded that the risk of relapse with newer SGAs is similar to that associated with older drugs.[3] (Note that lack of relapse is not the same as good functioning.[37]) The proportion of patients with multi-episode schizophrenia who achieve remission is small and may differ between antipsychotic drugs. The CATIE study[38] reported that only 12% of patients treated with olanzapine achieved remission for at least 6 months, compared with 8% treated with quetiapine and 6% with risperidone. The advantage seen here for olanzapine is consistent with that seen in an acute efficacy network meta-analysis,[39] and in two recent meta-analyses of long-term efficacy.[40,41]

Adherence to antipsychotic treatment

Among people with schizophrenia, non-adherence to antipsychotic treatment is high. Only 10 days after discharge from hospital, up to 25% are partially or non-adherent, rising to 50% at 1 year and 75% at 2 years.[42] Not only does non-adherence increase the risk of relapse, it may also increase the severity of relapse and the duration of hospitalisation.[42] The risk of suicide attempts also increases four-fold[42] (see section on working towards adherence in Chapter 14). Given these low rates of adherence and the near certainty of relapse if antipsychotics are not taken, the use of oral antipsychotics is difficult to justify.

Dose for prophylaxis

Many patients probably receive higher doses than necessary (particularly of the older drugs) when acutely psychotic.[43,44] In the longer term, a balance needs to be made between effectiveness and adverse effects. Lower doses of the older drugs (8mg haloperidol/day or equivalent) are, when compared with higher doses, associated with less severe adverse effects,[45] better subjective state and better community adjustment.[46] Very low doses increase the risk of psychotic relapse.[43,47,48] The largest meta-analysis showed very clearly that prophylactic efficacy begins to be lost at doses below around 5mg/day risperidone equivalents.[35]

Doses that are acutely effective should generally be continued as prophylaxis,[49,50] although an exception to this is prophylaxis after a first episode, where very careful dose reduction is probably supportable. There is some recent support for dose reduction in multi-episode schizophrenia.[51] The concept of guided antipsychotic dose reduction has gained attention in the past few years, following the apparent success of the famous Wunderink study.[14] Later studies have suggested that guided dose reduction is associated with a substantially greater risk of relapse compared with continuation.[52,53] However (and perhaps most importantly), guided dose reduction or stopping treatment does not result in relapse in everyone, at least over the time periods examined.[54] So some people (probably a small minority) appear to be able to stop antipsychotic treatment without relapsing.

How and when to stop[55]

The decision to stop antipsychotic drugs requires a thorough risk–benefit analysis for each patient. Withdrawal of antipsychotic drugs after long-term treatment should be gradual and closely monitored. The relapse rate in the first 6 months after abrupt withdrawal is double that seen after gradual withdrawal (defined as slow taper down over at least 3 weeks for oral antipsychotics or abrupt withdrawal of depot preparations).[56] One analysis of incidence of relapse after switch to placebo found time to relapse to be very much longer for 3-monthly paliperidone than for 1-monthly and oral.[57] Overall percentage relapse was also reduced. Abrupt withdrawal of oral treatment may also lead to discontinuation symptoms (e.g. headache, nausea, insomnia) in some patients.[58]

The following factors should be considered:[55]

- Is the patient symptom-free and, if so, for how long? Long-standing, non-distressing symptoms which have not previously been responsive to medication may be excluded.
- What is the severity of adverse effects (EPS, TD, sedation, obesity, etc.)?
- What was the previous pattern of illness? Consider the speed of onset, duration and severity of episodes and any danger posed to self and others.
- Has dosage reduction been attempted before and, if so, what was the outcome?
- What are the patient's current social circumstances? Is it a period of relative stability or are stressful life events anticipated?
- What is the social cost of relapse (e.g. is the patient the sole breadwinner for a family)?
- Is the patient/carer able to monitor symptoms and, if so, will they seek help?

As with patients having their first episode, patients, carers and keyworkers should be aware of the early signs of relapse and how to access help. Be aware that targeted relapse treatment is much less effective than continuous prophylaxis.[10] Those with a history of aggressive behaviour or serious suicide attempts and those with residual psychotic symptoms should be considered for life-long treatment.

Alternative views

While it is clear that antipsychotics effectively reduce symptom severity and rates of relapse, a minority view is that antipsychotics might also sensitise patients to psychosis. The hypothesis is that relapse on withdrawal can be seen as a type of discontinuation reaction resulting from super-sensitivity of dopamine receptors, although the evidence for this remains uncertain.[59] This phenomenon might explain better outcomes seen in patients with first-episode schizophrenia who receive lower doses of antipsychotics, but it also suggests the possibility that the use of antipsychotics might ultimately worsen outcomes. It might also explain the poor outcomes seen with abrupt discontinuation of antipsychotics.[56] This observation in turn leads some to question the validity of long-term studies in which active and successful treatment is abruptly stopped, since rebound phenomena and withdrawal reactions may account for at least some of the observed high relapse rates.[60]

The concept of 'super-sensitivity psychosis' was much discussed decades ago[61,62] and has more recently seen a resurgence.[59,63] It is striking that dopamine antagonists used for non-psychiatric conditions can induce withdrawal psychosis.[64–66] While these theories and observations do not alter recommendations made in this section, they do emphasise the need for using the lowest possible dose of antipsychotic in all patients and the balancing of observed benefit with adverse outcomes, including those that might be less clinically obvious (e.g. the possibility of structural brain changes).[67] Clinicians should remain open-minded about the possibility that long-term antipsychotics may worsen, or at least not improve, outcomes in some people with schizophrenia.

References

1. Karson C, et al. Long-term outcomes of antipsychotic treatment in patients with first-episode schizophrenia: a systematic review. *Neuropsychiatr Dis Treat* 2016; **12**:57–67.

2. Taylor M, et al. Are we getting any better at staying better? The long view on relapse and recovery in first episode nonaffective psychosis and schizophrenia. *Ther Adv Psychopharmacol* 2019; **9**:2045125319870033.

3. Leucht S, et al. Antipsychotic drugs versus placebo for relapse prevention in schizophrenia: a systematic review and meta-analysis. *Lancet* 2012; **379**:2063–2071.

4. American Psychiatric Association. *Practice Guideline for the Treatment of Patients with Schizophrenia*, 3rd edn. Washington, DC: APA; 2020 (last accessed December 2024); https://psychiatryonline.org/doi/book/10.1176/appi.books.9780890424841.

5. Sheitman BB, et al. The evaluation and treatment of first-episode psychosis. *Schizophrenia Bulletin* 1997; **23**:653–661.

6. Gitlin M, et al. Clinical outcome following neuroleptic discontinuation in patients with remitted recent-onset schizophrenia. *Am J Psychiatry* 2001; **158**:1835–1842.

7. Hayes JF, et al. Psychiatric hospitalization following antipsychotic medication cessation in first episode psychosis. *J Psychopharmacol* 2019; **33**:532–534.

8. Wunderink L, et al. Guided discontinuation versus maintenance treatment in remitted first-episode psychosis: relapse rates and functional outcome. *J Clin Psychiatry* 2007; **68**:654–661.

9. Chen EY, et al. Maintenance treatment with quetiapine versus discontinuation after one year of treatment in patients with remitted first episode psychosis: randomised controlled trial. *BMJ* 2010; **341**:c4024.

10. Gaebel W, et al. Relapse prevention in first-episode schizophrenia. Maintenance vs intermittent drug treatment with prodrome-based early intervention: results of a randomized controlled trial within the German Research Network on Schizophrenia. *J Clin Psychiatry* 2011; **72**:205–218.

11. Caseiro O, et al. Predicting relapse after a first episode of non-affective psychosis: a three-year follow-up study. *J Psychiatr Res* 2012; **46**:1099–1105.

12. Emsley R, et al. Symptom recurrence following intermittent treatment in first-episode schizophrenia successfully treated for 2 years: a 3-year open-label clinical study. *J Clin Psychiatry* 2012; **73**:e541–e547.

13. Kishi T, et al. Effect of discontinuation v. maintenance of antipsychotic medication on relapse rates in patients with remitted/stable first-episode psychosis: a meta-analysis. *Psychol Med* 2019; **49**:772–779.

14. Wunderink L, et al. Recovery in remitted first-episode psychosis at 7 years of follow-up of an early dose reduction/discontinuation or maintenance treatment strategy: long-term follow-up of a 2-year randomized clinical trial. *JAMA Psychiatry* 2013; **70**:913–920.

15. Correll CU, et al. What is the risk-benefit ratio of long-term antipsychotic treatment in people with schizophrenia? *World Psychiatry* 2018; **17**:149–160.

16. Boonstra G, et al. Antipsychotic prophylaxis is needed after remission from a first psychotic episode in schizophrenia patients: results from an aborted randomised trial. *Int J Psychiatry Clin Pract* 2011; **15**:128–134.

17. Murray RM, et al. Should psychiatrists be more cautious about the long-term prophylactic use of antipsychotics? *Br J Psychiatry* 2016; **209**:361–365.

18. Bowtell M, et al. Rates and predictors of relapse following discontinuation of antipsychotic medication after a first episode of psychosis. *Schizophr Res* 2018; **195**:231–236.

19. Emsley R, et al. How long should antipsychotic treatment be continued after a single episode of schizophrenia? *Curr Opin Psychiatry* 2016; **29**:224–229.

20. Horowitz MA, et al. Tapering antipsychotic treatment. *JAMA Psychiatry* 2020; **78**:125–126.

21. Liu CC, et al. Achieving the lowest effective antipsychotic dose for patients with remitted psychosis: a proposed guided dose-reduction algorithm. *CNS Drugs* 2020; **34**:117–126.

22. Girgis RR, et al. Clozapine v. chlorpromazine in treatment-naive, first-episode schizophrenia: 9-year outcomes of a randomised clinical trial. *Br J Psychiatry* 2011; **199**:281–288.

23. Tiihonen J, et al. A nationwide cohort study of oral and depot antipsychotics after first hospitalization for schizophrenia. *Am J Psychiatry* 2011; **168**:603–609.

24. Subotnik KL, et al. Long-acting injectable risperidone for relapse prevention and control of breakthrough symptoms after a recent first episode of schizophrenia. a randomized clinical trial. *JAMA Psychiatry* 2015; **72**:822–829.

25. Schreiner A, et al. Paliperidone palmitate versus oral antipsychotics in recently diagnosed schizophrenia. *Schizophr Res* 2015; **169**:393–399.

26. Kahn RS, et al. Amisulpride and olanzapine followed by open-label treatment with clozapine in first-episode schizophrenia and schizophreniform disorder (OPTiMiSE): a three-phase switching study. *Lancet Psychiatry* 2018; **5**:797–807.

27. Johnson DAW, et al. Professional attitudes in the UK towards neuroleptic maintenance therapy in schizophrenia. *Psychiatr Bull* 1997; **21**:394–397.

28. National Institute for Health and Care Excellence. Psychosis and schizophrenia in adults: prevention and management. Clinical guideline [CG178]. 2014 (last checked November 2024); https://www.nice.org.uk/guidance/cg178.

29. Schennach R, et al. Predictors of relapse in the year after hospital discharge among patients with schizophrenia. *Psychiatr Serv* 2012; **63**:87–90.

30. Wyatt RJ. Neuroleptics and the natural course of schizophrenia. *Schizophrenia Bulletin* 1991; **17**:325–351.

31. Almerie MQ, et al. Cessation of medication for people with schizophrenia already stable on chlorpromazine. *Schizophr Bull* 2008; **34**:13–14.

32. Jolley AG, et al. Trial of brief intermittent neuroleptic prophylaxis for selected schizophrenic outpatients: clinical and social outcome at two years. *BMJ* 1990; **301**:837–842.

33. Herz MI, et al. Intermittent vs maintenance medication in schizophrenia: two-year results. *Arch Gen Psychiatry* 1991; **48**:333–339.

34. Schooler NR, et al. Relapse and rehospitalization during maintenance treatment of schizophrenia. The effects of dose reduction and family treatment. *Arch Gen Psychiatry* 1997; **54**:453–463.

35. Leucht S, et al. Examination of dosing of antipsychotic drugs for relapse prevention in patients with stable schizophrenia: a meta-analysis. *JAMA Psychiatry* 2021; **78**:1238–1248.

36. Leucht C, et al. Oral versus depot antipsychotic drugs for schizophrenia—a critical systematic review and meta-analysis of randomised long-term trials. *Schizophr Res* 2011; **127**:83–92.

37. Schooler NR. Relapse prevention and recovery in the treatment of schizophrenia. *J Clin Psychiatry* 2006; **67** Suppl 5:19–23.

38. Levine SZ, et al. Extent of attaining and maintaining symptom remission by antipsychotic medication in the treatment of chronic schizophrenia: evidence from the CATIE study. *Schizophr Res* 2011; **133**:42–46.

39. Leucht S, et al. Comparative efficacy and tolerability of 15 antipsychotic drugs in schizophrenia: a multiple-treatments meta-analysis. *Lancet* 2013; **382**:951–962.

40. Leucht S, et al. Long-term efficacy of antipsychotic drugs in initially acutely ill adults with schizophrenia: systematic review and network meta-analysis. *World Psychiatry* 2023; **22**:315–324.

41. Ostuzzi G, et al. Oral and long-acting antipsychotics for relapse prevention in schizophrenia-spectrum disorders: a network meta-analysis of 92 randomized trials including 22,645 participants. *World Psychiatry* 2022; **21**:295–307.

42. Leucht S, et al. Epidemiology, clinical consequences, and psychosocial treatment of nonadherence in schizophrenia. *J Clin Psychiatry* 2006; **67** Suppl 5:3–8.

43. Baldessarini RJ, et al. Significance of neuroleptic dose and plasma level in the pharmacological treatment of psychoses. *Arch Gen Psychiatry* 1988; **45**:79–90.

44. Harrington M, et al. The results of a multi-centre audit of the prescribing of antipsychotic drugs for in-patients in the UK. *Psychiatr Bull* 2002; **26**:414–418.

45. Geddes J, et al. Atypical antipsychotics in the treatment of schizophrenia: systematic overview and meta-regression analysis. *BMJ* 2000; **321**:1371–1376.

46. Hogarty GE, et al. Dose of fluphenazine, familial expressed emotion, and outcome in schizophrenia. Results of a two-year controlled study. *Arch Gen Psychiatry* 1988; **45**:797–805.

47. Marder SR, et al. Low- and conventional-dose maintenance therapy with fluphenazine decanoate. Two-year outcome. *Arch Gen Psychiatry* 1987; **44**:518–521.

48. Uchida H, et al. Low dose vs standard dose of antipsychotics for relapse prevention in schizophrenia: meta-analysis. *Schizophr Bull* 2011; **37**:788–799.

49. Rouillon F, et al. Strategies of treatment with olanzapine in schizophrenic patients during stable phase: results of a pilot study. *Eur Neuropsychopharmacol* 2008; **18**:646–652.

50. Wang CY, et al. Risperidone maintenance treatment in schizophrenia: a randomized, controlled trial. *Am J Psychiatry* 2010; **167**:676–685.

51. Huhn M, et al. Reducing antipsychotic drugs in stable patients with chronic schizophrenia or schizoaffective disorder: a randomized controlled pilot trial. *Eur Arch Psychiatry Clin Neurosci* 2021; **271**:293–302.

52. Liu CC, et al. Guided antipsychotic reduction to reach minimum effective dose (GARMED) in patients with remitted psychosis: a 2-year randomized controlled trial with a naturalistic cohort. *Psychol Med* 2023; **53**:7078–7086.

53. Moncrieff J, et al. Antipsychotic dose reduction and discontinuation versus maintenance treatment in people with schizophrenia and other recurrent psychotic disorders in England (the RADAR trial): an open, parallel-group, randomised controlled trial. *Lancet Psychiatry* 2023; **10**:848–859.

54. Ostuzzi G, et al. Continuing, reducing, switching, or stopping antipsychotics in individuals with schizophrenia-spectrum disorders who are clinically stable: a systematic review and network meta-analysis. *Lancet Psychiatry* 2022; **9**:614–624.

55. Wyatt RJ. Risks of withdrawing antipsychotic medications. *Arch Gen Psychiatry* 1995; **52**:205–208.

56. Viguera AC, et al. Clinical risk following abrupt and gradual withdrawal of maintenance neuroleptic treatment. *Arch Gen Psychiatry* 1997; **54**:49–55.

57. Weiden PJ, et al. Does half-life matter after antipsychotic discontinuation? A relapse comparison in schizophrenia with 3 different formulations of paliperidone. *J Clin Psychiatry* 2017; **78**:e813–e820.

58. Chouinard G, et al. Withdrawal symptoms after long-term treatment with low-potency neuroleptics. *J Clin Psychiatry* 1984; **45**:500–502.

59. Yin J, et al. Antipsychotic induced dopamine supersensitivity psychosis: a comprehensive review. *Curr Neuropharmacol* 2017; **15**:174–183.

60. Cohen D, et al. Discontinuing psychotropic drugs from participants in randomized controlled trials: a systematic review. *Psychother Psychosom* 2019; **88**:96–104.

61. Chouinard G, et al. Neuroleptic-induced supersensitivity psychosis: clinical and pharmacologic characteristics. *Am J Psychiatry* 1980; **137**:16–21.

62. Kirkpatrick B, et al. The concept of supersensitivity psychosis. *J Nerv Ment Dis* 1992; **180**:265–270.

63. Lugg W. Antipsychotic-induced supersensitivity: a reappraisal. *Aust N Z J Psychiatry* 2022; **56**:437–444.

64. Chaffin DS. Phenothiazine-induced acute psychotic reaction: the 'psychotoxicity' of a drug. *Am J Psychiatry* 1964; **121**:26–32.

65. Lu ML, et al. Metoclopramide-induced supersensitivity psychosis. *Ann Pharmacother* 2002; **36**:1387–1390.

66. Roy-Desruisseaux J, et al. Domperidone-induced tardive dyskinesia and withdrawal psychosis in an elderly woman with dementia. *Ann Pharmacother* 2011; **45**:e51.

67. Huhtaniska S, et al. Long-term antipsychotic use and brain changes in schizophrenia - a systematic review and meta-analysis. *Hum Psychopharmacol* 2017; **32**:e2574.

Negative symptoms

Negative symptoms in schizophrenia represent the absence or diminution of normal behaviours and functions and constitute an important dimension of psychopathology. A subdomain of 'expressive deficits' manifests as a decrease in verbal output and verbal expressiveness, and flattened or blunted affect, which is assessed by diminished facial emotional expression, poor eye contact, decreased spontaneous movement and lack of spontaneity. A second 'avolition/amotivation' subdomain is characterised by a subjective reduction in interests, desires and goals, and a behavioural reduction in purposeful acts, including a lack of self-initiated social interactions.[1,2] While there is some consensus around this two-dimensional model, five-factor models of negative symptoms have also been propounded.[3,4]

Persistent negative symptoms are held to account for much of the long-term morbidity and poor functional outcome of patients with schizophrenia.[5-8] The aetiology of negative symptoms is complex, and it is important to determine the most likely cause in any individual case before embarking on a treatment regimen. An important clinical distinction is between primary negative symptoms, which constitute an enduring deficit state, predict a poor prognosis and are stable over time, and secondary negative symptoms, which are consequent upon positive psychotic symptoms, depression or demoralisation, or adverse medication effects, such as dysphoria and bradykinesia as part of drug-induced parkinsonism.[7,9] Other sources of secondary negative symptoms may include chronic substance or alcohol use, high-dose antipsychotic medication, social deprivation, lack of stimulation and hospitalisation.[10] Secondary negative symptoms may be best tackled by treating the relevant underlying cause. In people with established schizophrenia, prominent, clinically relevant negative symptoms are seen in around 60%, with up to 20% judged to have persistent, primary negative symptoms.[11-13]

The literature pertaining to the pharmacological treatment of negative symptoms partly comprises sub-analyses of acute efficacy studies, correlational analyses and path analyses.[14] There is often no reliable distinction between primary and secondary negative symptoms or between the two subdomains of expressive deficits and avolition/amotivation, and relatively few studies specifically recruit patients with persistent or predominant negative symptoms. While the evidence suggests short- and medium-term efficacy for a few interventions, there is no widely accepted evidence for an effective treatment for persistent primary negative symptoms.

Pharmacological treatment of negative symptoms

- In first-episode psychosis, the presence of negative symptoms is related to poor outcome in terms of recovery and level of social functioning.[6,11] There is evidence to suggest that the earlier a psychotic illness is effectively treated, the less likely is the development of negative symptoms over time.[15-17] However, when interpreting such data, it should be borne in mind that an early clinical picture characterised by negative symptoms, being a less socially disruptive and more subtle signal of psychotic illness than positive symptoms, may contribute to delay in presentation to clinical services and thus be associated with a longer duration of untreated psychosis. In other words, patients with an inherently poorer prognosis in terms of persistent negative symptoms may be diagnosed and treated later.

- While antipsychotic medication has been shown to improve negative symptoms, this benefit has mainly been shown in secondary negative symptoms in acute psychotic episodes.[18] Against expectations, there is no consistent evidence for the superiority of SGAs over FGAs in the treatment of negative symptoms.[19–23] Similarly, early analyses found no consistent evidence for the superiority of any individual SGA.[24] A 2015 meta-analysis of 38 RCTs found a statistically significant reduction in negative symptoms with SGAs, but the effect size did not reach a threshold for 'minimally detectable clinical improvement over time'.[25]

- There are some relatively robust data suggesting superior efficacy for negative symptoms with certain antipsychotics, such as **cariprazine**,[26–28] **aripiprazole** and **amisulpride**, and single trials suggesting that **olanzapine** and **quetiapine** may be more effective than risperidone.[26,29–37] A 2023 review included **amisulpride** and **cariprazine** among the medications considered to have the most promise as treatments for primary negative symptoms.[38]

- While **clozapine** remains the only medication with convincing superiority for TRS, whether or not it has superior efficacy for negative symptoms in such cases, at least in the short term, remains uncertain.[39–41] One potential confound in studies of clozapine for negative symptoms is that the medication has a low liability for parkinsonian adverse effects, including bradykinesia. These are symptoms which have a phenomenological overlap with negative symptoms, particularly the subdomain of expressive deficits. There is some evidence to suggest that for patients being treated with clozapine who have residual negative symptoms, the addition of cariprazine may help.[42,43]

- With respect to the effect of decreasing glutamate transmission on negative symptoms, three meta-analyses have suggested a beneficial response with add-on **memantine**[44–46] but there have been inconsistent meta-analysis findings for lamotrigine augmentation of clozapine.[47,48] Adding **minocycline**, an antibiotic and inflammatory drug, initially showed promise[46,49,50] but a relatively large RCT of adjunctive minocycline found it was not efficacious in treating negative symptoms.[51] Further, the BeneMin study,[49] which was designed to determine whether adjunctive minocycline, administered early in the course of schizophrenia, protected against the development of negative symptoms over a year, also failed to find any evidence of clinical benefit. The glutamate antagonist **topiramate** may have some efficacy for symptom reduction in schizophrenia spectrum disorders, including negative symptoms.[52]

- A 2006 Cochrane review concluded that **antidepressant augmentation** of an antipsychotic for negative symptoms may be an effective strategy for reducing affective flattening, alogia and avolition.[53] RCTs and meta-analyses addressing antidepressant augmentation of antipsychotic medication have yielded somewhat inconsistent evidence of modest efficacy.[54–59] One meta-analysis of placebo-controlled studies in people with established schizophrenia found that adjunctive antidepressant treatment was associated with a limited reduction in negative symptoms, and only when added to treatment with FGAs.[58] Another review of meta-analyses concluded that the evidence suggested a beneficial effect for some SSRIs, such as **fluvoxamine**, **citalopram**, and the α_2 receptor antagonists **mirtazapine** and **mianserin**.[18] **Reboxetine** (a noradrenaline reuptake inhibitor) may also have some activity.[60]

- A host of other augmentation agents have been tested.[46,61,62] For example, meta-analyses provide some support for adjunctive treatment with **Ginkgo biloba**[63] and a **COX-2 (cyclooxygenase-2) inhibitor** (albeit with a small effect size),[64] while small

RCTs have demonstrated some benefit for **selegiline**,[65,66] **pramiprexole**,[67] **topical testosterone**,[68] **ondansetron**,[69] **granisetron**,[70] **palmitoylethanolamide** (an endogenous analogue of anandamide, an endocannabinoid) added to risperidone[71] and **pimavanserin**, a potent $5\text{-}HT_{2A}$ inverse agonist and antagonist.[72,73] The $5HT_2$ antagonist **roluperidone** may also be effective.[74,75]

- Other experimental treatments for which promising data exist include **pregnenolone**,[76] **raloxifene** (in women),[77] **levetiracetam**,[78] **clonidine**,[79] **nanocurcumin**,[80] **xanomeline** (as Cobenfy)[81] and the anti-inflammatory drugs **berberine**[82] and **fingolimod.**[61]
- The findings from studies of repetitive transcranial magnetic stimulation (**rTMS**) are mixed but promising.[83] Transcranial direct current stimulation (**tDCS**) may also have some potential as a treatment for negative symptoms, but the evidence thus far is limited and rather inconsistent.[18,84–87]

Patients who misuse psychoactive substances may experience less severe negative symptoms than patients who do not.[88] But rather than any pharmacological effect, it may be that this association at least partly reflects that those people who develop psychosis in the context of substance use, specifically cannabis, have fewer neurodevelopmental risk factors and thus better cognitive and social function.[89,90]

Summary and recommendations

These recommendations are derived from the British Association for Psychopharmacology (BAP) schizophrenia guideline (2020),[91] Galderisi et al. (2021),[87] Veerman et al. (2017),[10] Aleman et al. (2017)[18] and Howes et al. (2023).[38]

- There are no well-replicated, large trials or meta-analyses of trials with negative symptoms as the primary outcome measure that have yielded convincing evidence for enduring and clinically significant benefit.
- Where some improvement has been demonstrated in clinical trials, this may be limited to secondary negative symptoms.
- Psychotic illness should be identified and treated as early as possible, as this may offer some protection against the development of negative symptoms.
- For any given patient, the antipsychotic medication that provides the best balance between overall efficacy and adverse effects should be used, at the lowest dose that maintains control of positive symptoms.
- Where negative symptoms persist beyond an acute episode of psychosis:
  - Ensure that EPS (specifically bradykinesia) and depression are detected and treated if present, and consider the contribution of the environment to negative symptoms (e.g. institutionalisation, lack of stimulation).
  - There is insufficient evidence at present to support a recommendation for any specific pharmacological treatment for negative symptoms. Nevertheless, a trial of add-on medication for which there is some RCT evidence for efficacy, such as an antidepressant or an antipsychotic, may be worth considering in some cases, ensuring that the choice of the augmenting agent is based on minimising the potential for compounding adverse effects through pharmacokinetic or pharmacodynamic drug interactions.

References

1. Messinger JW, et al. Avolition and expressive deficits capture negative symptom phenomenology: implications for DSM-5 and schizophrenia research. *Clin Psychol Rev* 2011; **31**:161–168.

2. Foussias G, et al. Dissecting negative symptoms in schizophrenia: opportunities for translation into new treatments. *J Psychopharmacol* 2015; **29**:116–126.

3. Strauss GP, et al. Reconsidering the latent structure of negative symptoms in schizophrenia: a review of evidence supporting the 5 consensus domains. *Schizophr Bull* 2019; **45**:725–729.

4. Rucci P, et al. The structure stability of negative symptoms: longitudinal network analysis of the Brief Negative Symptom Scale in people with schizophrenia. *BJPsych Open* 2023; **9**:e168.

5. Carpenter WT. The treatment of negative symptoms: pharmacological and methodological issues. *Br J Psychiatry* 1996; **168**:17–22.

6. Galderisi S, et al. Persistent negative symptoms in first episode patients with schizophrenia: results from the European First Episode Schizophrenia Trial. *Eur Neuropsychopharmacol* 2013; **23**:196–204.

7. Buchanan RW. Persistent negative symptoms in schizophrenia: an overview. *Schizophr Bull* 2007; **33**:1013–1022.

8. Rabinowitz J, et al. Negative symptoms have greater impact on functioning than positive symptoms in schizophrenia: analysis of CATIE data. *Schizophr Res* 2012; **137**:147–150.

9. Barnes TR, et al. How to distinguish between the neuroleptic-induced deficit syndrome, depression and disease-related negative symptoms in schizophrenia. *Int Clin Psychopharmacol* 1995; **10** Suppl 3:115–121.

10. Veerman SRT, et al. Treatment for negative symptoms in schizophrenia: a comprehensive review. *Drugs* 2017; **77**:1423–1459.

11. Rammou A, et al. Negative symptoms in first-episode psychosis: clinical correlates and 1-year follow-up outcomes in London Early Intervention Services. *Early Interv Psychiatry* 2019; **13**:443–452.

12. Bobes J, et al. Prevalence of negative symptoms in outpatients with schizophrenia spectrum disorders treated with antipsychotics in routine clinical practice: findings from the CLAMORS study. *J Clin Psychiatry* 2010; **71**:280–286.

13. Correll CU, et al. Negative symptoms in schizophrenia: a review and clinical guide for recognition, assessment, and treatment. *Neuropsychiatr Dis Treat* 2020; **16**:519–534.

14. Buckley PF, et al. Pharmacological treatment of negative symptoms of schizophrenia: therapeutic opportunity or cul-de-sac? *Acta Psychiatr Scand* 2007; **115**:93–100.

15. Waddington JL, et al. Sequential cross-sectional and 10-year prospective study of severe negative symptoms in relation to duration of initially untreated psychosis in chronic schizophrenia. *Psychol Med* 1995; **25**:849–857.

16. Melle I, et al. Prevention of negative symptom psychopathologies in first-episode schizophrenia: two-year effects of reducing the duration of untreated psychosis. *Arch Gen Psychiatry* 2008; **65**:634–640.

17. Perkins DO, et al. Relationship between duration of untreated psychosis and outcome in first-episode schizophrenia: a critical review and meta-analysis. *Am J Psychiatry* 2005; **162**:1785–1804.

18. Aleman A, et al. Treatment of negative symptoms: where do we stand, and where do we go? *Schizophr Res* 2017; **186**:55–62.

19. Darbà J, et al. Efficacy of second-generation-antipsychotics in the treatment of negative symptoms of schizophrenia: a meta-analysis of randomized clinical trials. *Rev Psiquiatr Salud Ment* 2011; **4**:126–143.

20. Leucht S, et al. Second-generation versus first-generation antipsychotic drugs for schizophrenia: a meta-analysis. *Lancet* 2009; **373**:31–41.

21. Erhart SM, et al. Treatment of schizophrenia negative symptoms: future prospects. *Schizophr Bull* 2006; **32**:234–237.

22. Harvey RC, et al. A systematic review and network meta-analysis to assess the relative efficacy of antipsychotics for the treatment of positive and negative symptoms in early-onset schizophrenia. *CNS Drugs* 2016; **30**:27–39.

23. Zhang JP, et al. Efficacy and safety of individual second-generation vs. first-generation antipsychotics in first-episode psychosis: a systematic review and meta-analysis. *Int J Neuropsychopharmacol* 2013; **16**:1205–1218.

24. Leucht S, et al. A meta-analysis of head-to-head comparisons of second-generation antipsychotics in the treatment of schizophrenia. *Am J Psychiatry* 2009; **166**:152–163.

25. Fusar-Poli P, et al. Treatments of negative symptoms in schizophrenia: meta-analysis of 168 randomized placebo-controlled trials. *Schizophr Bull* 2015; **41**:892–899.

26. Németh G, et al. Cariprazine versus risperidone monotherapy for treatment of predominant negative symptoms in patients with schizophrenia: a randomised, double-blind, controlled trial. *Lancet* 2017; **389**:1103–1113.

27. Ivanov SV, et al. Early clinical effects of novel partial D3/D2 agonist cariprazine in schizophrenia patients with predominantly negative symptoms (open-label, non-controlled study). *Front Psychiatry* 2021; **12**:770592.

28. Németh G, et al. Addressing negative symptoms of schizophrenia pharmacologically with cariprazine: evidence from clinical trials, a real-world study, and clinical cases. *Expert Opin Pharmacother* 2022; **23**:1467–1468.

29. Speller JC, et al. One-year, low-dose neuroleptic study of in-patients with chronic schizophrenia characterised by persistent negative symptoms: amisulpride v. haloperidol. *Br J Psychiatry* 1997; **171**:564–568.

30. Krause M, et al. Antipsychotic drugs for patients with schizophrenia and predominant or prominent negative symptoms: a systematic review and meta-analysis. *Eur Arch Psychiatry Clin Neurosci* 2018; **268**:625–639.

31. Danion JM, et al. Improvement of schizophrenic patients with primary negative symptoms treated with amisulpride. Amisulpride Study Group. *Am J Psychiatry* 1999; **156**:610–616.

32. Leucht S, et al. Amisulpride, an unusual 'atypical' antipsychotic: a meta-analysis of randomized controlled trials. *Am J Psychiatry* 2002; **159**:180–190.

33. Liang Y, et al. Effectiveness of amisulpride in Chinese patients with predominantly negative symptoms of schizophrenia: a subanalysis of the ESCAPE study. *Neuropsychiatr Dis Treat* 2017; **13**:1703–1712.

34. Zheng W, et al. Efficacy and safety of adjunctive aripiprazole in schizophrenia: meta-analysis of randomized controlled trials. *J Clin Psychopharmacol* 2016; **36**:628–636.

35. Galling B, et al. Antipsychotic augmentation vs. monotherapy in schizophrenia: systematic review, meta-analysis and meta-regression analysis. *World Psychiatry* 2017; **16**:77–89.

36. Earley W, et al. Efficacy of cariprazine on negative symptoms in patients with acute schizophrenia: a post hoc analysis of pooled data. *Schizophr Res* 2019; **204**:282–288.

37. Brasso C, et al. Efficacy of serotonin and dopamine activity modulators in the treatment of negative symptoms in schizophrenia: a rapid review. *Biomedicines* 2023; **11**:921.

38. Howes O, et al. Treating negative symptoms of schizophrenia: current approaches and future perspectives. *Br J Psychiatry* 2023; **223**:332–335.

39. Siskind D, et al. Clozapine v. first- and second-generation antipsychotics in treatment-refractory schizophrenia: systematic review and meta-analysis. *Br J Psychiatry* 2016; **209**:385–392.

40. Souza JS, et al. Efficacy of olanzapine in comparison with clozapine for treatment-resistant schizophrenia: evidence from a systematic review and meta-analyses. *CNS Spectr* 2013; **18**:82–89.

41. Asenjo Lobos C, et al. Clozapine versus other atypical antipsychotics for schizophrenia. *Cochrane Database Syst Rev* 2010; (11):CD006633.

42. Oloyede E, et al. Clozapine augmentation with cariprazine for negative symptoms: a case series and literature review. *Ther Adv Psychopharmacol* 2022; **12**:20451253211066642.

43. Siwek M, et al. Cariprazine augmentation of clozapine in schizophrenia: a retrospective chart review. *Front Pharmacol* 2023; **14**:1321112.

44. Kishi T, et al. Memantine add-on to antipsychotic treatment for residual negative and cognitive symptoms of schizophrenia: a meta-analysis. *Psychopharmacology (Berl)* 2017; **234**:2113–2125.

45. Zheng W, et al. Adjunctive memantine for schizophrenia: a meta-analysis of randomized, double-blind, placebo-controlled trials. *Psychol Med* 2018; **48**:72–81.

46. Etchecopar-Etchart D, et al. Comprehensive evaluation of 45 augmentation drugs for schizophrenia: a network meta-analysis. *EClinicalMedicine* 2024; **69**:102473.

47. Tiihonen J, et al. The efficacy of lamotrigine in clozapine-resistant schizophrenia: a systematic review and meta-analysis. *Schizophr Res* 2009; **109**:10–14.

48. Veerman SR, et al. Clozapine augmented with glutamate modulators in refractory schizophrenia: a review and metaanalysis. *Pharmacopsychiatry* 2014; **47**:185–194.

49. Oya K, et al. Efficacy and tolerability of minocycline augmentation therapy in schizophrenia: a systematic review and meta-analysis of randomized controlled trials. *Hum Psychopharmacol* 2014; **29**:483–491.

50. Xiang YQ, et al. Adjunctive minocycline for schizophrenia: a meta-analysis of randomized controlled trials. *Eur Neuropsychopharmacol* 2017; **27**:8–18.

51. Weiser M, et al. The effect of minocycline on symptoms in schizophrenia: results from a randomized controlled trial. *Schizophr Res* 2019; **206**:325–332.

52. Afshar H, et al. Topiramate add-on treatment in schizophrenia: a randomised, double-blind, placebo-controlled clinical trial. *J Psychopharmacol* 2009; **23**:157–162.

53. Rummel C, et al. Antidepressants for the negative symptoms of schizophrenia. *Cochrane Database Syst Rev* 2006; (3):CD005581.

54. Kishi T, et al. Meta-analysis of noradrenergic and specific serotonergic antidepressant use in schizophrenia. *Int J Neuropsychopharmacol* 2014; **17**:343–354.

55. Sepehry AA, et al. Selective serotonin reuptake inhibitor (SSRI) add-on therapy for the negative symptoms of schizophrenia: a meta-analysis. *J Clin Psychiatry* 2007; **68**:604–610.

56. Singh SP, et al. Efficacy of antidepressants in treating the negative symptoms of chronic schizophrenia: meta-analysis. *Br J Psychiatry* 2010; **197**:174–179.

57. Barnes TR, et al. Antidepressant Controlled Trial For Negative Symptoms In Schizophrenia (ACTIONS): a double-blind, placebo-controlled, randomised clinical trial. *Health Technol Assess* 2016; **20**:1–46.

58. Galling B, et al. Efficacy and safety of antidepressant augmentation of continued antipsychotic treatment in patients with schizophrenia. *Acta Psychiatr Scand* 2018; **137**:187–205.

59. Helfer B, et al. Efficacy and safety of antidepressants added to antipsychotics for schizophrenia: a systematic review and meta-analysis. *Am J Psychiatry* 2016; **173**:876–886.

60. Zheng W, et al. Adjunctive reboxetine for schizophrenia: meta-analysis of randomized double-blind, placebo-controlled trials. *Pharmacopsychiatry* 2020; **53**:5–13.

61. Karbalaee M, et al. Efficacy and safety of adjunctive therapy with fingolimod in patients with schizophrenia: a randomized, double-blind, placebo-controlled clinical trial. *Schizophr Res* 2023; **254**:92–98.

62. Correll CU, et al. Efficacy of 42 pharmacologic cotreatment strategies added to antipsychotic monotherapy in schizophrenia: systematic overview and quality appraisal of the meta-analytic evidence. *JAMA Psychiatry* 2017; **74**:675–684.

63. Singh V, et al. Review and meta-analysis of usage of ginkgo as an adjunct therapy in chronic schizophrenia. *Int J Neuropsychopharmacol* 2010; **13**:257–271.

64. Sommer IE, et al. Nonsteroidal anti-inflammatory drugs in schizophrenia: ready for practice or a good start? A meta-analysis. *J Clin Psychiatry* 2012; **73**:414–419.

65. Amiri A, et al. Efficacy of selegiline add on therapy to risperidone in the treatment of the negative symptoms of schizophrenia: a double-blind randomized placebo-controlled study. *Hum Psychopharmacol* 2008; **23**:79–86.

66. Bodkin JA, et al. Double-blind, placebo-controlled, multicenter trial of selegiline augmentation of antipsychotic medication to treat negative symptoms in outpatients with schizophrenia. *Am J Psychiatry* 2005; **162**:388–390.

67. Kelleher JP, et al. Pilot randomized, controlled trial of pramipexole to augment antipsychotic treatment. *Eur Neuropsychopharmacol* 2012; 22:415–418.

68. Ko YH, et al. Short-term testosterone augmentation in male schizophrenics: a randomized, double-blind, placebo-controlled trial. *J Clin Psychopharmacol* 2008; 28:375–383.

69. Zhang ZJ, et al. Beneficial effects of ondansetron as an adjunct to haloperidol for chronic, treatment-resistant schizophrenia: a double-blind, randomized, placebo-controlled study. *Schizophr Res* 2006; 88:102–110.

70. Khodaie-Ardakani MR, et al. Granisetron as an add-on to risperidone for treatment of negative symptoms in patients with stable schizophrenia: randomized double-blind placebo-controlled study. *J Psychiatr Res* 2013; 47:472–478.

71. Salehi A, et al. Adjuvant palmitoylethanolamide therapy with risperidone improves negative symptoms in patients with schizophrenia: a randomized, double-blinded, placebo-controlled trial. *Psychiatry Res* 2022; 316:114737.

72. Bugarski-Kirola D, et al. Pimavanserin for negative symptoms of schizophrenia: results from the ADVANCE phase 2 randomised, placebo-controlled trial in North America and Europe. *Lancet Psychiatry* 2022; 9:46–58.

73. Davis J, et al. Evaluating pimavanserin as a treatment for psychiatric disorders: a pharmacological property in search of an indication. *Expert Opin Pharmacother* 2021; 22:1651–1660.

74. Davidson M, et al. Efficacy and safety of roluperidone for the treatment of negative symptoms of schizophrenia. *Schizophr Bull* 2022; 48:609–619.

75. Romeo B, et al. Efficacy of 5-HT2A antagonists on negative symptoms in patients with schizophrenia: a meta-analysis. *Psychiatry Res* 2023; 321:115104.

76. Ritsner MS, et al. Pregnenolone treatment reduces severity of negative symptoms in recent-onset schizophrenia: an 8-week, double-blind, randomized add-on two-center trial. *Psychiatry Clin Neurosci* 2014; 68:432–440.

77. Brand BA, et al. The direct and long-term effects of raloxifene as adjunctive treatment for schizophrenia-spectrum disorders: a double-blind, randomized clinical trial. *Schizophr Bull* 2023; 49:1579–1590.

78. Behdani F, et al. Can levetiracetam improve clinical symptoms in schizophrenic patients? A randomized placebo-controlled clinical trial. *Int Clin Psychopharmacol* 2022; 37:159–165.

79. Kruiper C, et al. Clonidine augmentation in patients with schizophrenia: a double-blind, randomized placebo-controlled trial. *Schizophr Res* 2023; 255:148–154.

80. Hosseininasab M, et al. Nanocurcumin as an add-on to antipsychotic drugs for treatment of negative symptoms in patients with chronic schizophrenia: a randomized, double-blind, placebo-controlled study. *J Clin Psychopharmacol* 2021; 41:25–30.

81. Kaul I, et al. Efficacy and safety of the muscarinic receptor agonist KarXT (xanomeline-trospium) in schizophrenia (EMERGENT-2) in the USA: results from a randomised, double-blind, placebo-controlled, flexible-dose phase 3 trial. *Lancet* 2024; 403:160–170.

82. Li M, et al. Improvement of adjunctive berberine treatment on negative symptoms in patients with schizophrenia. *Eur Arch Psychiatry Clin Neurosci* 2022; 272:633–642.

83. Yi S, et al. Efficacy of repetitive transcranial magnetic stimulation (rTMS) on negative symptoms and cognitive functioning in schizophrenia: an umbrella review of systematic reviews and meta-analyses. *Psychiatry Res* 2024; 333:115728.

84. Mondino M, et al. Transcranial direct current stimulation for the treatment of refractory symptoms of schizophrenia. Current evidence and future directions. *Curr Pharm Des* 2015; 21:3373–3383.

85. Kim J, et al. A meta-analysis of transcranial direct current stimulation for schizophrenia: 'is more better?' *J Psychiatr Res* 2019; 110:117–126.

86. Galderisi S, et al. EPA guidance on treatment of negative symptoms in schizophrenia. *Eur Psychiatry* 2021; 64:e21.

87. Valiengo L, et al. Efficacy and safety of transcranial direct current stimulation for treating negative symptoms in schizophrenia: a randomized clinical trial. *JAMA Psychiatry* 2020; 77:121–129.

88. Potvin S, et al. A meta-analysis of negative symptoms in dual diagnosis schizophrenia. *Psychol Med* 2006; 36:431–440.

89. Arndt S, et al. Comorbidity of substance abuse and schizophrenia: the role of pre-morbid adjustment. *Psychol Med* 1992; 22:379–388.

90. Leeson VC, et al. The effect of cannabis use and cognitive reserve on age at onset and psychosis outcomes in first-episode schizophrenia. *Schizophr Bull* 2012; 38:873–880.

91. Barnes T, et al. Evidence-based guidelines for the pharmacological treatment of schizophrenia: updated recommendations from the British Association for Psychopharmacology. *J Psychopharm* 2020; 34:3–78.

Monitoring

Table 1.6 summarises suggested monitoring for those receiving antipsychotic medication.[1] Monitoring of people taking antipsychotics is very poor in most countries.[2–5] The guidance given here is strongly recommended to ensure safer use of these drugs. Other sections in this chapter provide further background information and relevant references. This table is a summary; see the individual sections for details and discussion.

Table 1.6 Suggested monitoring for people receiving antipsychotic medication.

Parameter/test	Suggested frequency	Action to be taken if results outside reference range	Medications with special precautions	Medications for which monitoring is not required
Urea and electrolytes (including creatinine or eGFR)	Baseline, then yearly as part of a routine physical health check	Investigate all abnormalities detected	Amisulpride and sulpiride renally excreted – consider reducing dose if eGFR reduced	None
Full blood count[6–8]	Baseline, then yearly as part of a routine physical health check and to detect chronic bone marrow suppression (small risk associated with some antipsychotic medications)	Stop suspect medication if neutrophils fall below 1.5×10⁹/L (unless diagnosed with BEN). Refer to specialist medical care if neutrophils below 0.5×10⁹/L.	Clozapine FBC weekly for 18 weeks, then 2-weekly up to 1 year, then monthly (schedule varies from country to country)	None
Blood lipids[9,10] (cholesterol, triglycerides; fasting sample, if possible)	Baseline, at 3 months, then yearly to detect antipsychotic-induced changes and to generally monitor physical health	Offer lifestyle advice. Consider changing antipsychotic medication and/or initiating statin therapy.	Clozapine, olanzapine: 3-monthly for first year, then yearly	Some antipsychotic medications (e.g. aripiprazole, brexpiprazole cariprazine,[11] lurasidone) not clearly associated with dyslipidaemia but prevalence is high in this patient group[12–14] so all patients should be monitored
Weight[9,10,14] (include waist size and BMI, if possible)	Baseline, frequently for 3 months, then yearly to detect antipsychotic-induced changes and generally monitor physical health	Offer lifestyle advice. Consider changing antipsychotic medication and/or dietary/ pharmacological intervention.	Clozapine, olanzapine – frequently for 3 months then 3-monthly for first year, then yearly	Aripiprazole, ziprasidone, brexpiprazole, cariprazine and lurasidone not clearly associated with weight gain but monitoring strongly recommended
Plasma glucose (fasting sample, if possible)	Baseline, at 4–6 months, then yearly to detect antipsychotic-induced changes and generally monitor physical health	Offer lifestyle advice. Obtain fasting sample or non-fasting and HbA₁C. Refer to GP or specialist.	Clozapine, olanzapine, chlorpromazine – test at baseline, one month, then 4–6 monthly	Some antipsychotic medications not clearly associated with IFG but prevalence is high,[15,16] so all patients should be monitored

(Continued)

Table 1.6 (*Continued*)

CHAPTER 1

Parameter/test	Suggested frequency	Action to be taken if results outside reference range	Medications with special precautions	Medications for which monitoring is not required
ECG[17,18]	Baseline, when the target dose is reached (ECG changes are rare in practice),[19] on admission to hospital, if there are cardiac symptoms, or when medication is changed (e.g. to high-dose or combined antipsychotic medications)[17]	Discuss with/refer to cardiologist if abnormality detected	Haloperidol, pimozide, sertindole – ECG mandatory Ziprasidone – ECG mandatory in some situations Pimavanserin – ECG strongly recommended	Risk of sudden cardiac death increased with most antipsychotic medications.[20] Ideally, all patients should be offered an ECG at least yearly.
Blood pressure	Baseline and then frequently during dose titration and after dosage changes	If severe hypotension or hypertension (clozapine) observed, slow rate of titration. Consider switching to another antipsychotic if symptomatic postural hypotension. Treat hypertension in line with national guidelines.	Clozapine, chlorpromazine and quetiapine most likely to be associated with postural hypotension	Amisulpride, aripiprazole, brexpiprazole, cariprazine, lumateperone, lurasidone, trifluoperazine, sulpiride
Prolactin	Baseline, at 6 months, then yearly	Switch medications if hyperprolactinaemia confirmed and symptomatic. Consider tests of bone mineral density (e.g. DEXA) for those with chronically raised prolactin.	Amisulpride, sulpiride, risperidone and paliperidone particularly associated with hyperprolactinaemia	Asenapine, aripiprazole, brexpiprazole, cariprazine, clozapine, lumateperone, lurasidone, quetiapine, olanzapine (low dose), xanomeline and ziprasidone do not usually elevate plasma prolactin, but measure if symptoms arise
Liver function tests[21–23]	Baseline, then yearly as part of a routine physical health check	Stop suspect medication if LFTs indicate hepatitis (transaminases × 3 normal) or functional damage (PT/albumin change)	Clozapine and chlorpromazine associated with hepatic failure	Amisulpride, sulpiride
Creatinine phosphokinase	Baseline, then if NMS suspected	See section on NMS in this chapter	NMS most likely with high-potency FGAs but can occur with any dopamine antagonist or partial agonist	None
Other tests	Patients on clozapine may benefit from an **EEG**[24,25] as this may help determine the need for antiseizure treatment (although interpretation is obviously complex). Those on quetiapine should have **thyroid** function tests yearly, although the risk of abnormality is very small.[26,27]			

BEN, benign ethnic neutropenia; BMI, body mass index; DEXA, dual-energy x-ray absorptiometry; eGFR, estimated glomerular filtration rate; FGA, first-generation antipsychotic; HbA$_{1c}$, glycated haemoglobin; IFG, impaired fasting glucose; NMS, neuroleptic malignant syndrome; PT, prothrombin time.

References

1. National Institute for Health and Care Excellence. Clinical Knowledge Summaries. Psychosis and schizophrenia: what monitoring is required? 2014 (last revised November 2021, checked January 2024); https://cks.nice.org.uk/topics/psychosis-schizophrenia/prescribing-information/monitoring/#:~:text=References,What%20monitoring%20is%20required%3F,stabilized%20(whichever%20is%20longer).

2. Bulteau S, et al. Advocacy for better metabolic monitoring after antipsychotic initiation: based on data from a French health insurance database. *Expert Opin Drug Saf* 2021; **20**:225–233.

3. Lydon A, et al. Routine screening and rates of metabolic syndrome in patients treated with clozapine and long-acting injectable antipsychotic medications: a cross-sectional study. *Ir J Psychol Med* 2021; **38**:40–48.

4. Poojari PG, et al. Identification of risk factors and metabolic monitoring practices in patients on antipsychotic drugs in South India. *Asian J Psychiatr* 2020; **53**:102186.

5. Perry BI, et al. Prolactin monitoring in the acute psychiatry setting. *Psychiatry Res* 2016; **235**:104–109.

6. Burckart GJ, et al. Neutropenia following acute chlorpromazine ingestion. *Clin Toxicol* 1981; **18**:797–801.

7. Montgomery J. Ziprasidone-related agranulocytosis following olanzapine-induced neutropenia. *Gen Hosp Psychiatry* 2006; **28**:83–85.

8. Cowan C, et al. Leukopenia and neutropenia induced by quetiapine. *Prog Neuropsychopharmacol Biol Psychiatry* 2007; **31**:292–294.

9. Marder SR, et al. Physical health monitoring of patients with schizophrenia. *Am J Psychiatry* 2004; **161**:1334–1349.

10. Fenton WS, et al. Medication-induced weight gain and dyslipidemia in patients with schizophrenia. *Am J Psychiatry* 2006; **163**:1697–1704.

11. Taylor D, et al. Dopamine partial agonists: a discrete class of antipsychotics. *Int J Psychiatry Clin Pract* 2023; **27**:272–284.

12. Weissman EM, et al. Lipid monitoring in patients with schizophrenia prescribed second-generation antipsychotics. *J Clin Psychiatry* 2006; **67**:1323–1326.

13. Cohn TA, et al. Metabolic monitoring for patients treated with antipsychotic medications. *Can J Psychiatry* 2006; **51**:492–501.

14. Paton C, et al. Obesity, dyslipidaemias and smoking in an inpatient population treated with antipsychotic drugs. *Acta Psychiatr Scand* 2004; **110**:299–305.

15. Taylor D, et al. Undiagnosed impaired fasting glucose and diabetes mellitus amongst inpatients receiving antipsychotic drugs. *J Psychopharmacol* 2005; **19**:182–186.

16. Citrome L, et al. Incidence, prevalence, and surveillance for diabetes in New York State psychiatric hospitals, 1997–2004. *Psychiatr Serv* 2006; **57**:1132–1139.

17. Barnes T, et al. Evidence-based guidelines for the pharmacological treatment of schizophrenia: updated recommendations from the British Association for Psychopharmacology. *J Psychopharm* 2020; **34**:3–78.

18. Shah AA, et al. QTc prolongation with antipsychotics: is routine ECG monitoring recommended? *J Psychiatr Pract* 2014; **20**:196–206.

19. Novotny T, et al. Monitoring of QT interval in patients treated with psychotropic drugs. *Int J Cardiol* 2007; **117**:329–332.

20. Ray WA, et al. Atypical antipsychotic drugs and the risk of sudden cardiac death. *N Engl J Med* 2009; **360**:225–235.

21. Hummer M, et al. Hepatotoxicity of clozapine. *J Clin Psychopharmacol* 1997; **17**:314–317.

22. Erdogan A, et al. Management of marked liver enzyme increase during clozapine treatment: a case report and review of the literature. *Int J Psychiatry Med* 2004; **34**:83–89.

23. Regal RE, et al. Phenothiazine-induced cholestatic jaundice. *Clin Pharm* 1987; **6**:787–794.

24. Centorrino F, et al. EEG abnormalities during treatment with typical and atypical antipsychotics. *Am J Psychiatry* 2002; **159**:109–115.

25. Gross A, et al. Clozapine-induced QEEG changes correlate with clinical response in schizophrenic patients: a prospective, longitudinal study. *Pharmacopsychiatry* 2004; **37**:119–122.

26. Twaites BR, et al. The safety of quetiapine: results of a post-marketing surveillance study on 1728 patients in England. *J Psychopharmacol* 2007; **21**:392–399.

27. Kelly DL, et al. Thyroid function in treatment-resistant schizophrenia patients treated with quetiapine, risperidone, or fluphenazine. *J Clin Psychiatry* 2005; **66**:80–84.

Relative adverse effects – a rough guide

Table 1.7 provides approximate estimates of relative incidence and severity of adverse effects. It serves as a rough guide and does not replace the detailed and referenced sections included elsewhere. For further details, refer to the dedicated sections in this chapter. Other adverse effects not mentioned in this table also occur.

Table 1.7 Approximate estimates of relative incidence and severity of adverse effects.

Drug	Sedation	Weight gain	Akathisia	Parkinsonism	Anticholinergic	Hypotension	Prolactin elevation	Prolonged QT interval
Amisulpride	–	+	+	+	–	–	+++	++
Aripiprazole	–	+	+	–	–	–	–	–
Asenapine	+	+	+	+	–	–	+	–
Benperidol	+	+	+	+++	+	+	+++	+
Blonanserin	–	–	+	–	–	–	+	–
Brexpiprazole	–	+	+	–	–	–	–	–
Cariprazine	–	+	+	–	–	–	–	–
Chlorpromazine	+++	++	+	++	++	+++	++	++
Clozapine	+++	+++	–	–	+++	+++	–	+++
Flupentixol	+	++	++	++	++	+	+++	–
Fluphenazine	+	+	++	+++	+	+	+++	+
Haloperidol	+	+	+++	+++	–	+	+++	++
Iloperidone	–	++	+	+	–	+	–	++
Levomepromazine	+++	+	+	+	++	++	++	+
Lumateperone	++	–	–	–	–	–	–	–
Loxapine	++	+	+	++	+	++	+++	–
Lurasidone	+	+	+	+	–	–	–	–
Olanzapine	+++	+++	+	–	+	+	+	+
Paliperidone	+	++	++	+	–	++	+++	+
Penfluridol	–	++	++	++	++	+	+++	++
Perphenazine	+	+	++	+++	+	+	+++	+
Pimavanserin	–	–	–	–	–	–	–	++
Pimozide	+	++	++	+	++	+	+++	+++
Promazine	+++	++	+	+	++	++	+	++
Quetiapine	+++	++	+	–	+	++	–	++
Risperidone	+	++	++	+	–	++	+++	+
Sertindole	–	+	+	–	–	+++	–	+++
Sulpiride	–	+	+	+	–	–	+++	+

(Continued)

CHAPTER 1

Table 1.7 (*Continued*)

Drug	Sedation	Weight gain	Akathisia	Parkinsonism	Anticholinergic	Hypotension	Prolactin elevation	Prolonged QT interval
Thiothixene	++	++	+	+	++	++	+	+
Trifluoperazine	+	+	+	+++	+	+	+++	?
Xanomeline	–	–	–	–	–	–	–	+
Ziprasidone	+	–	+	–	–	+	–	++
Zuclopenthixol	++	++	++	++	++	+	+++	+

Key: +++ high incidence/severity, ++ moderate, + low, – very low/zero.

Treatment algorithms for schizophrenia

First-episode schizophrenia

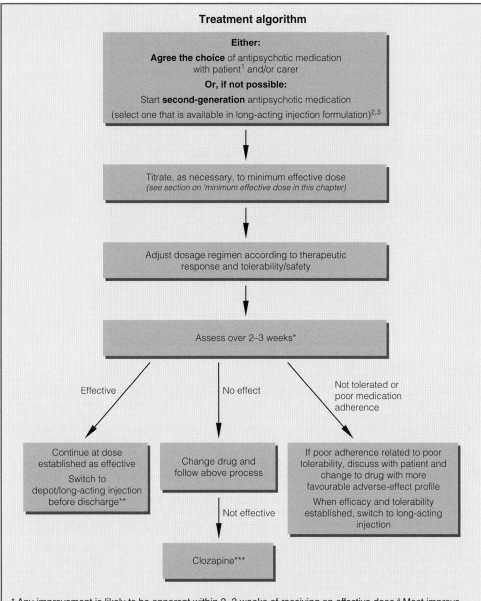

Treatment algorithm

Either:
Agree the choice of antipsychotic medication with patient[1] and/or carer
Or, if not possible:
Start **second-generation** antipsychotic medication
(select one that is available in long-acting injection formulation)[2,3]

↓

Titrate, as necessary, to minimum effective dose
(see section on 'minimum effective dose in this chapter)

↓

Adjust dosage regimen according to therapeutic response and tolerability/safety

↓

Assess over 2–3 weeks*

Effective / No effect / Not tolerated or poor medication adherence

Effective:
Continue at dose established as effective
Switch to depot/long-acting injection before discharge**

No effect:
Change drug and follow above process
↓
Not effective
↓
Clozapine***

Not tolerated or poor medication adherence:
If poor adherence related to poor tolerability, discuss with patient and change to drug with more favourable adverse-effect profile
When efficacy and tolerability established, switch to long-acting injection

* Any improvement is likely to be apparent within 2–3 weeks of receiving an effective dose.[4] Most improvement occurs during this period.[5] If *no* effect by 2–3 weeks, increase the dose or change the drug. If some response detected, continue for a total of 10 weeks before abandoning treatment.[6]
** Relapse and readmission rates are vastly reduced by early use of depot/long-acting injections in this patient group.[7–9] Patients with first-episode schizophrenia will accept long-acting injections.[10]
*** Early use of clozapine much more likely than anything else to be successful.[6,11] Reluctance to use clozapine is associated with poor outcomes.[12] Delaying the use of clozapine diminishes response to clozapine.[13]

Relapse or acute exacerbation of schizophrenia

(full adherence to medication confirmed)*

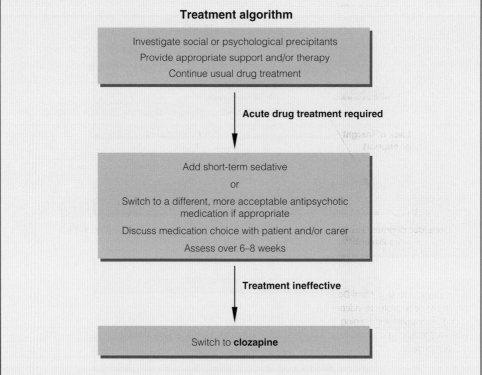

Treatment algorithm

Investigate social or psychological precipitants
Provide appropriate support and/or therapy
Continue usual drug treatment

Acute drug treatment required

Add short-term sedative

or

Switch to a different, more acceptable antipsychotic medication if appropriate

Discuss medication choice with patient and/or carer

Assess over 6–8 weeks

Treatment ineffective

Switch to **clozapine**

Notes

■ First-generation drugs may be slightly less efficacious than some SGAs.[14,15] FGAs should probably be reserved for second- or third-line use (or not used at all) because of the possibility of poorer outcome compared with SGAs and the higher risk of movement disorder, particularly TD.[16,17]

■ Choice should be based largely on comparative adverse-effect profile and relative toxicity. Patients seem able to make informed choices based on these factors,[18,19] although in practice they are rarely involved in drug choice.[20] Allowing patients informed choice seems to improve outcomes.[1]

■ Where there is prior treatment failure (but not confirmed treatment refractoriness), olanzapine or risperidone may be better options than quetiapine.[21] Olanzapine, because of the wealth of evidence suggesting slight superiority over other antipsychotics, should probably be tried before clozapine unless contraindicated.[22–25] However, one RCT[6] found that continuing with amisulpride was as effective as switching to olanzapine.

■ Before considering clozapine, ensure adherence to prior therapy using depot/LAI formulation or plasma drug level monitoring of oral treatment. Most non-adherence is undetected in practice,[21,26] and apparent treatment resistance may simply be a result of inadequate treatment.[27]

■ Time to response is increased and total response decreased in exacerbations of multi-episode schizophrenia.[28]

■ Where there is confirmed treatment resistance (failure to respond to adequate trials of at least two antipsychotic medications), evidence supporting the use of clozapine (and only clozapine) is overwhelming.[29,30]

* In patients taking oral antipsychotics, non-compliance often goes undetected.[26] Absolute non-compliance (blood levels of zero) is surprisingly common.[27]

Relapse or acute exacerbation of schizophrenia

(adherence doubtful or known to be poor)

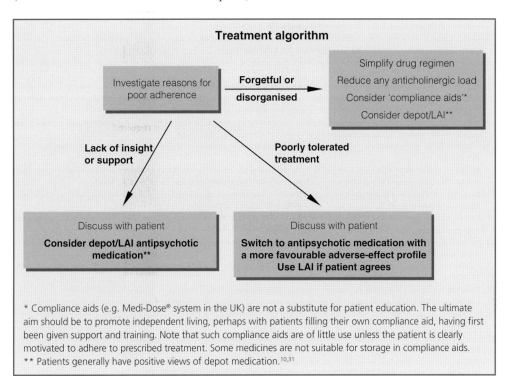

Treatment algorithm

Investigate reasons for poor adherence

Forgetful or disorganised

Simplify drug regimen
Reduce any anticholinergic load
Consider 'compliance aids'*
Consider depot/LAI**

Lack of insight or support

Poorly tolerated treatment

Discuss with patient
Consider depot/LAI antipsychotic medication**

Discuss with patient
**Switch to antipsychotic medication with a more favourable adverse-effect profile
Use LAI if patient agrees**

* Compliance aids (e.g. Medi-Dose® system in the UK) are not a substitute for patient education. The ultimate aim should be to promote independent living, perhaps with patients filling their own compliance aid, having first been given support and training. Note that such compliance aids are of little use unless the patient is clearly motivated to adhere to prescribed treatment. Some medicines are not suitable for storage in compliance aids.
** Patients generally have positive views of depot medication.[10,31]

References

1. Robinson DG, et al. Psychopharmacological treatment in the RAISE-ETP study: outcomes of a manual and computer decision support system based intervention. *Am J Psychiatry* 2018; **175**:169–179.
2. Zhu Y, et al. Antipsychotic drugs for the acute treatment of patients with a first episode of schizophrenia: a systematic review with pairwise and network meta-analyses. *Lancet Psychiatry* 2017; **4**:694–705.
3. Zhang JP, et al. Efficacy and safety of individual second-generation vs. first-generation antipsychotics in first-episode psychosis: a systematic review and meta-analysis. *Int J Neuropsychopharmacol* 2013; **16**:1205–1218.
4. Leucht S, et al. Early-onset hypothesis of antipsychotic drug action: a hypothesis tested, confirmed and extended. *Biol Psychiatry* 2005; **57**:1543–1549.
5. Agid O, et al. The 'delayed onset' of antipsychotic action: an idea whose time has come and gone. *J Psychiatry Neurosci* 2006; **31**:93–100.
6. Kahn RS, et al. Amisulpride and olanzapine followed by open-label treatment with clozapine in first-episode schizophrenia and schizophreniform disorder (OPTiMiSE): a three-phase switching study. *Lancet Psychiatry* 2018; **5**:797–807.
7. Subotnik KL, et al. Long-acting injectable risperidone for relapse prevention and control of breakthrough symptoms after a recent first episode of schizophrenia. A randomized clinical trial. *JAMA Psychiatry* 2015; **72**:822–829.
8. Schreiner A, et al. Paliperidone palmitate versus oral antipsychotics in recently diagnosed schizophrenia. *Schizophr Res* 2015; **169**:393–399.
9. Alphs L, et al. Treatment effect with paliperidone palmitate compared with oral antipsychotics in patients with recent-onset versus more chronic schizophrenia and a history of criminal justice system involvement. *Early Interv Psychiatry* 2018; **12**:55–65.
10. Kane JM, et al. Patients with early-phase schizophrenia will accept treatment with sustained-release medication (long-acting injectable antipsychotics): results from the recruitment phase of the PRELAPSE trial. *J Clin Psychiatry* 2019; **80**:18m12546.
11. Agid O, et al. An algorithm-based approach to first-episode schizophrenia: response rates over 3 prospective antipsychotic trials with a retrospective data analysis. *J Clin Psychiatry* 2011; **72**:1439–1444.
12. Drosos P, et al. One-year outcome and adherence to pharmacological guidelines in first-episode schizophrenia: results from a consecutive cohort study. *J Clin Psychopharmacol* 2020; **40**:534–540.
13. Rajalingham K. Clozapine delay results in poorer outcomes for treatment-resistant schizophrenia patients. *Psiquiatría Biológica* 2024; **31**:100493.
14. Davis JM, et al. A meta-analysis of the efficacy of second-generation antipsychotics. *Arch Gen Psychiatry* 2003; **60**:553–564.
15. Leucht S, et al. Second-generation versus first-generation antipsychotic drugs for schizophrenia: a meta-analysis. *Lancet* 2009; **373**:31–41.
16. Schooler N, et al. Risperidone and haloperidol in first-episode psychosis: a long-term randomized trial. *Am J Psychiatry* 2005; **162**:947–953.
17. Oosthuizen PP, et al. Incidence of tardive dyskinesia in first-episode psychosis patients treated with low-dose haloperidol. *J Clin Psychiatry* 2003; **64**:1075–1080.
18. Whiskey E, et al. Evaluation of an antipsychotic information sheet for patients. *Int J Psychiatry Clin Pract* 2005; **9**:264–270.
19. Stroup TS, et al. Results of phase 3 of the CATIE schizophrenia trial. *Schizophr Res* 2009; **107**:1–12.
20. Olofinjana B, et al. Antipsychotic drugs: information and choice: a patient survey. *Psychiatr Bull* 2005; **29**:369–371.
21. Stroup TS, et al. Effectiveness of olanzapine, quetiapine, risperidone, and ziprasidone in patients with chronic schizophrenia following discontinuation of a previous atypical antipsychotic. *Am J Psychiatry* 2006; **163**:611–622.
22. Haro JM, et al. Remission and relapse in the outpatient care of schizophrenia: three-year results from the Schizophrenia Outpatient Health Outcomes study. *J Clin Psychopharmacol* 2006; **26**:571–578.
23. Novick D, et al. Recovery in the outpatient setting: 36-month results from the Schizophrenia Outpatients Health Outcomes (SOHO) study. *Schizophr Res* 2009; **108**:223–230.
24. Tiihonen J, et al. Effectiveness of antipsychotic treatments in a nationwide cohort of patients in community care after first hospitalisation due to schizophrenia and schizoaffective disorder: observational follow-up study. *BMJ* 2006; **333**:224.
25. Leucht S, et al. A meta-analysis of head-to-head comparisons of second-generation antipsychotics in the treatment of schizophrenia. *Am J Psychiatry* 2009; **166**:152–163.
26. Remington G, et al. The use of electronic monitoring (MEMS) to evaluate antipsychotic compliance in outpatients with schizophrenia. *Schizophr Res* 2007; **90**:229–237.
27. McCutcheon R, et al. Antipsychotic plasma levels in the assessment of poor treatment response in schizophrenia. *Acta Psychiatr Scand* 2018; **137**:39–46.
28. Takeuchi H, et al. Does relapse contribute to treatment resistance? Antipsychotic response in first- vs. second-episode schizophrenia. *Neuropsychopharmacology* 2019; **44**:1036–1042.
29. McEvoy JP, et al. Effectiveness of clozapine versus olanzapine, quetiapine, and risperidone in patients with chronic schizophrenia who did not respond to prior atypical antipsychotic treatment. *Am J Psychiatry* 2006; **163**:600–610.
30. Lewis SW, et al. Randomized controlled trial of effect of prescription of clozapine versus other second-generation antipsychotic drugs in resistant schizophrenia. *Schizophr Bull* 2006; **32**:715–723.
31. Mace S, et al. Positive views on antipsychotic long-acting injections: results of a survey of community patients prescribed antipsychotics. *Ther Adv Psychopharmacol* 2019; **9**:2045125319860977.

First-generation antipsychotics – place in therapy

Nomenclature

First-generation ('typical') and second-generation ('atypical') antipsychotic medications are not categorically differentiated. Drugs in both groups differ substantially in pharmacological and adverse-effect profiles and there is some overlap between the two groups in pharmacological characteristics. FGA medications were introduced before 1990 and tend to be associated with acute EPS, hyperprolactinaemia and, in the longer term, TD. It might be expected that these adverse effects are less likely or absent with SGA medications (introduced after 1990), although in practice most SGAs show dose-related EPS, some induce hyperprolactinaemia (some to a greater extent than FGAs) and all will give rise to TD, albeit at a lower incidence than FGAs. SGA medications tend to be associated with metabolic and cardiac complications,[1–3] although this is *not* true of all SGAs and it *is* true of some FGAs. To complicate matters further, it has been suggested that the therapeutic and adverse effects of FGAs can be separated by careful dosing.[4] That is, FGAs can be indistinguishable from SGAs if used in small enough doses (there is much evidence to the contrary).[5–7]

Given these observations, it seems unwise and unhelpful to consider so-called FGAs and SGAs as distinct groups of drugs. Perhaps the essential difference between the two groups is the size of the therapeutic index in relation to acute EPS. For instance, haloperidol has an extremely narrow range of doses at which it is effective but does not cause EPSEs (perhaps 4.0–4.5mg/day) whereas olanzapine has a wide range of therapeutic doses (5–40mg/day) at which it does not generally cause such adverse effects.

The use of NbN[1,2] (for which there is a free application for smartphones and other devices) obviates the need for classification into an FGA or SGA and describes individual drug by their pharmacological activity. NbN is certainly a useful alternative to standard classifications, but one possible limitation is that it preselects specific pharmacological features to create categories while ignoring others, based on the opinion of experts that these features are essential to drug action (despite exact mechanisms of action being unknown). In 2023, a different approach based on in vitro binding profiles was proposed.[3] Four clusters of effects were identified, one with high affinity for muscarinic receptors (e.g. olanzapine and quetiapine), one with relatively low antagonism of the dopamine D2 receptor (e.g. the partial agonists and lurasidone), one with serotonergic antagonism (e.g. risperidone) and one with relatively pure dopaminergic antagonism (e.g. amisulpride). These clusters mapped to adverse-effect profiles with greater accuracy than the other classification systems. One possible disadvantage of this so-called data-driven approach is that all receptors are assigned an equal level of importance regardless of their magnitude of impact in producing clinically relevant effects. The wider use of NbN or the data-driven approach will undoubtedly improve understanding of individual drug effects and perhaps forestall future redundant categorisation.

Role of older antipsychotics

FGAs still play an important role in schizophrenia. For example, haloperidol is a frequent choice for 'when necessary' medication and depot preparations of haloperidol, zuclopenthixol and flupentixol are still commonly prescribed. FGAs can offer a valid alternative to SGAs where SGAs are poorly tolerated (usually because of metabolic changes) or where FGAs are preferred by patients themselves. Some FGAs may be less effective than some non-clozapine SGAs (amisulpride, olanzapine and risperidone may be slightly more efficacious)[4,5] but any differences in therapeutic efficacy seem to be modest. Two large, independent and pragmatic studies, CATIE[6] and CUtLASS,[7] found few important differences between SGAs and FGAs (mainly perphenazine and sulpiride, respectively).

The main drawbacks of FGAs are acute EPS, hyperprolactinaemia and TD. Hyperprolactinaemia is probably unavoidable in practice because the dose that achieves efficacy is too close to the dose that causes hyperprolactinaemia. Even when not symptomatic, hyperprolactinaemia may grossly affect hypothalamic function.[8] Raised prolactin is also associated with sexual dysfunction,[9] as are the autonomic effects of some SGAs.[10] Notably, some SGAs (risperidone, paliperidone, amisulpride) increase prolactin to a greater extent than FGAs.[11]

All FGAs are potent dopamine antagonists, which are liable to induce dysphoria.[12] Perhaps as a consequence, some FGAs may produce smaller benefits in quality of life than some SGAs.[6]

Tardive dyskinesia very probably occurs more frequently with FGAs than SGAs[13–16] (notwithstanding difficulties in defining what is 'atypical'), although there remains some uncertainty[16–18] and the dose of FGA used is a crucial factor.[19] A complicating aspect is the occurrence of TD in untreated schizophrenia,[20] which may mean that antipsychotics do not necessarily cause TD but simply fail to suppress it to varying degrees. Among SGAs, partial agonists may have the lowest risk of TD.[21] Careful observation of patients and the prescribing of the lowest effective dose are essential to help reduce the risk of this serious adverse event.[22,23] Even with these precautions, the risk of TD with some FGAs may be unacceptably high.[24]

A good example of the relative merits of SGAs and a carefully dosed FGA comes from a trial comparing paliperidone palmitate with low-dose haloperidol decanoate.[25] Paliperidone produced more weight gain and prolactin change but haloperidol was associated with significantly more frequent akathisia and parkinsonism, and, numerically, a higher incidence of TD. Efficacy was identical.

References

1. Blier P, et al. Progress on the Neuroscience-Based Nomenclature (NbN) for psychotropic medications. *Neuropsychopharmacology* 2017; 42:1927–1928.
2. Caraci F, et al. A new nomenclature for classifying psychotropic drugs. *Br J Clin Pharmacol* 2017; 83:1614–1616.
3. McCutcheon RA, et al. Data-driven taxonomy for antipsychotic medication: a new classification system. *Biol Psychiatry* 2023; 94:561–568.
4. Davis JM, et al. A meta-analysis of the efficacy of second-generation antipsychotics. *Arch Gen Psychiatry* 2003; 60:553–564.
5. Leucht S, et al. Second-generation versus first-generation antipsychotic drugs for schizophrenia: a meta-analysis. *Lancet* 2009; 373:31–41.
6. Grunder G, et al. Effects of first-generation antipsychotics versus second-generation antipsychotics on quality of life in schizophrenia: a double-blind, randomised study. *Lancet Psychiatry* 2016; 3:717–729.
7. Jones PB, et al. Randomized controlled trial of the effect on quality of life of second- vs first-generation antipsychotic drugs in schizophrenia: Cost Utility of the Latest Antipsychotic Drugs in Schizophrenia Study (CUtLASS 1). *Arch Gen Psychiatry* 2006; 63:1079–1087.
8. Smith S, et al. The effects of antipsychotic-induced hyperprolactinaemia on the hypothalamic-pituitary-gonadal axis. *J Clin Psychopharmacol* 2002; 22:109–114.
9. Smith SM, et al. Sexual dysfunction in patients taking conventional antipsychotic medication. *Br J Psychiatry* 2002; 181:49–55.
10. Aizenberg D, et al. Comparison of sexual dysfunction in male schizophrenic patients maintained on treatment with classical antipsychotics versus clozapine. *J Clin Psychiatry* 2001; 62:541–544.
11. Leucht S, et al. Comparative efficacy and tolerability of 15 antipsychotic drugs in schizophrenia: a multiple-treatments meta-analysis. *Lancet* 2013; 382:951–962.

12. King DJ, et al. Antipsychotic drug-induced dysphoria. *Br J Psychiatry* 1995; **167**:480–482.

13. Tollefson GD, et al. Blind, controlled, long-term study of the comparative incidence of treatment-emergent tardive dyskinesia with olanzapine or haloperidol. *Am J Psychiatry* 1997; **154**:1248–1254.

14. Beasley C, et al. Randomised double-blind comparison of the incidence of tardive dyskinesia in patients with schizophrenia during long-term treatment with olanzapine or haloperidol. *Br J Psychiatry* 1999; **174**:23–30.

15. Correll CU, et al. Lower risk for tardive dyskinesia associated with second-generation antipsychotics: a systematic review of 1-year studies. *Am J Psychiatry* 2004; **161**:414–425.

16. Novick D, et al. Tolerability of outpatient antipsychotic treatment: 36-month results from the European Schizophrenia Outpatient Health Outcomes (SOHO) study. *Eur Neuropsychopharmacol* 2009; **19**:542–550.

17. Halliday J, et al. Nithsdale Schizophrenia Surveys 23: movement disorders. 20-year review. *Br J Psychiatry* 2002; **181**:422–427.

18. Miller DD, et al. Extrapyramidal side-effects of antipsychotics in a randomised trial. *Br J Psychiatry* 2008; **193**:279–288.

19. Takeuchi H, et al. Pathophysiology, prognosis and treatment of tardive dyskinesia. *Ther Adv Psychopharmacol* 2022; **12**:20451253221117313.

20. Kalniunas A, et al. Prevalence of spontaneous movement disorders (dyskinesia, parkinsonism, akathisia and dystonia) in never-treated patients with chronic and first-episode psychosis: a systematic review and meta-analysis. *BMJ Ment Health* 2024; **27**:e301184.

21. Carbon M, et al. Tardive dyskinesia prevalence in the period of second-generation antipsychotic use: a meta-analysis. *J Clin Psychiatry* 2017; **78**:e264–e278.

22. Jeste DV, et al. Tardive dyskinesia. *Schizophr Bull* 1993; **19**:303–315.

23. Cavallaro R, et al. Recognition, avoidance, and management of antipsychotic-induced tardive dyskinesia. *CNS Drugs* 1995; **4**:278–293.

24. Oosthuizen P, et al. A randomized, controlled comparison of the efficacy and tolerability of low and high doses of haloperidol in the treatment of first-episode psychosis. *Int J Neuropsychopharmacol* 2004; **7**:125–131.

25. McEvoy JP, et al. Effectiveness of paliperidone palmitate vs haloperidol decanoate for maintenance treatment of schizophrenia: a randomized clinical trial. *JAMA* 2014; **311**:1978–1987.

NICE guidelines for the treatment of schizophrenia[1]

The UK NICE guidelines[1] were published in February 2014 and last reviewed in September 2024 but have remained largely unchanged.

NICE guidelines – a summary

First-episode psychosis

For people with newly diagnosed schizophrenia, offer oral antipsychotic medication as well as psychological interventions (cognitive behavioural therapy [CBT] or family intervention). Provide information and discuss the benefits and adverse-effect profile of each drug with the service user.

The choice of drug should be made by the service user and healthcare professional together, considering:

- the relative potential of individual antipsychotic drugs to cause extrapyramidal adverse effects (EPSEs; including akathisia), cardiovascular adverse effects, metabolic adverse effects (including weight gain), hormonal adverse effects (including raised prolactin levels) and other adverse effects (including unpleasant subjective experiences)
- the views of the carer where the service user agrees.

Before starting antipsychotic medication, undertake a thorough assessment of physical health and offer an ECG if specified in the summary of product characteristics (SPC) or clinically indicated.

Treatment with antipsychotic medication should be considered an explicit individual therapeutic trial and the following should be considered:

- Recording of indications and expected benefits and risks of oral antipsychotic medication, and the expected time for a change in symptoms and appearance of adverse effects.
- At the start of treatment, give a dose at the lower end of the licensed range and slowly titrate upwards within the dose range given in the BNF or SPC.
- Justify and record reasons for dosages outside the range given in the BNF or SPC.
- Record the rationale for continuing, changing or stopping medication and the effects of such changes.
- Carry out a trial of medication at optimum dosage for 4–6 weeks (although half of this period is probably sufficient if no effect at all is seen).
- Monitor and record the following regularly and systematically throughout treatment, but especially during titration:
  - efficacy, including changes in symptoms and behaviour
  - adverse effects of treatment, taking into account overlap between certain adverse effects and clinical features of schizophrenia (e.g. the overlap between akathisia and agitation or anxiety)
  - adherence
  - weight, weekly for the first 6 weeks, then at 12 weeks, 1 year and annually
  - waist circumference annually

- pulse and blood pressure at 12 weeks, 1 year and annually
- fasting blood glucose, HbA_{1c} and blood lipids at 12 weeks, 1 year and annually
- nutritional status, diet and physical activity.
- Physical monitoring is to be the responsibility of the secondary care team for 1 year or until the patient is stable.
- Discuss the use of alcohol, tobacco, prescription and non-prescription medication, as well as the use of illicit drugs, with the service user and carer if appropriate. Discuss their potential interactions with the prescribed therapy and psychological treatments.
- Do not use a loading dose of antipsychotic medication (note that this does not apply to loading doses of depot forms of olanzapine and paliperidone).
- Do not routinely initiate regular combined antipsychotic medication, except for short periods (e.g. when changing medication).

Subsequent episodes of psychosis/maintenance treatment of schizophrenia

- Consider the clinical response and adverse effects of the service user's current and previous medication.
- Consider offering depot/LAI antipsychotic medication to people with schizophrenia:
  - who would prefer such treatment after an acute episode
  - known to be non-adherent to oral treatment and/or those who prefer this method of administration.

GPs and other primary healthcare professionals should monitor the physical health of people with psychosis or schizophrenia when responsibility for monitoring is first transferred from secondary care, and then at least annually. The health check should be comprehensive, focusing on physical health problems that are common in people with psychosis and schizophrenia.

Treatment-resistant schizophrenia

Offer clozapine to people with schizophrenia whose illness has not responded adequately to treatment despite the sequential use of adequate doses of at least two different anti-psychotic drugs alongside psychological therapies. The misuse of illicit substances (including alcohol) and the use of other prescribed medication or physical illness should be excluded. At least one of the drugs should be a non-clozapine SGA (see section on treatment algorithms for schizophrenia in this chapter – we recommend that one of the drugs should be olanzapine).

For people with schizophrenia whose illness has not responded adequately to clozapine at an optimised dose, healthcare professionals should establish prior compliance with opti-mised antipsychotic treatment (including measuring drug levels) and engagement with psychological treatment before adding a second antipsychotic to augment treatment with clozapine. An adequate trial of such an augmentation may need to be up to 8–10 weeks. Choose a drug that does not compound the common adverse effects of clozapine.

There are some notable differences with some more recently published guidelines. In first-episode psychosis, NICE makes no specific antipsychotic recommendation, whereas the Royal Australian and New Zealand College of Psychiatrists (RANZCP)[2] guidelines recommend atypical antipsychotics. They also explicitly suggest or at least allow the use of long-acting agents, as do the BAP guidelines.[3] The duration of antipsychotic treatment in first episode is not clearly defined in the NICE guidelines. The Canadian Psychiatric Association guidelines[4] recommend at least 18 months, the BAP at least 2 years, and RANZCP 2–5 years. There is scant mention of the treatment of negative symptoms in any of the guidelines. UK NICE guidelines recommend psychological approaches while RANZCP tentatively recommends rTMS. Reflecting the paucity of evidence in clozapine-resistant schizophrenia there is little detail or difference in guideline recommendations – all suggest adding a second antipsychotic.

References

1. National Institute for Health and Care Excellence. Psychosis and schizophrenia in adults: prevention and management. Clinical guideline [CG178]. 2014 (last checked November 2024); https://www.nice.org.uk/guidance/cg178.

2. Galletly C, et al. Royal Australian and New Zealand College of Psychiatrists clinical practice guidelines for the management of schizophrenia and related disorders. *Aust N Z J Psychiatry* 2016; 50:410–472.

3. Barnes T, et al. Evidence-based guidelines for the pharmacological treatment of schizophrenia: updated recommendations from the British Association for Psychopharmacology. *J Psychopharmacol* 2020; 34:3–78.

4. Remington G, et al. Guidelines for the pharmacotherapy of schizophrenia in adults. *Can J Psychiatry* 2017; 62:604–616.

Antipsychotic response – to increase the dose, to switch, to add or just wait – what is the right move?

For any clinician actively involved in the care of people with schizophrenia, perhaps the single most common clinical dilemma is what to do when treatment with the current antipsychotic medication seems to be suboptimal (symptoms are well controlled but adverse effects are problematic or the therapeutic response is inadequate). Fortunately, with regard to poor tolerability, the diversity of the available antipsychotic medications means that it is usually possible to find one that has an adverse-effect profile that is more appropriate and more tolerable. With regard to inadequate symptom response, what to do next is a more difficult question. If the illness has not shown sufficient improvement despite serial adequate trials, in terms of dosage, duration and adherence, of at least two antipsychotic medications, then a trial of clozapine should be considered. However, should the person be reluctant to try clozapine, the clinician has four main options: to increase the dose of the current medication, to switch to another antipsychotic medication, to add an adjunctive medication, or just to monitor the illness in the hope that changing external factors will allow recovery. Unfortunately, the evidence base supporting these management options is limited.[1–3]

Optimal dosage

While the optimal doses for FGAs were always a matter of debate, the recommended doses of the SGAs are generally based on careful and extensive (fixed-dose) clinical trials. Despite this, the consensus on optimal SGA dosages has changed over time. For example, when risperidone was first introduced it was suggested that the optimal dose was 6mg or more for all patients. However, subsequently clinical practice moved towards the use of lower doses.[4] On the other hand, when quetiapine was introduced, 300mg was considered the optimal dose. The overall consensus now is towards higher doses,[5] although RCT and other evidence does not consistently support this shift.[5,6] Nonetheless, most clinicians feel comfortable in navigating within the recommended clinical dose ranges for the SGAs. The more critical question is what should be done if the upper limit of the dose range has been reached and, while the individual is tolerating the medication well, there is only limited benefit.

High dosage

For antipsychotic medications, the dose–response relationships for the treatment of schizophrenia are not that well defined. Davis and Chen[7] performed the first comprehensive systematic meta-analysis of relevant dose–response data available up to 2004 and concluded that the average dose that produces maximal benefit was 4mg for risperidone, 16mg olanzapine, 120mg ziprasidone and 10–15mg aripiprazole (they could not determine such a dose for quetiapine using their method). In 2020, Leucht and colleagues[8] carried out a similar meta-analysis of dose–response in acute schizophrenia and concluded that doses higher than standard doses were not more efficacious. However, they did suggest that for a few medications (such as olanzapine, lurasidone, ziprasidone) with clearly increasing dose curves (i.e. did not plateau), it might be worth testing higher-than-licensed doses in clinical trials. For example, the findings of a network meta-analysis of the dose–response effects of lurasidone in acute schizophrenia suggested that 160mg/day might be the most effective and acceptable dose.[9]

Several trials have tried to compare high-dose antipsychotic medication with standard dosage. For example, one study[10] explored the dose–response relationship of olanzapine in a randomised, double-blind, 8-week, fixed-dose study, comparing doses of 10mg, 20mg and 40mg. While no additional benefit was found with the higher doses (i.e. 40mg was no better than 10mg), there was clear evidence of a greater adverse-effect burden (weight gain and raised plasma prolactin level). Similarly, early studies of risperidone[11] compared the usual daily doses of 2mg and 6mg with higher doses, up to 16mg. There was no additional benefit with the higher doses but a clear signal for a greater risk of adverse effects (EPS and raised plasma prolactin). The findings of these studies are in accord with older studies involving fixed doses of haloperidol,[12] where 8mg/day is clearly the dose above which no additional benefit is seen.[13] Interestingly, the likelihood of inducing EPSEs is not constrained by dose in the same way – the frequency of EPS continues to increase at doses well beyond standard or even high doses.[14]

Despite the lack of evidence for the benefit of higher doses, it is important to keep in mind that these doses are extracted from group evidence where patients are assigned to different doses, which is a different situation from the clinical one where the prescriber considers increasing the dose only in those patients whose illnesses have failed to respond to the initial dosage regimen. In 1993, Kinon and colleagues[15] examined patients who failed to respond to the (then) standard dose of fluphenazine (20mg) and tested three strategies: increasing the dose to 80mg, switching to haloperidol or watchful waiting (on the original dose). All three strategies proved to be equivalent in terms of efficacy. These findings provide little supportive evidence at a group level (as opposed to an individual level) for treatment beyond the recommended dose range. Such RCT evidence is corroborated by the clinical practice norms – Hermes and colleagues examined the CATIE data to identify clinical factors that predicted a prescriber's decision to increase the dose (within the standard ranges) and found that such decisions were only weakly associated with clinical measures.[16] A later trial of lurasidone[17] for early, non-responsive schizophrenia showed that after 2 weeks on lurasidone 80mg/day, a dose increase to 160mg/day was associated with significant symptom improvement compared with continuing on lurasidone 80mg/day. However, the clinical implications of these findings are uncertain, given the limitations of the trial: it lasted only 4 weeks, and there was no testing of the intermediate dose of 120mg/day.

A 2018 Cochrane systematic review of relevant studies concluded that there was no good-quality evidence that for illness not responding to initial antipsychotic treatment there was any difference between increasing the antipsychotic dose and continuing antipsychotic treatment at the same dose.[1] A similar meta-analysis in 2023[3] concluded that, for early non-responsive schizophrenia, the evidence for treatment strategies such as dose escalation or switching antipsychotic medication was too limited to allow for any strong clinical recommendations.

Plasma level variations

There are significant inter-individual variations in plasma drug levels in patients treated with antipsychotic medication. Patients may be encountered who, when receiving medication at the higher end of the dose range (say 6mg of risperidone or 20mg of olanzapine), have plasma drug levels that are well below the range expected for 2mg risperidone or 10mg olanzapine, and these levels may not reach the threshold required for a therapeutic effect. In such patients, a rational case could be made for increasing the dose, provided the patient is informed and the adverse effects are tolerable, to bring the plasma levels into the optimal range for the particular medication. Genetic analysis is helpful in identifying ultrafast metabolisers of aripiprazole, risperidone[18] and clozapine.[19]

Treatment options for schizophrenia that is poorly responsive to standard antipsychotic treatment

So what are the treatment possibilities when a lack of therapeutic response is encountered despite a patient's adherence to their medication regimen, the prescription of a dosage at the top of the recommended range, and apparently sufficient plasma drug levels? There are essentially three options: a trial of clozapine, switching to another antipsychotic medication or adding another (non-clozapine) antipsychotic medication. If the patient meets the criteria for clozapine treatment, this is undoubtedly the preferred option. Yet, in a clinical audit of community (not inpatient) practice in the UK, covering some 5,000 patients in 60 different NHS trusts, it was found that 40% of the patients whose illnesses met the criteria for TRS had not received clozapine. For the vast majority (85%) of those who had started clozapine, this had been delayed after the failure of two serial trials of antipsychotic medication for much longer than is advised in most guidelines.[20] Significant delay in the commencement of clozapine treatment has also been found in early intervention in psychosis services.[21] However, when reflecting on the findings suggesting delay or underuse of clozapine, it should be borne in mind that among those patients with a diagnosis of treatment-resistant illness who have not had a trial of clozapine, there will be some who have declined this treatment, some who have yet to be persuaded, and some for whom the prescribing clinician considers, perhaps because of factors such as comorbid physical illness, substance use or adverse social circumstances, that another intervention has a more favourable risk–benefit balance.[22]

Some patients may be averse to the mandatory regular blood testing, the adverse effects and the regular appointments required as part of the clozapine regimen. In such patients, the options are switching to another antipsychotic medication or adding one. The data on switching are sparse. While almost every clinical trial in patients with established schizophrenia has entailed the patient switching from one antipsychotic medication to another, there are no rigorous studies addressing preferred medication switches (e.g. if risperidone fails – what next? Olanzapine, quetiapine, aripiprazole or ziprasidone?). If one looks at only the switching trials which have been sponsored by the drug companies it leads to a rather confusing picture, with the trial results being very closely linked to the sponsors' interest (see 'Why olanzapine beats risperidone, risperidone beats quetiapine, and quetiapine beats olanzapine: an exploratory analysis of head-to-head comparison studies of second-generation antipsychotics').[23] Further, switching can be associated with destabilisation of the illness and the emergence of adverse effects, which may be a consequence of stopping the original antipsychotic medication and/or a response to the subsequent medication and/or differences between the pharmacological profiles of the two medications. The extent to which the management of a switch can minimise such problems is not entirely clear, but a gradual cross-tapering approach is usually recommended.[24–26]

CATIE, the major US-based publicly funded comparative trial, examined partici-pants whose illness had failed to respond to a first SGA and were then randomly assigned to a different second one.[27] Participants switched to olanzapine and risperi-done did better than those switched to quetiapine and ziprasidone. This greater effec-tiveness is supported by a meta-analysis that compared a number of SGAs with FGAs and concluded that, other than clozapine, only amisulpride, risperidone and olanzapine were superior to FGAs in efficacy.[28] Further, the findings of a meta-analysis comparing SGAs among themselves suggested that olanzapine and risperidone (in that order) may be modestly more effective than the others.[29] Thus, if olanzapine or risperidone have not yet been tried, it would be a reasonable decision to switch to these medications, provided the risk–benefit balance was considered likely to be favourable for the par-ticular patient. Comparing these two medications, the data are somewhat limited. However, a number of controlled and open-label studies do show an asymmetrical advantage, with a switch to olanzapine being more effective than to risperidone.[30,31] Such findings have been reinforced recently: a systematic review[32] found high-dose olanzapine to be superior to other commonly used FGAs and SGAs, including risperi-done, for TRS, while a network meta-analysis[33] confirmed olanzapine as the second most effective antipsychotic, behind clozapine, for such illness.

The best medication regimen (aside from clozapine) to choose for a patient whose illness has failed trials of olanzapine and risperidone remains unclear. Should one switch to, say, aripiprazole or ziprasidone or even an older FGA, or should another antipsy-chotic medication be added? Interestingly, studies that have switched patients to ari-piprazole for reasons of tolerability (weight gain, etc.) find either no loss of efficacy[34,35] or an improvement in symptom severity.[24,36]

After switching, adding another antipsychotic is probably the most common clinical strategy chosen. A 2022 clinical audit in the UK[37] found that of 4,156 people on acute adult psychiatric wards, 14% were prescribed more than one antipsychotic medication. By far the most common reason for such a prescription was an insufficient response of symptoms and/or behavioural disturbance with antipsychotic monotherapy at standard dosage. A second antipsychotic may also be added for additional properties (e.g. que-tiapine for sedation or aripiprazole to decrease plasma prolactin – these matters are discussed elsewhere) but here we are concerned solely with the use of combined anti-psychotic medications to increase efficacy. From a theoretical point of view, since all currently available antipsychotic medications (with xanomeline and pimavanserin as exceptions) block D_2 receptors (unlike, say, antihypertensive drugs which use different mechanisms) there is a limited rationale for addition. Studies of add-ons have often chosen combinations on the basis of convenience or clinical lore and perhaps the most systematic evidence is available for the addition of a second antipsychotic to clozap-ine,[38–40] a strategy that may be supported by the rationale that since clozapine has rela-tively low D_2 occupancy, increasing its D_2 occupancy may yield additional benefits.[41] However, a meta-analysis of RCTs comparing augmentation with a second antipsy-chotic with continuing monotherapy in schizophrenia[42] found a lack of double-blind/high-quality evidence for efficacy, in terms of treatment response and symptom improvement, for a range of antipsychotic combinations. Further, compared with antipsychotic mono-therapy, combined antipsychotics seem to be associated with an increased adverse-effect burden and a greater risk of high-dose prescribing.[43,44] Nonetheless, at a population level, antipsychotic polypharmacy does not appear to result in increased rates of hospitalisation for either physical or specifically cardiovascular illness.[45]

While augmentation with another antipsychotic medication as a treatment strategy should probably be avoided, under some conditions of acute exacerbation or agitation the prescriber may see this as the only practicable solution. Or quite often the prescriber may inherit the care of a patient on antipsychotic polypharmacy. Most RCT evidence suggests that such a regimen can be safely switched back to antipsychotic monotherapy without symptom exacerbation, at least in the majority of patients,[46–48] although this is not a universal finding.[49] Essock and co-workers[48] conducted a trial involving 127 patients with schizophrenia who were stable on antipsychotic polypharmacy. Over a 12-month period, a switch to monotherapy was successful in about two-thirds of the participants in whom it was tested. And in those cases where the move to monotherapy resulted in a return of symptoms, the most common recourse was a return to the original polypharmacy. This was achieved without any significant worsening in this group. The advantages for the monotherapy group were exposure to less medication, equivalent symptom severity and some loss of weight.

So when should the prescriber just continue with the current regimen? The evidence reviewed above suggests that no one strategy, such as increasing the dose, switching to another antipsychotic medication or augmentation with a second antipsychotic medication, is the clear winner in all situations. But increasing the dose if plasma drug levels are low, switching to olanzapine if this has not been tried, or augmentation if there is insufficient response to clozapine may be beneficial in some cases. Given the limited efficacy of these manoeuvres perhaps an equally important call by the treating doctor is when to just stay with the current pharmacotherapy and focus on non-pharmacological means: engagement in case management, targeted psychological treatments and vocational rehabilitation as means of enhancing patient well-being. While it may seem a passive option, staying with the current medication regimen may often do less harm than aimless switching and dosage increments.

Summary

When treatment fails
■ If the dose of antipsychotic medication has been optimised, consider watchful waiting.   ■ Consider increasing the antipsychotic dose according to tolerability and plasma levels (little supporting evidence for most drugs).[2,50]   ■ If this fails, consider switching to olanzapine or risperidone (if not already used).   ■ If this fails, use clozapine (supporting evidence very strong).   ■ If clozapine fails, use time-limited augmentation strategies (supporting evidence variable).

References

1. Samara MT, et al. Increasing antipsychotic dose versus switching antipsychotic for non response in schizophrenia. *Cochrane Database Syst Rev* 2018; (5):CD011884.
2. Barnes T, et al. Evidence-based guidelines for the pharmacological treatment of schizophrenia: updated recommendations from the British Association for Psychopharmacology. *J Psychopharmacol* 2020; 34:3–78.
3. Rubio JM, et al. Early non-response to antipsychotic treatment in schizophrenia: a systematic review and meta-analysis of evidence-based management options. *CNS Drugs* 2023; 37:499–512.
4. Ezewuzie N, et al. Establishing a dose–response relationship for oral risperidone in relapsed schizophrenia. *J Psychopharm* 2006; 20:86–90.
5. Sparshatt A, et al. Quetiapine: dose–response relationship in schizophrenia. *CNS Drugs* 2008; 22:49–68.
6. Honer WG, et al. A randomized, double-blind, placebo-controlled study of the safety and tolerability of high-dose quetiapine in patients with persistent symptoms of schizophrenia or schizoaffective disorder. *J Clin Psychiatry* 2012; 73:13–20.
7. Davis JM, et al. Dose response and dose equivalence of antipsychotics. *J Clin Psychopharmacol* 2004; 24:192–208.
8. Leucht S, et al. Dose–response meta-analysis of antipsychotic drugs for acute schizophrenia. *Am J Psychiatry* 2020; 177:342–353.
9. Srisurapanont M, et al. A network meta-analysis of the dose-response effects of lurasidone on acute schizophrenia. *Sci Rep* 2021; 11:5571.
10. Kinon BJ, et al. Standard and higher dose of olanzapine in patients with schizophrenia or schizoaffective disorder: a randomized, double-blind, fixed-dose study. *J Clin Psychopharmacol* 2008; 28:392–400.
11. Marder SR, et al. Risperidone in the treatment of schizophrenia. *Am J Psychiatry* 1994; 151:825–835.
12. Van Putten T, et al. A controlled dose comparison of haloperidol in newly admitted schizophrenic patients. *Arch Gen Psychiatry* 1990; 47:754–758.
13. Zimbroff DL, et al. Controlled, dose-response study of sertindole and haloperidol in the treatment of schizophrenia. Sertindole Study Group. *Am J Psychiatry* 1997; 154:782–791.
14. Siafis S, et al. Antipsychotic dose, dopamine D2 receptor occupancy and extrapyramidal side-effects: a systematic review and dose–response meta-analysis. *Mol Psychiatry* 2023; 28:3267–3277.
15. Kinon BJ, et al. Treatment of neuroleptic-resistant schizophrenic relapse. *Psychopharmacol Bull* 1993; 29:309–314.
16. Hermes E, et al. Predictors of antipsychotic dose changes in the CATIE schizophrenia trial. *Psychiatry Res* 2012; 199:1–7.
17. Loebel A, et al. Lurasidone dose escalation in early nonresponding patients with schizophrenia: a randomized, placebo-controlled study. *J Clin Psychiatry* 2016; 77:1672–1680.
18. Jukic MM, et al. Effect of CYP2D6 genotype on exposure and efficacy of risperidone and aripiprazole: a retrospective, cohort study. *Lancet Psychiatry* 2019; 6:418–426.
19. Taylor D, et al. Predicting clozapine dose required to achieve a therapeutic plasma concentration: a comparison of a population algorithm and three algorithms based on gene variant models. *J Psychopharmacol* 2023; 37:1030–1039.
20. Patel MX, et al. Quality of prescribing for schizophrenia: evidence from a national audit in England and Wales. *Eur Neuropsychopharmacol* 2014; 24:499–509.
21. Stokes I, et al. Prevalence of treatment resistance and clozapine use in early intervention services. *BJPsych Open* 2020; 6:e107.
22. Paton C, et al. Is clozapine really under-used? Investigating clinical practice in a community psychosis team. *J Psychiatry Behav Sci* 2023; 6:1089.
23. Heres S, et al. Why olanzapine beats risperidone, risperidone beats quetiapine, and quetiapine beats olanzapine: an exploratory analysis of head-to-head comparison studies of second-generation antipsychotics. *Am J Psychiatry* 2006; 163:185–194.
24. Obayashi Y, et al. Switching strategies for antipsychotic monotherapy in schizophrenia: a multi-center cohort study of aripiprazole. *Psychopharmacology (Berl)* 2020; 237:167–175.
25. Lambert TJ. Switching antipsychotic therapy: what to expect and clinical strategies for improving therapeutic outcomes. *J Clin Psychiatry* 2007; 68 Suppl 6:10–13.
26. Takeuchi H, et al. Immediate vs gradual discontinuation in antipsychotic switching: a systematic review and meta-analysis. *Schizophr Bull* 2017; 43:862–871.
27. Stroup TS, et al. Effectiveness of olanzapine, quetiapine, risperidone, and ziprasidone in patients with chronic schizophrenia following discontinuation of a previous atypical antipsychotic. *Am J Psychiatry* 2006; 163:611–622.
28. Leucht S, et al. Second-generation versus first-generation antipsychotic drugs for schizophrenia: a meta-analysis. *Lancet* 2009; 373:31–41.
29. Leucht S, et al. A meta-analysis of head-to-head comparisons of second-generation antipsychotics in the treatment of schizophrenia. *Am J Psychiatry* 2009; 166:152–163.
30. Hong J, et al. Clinical consequences of switching from olanzapine to risperidone and vice versa in outpatients with schizophrenia: 36-month results from the Worldwide Schizophrenia Outpatients Health Outcomes (W-SOHO) study. *BMC Psychiatry* 2012; 12:218.
31. Agid O, et al. Antipsychotic response in first-episode schizophrenia: efficacy of high doses and switching. *Eur Neuropsychopharmacol* 2013; 23:1017–1022.
32. Gannon L, et al. High-dose olanzapine in treatment-resistant schizophrenia: a systematic review. *Ther Adv Psychopharmacol* 2023; 13:20451253231168788.
33. Dong S, et al. A network meta-analysis of efficacy, acceptability, and tolerability of antipsychotics in treatment-resistant schizophrenia. *Eur Arch Psychiatry Clin Neurosci* 2023; 274:917–928.
34. Stroup TS, et al. A randomized trial examining the effectiveness of switching from olanzapine, quetiapine, or risperidone to aripiprazole to reduce metabolic risk: comparison of antipsychotics for metabolic problems (CAMP). *Am J Psychiatry* 2011; 168:947–956.
35. Montastruc F, et al. Association of aripiprazole with the risk for psychiatric hospitalization, self-harm, or suicide. *JAMA Psychiatry* 2019; 76:409–417.

36. Pae CU, et al. Effectiveness and tolerability of switching to aripiprazole once monthly from antipsychotic polypharmacy and/or other long acting injectable antipsychotics for patients with schizophrenia in routine practice: a retrospective, observation study. *Clin Psychopharmacol Neurosc* 2020; **18**:153–158.

37. Prescribing Observatory for Mental Health. Topic 1h & 3e: Prescribing of antipsychotic medication in adult mental health services, including high dose, combined, and PRN. CCQI 422. 2022 (last accessed February 2025); https://www.rcpsych.ac.uk/improving-care/ccqi/national-clinical-audits/pomh.

38. Wagner E, et al. Clozapine combination and augmentation strategies in patients with schizophrenia - recommendations from an international expert survey among the Treatment Response and Resistance in Psychosis (TRRIP) working group. *Schizophr Bull* 2020; **46**:1459–1470.

39. Taylor DM, et al. Augmentation of clozapine with a second antipsychotic: a meta-analysis of randomized, placebo-controlled studies. *Acta Psychiatr Scand* 2009; **119**:419–425.

40. Grover S, et al. Augmentation strategies for clozapine resistance: a systematic review and meta-analysis. *Acta Neuropsychiatr* 2023; **35**:65–75.

41. Kapur S, et al. Increased dopamine D2 receptor occupancy and elevated prolactin level associated with addition of haloperidol to clozapine. *Am J Psychiatry* 2001; **158**:311–314.

42. Galling B, et al. Antipsychotic augmentation vs. monotherapy in schizophrenia: systematic review, meta-analysis and meta-regression analysis. *World Psychiatry* 2017; **16**:77–89.

43. Gallego JA, et al. Safety and tolerability of antipsychotic polypharmacy. *Expert Opin Drug Saf* 2012; **11**:527–542.

44. Barnes T, et al. Antipsychotic polypharmacy in schizophrenia: benefits and risks. *CNS Drugs* 2011; **25**:383–399.

45. Taipale H, et al. Safety of antipsychotic polypharmacy versus monotherapy in a nationwide cohort of 61,889 patients with schizophrenia. *Am J Psychiatry* 2023; **180**:377–385.

46. Borlido C, et al. Switching from 2 antipsychotics to 1 antipsychotic in schizophrenia: a randomized, double-blind, placebo-controlled study. *J Clin Psychiatry* 2016; **77**:e14–e20.

47. Hori H, et al. Switching to antipsychotic monotherapy can improve attention and processing speed, and social activity in chronic schizophrenia patients. *J Psychiatr Res* 2013; **47**:1843–1848.

48. Essock SM, et al. Effectiveness of switching from antipsychotic polypharmacy to monotherapy. *Am J Psychiatry* 2011; **168**:702–708.

49. Constantine RJ, et al. The risks and benefits of switching patients with schizophrenia or schizoaffective disorder from two to one antipsychotic medication: a randomized controlled trial. *Schizophr Res* 2015; **166**:194–200.

50. Royal College of Psychiatrists. *The Risks and Benefits of High-Dose Antipsychotic Medication*. College Report CR190. London: Royal College of Psychiatrists; 2014.

Acutely disturbed or violent behaviour

Acute behavioural disturbance can occur in the context of psychiatric illness, physical illness, substance abuse or personality disorder. Psychotic symptoms are common and the patient may be aggressive towards others secondary to persecutory delusions or auditory, visual or tactile hallucinations. This section deals with behavioural disturbance in the context of severe mental illness. Agitated states caused by illicit substance misuse are dealt with in Chapter 9.

The clinical practice of rapid tranquillisation is used when appropriate psychological and behavioural approaches have failed to de-escalate acutely disturbed behaviour. It is, essentially, a treatment of last resort. Patients who require rapid tranquillisation (RT) are often too disturbed to give informed consent and therefore participate in RCTs but, with the use of a number of creative methodologies, the evidence base with respect to the efficacy and tolerability of pharmacological strategies has grown substantially. A comprehensive and up-to-date consensus guideline was published in 2018[1] and, more recently, a systematic review and meta-analysis.[2] A network meta-analysis of RT in the emergency department has also been published.[3]

Oral/inhaled treatment

Several studies supporting the efficacy of oral SGAs have been conducted.[4–7] The level of behavioural disturbance exhibited by the patients in these studies was moderate at most, and all participants accepted oral treatment (this degree of compliance would be unusual in clinical practice). Patients recruited to these studies received the SGA as antipsychotic monotherapy. The efficacy and safety of adding a second antipsychotic as a 'when necessary' treatment have not been explicitly tested in formal RCTs.

A single-dose RCT showed sublingual asenapine to be more effective than placebo for acute agitation.[8] The efficacy of inhaled loxapine in behavioural disturbance that is moderate in severity is also supported by RCTs.[9–11] The use of this preparation is now restricted in many countries owing to the risk of bronchospasm.

Dexmedetomidine, an α_2 receptor agonist used in anaesthesia, has been developed as a sublingual film. It seems to be rapidly effective in acute agitation.[12]

Parenteral treatment

Large, placebo-controlled RCTs support the efficacy of IM preparations of olanzapine, ziprasidone and aripiprazole. When considered together, these trials suggested that IM olanzapine is more effective than IM haloperidol, which in turn is more effective than IM aripiprazole, which itself is more effective than ziprasidone.[2,13,14] The level of behavioural disturbance in these studies was moderate at most and differences between treatments small.

A large observational study supported the efficacy and tolerability of IM olanzapine in clinical emergencies (where disturbance was severe).[15] A study comparing IM haloperidol with a combination of IM midazolam and IM haloperidol found the combination more effective than haloperidol alone for controlling agitation in palliative care patients.[16]

Several RCTs have investigated the effectiveness of parenteral medication in 'real-life' acutely disturbed patients. Overall:

- Compared with IV midazolam alone, a combination of IV olanzapine or IV droperidol with IV midazolam was more rapidly effective and resulted in fewer subsequent doses of medication being required.[17]
- IM midazolam 7.5–15mg was more rapidly sedating than a combination of haloperidol 5–10mg and promethazine 50mg (TREC 1).[18]
- Olanzapine 10mg was as effective as a combination of haloperidol 10mg and promethazine 25–50mg in the short term, but the effect did not last as long (TREC 4).[19]
- A combination of haloperidol 5–10mg and promethazine 50mg was more effective and better tolerated than haloperidol 5–10mg alone; 6% of patients had an acute dystonic reaction (TREC 3).[20]
- A combination of haloperidol 10mg and promethazine 25–50mg was more effective than lorazepam 4mg (TREC 2).[21]
- A combination of IM chlorpromazine 100mg, haloperidol 5mg and promethazine 25mg was no better than IM haloperidol 5mg plus promethazine 25mg (TREC Lebanon).[22]
- A combination of IV midazolam and IV droperidol was more rapidly sedating than either IV droperidol or IV olanzapine alone. Fewer patients in the midazolam–droperidol group required additional medication doses to achieve sedation.[23]
- IM olanzapine was more effective than IM aripiprazole in the treatment of agitation in schizophrenia in the short-term (at 2 hours) but there was no significant difference between treatments at 24 hours.[24]
- IM midazolam 5mg was faster acting and more effective than olanzapine 10mg, ziprasidone 20mg and both 5 and 10mg haloperidol in a large ($n = 737$) emergency room study.[25]
- In an open-label study, the combination of IM haloperidol and IM lorazepam was found to be similar in efficacy to IM olanzapine.[26]
- IM droperidol and IM haloperidol were equally effective.[27]
- IM droperidol with IM midazolam was more effective than IM haloperidol with IM lorazepam.[28]

Nearly 10 years ago, Cochrane concluded that haloperidol alone is effective in the management of acute behavioural disturbance but poorly tolerated, and that co-administration of promethazine (but not lorazepam) improves tolerability.[29,30] However NICE considers the evidence relating to the use of promethazine for this purpose to be inconclusive.[31] The authors also stated that 'haloperidol used on its own without something to offset its frequent and serious adverse effects is difficult to justify'.[32]

A systematic review and meta-analysis of IM olanzapine for agitation found IM olanzapine and IM haloperidol to be equally effective, but IM olanzapine was associated with a lower incidence of EPSEs.[33] Cochrane suggests that droperidol is effective and may be used to control disturbed and aggressive behaviours caused by psychosis.[34] Droperidol has seen a resurgence in use in some countries having become available again (its initial withdrawal was voluntary, so reintroduction is not prohibited).

In a meta-analysis that examined the tolerability of IM antipsychotics when used for the treatment of agitation, the incidence of acute dystonia with haloperidol was reported to be 5%, with SGAs performing considerably better.[35] Acute EPSEs may adversely affect longer-term compliance.[36] In addition, the formal prescribing information in most countries for haloperidol calls for a pretreatment ECG[37,38] and recommends that concomitant antipsychotics are not prescribed. The mean increase in QTc after 10mg IM haloperidol can be up to 15ms but the range is wide.[39]

Promethazine may inhibit the metabolism of haloperidol;[40] a pharmacokinetic interaction that is potentially clinically significant given the potential of haloperidol to prolong QTc. While this is unlikely to be problematic if a single dose is administered, repeat dosing may confer risk.

Droperidol is also associated with QT changes (the reason for its withdrawal). In an observational study set in hospital emergency departments, of the 1,009 patients administered parenteral droperidol, only 13 patients (1.28%) had an abnormal QT after dose administration. In seven of these cases, another contributory factor was identified. There were no cases of torsades de pointes (TdP).[27] In all RT studies of IM droperidol, the overall rate of QTc measurements greater than 500ms was less than 2%.[2]

Intravenous treatment is now rarely used in RT but where benefits are thought to outweigh risks it may be considered as a last resort. A small study comparing high-dose IV haloperidol with IV diazepam found both drugs to be effective at 24 hours.[41] Two large observational studies have examined the safety of IV olanzapine when used in the emergency department. The indications for its use varied, agitation being the most common. In one study,[42] in the group treated for agitation ($n = 265$), over a third of patients required an additional sedative dose after the initial IV olanzapine dose. Hypoxia was reported in 17.7% of patients and supplemental oxygen was used in 20.4%. Six patients required intubation (two of these because of olanzapine treatment). In the other study,[43] IV olanzapine ($n = 295$) was compared with IM olanzapine ($n = 489$). Additional doses were not required for 81% of patients in the IV group and 84% of patients in the IM group. Respiratory depression was more commonly observed in the group receiving IV olanzapine. Five patients in the IM group and two in the IV group required intubation.

In an acute psychiatric setting, 'high-dose sedation' (defined as a dose of more than 10mg of haloperidol, droperidol or midazolam) was not more effective than lower doses but was associated with more adverse effects (hypotension and oxygen desaturation).[44] Consistent with this, a small RCT supports the efficacy of low-dose haloperidol, although both efficacy and tolerability were superior when midazolam was co-prescribed.[45] These data broadly support the use of standard doses in clinical emergencies but the need for further physical restraint after lower doses needs to be considered.

A small observational study supported the effectiveness of buccal midazolam in a PICU setting.[46] Parenteral administration of midazolam, particularly in higher doses, may cause over-sedation accompanied by respiratory depression.[47] Lorazepam IM is an established treatment and TREC 2[21] supports its efficacy, although combining all results from the TREC studies suggests that midazolam 7.5–15mg is probably more effective. More recent studies have used 5mg IM midazolam and found it to be rapidly effective.[28,48] A Cochrane review of benzodiazepines for psychosis-induced aggression and agitation concluded that most trials were too small to highlight differences in either positive or negative effects and while adding a benzodiazepine to another drug may not be clearly advantageous it may lead to unnecessary adverse effects.[49]

With respect to those who are behaviourally disturbed secondary to acute intoxication with alcohol or illicit drugs, there are fewer data to guide practice. A large observational study of IV sedation in patients intoxicated with alcohol found that combination treatment (most commonly haloperidol 5mg and lorazepam 2mg) was more effective and reduced the need for subsequent sedation than either drug given alone.[50] A case series (*n* = 59) of patients who received modest doses of oral, IM or IV haloperidol to manage behavioural disturbance in the context of phencyclidine consumption showed that haloperidol was effective and well tolerated (one case each of mild hypotension and mild hypoxia).[51] A section on the treatment of behavioural disturbance caused by substance misuse is included in Chapter 9.

Ketamine is widely used for agitation in hospital emergency departments. In a systematic review of 18 studies of ketamine,[52] a mean dose of 315mg IM ketamine achieved adequate sedation in an average of 7.2 minutes. Over 30% of 650 patients were eventually intubated and more than 1% experienced laryngospasm. Ketamine is not suitable for RT where facilities for intubation are not available, although it may be the most effective treatment.[3]

Overall, the current broad consensus is that midazolam and droperidol are the fastest-acting single-drug, intramuscular treatments[53] and that haloperidol alone should be avoided and perhaps abandoned completely even in combination.[54] Second-line treatments are combinations of benzodiazepines and antipsychotics and third line would probably be intravenous benzodiazepines and then ketamine (2–5mg/kg IM), assuming intubation facilities are available.

Practical measures

Plans for the management of individual patients should ideally be made in advance. The aim is to prevent disturbed behaviour and reduce risk of violence. Nursing interventions (de-escalation, time out, seclusion),[55] increased nursing levels, transfer of the patient to a psychiatric intensive care unit and pharmacological management are options that may be employed. Care should be taken to avoid combinations and high cumulative doses of antipsychotic drugs. The monitoring of routine physical observations after RT is essential. RT is often, of course, viewed as punitive by patients. There is little research into the patient experience of RT. The aims of RT are threefold:

- To reduce suffering for the patient: psychological or physical (through self-harm or accidents).
- To reduce risk of harm to others by maintaining a safe environment.
- To do no harm (by prescribing safe regimens and monitoring physical health).

Note: Despite the need for rapid and effective treatment, concomitant use of two or more antipsychotics (antipsychotic polypharmacy) should be avoided on the basis of risk associated with QT prolongation (common to almost all antipsychotics). This is a particularly important consideration in RT, where the patient's physical state predisposes to cardiac arrhythmia.

66 The Maudsley® Prescribing Guidelines in Psychiatry

CHAPTER 1

Zuclopenthixol acetate

Zuclopenthixol acetate (ZA) is widely used in the UK and elsewhere in Europe, and is best known by its trade name Acuphase®. Zuclopenthixol itself is a thioxanthene dopamine antagonist first introduced in the early 1960s. ZA is not a rapidly tranquillising agent. Its elimination half-life is around 20 hours. IM injection of zuclopenthixol base results in rapid absorption and a duration of action of 12–24 hours. By slowing absorption after IM injection, the biological half-life (and so duration of action) becomes dependent on the rate of release from the IM reservoir. This can be achieved by esterification of the zuclopenthixol molecule, the rate of release being broadly proportional to the length of the ester carbon chain. Thus, zuclopenthixol decanoate is slow to act but very long-acting as a result of retarded release after IM injection. ZA (with eight carbon atoms fewer) would be expected to provide relatively prompt release but with an intermediate duration of action. The intention of the manufacturers was that the use of ZA would obviate the need for repeated IM injections in disturbed patients.

An initial pharmacokinetic study of ZA included 19 patients 'in whom calming effect by parenteral neuroleptic was considered necessary'.[56] Zuclopenthixol was detectable in the plasma after 1–2 hours but did not reach peak concentrations until around 36 hours after dosing. At 72 hours, plasma levels were around one-third of those at 36 hours. The clinical effect of ZA was not rapid – 10 of 17 patients exhibited minimal or no change in psychotic symptoms at 4 hours. Sedation was evident at 4 hours but it had effectively abated by 72 hours.

A follow-up study by the same research group[57] examined more closely the clinical effects of ZA in 83 patients. The authors concluded that ZA produced 'pronounced and rapid reduction in psychotic symptoms'. In fact, psychotic symptoms were first assessed only after 24 hours and so a claim of rapid effect is not reasonably supported. Sedative effects were measured after 2 hours when a statistically significant effect was observed – at baseline mean sedation score was 0.0 (0 = no sign of sedation) and at 2 hours 0.6 (1 = slightly sedated). Maximum sedation was observed at 8 hours (mean score 2.2; 2 = moderately sedated). At 72 hours mean score was 1.1. Dystonia and rigidity were the most commonly reported adverse effects.

Two independently conducted open studies produced similar results – a slow onset of effect peaking at 24 hours and still being evident at 72 hours.[58,59] The first UK study was reported in 1990.[60] In the trial, a significant reduction in psychosis score was first evident at 8 hours and scores continued to fall until the last measurement at 72 hours. Of 25 patients assessed only 4 showed signs of tranquillisation at 1 hour (19 at 2 hours and 22 at 24 hours).

A comparative trial of ZA[61] examined its effects and those of IM/oral haloperidol and IM/oral zuclopenthixol base (in multiple doses over 6 days). The two non-ester, IM/oral preparations produced a greater degree of sedation at 2 hours than did ZA but the effect of ZA and zuclopenthixol was more sustained than with haloperidol over 144 hours (although patients received more zuclopenthixol doses). No clear differences between treatments were detected, with the exception of the slow onset of effect of ZA. The number of doses given varied substantially: ZA 1–4; haloperidol 1–26; and zuclopenthixol 1–22. This is the key (and perhaps unique) advantage of ZA – it reduces the need for repeat doses in acute psychosis. Indeed, this was the principal finding of the first double-blind study of ZA.[62] Participants were given either ZA or haloperidol IM and assessed over 3 days. Changes in Brief Psychiatric Rating Scale and Clinical Global Impression scores were near identical on each daily assessment. However, only 1 of 23 patients taking ZA required a second injection, whereas 7 of 21 required a repeat dose of haloperidol. Speed of onset was not examined. Similar findings were reported by Thai researchers comparing the same treatments[63] and in three other studies of moderate size ($n = 44$,[64] $n = 40$,[65] $n = 50$[66]). In each study, the timing of assessments was such that time to onset of effect could not be determined.

Overall, the utility of ZA in rapid tranquillisation is limited by a somewhat delayed onset of both sedative and antipsychotic actions. Sedation may be apparent in a minority of patients after 2–4 hours, but antipsychotic action is evident only after 8 hours. If ZA is given to a restrained patient, their behaviour on release from restraint is likely to be unchanged and will remain as such for several hours. ZA has a role in reducing the number of restraints for IM injection but it has no role in rapid tranquillisation.

Guidelines for the use of zuclopenthixol acetate (Acuphase)

- ZA is not a rapidly tranquillising agent. It should be used only after an acutely psychotic patient has required (or is likely to require) *repeated* injections of short-acting antipsychotic drugs such as haloperidol or olanzapine, or sedative drugs such as lorazepam. It is perhaps best reserved for those few patients who have a prior history of good response to Acuphase.
- ZA should be given only when enough time has elapsed to assess the full response to previously injected drugs: allow 15 minutes after IV injections; 60 minutes after IM.
- ZA should never be administered for rapid tranquillisation (the onset of effect is too slow) or to a patient who is physically resistant (risk of intravasation and oil embolus) or to neuroleptic-naïve patients (risk of prolonged EPSEs).

Rapid tranquillisation summary

In an emergency situation: Assess whether there may be a medical cause.[67] Optimise regular prescription. The aim of pharmacological treatment is to calm the patient but not to over-sedate. Note that lower doses should be used for children, adolescents and older adults. Patients' levels of consciousness and physical health should be monitored after administration of parenteral medication (see protocol).

Step intervention

1 De-escalation, time out, placement, etc., as appropriate

2 Offer oral treatment

If patient is prescribed a regular antipsychotic:

Lorazepam 1–2mg
Promethazine 25–50mg
Monotherapy with **buccal midazolam** may avoid the need for IM treatment
Dose: 10mg
Note that this preparation is unlicensed

If patient is not already taking a regular oral or LAI antipsychotic:
- **Olanzapine** 10mg or
- **Risperidone** 1–2mg or
- **Quetiapine** 50–100mg or
- **Haloperidol** 5mg (with promethazine 25mg). ECG is required in UK/EU

Repeat after 45–60 minutes, if necessary. Consider combining sedative and antipsychotic treatment.
Go to step 3 if two doses fail or sooner if the patient is placing themselves or others at significant risk.

3 Consider IM treatment

Lorazepam 2mg[a,b]	Have flumazenil to hand in case of benzodiazepine-induced respiratory depression
Promethazine 50mg	IM promethazine is a useful option in a benzodiazepine-tolerant patient
Olanzapine 10mg[d]	IM olanzapine should not be combined with an IM benzodiazepine, particularly if alcohol has been consumed[68]
Aripiprazole 9.75mg	Less hypotension than olanzapine, but less effective[6,13,69]
Haloperidol 5mg	**Haloperidol should be the last drug considered.** The incidence of acute dystonia is high; combine with IM promethazine and ensure IM procyclidine is available. Pretreatment ECG required

Repeat after 30–60 minutes if insufficient effect. Combinations of haloperidol and lorazepam or haloperidol and promethazine may be considered if single drug treatment fails. Drugs must not be mixed in the same syringe. IM olanzapine must never be combined with IM benzodiazepine.

4 Consider IV treatment

Diazepam 10mg over at least 2 minutes[b,e]
Repeat after 5–10 minutes if insufficient effect (up to 3 times)
Have flumazenil to hand

5 Seek expert advice[f]
Consider transfer to medical unit for administration of **IM ketamine**

Notes

a. Carefully check administration and dilution instructions, which differ between manufacturers. Many centres use 4mg. An alternative is IM midazolam 5–15mg. 5mg is usually sufficient. The risk of respiratory depression is dose-related with both drugs but generally greater with midazolam.
b. Caution in the very young and elderly and those with pre-existing brain damage or impulse control problems, as disinhibition reactions are more likely.[70]

(Continued)

Rapid tranquillisation summary   *(Continued)*

c. Promethazine has a slow onset of action but is often an effective sedative. Dilution is not required before IM injection. May be repeated up to a maximum of 100mg/day. Wait 1–2 hours after injection to assess response. Note that promethazine alone has been reported, albeit very rarely, to cause NMS,[71] although it is an extremely weak dopamine antagonist. Note also the potential pharmacokinetic interaction between promethazine and haloperidol (reduced metabolism of haloperidol) which may confer risk if repeated doses of both are administered.

d. Recommended by NICE only for moderate behavioural disturbance, but data from a large observational study also support efficacy in clinical emergencies.

e. Use diazepam to avoid injection site reactions. Lorazepam can also be given IV. IV therapy may be used instead of IM when a very rapid effect is required. IV therapy also ensures near immediate delivery of the drug to its site of action and effectively avoids the danger of inadvertent accumulation of slowly absorbed IM doses. IV doses can be repeated after only 5–10 minutes if no effect is observed. Midazolam can also be used IV but respiratory depression is common.[1]

f. Options at this point are limited, although the wider use of IM ketamine has improved the range of options available. IM amylobarbitone and IM paraldehyde have been used in the past but are used now only extremely rarely and are generally not easy to obtain. IV olanzapine, IV droperidol and IV haloperidol are possible but adverse effects are fairly common. ECT is also an option.

Rapid tranquillisation – physical monitoring

After any parenteral drug administration, monitor as follows:

- **Temperature**
- **Pulse**
- **Blood pressure**
- **Respiratory rate**

Every 15 minutes for 1 hour and then hourly until the patient is ambulatory. Patients who refuse to have their vital signs monitored or who remain too behaviourally disturbed to be approached should be observed for signs/symptoms of pyrexia, hypoxia, hypotension, over-sedation and general physical well-being.

All patients should be continuously observed ('in sight') for at least 1 hour and until clearly ambulatory.

If the patient is asleep or **unconscious**, the continuous use of pulse oximetry to measure oxygen saturation is desirable. A nurse should remain with the patient until ambulatory.

ECG and haematological monitoring are also strongly recommended when parenteral antipsychotics are given, especially when higher doses are used.[72,73] Hypokalaemia, stress and agitation place the patient at risk of cardiac arrhythmia[74] (see section on 'QT prolongation'). ECG monitoring is formally recommended for all patients who receive haloperidol.

Remedial measures in rapid tranquillisation

Problem	Remedial measures
Acute dystonia (including oculogyric crises)	Give **procyclidine** 5–10mg IM or IV
Reduced respiratory rate (<10/minute) or oxygen saturation (<90%)	Give oxygen, raise legs, ensure patient is not lying face down
	Give **flumazenil** if benzodiazepine-induced respiratory depression suspected (see protocol)
	If induced by any other sedative agent:
	transfer to a medical bed and ventilate mechanically
Irregular or slow (<50/minute) **pulse**	**Refer** to specialist medical care immediately
Fall in blood pressure (>30mmHg orthostatic drop or <50mmHg diastolic)	**Have patient lie flat**, tilt bed towards head Monitor closely
Increased temperature	Risk of NMS and perhaps arrhythmia; check creatine kinase urgently

Guidelines for the use of flumazenil

Indication for use	If, after the administration of lorazepam, midazolam or diazepam, respiratory rate falls below 10/minute
Contraindications	Patients with epilepsy who have been receiving long-term benzodiazepines
Caution	Dose should be carefully titrated in hepatic impairment
Dose and route of administration	*Initial:* 200mcg *intravenously* over 15 seconds if required level of consciousness not achieved after 60 seconds, then *Subsequent dose:* 100mcg over 15 seconds
Time before dose can be repeated	60 seconds
Maximum dose	1mg in 24 hours (one initial dose and eight subsequent doses)
Adverse effects[75]	Patients may become agitated, anxious or fearful on awakening. Seizures may occur in regular benzodiazepine users. Cardiac arrhythmia (supraventricular tachycardia)
Management	Adverse effects usually subside
Monitoring:	
■ **What to monitor?**	Respiratory rate
■ **How often?**	Continuously until respiratory rate returns to baseline level Flumazenil has a short half-life (much shorter than diazepam) and respiratory function may recover and then deteriorate again

Note: If respiratory rate does not return to normal or patient is not alert after initial doses given, assume that sedation is from some other cause

References

1. Patel MX, et al. Joint BAP NAPICU evidence-based consensus guidelines for the clinical management of acute disturbance: de-escalation and rapid tranquillisation. *J Psychopharmacol* 2018; **32**:601–640.

2. Bak M, et al. The pharmacological management of agitated and aggressive behaviour: a systematic review and meta-analysis. *Eur Psychiatry* 2019; **57**:78–100.

3. deSouza IS, et al. Rapid tranquilization of the agitated patient in the emergency department: a systematic review and network meta-analysis. *Am J Emerg Med* 2022; **51**:363–373.

4. Currier GW, et al. Acute treatment of psychotic agitation: a randomized comparison of oral treatment with risperidone and lorazepam versus intramuscular treatment with haloperidol and lorazepam. *J Clin Psychiatry* 2004; **65**:386–394.

5. Ganesan S, et al. Effectiveness of quetiapine for the management of aggressive psychosis in the emergency psychiatric setting: a naturalistic uncontrolled trial. *Int J Psychiatry Clin Pract* 2005; **9**:199–203.

6. Simpson JR, Jr., et al. Impact of orally disintegrating olanzapine on use of intramuscular antipsychotics, seclusion, and restraint in an acute inpatient psychiatric setting. *J Clin Psychopharmacol* 2006; **26**:333–335.

7. Hsu WY, et al. Comparison of intramuscular olanzapine, orally disintegrating olanzapine tablets, oral risperidone solution, and intramuscular haloperidol in the management of acute agitation in an acute care psychiatric ward in Taiwan. *J Clin Psychopharmacol* 2010; **30**:230–234.

8. Pratts M, et al. A single-dose, randomized, double-blind, placebo-controlled trial of sublingual asenapine for acute agitation. *Acta Psychiatr Scand* 2014; **130**:61–68.

9. Lesem MD, et al. Rapid acute treatment of agitation in individuals with schizophrenia: multicentre, randomised, placebo-controlled study of inhaled loxapine. *Br J Psychiatry* 2011; **198**:51–58.

10. Kwentus J, et al. Rapid acute treatment of agitation in patients with bipolar I disorder: a multicenter, randomized, placebo-controlled clinical trial with inhaled loxapine. *Bipolar Disord* 2012; **14**:31–40.

11. Allen MH, et al. Efficacy and safety of loxapine for inhalation in the treatment of agitation in patients with schizophrenia: a randomized, double-blind, placebo-controlled trial. *J Clin Psychiatry* 2011; **72**:1313–1321.

12. Karlin DM, et al. Dexmedetomidine sublingual film: a new treatment to reduce agitation in schizophrenia and bipolar disorders. *Ann Pharmacother* 2024; **58**:54–64.

13. Citrome L. Comparison of intramuscular ziprasidone, olanzapine, or aripiprazole for agitation: a quantitative review of efficacy and safety. *J Clin Psychiatry* 2007; **68**:1876–1885.

14. Paris G, et al. Short-acting intramuscular second-generation antipsychotic drugs for acutely agitated patients with schizophrenia spectrum disorders: a systematic review and network meta-analysis. *Schizophr Res* 2021; **229**:3–11.

15. Perrin E, et al. A prospective, observational study of the safety and effectiveness of intramuscular psychotropic treatment in acutely agitated patients with schizophrenia and bipolar mania. *Eur Psychiatry* 2012; **27**:234–239.

16. Ferraz Goncalves JA, et al. Comparison of haloperidol alone and in combination with midazolam for the treatment of acute agitation in an inpatient palliative care service. *J Pain Palliat Care Pharmacother* 2016; **30**:284–288.

17. Chan EW, et al. Intravenous droperidol or olanzapine as an adjunct to midazolam for the acutely agitated patient: a multicenter, randomized, double-blind, placebo-controlled clinical trial. *Ann Emerg Med* 2013; **61**:72–81.

18. TREC Collaborative Group. Rapid tranquillisation for agitated patients in emergency psychiatric rooms: a randomised trial of midazolam versus haloperidol plus promethazine. *BMJ* 2003; **327**:708–713.

19. Raveendran NS, et al. Rapid tranquillisation in psychiatric emergency settings in India: pragmatic randomised controlled trial of intramuscular olanzapine versus intramuscular haloperidol plus promethazine. *BMJ* 2007; **335**:865.

20. Huf G, et al. Rapid tranquillisation in psychiatric emergency settings in Brazil: pragmatic randomised controlled trial of intramuscular haloperidol versus intramuscular haloperidol plus promethazine. *BMJ* 2007; **335**:869.

21. Alexander J, et al. Rapid tranquillisation of violent or agitated patients in a psychiatric emergency setting. Pragmatic randomised trial of intramuscular lorazepam v. haloperidol plus promethazine. *Br J Psychiatry* 2004; **185**:63–69.

22. Dib JE, et al. Rapid tranquillisation in a psychiatric emergency hospital in Lebanon: TREC-Lebanon: a pragmatic randomised controlled trial of intramuscular haloperidol and promethazine v. intramuscular haloperidol, promethazine and chlorpromazine. *Psychol Med* 2022; **52**:2751–2759.

23. Taylor DM, et al. Midazolam–droperidol, droperidol, or olanzapine for acute agitation: a randomized clinical trial. *Ann Emerg Med* 2017; **69**:318–326.e1.

24. Kittipeerachon M, et al. Intramuscular olanzapine versus intramuscular aripiprazole for the treatment of agitation in patients with schizophrenia: a pragmatic double-blind randomized trial. *Schizophr Res* 2016; **176**:231–238.

25. Klein LR, et al. Intramuscular midazolam, olanzapine, ziprasidone, or haloperidol for treating acute agitation in the emergency department. *Ann Emerg Med* 2018; **72**:374–385.

26. Huang CL, et al. Intramuscular olanzapine versus intramuscular haloperidol plus lorazepam for the treatment of acute schizophrenia with agitation: an open-label, randomized controlled trial. *J Formos Med Assoc* 2015; **114**:438–445.

27. Calver L, et al. The safety and effectiveness of droperidol for sedation of acute behavioral disturbance in the emergency department. *Ann Emerg Med* 2015; **66**:230-238.e1.

28. Thiemann P, et al. Prospective study of haloperidol plus lorazepam versus droperidol plus midazolam for the treatment of acute agitation in the emergency department. *Am J Emerg Med* 2022; **55**:76–81.

29. Powney MJ, et al. Haloperidol for psychosis-induced aggression or agitation (rapid tranquillisation). *Cochrane Database Syst Rev* 2012; **11**:CD009377.

30. Ostinelli EG, et al. Haloperidol for psychosis-induced aggression or agitation (rapid tranquillisation). *Cochrane Database Syst Rev* 2017; **7**:CD009377.

31. National Institute for Health and Care Excellence. Violence and aggression: short-term management in mental health, health and community settings. NICE guideline [NG10]. 2015 (reviewed May 2023, last checked December 2024); https://www.nice.org.uk/guidance/NG10.

32. Huf G, et al. Haloperidol plus promethazine for psychosis-induced aggression. *Cochrane Database Syst Rev* 2016; **11**:CD005146.

33. Kishi T, et al. Intramuscular olanzapine for agitated patients: a systematic review and meta-analysis of randomized controlled trials. *J Psychiatr Res* 2015; **68**:198–209.

34. Khokhar MA, et al. Droperidol for psychosis-induced aggression or agitation. *Cochrane Database Syst Rev* 2016; **12**:CD002830.

35. Satterthwaite TD, et al. A meta-analysis of the risk of acute extrapyramidal symptoms with intramuscular antipsychotics for the treatment of agitation. *J Clin Psychiatry* 2008; **69**:1869–1879.

36. van Harten PN, et al. Acute dystonia induced by drug treatment. *BMJ* 1999; **319**:623–626.

37. Pharmacovigilance Working Party. Public Assessment Report on Neuroleptics and Cardiac safety, in particular QT prolongation, cardiac arrhythmias, ventricular tachycardia and torsades de pointes. 2006.

38. Essential Pharma Ltd (Malta). Summary of Product Characteristics. HALDOL Decanoate (haloperidol decanoate) 100 mg/ml solution for injection. 2023 (last checked December 2024); https://www.medicines.org.uk/emc/product/15246/smpc.

39. Miceli JJ, et al. Effects of high-dose ziprasidone and haloperidol on the QTc interval after intramuscular administration: a randomized, single-blind, parallel-group study in patients with schizophrenia or schizoaffective disorder. *Clin Ther* 2010; **32**:472–491.

40. Suzuki A, et al. Histamine H1-receptor antagonists, promethazine and homochlorcyclizine, increase the steady-state plasma concentrations of haloperidol and reduced haloperidol. *Ther Drug Monit* 2003; **25**:192–196.

41. Lerner Y, et al. Acute high-dose parenteral haloperidol treatment of psychosis. *Am J Psychiatry* 1979; **136**:1061–1064.

42. Martel ML, et al. A large retrospective cohort of patients receiving intravenous olanzapine in the emergency department. *Acad Emerg Med* 2016; **23**:29–35.

43. Cole JB, et al. A prospective observational study of patients receiving intravenous and intramuscular olanzapine in the emergency department. *Ann Emerg Med* 2017; **69**:327–336.e2.

44. Calver L, et al. A prospective study of high dose sedation for rapid tranquilisation of acute behavioural disturbance in an acute mental health unit. *BMC Psychiatry* 2013; **13**:225.

45. Mantovani C, et al. Are low doses of antipsychotics effective in the management of psychomotor agitation? A randomized, rated-blind trial of 4 intramuscular interventions. *J Clin Psychopharmacol* 2013; **33**:306–312.

46. Taylor D, et al. Buccal midazolam for rapid tranquillisation. *Int J Psychiatry Clin Pract* 2008; **12**:309–311.

47. Spain D, et al. Safety and effectiveness of high-dose midazolam for severe behavioural disturbance in an emergency department with suspected psychostimulant-affected patients. *Emerg Med Australas* 2008; **20**:112–120.

48. Chan EW, et al. Intramuscular midazolam, olanzapine, or haloperidol for the management of acute agitation: a multi-centre, double-blind, randomised clinical trial. *EClinicalMedicine* 2021; **32**:100751.

49. Zaman H, et al. Benzodiazepines for psychosis-induced aggression or agitation. *Cochrane Database Syst Rev* 2017; **12**:CD003079.

50. Li SF, et al. Safety and efficacy of intravenous combination sedatives in the ED. *Am J Emerg Med* 2013; **31**:1402–1404.

51. MacNeal JJ, et al. Use of haloperidol in PCP-intoxicated individuals. *Clin Toxicol (Phila)* 2012; **50**:851–853.

52. Mankowitz SL, et al. Ketamine for rapid sedation of agitated patients in the prehospital and emergency department settings: a systematic review and proportional meta-analysis. *J Emerg Med* 2018; **55**:670–681.

53. Kim HK, et al. Safety and efficacy of pharmacologic agents used for rapid tranquilization of emergency department patients with acute agitation or excited delirium. *Expert Opin Drug Saf* 2021; **20**:123–138.

54. Pierre JM. Time to retire haloperidol? For emergency agitation, evidence suggests newer alternatives may be a better choice. *Current Psychiatry* 2020; **19**:18–28.

55. Huf G, et al. Physical restraints versus seclusion room for management of people with acute aggression or agitation due to psychotic illness (TREC-SAVE): a randomized trial. *Psychol Med* 2012; **42**:2265–2273.

56. Amdisen A, et al. Serum concentrations and clinical effect of zuclopenthixol in acutely disturbed, psychotic patients treated with zuclopenthixol acetate in Viscoleo. *Psychopharmacology (Berl)* 1986; **90**:412–416.

57. Amdisen A, et al. Zuclopenthixol acetate in viscoleo: a new drug formulation. An open Nordic multicentre study of zuclopenthixol acetate in Viscoleo in patients with acute psychoses including mania and exacerbation of chronic psychoses. *Acta Psychiatr Scand* 1987; **75**:99–107.

58. Lowert AC, et al. Acute psychotic disorders treated with 5% zuclopenthixol acetate in 'Viscoleo' ('Cisordinol-Acutard'), a global assessment of the clinical effect: an open multi-centre study. *Pharmatherapeutica* 1989; **5**:380–386.

59. Balant LP, et al. Clinical and pharmacokinetic evaluation of zuclopenthixol acetate in Viscoleo. *Pharmacopsychiatry* 1989; **22**:250–254.

60. Chakravarti SK, et al. Zuclopenthixol acetate (5% in 'Viscoleo'): single-dose treatment for acutely disturbed psychotic patients. *Curr Med Res Opin* 1990; **12**:58–65.

61. Baastrup PC, et al. A controlled Nordic multicentre study of zuclopenthixol acetate in oil solution, haloperidol and zuclopenthixol in the treatment of acute psychosis. *Acta Psychiatr Scand* 1993; **87**:48–58.

62. Chin CN, et al. A double blind comparison of zuclopenthixol acetate with haloperidol in the management of acutely disturbed schizophrenics. *Med J Malaysia* 1998; **53**:365–371.

63. Taymeeyapradit U, et al. Comparative study of the effectiveness of zuclopenthixol acetate and haloperidol in acutely disturbed psychotic patients. *J Med Assoc Thai* 2002; **85**:1301–1308.

64. Brook S, et al. A randomized controlled double blind study of zuclopenthixol acetate compared to haloperidol in acute psychosis. *Hum Psychopharmacol* 1998; **13**:17–20.

65. Chouinard G, et al. A double-blind controlled study of intramuscular zuclopenthixol acetate and liquid oral haloperidol in the treatment of schizophrenic patients with acute exacerbation. *J Clin Psychopharmacol* 1994; **14**:377–384.

66. Al-Haddad MK, et al. Zuclopenthixol versus haloperidol in the initial treatment of schizophrenic psychoses, affective psychoses and paranoid states: a controlled clinical trial. *Arab J Psychiatry* 1996; **7**:44–54.

67. Garriga M, et al. Assessment and management of agitation in psychiatry: expert consensus. *World J Biol Psychiatry* 2016; **17**:86–128.

68. Wilson MP, et al. Potential complications of combining intramuscular olanzapine with benzodiazepines in emergency department patients. *J Emerg Med* 2012; **43**:889–896.

69. Villari V, et al. Oral risperidone, olanzapine and quetiapine versus haloperidol in psychotic agitation. *Prog Neuropsychopharmacol Biol Psychiatry* 2008; **32**:405–413.

70. Paton C. Benzodiazepines and disinhibition: a review. *Psychiatr Bull* 2002; **26**:460–462.

71. Chan-Tack KM. Neuroleptic malignant syndrome due to promethazine. *South Med J* 1999; **92**:1017–1018.

72. Appleby L, et al. Sudden unexplained death in psychiatric in-patients. *Br J Psychiatry* 2000; **176**:405–406.

73. Yap YG, et al. Risk of torsades de pointes with non-cardiac drugs. Doctors need to be aware that many drugs can cause QT prolongation. *BMJ* 2000; **320**:1158–1159.

74. Taylor DM. Antipsychotics and QT prolongation. *Acta Psychiatr Scand* 2003; **107**:85–95.

75. Penninga EI, et al. Adverse events associated with flumazenil treatment for the management of suspected benzodiazepine intoxication: a systematic review with meta-analyses of randomised trials. *Basic Clin Pharmacol Toxicol* 2016; **118**:37–44.

Antipsychotic depots/long-acting injections

Long-acting injectable preparations of antipsychotic medication are commonly prescribed in clinical practice, especially in the UK, Australasia and the EU. Real-world, observational studies of patients with schizophrenia have confirmed that continued treatment with such medication is associated with fewer relapses and readmissions to hospital compared with oral antipsychotic treatment,[1–5] although there are confounding factors in such studies, such as indication bias.

A 2020 Cochrane systematic review of RCTs comparing antipsychotic maintenance treatment with placebo for people with schizophrenia found that LAI antipsychotic medications (in particular, LAI haloperidol and LAI fluphenazine) were more effective than oral antipsychotic medications.[6] However, the authors noted that only head-to-head comparisons of LAI and oral antipsychotic medications can determine whether the former are more effective. The findings of such RCTs have generally failed to show the superiority of LAI antipsychotic medications that is apparent in real-world studies,[7–9] and it has been postulated that this is partly related to study design and methodology issues.[2] Specifically, double-blind RCTs are generally relatively short term and the study samples will tend to be biased towards patients with rather less severe illness, fewer comorbid conditions and better adherence to medication.[10,11] Nevertheless, a 2021 systematic review and meta-analysis of RCTs, observational cohort studies and pre–post (mirror-image) studies comparing LAIs with oral antipsychotic medications found that LAIs were associated with a lower risk of hospitalisation or relapse, across all the study designs.[12] There are also hints from meta-analyses of relevant RCTs that some adverse effects are less frequent with LAIs than with their oral counterparts.[8,13]

While it is generally accepted that treatment with LAI antipsychotic medication reduces the risk of relapse, the findings of studies of all designs suggest that treatment with LAIs does not confer complete protection against relapse.[14] In clinical practice, relapse is strongly linked to delayed or missed doses of LAIs. Two UK studies showed that patients receiving 10 doses a year (or fewer) of monthly paliperidone palmitate were at a substantially higher risk of relapse than those receiving 11 or 12 doses.[15,16] Very long-acting injections given consistently on time may offer better protection against relapse.[17–19]

LAI antipsychotic medication is recommended for all patients, but especially where a patient has expressed a preference for such a formulation because of its convenience or where avoidance of covert non-adherence is considered a clinical priority.[10,20,21] While LAI medication does not ensure adherence, it does ensure clinical awareness of adherence, unlike the use of oral medication. Thus, failure to adhere, which may be a sign of relapse or a potential cause, will be signalled by delayed attendance for, or refusal of, an injection, allowing the clinical team to intervene promptly. Another advantage for LAI antipsychotic medication is that its use may help clarify whether an unsatisfactory therapeutic response to antipsychotic medication is because of adherence problems or treatment resistance. Patients with an apparently refractory illness may simply be non-adherent to their oral medication, sometimes completely so.[22] Further, an LAI antipsychotic regimen provides the opportunity for regular scrutiny of a patient's mental state and adverse effects.[23]

The proportion of patients with schizophrenia prescribed LAI antipsychotic medications varies between and across countries, suggesting that the use of such medication is influenced by factors beyond the extent of poor adherence. Greater understanding of these factors might allow for possible barriers to the optimal implementation of this treatment to be identified.[24–26] A study in the USA found that patients with first-episode schizophrenia were largely willing to accept long-acting treatment.[27] This suggests that the relatively low usage of LAIs in the USA might be partly a result of reluctance on the part of clinicians, rather than resistance from patients.[28,29]

Advice on prescribing LAIs

- Test doses
  Because of its long half-life, any adverse effects that result from the administration of LAI antipsychotic medication are likely to be long lived. Therefore, such treatment should be avoided in patients with a history of serious adverse effects that would warrant immediate discontinuation of the medication, such as neuroleptic malignant syndrome (NMS). For LAI FGAs, a test dose, consisting of a small dose of active drug in a small volume of oil, serves a dual purpose: it is a test of the patient's sensitivity to EPS and of any sensitivity to the base oil. For LAI SGAs, test doses may not be required (there is a lower propensity to cause EPS and the aqueous base is not known to be allergenic), although they could be considered appropriate where a patient is suspected of being non-adherent to oral antipsychotic medication and the LAI preparation will be the first exposure to guaranteed antipsychotic medication delivery. For both LAI FGAs and SGAs, prior treatment with the equivalent oral formulation, establishing the optimally effective and tolerated dose, is advised,[30] but may not be necessary from a pharmacokinetic viewpoint. Most LAI SGAs can be used as sole treatment from the outset, although loading doses are usually necessary (e.g. for paliperidone and aripiprazole).

- Begin with the lowest therapeutic dose
  For LAI FGA medications, there is limited evidence for a clear dose–response effect and a near absence of data on optimal dosing. However, low doses (within the licensed range) may be at least as effective as higher ones.[31–34] For the LAI antipsychotic medications that are commonly used, it remains uncertain that the dosages and frequency of injections achieve the optimal benefit–risk balance.[35–37]

- Administer at the longest possible licensed interval
  All LAI antipsychotic medications can be safely administered at their licensed dosing intervals, bearing in mind the maximum recommended single dose. There is no evidence to suggest that shortening the dose interval improves efficacy. Moreover, less frequent administration may be desirable, as the IM injection site can be a cause of discomfort and pain; these reactions may be more common with LAIs that have oil-based formulations.[38,39]

  Although there are reports of illness deterioration in some patients in the days before their next injection is due, plasma drug concentrations may continue to fall for some hours (or even days with some preparations) after each injection. In this context, a patient's apparent recovery soon after the injection makes little sense. More importantly, at steady state, trough plasma levels (immediately before and after the dose) are usually substantially above the threshold concentration required for therapeutic effect.[30,40,41]

■ **Adjust doses only after an adequate period of assessment**

Attainment of peak plasma levels, therapeutic effect and steady-state plasma levels are all delayed with LAI antipsychotic medications, compared with oral antipsychotics. Doses may be *reduced* if adverse effects occur but should only be increased after careful assessment over at least 1 month, and preferably longer. Note that with most LAI antipsychotic preparations, at the start of treatment, plasma drug levels increase over several weeks to months without any increase in the dosage. This is due to accumulation: steady state is only achieved after at least 6–8 weeks. Dose increases during this initial period are therefore illogical and impossible to evaluate properly. With continued LAI antipsychotic treatment, the monitoring and recording of therapeutic efficacy, adverse effects and any impact on physical health are recommended, although in clinical practice there seems to be a relatively low frequency of assessment of adverse effects.[42]

Table 1.8 gives doses and frequencies for LAI antipsychotic medications for adults.

■ **Adding an oral antipsychotic medication risks a high-dose prescription**

The regular prescription of an oral antipsychotic medication in addition to an LAI antipsychotic preparation was once common with LAI FGAs.[22,43] While this may be a possible strategy for the control of breakthrough symptoms and may offer greater flexibility in dosage titration, the safety and tolerability of such a combination are uncertain, particularly over the longer term.[44] The co-prescription of an LAI and oral antipsychotic medication may well result in a possibly inadvertent high-dose prescription, with an increased adverse effect burden and implications for physical health monitoring.[10,23]

Differences between LAIs

A 2021 network meta-analysis of 86 RCTs[45] comparing LAIs with each other, with placebo or with oral antipsychotic medication concluded that the LAI formulations of paliperidone (3-month formulation), aripiprazole, olanzapine and paliperidone (1-month formulation) had the largest effect sizes and greater certainty of evidence for both relapse prevention and acceptability. The LAI SGAs, aripiprazole, paliperidone, risperidone and olanzapine, have generally been reported to have comparable efficacy, although they vary in their liability for particular adverse effects, such as weight gain, metabolic effects, EPS and raised plasma prolactin.[46–49] For example, LAI paliperidone is associated with substantial increases in serum prolactin[48] and LAI olanzapine can cause significant weight gain and is associated with a post-injection delirium/sedation syndrome, assumed to be caused by unintended partial intravascular injection or blood vessel injury.[50,51] Details on dosing of individual SGAs are given elsewhere in this chapter.

Table 1.8 Long-acting injectable antipsychotic medications – doses and frequencies.*

Drug	UK trade name	Licensed injection site	Test dose (mg)	Dose range (mg/day or week or month)	Dosing interval (weeks)	Comments
Aripiprazole	Abilify Maintena	Buttock	Not required**	300–400mg monthly	Monthly	Does not increase prolactin
Aripiprazole	Abilify Asimtufil	Gluteal	Not required**	720–960mg every 2 months	8	Can be started after oral loading or as continuation of monthly injections
Aripiprazole	Aristada Initio	Deltoid or gluteal	Not required**	675mg	Single dose, not for repeat dosing	Given together with 30mg dose of oral aripiprazole. The first Aristata injection can be given on the same day or up to 10 days after Aristada Initio.
Aripiprazole	Aristada	Deltoid[†] or gluteal	Not required**	441mg, 662mg monthly, 882mg every 4–6 weeks and 1062mg every 2 months	4–8	Can be given with 30mg dose of oral aripiprazole and 675mg Aristada Initio *or* continue with oral aripiprazole for 21 consecutive days
Flupentixol decanoate	Depixol	Buttock or thigh	20	50mg every 4 weeks to 400mg a week	2–4	Maximum licensed dose is high relative to other LAIs
Fluphenazine decanoate	Modecate	Gluteal region	12.5	12.5mg every 2 weeks to 100mg every 2 weeks	2–5	High risk of EPS
Haloperidol decanoate	Haldol	Gluteal region	25[††]	50–300mg every 4 weeks	4	High risk of EPS
Olanzapine pamoate	ZypAdhera	Gluteal	Not required**	150mg every 4 weeks to 300mg every 2 weeks	2–4	Risk of post-injection syndrome
Paliperidone palmitate (monthly)	Xeplion	Deltoid or gluteal	Not required**	50–150mg monthly	Monthly	Loading dose required at treatment initiation
Paliperidone palmitate (3-monthly)	Trevicta	Deltoid or gluteal	Not required[‡]	175–525mg every 3 months	3 months	Not suitable for acutely agitated patients
Paliperidone palmitate (6-monthly)	Byannli	Gluteal region	Not required[§]	700–1000mg every 6 months	6 months	Contraindicated in mild renal impairment (creatinine clearance ≥50 to ≤80 mL/minute)

(*Continued*)

Table 1.8 (*Continued*)

Drug	UK trade name	Licensed injection site	Test dose (mg)	Dose range (mg/day or week or month)	Dosing interval (weeks)	Comments
Pipothiazine palmitate	Piportil	Gluteal region	25	50–200mg every 4 weeks	4	Lower incidence of EPS (relative to other FGAs)
Risperidone microspheres	Risperidal Consta	Deltoid or gluteal	Not required**	25–50mg every 2 weeks	2	Drug release delayed for 2–3 weeks – oral therapy required
Risperidone	Perseris	Abdomen	Not required**	90–120mg every month	4	Given subcutaneously in the abdomen
Risperidone	Okedi	Deltoid or gluteal	Not required**	75–100mg every 28 days	4	Loading dose not required at treatment initiation
Zuclopenthixol decanoate	Clopixol	Buttock or thigh	100	200mg every 3 weeks to 600mg/week	2–4	High risk of EPS

* Refer to manufacturer's official documentation for full details.

** Tolerability and response to the oral preparation should be established before administering the LAI. With respect to paliperidone LAI, oral risperidone can be used for this purpose.

† Aripiprazole 441mg dose only.

†† Test dose not stated by manufacturer.

‡ May not be started until the completion of 4 months' treatment with monthly LAI.

§ For patients stabilised on 100mg or 150mg of monthly LAI for at least 4 months or for patients given at least one injection of 350mg or 525mg of 3-monthly LAI.

EPS, extrapyramidal symptoms; FGA, first-generation antipsychotic; LAI, long-acting injection.

Notes:

The doses in this table are for adults. Check formal labelling for appropriate doses in the elderly.

After a test dose, wait 4–10 days then titrate to maintenance dose according to response (see product information for individual drugs).

Avoid using shorter dose intervals than those recommended except in exceptional circumstances (e.g. long interval necessitates high volume [>3–4 mL?] injection). Maximum licensed single dose overrides longer intervals and lower volumes.

For example, zuclopenthixol 500mg every week is licensed whereas 1000mg every 2 weeks is not (more than the licensed maximum of 600mg is administered). Always check official manufacturer's information.

References

1. Tiihonen J, et al. Real-world effectiveness of antipsychotic treatments in a nationwide cohort of 29823 patients with schizophrenia. *JAMA Psychiatry* 2017; **74**:686–693.

2. Kirson NY, et al. Efficacy and effectiveness of depot versus oral antipsychotics in schizophrenia: synthesizing results across different research designs. *J Clin Psychiatry* 2013; **74**:568–575.

3. Marcus SC, et al. Antipsychotic adherence and rehospitalization in schizophrenia patients receiving oral versus long-acting injectable antipsychotics following hospital discharge. *J Manag Care Spec Pharm* 2015; **21**:754–768.

4. Nielsen RE, et al. Second-generation LAI are associated to favorable outcome in a cohort of incident patients diagnosed with schizophrenia. *Schizophr Res* 2018; **202**:234–240.

5. Kishimoto T, et al. Effectiveness of long-acting injectable vs oral antipsychotics in patients with schizophrenia: a meta-analysis of prospective and retrospective cohort studies. *Schizophr Bull* 2018; **44**:603–619.

6. Ceraso A, et al. Maintenance treatment with antipsychotic drugs for schizophrenia. *Cochrane Database Syst Rev* 2020; **8**:CD008016.

7. Ostuzzi G, et al. Oral and long-acting antipsychotics for relapse prevention in schizophrenia-spectrum disorders: a network meta-analysis of 92 randomized trials including 22,645 participants. *World Psychiatry* 2022; **21**:295–307.

8. Wang D, et al. Long-acting injectable second-generation antipsychotics vs placebo and their oral formulations in acute schizophrenia: a systematic review and meta-analysis of randomized-controlled-trials. *Schizophr Bull* 2024; **50**:132–144.

9. Efthimiou O, et al. Efficacy and effectiveness of antipsychotics in schizophrenia: network meta-analyses combining evidence from randomised controlled trials and real-world data. *Lancet Psychiatry* 2024; **11**:102–111.

10. Barnes T, et al. Evidence-based guidelines for the pharmacological treatment of schizophrenia: updated recommendations from the British Association for Psychopharmacology. *J Psychopharm* 2020; **34**:3–78.

11. Kane JM, et al. Optimizing treatment choices to improve adherence and outcomes in schizophrenia. *J Clin Psychiatry* 2019; **80**:IN18031AH18031C.

12. Kishimoto T, et al. Long-acting injectable versus oral antipsychotics for the maintenance treatment of schizophrenia: a systematic review and comparative meta-analysis of randomised, cohort, and pre-post studies. *Lancet Psychiatry* 2021; **8**:387–404.

13. Wang D, et al. Efficacy, acceptability and side-effects of oral versus long-acting - injectables antipsychotics: systematic review and network meta-analysis. *Eur Neuropsychopharmacol* 2024; **83**:11–18.

14. Rubio JM, et al. Psychosis relapse during treatment with long-acting injectable antipsychotics in individuals with schizophrenia-spectrum disorders: an individual participant data meta-analysis. *Lancet Psychiatry* 2020; **7**:749–761.

15. Laing E, et al. Relapse and frequency of injection of monthly paliperidone palmitate—a retrospective case-control study. *Eur Psychiatry* 2021; **64**:e11.

16. Pappa S, et al. Partial compliance with long-acting paliperidone palmitate and impact on hospitalization: a 6-year mirror-image study. *Ther Adv Psychopharmacol* 2020; **10**:2045125320924789.

17. Turkoz I, et al. Comparative effectiveness study of paliperidone palmitate 6-month with a real-world external comparator arm of paliperidone palmitate 1-month or 3-month in patients with schizophrenia. *Ther Adv Psychopharmacol* 2023; **13**:20451253231200258.

18. Clark I, et al. Clinical outcomes with paliperidone palmitate 3-monthly injection as monotherapy: observational 3-year follow-up of patients with schizophrenia. *Eur Psychiatry* 2024; **67**:e15.

19. Clark I, et al. Long term impact of 3-monthly paliperidone palmitate on hospitalisation in patients with schizophrenia: six-year mirror image study. *Acta Psychiatr Scand* 2024; **150**:48–50.

20. National Institute for Health and Care Excellence. Psychosis and schizophrenia in adults: prevention and management. Clinical guideline [CG178] 2014 (last checked February 2024); https://www.nice.org.uk/guidance/cg178.

21. Boyer L, et al. Real-world effectiveness of long-acting injectable antipsychotic treatments in a nationwide cohort of 12,373 patients with schizophrenia-spectrum disorders. *Mol Psychiatry* 2023; **28**:3709–3716.

22. McCutcheon R, et al. Antipsychotic plasma levels in the assessment of poor treatment response in schizophrenia. *Acta Psychiatr Scand* 2018; **137**:39–46.

23. Barnes T, et al. Antipsychotic long acting injections: prescribing practice in the UK. *Br J Psychiatry Suppl* 2009; **52**:S37–S42.

24. Brissos S, et al. The role of long-acting injectable antipsychotics in schizophrenia: a critical appraisal. *Ther Adv Psychopharmacol* 2014; **4**:198–219.

25. Lambert P. Prescribing patterns and determinants of use of antipsychotic long-acting injections: an international perspective. In: *Antipsychotic Long-Acting Injections*, 2nd edn. Oxford: Oxford University Press; 2016:279–310.

26. Patel MX, et al. Attitudes of European physicians towards the use of long-acting injectable antipsychotics. *BMC Psychiatry* 2020; **20**:123.

27. Kane JM, et al. Patients with early-phase schizophrenia will accept treatment with sustained-release medication (long-acting injectable antipsychotics): results from the recruitment phase of the PRELAPSE trial. *J Clin Psychiatry* 2019; **80**:18m12546.

28. Iyer S, et al. A qualitative study of experiences with and perceptions regarding long-acting injectable antipsychotics: part II-physician perspectives. *Can J Psychiatry* 2013; **58**:23s–29s.

29. Kane JM, et al. Treatment journey from diagnosis to the successful implementation of a long-acting injectable antipsychotic agent in young adults with schizophrenia. *J Clin Psychiatry* 2023; **84**:22m14544.

30. Correll CU, et al. Pharmacokinetic characteristics of long-acting injectable antipsychotics for schizophrenia: an overview. *CNS Drugs* 2021; **35**:39–59.

31. Kane JM, et al. A multidose study of haloperidol decanoate in the maintenance treatment of schizophrenia. *Am J Psychiatry* 2002; **159**:554–560.

32. Taylor D. Establishing a dose–response relationship for haloperidol decanoate. *Psychiatr Bull* 2005; **29**:104–107.

33. McEvoy JP, et al. Effectiveness of paliperidone palmitate vs haloperidol decanoate for maintenance treatment of schizophrenia: a randomized clinical trial. *JAMA* 2014; **311**:1978–1987.

34. Bailey L, et al. Estimating the optimal dose of flupentixol decanoate in the maintenance treatment of schizophrenia: a systematic review of the literature. *Psychopharmacology (Berl)* 2019; **236**:3081–3092.

35. Uchida H, et al. Monthly administration of long-acting injectable risperidone and striatal dopamine D2 receptor occupancy for the management of schizophrenia. *J Clin Psychiatry* 2008; **69**:1281–1286.

36. Ikai S, et al. Plasma levels and estimated dopamine D(2) receptor occupancy of long-acting injectable risperidone during maintenance treatment of schizophrenia: a 3-year follow-up study. *Psychopharmacology (Berl)* 2016; **233**:4003–4010.

37. Hill AL, et al. Dose-associated changes in safety and efficacy parameters observed in a 24-week maintenance trial of olanzapine long-acting injection in patients with schizophrenia. *BMC Psychiatry* 2011; **11**:28.

38. Jones JC, et al. Investigation of depot neuroleptic injection site reactions. *Psychiatr Bull* 1998; **22**:605–607.

39. Zolezzi M, et al. Long-acting injectable antipsychotics: a systematic review of their non-systemic adverse effect profile. *Neuropsychiatr Dis Treat* 2021; **17**:1917–1926.

40. Coppola D, et al. A one-year prospective study of the safety, tolerability and pharmacokinetics of the highest available dose of paliperidone palmitate in patients with schizophrenia. *BMC Psychiatry* 2012; **12**:26.

41. Mallikaarjun S, et al. Pharmacokinetics, tolerability and safety of aripiprazole once-monthly in adult schizophrenia: an open-label, parallel-arm, multiple-dose study. *Schizophr Res* 2013; **150**:281–288.

42. Paton C, et al. Side-effect monitoring of continuing LAI antipsychotic medication in UK adult mental health services. *Ther Adv Psychopharmacol* 2021; **11**:2045125321991278.

43. Doshi JA, et al. Concurrent oral antipsychotic drug use among schizophrenia patients initiated on long-acting injectable antipsychotics post-hospital discharge. *J Clin Psychopharmacol* 2015; **35**:442–446.

44. Correll CU, et al. Practical considerations for managing breakthrough psychosis and symptomatic worsening in patients with schizophrenia on long-acting injectable antipsychotics. *CNS Spectr* 2019; **24**:354–370.

45. Ostuzzi G, et al. Maintenance treatment with long-acting injectable antipsychotics for people with nonaffective psychoses: a network meta-analysis. *Am J Psychiatry* 2021; **178**:424–436.

46. Jann MW, et al. Long-acting injectable second-generation antipsychotics: an update and comparison between agents. *CNS Drugs* 2018; **32**:241–257.

47. Correll CU, et al. The use of long-acting injectable antipsychotics in schizophrenia: evaluating the evidence. *J Clin Psychiatry* 2016; **77**:1–24.

48. Nussbaum AM, et al. Paliperidone palmitate for schizophrenia. *Cochrane Database Syst Rev* 2012; (6):CD008296.

49. Sampson S, et al. Risperidone (depot) for schizophrenia. *Cochrane Database Syst Rev* 2016; **4**:CD004161.

50. Citrome L. Olanzapine pamoate: a stick in time? *Int J Clin Pract* 2009; **63**:140–150.

51. Luedecke D, et al. Post-injection delirium/sedation syndrome in patients treated with olanzapine pamoate: mechanism, incidence, and management. *CNS Drugs* 2015; **29**:41–46.

52. Harrison TS, et al. Long-acting risperidone: a review of its use in schizophrenia. *CNS Drugs* 2004; **18**:113–132.

53. Knox ED, et al. Clinical review of a long-acting, injectable formulation of risperidone. *Clin Ther* 2004; **26**:1994–2002.

Depot antipsychotics – summary of pharmacokinetics

Table 1.9 provides a summary of the pharmacokinetics of depot antipsychotic medications.

Table 1.9 Depot antipsychotics – summary of pharmacokinetics.

Drug	UK trade name	Time to peak (days)*	Plasma half-life (days)	Time to steady state (weeks or months)**
Aripiprazole[1–3]	Abilify Maintena	Deltoid: 4 Gluteal: 5–7	27	~20 weeks
Aripiprazole 2-monthly injection[3–6]	Abilify Maintena	28	~29	~6 months
Aripiprazole lauroxil[2]	Aristada in USA	44–50	~54–57	~4 months
Aripiprazole lauroxil nanocrystal[2,7†]	Aristada Initio in USA	4	~15–18	
Flupentixol decanoate[8,9]	Depixol	4–7	8–17	~8–12 weeks
Fluphenazine decanoate[2,10–12]	Modecate	8–12d[††]	7–10	~8 weeks
Haloperidol decanoate[2]	Haldol	3–9	21	~14 weeks
Olanzapine pamoate[2,13]	ZypAdhera	2–6	30	~12 weeks
Paliperidone palmitate[2] (monthly)	Xeplion	13	25–49	~20 weeks
Paliperidone palmitate[14,15] (3-monthly)	Trevicta	25	Deltoid: 84–95 Gluteal: 118–139	~52 weeks
Paliperidone palmitate (6-monthly)[16]	Byannli	700mg: 29 1000mg: 32	700mg: 148 1000mg: 159	Not known
Pipotiazine palmitate[17,18]	Piportil	7–14	15	~9 weeks
RBP-7000[2,19] (risperidone SC monthly)	Perseris in USA	1st peak ~1 2nd peak ~11	~8–9	~8 weeks
Risperidone extended-release injectable suspension[20,21]	Rykindo in USA	25mg: 14 50mg: 17	3–6	~4 weeks
Risperidone in situ microimplants (ISM)[22,23]	Okedi	1st peak: 1–2 2nd peak: 18–25	7–9	~4 weeks
Risperidone microspheres[2]	Risperidal Consta	~28	3–6	~8 weeks
TV-46000[24] (risperidone SC)	Uzedy in USA	8–14	14–22	~2 months
Zuclopenthixol decanoate[2,8,17,25]	Clopixol	4–7	19	~12 weeks

* Time to peak is not the same as time to reach therapeutic plasma concentration but both are dependent on dose. For large (loading) doses, therapeutic activity is often seen before attaining peak levels. For low (test) doses, the initial peak level may be subtherapeutic.

** Attainment of steady state (SS) follows logarithmic, not linear characteristics: nearly 90% of SS levels are achieved in three half-lives. Time to attain steady state is independent of dose and dosing frequency (i.e. you cannot hurry it up by giving more, more often). Loading doses can be used to produce prompt therapeutic plasma levels but time to SS remains the same. SS is not the same as the concentration required for therapeutic effect. For most depots, SS concentrations during the dosing interval are some way above the concentration needed to give a therapeutic response.

† Used to initiate treatment with Aristada, IM injection with one 30mg oral dose of aripiprazole; not designed for repeat dosing.

†† Some estimates suggest peak concentrations after only a few hours.[25,26] It is likely that fluphenazine decanoate produces two peaks – one on the day of injection and a second slightly higher peak a week or so later.

References

1. Mallikaarjun S, et al. Pharmacokinetics, tolerability and safety of aripiprazole once-monthly in adult schizophrenia: an open-label, parallel-arm, multiple-dose study. *SchizophrRes* 2013; **150**:281–288.

2. Correll CU, et al. Pharmacokinetic characteristics of long-acting injectable antipsychotics for schizophrenia: an overview. *CNS Drugs* 2021; **35**:39–59.

3. Wang Y, et al. Population pharmacokinetics and dosing simulations for aripiprazole 2-month ready-to-use long-acting injectable in adult patients with schizophrenia or bipolar I disorder. *Clin Pharmacol Drug Dev* 2024; **13**:631–643.

4. Otsuka Pharmaceutical Co Ltd. Highlights of Prescribing Information. ABILIFY ASIMTUFII® (aripiprazole) extended-release injectable suspension for intramuscular use. 2023 (last accessed November 2024); https://www.accessdata.fda.gov/drugsatfda_docs/label/2023/217006s000lbl.pdf.

5. Harlin M, et al. A randomized, open-label, multiple-dose, parallel-arm, pivotal study to evaluate the safety, tolerability, and pharmacokinetics of aripiprazole 2-month long-acting injectable in adults with schizophrenia or bipolar I disorder. *CNS Drugs* 2023; **37**:337–350.

6. Baune BT. Aripiprazole 2-month ready-to-use 960 mg (Ari 2MRTU): review of its possible role in schizophrenia therapy. *Curr Med Res Opin* 2024; **40**:87–96.

7. Alkermes Inc. ARISTADA INITIO™ (aripiprazole lauroxil) extended-release injectable suspension [product monograph]. 2020 (last accessed February 2025); https://www.aristadacaresupport.com/downloadables/ARISTADA-INITIO-ARISTADA-Payer-Hospital-Monograph.pdf.

8. Jann MW, et al. Clinical pharmacokinetics of the depot antipsychotics. *Clin Pharmacokinet* 1985; **10**:315–333.

9. Bailey L, et al. Estimating the optimal dose of flupentixol decanoate in the maintenance treatment of schizophrenia: a systematic review of the literature. *Psychopharmacology* 2019; **236**:3081–3092.

10. Simpson GM, et al. Single-dose pharmacokinetics of fluphenazine after fluphenazine decanoate administration. *J Clin Psychopharmacol* 1990; **10**:417–421.

11. Balant-Gorgia AE, et al. Antipsychotic drugs: clinical pharmacokinetics of potential candidates for plasma concentration monitoring. *Clin Pharmacokinet* 1987; **13**:65–90.

12. Gitlin MJ, et al. Persistence of fluphenazine in plasma after decanoate withdrawal. *J Clin Psychopharmacol* 1988; **8**:53–56.

13. Heres S, et al. Pharmacokinetics of olanzapine long-acting injection: the clinical perspective. *Int Clin Psychopharmacol* 2014; **29**:299–312.

14. Ravenstijn P, et al. Pharmacokinetics, safety, and tolerability of paliperidone palmitate 3-month formulation in patients with schizophrenia: a phase-1, single-dose, randomized, open-label study. *J Clin Pharmacol* 2016; **56**:330–339.

15. Janssen Pharmaceuticals Inc. Highlights of Prescribing Information. INVEGA TRINZA® (paliperidone palmitate) extended-release injectable suspension for intramuscular use. 2024 (last checked November 2024); https://www.janssenlabels.com/package-insert/product-monograph/prescribing-information/INVEGA+TRINZA-pi.pdf.

16. Janssen Pharmaceuticals Ltd. Highlights of Prescribing Information: INVEGA HAFYERA™ (paliperidone palmitate) extended-release injectable suspension, for gluteal intramuscular use. 2021 (last checked November 2024); https://www.accessdata.fda.gov/drugsatfda_docs/label/2021/207946s010lbl.pdf.

17. Barnes TR, et al. Long-term depot antipsychotics. A risk-benefit assessment. *Drug Saf* 1994; **10**:464–479.

18. Ogden DA, et al. Determination of pipothiazine in human plasma by reversed-phase high-performance liquid chromatography. *J Pharm Biomed Anal* 1989; **7**:1273–1280.

19. US Center for Drug Evaluation and Research. Clinical Pharmacology and Biopharmaceutics Review(s). PERSERIS (Risperidone, RBP-7000, Risperidone ATRIGEL). 2018 (last checked February 2025); https://www.accessdata.fda.gov/drugsatfda_docs/nda/2018/210655Orig1s000ClinPharmR.pdf.

20. Shandong Luye Pharmaceutical Co Ltd. Highlights of Prescribing Information. RYKINDO® (risperidone) for extended-release injectable suspension for intramuscular use. 2023 (last checked November 2024); https://www.accessdata.fda.gov/drugsatfda_docs/label/2023/212849s000lbl.pdf.

21. Walling DP, et al. Pharmacokinetics and safety of a novel extended-release microsphere formulation of risperidone in patients with schizophrenia or schizoaffective disorder. *J Clin Pharmacology* 2024; doi: 10.1002/jcph.6143.

22. Laboratorios Farmacéuticos Rovi S A Madrid Spain. Highlights of Prescribing Information. RISVAN® (risperidone) for extended-release injectable suspension for intramuscular use. 2024 (last checked November 2024); https://www.accessdata.fda.gov/drugsatfda_docs/label/2024/214835s000lbl.pdf.

23. Laveille C, et al. Development of a population pharmacokinetic model for the novel long-acting injectable antipsychotic risperidone ISM®. *Br J Clin Pharmacol* 2024; **90**:2256–2270.

24. Teva Neuroscience Inc. Highlights of Prescribing Information. UZEDY (risperidone) extended-release injectable suspension for subcutaneous use. 2023 (last checked November 2024); https://www.accessdata.fda.gov/drugsatfda_docs/label/2023/213586s000lbl.pdf.

25. Viala A, et al. Comparative study of the pharmacokinetics of zuclopenthixol decanoate and fluphenazine decanoate. *Psychopharmacology (Berl)* 1988; **94**:293–297.

26. Soni SD, et al. Plasma levels of fluphenazine decanoate. Effects of site of injection, massage and muscle activity. *Br J Psychiatry* 1988; **153**:382–384.

Management of patients on long-term treatment with long-acting injectable antipsychotic medication

For people with multi-episode schizophrenia prescribed maintenance LAI antipsychotic treatment, long-term follow-up is essential. Treatment and progress should be reviewed at least once a year (ideally more frequently) by the responsible psychiatrist, including a systematic assessment of the efficacy, tolerability and safety of the medication. The assessment of adverse effects should include cardiovascular and metabolic adverse effects, and EPS (principally parkinsonism, akathisia and TD).[1-3] Whether LAI antipsychotic medications are more or less likely to be associated with TD than oral antipsychotic medications remains uncertain,[4-7] but the risk of TD does not appear to be different when the LAI and oral formulations of the same antipsychotic medication are compared.[8,9]

Any reduction in dosage should be cautious and closely monitored, given the increased risk of relapse and rehospitalisation with lower than standard doses,[2,10,11] particularly in the longer term.[12-15] In a 2022 naturalistic study[16] of the risk of rehospitalisation associated with maintenance treatment with a range of antipsychotic medications, both oral and LAI formulations, in a nationwide cohort ($n = 61,889$), the risk of severe relapse was lowest with continuing standard dose LAI, two exceptions being better outcomes for high-dose olanzapine LAI and relatively low-dose oral perphenazine.

There is no simple formula for deciding when or whether to reduce the dose of continuing LAI antipsychotic treatment, so a risk–benefit analysis must be carried out for every patient. Many patients, it should be noted, prefer LAI antipsychotic preparations to oral medication.[9,17] When considering dose reduction, the patient's individual circumstances should be considered, including the severity of the illness, the risk of relapse and its possible consequences, their response to treatment and their social situation:[1,2]

- Is the patient symptom-free and, if so, for how long?
- How severe, tolerable, distressing and disabling are the current adverse effects?
- What is the previous pattern of illness? Consider the speed of onset, duration and severity of past relapses and any dangers or risks posed to self or others.
- Has dosage reduction been attempted before? If so, what was the outcome?
- What are the patient's current social circumstances? Is it a period of relative stability or should stressful life events be anticipated?
- What is the potential social cost of relapse (e.g. is the patient the sole breadwinner for a family)?
- Is the patient able to monitor their own symptoms? If so, will they seek appropriate help?

If, after consideration of the above, the decision is taken to reduce the medication dose, the patient's family should be involved, and a clear explanation given of what should be done if and when symptoms return or worsen.

If it has not already been done, any co-prescribed oral antipsychotic medication should be discontinued.

- Where the product labelling allows, the interval between injections should be increased to 4 weeks before starting to decrease the dose given each time.
- The dose should be reduced by no more than a third of the previous dose at any one time.
- Decrements should, if possible, be made no more frequently than every 3 months, preferably every 6 months or more.

- Discontinuation of medication should not be seen as the ultimate aim of the above process although it sometimes results.
- Because of their longer half-lives, relapse following discontinuation of LAI antipsychotic formulations may be delayed compared with their oral equivalents and shorter-acting LAIs, probably because of longer exposure and prolonged dopamine receptor blockade following discontinuation.[18]
- While an intermittent, targeted (i.e. symptom-triggered) treatment approach with antipsychotic medication is not as effective as continuous treatment, it may be preferable to no treatment.[2,19,20]
- If a patient becomes symptomatic following antipsychotic dose reduction, this should be seen as information relevant to the determination of the minimum effective dose for that patient.
- Complex hyperbolic tapering regimens have been proposed[21] and these may offer protection against relapse.

For more discussion, see the section on antipsychotic prophylaxis in this chapter.

References

1. Galletly C, et al. Royal Australian and New Zealand College of Psychiatrists clinical practice guidelines for the management of schizophrenia and related disorders. *Aust N Z J Psychiatry* 2016; **50**:410–472.
2. Barnes T, et al. Evidence-based guidelines for the pharmacological treatment of schizophrenia: updated recommendations from the British Association for Psychopharmacology. *J Psychopharm* 2020; **34**:3–78.
3. Arango C, et al. Delphi panel to obtain clinical consensus about using long-acting injectable antipsychotics to treat first-episode and early-phase schizophrenia: treatment goals and approaches to functional recovery. *BMC Psychiatry* 2023; **23**:453.
4. Novick D, et al. Incidence of extrapyramidal symptoms and tardive dyskinesia in schizophrenia: thirty-six-month results from the European schizophrenia outpatient health outcomes study. *J Clin Psychopharmacol* 2010; **30**:531–540.
5. Barnes TR, et al. Long-term depot antipsychotics: a risk-benefit assessment. *Drug Saf* 1994; **10**:464–479.
6. Baldessarini RJ, et al. Incidence of extrapyramidal syndromes and tardive dyskinesia. *J Clin Psychopharmacol* 2011; **31**:382–384; author reply 384–385.
7. Misawa F, et al. Tardive dyskinesia and long-acting injectable antipsychotics: analyses based on a spontaneous reporting system database in Japan. *J Clin Psychiatry* 2022; **83**:21m14304.
8. Gopal S, et al. Incidence of tardive dyskinesia: a comparison of long-acting injectable and oral paliperidone clinical trial databases. *Int J Clin Pract* 2014; **68**:1514–1522.
9. Patel MX, et al. Why aren't depot antipsychotics prescribed more often and what can be done about it? *Adv Psychiatr Treat* 2005; **11**:203–211.
10. Correll CU, et al. What is the risk–benefit ratio of long-term antipsychotic treatment in people with schizophrenia? *World Psychiatry* 2018; **17**:149–160.
11. Rodolico A, et al. Antipsychotic dose reduction compared to dose continuation for people with schizophrenia. *Cochrane Database Syst Rev* 2022; **11**:CD014384.
12. Marder SR, et al. Low- and conventional-dose maintenance therapy with fluphenazine decanoate: two-year outcome. *Arch Gen Psychiatry* 1987; **44**:518–521.
13. Kane JM, et al. Low-dose neuroleptic treatment of outpatient schizophrenics: I. preliminary results for relapse rates. *Arch Gen Psychiatry* 1983; **40**:893–896.
14. Kane JM, et al. A multidose study of haloperidol decanoate in the maintenance treatment of schizophrenia. *Am J Psychiatry* 2002; **159**:554–560.
15. Højlund M, et al. Standard versus reduced dose of antipsychotics for relapse prevention in multi-episode schizophrenia: a systematic review and meta-analysis of randomised controlled trials. *Lancet Psychiatry* 2021; **8**:471–486.
16. Taipale H, et al. Optimal doses of specific antipsychotics for relapse prevention in a nationwide cohort of patients with schizophrenia. *Schizophr Bull* 2022; **48**:774–784.
17. Heres S, et al. The attitude of patients towards antipsychotic depot treatment. *Int Clin Psychopharmacol* 2007; **22**:275–282.
18. Weiden PJ, et al. Does half-life matter after antipsychotic discontinuation? A relapse comparison in schizophrenia with 3 different formulations of paliperidone. *J Clin Psychiatry* 2017; **78**:e813–e820.
19. National Institute for Health and Care Excellence. Psychosis and schizophrenia in adults: prevention and management. Clinical guideline [CG178]. 2014 (last checked February 2024); https://www.nice.org.uk/guidance/cg178.
20. Sampson S, et al. Intermittent drug techniques for schizophrenia. *Cochrane Database Syst Rev* 2013; (7):CD006196.
21. O'Neill JR, et al. Implementing gradual, hyperbolic tapering of long-acting injectable antipsychotics by prolonging the inter-dose interval: an in silico modelling study. *Ther Adv Psychopharmacol* 2023; **13**:20451253231198463.

Aripiprazole long-acting injection

Aripiprazole 1-monthly

Aripiprazole lacks the prolactin-related and metabolic adverse effects of other SGA LAIs and so is a useful alternative to them. Placebo-controlled studies show a good acute and longer-term effect in the treatment of schizophrenia.[1] In the USA, aripiprazole long-acting injection (ALAI) is approved for maintenance monotherapy in bipolar I disorder in adults.[2] In the UK and some other countries, the use of aripiprazole LAI in bipolar is off-label.

Oral aripiprazole 10–20mg/day should be given for 14 days to establish tolerability and response. This oral run-in is also a vital part of the loading process.[3] In patients switching from another oral antipsychotic to ALAI, aripiprazole should have been effective and tolerated in the past. The current antipsychotic should be continued for the first 14 days following the initial ALAI administration.[2]

One of the following two regimens may be followed for administering the starting dose of aripiprazole LAI.[4]

One-injection start

On the day of initiation, administer one injection of 400mg aripiprazole LAI and continue treatment with 10–20mg/day oral aripiprazole for 14 consecutive days (i.e. 28 days in total) to maintain therapeutic aripiprazole concentrations during initiation. In the absence of the 14-day oral overlap, plasma levels may not be sufficient to afford a therapeutic effect.[3]

Two-injection start

On the day of initiation, administer two separate injections of 400mg aripiprazole LAI at separate injection sites in two different muscles (separate gluteal, separate deltoid or gluteal and deltoid injection sites), together with one 20mg dose of oral aripiprazole. Oral therapy should not continue after this point. The necessity for the single oral dose is doubtful, given it represents only 2.5% of the total dose given.

One month after the day of initiation, begin a regimen of 400mg each month (the manufacturer appears to define 'monthly' as every 28 days).[4] A monthly dose of 400mg aripiprazole is equivalent to 15–20mg of daily aripiprazole.[5]

After the one-injection plus oral starting regimen, peak plasma levels are reached 7 days post-injection, with trough levels occurring at 4 weeks.[6] After two-injection start, peak plasma concentration is observed at 5–7 days when administered in the gluteal muscle and at 4 days for the deltoid muscle.[7] Steady-state plasma levels are achieved after the fourth IM injection for both administration sites (see Table 1.10 for missed doses).[7]

A lower dose of 300mg a month can be used in those not tolerating 400mg or for those who are poor metabolisers via CYP2D6. A dose of 200mg/month may only be used for those patients receiving particular enzyme-inhibiting drugs. Most common adverse events are increased weight, akathisia, insomnia and injection site pain.[4,7]

Table 1.10 Delayed doses of aripiprazole long-acting injection.[4]

ALAI dose missed	Regimen
2nd or 3rd ALAI dose is missed and time since last injection is >4 weeks and <5 weeks	Administer as soon as possible
2nd or 3rd ALAI is missed and time since last injection is >5 weeks	Give oral aripiprazole for 14 days and one dose of ALAI *or* Give two ALAI injections at different sites + single dose 20mg aripiprazole
If ≥4th ALAI is missed and time since last injection is >4 weeks and <6 weeks	Administer as soon as possible
If ≥4th ALAI is missed and time since last injection is >6 weeks	Give oral aripiprazole for 14 days and one dose of ALAI *or* Give two ALAI injections at different sites + single dose 20mg aripiprazole

ALAI, aripiprazole long-acting injection.

While there are no official guidelines for switching to aripiprazole, the recommendations in Table 1.11 are based on our interpretation of existing pharmacokinetic data.

Table 1.11 Switching to 1-monthly aripiprazole long-acting injection.

Switching from	Aripiprazole LAI regimen
Oral antipsychotics	Cross-taper antipsychotic with oral aripiprazole* over 2 weeks **One-injection start** Start aripiprazole LAI, continue aripiprazole oral for another 2 weeks then stop **Two-injection start** Start aripiprazole LAI as indicated above after 2 weeks of oral aripiprazole, then stop oral treatment**
Depot antipsychotics (not Risperidone Consta)	Start oral aripiprazole* on day the last depot injection was due **One-injection start** Start aripiprazole LAI after 2 weeks then stop oral aripiprazole 2 weeks later **Two-injection start** Start aripiprazole LAI as indicated above after 2 weeks of oral aripiprazole, then stop oral treatment**
Risperidone Consta	Start oral aripiprazole* 4–5 weeks after the last risperidone injection **One-injection start** Start aripiprazole LAI 2 weeks later; discontinue oral aripiprazole 2 weeks after that **Two-injection start** Start aripiprazole LAI as indicated above after 2 weeks of oral aripiprazole, then stop oral treatment**

* If prior response and tolerability to aripiprazole are known, pre-injection oral aripiprazole may not be strictly required. However, attainment of effective aripiprazole plasma levels is dependent upon 4 weeks of oral supplementation for the one-injection start regimen. Similarly, for the two-injection start regimen, the pharmacokinetic modelling study was based on plasma levels from oral aripiprazole being at (therapeutic) steady state on the day of initiation. It may be sufficient to start aripiprazole LAI in the absence of prior oral aripiprazole where the prior antipsychotic is at a therapeutic level. Continuation for 14 days is presumably also required.
** If oral aripiprazole cannot be given at all (e.g. patient refusal) always use the two-injection starting regimen. This 800mg dose is likely to afford sustained therapeutic plasma concentrations even in the absence of prior oral treatment.
LAI, long-acting injection.

Aripiprazole 2-monthly[8,9]

Two-monthly ALAI (Aripiprazole 2-Month Ready-to-Use 960mg [Ari2MRTU]) is indicated for maintenance treatment of schizophrenia (in the USA it is also licensed for maintenance monotherapy treatment of bipolar-1 disorder[9]). It is available as 720mg and 960mg formulations and should only be administered into the gluteal muscle. The 960mg dose is equivalent to 10–20mg daily of oral aripiprazole. The initiation regimen is shown in Table 1.12.

The maintenance dose of Ari 2MRTU should be administered into the gluteal muscle every 56 days (this seems to be the manufacturer's definition of '2-monthly'). It may be given up to 2 weeks before or 2 weeks after the scheduled injection due date.[8] Table 1.13 gives recommendations in the event of a missed or delayed maintenance dose of Ari 2MRTU.

In the event of an adverse reaction, reduce the maintenance dose to 720mg every 2 months. For patients on concomitant treatment with CYP2D6 or CYP3A4 inhibitors or those who are confirmed CYP2D6 poor metabolisers, the 720mg dose is considered more appropriate.[9] Ari 2MRTU 960 is generally well tolerated, with safety, tolerability, efficacy and pharmacokinetic profiles similar to those of the 1-monthly ALAI (400mg).[10–13]

Table 1.12 Aripiprazole 2-month ready-to-use initiation regimen.[8]

Switching from	Initiation regimen
Oral antipsychotics	Establish tolerability with aripiprazole before initiating ALAI treatment
	One-injection start Administer one 960mg injection + give 10–20mg oral aripiprazole for 14 consecutive days
	Two-injection start Administer one 960mg injection and one 400mg injection at two different injection sites + give one 20mg dose of oral aripiprazole
400mg ALAI	Initiate 960mg no sooner than 26 days after the last 400mg ALAI

Table 1.13 Recommendations for delayed maintenance dose of Ari 2MRTU.

Missed maintenance dose[8]	Recommendations
>8weeks and <14 weeks since last injection	Administer 960mg or 720mg as soon as possible
>14 weeks since last injection	Administer 960mg or 720mg + oral aripiprazole for 14 days
	or
	Maintenance dose 960mg: Administer 960mg + 400mg + one dose of 20mg oral aripiprazole
	Maintenance dose 720mg: Administer 720mg + 300mg + one dose of 20mg oral aripiprazole
	Resume 2-monthly dosing schedule

Other LAI aripiprazole brands

Another two long-acting formulations of aripiprazole lauroxil (Aristada Initio and Aristada) are approved by the US Food and Drug Administration (FDA) for the treatment of schizophrenia.[14] Aristada Initio is given as a single 675mg IM injection to initiate treatment (Table 1.14). Aristada is administered at 1-monthly, 6-weekly or 2-monthly intervals by IM injection into the deltoid or gluteal muscle, depending on the dose (Table 1.15).[15,16] It is available in four strengths (441mg, 662mg, 882mg and 1064mg doses to deliver 300mg, 450mg, 600mg and 724mg of aripiprazole, respectively).[17] The most commonly reported adverse reaction is akathisia.[14]

The 1-day initiation regimen with 1064mg Aristada did not demonstrate any new safety or tolerability concerns and its adverse-effect profile was comparable to that of paliperidone palmitate 1-monthly injection.[13,18] Most adverse reactions occurred within the first 4 weeks of treatment (injection-site pain, akathisia, increased weight).[18]

Aristada 1064mg and Ari 2MRTU both give therapeutic plasma levels over the entire 2-month dosing interval.[19] The key differences between the two formulations lie in their dosing and the licensed indications. Aristada 1064mg corresponds to 15mg daily oral aripiprazole, while Ari 2MRTU is claimed to be suitable for patients taking 10–20mg of oral aripiprazole daily. While both formulations are licensed for the treatment of schizophrenia, Ari 2MRTU is also approved for the maintenance treatment of bipolar I disorder in the USA.

Table 1.14 Starting treatment with Aristada.[17]

1-day initiation regimen	Second option
Establish tolerability with oral aripiprazole before initiating treatment	Establish tolerability with oral aripiprazole before initiating treatment
Give single dose of 675mg IM Aristada Initio* into the gluteal muscle	Give IM Aristada on day one** and continue oral aripiprazole for 21 days
Give single dose of 30mg aripiprazole	
Give IM Aristada on the same day or up to 10 days after initiation**	

* Avoid giving Aristada Initio and Aristada into the same muscle.
** Only the 441mg dose can be given in the deltoid muscle; 662mg, 882mg and 1064mg must be given into the gluteal muscle.

Table 1.15 Equivalent doses and sites of administration for Aristada.[17]

Aripiprazole oral (mg/day)	Aripiprazole lauroxil dose (mg)	Dosing interval	Site of IM administration
10	441	Monthly	Deltoid or gluteal
15	662	Monthly	Gluteal
≥20	882	Monthly	Gluteal
15	882	Every 6 weeks	Gluteal
15	1064	Every 2 months	Gluteal

References

1. Shirley M, et al. Aripiprazole (ABILIFY MAINTENA®): a review of its use as maintenance treatment for adult patients with schizophrenia. *Drugs* 2014; **74**:1097–1110.

2. US Food and Drug Administration. Highlights of Prescribing Information. Abilify Maintena (aripiprazole) for extended-release suspension for intramuscular use. 2020 (last accessed August 2024); https://www.accessdata.fda.gov/drugsatfda_docs/label/2020/202971s013lbl.pdf.

3. Raoufinia A, et al. Initiation of aripiprazole once-monthly in patients with schizophrenia. *Curr Med Res Opin* 2015; **31**:583–592.

4. Otsuka Pharmaceuticals (UK) Ltd. Summary of Product Characteristics. Abilify Maintena 400 mg powder and solvent for prolonged-release suspension for injection. 2024 (last accessed October 2024); https://www.medicines.org.uk/emc/product/7965/smpc.

5. Raoufinia A, et al. Aripiprazole once-monthly 400 mg: comparison of pharmacokinetics, tolerability, and safety of deltoid versus gluteal administration. *Int J Neuropsychopharmacol* 2017; **20**:295–304.

6. Mallikaarjun S, et al. Pharmacokinetics, tolerability and safety of aripiprazole once-monthly in adult schizophrenia: an open-label, parallel-arm, multiple-dose study. *Schizophr Res* 2013; **150**:281–288.

7. Otsuka Pharmaceutical Co Ltd. Highlights of Prescribing Information. ABILIFY MAINTENA® (aripiprazole) for extended-release injectable suspension, for intramuscular use. 2017 (last accessed October 2024); https://www.accessdata.fda.gov/drugsatfda_docs/label/2020/202971s013lbl.pdf.

8. Otsuka Pharmaceuticals (UK) Ltd. Summary of Product Characteristics. Abilify Maintena 960 mg prolonged-release suspension for injection in pre-filled syringe. 2024 (last accessed October 2024); https://www.medicines.org.uk/emc/product/15679/smpc.

9. Otsuka Pharmaceutical Co Ltd. Highlights of Prescribing Information. ABILIFY ASIMTUFII® (aripiprazole) extended-release injectable suspension for intramuscular use. 2023 (last accessed October 2024); https://www.accessdata.fda.gov/drugsatfda_docs/label/2023/217006s000lbl.pdf.

10. Citrome L, et al. Safety and efficacy of aripiprazole 2-month ready-to-use 960 mg: secondary analysis of outcomes in adult patients with schizophrenia in a randomized, open-label, parallel-arm, pivotal study. *J Clin Psychiatry* 2023; **84**:23m14873.

11. Harlin M, et al. A randomized, open-label, multiple-dose, parallel-arm, pivotal study to evaluate the safety, tolerability, and pharmacokinetics of aripiprazole 2-month long-acting injectable in adults with schizophrenia or bipolar I disorder. *CNS Drugs* 2023; **37**:337–350.

12. McIntyre RS, et al. Safety and efficacy of aripiprazole 2-month ready-to-use 960 mg: secondary analysis of outcomes in adult patients with bipolar I disorder in a randomized, open-label, parallel-arm, pivotal study. *Curr Med Res Opin* 2023; **39**:1021–1030.

13. Samalin L, et al. Evaluating the efficacy and safety of the currently available once-every-two months long-acting injectable formulations of aripiprazole for the treatment of schizophrenia or as a maintenance monotherapy for bipolar I disorder in adults. *Expert Rev Neurother* 2024; **24**:291–298.

14. Alkermes Inc. ARISTADA INITIO™ (aripiprazole lauroxil) extended-release injectable suspension [product monograph]. 2020 (last accessed October 2024); https://www.aristadacaresupport.com/downloadables/ARISTADA-INITIO-ARISTADA-Payer-Hospital-Monograph.pdf.

15. Hard ML, et al. Aripiprazole lauroxil: pharmacokinetic profile of this long-acting injectable antipsychotic in persons with schizophrenia. *J Clin Psychopharmacol* 2017; **37**:289–295.

16. Turncliff R, et al. Relative bioavailability and safety of aripiprazole lauroxil, a novel once-monthly, long-acting injectable atypical antipsychotic, following deltoid and gluteal administration in adult subjects with schizophrenia. *Schizophr Res* 2014; **159**:404–410.

17. Alkermes Inc. Highlights of Prescribing Information. ARISTADA® (aripiprazole lauroxil) extended-release injectable suspension for intramuscular use. 2018 (last accessed October 2024); https://www.accessdata.fda.gov/drugsatfda_docs/label/2018/207533s013lbl.pdf.

18. Citrome L, et al. Safety and tolerability of starting aripiprazole lauroxil with aripiprazole lauroxil nanocrystal dispersion in 1 day followed by aripiprazole lauroxil every 2 months using paliperidone palmitate monthly as an active control in patients with schizophrenia: a post hoc analysis of a randomized controlled trial. *J Clin Psychiatry* 2024; **85**:23m15095.

19. Harlin M, et al. Aripiprazole plasma concentrations delivered from two 2-month long-acting injectable formulations: an indirect comparison. *Neuropsychiatr Dis Treat* 2023; **19**:1409–1416.

Olanzapine long-acting injection

Olanzapine pamoate (embonate, in some countries) is a very poorly water-soluble salt ester of olanzapine. An aqueous suspension of olanzapine pamoate, when injected deep in the gluteal muscle, affords both prompt and sustained release of olanzapine. Peak plasma levels are seen within 1 week of injection (in most people within 2–4 days)[1,2] and efficacy can be demonstrated after only 3 days.[3] Only gluteal injection is licensed – deltoid injection is less effective.[2] Olanzapine LAI is effective when given every 4 weeks, with 2-weekly administrations only required when the highest dose is prescribed. Half-life is 30 days.[1,4] Olanzapine has not been compared with other LAIs in RCTs, but naturalistic data suggest similar effectiveness to paliperidone LAI.[5,6] Loading doses are recommended in some dose regimens (Table 1.16). The manufacturer recommends that patients be given oral olanzapine first to assess response and tolerability. Oral supplementation after the first depot injection is not necessary.

Table 1.16 Dosing regimen for olanzapine.

Oral olanzapine (mg/day)	Starting dose	Maintenance dose (given 8 weeks after the first dose)
10	210mg every 2 weeks or 405mg every 4 weeks	300mg/4 weeks (or 150mg every 2 weeks)
15	300mg every 2 weeks	405mg/4 weeks (or 210mg every 2 weeks)
20	300mg every 2 weeks	300mg every 2 weeks

Switching

Direct switching to olanzapine LAI, ideally following an oral trial, is usually possible. When switching from another LAI, olanzapine oral or LAI can be started on the day the last LAI was due. Likewise, for switching from oral treatment, a direct switch is possible, but prior antipsychotics are probably best reduced slowly after starting olanzapine. When switching from risperidone Consta, olanzapine should be started, we suggest, 2 weeks after the last Consta injection was due. That is, 4 weeks after the last Consta injection (peak risperidone plasma levels occur 4–5 weeks after the last injection).

Stopping

Clinicians should consider the gradual release of olanzapine from the pamoate salt when discontinuing treatment. There are various methods of ensuring a linear reduction in drug activity.[7] Olanzapine may remain detectable in the bloodstream for up to 8 months following the last dose.[4]

Post-injection delirium sedation syndrome

Although the precise mechanism of post-injection delirium sedation syndrome (PDSS) remains unclear, it is thought to occur when the pamoate salt of olanzapine is inadvertently exposed to a large volume of blood or plasma, such as through IV injection or a blood vessel injury.[8,9] This exposure can cause the salt to dissolve more rapidly and release a large amount of olanzapine into the circulation.[8] Olanzapine plasma levels may reach over 800mcg/L and confusion, delirium and somnolence result.[10,11] Treatment is supportive and outcomes invariably good.[9] The incidence of PDSS is less than 0.1% of injections and almost all reactions (86%) occur within 1 hour of injection (mean time is 30 minutes)[12] and fully resolve within 72 hours.[8,9,13] One study suggested an incidence of 0.044% of injections (less than 1 in 2,000) with 91% of reactions being apparent within 1 hour.[14] There are very rare reports of events occurring after 3 hours, including one case where the reaction occurred 12 hours after the injection.[15]

In most countries, olanzapine LAI may only be given in healthcare facilities under supervision and patients need to be kept under observation for 3 hours after the injection is given. Given the tiny number of cases appearing only after 2 hours, a good case can be made for shortening the observation period to 2 hours (as in Australia, New Zealand[16,17] and some other countries). Shorter monitoring periods were also employed during the COVID-19 pandemic.[18] However, it is worth emphasising that PDSS may occur at any time and has no clear predictive risk factors,[8] even after several uses in the same patient. That is to say, prior safe use of olanzapine LAI in an individual does not imply low risk of PDSS. The risk may be reduced in patients on 1-monthly injection intervals,[8,19] presumably because they receive relatively fewer injections.

In the EU and UK, the exact wording of the SPC[4] is as follows:

After each injection, patients should be observed in a healthcare facility by appropriately qualified personnel for at least 3 hours for signs and symptoms consistent with olanzapine overdose.

Immediately prior to leaving the healthcare facility, it should be confirmed that the patient is alert, oriented, and absent of any signs and symptoms of overdose. If an overdose is suspected, close medical supervision and monitoring should continue until examination indicates that signs and symptoms have resolved. The 3-hour observation period should be extended as clinically appropriate for patients who exhibit any signs or symptoms consistent with olanzapine overdose.

For the remainder of the day after injection, patients should be advised to be vigilant for signs and symptoms of overdose secondary to post-injection adverse reactions, be able to obtain assistance if needed, and should not drive or operate machinery.

This monitoring requirement has undoubtedly adversely affected the popularity of olanzapine LAI. Interestingly some patients continue treatment even after an episode of post-injection syndrome.[20]

As stated, no patient or medical factor has been identified which definitively predicts PDSS,[10] except perhaps that those experiencing the syndrome are somewhat more likely to have previously had an injection site-related adverse effect.[21] Male gender and higher doses have also been suggested to be risk factors for PDSS.[12,14]

References

1. Heres S, et al. Pharmacokinetics of olanzapine long-acting injection: the clinical perspective. *Int Clin Psychopharmacol* 2014; **29**:299–312.

2. Mitchell M, et al. Single- and multiple-dose pharmacokinetic, safety, and tolerability profiles of olanzapine long-acting injection: an open-label, multicenter, nonrandomized study in patients with schizophrenia. *Clin Ther* 2013; **35**:1890–1908.

3. Lauriello J, et al. An 8-week, double-blind, randomized, placebo-controlled study of olanzapine long-acting injection in acutely ill patients with schizophrenia. *J Clin Psychiatry* 2008; **69**:790–799.

4. Eli Lily and Company Limited. Summary of Product Characteristics. Zypadhera (olanzapine pamoate monohydrate) 210mg powder and solvent for prolonged release suspension for injection. 2023 (last accessed August 2024); https://www.medicines.org.uk/emc/product/6429/smpc.

5. Denee TR, et al. Treatment continuation and treatment characteristics of four long acting antipsychotic medications (paliperidone palmitate, risperidone microspheres, olanzapine pamoate and haloperidol decanoate) in the Netherlands. *Value Health* 2015; **18**:A407.

6. Taipale H, et al. Comparative effectiveness of antipsychotic drugs for rehospitalization in schizophrenia-a nationwide study with 20-year follow-up. *Schizophr Bull* 2017; **44**:1381–1387.

7. O'Neill JR, et al. Implementing gradual, hyperbolic tapering of long-acting injectable antipsychotics by prolonging the inter-dose interval: an in silico modelling study. *Ther Adv Psychopharmacol* 2023; **13**:20451253231198463.

8. Citrome L. Long-acting injectable antipsychotics: what, when, and how. *CNS Spectr* 2021; **26**:118–129.

9. Kochen SA, et al. Olanzapine postinjection delirium/sedation syndrome after long-acting olanzapine depot injection presenting to the emergency department: practical guidelines for diagnosis and management. *Emerg Med J* 2024; **41**:759–763.

10. McDonnell DP, et al. Post-injection delirium/sedation syndrome in patients with schizophrenia treated with olanzapine long-acting injection, II: investigations of mechanism. *BMC Psychiatry* 2010; **10**:45.

11. Podgorná G, et al. Post-injection delirium/sedation syndrome: a case report and 2-year follow-up. *Am J Case Rep* 2022; **23**:e937579.

12. Seebaluck J, et al. Case series profile of olanzapine post-injection delirium/sedation syndrome. *Br J Clin Pharmacol* 2023; **89**:903–907.

13. Bushes CJ, et al. Olanzapine long-acting injection: review of first experiences of post-injection delirium/sedation syndrome in routine clinical practice. *BMC Psychiatry* 2015; **15**:65.

14. Meyers KJ, et al. Postinjection delirium/sedation syndrome in patients with schizophrenia receiving olanzapine long-acting injection: results from a large observational study. *BJPsych Open* 2017; **3**:186–192.

15. Garg S, et al. Delayed onset postinjection delirium/sedation syndrome associated with olanzapine pamoate: a case report. *J Clin Psychopharmacol* 2019; **39**:523–524.

16. Eli Lilly Australia Pty Ltd. Consumer Medicine Information: ZYPREXA RELPREVV® (olanzapine pamoate monohydrate). 2024 (last accessed August 2024); https://www.ebs.tga.gov.au/ebs/picmi/picmirepository.nsf/pdf?OpenAgent&id=CP-2024-CMI-01649-1&d=20240807172310101.

17. Pharmaco (N.Z.) Ltd. Consumer Medicine Information: ZYPREXA RELPREVV® (olanzapine pamoate monohydrate). 2023 (last accessed August 2024); https://www.medsafe.govt.nz/consumers/cmi/z/zyprexarelprevvinj.pdf.

18. Siskind D, et al. Monitoring for post-injection delirium/sedation syndrome with long-acting olanzapine during the COVID-19 pandemic. *Aust N Z J Psychiatry* 2020; **54**:759–761.

19. Venkatesan V, et al. Postinjection delirium/sedation syndrome after 31st long-acting olanzapine depot injection. *Clin Neuropharmacol* 2019; **42**:64–65.

20. Anand E, et al. A 6-year open-label study of the efficacy and safety of olanzapine long-acting injection in patients with schizophrenia: a post hoc analysis based on the European label recommendation. *Neuropsychiatr Dis Treat* 2015; **11**:1349–1357.

21. Atkins S, et al. A pooled analysis of injection site-related adverse events in patients with schizophrenia treated with olanzapine long-acting injection. *BMC Psychiatry* 2014; **14**:7.

Paliperidone palmitate long-acting injection

Paliperidone (9-hydroxyrisperidone) is the major active metabolite of risperidone. Paliperidone palmitate is the ester prodrug of paliperidone. It is available as a monthly, 3-monthly and 6-monthly LAI. The ester is an aqueous nanosuspension, which is hydrolysed to paliperidone after IM administration and slowly absorbed into the circulatory system.[1,2]

Paliperidone long-acting injection 1-monthly

After the recommended initial loading dose of paliperidone LAI 1-monthly (PP1M), active paliperidone plasma levels are seen within a few days, so co-administration of oral paliperidone or risperidone during initiation is not required from a pharmacokinetic viewpoint but some patients may benefit from gradual withdrawal.[3] Dosing consists of two initiation doses (deltoid) followed by monthly maintenance doses (deltoid or gluteal). Administering a single IM dose to the deltoid muscle results in an average 28% higher peak concentration compared with IM injection to the gluteal muscle.[3] Therefore, the two deltoid muscle injections on days 1 and 8 help to attain therapeutic drug concentration quickly. Improvement in psychotic symptoms has been observed as early as day 4.[3] Table 1.17 gives information on dose and administration of PP1M. Table 1.19, later in this section, provides guidance on how to switch to PP1M.[3]

Table 1.17 Paliperidone dose and administration information.[3]

	Dose	Route
Initiation		
Day 1	150mg IM	Deltoid only
Day 8 (±4 days)	100mg IM	Deltoid only
Maintenance		
Every month (±7 days) thereafter	50–150mg IM*	Deltoid or gluteal**

*The maintenance dose is perhaps best judged by consideration of what might be a suitable dose of oral risperidone and then giving paliperidone palmitate in an equivalent dose (Table 1.18). Pre-treatment with oral risperidone is helpful in establishing efficacy and tolerability of a given dose.
**Continuation with deltoid injections for the first 6 months may be considered in some patients who switch from higher doses of oral paliperidone or risperidone.[3]

The second initiation dose may be given 4 days before or after day 8 (after the first initiation dose on day 1).[3] The manufacturer recommends that patients may be given maintenance doses up to 7 days before or after the monthly time point.[3] This flexibility should help to minimise the number of missed doses. See the manufacturer's information for full recommendations regarding missed doses.[3]

Points to note

- No test dose is necessary for paliperidone palmitate. However, patients should ideally be stabilised on or have previously responded to oral paliperidone or risperidone.
- After a single IM injection, paliperidone is continuously released into the systemic circulation from day 1 for at least 4 months.[3]

- The median time to maximum plasma concentration is 13 days,[3] and half-life ranges from 25 to 49 days.
- Patients receiving fewer than 12 injections a year have an increased risk of relapse – correct dosing is critical to the effectiveness of paliperidone monthly.[4,5]

Table 1.18 Approximate dose equivalence for paliperidone and risperidone.[3,6]

Risperidone oral (mg/day) (bioavailability = 70%)[7]	Paliperidone oral (mg/day) (bioavailability = 28%)[8]	Risperidone LAI (Consta) (mg/2 weeks)	Paliperidone palmitate (mg/monthly) (bioavailability = 100%)[3]
2	3	25	50
3	6	37.5	75
4	9	50	100
6	12	–	150

Paliperidone LAI has been compared with haloperidol depot given in a loading dose schedule matching that of paliperidone.[9] The two formulations were equally effective in preventing relapse but paliperidone increased prolactin to a greater extent and caused more weight gain. Haloperidol caused more akathisia and more acute movement disorder, and there was a trend for a higher incidence of tardive dyskinesia. The average dose of haloperidol was around 75mg a month, a dose rarely used in practice.

There are two studies comparing monthly paliperidone LAI with aripiprazole LAI. The first was a 28-week randomised head-to-head trial that found aripiprazole monthly injection superior in the improvement of quality of life and functioning in the short term, although the aripiprazole group included more younger patients.[10] The second study compared the two LAIs in patients with psychosis and comorbid substance use disorder. Improvement in quality of life and reduced substance cravings were seen with both LAIs, although aripiprazole fared better. Overall, there was no clear clinically meaningful superiority for aripiprazole over paliperidone in either of these studies.[11]

Table 1.19 Switching to paliperidone palmitate 1-monthly.[3]

Switching from	Recommended method of switching	Comments
No treatment	Give the two initiation doses: 150mg IM deltoid on day 1 and 100mg IM deltoid on day 8	The manufacturer recommends a dose of 75mg monthly for the general adult population.[12] This is approximately equivalent to 3mg/day oral risperidone (Table 1.18). In practice, the modal dose is 100mg/month.[13]
	Maintenance dose starts 1 month later	Maintenance dose adjustments should be made monthly. However, the full effect of the dose adjustment may not be apparent for several months.[3]
Oral paliperidone/ risperidone	Give the two initiation doses followed by the maintenance dose (see Table 1.18 and prescribe equivalent dose)	Oral paliperidone/risperidone can be discontinued at the time of initiation; some patients may benefit from a gradual withdrawal

(Continued)

Table 1.19 (*Continued*)

Switching from	Recommended method of switching	Comments
Oral antipsychotics	Reduce the dose of the oral antipsychotic over 1–2 weeks following the first injection of paliperidone. Give the two initiation doses followed by the maintenance dose.	
Depot antipsychotic	Start paliperidone (at the maintenance dose) when the next injection is due	Doses of paliperidone palmitate IM are difficult to predict from the dose of FGA depots. The manufacturer recommends a dose of 75mg monthly for the general adult population but in practice 100mg and 150mg are more often prescribed.[13,14] If switching from risperidone LAI see Table 1.18 and prescribe equivalent dose.
	NB No initiation doses are required	Maintenance dose adjustments should be made monthly. However, the full effect of the dose adjustment may not be apparent for several months.[3]
Antipsychotic polypharmacy with depot	Start paliperidone (at the maintenance dose) when the next injection is due NB No initiation doses are required	Aim to treat the patient with paliperidone palmitate IM as the sole antipsychotic
	Reduce the dose of the oral antipsychotic over 1–2 weeks following the first injection of paliperidone	The maintenance dose should be governed as far as possible by the total dose of oral and injectable antipsychotic (see section on dose equivalence in this chapter)

Paliperidone long-acting injection 3-monthly

Paliperidone LAI 3-monthly (PP3M) is indicated for patients who are clinically stable on PP1M and do not require dose adjustment.[15] It is recommended that before switching to PP3M, patients be treated for 4 months or more with PP1M and that the last two doses of PP1M are the same.

PP3M is generally well tolerated, with a tolerability and safety profile similar to the 1-monthly preparation.[16,17] PP3M has a lower risk of hospitalisations and emergency department visits compared with PP1M.[18]

Patient and family perspective of PP3M have been systematically examined.[19] In this study, PP3M was reported to be as effective, or even more effective, than PP1M and had similar or fewer adverse effects. The majority of patients preferred PP3M over PP1M. The advantages for the patients included less frequent and painful injections, less travelling and fewer moments of experiencing shame. The switch did not influence the frequency of their interaction with healthcare professionals.

Practical experience suggests that contacts with healthcare staff are reduced when LAIs are used. Healthcare workers should probably work towards ensuring that contact with patients is not reduced just because there are fewer antipsychotic administrations.

When initiating PP3M, give the first dose in place of the next scheduled dose of PP1M (±7 days). The dose of PP3M should be based on the previous PP1M dose

(Table 1.20). Dose adjustments should not be necessary but may be made at 3-monthly intervals thereafter; however, the full response to the new dose may not be apparent for several months.[15]

The administration process is important for avoiding incomplete administration of the suspension. This requires shaking vigorously the prefilled syringe with the cap and a loose wrist, in a vertical motion for at least 15 seconds to ensure an evenly distributed suspension.[15]

Table 1.20 Dosing of paliperidone long-acting injection 3-monthly.[15]

Dose of PP1M	Dose of PP3M
50mg	175mg
75mg	263mg
100mg	350mg
150mg	525mg

Points to note

- Patients should be on a stable and effective therapeutic dose of PP1M before changing to PP3M to ensure optimal dosing and avoid relapse and hospital admissions.[14,20–22]
- PP3M should be given in place of the next PP1M injection at an equivalent dose.
- The median time to maximum plasma concentration is 30–33 days.[15]
- The median half-life for deltoid injection is 84–95 days and for gluteal injection is 118–139 days.
- After IM injection of PP3M into the deltoid muscle, there was an average increase of 11–12% maximum concentration in plasma compared with gluteal injection.

Paliperidone LAI 6-monthly (PP6M)

PP6M is indicated for patients on maintenance treatment with 100mg or 150mg of PP1M (ideally for 4 months or more, same dose for the last two injections) or patients who have had at least one injection of 350mg or 525mg of PP3M and do not require any dose changes. It is designed to be given once every 6 months into the gluteal muscle. It should not be administered via any other route. There are no corresponding PP6M doses for 25mg, 50mg, 75mg of PP1M or for 263mg and 350mg of PP3M.[23] Table 1.21 gives equivalent doses for paliperidone LAI.

Table 1.21 Paliperidone long-acting injection – equivalent doses.

Dose of PP1M (mg)	Dose of PP3M (mg)	Dose of PP6M (mg)
100	350	700
150	525	1000

CHAPTER 1

PP6M is generally well tolerated and has a tolerability profile similar to PP3M and PP1M.[24] The most common adverse effect in one phase 3 trial was the injection site pain (which can be attributed to the large injection volume: 3.5mL or 5mL), followed by weight gain.[24] Patients and clinicians seem to prefer PP6M over PP3M.[25] Table 1.22 gives the regimen for switching to PP6M.

Table 1.22 Switching to paliperidone 6-monthly.[23]

Switching from	Recommended method of switching	Comments
100mg PP1M	Give 700mg of PP6M in place of the next scheduled dose of 100mg PP1M	PP6M can be initiated ±7 days of the PP1M due date
150mg PP1M	Give 1000mg of PP6M in place of the next scheduled dose of 150mg PP1M	
350mg PP3M	Give 700mg of PP6M in place of the next scheduled dose of 350mg PP3M	PP6M can be initiated ±14 days of the PP3M due date
525mg PP3M	Give 1000mg of PP6M in place of the next scheduled dose of 525mg PP3M	

Dose adjustments should not be needed but can be made every 6 months based on patient response and tolerability. Any dose change may not be apparent in respect to clinical effects for several months owing to the long-acting nature of PP6M and the time needed for a new steady-state level to be reached.[23]

Points to note

- PP6M is suitable for patients who are stable in their mental state and do not require any dose adjustments.
- PP6M should be given only into the upper-outer quadrant of the gluteal muscle.
- Before IM administration, the vial requires extensive and rapid shaking for a minimum of 30 seconds.
- The median half-life is 148–159 days or longer.[23,24]

See the manufacturer's information for full information on missed doses and re-initiation regimens.

References

1. Cleton A, et al. A single-dose, open-label, parallel, randomized, dose-proportionality study of paliperidone after intramuscular injections of paliperidone palmitate in the deltoid or gluteal muscle in patients with schizophrenia. *J Clin Pharmacol* 2014; **54**:1048–1057.
2. Lopez A, et al. Role of paliperidone palmitate 3-monthly in the management of schizophrenia: insights from clinical practice. *Neuropsychiatr Dis Treat* 2019; **15**:449–456.
3. Janssen-Cilag Ltd. Summary of Product Characteristics. Xeplion (paliperidone) 25 mg, 50 mg, 75 mg, 100 mg, and 150 mg prolonged-release suspension for injection. 2023 (last accessed May 2024); https://www.medicines.org.uk/emc/product/7652/smpc.
4. Pappa S, et al. Partial compliance with long-acting paliperidone palmitate and impact on hospitalization: a 6-year mirror-image study. *Ther Adv Psychopharmacol* 2020; **10**:2045125320924789.
5. Laing E, et al. Relapse and frequency of injection of monthly paliperidone palmitate—a retrospective case-control study. *Eur Psychiatry* 2021; **64**:e11.

6. Russu A, et al. Maintenance dose conversion between oral risperidone and paliperidone palmitate 1 month: practical guidance based on pharmacokinetic simulations. *Int J Clin Pract* 2018; **72**:e13089.
7. Dexcel Pharma Ltd. Summary of Product Characteristics. Risperidone 1mg Film-Coated Tablets. 2023 (last checked May 2024); https://www.medicines.org.uk/emc/product/8207/smpc.
8. Janssen-Cilag Limited. Summary of Product Characteristics. Invega (paliperidone) 3 mg prolonged-release tablets. 2021 (last checked May 2024); https://www.medicines.org.uk/emc/product/6816.
9. McEvoy JP, et al. Effectiveness of paliperidone palmitate vs haloperidol decanoate for maintenance treatment of schizophrenia: a randomized clinical trial. *JAMA* 2014; **311**:1978–1987.
10. Naber D, et al. Qualify: a randomized head-to-head study of aripiprazole once-monthly and paliperidone palmitate in the treatment of schizophrenia. *Schizophr Res* 2015; **168**:498–504.
11. Cuomo I, et al. Head-to-head comparison of 1-year aripiprazole long-acting injectable (LAI) versus paliperidone LAI in comorbid psychosis and substance use disorder: impact on clinical status, substance craving, and quality of life. *Neuropsychiatr Dis Treat* 2018; **14**:1645–1656.
12. Janssen Pharmaceuticals Inc. Highlights of Prescribing Information. INVEGA SUSTENNA (paliperidone palmitate) extended-release injectable suspension, for intramuscular use. 2022 (last accessed May 2024); http://www.janssenlabels.com/package-insert/product-monograph/prescribing-information/INVEGA+SUSTENNA-pi.pdf.
13. Taylor DM, et al. Paliperidone palmitate: factors predicting continuation with treatment at 2 years. *Eur Neuropsychopharmacol* 2016; **26**:2011–2017.
14. Clark I, et al. Clinical outcomes with paliperidone palmitate 3-monthly injection as monotherapy: observational 3-year follow-up of patients with schizophrenia. *Eur Psychiatry* 2024; **67**:e15.
15. Janssen-Cilag Limited. Summary of Product Characteristics. TREVICTA (paliperidone) 175mg, 263mg, 350mg, 525mg prolonged release suspension for injection. 2023 (last accessed May 2024); https://www.medicines.org.uk/cmc/medicine/32050.
16. Ravenstijn P, et al. Pharmacokinetics, safety, and tolerability of paliperidone palmitate 3-month formulation in patients with schizophrenia: a phase-1, single-dose, randomized, open-label study. *J Clin Pharmacol* 2016; **56**:330–339.
17. Cicala G, et al. Tolerability profile of paliperidone palmitate formulations: a pharmacovigilance analysis of the EUDRAVigilance database. *Front Psychiatry* 2023; **14**:1130636.
18. Gutiérrez-Rojas L, et al. Impact of 3-monthly long-acting injectable paliperidone palmitate in schizophrenia: a retrospective, real-world analysis of population-based health records in Spain. *CNS Drugs* 2022; **36**:517–527.
19. Spoelstra SK, et al. One-month versus three-month formulation of paliperidone palmitate treatment in psychotic disorders: patients', relatives', and mental health professionals' perspectives. *Patient Prefer Adherence* 2022; **16**:615–624.
20. Clark I, et al. Long term impact of 3-monthly paliperidone palmitate on hospitalisation in patients with schizophrenia: six-year mirror image study. *Acta Psychiatr Scand* 2024; **150**:48–50.
21. Turkoz I, et al. Comparing relapse rates in real-world patients with schizophrenia who were adequately versus not adequately treated with paliperidone palmitate once-monthly injections before transitioning to once-every-3-months injections. *Neuropsychiatr Dis Treat* 2022; **18**:1927–1937.
22. O'Donnell A, et al. Defining 'adequately treated': a post hoc analysis examining characteristics of patients with schizophrenia successfully transitioned from once-monthly paliperidone palmitate to once-every-3-months paliperidone palmitate. *Neuropsychiatr Dis Treat* 2021; **17**:1–9.
23. Janssen-Cilag Ltd. Summary of Product Characteristics. Byannli 700mg prolonged-release suspension for injection in pre-filled syringe (paliperidone). 2023 (last accessed February 2025); https://www.medicines.org.uk/emc/product/13307/smpc.
24. Cirnigliaro G, et al. Evaluating the 6-month formulation of paliperidone palmitate: a twice-yearly injectable treatment for schizophrenia in adults. *Expert Rev Neurother* 2024; **24**:325–332.
25. García-Carmona JA, et al. Preliminary data from a 4-year mirror-image and multicentre study of patients initiating paliperidone palmitate 6-monthly long-acting injectable antipsychotic: the Paliperidone 2 per Year study. *Ther Adv Psychopharmacol* 2023; **13**:20451253231220907.

Risperidone long-acting injection

In this section we give brief details on the range of risperidone LAIs (RLAIs) available around the world in 2024. We have done our best to identify each formulation by some unique property and by a trade name. These trade names do vary somewhat by country. Readers are directed to formal product information for full details of each formulation.

Risperidone intramuscular long-acting injections

Risperdal Consta – risperidone 2-weekly long-acting injection

RLAI is now very rarely initiated in practice and here we give no information on starting doses or its therapeutic uses. It has been superseded by longer-acting risperidone and paliperidone injections with less complex pharmacokinetic profiles. Here we provide information on stopping RLAI and on switching to other formulations. In doing this, we have relied upon the following assumptions:[1]

Timescale of plasma concentrations after last dose of RLAI	
4–5 weeks	Peak plasma concentration from last dose reached
6 weeks	Plasma levels fall below threshold for therapeutic effect
7–8 weeks	Plasma concentrations approach zero

Switching from RLAI is complicated because, in regular dosing, plasma concentrations remain therapeutic for around 6 weeks following the last injection. Two weeks after the last injection (i.e. the time of the first missed injection) plasma levels are yet to peak and will in fact reach a peak on two occasions after this time (Figure 1.1).

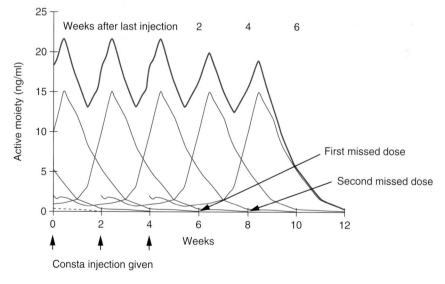

Figure 1.1 Blood levels following discontinuation of treatment with 25mg every 2 weeks: last injection at week 4. Source: reproduced with permission from Wilson (2004).[2]

Table 1.23 provides general recommendations when switching from RLAI. These suggestions are aimed at ensuring that, when switching someone who is responsive to RLAI, a therapeutic plasma concentration of the new antipsychotic is established before risperidone concentrations become subtherapeutic. A further aim is to ensure that therapeutic levels of the new drug will be maintained during the first dosing interval.

Table 1.23 Switching from risperidone long-acting injections.[3,4]

Switching to	Recommended method of switching	Comments
Oral risperidone	Start oral tablets 4–5 weeks after the last RLAI injection	25mg/2 weeks = 2mg/day 37.5mg/2 weeks = 3mg/day 50mg/2 weeks = 4 mg/day[5]
Oral antipsychotic (not risperidone)	Start oral antipsychotic 4–5 weeks after the last RLAI injection	Monitor for adverse effects
Paliperidone LAI[6]	Initiate the equivalent dose of the paliperidone LAI in place of the next scheduled dose of RLAI, then continue monthly administration (a second loading dose is not required and should not be given)	25mg/2 weeks = 50mg/monthly 37.5mg/2 weeks = 75mg/monthly 50mg/2 weeks = 100mg/monthly
Risperidone ISM®* (Okedi, Risvan, and others)[7]	Initiate the equivalent dose of risperidone ISM in place of the next scheduled dose of RLAI and continue risperidone ISM at 28-day intervals	37.5mg/2 weeks = 75mg/28 days 50mg/2 weeks = 100mg/28 days
Aripiprazole LAI	Start oral aripiprazole 4–5 weeks after the last RLAI dose. Initiate ALAI 2 weeks after starting oral aripiprazole.	Note that aripiprazole LAI can be initiated in two ways. For more information refer to the relevant section of this book and manufacturer's advice.
Antipsychotic LAI (not paliperidone or risperidone ISM)	Start the new LAI 4–5 weeks after the last RLAI	For some LAIs, oral trial and/or test dose may be required to establish response and tolerability

* Formal recommendations recommend giving risperidone ISM in place of the next RLAI injection; i.e. 2 weeks after the last injection. A 4-week interval makes more sense because risperidone ISM will then be given shortly before the time of peak plasma levels from the last RLAI injection.

Rykindo®

Rykindo is a 2-weekly injectable suspension of risperidone given in the gluteal muscle to patients who have previously responded and tolerated risperidone.[8] After IM injection risperidone blood concentration peaks at 14 days and reaches steady state after two administrations. Oral supplementation is required for the first 7 days of treatment. The recommended starting dose is 25mg every 2 weeks, with a maximum dose of 50mg every 2 weeks. Dose adjustments can be made every 4 weeks.

Patients on Consta can switch directly to Rykindo without needing oral supplementation. The first IM injection should be given 4–5 weeks after the last Consta administration (refer to Table 1.25 later in this section for equivalent doses). Like Consta, Rykindo must be stored in the refrigerator and allowed to sit at room temperature for at least 30 minutes before reconstitution. The reconstitution process is similar to that for Consta. Please refer to manufacturer's advice for further details.

Risperidone ISM® (Risvan, Okedi)

Risperidone ISM is an injectable suspension of risperidone suitable for stable patients who have previously responded and tolerated risperidone.[7] Risperidone ISM employs in situ microparticle technology (ISM) to provide effective plasma levels as early as 2 hours following IM administration without requiring a loading dose or oral supplementation. An initial peak in plasma concentration is seen within 24–48 hours of administration with a second peak appearing between days 18 and 25. The delayed appearance of the second peak should be noted when assessing clinical efficacy, tolerability and when making changes to dose.[7] The dosing interval for the injection is every 28 days (Table 1.24).

Table 1.24 Initiation of risperidone ISM.

	Dose	Route
Initiation		
Day 1*	75mg or 100mg IM	Deltoid or gluteal
Maintenance		
Every 28 days (±3 days) thereafter	75mg IM or 100mg** IM	Deltoid or gluteal

* No loading dose is required but response and tolerability to oral risperidone must be assured by prior oral supplementation for at least 14 days.
** 75mg risperidone ISM is recommended as maintenance treatment by the manufacturer. It seems likely that 100mg will be required by most people (equivalent to 4mg/day oral risperidone).

Risperidone ISM is effective both as an acute[9] and maintenance[10] treatment and is generally well tolerated, although increased prolactin is common, as with all risperidone formulations.[9] An indirect comparison with other SGA LAIs suggested somewhat better tolerability for risperidone ISM, but this study was authored by researchers linked to risperidone ISM's manufacturers.[11] Its main advantages are the absence of a loading dose requirement and the 28-day administration interval. The main disadvantages of risperidone ISM are that it is not suitable for patients requiring 2mg or 6mg/day of oral risperidone and that it may not be given to patients with a creatinine clearance of less than 60mL/minute.

Risperidone subcutaneous long-acting injections

Perseris®

RBP-7000 (Perseris) is SC risperidone LAI that is available in 90mg and 120mg dosage forms. It is given every 28 days. The lower dose is equivalent to 3mg/day oral risperidone and the higher dose 4mg/day.[12] There are no specific formulations corresponding to 2mg or 6mg/day of oral risperidone. However, two SC injections of 90mg RBP-7000 can be given to afford a similar plasma concentration to 6mg oral risperidone.[13]

RBP-7000 is suitable for SC administration in the abdominal region or back of the upper arm.[14] It has a biphasic release pattern, with the first peak occurring 4–6 hours after administration and the second at 10–14 days post-dose.[15] The active metabolite, paliperidone, has its first peak at 4–48 hours post-injection and the second at 7–11 days. Steady state is achieved after the second SC injection.[16]

The injection is acutely effective at both licensed doses (although 120mg may be better than 90mg), without the need for oral pre-treatment or oral supplementation, although tolerability with oral risperidone should be established before commencing treatment.[17,18] In the longer term, monthly doses of 120mg are effective in maintaining response.[19,20]

RBP-7000 is rapidly active, achieving therapeutic plasma concentration on the first day.[21] Disadvantages include the need for refrigerated storage and a complex multi-step injection procedure. The complexity of preparation and subcutaneous administration are new to psychiatry and failure to follow the instructions might result in dosage errors.[14,21,22] RBP-7000 appears to be well tolerated and has a safety profile similar to that of oral risperidone. In clinical trials, the most commonly reported adverse effects were injection site pain and weight gain.[16,19] See manufacturer's advice on how to initiate RBP-7000.[21]

Uzedy® (TV-46000)

Uzedy is a risperidone extended-release injectable suspension licensed for SC administration in the abdominal region or upper arm. It is available as a 1- or 2-monthly injection (see Table 1.25 for equivalent doses).[23] Uzedy does not require oral supplementation or loading doses but response and tolerability to oral risperidone should be established before initiating treatment. The pre-filled syringe must be stored in the fridge and allowed to sit at room temperature for at least 30 minutes before administration. The syringe content is solid at refrigerated temperatures and converts to liquid at 20–25°C.

Steady-state plasma level of Uzedy is reached after two SC injections. Therapeutic concentrations are seen on day one. Like other risperidone injections, Uzedy has a biphasic release pattern with two peak levels.

In clinical trials,[24–26] Uzedy was effective both acutely and as relapse prevention. One-monthly administration afforded numerically better protection against relapse than two-monthly injections.[27] The most commonly reported adverse effects were injection site pain, injection site nodules, weight gain and EPSEs. Most participants had an F20 diagnosis for 20 years and were stabilised on oral risperidone for at least 12 weeks before trial entry.

Table 1.25 Equivalent doses – risperidone-based long-acting injections. [6,7,28-33]

Risperidone oral (mg/day) (bioavailability = 70%)	Paliperidone oral (mg/day) (bioavailability = 28%)	Risperidone LAI						Paliperidone palmitate** (mg/monthly)	Paliperidone palmitate** (mg/3-monthly)
		(Consta)* (mg/2weeks)	Rykindo* (mg/2 weeks)	Risperidone ISM† (mg/28 days)	RBP-7000* (mg/28 days)	Uzedy* (mg/ monthly)	Uzedy* (mg/2 monthly)		
1	–	–	12.5***	–	–	–	–	–	–
2	3	25	25	–	–	50	100	50	175
3	6	37.5	37.5	75	90	75	150	75	263
4	9	50	50	100	120	100	200	100	350
6	12	–	–	–	–††	125	250	150	525

* Bioavailability assumed to be 100%.

** Bioavailability has been confirmed to be 100%.

*Initiate risperidone ISM 24 hours after the last oral dose of risperidone.

† Recommended starting dose for patients with renal or hepatic impairment[8] or poor antipsychotic tolerability, not studied in clinical trials.[34]

†† 180mg (two SC injections of 90mg) of RBP-7000 is equivalent to 6mg daily risperidone dose.

References

1. Knox ED, et al. Clinical review of a long-acting, injectable formulation of risperidone. *Clin Ther* 2004; **26**:1994–2002.

2. Wilson WH. A visual guide to expected blood levels of long-acting injectable risperidone in clinical practice. *J Psychiatr Pract* 2004; **10**:393–401.

3. Royal Pharmaceutical Society. *Psychotropic Drug Directory*. Pharmaceutical Press; 2024 (last accessed May 2024); https://www.pharmaceuticalpress.com/products/psychotropic-drug-directory.

4. Datapharm. *Electronic Medicines Compendium*. 2024 (last accessed February 2025); https://www.medicines.org.uk/emc.

5. Nesvag R, et al. Serum concentrations of risperidone and 9-OH risperidone following intramuscular injection of long-acting risperidone compared with oral risperidone medication. *Acta Psychiatr Scand* 2006; **114**:21–26.

6. Janssen-Cilag Ltd. Summary of Product Characteristics. Xeplion (paliperidone) 25 mg, 50 mg, 75 mg, 100 mg, and 150 mg prolonged-release suspension for injection. 2023 (last accessed May 2024); https://www.medicines.org.uk/emc/product/7652/smpc.

7. ROVI Biotech Limited. Summary of Product Characteristics. Okedi (risperidone) 100mg powder and solvent for prolonged-release suspension for injection pre-filled syringes. 2023 (last accessed August 2024); https://www.medicines.org.uk/emc/product/13778/smpc.

8. Shandong Luye Pharmaceutical Co Ltd. Highlights of Prescribing Information. RYKINDO® (risperidone) for extended-release injectable suspension for intramuscular use. 2023 (last checked June 2024); https://www.accessdata.fda.gov/drugsatfda_docs/label/2023/212849s000lbl.pdf.

9. Correll CU, et al. Efficacy and safety of once-monthly Risperidone ISM(®) in schizophrenic patients with an acute exacerbation. *NPJ Schizophr* 2020; **6**:37.

10. Álamo C. Risperidone ISM as a new option in the clinical management of schizophrenia: a narrative review. *Adv Ther* 2022; **39**:4875–4891.

11. Sánchez P, et al. Extrapyramidal adverse events and anticholinergics use after the long-term treatment of patients with schizophrenia with the new long-acting antipsychotic Risperidone ISM(®): results from matching-adjusted indirect comparisons versus once-monthly formulations of paliperidone palmitate and aripiprazole monohydrate in 52-week studies. *Ann Gen Psychiatry* 2023; **22**:33.

12. US Food and Drug Administration. Cross-Discipline Team Leader Review. RBP-7000 (risperidone-ATRIGEL). 2018 (last accessed February 2025); https://www.accessdata.fda.gov/drugsatfda_docs/nda/2018/210655Orig1s000SumR.pdf.

13. Walling DP, et al. An open-label study to assess monthly risperidone injections (180 mg) following switch from daily oral risperidone (6 mg) in stable schizophrenic patients. *Clin Drug Investig* 2024; **44**:251–260.

14. Invidior UK Limited. Highlights of Prescribing Information. Perseris (risperidone) for extended-release suspension, for subcutaneous use. 2022 (last checked June 2024); https://www.perserishcp.com/prescribing-information.pdf.

15. Højlund M, et al. Switching to long-acting injectable antipsychotics: pharmacological considerations and practical approaches. *Expert Opin Pharmacother* 2023; **24**:1463–1489.

16. Tchobaniouk LV, et al. Once-monthly subcutaneously administered risperidone in the treatment of schizophrenia: patient considerations. *Patient Prefer Adherence* 2019; **13**:2233–2241.

17. Nasser AF, et al. Efficacy, safety, and tolerability of rbp-7000 once-monthly risperidone for the treatment of acute schizophrenia: an 8-week, randomized, double-blind, placebo-controlled, multicenter phase 3 study. *J Clin Psychopharmacol* 2016; **36**:130–140.

18. Le Moigne A, et al. Reanalysis of a phase 3 trial of a monthly extended-release risperidone injection for the treatment of acute schizophrenia. *J Clin Psychopharmacol* 2021; **41**:76–77.

19. Andorn A, et al. Monthly extended-release risperidone (rbp-7000) in the treatment of schizophrenia: results from the phase 3 program. *J Clin Psychopharmacol* 2019; **39**:428–433.

20. Le Moigne A, et al. PANSS individual item and marder dimension analyses from a pivotal trial of RBP-7000 (monthly extended-release risperidone) in schizophrenia patients. *J Clin Psychiatry* 2021; **82**:21m13906.

21. Indivior UK Limited. Highlights of Prescribing Information: Perseris (risperidone) for extended-release injectable suspension, for subcutaneous use. 2018 (last accessed June 2024); https://www.accessdata.fda.gov/drugsatfda_docs/label/2018/210655s000lbl.pdf.

22. Citrome L. Sustained-release risperidone via subcutaneous injection: a systematic review of RBP-7000 (PERSERIS™) for the treatment of schizophrenia. *Clin Schizophr Relat Psychoses* 2018; **12**:130–141.

23. Teva Neuroscience Inc. Highlights of Prescribing Information. UZEDY (risperidone) extended-release injectable suspension for subcutaneous use. 2024 (last checked June 2024); https://www.uzedy.com/globalassets/uzedy/prescribing-information.pdf.

24. Clinical Trials.gov. Study to Evaluate TV-46000 as Maintenance Treatment in Adult and Adolescent Participants With Schizophrenia (RISE). 2023 (last accessed February 2025); https://clinicaltrials.gov/study/NCT03503318.

25. Clinical Trials.gov. A Study to Test if TV-46000 is Safe for Maintenance Treatment of Schizophrenia (SHINE). 2022 (last accessed February 2025); https://classic.clinicaltrials.gov/ct2/show/NCT03893825.

26. Kane JM, et al. A long-term safety and tolerability study of tv-46000 for subcutaneous use in patients with schizophrenia: a phase 3, randomized, double-blinded clinical trial. *CNS Drugs* 2024; **38**:625–636.

27. Kane JM, et al. Efficacy and safety of TV-46000, a long-acting, subcutaneous, injectable formulation of risperidone, for schizophrenia: a randomised clinical trial in the USA and Bulgaria. *Lancet Psychiatry* 2023; **10**:934–943.

28. Karas A, et al. Perseris(TM): A new and long-acting, atypical antipsychotic drug-delivery system. *P T* 2019; **44**:460–466.

29. Dexcel Pharma Ltd. Summary of Product Characteristics. Risperidone 1mg Film-Coated Tablets. 2023 (last checked May 2024); https://www.medicines.org.uk/emc/product/8207/smpc.

30. Janssen Pharmaceutical Companies. Highlights of Prescribing Information: RISPERDAL® (risperidone) tablets, RISPERDAL® (risperidone) oral solution, RISPERDAL® M-TAB® (risperidone) orally disintegrating tablets. 2019 (last checked May 2024); https://www.accessdata.fda.gov/drugsatfda_docs/label/2019/020272s082,020588s070,021444s056lbl.pdf.

31. Janssen-Cilag Limited. Summary of Product Characteristics. Invega (paliperidone) 3 mg prolonged-release tablets. 2021 (last checked May 2024); https://www.medicines.org.uk/emc/product/6816.

32. Walling DP, et al. The steady-state comparative bioavailability of intramuscular risperidone ISM and oral risperidone: an open-label, one-sequence study. *Drug Des Devel Ther* 2021; **15**:4371–4382.

33. Perlstein I, et al. Population pharmacokinetic modeling and simulation of tv-46000: a long-acting injectable formulation of risperidone. *Clin Pharmacol Drug Dev* 2022; **11**:865–877.

34. Drugs.com. Risperidone Dosage. 2023 (last accessed June 2024); https://www.drugs.com/dosage/risperidone.html.

CHAPTER 1

Penfluridol weekly

Background

Penfluridol is a diphenylbutylpiperidine FGA available in countries such as Brazil, China, India, Israel and the Netherlands and can be imported to other countries.

Penfluridol is unusual in having a very long plasma half-life – at least 60 hours.[1] After oral administration, peak levels are reached within 12 hours and drug can still be detected 168 hours after a single oral dose.[2] Its long duration of action seems to be a result of rapid distribution into fat tissue which acts as a drug reservoir.[3] This property allows penfluridol to be used as a once-weekly oral therapy for supervised ingestion – an alternative to long-acting injectable antipsychotics.

Clinical effectiveness

Several trials have examined the use of once-weekly oral penfluridol, in doses ranging from 5mg to 160mg per week.[4] When given in this manner it is at least as effective as depot FGAs[5,6] and may be better tolerated overall.[4] A Dutch retrospective cohort study ($n = 8,257$) found that discontinuation trends for oral penfluridol and depot formulations were similar.[7] In a small retrospective observational study of 19 patients (most of whom were treatment resistant), Dunnett and colleagues found just over half of the people prescribed penfluridol ($n = 9$) continued taking it during a 1-year follow-up,[8] suggesting some efficacy in these patients.

Although the dose–response relationship remains unclear, a weekly dose of 30mg is thought to be adequately effective,[9] although a dose of 120mg a day (that is, a total of 840mg a week) has been used.[10] Steady-state levels and plasma elimination half-lives of people taking penfluridol can vary significantly, probably because of differences in adiposity.[3] An early study found that a loading dose regimen (first dose 80mg; a total of 200mg over the first week) is effective and well tolerated[11] but this regimen remains unlicensed and untested in larger studies. Penfluridol is probably underused considering the high rates of non-adherence with oral antipsychotics and the reluctance to prescribe depots.[12]

Adverse effects

Adverse effects include acute EPS, increased prolactin and TD, as might be expected.[8] It is usually not sedative. Like pimozide (another diphenylbutylpiperidine), penfluridol appears to prolong the QT interval.[13] Penfluridol is a cytotoxic agent which may have anticancer properties.[14]

Summary

- Penfluridol can be given orally once a week.
- Supervised weekly administration is at least as effective as long-acting injections.
- The usual dose is 20–40mg a week, but much higher doses have been used.
- Adverse effects are those common to FGAs and include QT prolongation.
- Sedation is minimal.

In practice, penfluridol is usually started at a dose of 20mg and increased to a maximum of 40mg after assessment. Steady-state levels are effectively reached after 2–3 weeks. Monitoring includes investigations of renal and hepatic function, changes in cardio-metabolic parameter such as lipids, blood glucose, ECG and general adverse effect screening.

Other antipsychotics which may be suitable for once-weekly oral administration include pimozide, aripiprazole and cariprazine.[12]

References

1. Janssen PA, et al. The pharmacology of penfluridol (R 16341) a new potent and orally long-acting neuroleptic drug. *Eur J Pharmacol* 1970; 11:139–154.
2. Cooper SF, et al. Penfluridol steady-state kinetics in psychiatric patients. *Clin Pharmacol Ther* 1975; 18:325–329.
3. Migdalof BH, et al. Penfluridol: a neuroleptic drug designed for long duration of action. *Drug Metab Rev* 1979; 9:281–299.
4. Soares BG, et al. Penfluridol for schizophrenia. *Cochrane Database Syst Rev* 2006; (2):CD002923.
5. Iqbal MJ, et al. A long term comparative trial of penfluridol and fluphenazine decanoate in schizophrenic outpatients. *J Clin Psychiatry* 1978; 39:375–379.
6. Quitkin F, et al. Long-acting oral vs injectable antipsychotic drugs in schizophrenics: a one-year double-blind comparison in multiple episode schizophrenics. *Arch Gen Psychiatry* 1978; 35:889–892.
7. van der Lee APM, et al. The impact of antipsychotic formulations on time to medication discontinuation in patients with schizophrenia: a Dutch registry-based retrospective cohort study. *CNS Drugs* 2021; 35:451–460.
8. Dunnett D, et al. Evaluation of the effectiveness and acceptability of the long-acting oral antipsychotic penfluridol: illustrative case series. *J Psychopharmacol* 2021; 36:223–231.
9. van Praag HM, et al. Controlled trial of penfluridol in acute psychosis. *Br Med J* 1971; 4:710–713.
10. Shopsin B, et al. Penfluridol: an open phase III study in acute newly admitted hospitalized schizophrenic patients. *Psychopharmacology (Berl)* 1977; 55:157–164.
11. Munitz H, et al. Loading: a beneficial therapeutic effect using an oral long-acting drug, Penfluridol (SEMAP). A pilot study. *Isr J Psychiatry Relat Sci* 1986; 23:215–220.
12. Brissos S, et al. Weekly supervised administration of oral antipsychotics: an alternative to long-acting injections? *CNS Drugs* 2022; 36:315–325.
13. Bhattacharyya R, et al. Resurgence of penfluridol: merits and demerits. *Eastern J Psychiatry* 2015; 18:23–29.
14. Ashraf-Uz-Zaman M, et al. Analogs of penfluridol as chemotherapeutic agents with reduced central nervous system activity. *Bioorg Med Chem Lett* 2018; 28:3652–3657.

CHAPTER 1

Electroconvulsive therapy and psychosis

Evidence from prospective RCTs and retrospective studies suggests that ECT augmentation of antipsychotic medication can have a beneficial effect on persistent positive symptoms in schizophrenia, including medication-resistant schizophrenia.[1-7] However, there is a relative lack of data on long-term effectiveness and efficacy, cognitive deficits and quality of life.

A 2005 Cochrane systematic review[8] assessed RCTs that had compared ECT with placebo, sham ECT, non-pharmacological interventions and antipsychotic medication for patients with schizophrenia, schizoaffective disorder or chronic mental disorder. In studies where ECT was compared with placebo or sham ECT, more participants improved in the real ECT group and there was a suggestion that real ECT resulted in fewer relapses in the short term and a greater likelihood of being discharged from hospital. The review concluded that ECT combined with continuing antipsychotic medication is a valid treatment option for schizophrenia, particularly when rapid global improvement and reduction of symptoms are desired (for example, treating patients with a high risk of aggression or self-harm),[9] and where the illness has shown only a limited response to medication alone.

A naturalistic, mirror-image study compared 2,074 people with schizophrenia on antipsychotic medication who had received ECT with a control group of patients prescribed continuing antipsychotic medication.[10] The rate of psychiatric hospitalisation over a 1-year post-treatment period decreased in those treated with ECT, but not in the control group. The effectiveness of ECT was more pronounced among those treated with clozapine or a medium to high antipsychotic dosage.

Treatment-refractory schizophrenia

The benefits and harms of adding ECT to standard care for people with TRS were examined in a 2019 Cochrane systematic review.[6] The investigators were able to reach the limited conclusion that the moderate-quality RCT evidence available suggested a positive effect for ECT on medium-term clinical response. It was noted that further evidence of better quality was required before a stronger conclusion could be made.

Several studies have focused on ECT augmentation of antipsychotic medication for TRS.[1-3,11,12] For example, in a small sample of patients with TRS characterised by 'dominant negative symptoms', ECT augmentation of a variety of antipsychotic medications produced a significant decrease in symptom severity.[13] A 2016 meta-analysis of RCTs[3] in TRS that examined the efficacy of the combination of ECT and (non-clozapine) antipsychotic medication versus the same antipsychotic medication as monotherapy found that the combination proved to be superior in terms of symptom improvement, study-defined response and remission rate.

ECT augmentation of clozapine may be at least as effective as ECT augmentation of other antipsychotic medications, if not more so.[4,12,14-16] Response is probably unrelated to post-ECT changes in clozapine levels.[17] In a retrospective study[1] assessing the effectiveness and safety of the combination of clozapine and ECT in a sample of patients with TRS, almost two-thirds were responders (defined as a 30% or greater reduction in Positive and Negative Syndrome Scale [PANSS] total score).[18] Follow-up data on a subsample of these patients over a mean of 30 months revealed that the majority had maintained their symptomatic improvement or improved further. Another small retrospective study of ECT augmentation of clozapine reported an acute response (defined as improvement rated on the Clinical Global Impression Improvement scale)[19] in around three-quarters of the patient sample, and three-quarters of the responders remained out of hospital over a 1-year follow-up period.[20] In a randomised, single-blind study,[2] participants with clozapine-refractory schizophrenia either continued solely on their clozapine treatment or had it augmented with a course of bilateral ECT. After 8 weeks, a predefined response criterion (which included a 40% or greater reduction in the psychotic symptom subscale of the Brief Psychiatric Rating Scale)[21] was met by half the participants receiving clozapine plus ECT but none of the group on clozapine alone. When the non-responders from the clozapine-alone group crossed over to an 8-week, open trial of ECT, nearly half met the response criterion.

A 2016 systematic review and meta-analysis[22] looking specifically at ECT augmentation of clozapine treatment found a paucity of controlled studies, although the authors acknowledged the methodological challenges of such investigations. They concluded that ECT may be an effective augmentation strategy for schizophrenia that has failed to respond to clozapine monotherapy, but that further research was required to determine the place of such a strategy in any TRS treatment algorithm. A subsequent meta-analysis of RCTs addressing ECT augmentation for clozapine-resistant schizophrenia noted the lack of studies with sham ECT as a control, but reached the conclusion that such a treatment strategy was effective and relatively safe.[23] In 2021, Chakrabarti[9] reinforced the point that such meta-analyses were based on limited and low-quality evidence and only addressed the short-term efficacy of ECT augmentation. Counter to the relatively encouraging conclusions of these meta-analyses, in a more recent, 10-week RCT[24] involving 40 participants with clozapine-resistant schizophrenia, augmentation with real ECT was not found to be superior to sham treatment in terms of symptom response. The primary outcome was a 50% reduction in PANSS total score, but this was achieved for only one participant (in the real ECT group). There is some provisional evidence that maintenance ECT may be effective when combined with clozapine.[25]

Adverse effects

Although ECT augmentation of continuing antipsychotic medication appears to be generally well tolerated, adverse effects such as transient retrograde and anterograde amnesia, drowsiness, headaches and nausea have been reported for a minority of cases[3,12,13,24,26] and there are reports of an increase in blood pressure after ECT and prolonged seizures.[1] The cognitive adverse effects are generally considered to be mild and transient.[20,23,27]

Summary

While the evidence remains rather inconclusive, it tends to support ECT augmentation of antipsychotic treatment, particularly clozapine, as a potentially efficacious and relatively safe augmentation strategy in TRS.[7,28–30] However, further, well-controlled trials are required to establish the clinical benefit–risk balance of such a treatment strategy in both the short and long term.

References

1. Grover S, et al. Effectiveness of electroconvulsive therapy in patients with treatment resistant schizophrenia: a retrospective study. *Psychiatry Res* 2017; **249**:349–353.

2. Petrides G, et al. Electroconvulsive therapy augmentation in clozapine-resistant schizophrenia: a prospective, randomized study. *Focus* 2019; **17**:76–82.

3. Zheng W, et al. Electroconvulsive therapy added to non-clozapine antipsychotic medication for treatment resistant schizophrenia: meta-analysis of randomized controlled trials. *PLoS One* 2016; **11**:e0156510.

4. Kim HS, et al. Effectiveness of electroconvulsive therapy augmentation on clozapine-resistant schizophrenia. *Psychiatry Investig* 2017; **14**:58–62.

5. Vuksan Ćusa B, et al. The effects of electroconvulsive therapy augmentation of antipsychotic treatment on cognitive functions in patients with treatment-resistant schizophrenia. *J ECT* 2018; **34**:31–34.

6. Sinclair DJM, et al. Electroconvulsive therapy for treatment-resistant schizophrenia. *Schizophr Bull* 2019; **45**:730–732.

7. Grover S, et al. ECT in schizophrenia: a review of the evidence. *Acta Neuropsychiatr* 2019; **31**:115–127.

8. Tharyan P, et al. Electroconvulsive therapy for schizophrenia. *Cochrane Database Syst Rev* 2005; (2):CD000076.

9. Chakrabarti S. Clozapine resistant schizophrenia: newer avenues of management. *World J Psychiatry* 2021; **11**:429–448.

10. Lin HT, et al. Impacts of electroconvulsive therapy on 1-year outcomes in patients with schizophrenia: a controlled, population-based mirror-image study. *Schizophr Bull* 2018; **44**:798–806.

11. Masoudzadeh A, et al. Comparative study of clozapine, electroshock and the combination of ECT with clozapine in treatment-resistant schizophrenic patients. *Pak J Biol Sci* 2007; **10**:4287–4290.

12. Kaster TS, et al. Clinical effectiveness and cognitive impact of electroconvulsive therapy for schizophrenia: a large retrospective study. *J Clin Psychiatry* 2017; **78**:e383–e389.

13. Pawełczyk T, et al. Augmentation of antipsychotics with electroconvulsive therapy in treatment-resistant schizophrenia patients with dominant negative symptoms: a pilot study of effectiveness. *Neuropsychobiology* 2014; **70**:158–164.

14. Ahmed S, et al. Combined use of electroconvulsive therapy and antipsychotics (both clozapine and non-clozapine) in treatment resistant schizophrenia: a comparative meta-analysis. *Heliyon* 2017; **3**:e00429.

15. Grover S, et al. Augmentation strategies for clozapine resistance: a systematic review and meta-analysis. *Acta Neuropsychiatr* 2023; **35**:65–75.

16. Yeh TC, et al. Pharmacological and nonpharmacological augmentation treatments for clozapine-resistant schizophrenia: a systematic review and network meta-analysis with normalized entropy assessment. *Asian J Psychiatr* 2023; **79**:103375.

17. Schoretsanitis G, et al. Lack of ECT effects on clozapine plasma levels in patients with treatment-resistant schizophrenia: pharmacokinetic evidence from a randomized clinical trial. *Schizophr Res* 2020; **218**:309–311.

18. Kay SR, et al. The positive and negative syndrome scale (PANSS) for schizophrenia. *Schizophr Bull* 1987; **13**:261–276.

19. Guy W. *ECDEU Assessment Manual for Psychopharmacology*. Rockville, MD: US Department of Health, Education, and Welfare, Public Health Service, Alcohol, Drug Abuse, and Mental Health Administration, National Institute of Mental Health, Psychopharmacology Research Branch, Division of Extramural Research Programs; 1976.

20. Lally J, et al. Augmentation of clozapine with ECT: a retrospective case analysis. *Acta Neuropsychiatr* 2021; **33**:31–36.

21. Overall JE, et al. The Brief Psychiatric Rating Scale. *Psychol Rep* 1962; **10**:812.

22. Lally J, et al. Augmentation of clozapine with electroconvulsive therapy in treatment resistant schizophrenia: a systematic review and meta-analysis. *Schizophr Res* 2016; **171**:215–224.

23. Wang G, et al. ECT augmentation of clozapine for clozapine-resistant schizophrenia: a meta-analysis of randomized controlled trials. *J Psychiatr Res* 2018; **105**:23–32.

24. Melzer-Ribeiro DL, et al. Randomized, double-blind, sham-controlled trial to evaluate the efficacy and tolerability of electroconvulsive therapy in patients with clozapine-resistant schizophrenia. *Schizophr Res* 2023; **268**:252–260.

25. George R, et al. Examining the clinical effectiveness of continuation and maintenance electroconvulsive therapy in schizophrenia. *Asian J Psychiatr* 2024; **92**:103895.

26. Zheng W, et al. Memory impairment following electroconvulsive therapy in Chinese patients with schizophrenia: meta-analysis of randomized controlled trials. *Perspect Psychiatr Care* 2018; **54**:107–114.

27. Sanghani SN, et al. Electroconvulsive therapy (ECT) in schizophrenia: a review of recent literature. *Curr Opin Psychiatry* 2018; **31**:213–222.

28. Zervas IM, et al. Using ECT in schizophrenia: a review from a clinical perspective. *World J Biol Psychiatry* 2012; **13**:96–105.

29. Wagner E, et al. Clozapine combination and augmentation strategies in patients with schizophrenia-recommendations from an international expert survey among the Treatment Response and Resistance in Psychosis (TRRIP) working group. *Schizophr Bull* 2020; **46**:1459–1470.

30. Arumugham SS, et al. Efficacy and safety of combining clozapine with electrical or magnetic brain stimulation in treatment-refractory schizophrenia. *Expert Rev Clin Pharmacol* 2016; **9**:1245–1252.

Omega-3 fatty acid (fish oils) in schizophrenia

Fish oils contain the omega-3 fatty acids, eicosapentaenoic acid (EPA) and docosahexanoic acid (DHA) – also known as polyunsaturated fatty acids or PUFAs. These compounds are thought to be involved in maintaining neuronal membrane structure, in the modulation of membrane proteins and in the production of prostaglandins and leukotrienes.[1] Imaging studies suggest that the ratio between omega-6 and omega-3 may be relevant in the development of psychotic disorders.[2] One genetic study has suggested that people with schizophrenia may have difficulty converting short-chain fatty acids to long-chain polyunsaturated fatty acids.[3] High dietary intake of PUFAs may protect against psychosis[4] and antipsychotic treatment seems to normalise PUFA deficits.[5] Animal models suggest a protective effect for PUFAs.[6] They have been suggested as treatments for a variety of psychiatric illnesses.[7,8] In schizophrenia, case reports,[9–12] case series[13] and prospective trials originally suggested useful efficacy.[14–18]

Treatment

A 2012 meta-analysis of these RCTs[19] concluded that EPA had 'no beneficial effect in established schizophrenia'. Since then, an RCT comprising 71 patients with first-episode schizophrenia given 2.2g EPA + DHA daily for 6 months showed a reduction in symptom severity for patients in the active arm, finding a number needed to treat (NNT) of 4 to produce a 50% reduction in symptoms measured by PANSS.[20] However, a further RCT of 97 patients in acute psychosis showed no advantage for EPA 2g daily[21] and a relapse prevention study of EPA 2g + DHA 1g/day failed to demonstrate any value for PUFAs over placebo (relapse rate was 90% with PUFAs, 75% with placebo).[22] The limitations affecting the published data in this area (small sample sizes, heterogeneity of diagnosis and stage of illness, differences in intervention combinations and doses) mean that overall findings remain at best inconclusive.[23,24] A 2019 meta-review of published meta-analyses found no evidence for the use of PUFAs in the treatment of schizophrenia.[25]

On balance, evidence now suggests that EPA (2–3g daily) is unlikely to be a worthwhile option in schizophrenia when added to standard treatment. Omega-3 fatty acids are not recommended by the World Federation of Societies of Biological Psychiatry for use in schizophrenia.[26] Set against doubts over efficacy are the facts that fish oils are relatively cheap, well tolerated[27] (mild gastrointestinal [GI] symptoms may occur) and benefit physical health.[1,28–32] A few small RCTs suggest some benefit to neurocognition (social cognition),[33] verbal fluency and working memory[34] in recent-onset psychosis or young people at ultra-high risk of psychosis. Other studies have failed to show any benefit on aggressive behaviour.[35]

Prevention

The Vienna High Risk study (VHR) gave 700mg EPA + 480mg DHA to adolescents and young adults at high risk of psychosis, and showed that such treatment greatly reduced emergence of psychotic symptoms compared with placebo[36] (although a review described this study as 'very low quality evidence').[37] Since publication of this single-site study, the large, multi-site NEURAPRO trial[38] gave adult patients at high risk of psychosis 840mg EPA + 560mg DHA for 6 months and failed to find any evidence of efficacy either for reduction in transition to psychosis or improvement in symptoms. From these RCTs, Cochrane concluded that omega-3 fatty acids 'may' prevent transition to psychosis in the prodromal phase, but that the evidence is of low quality and this conclusion unconfirmed.[39] The non-randomised North American Prodromal Longitudinal Studies (NAPLS)[40] found a positive correlation between functional improvement and frequency of dietary intake of EPA. The Program of Rehabilitation and Therapy (PORT) study[41] found that young people at ultra-high risk of psychosis who then developed the condition had lower dietary intake of omega-3 and higher consumption of omega-6 fatty acids compared with healthy controls. Taken together, these two RCTs (VHR and NEURAPRO) and two non-randomised trials (PORT and NAPLS) indicate a possible positive correlation between dietary omega-3 and functional status, but more studies are required before a clinical benefit can be confirmed.[42] A 2024 network meta-analysis concluded that omega-3 fatty acids are correlated with a lower risk of transition to psychosis compared with placebo, antipsychotics, mood stabilisers or antidepressants.[43] However, this result was derived from only two studies (VHR and NEURAPRO) and just 194 participants.

Overall

PUFAs are no longer recommended for the treatment of residual symptoms of schizophrenia or for the prevention of transition to psychosis in young people at high risk.[25,44–46] If used, careful assessment of response is important and fish oils should be withdrawn if no effect is observed after 3 months' treatment, unless required for their beneficial metabolic effects.

Summary recommendations – fish oils (PUFAs)

- Patients at high risk of first-episode psychosis:
  - Not recommended. If used, suggest **EPA 700mg/day**.
- Residual symptoms of multi-episode schizophrenia (added to antipsychotic):
  - Not recommended. If used, suggest dose of **EPA 2g/day**.

References

1. Fenton WS, et al. Essential fatty acids, lipid membrane abnormalities, and the diagnosis and treatment of schizophrenia. *Biol Psychiatry* 2000; 47:8–21.
2. Mongan D, et al. Plasma polyunsaturated fatty acids and mental disorders in adolescence and early adulthood: cross-sectional and longitudinal associations in a general population cohort. *Transl Psychiatry* 2021; 11:321.
3. Jones HJ, et al. Associations between plasma fatty acid concentrations and schizophrenia: a two-sample Mendelian randomisation study. *Lancet Psychiatry* 2021; 8:1062–1070.
4. Hedelin M, et al. Dietary intake of fish, omega-3, omega-6 polyunsaturated fatty acids and vitamin D and the prevalence of psychotic-like symptoms in a cohort of 33,000 women from the general population. *BMC Psychiatry* 2010; 10:38.
5. Sethom MM, et al. Polyunsaturated fatty acids deficits are associated with psychotic state and negative symptoms in patients with schizophrenia. *Prostaglandins Leukot Essent Fatty Acids* 2010; 83:131–136.
6. Zugno AI, et al. Omega-3 prevents behavior response and brain oxidative damage in the ketamine model of schizophrenia. *Neuroscience* 2014; 259:223–231.
7. Freeman MP. Omega-3 fatty acids in psychiatry: a review. *Ann Clin Psychiatry* 2000; 12:159–165.
8. Ross BM, et al. Omega-3 fatty acids as treatments for mental illness: which disorder and which fatty acid? *Lipids Health Dis* 2007; 6:21.
9. Richardson AJ, et al. Red cell and plasma fatty acid changes accompanying symptom remission in a patient with schizophrenia treated with eicosapentaenoic acid. *Eur Neuropsychopharmacol* 2000; 10:189–193.

10. Puri BK, et al. Eicosapentaenoic acid treatment in schizophrenia associated with symptom remission, normalisation of blood fatty acids, reduced neuronal membrane phospholipid turnover and structural brain changes. *Int J Clin Pract* 2000; **54**:57–63.

11. Su KP, et al. Omega-3 fatty acids as a psychotherapeutic agent for a pregnant schizophrenic patient. *Eur Neuropsychopharmacol* 2001; **11**:295–299.

12. Cuéllar-Barboza AB, et al. Use of omega-3 polyunsaturated fatty acids as augmentation therapy in treatment-resistant schizophrenia. *Prim Care Companion CNS Disord* 2017; **19**:16l02040.

13. Sivrioglu EY, et al. The impact of omega-3 fatty acids, vitamins E and C supplementation on treatment outcome and side effects in schizophrenia patients treated with haloperidol: an open-label pilot study. *Prog Neuropsychopharmacol Biol Psychiatry* 2007; **31**:1493–1499.

14. Mellor JE, et al. Schizophrenic symptoms and dietary intake of n-3 fatty acids. *Schizophr Res* 1995; **18**:85–86.

15. Peet M, et al. Two double-blind placebo-controlled pilot studies of eicosapentaenoic acid in the treatment of schizophrenia. *Schizophr Res* 2001; **49**:243–251.

16. Fenton WS, et al. A placebo-controlled trial of omega-3 fatty acid (ethyl eicosapentaenoic acid) supplementation for residual symptoms and cognitive impairment in schizophrenia. *Am J Psychiatry* 2001; **158**:2071–2074.

17. Emsley R, et al. Randomized, placebo-controlled study of ethyl-eicosapentaenoic acid as supplemental treatment in schizophrenia. *Am J Psychiatry* 2002; **159**:1596–1598.

18. Berger GE, et al. Ethyl-eicosapentaenoic acid in first-episode psychosis: a randomized, placebo-controlled trial. *J Clin Psychiatry* 2007; **68**:1867–1875.

19. Fusar-Poli P, et al. Eicosapentaenoic acid interventions in schizophrenia: meta-analysis of randomized, placebo-controlled studies. *J Clin Psychopharmacol* 2012; **32**:179–185.

20. Pawelczyk T, et al. A randomized controlled study of the efficacy of six-month supplementation with concentrated fish oil rich in omega-3 polyunsaturated fatty acids in first episode schizophrenia. *J Psychiatr Res* 2016; **73**:34–44.

21. Bentsen H, et al. A randomized placebo-controlled trial of an omega-3 fatty acid and vitamins E+C in schizophrenia. *Transl Psychiatry* 2013; **3**:e335.

22. Emsley R, et al. A randomized, controlled trial of omega-3 fatty acids plus an antioxidant for relapse prevention after antipsychotic discontinuation in first-episode schizophrenia. *Schizophr Res* 2014; **158**:230–235.

23. Bozzatello P, et al. Polyunsaturated fatty acids: what is their role in treatment of psychiatric disorders? *Int J Mol Sci* 2019; **20**:5257.

24. Hsu MC, et al. Beneficial effects of omega-3 fatty acid supplementation in schizophrenia: possible mechanisms. *Lipids Health Dis* 2020; **19**:159.

25. Firth J, et al. The efficacy and safety of nutrient supplements in the treatment of mental disorders: a meta-review of meta-analyses of randomized controlled trials. *World Psychiatry* 2019; **18**:308–324.

26. Sarris J, et al. Clinician guidelines for the treatment of psychiatric disorders with nutraceuticals and phytoceuticals: the World Federation of Societies of Biological Psychiatry (WFSBP) and Canadian Network for Mood and Anxiety Treatments (CANMAT) Taskforce. *World J Biol Psychiatry* 2022; **23**:424–455.

27. Schlögelhofer M, et al. Polyunsaturated fatty acids in emerging psychosis: a safer alternative? *Early Interv Psychiatry* 2014; **8**:199–208.

28. Scorza FA, et al. Omega-3 fatty acids and sudden cardiac death in schizophrenia: if not a friend, at least a great colleague. *Schizophr Res* 2007; **94**:375–376.

29. Caniato RN, et al. Effect of omega-3 fatty acids on the lipid profile of patients taking clozapine. *Aust N Z J Psychiatry* 2006; **40**:691–697.

30. Emsley R, et al. Safety of the omega-3 fatty acid, eicosapentaenoic acid (EPA) in psychiatric patients: results from a randomized, placebo-controlled trial. *Psychiatry Res* 2008; **161**:284–291.

31. Das UN. Essential fatty acids and their metabolites could function as endogenous HMG-CoA reductase and ACE enzyme inhibitors, anti-arrhythmic, anti-hypertensive, anti-atherosclerotic, anti-inflammatory, cytoprotective, and cardioprotective molecules. *Lipids Health Dis* 2008; **7**:37.

32. Pawelczyk T, et al. Omega-3 fatty acids reduce cardiometabolic risk in first-episode schizophrenia patients treated with antipsychotics: findings from the OFFER randomized controlled study. *Schizophr Res* 2021; **230**:61–68.

33. Szeszko PR, et al. Longitudinal investigation of the relationship between omega-3 polyunsaturated fatty acids and neuropsychological functioning in recent-onset psychosis: a randomized clinical trial. *Schizophr Res* 2021; **228**:180–187.

34. McLaverty A, et al. Omega-3 fatty acids and neurocognitive ability in young people at ultra-high risk for psychosis. *Early Interv Psychiatry* 2021; **15**:874–881.

35. de Bles NJ, et al. Effects of multivitamin, mineral and n-3 polyunsaturated fatty acid supplementation on aggression among long-stay psychiatric in-patients: randomised clinical trial. *BJPsych Open* 2022; **8**:e42.

36. Amminger GP, et al. Long-chain omega-3 fatty acids for indicated prevention of psychotic disorders: a randomized, placebo-controlled trial. *Arch Gen Psychiatry* 2010; **67**:146–154.

37. Stafford MR, et al. Early interventions to prevent psychosis: systematic review and meta-analysis. *BMJ* 2013; **346**:f185.

38. McGorry PD, et al. Effect of omega-3 polyunsaturated fatty acids in young people at ultrahigh risk for psychotic disorders: the NEURAPRO randomized clinical trial. *JAMA Psychiatry* 2017; **74**:19–27.

39. Bosnjak Kuharic D, et al. Interventions for prodromal stage of psychosis. *Cochrane Database Syst Rev* 2019; (11):CD012236.

40. Cadenhead KS, et al. Metabolic abnormalities and low dietary omega 3 are associated with symptom severity and worse functioning prior to the onset of psychosis: findings from the North American Prodrome Longitudinal Studies Consortium. *Schizophr Res* 2019; **204**:96–103.

41. Kotlicka-Antczak M, et al. PORT (Programme of Recognition and Therapy): the first Polish recognition and treatment programme for patients with an at-risk mental state. *Early Interv Psychiatry* 2015; **9**:339–342.

42. Susai SR, et al. Omega-3 fatty acid in ultra-high-risk psychosis: a systematic review based on functional outcome. *Early Interv Psychiatry* 2022; **16**:3–16.

43. Chen C, et al. Network meta-analysis indicates superior effects of omega-3 polyunsaturated fatty acids in preventing the transition to psychosis in individuals at clinical high-risk. *Int J Neuropsychopharmacol* 2024; **27**:pyae014.

44. Devoe DJ, et al. Attenuated psychotic symptom interventions in youth at risk of psychosis: a systematic review and meta-analysis. *Early Interv Psychiatry* 2019; **13**:3–17.

45. Nasir M, et al. Trim the fat: the role of omega-3 fatty acids in psychopharmacology. *Ther Adv Psychopharmacol* 2019; **9**:2045125319869791.

46. Cho M, et al. Adjunctive use of anti-inflammatory drugs for schizophrenia: a meta-analytic investigation of randomized controlled trials. *Aust N Z J Psychiatry* 2019; **53**:742–759.

Alternative routes of administration

The main routes of administration for antipsychotics are oral or intramuscular. Preparations formulated for these routes of administration are readily available and discussed elsewhere in the *Guidelines*. There may be some rare circumstances where these routes of administration are unsuitable, for example due to medical illness or surgery affecting the GI tract and/or patient preference. Below and in Table 1.26 we list some alternative routes of administration and the drugs available in formulations suitable for these routes.

Table 1.26 Alternative formulations and routes of administration of antipsychotics.

Drug name and route	Dosing information	Manufacturer	Notes
Inhaled			
Loxapine inhaled (Adasuve)	9.1mg (10mg), can be repeated after 2 hours	Angelini Pharma (UK) Teva (USA)	■ Licensed for the rapid control of mild to moderate agitation in patients with schizophrenia or bipolar disorder in the UK and USA ■ Administration requires co-operation of the patient ■ Associated with increased risk of bronchospasms
Intranasal			
Droperidol IV	5–10mg (higher doses have been used)	Off-label, see notes	■ ECG monitoring is recommended
Haloperidol IV	5–10mg (higher doses have been used)	Off-label, see notes	■ Used off-label for acute disturbance, limited evidence ■ ECG monitoring is recommended ■ EPSEs reported in case studies
Olanzapine IV	1.25–30mg	Off-label, see notes	■ Used off-label for acute disturbance, limited evidence ■ Hypoxia, respiratory depression and bradycardia reported
Sublingual			
Asenapine sublingual (Sycrest, Saphris)	5mg twice daily, up to a maximum dose of 10mg twice daily	Organon Pharma (UK)	■ Licensed for moderate to severe manic episodes associated with bipolar disorder in the UK ■ Licensed for schizophrenia and bipolar disorder in the USA ■ Eating and drinking should be avoided for 10 minutes after administration

(Continued)

CHAPTER 1

Table 1.26 *(Continued)*

Drug name and route	Dosing information	Manufacturer	Notes
Transdermal			
Asenapine transdermal patch (Secuado)	Starting dose 3.8mg/24 hr, may increase to 5.7mg/24 hr or 7.6mg/24 hr after 1 week	Noven Pharmaceuticals Inc (USA)	▪ Licensed in the USA ▪ Can be applied to upper arm, upper back, abdomen and hip ▪ Patients may shower with the patch on. Avoid bathing or swimming.
Blonanserin transdermal patch (Lonasen)	Starting dose 40mg/24 hr up to 80mg/24 hr	Sumitomo Pharma	▪ Licensed in China, Japan and South Korea ▪ Can be applied to upper arm, upper back, abdomen and hip ▪ Patients may shower with the patch on. However, avoid bathing or swimming.
Rectal			
Chlorpromazine rectal	100mg every 6–8 hr	Special order	▪ 25mg and 100mg suppositories available. Limited information about this route for the treatment of psychosis.
Olanzapine rectal	2.5–10mg suppositories used	Suppositories have been manufactured by pharmacies	▪ Has been used for delirium, nausea and vomiting in terminally ill patients rather than for psychosis
Prochlorperazine rectal	25mg every 12 hr	Suppositories available in some countries	▪ Case report only

Inhaled

Loxapine is the only antipsychotic licensed as an inhalation powder. It is indicated for adults with mild to moderate agitation associated with schizophrenia and bipolar disorder in the hospital setting. It was licensed in Europe and the USA in 2013 but has since been discontinued in the UK. Inhaled loxapine remains available in the EU and USA but use is restricted. Onset of tranquillising effect is around 10 minutes. Administration requires co-operation with the patient, which may not be possible in medically unwell patients. It is not clear if repeated administration of inhaled loxapine has an antipsychotic effect.

Intranasal

There are no commercially available preparations designed for intranasal and clinical investigations in humans are limited.[1] Nanotechnology delivery systems have been developed for intranasal delivery of various antipsychotics, but this system remains clinically untested.[2–4] One small study compared the pharmacokinetics of intranasal and intramuscular haloperidol in healthy volunteers.[5] Using a compounded nasal spray, intranasal haloperidol had a shorter time to peak levels (15 minutes) and a bioavailability comparable to oral routes of administration. Similar findings have been reported with droperidol.[6]

Intravenous

Intravenous haloperidol is often used off-label to manage acute behavioural disturbance or agitation and psychosis in patients with delirium in a general hospital setting. However, antipsychotics are probably not effective in delirium. A large clinical trial ($n = 566$) showed no evidence that either IV haloperidol or ziprasidone provided benefit over placebo in patients with delirium in intensive care.[7] Other studies have reported similar findings.[8]

In respect to toxicity, a systematic review found that IV haloperidol did not cause greater QT prolongation than placebo, but close ECG monitoring is officially advised for IV haloperidol.[9] Doses between 5 and 10mg are typically recommended but doses in the literature have ranged from 50 to 1500mg (over hours to days).[9] A review of observational studies reported effectiveness of off-label IV olanzapine.[10] Bolus doses from 2.5 to 10mg (maximum dose of 30mg/day) have apparently been safely administered. IV droperidol is used off-label to manage acute behavioural disturbance. Low-dose IV prochlorperazine (a piperazine phenothiazine)[11] has been used in migraine.[12]

Sublingual

Asenapine is the only commercially available antipsychotic designed for sublingual use. When used sublingually, the bioavailability of asenapine is 35%, compared with only 2% when taken orally.[13] Other drugs may be absorbed sublingually but this has not been investigated. Dexmedetomidine is used sublingually in acute agitation.[14,15]

Buccal

Buccally administered drugs are absorbed through the lining of the cheek. Compared with sublingual use, buccal administration results in somewhat slower absorption.[13] There are no commercially available preparations licensed for buccal use and there has been little clinical investigation into this route of administration for antipsychotics. Prochlorperazine is available in the UK as a buccal tablet[16] but it is indicated for the treatment of nausea and vomiting associated with migraines.[17] Prochlorperazine is now rarely used for psychiatric indications and the dose needed for an antipsychotic effect (75–100mg a day) is much greater than that used for nausea.

Transdermal

Asenapine is available in the USA as a daily transdermal patch (Secuado) for treatment of adults with schizophrenia. Blonanserin (Lonasen) is commercially available as a daily transdermal patch in China, Japan and South Korea. Transdermal drug delivery minimises fluctuations in plasma drug concentrations and allows for lower doses (by bypassing first-pass metabolism) and possibly reduced systemic adverse effects. At the time of writing, proof of concept clinical trials of once-weekly aripiprazole transdermal patch had been successfully conducted.[18] Chlorpromazine, haloperidol, olanzapine, prochlorperazine, quetiapine and risperidone have been developed as transdermal delivery systems but are not commercially available.[19,20]

Rectal

Chlorpromazine suppositories are available from specials manufacturers in the UK in 25mg and 100mg strengths.[21] The rectal route is not licensed in adults.[17] 100mg given rectally as a suppository is approximately equivalent to 20–25mg chlorpromazine hydrochloride given by IM injection or 40–50mg of chlorpromazine base or hydrochloride given orally.[17] Prochlorperazine suppositories were used successfully short term for the treatment of psychosis in one case report.[22] Olanzapine suppositories have been manufactured by a hospital pharmacy and administered for the treatment of delirium or nausea and vomiting in terminally ill patients.[23]

References

1. Katare YK, et al. Intranasal delivery of antipsychotic drugs. *Schizophr Res* 2017; **184**:2–13.
2. Majcher MJ, et al. In situ-gelling starch nanoparticle (SNP)/O-carboxymethyl chitosan (CMCh) nanoparticle network hydrogels for the intranasal delivery of an antipsychotic peptide. *J Control Release* 2021; **330**:738–752.
3. Pandey M, et al. Advances and challenges in intranasal delivery of antipsychotic agents targeting the central nervous system. *Front Pharmacol* 2022; **13**:865590.
4. Pires PC, et al. Antipsychotics-loaded nanometric emulsions for brain delivery. *Pharmaceutics* 2022; **14**:2174.
5. Miller JL, et al. Comparison of intranasal administration of haloperidol with intravenous and intramuscular administration: a pilot pharmacokinetic study. *Pharmacotherapy* 2008; **28**:875–882.
6. Cooper I, et al. The pharmacokinetics of intranasal droperidol in volunteers characterised via population modelling. *SAGE Open Med* 2018; **6**:2050312118813283.
7. Bleck TP. Dopamine antagonists in ICU delirium. *N Engl J Med* 2018; **379**:2569–2570.
8. Smit L, et al. Efficacy of haloperidol to decrease the burden of delirium in adult critically ill patients: the EuRIDICE randomized clinical trial. *Crit Care* 2023; **27**:413.
9. Beach SR, et al. Intravenous haloperidol: a systematic review of side effects and recommendations for clinical use. *Gen Hosp Psychiatry* 2020; **67**:42–50.
10. Khorassani F, et al. Intravenous olanzapine for the management of agitation: review of the literature. *Ann Pharmacother* 2019; **53**:853–859.
11. Wilson IC, et al. A double-blind trial to investigate the effects of Thorazine (Largactil, chlorpromazine), Compazine (Stemetil, prochlorperazine) and Stelazine (trifluoperazine) in paranoid schizophrenia. *J Ment Sci* 1961; **107**:90–99.
12. Kostic MA, et al. A prospective, randomized trial of intravenous prochlorperazine versus subcutaneous sumatriptan in acute migraine therapy in the emergency department. *Ann Emerg Med* 2010; **56**:1–6.
13. Kaminsky BM, et al. Alternate routes of administration of antidepressant and antipsychotic medications. *Ann Pharmacother* 2015; **49**:808–817.
14. Karlin DM, et al. Dexmedetomidine sublingual film: a new treatment to reduce agitation in schizophrenia and bipolar disorders. *Ann Pharmacother* 2024; **58**:54–64.
15. Citrome L, et al. Sublingual dexmedetomidine for the treatment of acute agitation in adults with schizophrenia or schizoaffective disorder: a randomized placebo-controlled trial. *J Clin Psychiatry* 2022; **83**:22m14447.
16. Fernando T, et al. Buccally absorbed vs intravenous prochlorperazine for treatment of migraines headaches. *Acta Neurol Scand* 2019; **140**:72–77.
17. National Institute for Health and Care Excellence. *British National Formulary* (BNF). 2024; https://bnf.nice.org.uk.
18. Citrome L, et al. Patches: established and emerging transdermal treatments in psychiatry. *J Clin Psychiatry* 2019; **80**:18nr12554.
19. Abruzzo A, et al. Transdermal delivery of antipsychotics: rationale and current status. *CNS Drugs* 2019; **33**:849–865.
20. El-Tokhy FSe, et al. Transdermal delivery of second-generation antipsychotics for management of schizophrenia; disease overview, conventional and nanobased drug delivery systems. *J Drug Delivery Sci Technol* 2021; **61**:102104.
21. National Health Service UK. dm+d browser. 2024; https://dmd-browser.nhsbsa.nhs.uk.
22. Servis M, et al. Treatment of psychosis with prochlorperazine in the ICU setting. *Psychosomatics* 1997; **38**:589–590.
23. Matsumoto K, et al. Pharmaceutical studies on and clinical application of olanzapine suppositories prepared as a hospital preparation. *J Pharm Health Care Sci* 2016; **2**:20.

Stopping antipsychotics

Antipsychotics are recommended for long-term treatment of schizophrenia because they reduce symptoms and lessen the risk of relapse.[1] However, antipsychotics have many adverse effects, including metabolic complications, TD, emotional blunting and anatomical brain changes.[2] There is some (hotly disputed) evidence that reducing or stopping antipsychotics may improve social functioning (relationships, education or employment, independent living) without worsening the rate of relapse or symptom burden in the medium term,[3] although it might increase risk of relapse in the short term.[4,5] Reducing antipsychotic burden may also improve cognitive functioning.[6]

It is also worth considering that much of the evidence for the relapse prevention properties of antipsychotics relies on discontinuation trials in which antipsychotics are stopped quickly (over a matter of weeks), and that process may have elevated the apparent rate of relapse in the discontinuation group, so exaggerating the relapse prevention properties of antipsychotics.[7] Patients often ask to reduce or stop medication and, in light of the above, this may be a reasonable course of action. Cautious deprescribing should be a component of high-quality prescribing practice, depending on the condition being treated. More than half of antipsychotic prescriptions in the UK are given to patients without a psychotic or manic disorder and instead are prescribed for insomnia, anxiety, personality disorders and symptoms of dementia.[8] In the UK, NICE strongly cautions against medium- or long-term use of antipsychotics in personality disorder,[9] and only limited use in dementia.[10] The principles for deprescribing outlined below also apply to these patients.

Withdrawal effects of antipsychotics

Stopping or reducing the dose of an antipsychotic can cause a variety of withdrawal symptoms reflecting their various actions (blocking dopamine, histamine, acetylcholine, serotonin and noradrenaline receptors).[11,12] Symptoms are listed in Figure 1.2.[11-15]

Importantly, withdrawal/discontinuation symptoms from antipsychotics can include psychotic symptoms.[12,16] This is suggested by a number of case studies in which people without a psychotic disorder treated with dopamine antagonists for reasons such as nausea or lactation difficulties develop psychotic symptoms when these medications are abruptly stopped.[17-19] Non-psychotic withdrawal effects (e.g. insomnia, agitation and anxiety) may also precipitate genuine relapse that would not have occurred in the absence of antipsychotic dose reduction (perhaps clumsily named withdrawal-associated relapse).[20]

In patients with psychotic disorders, relapse often occurs when antipsychotics are withdrawn. This has been widely thought to represent an unmasking of the underlying chronic illness, but the nature of the process of withdrawing antipsychotics may itself be causally related to relapse.[7] This suggestion is supported by the marked preponderance of relapses soon after abrupt antipsychotic cessation in patients with schizophrenia. In one analysis 60% of all relapses over 4 years occurred within 3 months of drug cessation,[21] the time most likely for withdrawal effects to be evident. The idea that speed of stopping is an influence on relapse is also supported by evidence that slower tapering can reduce the rate of relapse.[22,23] Withdrawal effects can be delayed in onset for weeks and sometimes months, for reasons that are poorly understood.[20]

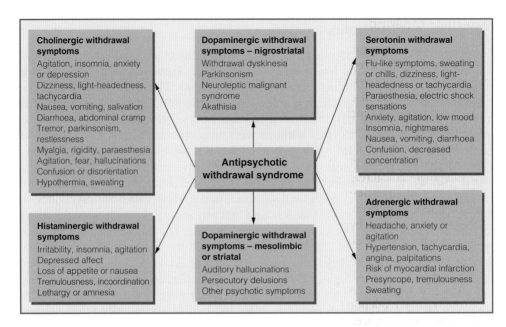

Figure 1.2 Antipsychotic withdrawal symptoms. Source: adapted from Chouinard et al. (2017).[12]

Neurobiology of withdrawal

Withdrawal-associated relapse has been attributed to neural adaptations to long-term antipsychotic treatment (dopaminergic hypersensitivity, among other effects) that persist after antipsychotic cessation.[24] Indeed, molecular imaging studies in schizophrenia have found increased D_2/D_3 receptor availability in those patients who had been exposed to antipsychotic medication but not in antipsychotic-naïve patients.[25] This hypersensitivity to dopamine may render patients more susceptible to psychotic relapse when D_2 blockade is diminished by antipsychotic dose reduction.[11,24]

There are converging lines of evidence that suggest that the neuroadaptive effects of antipsychotics can persist for months or years after stopping. Dopaminergic hypersensitivity in animals persists for the equivalent of a human year after treatment is stopped.[26,27] TD – widely attributed to dopaminergic hypersensitivity – can persist for years after antipsychotic medication has been ceased.[28] There is also evidence that patients who have discontinued antipsychotics have increased rates of relapse for 3 years compared with people maintained on their antipsychotics, after which relapse rates converge,[1] perhaps suggesting that adaptations may have resolved by this point. Persisting dopaminergic hypersensitivity may lower the threshold for precipitating relapse from other triggers for as long as they persist (which may be months or years).[20]

It follows that the risk of relapse on cessation of antipsychotics might be minimised by more gradual dose tapering because these neuroadaptations would then have time to resolve during the tapering process and the rate of decline of receptor antagonism is more modest.[20] Studies in which antipsychotics are tapered over months or years show reduced rates of relapse compared with relatively faster tapers,[23,29,30] with one study finding that reducing dose over a year reduced the hazard rate of relapse by 3.5-fold compared with reducing over days.[29]

Pattern of tapering

Positron emission tomography demonstrates a hyperbolic relationship between dose of antipsychotic and D_2 receptor occupancy.[31] This hyperbolic relationship applies to other receptor targets of antipsychotics as well (including histaminergic, cholinergic and serotonergic receptors) because it arises from the law of mass action (whereby each additional molecule of a drug has incrementally less effect as receptor targets become saturated).[32] The nature of this relationship is often obscured by the habit of plotting dose–response curves on semi-logarithmic axes.[32] A hyperbolic relationship between dose of antipsychotic and its therapeutic effects (as measured by symptoms scales) has also been shown,[33] suggesting that clinical response mirrors the neurobiological pattern of effects.

This brings into question the rationale for a linear reduction of antipsychotic dose – for example, a reduction from 20 to 15 to 10 to 5 to 0mg of olanzapine. Although this regimen appears logical, the hyperbolic relationship between dose and effect on D_2 blockade dictates that these linear dose decreases will produce increasingly larger reductions of D_2 blockade (and there may be clinical consequences of this; Figure 1.3a). Indeed, the reduction of dose from 5 to 0mg will produce a reduction in D_2 blockade (52.6%) that is larger than that produced by the reduction from 40 to 5mg of olanzapine (37.3%). These increasingly large reductions in D_2 blockade are more likely to provoke relapse.[34,35]

Linear or 'evenly spaced' reductions in D_2 blockade require hyperbolically reducing doses of antipsychotic (Figure 1.3b).[36] These hyperbolic reductions are approximated by sequential halving of dose: for example, olanzapine doses of 20mg, 10mg, 5mg, 2.5mg, 1.25mg, 0.6mg, 0.3mg, 0mg produce roughly 15 percentage point reductions in D_2 blockade. This pattern of reduction may be less likely to provoke relapse because it avoids large increases in dopaminergic signalling. Example regimens are shown in Table 1.27 and Box 1.1. Preliminary support for this approach comes from a study in which antipsychotics were reduced hyperbolically by on average 40% in people with chronic psychotic disorders, with no difference in relapse rates from the maintenance group but improved clinical outcomes.[30]

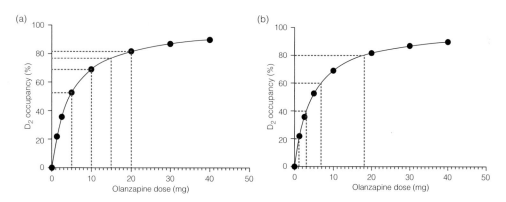

Figure 1.3 (a) Linear dose reductions of olanzapine cause increasingly large reductions in D_2 dopaminergic receptor blockade. The relationship between dose of olanzapine and D_2 blockade is derived from the line of best fit from meta-analysis of positron emission tomography studies.[31] (b) Linear reductions of D_2 dopaminergic occupancy (in this case 20% reductions) correspond to hyperbolically decreasing doses of olanzapine. The doses in this case correspond to 6.9mg (80% D_2 occupancy), 2.0mg (60% D_2 occupancy), 0.82 mg (40% D_2 occupancy) and 0.30mg (20% D_2 occupancy). Approximations to this regimen that correspond to available formulations are given in the text.

Table 1.27 Reductions of olanzapine dose by up to 5 percentage points of D_2 occupancy at each step, adjusted to allow use of quarter tablets. Liquid versions of drug will be needed for smaller doses.

Period	Olanzapine dose (mg)	D_2 occupancy (%)	Period	Olanzapine dose (mg)	D_2 occupancy (%)
1	20	72.9	11	4.375	37.5
2	17.5	70.9	12	3.75	34.0
3	15	66.9	13	3.125	30.4
4	12.5	62.8	14	2.5	26.3
5	10	58.8	15	2	22.3
6	8.75	54.7	16	1.5	17.3
7	7.5	50.7	17	1.1	13.1
8	6.25	46.6	18	0.7	9.1
9	5.625	43.5	19	0.35	4.0
10	5	40.5	20	0	0

Box 1.1 A summary of a slow hyperbolic reduction schedule for olanzapine

Reduce olanzapine by 5–10mg every 1–3 months until reaching 20mg per day, *then*
Reduce dose by 2.5–5mg every 1–3 months until reaching 10mg per day, *then*
Reduce dose by 1.25–2.5mg every 1–3 months until reaching 5mg per day, *then*
Reduce dose by 0.6–1.25mg every 1–3 months until reaching 2.5mg per day, *then*
Reduce dose by 0.3–0.6mg every 1–3 months until reaching 1.25mg per day, *then*
Reduce dose by 0.15–0.3mg every 1–3 months until reaching 0.6mg per day, *then*
Reduce dose by 0.07–0.15mg every 1–3 months until olanzapine is **completely stopped**.

This process could take 12–48 months, depending on how the patient tolerates the reductions. Liquid versions of drug or other options will be required for smaller doses.

Exponentially reducing regimens (reducing by a fixed proportion of the most recent dose, e.g. 10%) will produce roughly linear reductions at all receptor targets of antipsychotics, making it applicable to a wide range of antipsychotic medication.

Tapering in practice

All patients should be informed of the risk of withdrawal symptoms on stopping or reducing the dose of any antipsychotic, including insomnia and a potential increase in psychotic symptoms.

Patients should be warned not to stop antipsychotics abruptly or too quickly, because this is the method thought to be most likely to precipitate a relapse and severe withdrawal effects.

When to attempt discontinuation

Longstanding or lifelong antipsychotic treatment is something of a modern-day phenomenon. In the 1960s, discontinuation of antipsychotics was usually attempted after acute response. There are currently no evidence-based recommendations for antipsychotic withdrawal but we suggest that it only be considered in patients who have been in remission for 6 months (first episode) or 1 year (multi-episode). Relapse rates using fast linear tapers generally exceed 90% for both groups of patients. This might suggest that abrupt tapering always precipitates relapse or that relapse is inevitable when antipsychotics are withdrawn. Certainly, some people (probably the majority with a schizophrenia diagnosis) will relapse no matter how the antipsychotic is stopped.

A cautious approach to antipsychotic reduction is recommended, especially in long-term users, where a test reduction of 5–10% of dose might be a sensible starting point. In people who have been on medication for shorter periods (e.g. <1 year) a reduction as large as 25% might be feasible.

The patient should then be monitored for several weeks following this reduction for any withdrawal symptoms or worsening of psychotic symptoms. These symptoms may be transitory withdrawal effects rather than signs of inevitable relapse necessitating reinstatement of the regular dose of medication.[20] If a patient tolerates this reduction with no significant effect on their overall mental state (or perhaps only mild symptoms) then further reductions could be made at the same rate (for example, a reduction of 10–25% of the dose every 2–3 months). Patients may require increased psychosocial support during this period of withdrawal.

If a patient experiences significant withdrawal symptoms or worsening of psychotic symptoms then an increase in dose back one or two steps or back to the original dose may be necessary.[20] This does not preclude further attempts at reduction, but these attempts should be delayed until stability is established and should be performed more gradually than previously attempted (some long-term users can only tolerate <5% dose reductions per month).

Final doses before complete cessation may need to be very small to prevent a large decrease in D_2 blockade. This may need to be as small as 1/80th the original therapeutic dose (for example, 0.25mg of olanzapine) or smaller. Delivery of these small doses will require splitting tablets or using liquid formulations of the medications. Use of adjunctive medication to manage withdrawal symptoms may lead to accumulation of further medications and so pausing or slowing the taper is generally more advisable.[20] Every-other-day dosing of antipsychotics with half-lives of less than 24 hours leads to fluctuating plasma levels, which can precipitate withdrawal effects and so should generally be avoided.

Reducing depot medication may facilitate gradual tapering because of the longer half-lives of elimination. However, depots cannot be said to be 'self-tapering' for long-term users because the time taken for elimination may be shorter than the time required for many patients to adapt to lower blood levels of medication, and will require switching from the lowest depot dose to oral medication in order to continue a gradual taper.[37,38] Example reducing regimens are presented in Table 1.27 and Box 1.1.

References

1. Leucht S, et al. Antipsychotic drugs versus placebo for relapse prevention in schizophrenia: a systematic review and meta-analysis. *Lancet* 2012; 379:2063–2071.
2. Murray RM, et al. Should psychiatrists be more cautious about the long-term prophylactic use of antipsychotics? *Br J Psychiatry* 2016; 209:361–365.
3. Wunderink L, et al. Recovery in remitted first-episode psychosis at 7 years of follow-up of an early dose reduction/discontinuation or maintenance treatment strategy: long-term follow-up of a 2-year randomized clinical trial. *JAMA Psychiatry* 2013; 70:913–920.
4. Wunderink L, et al. Guided discontinuation versus maintenance treatment in remitted first-episode psychosis: relapse rates and functional outcome. *J Clin Psychiatry* 2007; 68:654–661.
5. Moncrieff J, et al. Antipsychotic dose reduction and discontinuation versus maintenance treatment in people with schizophrenia and other recurrent psychotic disorders in England (the RADAR trial): an open, parallel-group, randomised controlled trial. *Lancet Psychiatry* 2023; 10:848–859.
6. Omachi Y, et al. Dose reduction/discontinuation of antipsychotic drugs in psychosis; effect on cognition and functional outcomes. *Front Psychiatry* 2018; 9:447.
7. Moncrieff J. Antipsychotic maintenance treatment: time to rethink? *PLoS Med* 2015; 12:e1001861.
8. Marston L, et al. Prescribing of antipsychotics in UK primary care: a cohort study. *BMJ Open* 2014; 4:e006135.
9. National Institute for Health and Care Excellence. Borderline personality disorder: recognition and management. Clinical guideline [CG78]. 2009 (last checked April 2022, last accessed January 2024); https://www.nice.org.uk/guidance/CG78.
10. National Institute for Health and Care Excellence. Dementia: assessment, management and support for people living with dementia and their carers [NG97]. 2018 (last checked September 2023, last accessed December 2023); https://www.nice.org.uk/guidance/ng97.
11. Cerovecki A, et al. Withdrawal symptoms and rebound syndromes associated with switching and discontinuing atypical antipsychotics: theoretical background and practical recommendations. *CNS Drugs* 2013; 27:545–572.
12. Chouinard G, et al. Antipsychotic-induced dopamine supersensitivity psychosis: pharmacology, criteria, and therapy. *Psychother Psychosom* 2017; 86:189–219.
13. Brandt L, et al. Antipsychotic withdrawal symptoms: a systematic review and meta-analysis. *Front Psychiatry* 2020; 11:569912.
14. Brandt L, et al. Adverse events after antipsychotic discontinuation: an individual participant data meta-analysis. *Lancet Psychiatry* 2022; 9:232–242.
15. Morant N, et al. Experiences of reduction and discontinuation of antipsychotics: a qualitative investigation within the RADAR trial. *EClinicalMedicine* 2023; 64:102135.
16. Moncrieff J. Does antipsychotic withdrawal provoke psychosis? Review of the literature on rapid onset psychosis (supersensitivity psychosis) and withdrawal-related relapse. *Acta Psychiatr Scand* 2006; 114:3–13.
17. Lu ML, et al. Metoclopramide-induced supersensitivity psychosis. *Ann Pharmacother* 2002; 36:1387–1390.
18. Roy-Desruisseaux J, et al. Domperidone-induced tardive dyskinesia and withdrawal psychosis in an elderly woman with dementia. *Ann Pharmacother* 2011; 45:e51.
19. Seeman P. Breast is best but taper domperidone when stopping [e-letter]. *Br J Gen Pract* 2014; https://bjgp.org/content/yes-breast-best-taper-domperidone-when-stopping.
20. Horowitz MA, et al. Gradually tapering off antipsychotics: lessons for practice from case studies and neurobiological principles. *Curr Opin Psychiatry* 2024; 37:320–330.
21. Viguera AC, et al. Clinical risk following abrupt and gradual withdrawal of maintenance neuroleptic treatment. *Archives of General Psychiatry* 1997; 54:49–55.
22. Bogers JPAM, et al. Risk factors for psychotic relapse after dose reduction or discontinuation of antipsychotics in patients with chronic schizophrenia: a systematic review and meta-analysis. *Schizophr Bull Open* 2020; 50:722.
23. Bogers J, et al. Risk factors for psychotic relapse after dose reduction or discontinuation of antipsychotics in patients with chronic schizophrenia. A meta-analysis of randomized controlled trials. *Schizophr Bull* 2023; 49:11-23.
24. Chouinard G, et al. Atypical antipsychotics: CATIE study, drug-induced movement disorder and resulting iatrogenic psychiatric-like symptoms, supersensitivity rebound psychosis and withdrawal discontinuation syndromes. *Psychother Psychosom* 2008; 77:69–77.
25. Howes OD, et al. The nature of dopamine dysfunction in schizophrenia and what this means for treatment. *Arch Gen Psychiatry* 2012; 69:776–786.
26. Joyce JN. D2 but not D3 receptors are elevated after 9 or 11 months chronic haloperidol treatment: influence of withdrawal period. *Synapse* 2001; 40:137–144.
27. Quinn R. Comparing rat's to human's age: how old is my rat in people years? *Nutrition* 2005; 21:775–777.
28. Marsden CD. Is tardive dyskinesia a unique disorder? *Psychopharmacology Suppl* 1985; 2:64–71.
29. Schoretsanitis G, et al. Predictors of lack of relapse after random discontinuation of oral and long-acting injectable antipsychotics in clinically stabilized patients with schizophrenia: a re-analysis of individual participant data. *Schizophr Bull* 2022; 48:296–306.
30. Liu CC, et al. Guided antipsychotic reduction to reach minimum effective dose (GARMED) in patients with remitted psychosis: a 2-year randomized controlled trial with a naturalistic cohort. *Psychol Med* 2023; 53:7078–7086.
31. Lako IM, et al. Estimating dopamine D_2 receptor occupancy for doses of 8 antipsychotics: a meta-analysis. *J Clin Psychopharmacol* 2013; 33:675–681.
32. Holford N. Pharmacodynamic principles and the time course of delayed and cumulative drug effects. *Transl Clin Pharmacol* 2018; 26:56–59.
33. Leucht S, et al. Dose–response meta-analysis of antipsychotic drugs for acute schizophrenia. *Am J Psychiatry* 2020; 177:342–353.

34. Leucht S, et al. Examination of dosing of antipsychotic drugs for relapse prevention in patients with stable schizophrenia: a meta-analysis. *JAMA Psychiatry* 2021; **78**:1238–1248.

35. Horowitz MA, et al. Limitations in research on maintenance treatment for individuals with schizophrenia. *JAMA Psychiatry* 2022; **79**:83–85.

36. Horowitz MA, et al. Tapering antipsychotic treatment. *JAMA Psychiatry* 2020; **78**:125–126.

37. O'Neill JR, et al. Implementing gradual, hyperbolic tapering of long-acting injectable antipsychotics by prolonging the inter-dose interval: an in silico modelling study. *Ther Adv Psychopharmacol* 2023; **13**:20451253231198463.

38. O'Neill J, et al. Using in silico methods to determine optimal tapering regimens for decanoate-based long-acting injectable psychosis drugs. *Ther Adv Psychopharmacol* 2024; **14**:20451253241272790.

ANTIPSYCHOTIC ADVERSE EFFECTS

Extrapyramidal symptoms

The EPS associated with antipsychotic medication can be stigmatising, distressing, potentially disabling and act as a disincentive to taking medication.[1,2] EPS are commonly overlooked and underdiagnosed or misdiagnosed in clinical practice.[3,4] These movement disorders tend to be dose-related and are less likely to occur with SGAs, particularly clozapine, olanzapine, quetiapine and aripiprazole,[2,5] compared with FGAs such as haloperidol. Generally it is agreed that the greater use of SGAs has led to a reduction in the frequency of EPS,[6] although the prevalence of EPS of any description in community samples may exceed 30%.[7] The incidence of EPS is often steeply dose-related for most drugs (clozapine and quetiapine are possible exceptions) and this relationship extends beyond the licensed dose range for some drugs.[8]

Patients who experience one type of EPS may be more vulnerable to developing others.[9] Substance misuse increases the risk of dystonia, akathisia and TD,[10,11] and there is some evidence for an association between alcohol use and akathisia.[12,13] Vulnerability to EPS may be partly genetically determined.[14–16]

Establishing the prevalence of antipsychotic-induced EPS is problematic, given that similar movement disorders may be seen in never-medicated patients with schizophrenia.[17–19] In one study of such patients at first episode, 1% had dystonia, 8% parkinsonian symptoms and 11% akathisia.[19] Parkinsonian symptoms and other motor abnormalities in this context may be associated with cognitive impairment[19,20] and poor long-term psychosocial functioning.[21] In another study of never-treated patients with established psychotic illness, 9% exhibited spontaneous dyskinesias and 17% parkinsonian symptoms.[22] Table 1.28 details the most common EPSEs.

Table 1.28 Most common extrapyramidal side effects.

	Dystonia (uncontrolled muscular spasm)	Pseudoparkinsonism (bradykinesia, tremor, muscle rigidity, etc.)	Akathisia (restlessness)[23]	Tardive dyskinesia (TD) (abnormal involuntary movements)
Signs and symptoms[24]	■ Muscle spasm in any part of the body, e.g. ■ eyes rolling upwards (oculogyric spasm) ■ head and neck twisted to the side (torticollis) ■ The patient may be unable to swallow or speak clearly. In extreme cases, the back may arch or the jaw dislocate. ■ Acute dystonia can be both painful and very frightening	■ Tremor and/or rigidity ■ Bradykinesia (decreased facial expression, flat monotone voice, slow body movements, inability to initiate movement) ■ Bradyphrenia (slowed thinking) ■ Salivation ■ Pseudoparkinsonism can be mistaken for depression or negative symptoms of schizophrenia	■ A subjectively unpleasant state of inner restlessness with a desire or compulsion to move[23,25] ■ Foot stamping when seated ■ Constantly crossing/uncrossing legs ■ Rocking from foot to foot when standing ■ Constantly pacing up and down ■ Akathisia can be mistaken for psychotic agitation and has been linked with suicidal ideation[26] and aggression towards others[27]	■ A wide variety of movements can occur,[28] such as: ■ lip smacking or chewing ■ tongue protrusion ('fly catching') ■ choreiform hand movements ('piano playing') ■ dystonic and choreoathetoid movements of the limbs ■ Severe orofacial movements can lead to difficulty speaking, eating or breathing. Movements are worse when under stress.
Rating scales (see Martino et al. 2023)[29]	■ No specific scale ■ Small component of general EPS scales	■ Simpson–Angus EPS Rating Scale[30]	■ Barnes Akathisia Rating Scale[3,31]	■ Abnormal Involuntary Movement Scale[32,33]
Prevalence	■ Approximately 10%[34] but more common:[35] ■ in young males ■ in those who are antipsychotic-naïve with high-potency medications (e.g. haloperidol) ■ Dystonic reactions are rare in the elderly	■ Approximately 20%[36] but more common in: ■ elderly females ■ those with pre-existing neurological damage (head injury, stroke, etc.)	■ Wide variation but approximately 25%[37] for acute akathisia with FGAs, lower with SGAs ■ The relative liability of individual antipsychotic medications for akathisia is uncertain,[2] but there is consensus that the incidence is lowest for olanzapine, quetiapine and clozapine[38,39]	■ 5% of patients per year of antipsychotic exposure.[40] More common in respect to:[41] ■ age ■ affective illness ■ schizophrenia ■ higher doses ■ acute EPS early in treatment ■ Lower incidence in those on SGAs.[42,43] TD may be associated with neurocognitive deficits.[44]

(Continued)

Table 1.28 (Continued)

	Dystonia (uncontrolled muscular spasm)	Pseudoparkinsonism (bradykinesia, tremor, muscle rigidity, etc.)	Akathisia (restlessness)[3]	Tardive dyskinesia (TD) (abnormal involuntary movements)
Time taken to develop	▪ Acute dystonia can occur within hours of starting antipsychotic medication (minutes if the IM or IV route is used) ▪ TD occurs after months to years of antipsychotic treatment	▪ Days to weeks after the start of antipsychotic medication or an increase in dose	▪ Acute akathisia occurs within hours to weeks of starting antipsychotic medication or increasing the dose ▪ Akathisia that has persisted for several months or so is called 'chronic akathisia'. Tardive akathisia tends to occur later in treatment and may be exacerbated or provoked by antipsychotic dose reduction or withdrawal.[23]	▪ Months to years ▪ The proportion of cases showing reversibility on cessation of antipsychotic medication is unclear and may partly depend on age[28]
Treatment	▪ Anticholinergic drugs given orally, IM or IV depending on the severity of symptoms[35] ▪ Remember the patient may be unable to swallow ▪ Response to IV administration will be seen within 5 minutes ▪ Response to IM administration takes around 20 minutes ▪ TD may respond to ECT[45,46] ▪ Where severe symptoms do not respond to simpler measures including switching to an antipsychotic with a low propensity for EPS, botulinum toxin may be effective[47,48]	▪ Several options are available depending on the clinical circumstances: ▪ Reduce the antipsychotic dose ▪ Change to an antipsychotic medication with a lower propensity for pseudoparkinsonism (see section on relative liability of antipsychotic medications for adverse effects) ▪ Prescribe an anticholinergic. The majority of patients do not require long-term anticholinergic agents. Use should be reviewed at least every 3 months. Do not prescribe at night (symptoms usually absent during sleep).	▪ Reduce the antipsychotic dose ▪ Change to an antipsychotic drug with lower propensity for akathisia (see sections on akathisia and relative liability of antipsychotic medications for adverse effects) ▪ A reduction in symptoms may be seen with[25,49,50] low-dose propranolol, 30–80mg/day; clonazepam (low dose); $5HT_2$ antagonists such as cyproheptadine,[46] mirtazapine,[49] trazodone,[51,52] mianserin[53] and cyproheptadine[46] may help, as may possibly diphenhydramine[54] ▪ Note that all of the above medications are unlicensed for this indication ▪ Anticholinergics are generally unhelpful unless possibly if akathisia is part of a general EPS spectrum[55,56]	▪ Stop anticholinergic if prescribed ▪ Reduce dose of antipsychotic medication ▪ Change to an antipsychotic with lower propensity for TD;[57–60] note that data are conflicting[61,62] ▪ Clozapine is the antipsychotic most likely to be associated with resolution of symptoms.[63,64] Quetiapine may also be useful in this regard.[65] ▪ Both valbenazine[66] and deutetrabenazine[67–69] have a positive risk–benefit balance as add-on treatments.[67,70] There is also some evidence for tetrabenazine and Ginkgo biloba[71] as add-on treatments. For other treatment options,[72,73] see the review by the American Academy of Neurology[74] and the section on treatment of TD in this chapter.

References

1. Owens DGC. *A Guide to the Extrapyramidal Side-Effects of Antipsychotic Drugs*, 2nd edn. Cambridge: Cambridge University Press; 2014.

2. Martino D, et al. Movement disorders associated with antipsychotic medication in people with schizophrenia: an overview of Cochrane reviews and meta-analysis. *Can J Psychiatry* 2018; 63:706743718777392.

3. Barnes TRE. The Barnes akathisia scale – revisited. *J Psychopharm* 2003; 17:365–370.

4. Jouini L, et al. Akathisia among patients undergoing antipsychotic therapy: prevalence, associated factors, and psychiatric impact. *Clin Neuropharmacol* 2022; 45:89–94.

5. Leucht S, et al. Comparative efficacy and tolerability of 15 antipsychotic drugs in schizophrenia: a multiple-treatments meta-analysis. *Lancet* 2014; 382:951–962.

6. Misdrahi D, et al. Prevalence of and risk factors for extrapyramidal side effects of antipsychotics: results from the national FACE-SZ cohort. *J Clin Psychiatry* 2019; 80:18m12246.

7. Ali T, et al. Antipsychotic-induced extrapyramidal side effects: a systematic review and meta-analysis of observational studies. *PLoS One* 2021; 16:e0257319.

8. Siafis S, et al. Antipsychotic dose, dopamine D2 receptor occupancy and extrapyramidal side-effects: a systematic review and dose-response meta-analysis. *Mol Psychiatry* 2023; 28:3267–3277.

9. Kim JH, et al. Prevalence and characteristics of subjective akathisia, objective akathisia, and mixed akathisia in chronic schizophrenic subjects. *Clin Neuropharmacol* 2003; 26:312–316.

10. Potvin S, et al. Increased extrapyramidal symptoms in patients with schizophrenia and a comorbid substance use disorder. *J Neurol Neurosurg Psychiatry* 2006; 77:796–798.

11. Potvin S, et al. Substance abuse is associated with increased extrapyramidal symptoms in schizophrenia: a meta-analysis. *Schizophr Res* 2009; 113:181–188.

12. Hansen LK, et al. Movement disorders in patients with schizophrenia and a history of substance abuse. *Hum Psychopharmacol* 2013; 28:192–197.

13. Duke PJ, et al. South Westminster schizophrenia survey. Alcohol use and its relationship to symptoms, tardive dyskinesia and illness onset. *Br J Psychiatry* 1994; 164:630–636.

14. Zivkovic M, et al. The association study of polymorphisms in DAT, DRD2, and COMT genes and acute extrapyramidal adverse effects in male schizophrenic patients treated with haloperidol. *J Clin Psychopharmacol* 2013; 33:593–599.

15. Nedic Erjavec G, et al. SLC6A3, HTR2C and HTR6 gene polymorphisms and the risk of haloperidol-induced parkinsonism. *Biomedicines* 2022; 10:3237.

16. Kibitov AA, et al. The ANKK1/DRD2 gene TaqIA polymorphism (rs1800497) is associated with the severity of extrapyramidal side effects of haloperidol treatment in CYP2D6 extensive metabolizers with schizophrenia spectrum disorders. *Drug Metab Pers Ther* 2023; 38:133–142.

17. Cortese L, et al. Relationship of neuromotor disturbances to psychosis symptoms in first-episode neuroleptic-naive schizophrenia patients. *Schizophr Res* 2005; 75:65–75.

18. Puri BK, et al. Spontaneous dyskinesia in first episode schizophrenia. *J Neurol Neurosurg Psychiatry* 1999; 66:76–78.

19. Rybakowski JK, et al. Extrapyramidal symptoms during treatment of first schizophrenia episode: results from EUFEST. *Eur Neuropsychopharmacol* 2014; 24:1500–1505.

20. Cuesta MJ, et al. Spontaneous parkinsonism is associated with cognitive impairment in antipsychotic-naive patients with first-episode psychosis: a 6-month follow-up study. *Schizophr Bull* 2014; 40:1164–1173.

21. Cuesta MJ, et al. Motor abnormalities in first-episode psychosis patients and long-term psychosocial functioning. *Schizophr Res* 2018; 200:97–103.

22. Pappa S, et al. Spontaneous movement disorders in antipsychotic-naive patients with first-episode psychoses: a systematic review. *Psychol Med* 2009; 39:1065–1076.

23. Barnes TR, et al. Akathisia variants and tardive dyskinesia. *Arch Gen Psychiatry* 1985; 42:874–878.

24. Gervin M, et al. Assessment of drug-related movement disorders in schizophrenia. *Adv Psychiatr Treat* 2000; 6:332–341.

25. Pringsheim T, et al. The assessment and treatment of antipsychotic-induced akathisia. *Can J Psychiatry* 2018; 63:719–729.

26. Seemuller F, et al. Akathisia and suicidal ideation in first-episode schizophrenia. *J Clin Psychopharmacol* 2012; 32:694–698.

27. Leong GB, et al. Neuroleptic-induced akathisia and violence: a review. *J Forensic Sci* 2003; 48:187–189.

28. Owens DC. Tardive dyskinesia update: the syndrome. *BJPsych Advances* 2018; 25:57–69.

29. Martino D, et al. Scales for antipsychotic-associated movement disorders: systematic review, critique, and recommendations. *Mov Disord* 2023; 38:1008–1026.

30. Simpson GM, et al. A rating scale for extrapyramidal side effects. *Acta Psychiatr Scand* 1970; 212:11–19.

31. Barnes TRE. A rating scale for drug-induced akathisia. *BJPsychiatry* 1989; 154:672–676.

32. Guy W. Abnormal Involuntary Movement Scale (II7-AIMS). In: *ECDEU Assessment Manual for Psychopharmacology*. Washington, DC: US Department of Health, Education, and Welfare; 1976:534–537.

33. McEvoy JP. How to assess tardive dyskinesia symptom improvement with measurement-based care. *J Clin Psychiatry* 2020; 81:NU19047BR19044C.

34. American Psychiatric Association. Practice guideline for the treatment of patients with schizophrenia. *Am J Psychiatry* 1997; 154 Suppl 4:1–63.

35. van Harten PN, et al. Acute dystonia induced by drug treatment. *BMJ* 1999; 319:623–626.

36. Bollini P, et al. Antipsychotic drugs: is more worse? A meta-analysis of the published randomized control trials. *Psychol Med* 1994; 24:307–316.

37. Halstead SM, et al. Akathisia: prevalence and associated dysphoria in an in-patient population with chronic schizophrenia. *Br J Psychiatry* 1994; **164**:177–183.

38. Hirose S. The causes of underdiagnosing akathisia. *Schizophr Bull* 2003; **29**:547–558.

39. Juncal-Ruiz M, et al. Incidence and risk factors of acute akathisia in 493 individuals with first episode non-affective psychosis: a 6-week randomised study of antipsychotic treatment. *Psychopharmacology (Berl)* 2017; **234**:2563–2570.

40. Caligiuri M. Tardive dyskinesia: a task force report of the American Psychiatric Association. *Hosp Community Psychiatry* 1993; **44**:190.

41. Patterson-Lomba O, et al. Risk assessment and prediction of TD incidence in psychiatric patients taking concomitant antipsychotics: a retrospective data analysis. *BMC Neurol* 2019; **19**:174.

42. Widschwendter CG, et al. Antipsychotic-induced tardive dyskinesia: update on epidemiology and management. *Curr Opin Psychiatry* 2019; **32**:179–184.

43. Carbon M, et al. Tardive dyskinesia risk with first- and second-generation antipsychotics in comparative randomized controlled trials: a meta-analysis. *World Psychiatry* 2018; **17**:330–340.

44. Caroff SN, et al. Treatment outcomes of patients with tardive dyskinesia and chronic schizophrenia. *J Clin Psychiatry* 2011; **72**:295–303.

45. Yasui-Furukori N, et al. The effects of electroconvulsive therapy on tardive dystonia or dyskinesia induced by psychotropic medication: a retrospective study. *Neuropsychiatr Dis Treat* 2014; **10**:1209–1212.

46. Miller CH, et al. Managing antipsychotic-induced acute and chronic akathisia. *Drug Saf* 2000; **22**:73–81.

47. Havaki-Kontaxaki BJ, et al. Treatment of severe neuroleptic-induced tardive torticollis. *Ann Gen Hosp Psychiatry* 2003; **2**:9.

48. Hennings JM, et al. Successful treatment of tardive lingual dystonia with botulinum toxin: case report and review of the literature. *Prog Neuropsychopharmacol Biol Psychiatry* 2008; **32**:1167–1171.

49. Poyurovsky M, et al. Efficacy of low-dose mirtazapine in neuroleptic-induced akathisia: a double-blind randomized placebo-controlled pilot study. *J Clin Psychopharmacol* 2003; **23**:305–308.

50. Salem H, et al. Revisiting antipsychotic-induced akathisia: current issues and prospective challenges. *Curr Neuropharmacol* 2017; **15**:789–798.

51. Stryjer R, et al. Treatment of neuroleptic-induced akathisia with the 5-HT2A antagonist trazodone. *Clin Neuropharmacol* 2003; **26**:137–141.

52. Stryjer R, et al. Trazodone for the treatment of neuroleptic-induced acute akathisia: a placebo-controlled, double-blind, crossover study. *Clin Neuropharmacol* 2010; **33**:219–222.

53. Stryjer R, et al. Mianserin for the rapid improvement of chronic akathisia in a schizophrenia patient. *Eur Psychiatry* 2004; **19**:237–238.

54. Vinson DR. Diphenhydramine in the treatment of akathisia induced by prochlorperazine. *J Emerg Med* 2004; **26**:265–270.

55. Rathbone J, et al. Anticholinergics for neuroleptic-induced acute akathisia. *Cochrane Database Syst Rev* 2006; (3):CD003727.

56. Vanegas-Arroyave N, et al. An evidence-based update on anticholinergic use for drug-induced movement disorders. *CNS Drugs* 2024; **38**:239–254.

57. Glazer WM. Expected incidence of tardive dyskinesia associated with atypical antipsychotics. *J Clin Psychiatry* 2000; **61** Suppl 4:21–26.

58. Kinon BJ, et al. Olanzapine treatment for tardive dyskinesia in schizophrenia patients: a prospective clinical trial with patients randomized to blinded dose reduction periods. *Prog Neuropsychopharmacol Biol Psychiatry* 2004; **28**:985-996.

59. Bai YM, et al. Risperidone for severe tardive dyskinesia: a 12-week randomized, double-blind, placebo-controlled study. *J Clin Psychiatry* 2003; **64**:1342–1348.

60. Tenback DE, et al. Effects of antipsychotic treatment on tardive dyskinesia: a 6-month evaluation of patients from the European Schizophrenia Outpatient Health Outcomes (SOHO) Study. *J Clin Psychiatry* 2005; **66**:1130–1133.

61. Woods SW, et al. Incidence of tardive dyskinesia with atypical versus conventional antipsychotic medications: a prospective cohort study. *J Clin Psychiatry* 2010; **71**:463–474.

62. Pena MS, et al. Tardive dyskinesia and other movement disorders secondary to aripiprazole. *Mov Disord* 2011; **26**:147–152.

63. Stegmayer K, et al. Tardive dyskinesia associated with atypical antipsychotics: prevalence, mechanisms and management strategies. *CNS Drugs* 2018; **32**:135–147.

64. Simpson GM. The treatment of tardive dyskinesia and tardive dystonia. *J Clin Psychiatry* 2000; **61** Suppl 4:39–44.

65. Peritogiannis V, et al. Can atypical antipsychotics improve tardive dyskinesia associated with other atypical antipsychotics? Case report and brief review of the literature. *J Psychopharmacol* 2010; **24**:1121–1125.

66. Kishi T, et al. Valbenazine for tardive dyskinesia: a systematic review and network meta-analysis. *Int Clin Psychopharmacol* 2023; **38**:369–374.

67. Solmi M, et al. Treatment of tardive dyskinesia with VMAT-2 inhibitors: a systematic review and meta-analysis of randomized controlled trials. *Drug Des Devel Ther* 2018; **12**:1215–1238.

68. Hauser RA, et al. Long-term deutetrabenazine treatment for tardive dyskinesia is associated with sustained benefits and safety: a 3-year, open-label extension study. *Front Neurol* 2022; **13**:773999.

69. Frank S, et al. Clinical utility of deutetrabenazine as a treatment option for chorea associated with Huntington's disease and tardive dyskinesia. *Ther Clin Risk Manag* 2023; **19**:1019–1024.

70. Golsorkhi M, et al. Comparative analysis of deutetrabenazine and valbenazine as VMAT2 inhibitors for tardive dyskinesia: a systematic review. *Tremor Other Hyperkinet Mov* 2024; **14**:13.

71. Zhang WF, et al. Extract of ginkgo biloba treatment for tardive dyskinesia in schizophrenia: a randomized, double-blind, placebo-controlled trial. *J Clin Psychiatry* 2010; **72**:615–621.

72. Bergman H, et al. Systematic review of interventions for treating or preventing antipsychotic-induced tardive dyskinesia. *Health Technol Assess* 2017; **21**:1–218.

73. Ricciardi L, et al. Treatment recommendations for tardive dyskinesia. *Can J Psychiatry* 2019; **64**:388–399.

74. Bhidayasiri R, et al. Evidence-based guideline: treatment of tardive syndromes: report of the Guideline Development Subcommittee of the American Academy of Neurology. *Neurology* 2013; **81**:463–469.

Akathisia

Akathisia is a fairly common adverse effect of most antipsychotic medications, although the risk of developing akathisia varies markedly between such medications.[1-3] For example, a 2023 dose–response meta-analysis[4] investigating antipsychotic-induced akathisia with haloperidol and 16 SGAs (not including clozapine) found that the risk was minimal with sertindole and quetiapine but high with haloperidol and lurasidone. The risk of akathisia tended to increase with dose, but the dose–response curves differed between medications, plateauing at a certain dose with some medications, such as amisulpride, haloperidol and risperidone, but increasing beyond the licensed dose range with others, such as lurasidone and lumateperone. This meta-analysis[4] also confirmed the risk of akathisia with partial agonist to be greatest with cariprazine and lowest with brexpiprazole.

The core feature of akathisia is mental unease and dysphoria characterised by a sense of restlessness.[5,6] There is commonly a compulsion to move and a characteristic pattern of motor restlessness, which, when severe, can cause patients to pace up and down and be unable to stay seated for more than a short time.[5,6] There is a phenomenological overlap between antipsychotic-induced akathisia and the restless legs syndrome and possibly an overlap in pathophysiology.[7,8] The subjective experience of akathisia can be discomfiting and distressing; an association with suicidal ideation has been postulated[9,10] but remains uncertain.

There is some evidence to suggest that the risk of akathisia may be mitigated by avoiding high-dose antipsychotic medication, antipsychotic polypharmacy and a rapid increase in dosage.[5,11-13] There is limited evidence on the benefit–risk balance for pharmacological treatments of antipsychotic-induced akathisia, even those most commonly used, such as switching to an antipsychotic medication with a lower risk of akathisia or adding a beta-adrenergic blocker, 5-HT_{2A} antagonist or anticholinergic agent.[14,15] Nevertheless, a 2024 systematic review and meta-analysis of adjunctive treatments identified 15 eligible studies of 10 treatments.[16] Mirtazapine, biperiden and vitamin B6 emerged as the most efficacious, with vitamin B6 judged to have the most favourable efficacy and tolerability profile. Trazodone, mianserin and propranolol were considered effective alternative treatments, albeit with a slightly less favourable risk–benefit balance. However, given the lack of robust evidence of efficacy for such adjunctive treatments, particularly in the medium to long term, it is probably prudent to initially consider reduction of the antipsychotic dose or switching to an antipsychotic medication with a lower liability for the condition.

The following diagram suggests a programme of treatment options for persistent, antipsychotic-induced akathisia.

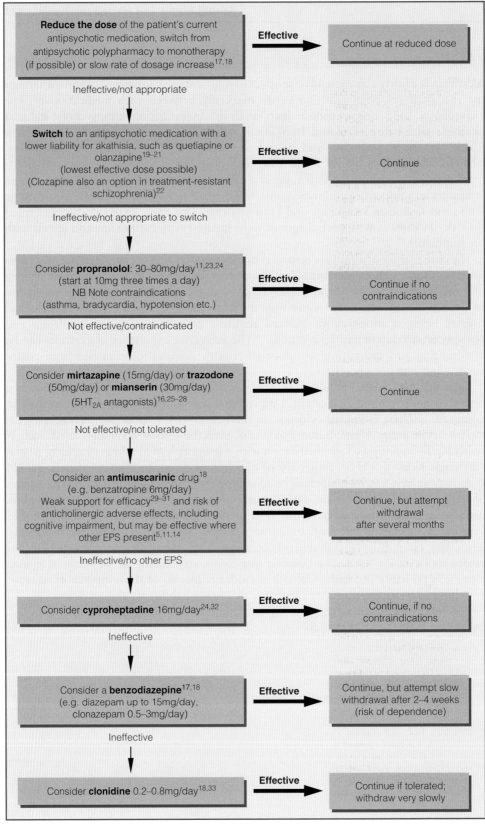

Effective → Continue at reduced dose

Reduce the dose of the patient's current antipsychotic medication, switch from antipsychotic polypharmacy to monotherapy (if possible) or slow rate of dosage increase[17,18]

Ineffective/not appropriate

Switch to an antipsychotic medication with a lower liability for akathisia, such as quetiapine or olanzapine[19-21] (lowest effective dose possible) (Clozapine also an option in treatment-resistant schizophrenia)[22]

Effective → Continue

Ineffective/not appropriate to switch

Consider **propranolol**: 30–80mg/day[11,23,24] (start at 10mg three times a day) NB Note contraindications (asthma, bradycardia, hypotension etc.)

Effective → Continue if no contraindications

Not effective/contraindicated

Consider **mirtazapine** (15mg/day) or **trazodone** (50mg/day) or **mianserin** (30mg/day) ($5HT_{2A}$ antagonists)[16,25-28]

Effective → Continue

Not effective/not tolerated

Consider an **antimuscarinic** drug[18] (e.g. benzatropine 6mg/day) Weak support for efficacy[29-31] and risk of anticholinergic adverse effects, including cognitive impairment, but may be effective where other EPS present[5,11,14]

Effective → Continue, but attempt withdrawal after several months

Ineffective/no other EPS

Consider **cyproheptadine** 16mg/day[24,32]

Effective → Continue, if no contraindications

Ineffective

Consider a **benzodiazepine**[17,18] (e.g. diazepam up to 15mg/day, clonazepam 0.5–3mg/day)

Effective → Continue, but attempt slow withdrawal after 2–4 weeks (risk of dependence)

Ineffective

Consider **clonidine** 0.2–0.8mg/day[18,33]

Effective → Continue if tolerated; withdraw very slowly

(Continued)

(Continued)

> **Notes**
>
> - Akathisia can be difficult to diagnose with certainty and is commonly overlooked or misdiagnosed in clinical practice. Clinical physical examination schedules for EPS and akathisia have been proposed.[34,35]
> - Evaluate the efficacy of each treatment option over at least 1 month if possible. Some effect may be seen after a few days, but it may take much longer to become apparent in those with chronic akathisia.
> - Withdraw previously ineffective add-on akathisia treatments before starting the next option in the algorithm.
> - Combinations of treatments may be considered for refractory cases, if carefully monitored.
> - Other possible treatments for acute akathisia that have been investigated include vitamin B6,[16,36,37] pregabalin,[38] diphenhydramine,[39] trazodone[25,40] and zolmitriptan.[41,42] Always read the primary literature before considering any of the treatment options.
> - Parenteral midazolam (1.5mg) has been successfully used to prevent akathisia associated with IV metoclopramide,[43] suggesting a specific therapeutic effect for midazolam against akathisia and perhaps benzodiazepines more generally.
> - In some cases where agitation/akathisia are recognised as short-lived effects of antipsychotic medication when initiated (e.g. with aripiprazole, cariprazine), prophylactic or rescue benzodiazepines may be prescribed for a limited period. Clinical experience suggests this practice can be effective.

References

1. Demyttenaere K, et al. Medication-induced akathisia with newly approved antipsychotics in patients with a severe mental illness: a systematic review and meta-analysis. *CNS Drugs* 2019; **33**:549–566.
2. Chow CL, et al. Akathisia and newer second-generation antipsychotic drugs: a review of current evidence. *Pharmacotherapy* 2020; **40**:565–574.
3. Martino D, et al. Movement disorders associated with antipsychotic medication in people with schizophrenia: an overview of Cochrane reviews and meta-analysis. *Can J Psychiatry* 2018; **63**:706743718777392.
4. Wu H, et al. Antipsychotic-induced akathisia in adults with acute schizophrenia: a systematic review and dose-response meta-analysis. *Eur Neuropsychopharmacol* 2023; **72**:40–49.
5. Braude WM, et al. Clinical characteristics of akathisia: a systematic investigation of acute psychiatric inpatient admissions. *Br J Psychiatry* 1983; **143**:139–150.
6. Barnes TRE. A rating scale for drug-induced akathisia. *Br J Psychiatry* 1989; **154**:672–676.
7. Ferré S, et al. Restless legs syndrome, neuroleptic-induced akathisia, and opioid-withdrawal restlessness: shared neuronal mechanisms? *Sleep* 2024; **47**:zsad273.
8. Walters AS. Restless legs syndrome, neuroleptic-induced akathisia, and the iron opioid dopamine link. *Sleep* 2024; **47**:zsae008.
9. Seemuller F, et al. Akathisia and suicidal ideation in first-episode schizophrenia. *J Clin Psychopharmacol* 2012; **32**:694–698.
10. Seemuller F, et al. The relationship of akathisia with treatment emergent suicidality among patients with first-episode schizophrenia treated with haloperidol or risperidone. *Pharmacopsychiatry* 2012; **45**:292–296.
11. Miller CH, et al. Managing antipsychotic-induced acute and chronic akathisia. *Drug Saf* 2000; **22**:73–81.
12. Berardi D, et al. Clinical correlates of akathisia in acute psychiatric inpatients. *Int Clin Psychopharmacol* 2000; **15**:215–219.
13. Yoshimura B, et al. Incidence and predictors of acute akathisia in severely ill patients with first-episode schizophrenia treated with aripiprazole or risperidone: secondary analysis of an observational study. *Psychopharmacology (Berl)* 2019; **236**:723–730.
14. Pringsheim T, et al. The assessment and treatment of antipsychotic-induced akathisia. *Can J Psychiatry* 2018; **63**:719–729.
15. Stroup TS. Management of common adverse effects of antipsychotic medications. *World Psychiatry* 2018; **17**:341–356.
16. Gerolymos C, et al. Drug efficacy in the treatment of antipsychotic-induced akathisia: a systematic review and network meta-analysis. *JAMA Netw Open* 2024; **7**:e241527.
17. Fleischhacker WW, et al. The pharmacologic treatment of neuroleptic-induced akathisia. *J Clin Psychopharmacol* 1990; **10**:12–21.
18. Sachdev P. The identification and management of drug-induced akathisia. *CNS Drugs* 1995; **4**:28–46.
19. Kumar R, et al. Akathisia and second-generation antipsychotic drugs. *Curr Opin Psychiatry* 2009; **22**:293–299.
20. Miller DD, et al. Extrapyramidal side-effects of antipsychotics in a randomised trial. *Br J Psychiatry* 2008; **193**:279–288.
21. Rummel-Kluge C, et al. Second-generation antipsychotic drugs and extrapyramidal side effects: a systematic review and meta-analysis of head-to-head comparisons. *Schizophr Bull* 2012; **38**:167–177.
22. Kane JM, et al. Akathisia: an updated review focusing on second-generation antipsychotics. *J Clin Psychiatry* 2009; **70**:627–643.
23. Adler L, et al. A controlled assessment of propranolol in the treatment of neuroleptic-induced akathisia. *Br J Psychiatry* 1986; **149**:42–45.
24. Fischel T, et al. Cyproheptadine versus propranolol for the treatment of acute neuroleptic-induced akathisia: a comparative double-blind study. *J Clin Psychopharmacol* 2001; **21**:612–615.
25. Laoutidis ZG, et al. 5-HT2A receptor antagonists for the treatment of neuroleptic-induced akathisia: a systematic review and meta-analysis. *Int J Neuropsychopharmacol* 2014; **17**:823–832.

26. Poyurovsky M, et al. Treatment of antipsychotic-induced akathisia: role of serotonin 5-HT(2a) receptor antagonists. *Drugs* 2020; 80:871–882.

27. Poyurovsky M. Acute antipsychotic-induced akathisia revisited. *Br J Psychiatry* 2010; **196**:89–91.

28. Shams-Alizadeh N, et al. Trazodone as an alternative treatment for neuroleptic-associated akathisia: a placebo-controlled, double-blind, clinical trial. *J Clin Psychopharmacol* 2020; **40**:611–614.

29. Rathbone J, et al. Anticholinergics for neuroleptic-induced acute akathisia. *Cochrane Database Syst Rev* 2006; (4):CD003727.

30. Baskak B, et al. The effectiveness of intramuscular biperiden in acute akathisia: a double-blind, randomized, placebo-controlled study. *J Clin Psychopharmacol* 2007; **27**:289–294.

31. Vanegas-Arroyave N, et al. An evidence-based update on anticholinergic use for drug-induced movement disorders. *CNS Drugs* 2024; **38**:239–254.

32. Weiss D, et al. Cyproheptadine treatment in neuroleptic-induced akathisia. *Br J Psychiatry* 1995; **167**:483–486.

33. Zubenko GS, et al. Use of clonidine in treating neuroleptic-induced akathisia. *Psychiatry Res* 1984; **13**:253–259.

34. Gervin M, et al. Assessment of drug-related movement disorders in schizophrenia. *Advances in Psychiatric Treatment* 2000; **6**:332–341.

35. Cunningham Owens D. *A Guide to the Extrapyramidal Side Effects of Antipsychotic Drugs.* Cambridge: Cambridge University Press; 1999.

36. Miodownik C, et al. Vitamin B6 versus mianserin and placebo in acute neuroleptic-induced akathisia: a randomized, double-blind, controlled study. *Clin Neuropharmacol* 2006; **29**:68–72.

37. Lerner V, et al. Vitamin B6 treatment in acute neuroleptic-induced akathisia: a randomized, double-blind, placebo-controlled study. *J Clin Psychiatry* 2004; **65**:1550–1554.

38. De BD, et al. Reversal of aripiprazole-induced tardive akathisia by addition of pregabalin. *J Neuropsychiatry Clin Neurosci* 2013; **25**:E9–E10.

39. Friedman BW, et al. A randomized trial of diphenhydramine as prophylaxis against metoclopramide-induced akathisia in nauseated emergency department patients. *Ann Emerg Med* 2009; **53**:379–385.

40. Stryjer R, et al. Trazodone for the treatment of neuroleptic-induced acute akathisia: a placebo-controlled, double-blind, crossover study. *Clin Neuropharmacol* 2010; **33**:219–222.

41. Gross-Isseroff R, et al. The 5-HT1D receptor agonist zolmitriptan for neuroleptic-induced akathisia: an open label preliminary study. *Int Clin Psychopharmacol* 2005; **20**:23–25.

42. Avital A, et al. Zolmitriptan compared to propranolol in the treatment of acute neuroleptic-induced akathisia: a comparative double-blind study. *Eur Neuropsychopharmacol* 2009; **19**:476–482.

43. Erdur B, et al. A trial of midazolam vs diphenhydramine in prophylaxis of metoclopramide-induced akathisia. *Am J Emerg Med* 2012; **30**:84–91.

Treatment of tardive dyskinesia

Tardive dyskinesia is a somewhat less commonly encountered problem now than in previous decades,[1,2] probably because of the more widespread use of SGAs,[3–6] which generally have a lower risk for the condition than FGAs. Treatment of established TD is often unsuccessful, so prevention, early detection and early remedial action are essential.[7,8] There is evidence to suggest that TD is associated with greater cognitive impairment,[7,9] more severe psychopathology[10,11] and higher mortality.[12,13] While the majority of patients seem to be unaware of the involuntary movements, the condition can still impose a substantial burden on physical, psychological and social well-being.[14–16]

While SGAs are less likely to cause TD,[17–23] the condition still occurs with these medications. An extensive meta-analysis of relevant studies found the annualised incidence of TD across all FGA treatment groups was 6.5%, while the respective figure for SGA treatment groups was 2.6%.[24] However, there is a significant variation in liability between individual SGA medications.[24–28] The risk of developing TD may be related to the extent of D2 receptor occupancy (greater occupancy, higher risk) with a medication,[29] although data from the meta-analysis mentioned above did not support the notion that the lower risk of TD with SGAs is a consequence of the use of relatively high equivalent doses of FGAs.[24] There is a hint that dopamine partial agonists (or, at least, aripiprazole) may have the lowest liability for TD.[24] Whether the risk of TD differs between LAI FGA and LAI SGA preparations is unclear[30] but there is one report suggesting that the risk of TD with LAI SGAs is lower than with the equivalent oral SGA preparations.[31]

TD can occur even with low doses of haloperidol (and in the absence of prior acute movement disorder)[32] and with the use of other dopamine antagonists such as metoclopramide.[33] The characteristic abnormal involuntary movements of TD have also been observed in never-medicated patients with both first-episode[34,35] and established[36] schizophrenia. This suggests that the use of antipsychotic medication adds to an inherent risk of TD that is present in people with a diagnosis of schizophrenia.

Treatment – first steps

Most authorities recommend the withdrawal of any co-prescribed anticholinergic agents and a reduction in the dose of antipsychotic medication (which may initially worsen TD) as initial steps in those with early signs of TD,[37,38] although there is a lack of robust evidence to support such a strategy.[14,39–41] Nevertheless, it is common practice to withdraw the antipsychotic prescribed when TD is first observed and to substitute it with an antipsychotic medication that is perceived to have a lower liability for the condition. However, the evidence for a beneficial effect on TD when switching to any particular SGA is limited.[42] Changing to clozapine[37,43] is probably best supported,[37,43–45] but quetiapine, another weak striatal dopamine antagonist, may also be effective.[46–52] Olanzapine[39–42,53,54] and aripiprazole[55] are also potential options.

Treatment – additional agents

Given that there is insufficient evidence to recommend dose reduction as a treatment for TD, and that switching or withdrawing antipsychotic medication is not always effective or advisable, add-on agents are often considered. Evidence-based, pharmacological treatment algorithms for TD have been published.[41,56] A 2020 meta-analysis[57] concluded that vesicular monoamine transporter 2 (VMAT-2) inhibitors (such as deutetrabenazine and valbenazine), vitamin E, amantadine and vitamin B6 (pyridoxine) are probably effective treatments. VMAT-2 inhibitors are considered agents of first choice, given the body of evidence supporting their use[58–60] and their additional antipsychotic action.[61] Table 1.29 describes the most frequently prescribed add-on medications for TD.

Table 1.29 First-choice agents prescribed for tardive dyskinesia (alphabetical order; no preference implied).

Drug	Comments
Amantadine[56,57,62–64]	Rarely used and evidence for efficacy is limited. Dose is 100–300mg/day.
Benzodiazepines[37,38]	Widely used for TD, but a Cochrane review considered that the limited evidence for efficacy was inconclusive.[65] Intermittent use may be necessary to avoid tolerance to effects. Most commonly used are clonazepam 1–4mg/day and diazepam 6–25mg/day, with better supporting evidence for clonazepam.[42,66]
Deutetrabenazine[8,56,58,60,67,68]	Deutetrabenazine (a VMAT-2 inhibitor) is effective as a treatment for TD. Licensed for TD in the USA.[69] Better supporting evidence than for tetrabenazine. Longer half-life than tetrabenazine but still needs to be taken twice a day (a once daily slow-release tablet is in development).[70] Low incidence of psychiatric and neurological effects. Dose is 12–48mg/day.
Ginkgo biloba[56,71,72]	Well tolerated. A Cochrane review concluded that while Ginkgo biloba could reduce TD symptoms, the available evidence did not justify its routine use as a treatment.[73] A meta-analysis of three Chinese RCTs showed a good effect with 240mg/day.[74]
Pyridoxine[75]	Supported by a Cochrane review[76] and a 2020 meta-analysis.[57] Dose is up to 400mg/day.
Tetrabenazine[77,78]	The only licensed treatment for moderate to severe TD in UK. Depression, drowsiness, parkinsonism and akathisia may occur.[66,79] Dose is 25–200mg/day. Reserpine (similar mode of action) also effective but rarely, if ever, used.
Valbenazine[8,59,67,73,80]	Evidence supports a favourable benefit–risk ratio for valbenazine (VMAT-2 inhibitor) as a treatment for TD. Licensed for TD in the USA.[81] A dose of 80mg once daily is effective. It has a benign cardiovascular profile and a low incidence of depression and akathisia.
Vitamin E[57,82]	Numerous studies but efficacy remains to be conclusively established. A Cochrane review suggested that there is evidence only for slowing the deterioration of TD,[8,83] but a 2022 meta-analysis also suggested a treatment effect.[84] Dose is in the range 400–1600 IU/day.

Treatment – other possible options

The large number of proposed treatments for TD undoubtedly reflects the somewhat limited effectiveness of standard remedies, at least before the introduction of valbenazine and deutetrabenazine.[14] Table 1.30 lists some of these putative treatments, most of which have a low level of evidence.[8,62]

Table 1.30 Other options for the treatment of tardive dyskinesia (in alphabetical order).

Drug	Comments
Amino acids[85]	Use is supported by a small randomised, placebo-controlled trial. Low risk of toxicity.
Botulinum toxin[86–89]	Case reports of success for localised dyskinesia. Probably now treatment of choice for disabling or distressing focal symptoms.
Calcium antagonists[90]	A few published studies but not widely used. A Cochrane review is dismissive.[91] A 2020 meta-analysis found no effect.[57]
DBS[8,92,93]	Reports refer most commonly to stimulation of the globus pallidus internus. The evidence is limited but DBS may potentially have a role when TD symptoms are severe and distressing and unresponsive to pharmacological treatment.
Donepezil[94–96]	Supported by a single open study and a case series. One very small, negative RCT. Dose is 10mg/day. No clear evidence of efficacy for rivastigmine or galantamine.[97]
Fish oils[98,99]	Very limited support for use of EPA at dose of 2g/day.
Fluvoxamine[100]	Three case reports. Dose is 100mg/day. Beware interactions.
Gabapentin[101]	Adds weight to the theory that GABAergic mechanisms improve TD. Dose is 900–1200mg/day. Inconclusive data on other GABA agonists.[102]
Levetiracetam[103–106]	Three published case studies. One RCT. Dose up to 3000mg/day.
Melatonin[107]	Use is supported by a meta-analysis of four trials.[108] Usually well tolerated. Dose is 10mg/day. Some evidence that melatonin receptor genotype determines risk of TD.[109]
Naltrexone[110]	May be effective when added to benzodiazepines. Well tolerated. Dose is 200mg/day.
Ondansetron[111,112]	Limited evidence but low toxicity. Dose is up to 12mg/day.
Propranolol[113–115]	Formerly a relatively widely used treatment. Open-label studies only but a prospective randomised trial is probably warranted. Dose is 40–120mg/day. Beware contraindications, such as asthma, bradycardia and hypotension.
Quercetin[116]	Plant compound which is thought to be an antioxidant. Some promising case reports.[116–118]
Sodium oxybate[119]	One case report. Dose was 8g/day.
rTMS[120,121]	RCT data on patients with 'tardive syndromes' suggest that bilateral hemispheric high-frequency rTMS has the potential to be a feasible treatment where TD is unresponsive to 'first-line' pharmacological treatment[120]
Zolpidem[122]	Three case reports. Dose is 10–30mg a day.

DBS, deep brain stimulation; EPA, eicosapentaenoic acid; GABA, gamma-aminobutyric acid; rTMS, repetitive transcranial magnetic stimulation.

References

1. Merrill RM, et al. Tardive and spontaneous dyskinesia incidence in the general population. *BMC Psychiatry* 2013; **13**:152.
2. Kane JM, et al. Tardive dyskinesia: prevalence, incidence, and risk factors. *J Clin Psychopharmacol* 1988; 8 4 Suppl:52s–56s.
3. de Leon J. The effect of atypical versus typical antipsychotics on tardive dyskinesia: a naturalistic study. *Eur Arch Psychiatry Clin Neurosci* 2007; **257**:169–172.
4. Halliday J, et al. Nithsdale Schizophrenia Surveys 23: movement disorders: 20-year review. *Br J Psychiatry* 2002; **181**:422–427.
5. Kane JM. Tardive dyskinesia circa 2006. *Am J Psychiatry* 2006; **163**:1316–1318.
6. Eberhard J, et al. Tardive dyskinesia and antipsychotics: a 5-year longitudinal study of frequency, correlates and course. *Int Clin Psychopharmacol* 2006; **21**:35–42.
7. Wu JQ, et al. Tardive dyskinesia is associated with greater cognitive impairment in schizophrenia. *Prog Neuropsychopharmacol Biol Psychiatry* 2013; **46**:71–77.

8. Ricciardi L, et al. Treatment recommendations for tardive dyskinesia. *Can J Psychiatry* 2019; **64**:388–399.

9. Strassnig M, et al. Tardive dyskinesia: motor system impairments, cognition and everyday functioning. *CNS Spectr* 2018; **23**:370–377.

10. Yuen O, et al. Tardive dyskinesia and positive and negative symptoms of schizophrenia: a study using instrumental measures. *Br J Psychiatry* 1996; **168**:702–708.

11. Ascher-Svanum H, et al. Tardive dyskinesia and the 3-year course of schizophrenia: results from a large, prospective, naturalistic study. *J Clin Psychiatry* 2008; **69**:1580–1588.

12. Dean CE, et al. Mortality and tardive dyskinesia: long-term study using the US National Death Index. *Br J Psychiatry* 2009; **194**:360–364.

13. Chong SA, et al. Mortality rates among patients with schizophrenia and tardive dyskinesia. *J Clin Psychopharmacol* 2009; **29**:5–8.

14. Caroff SN. Overcoming barriers to effective management of tardive dyskinesia. *Neuropsychiatr Dis Treat* 2019; **15**:785–794.

15. Barer Y, et al. The clinical and economic burden of tardive dyskinesia in Israel: real-world data analysis. *J Clin Psychopharmacol* 2022; **42**:454–460.

16. Jain R, et al. Impact of tardive dyskinesia on physical, psychological, social, and professional domains of patient lives: a survey of patients in the United States. *J Clin Psychiatry* 2023; **84**:22m14694.

17. Beasley C, et al. Randomised double-blind comparison of the incidence of tardive dyskinesia in patients with schizophrenia during long-term treatment with olanzapine or haloperidol. *Br J Psychiatry* 1999; **174**:23–30.

18. Glazer WM. Expected incidence of tardive dyskinesia associated with atypical antipsychotics. *J Clin Psychiatry* 2000; **61** Suppl 4:21–26.

19. Correll CU, et al. Lower risk for tardive dyskinesia associated with second-generation antipsychotics: a systematic review of 1-year studies. *Am J Psychiatry* 2004; **161**:414–425.

20. Dolder CR, et al. Incidence of tardive dyskinesia with typical versus atypical antipsychotics in very high risk patients. *Biol Psychiatry* 2003; **53**:1142–1145.

21. Correll CU, et al. Tardive dyskinesia and new antipsychotics. *Current Opin Psychiatry* 2008; **21**:151–156.

22. Carbon M, et al. Tardive dyskinesia prevalence in the period of second-generation antipsychotic use: a meta-analysis. *J Clin Psychiatry* 2017; **78**:e264–e278.

23. O'Brien A. Comparing the risk of tardive dyskinesia in older adults with first-generation and second-generation antipsychotics: a systematic review and meta-analysis. *Int J Geriatr Psychiatry* 2016; **31**:683–693.

24. Carbon M, et al. Tardive dyskinesia risk with first- and second-generation antipsychotics in comparative randomized controlled trials: a meta-analysis. *World Psychiatry* 2018; **17**:330–340.

25. Keck ME, et al. Ziprasidone-related tardive dyskinesia [Letter]. *Am J Psychiatry* 2004; **161**:175–176.

26. Maytal G, et al. Aripiprazole-related tardive dyskinesia. *CNS Spectr* 2006; **11**:435–439.

27. Fountoulakis KN, et al. Amisulpride-induced tardive dyskinesia. *Schizophr Res* 2006; **88**:232–234.

28. Sachdev P. Early extrapyramidal side-effects as risk factors for later tardive dyskinesia: a prospective study. *Aust N Z J Psychiatry* 2004; **38**:445–449.

29. Yoshida K, et al. Tardive dyskinesia in relation to estimated dopamine D2 receptor occupancy in patients with schizophrenia: analysis of the CATIE data. *Schizophr Res* 2014; **153**:184–188.

30. Saucedo Uribe E, et al. Preliminary efficacy and tolerability profiles of first versus second-generation Long-Acting Injectable antipsychotics in schizophrenia: a systematic review and meta-analysis. *J Psychiatr Res* 2020; **129**:222–233.

31. Misawa F, et al. Tardive dyskinesia and long-acting injectable antipsychotics: analyses based on a spontaneous reporting system database in Japan. *J Clin Psychiatry* 2022; **83**:21m14304.

32. Oosthuizen PP, et al. Incidence of tardive dyskinesia in first-episode psychosis patients treated with low-dose haloperidol. *J Clin Psychiatry* 2003; **64**:1075–1080.

33. Kenney C, et al. Metoclopramide, an increasingly recognized cause of tardive dyskinesia. *J Clin Pharmacol* 2008; **48**:379–384.

34. Pappa S, et al. Spontaneous movement disorders in antipsychotic-naive patients with first-episode psychoses: a systematic review. *Psychol Med* 2009; **39**:1065–1076.

35. Puri BK, et al. Spontaneous dyskinesia in first episode schizophrenia. *J Neurol Neurosurg Psychiatry* 1999; **66**:76–78.

36. McCreadie RG, et al. Spontaneous dyskinesia and parkinsonism in never-medicated, chronically ill patients with schizophrenia: 18-month follow-up. *Br J Psychiatry* 2002; **181**:135–137.

37. Duncan D, et al. Tardive dyskinesia: how is it prevented and treated? *Psychiatric Bulletin* 1997; **21**:422–425.

38. Simpson GM. The treatment of tardive dyskinesia and tardive dystonia. *J Clin Psychiatry* 2000; **61** Suppl 4:39–44.

39. Bergman H, et al. Antipsychotic reduction and/or cessation and antipsychotics as specific treatments for tardive dyskinesia. *Cochrane Database Syst Rev* 2018; **2**:CD000459.

40. Bergman H, et al. Anticholinergic medication for antipsychotic-induced tardive dyskinesia. *Cochrane Database Syst Rev* 2018; **1**:CD000204.

41. Owens DC. Tardive dyskinesia update: treatment and management. *BJPsych Advances* 2019; **25**:78–89.

42. Bhidayasiri R, et al. Evidence-based guideline: treatment of tardive syndromes: report of the Guideline Development Subcommittee of the American Academy of Neurology. *Neurology* 2013; **81**:463–469.

43. Pardis P, et al. Clozapine and tardive dyskinesia in patients with schizophrenia: a systematic review. *J Psychopharmacol* 2019; **33**:1187–1198.

44. Mentzel TQ, et al. Clozapine monotherapy as a treatment for antipsychotic-induced tardive dyskinesia: a meta-analysis. *J Clin Psychiatry* 2018; **79**:17r11852.

45. Wong J, et al. A systematic review on the use of clozapine in treatment of tardive dyskinesia and tardive dystonia in patients with psychiatric disorders. *Psychopharmacology (Berl)* 2022; **239**:3393–3420.

46. Vesely C, et al. Remission of severe tardive dyskinesia in a schizophrenic patient treated with the atypical antipsychotic substance quetiapine. *Int Clin Psychopharmacol* 2000; **15**:57–60.

47. Alptekin K, et al. Quetiapine-induced improvement of tardive dyskinesia in three patients with schizophrenia. *Int Clin Psychopharmacol* 2002; **17**:263–264.

48. Nelson MW, et al. Adjunctive quetiapine decreases symptoms of tardive dyskinesia in a patient taking risperidone. *Clin Neuropharmacol* 2003; **26**:297–298.

49. Emsley R, et al. A single-blind, randomized trial comparing quetiapine and haloperidol in the treatment of tardive dyskinesia. *J Clin Psychiatry* 2004; **65**:696–701.

50. Bressan RA, et al. Atypical antipsychotic drugs and tardive dyskinesia: relevance of D2 receptor affinity. *J Psychopharmacol* 2004; **18**:124–127.

51. Sacchetti E, et al. Quetiapine, clozapine, and olanzapine in the treatment of tardive dyskinesia induced by first-generation antipsychotics: a 124-week case report. *Int Clin Psychopharmacol* 2003; **18**:357–359.

52. Gourzis P, et al. Quetiapine in the treatment of focal tardive dystonia induced by other atypical antipsychotics: a report of 2 cases. *Clin Neuropharmacol* 2005; **28**:195–196.

53. Soutullo CA, et al. Olanzapine in the treatment of tardive dyskinesia: a report of two cases. *J Clin Psychopharmacol* 1999; **19**:100-101.

54. Kinon BJ, et al. Olanzapine treatment for tardive dyskinesia in schizophrenia patients: a prospective clinical trial with patients randomized to blinded dose reduction periods. *Prog Neuropsychopharmacol Biol Psychiatry* 2004; **28**:985–996.

55. Chan CH, et al. Switching antipsychotic treatment to aripiprazole in psychotic patients with neuroleptic-induced tardive dyskinesia: a 24-week follow-up study. *Int Clin Psychopharmacol* 2018; **33**:155–162.

56. Bhidayasiri R, et al. Updating the recommendations for treatment of tardive syndromes: a systematic review of new evidence and practical treatment algorithm. *J Neurol Sci* 2018; **389**:67–75.

57. Artukoglu BB, et al. Pharmacologic treatment of tardive dyskinesia: a meta-analysis and systematic review. *J Clin Psychiatry* 2020; **81**:19r12798.

58. Hauser RA, et al. Long-term deutetrabenazine treatment for tardive dyskinesia is associated with sustained benefits and safety: a 3-year, open-label extension study. *Front Neurol* 2022; **13**:773999.

59. Golsorkhi M, et al. Comparative analysis of deutetrabenazine and valbenazine as VMAT2 inhibitors for tardive dyskinesia: a systematic review. *Tremor Other Hyperkinet Mov* 2024; **14**:13.

60. Frank S, et al. Clinical utility of deutetrabenazine as a treatment option for chorea associated with Huntington's disease and tardive dyskinesia. *Ther Clin Risk Manag* 2023; **19**:1019–1024.

61. Connolly A, et al. Meta-analysis and systematic review of vesicular monoamine transporter (VMAT-2) inhibitors in schizophrenia and psychosis. *Psychopharmacology (Berl)* 2024; **241**:225–241.

62. Takeuchi H, et al. Pathophysiology, prognosis and treatment of tardive dyskinesia. *Ther Adv Psychopharmacol* 2022; **12**:20451253221117313.

63. Angus S, et al. A controlled trial of amantadine hydrochloride and neuroleptics in the treatment of tardive dyskinesia. *J Clin Psychopharmacol* 1997; **17**:88–91.

64. Pappa S, et al. Effects of amantadine on tardive dyskinesia: a randomized, double-blind, placebo-controlled study. *Clin Neuropharmacol* 2010; **33**:271–275.

65. Bergman H, et al. Benzodiazepines for antipsychotic-induced tardive dyskinesia. *Cochrane Database Syst Rev* 2018; **1**:CD000205.

66. Rana AQ, et al. New and emerging treatments for symptomatic tardive dyskinesia. *Drug Des Devel Ther* 2013; **7**:1329–1340.

67. Solmi M, et al. Treatment of tardive dyskinesia with VMAT-2 inhibitors: a systematic review and meta-analysis of randomized controlled trials. *Drug Des Devel Ther* 2018; **12**:1215–1238.

68. Claassen DO, et al. Deutetrabenazine for tardive dyskinesia and chorea associated with Huntington's disease: a review of clinical trial data. *Expert Opin Pharmacother* 2019; **20**:2209–2221.

69. Citrome L. Deutetrabenazine for tardive dyskinesia: a systematic review of the efficacy and safety profile for this newly approved novel medication. What is the number needed to treat, number needed to harm and likelihood to be helped or harmed? *Int J Clin Pract* 2017; **71**:e13030.

70. Sunzel EM, et al. A bioequivalence comparison between the once-daily extended-release tablet and the twice-daily tablet formulations of deutetrabenazine at steady state. *Clin Pharmacol Drug Dev* 2024; **13**:224–232.

71. Zhang WF, et al. Extract of Ginkgo biloba treatment for tardive dyskinesia in schizophrenia: a randomized, double-blind, placebo-controlled trial. *J Clin Psychiatry* 2011; **72**:615–621.

72. Petridis PD, et al. Tardive dyskinesia suppressed with Ginkgo biloba. *J Clin Psychopharmacol* 2023; **43**:549–551.

73. Soares-Weiser K, et al. Miscellaneous treatments for antipsychotic-induced tardive dyskinesia. *Cochrane Database Syst Rev* 2018; **3**:CD000208.

74. Zheng W, et al. Extract of ginkgo biloba for tardive dyskinesia: meta-analysis of randomized controlled trials. *Pharmacopsychiatry* 2016; **49**:107–111.

75. Lerner V, et al. Vitamin B(6) in the treatment of tardive dyskinesia: a double-blind, placebo-controlled, crossover study. *Am J Psychiatry* 2001; **158**:1511–1514.

76. Adelufosi AO, et al. Pyridoxal 5 phosphate for neuroleptic-induced tardive dyskinesia. *Cochrane Database Syst Rev* 2015; (4): CD010501.

77. Jankovic J, et al. Long-term effects of tetrabenazine in hyperkinetic movement disorders. *Neurology* 1997; **48**:358–362.

78. Leung JG, et al. Tetrabenazine for the treatment of tardive dyskinesia. *Ann Pharmacother* 2011; **45**:525–531.

79. Kenney C, et al. Long-term tolerability of tetrabenazine in the treatment of hyperkinetic movement disorders. *Mov Disord* 2007; **22**:193–197.

80. Kishi T, et al. Valbenazine for tardive dyskinesia: a systematic review and network meta-analysis. *Int Clin Psychopharmacol* 2023; **38**:369–374.

81. Citrome LL. Medication options and clinical strategies for treating tardive dyskinesia. *J Clin Psychiatry* 2020; **81**:TV18059BR18052C.

82. Zhang XY, et al. The effect of vitamin E treatment on tardive dyskinesia and blood superoxide dismutase: a double-blind placebo-controlled trial. *J Clin Psychopharmacol* 2004; **24**:83–86.

83. Soares-Weiser K, et al. Vitamin E for antipsychotic-induced tardive dyskinesia. *Cochrane Database Syst Rev* 2018; 1:CD000209.

84. Xu H, et al. Vitamin E in the treatment of tardive dyskinesia: a meta-analysis. *Int Clin Psychopharmacol* 2022; 37:60–66.

85. Richardson MA, et al. Efficacy of the branched-chain amino acids in the treatment of tardive dyskinesia in men. *Am J Psychiatry* 2003; 160:1117–1124.

86. Tarsy D, et al. An open-label study of botulinum toxin A for treatment of tardive dystonia. *Clin Neuropharmacol* 1997; 20:90–93.

87. Brashear A, et al. Comparison of treatment of tardive dystonia and idiopathic cervical dystonia with botulinum toxin type A. *Mov Disord* 1998; 13:158–161.

88. Hennings JM, et al. Successful treatment of tardive lingual dystonia with botulinum toxin: case report and review of the literature. *Prog Neuropsychopharmacol Biol Psychiatry* 2008; 32:1167–1171.

89. Beckmann YY, et al. Treatment of intractable tardive lingual dyskinesia with botulinum toxin. *J Clin Psychopharmacol* 2011; 31:250–251.

90. Essali A, et al. Calcium channel blockers for neuroleptic-induced tardive dyskinesia. *Cochrane Database Syst Rev* 2011; (11):CD000206.

91. Essali A, et al. Calcium channel blockers for antipsychotic-induced tardive dyskinesia. *Cochrane Database Syst Rev* 2018; 3:CD000206.

92. Macerollo A, et al. Deep brain stimulation for tardive syndromes: systematic review and meta-analysis. *J Neurol Sci* 2018; 389:55–60.

93. Szczakowska A, et al. Deep brain stimulation in the treatment of tardive dyskinesia. *J Clin Med* 2023; 12:1868.

94. Caroff SN, et al. Treatment of tardive dyskinesia with donepezil. *J Clin Psychiatry* 2001; 62:128–129.

95. Bergman J, et al. Beneficial effect of donepezil in the treatment of elderly patients with tardive movement disorders. *J Clin Psychiatry* 2005; 66:107–110.

96. Ogunmefun A, et al. Effect of donepezil on tardive dyskinesia. *J Clin Psychopharmacol* 2009; 29:102–104.

97. Tammenmaa-Aho I, et al. Cholinergic medication for antipsychotic-induced tardive dyskinesia. *Cochrane Database Syst Rev* 2018; 3:CD000207.

98. Emsley R, et al. The effects of eicosapentaenoic acid in tardive dyskinesia: a randomized, placebo-controlled trial. *Schizophr Res* 2006; 84:112–120.

99. Vaddadi K, et al. Tardive dyskinesia and essential fatty acids. *Int Rev Psychiatry* 2006; 18:133–143.

100. Albayrak Y, et al. Benefical effects of sigma-1 agonist fluvoxamine for tardive dyskinesia and tardive akathisia in patients with schizophrenia: report of three cases. *Psychiatry Investig* 2013; 10:417–420.

101. Hardoy MC, et al. Gabapentin in antipsychotic-induced tardive dyskinesia: results of 1-year follow-up. *J Affect Disord* 2003; 75:125–130.

102. Alabed S, et al. Gamma-aminobutyric acid agonists for antipsychotic-induced tardive dyskinesia. *Cochrane Database Syst Rev* 2018; 4:CD000203.

103. McGavin CL, et al. Levetiracetam as a treatment for tardive dyskinesia: a case report. *Neurology* 2003; 61:419.

104. Meco G, et al. Levetiracetam in tardive dyskinesia. *Clin Neuropharmacol* 2006; 29:265–268.

105. Woods SW, et al. Effects of levetiracetam on tardive dyskinesia: a randomized, double-blind, placebo-controlled study. *J Clin Psychiatry* 2008; 69:546–554.

106. Chen PH, et al. Rapid improvement of neuroleptic-induced tardive dyskinesia with levetiracetam in an interictal psychotic patient. *J Clin Psychopharmacol* 2010; 30:205–207.

107. Shamir E, et al. Melatonin treatment for tardive dyskinesia: a double-blind, placebo-controlled, crossover study. *Arch Gen Psychiatry* 2001; 58:1049–1052.

108. Sun CH, et al. Adjunctive melatonin for tardive dyskinesia in patients with schizophrenia: a meta-analysis. *Shanghai Arch Psychiatry* 2017; 29:129–136.

109. Lai IC, et al. Analysis of genetic variations in the human melatonin receptor (MTNR1A, MTNR1B) genes and antipsychotics-induced tardive dyskinesia in schizophrenia. *World J Biol Psychiatry* 2011; 12:143–148.

110. Wonodi I, et al. Naltrexone treatment of tardive dyskinesia in patients with schizophrenia. *J Clin Psychopharmacol* 2004; 24:441–445.

111. Sirota P, et al. Use of the selective serotonin 3 receptor antagonist ondansetron in the treatment of neuroleptic-induced tardive dyskinesia. *Am J Psychiatry* 2000; 157:287–289.

112. Naidu PS, et al. Reversal of neuroleptic-induced orofacial dyskinesia by 5-HT3 receptor antagonists. *Eur J Pharmacol* 2001; 420:113–117.

113. Perenyi A, et al. Propranolol in the treatment of tardive dyskinesia. *Biol Psychiatry* 1983; 18:391–394.

114. Pitts FN, Jr. Treatment of tardive dyskinesia with propranolol. *J Clin Psychiatry* 1982; 43:304.

115. Hatcher-Martin JM, et al. Propranolol therapy for tardive dyskinesia: a retrospective examination. *Parkinsonism Relat Disord* 2016; 32:124–126.

116. Naidu PS, et al. Reversal of haloperidol-induced orofacial dyskinesia by quercetin, a bioflavonoid. *Psychopharmacology (Berl)* 2003; 167:418–423.

117. Naidu PS, et al. Quercetin, a bioflavonoid, attenuates haloperidol-induced orofacial dyskinesia. *Neuropharmacology* 2003; 44:1100–1106.

118. Naidu PS, et al. Reversal of reserpine-induced orofacial dyskinesia and cognitive dysfunction by quercetin. *Pharmacology* 2004; 70:59–67.

119. Berner JE. A case of sodium oxybate treatment of tardive dyskinesia and bipolar disorder. *J Clin Psychiatry* 2008; 69:862.

120. Khedr EM, et al. Repetitive transcranial magnetic stimulation for treatment of tardive syndromes: double randomized clinical trial. *J Neural Transm (Vienna)* 2019; 126:183–191.

121. Brambilla P, et al. Transient improvement of tardive dyskinesia induced with rTMS. *Neurology* 2003; 61:1155.

122. Waln O, et al. Zolpidem improves tardive dyskinesia and akathisia. *Mov Disord* 2013; 28:1748–1749.

Antipsychotic-induced weight gain

Weight gain is a common adverse effect of antipsychotic medication.[1] This may reflect interference with the homeostatic control of appetite and metabolism, leading to increased food intake and reduced energy expenditure, although the various mechanisms involved are not well understood.[2-4] Factors such as $5HT_{2C}$ antagonism, H_1 antagonism, D_2 antagonism and increased serum leptin (leading to leptin desensitisation)[5-7] are commonly implicated, as well as, possibly, effects on gut microbiota.[8-11]

The risk of weight gain appears to be related to clinical response[12,13] (although the association may be too small to be clinically important)[14] and may have a genetic basis.[15] Weight gain may be more pronounced in antipsychotic-naïve patients and during the early stages of the treatment of psychotic illness[16-18] and women may be at greater risk than men.[19,20]

Almost all available antipsychotic medications have been associated with weight gain,[16] although the mean gain in body weight varies substantially between the medications. There is also marked inter-individual variation among those treated, with some losing weight, some gaining no weight and some gaining a great deal of weight. Thus, knowledge of the mean increase in weight reported for a particular medication may not be a helpful predictor of how much weight an individual might gain. Assessment of the relative liability for weight gain of different antipsychotic medications is based largely on short-term studies. Notwithstanding these limitations, the results of indirect and direct meta-analyses suggest that these medications can be clustered into three groups based on their relative risk of weight gain (Table 1.31).[21,22]

Table 1.31 Risk/extent of antipsychotic-induced weight gain (drugs in alphabetical order).[23-26]

Risk/extent of weight gain	Drug
High	Clozapine
	Olanzapine
Moderate	Chlorpromazine
	FGAs*
	Iloperidone
	Haloperidol
	Quetiapine
	Paliperidone
	Risperidone
	Sertindole

(Continued)

CHAPTER 1

Table 1.31 (Continued)

Risk/extent of weight gain	Drug
Low	Amisulpride
	Aripiprazole
	Asenapine
	Brexpiprazole
	Cariprazine
	Lumateperone
	Lurasidone
	Sulpiride
	Trifluoperazine
	Ziprasidone

*Data on individual FGAs other than chlorpromazine and haloperidol are scarce but one comprehensive analysis showed that FGAs (not including haloperidol) had a moderate risk of weight gain: 20–30% of people gained more than 7% of original body weight in the medium term.[16] Individual FGAs are likely to vary in their propensity for weight gain. Traditionally low-potency FGAs (e.g. chlorpromazine) were considered to have a higher risk of weight gain.

Time course

Antipsychotic-induced weight gain occurs primarily in the first few months of treatment but continues for many months or even years afterwards. In a 10-year study of patients with first-episode schizophrenia, the mean weight gain was 15kg. Most of this (9kg) was gained in the first year.[27] In those gaining the most weight, increase in weight continues at the same rate for at least 2 years.[28]

Dose–response

The relationship between dose and weight gain is complex and varies from one antipsychotic medication to another.[22,29] Two broad patterns have emerged: an increase in weight gained over a lower dose range, which then reaches a plateau (e.g. risperidone, haloperidol and quetiapine), and an increasing risk of weight gain up to and beyond the maximum dose (e.g. clozapine and olanzapine). Both patterns suggest that dose reduction might reverse or mitigate weight gain and there is some evidence that this is possible.[30] However, the dose–response relationships identified indicate that the risk of weight gain emerges at doses that are subtherapeutic for psychosis, meaning that there is no effective dose that does not carry a risk of weight gain.

See following section for advice on the treatment of antipsychotic-induced weight gain.

References

1. Barton BB, et al. Update on weight-gain caused by antipsychotics: a systematic review and meta-analysis. *Expert Opin Drug Saf* 2020; **19**:295–314.
2. Correll CU, et al. Antipsychotic drugs and obesity. *Trends Mol Med* 2011; **17**:97–107.
3. Stogios N, et al. Antipsychotic-induced weight gain in severe mental illness: risk factors and special considerations. *Curr Psychiatry Reps* 2023; **25**:707–721.
4. Cuerda C, et al. The effects of second-generation antipsychotics on food intake, resting energy expenditure and physical activity. *Eur J Clin Nutr* 2014; **68**:146–152.
5. Nielsen MO, et al. Striatal reward activity and antipsychotic-associated weight change in patients with schizophrenia undergoing initial treatment. *JAMA Psychiatry* 2016; **73**:121–128.
6. Ragguett RM, et al. Association between antipsychotic treatment and leptin levels across multiple psychiatric populations: an updated meta-analysis. *Hum Psychopharmacol* 2017; **32**:e2631.
7. Reynolds GP, et al. Mechanisms underlying metabolic disturbances associated with psychosis and antipsychotic drug treatment. *J Psychopharmacol* 2017; **31**:1430–1436.
8. Kanji S, et al. The microbiome–gut–brain axis: implications for schizophrenia and antipsychotic induced weight gain. *Eur Arch Psychiatry Clin Neurosci* 2018; **268**:3–15.
9. Qian L, et al. Longitudinal gut microbiota dysbiosis underlies olanzapine-induced weight gain. *Microbiol Spectr* 2023; **11**:e0005823.
10. Fang X, et al. The role of the gut microbiome in weight-gain in schizophrenia patients treated with atypical antipsychotics: evidence based on altered composition and function in a cross-sectional study. *Psychiatry Res* 2023; **328**:115463.
11. Ye W, et al. Mechanism and treatments of antipsychotic-induced weight gain. *Int J Obes (Lond)* 2023; **47**:423–433.
12. Garcia-Rizo C. Antipsychotic-induced weight gain and clinical improvement: a psychiatric paradox. *Front Psychiatry* 2020; **11**:560006.
13. Smith ECC, et al. Clinical improvement in schizophrenia during antipsychotic treatment in relation to changes in glucose parameters: a systematic review. *Psychiatry Res* 2023; **328**:115472.
14. Hermes E, et al. The association between weight change and symptom reduction in the CATIE schizophrenia trial. *Schizophr Res* 2011; **128**:166–170.
15. Zhang JP, et al. Pharmacogenetic associations of antipsychotic drug-related weight gain: a systematic review and meta-analysis. *Schizophr Bull* 2016; **42**:1418–1437.
16. Bak M, et al. Almost all antipsychotics result in weight gain: a meta-analysis. *PLoS One* 2014; **9**:e94112.
17. McEvoy JP, et al. Efficacy and tolerability of olanzapine, quetiapine, and risperidone in the treatment of early psychosis: a randomized, double-blind 52-week comparison. *Am J Psychiatry* 2007; **164**:1050–1060.
18. Vochoskova K, et al. Weight and metabolic changes in early psychosis—association with daily quantification of medication exposure during the first hospitalization. *Acta Psychiatr Scand* 2023; **148**:265–276.
19. Seeman MV. Secondary effects of antipsychotics: women at greater risk than men. *Schizophr Bull* 2009; **35**:937–948.
20. Stamoula E, et al. Weight gain, gender, and antipsychotics: a disproportionality analysis of the FDA Adverse Event Reporting System database (FAERS). *Expert Opin Drug Saf* 2024; **23**:239–245.
21. Cooper SJ, et al. BAP guidelines on the management of weight gain, metabolic disturbances and cardiovascular risk associated with psychosis and antipsychotic drug treatment. *J Psychopharmacol* 2016; **30**:717–748.
22. Sabé M, et al. Comparative effects of 11 antipsychotics on weight gain and metabolic function in patients with acute schizophrenia: a dose-response meta-analysis. *J Clin Psychiatry* 2023; **84**:22r14490.
23. Leucht S, et al. Comparative efficacy and tolerability of 15 antipsychotic drugs in schizophrenia: a multiple-treatments meta-analysis. *Lancet* 2013; **382**:951–962.
24. Leucht S, et al. Sixty years of placebo-controlled antipsychotic drug trials in acute schizophrenia: systematic review, Bayesian meta-analysis, and meta-regression of efficacy predictors. *Am J Psychiatry* 2017; **174**:927–942.
25. Musil R, et al. Weight gain and antipsychotics: a drug safety review. *Expert Opin Drug Saf* 2015; **14**:73–96.
26. Pillinger T, et al. Comparative effects of 18 antipsychotics on metabolic function in patients with schizophrenia, predictors of metabolic dysregulation, and association with psychopathology: a systematic review and network meta-analysis. *Lancet Psychiatry* 2020; **7**:64–77.
27. Vázquez-Bourgon J, et al. Pattern of long-term weight and metabolic changes after a first episode of psychosis: results from a 10-year prospective follow-up of the PAFIP program for early intervention in psychosis cohort. *Eur Psychiatry* 2022; **65**:e48.
28. Chua YC, et al. A retrospective database study on 2-year weight trajectories in first-episode psychosis. *Front Psychiatry* 2023; **14**:1185874.
29. Wu H, et al. Antipsychotic-induced weight gain: dose-response meta-analysis of randomized controlled trials. *Schizophr Bull* 2022; **48**:643–654.
30. Speyer H, et al. Reversibility of antipsychotic-induced weight gain: a systematic review and meta-analysis. *Front Endocrinol (Lausanne)* 2021; **12**:577919.

Treatment of antipsychotic-induced weight gain

Weight gain is an important adverse effect of nearly all antipsychotic medications.[1,2] Women may be at greater risk than men.[3] An increase in body weight has obvious consequences for self-image, morbidity and mortality, so prevention and treatment are matters of some clinical urgency.

Monitoring

Patients starting antipsychotic treatment or changing medication should, as an absolute minimum, have their body weight recorded in their clinical records. Ideally, BMI and waist circumference should also be recorded.[4,5] Early in treatment, monitoring of body weight every week or two is recommended, for at least the first 6 months.[5,6] Rapid weight gain in early treatment (e.g. an increase of $\geq 5\%$ above baseline after a month of treatment) strongly predicts long-term weight gain and should prompt consideration of preventative or remedial measures.[7–10] With continuing antipsychotic treatment, annual measurement of body weight is recommended as a minimum.[5,6,11]

In clinical practice, the monitoring of body weight and other metabolic adverse effects in people on continuing antipsychotic medication is inconsistent and limited, falling short of recommended best practice.[12–16]

Treatment and prevention

Most of the relevant literature in this area addresses attempts to reduce body weight gained during treatment with medication, although there are useful data suggesting that early interventions can prevent or mitigate weight gain.[17,18]

When weight gain occurs, initial options involve switching a patient's antipsychotic medication or instituting behavioural programmes (or both). Switching always presents a risk of relapse and treatment discontinuation,[19] but there is fairly strong support for switching to aripiprazole,[20] ziprasidone[21] or lurasidone as a method for reversing weight gain.[20,22,23] Another option is adjunctive aripiprazole:[5] weight loss has been observed when aripiprazole has been added to antipsychotic medications such as clozapine and olanzapine.[18,24]

Stopping antipsychotic treatment altogether can be associated with weight loss[25,26] but this course of action would not be clinically appropriate for the vast majority of people with multi-episode schizophrenia. Note that, while some switching and augmentation strategies may minimise further weight gain or facilitate weight loss, the overall effect is generally modest, and many patients continue to be overweight.[27] Additional lifestyle interventions are often required if BMI is to remain within or move towards the normal range.

A variety of lifestyle interventions have been proposed and evaluated with generally good results.[5,17,28–31] Interventions do vary, but they are mainly 'behavioural lifestyle programmes' aimed at improving diet and increasing physical activity. Meta-analyses of RCTs have generally found a positive effect for both prevention and intervention with these non-pharmacological interventions.[17,29,32,33]

Pharmacological methods should be considered only where behavioural treatment strategies or switching to a medication with a lower liability for weight gain have failed

CHAPTER 1

or where obesity presents a clear, immediate physical risk to the patient. Some drug treatment options for antipsychotic-induced weight gain are listed in Table 1.32.

Metformin is now probably considered to be the drug of choice for the prevention and treatment of antipsychotic-induced weight gain, although glucagon-like peptide-1 (GLP-1) agonists may ultimately prove to be more effective and better tolerated.[34] Bariatric surgery may have a role in a few rare, severe cases where all else has failed.[35] However, the efficacy of bariatric surgery for drug-induced weight gain is not known.[5]

Table 1.32 Drug treatment of antipsychotic-induced weight gain (alphabetical order).

Drug	Comments
Alpha-lipoic acid[36–38] (1200mg/day)	Supplementation may lead to a small, short-term, weight loss. Limited data for antipsychotic-induced weight gain. Not recommended.
Amantadine[39,40] (100–300mg/day)	May attenuate olanzapine-related weight gain. Seems to be well tolerated apart from insomnia and abdominal discomfort. May (theoretically, at least) exacerbate psychosis. Evidence base too limited to recommend.[5]
Aripiprazole augmentation[18,31,41] (5–15mg/day)	RCTs show beneficial effects on weight loss and possibly other metabolic parameters when used as an adjunct to clozapine or olanzapine. Adjunctive use appears to be safe and unlikely to worsen psychosis. Recommended as a possible option for weight gain associated with clozapine or olanzapine. Not recommended with other antipsychotic medications.
Betahistine[42,43] (48mg/day)	May attenuate olanzapine-induced weight gain. Limited data. Not recommended.
Bupropion[44,45] (formerly amfebutamone)	Seems to be effective in obesity when combined with calorie-restricted diets. Appears to not exacerbate psychosis symptoms, at least when used for smoking cessation.[46] One small (positive) RCT in antipsychotic-related weight gain.[47]
Bupropion + naltrexone (Contrave/Mysimba)[48]	Combination approved for weight management as an adjunct to diet and exercise. No data in drug-induced weight gain. Not recommended but should not be ruled out.
Fluvoxamine[49–51] (50mg/day)	Earlier conflicting data but one short-term RCT shows attenuated clozapine-induced weight gain (possibly related to a higher clozapine to norclozapine ratio). Co-administration markedly increases clozapine levels, requiring extreme caution. Evidence base is too limited to recommend.
Liraglutide[52–54] (3mg/day via SC injection)	GLP-1 agonist that was previously approved for type 2 diabetes and more recently approved as an anti-obesity agent in non-diabetic patients. Dose for weight loss (3mg/day) is higher than the dose used for diabetes ($\leq$1.8mg). Limited data in drug-induced weight gain. One RCT shows significant weight loss in overweight pre-diabetic patients stable on olanzapine or clozapine.[52] Beneficial effects on other metabolic parameters. Well tolerated but can cause GI disturbances. Recommended option in pre-diabetic/diabetic patients and clozapine-induced weight gain. Other GLP-1 agonists are currently only approved for diabetes and have a more limited dose range. Exenatide LA (a once-weekly GLP-1 agonist) may be effective for weight loss in clozapine-treated patients[55] but perhaps not with other antipsychotics.[56]

(Continued)

Table 1.32 (*Continued*)

Drug	Comments
Melatonin[57–59] (up to 5mg at night)	One small RCT showing attenuation of olanzapine-induced weight gain. Other studies show negative results. Effect, if any, is small.
Metformin[5,31,60–62] (500–2000mg/day)	There is a substantial database (in non-diabetic patients) supporting the use of metformin in both reducing and reversing weight gain caused by antipsychotic medications (mainly olanzapine). A Cochrane review in 2022 concluded that there was 'low-certainty evidence to suggest that metformin may be effective in preventing weight gain' in people with schizophrenia.[62] There may also be beneficial effects on other metabolic parameters. A later cohort study[63] showed that metformin prevented weight gain with clozapine. One positive RCT[64] and extension study[65] in children and adolescents with autism spectrum disorder. May be ideal for those with weight gain and diabetes or polycystic ovary syndrome. Note that metformin treatment increases the risk of vitamin B12 deficiency.[66]
Modafinil[67,68] (up to 300mg/day)	Limited positive data and one negative RCT for clozapine-induced weight gain. Not recommended.
Naltrexone[69,70] (25–50mg/day)	Some positive results but evidence is limited to two small pilot RCTs. Not recommended.
Orlistat[71–76] (120mg shortly before or after each meal). Official maximum is three times daily.	Reliable effect in obesity, especially when combined with calorie restriction. Few published data in medication-induced weight gain but widely used in practice with some success. In trials for clozapine or olanzapine-induced weight gain effect was only seen in men.[75,76] When used without calorie restriction in psychiatric patients, the effects are very limited. Failure to adhere to a low-fat diet will result in fatty diarrhoea and possible malabsorption of orally administered medication. Overall, a good choice for clozapine-induced weight gain where it reduces both weight and the incidence of constipation.[77]
Reboxetine[18] (4–8mg/day)	Attenuates olanzapine-induced weight gain. Reverses some metabolic changes.[78] Effective when combined with betahistine.
Samidorphan (μ–opioid receptor antagonist)[79–85]	There is good evidence from RCTs that the combination of samidorphan and olanzapine can mitigate olanzapine-associated weight gain. But these findings need to be confirmed 'through further high-quality research'.[83] The combination was approved by the US FDA in 2021 for indications including the treatment of schizophrenia and bipolar I disorder.
Semaglutide (weekly injectable, glucagon–like peptide-1RA)[86,87]	A small case series suggested that semaglutide, up to 2mg/week, might reduce antipsychotic-associated weight gain that had not responded to metformin.
Topiramate[31,58,88,89] (up to 300mg/day)	Reliably reduces weight even when medication induced. Meta-analyses of RCTs suggest a greater effect for prevention rather than treatment. Problems may arise because of topiramate's propensity for causing sedation, confusion and cognitive impairment. May have antipsychotic properties.
Zonisamide[90] (100–600mg/day)	Antiepileptic drug with weight-reducing properties. An RCT of 150mg/day showed significant weight reduction in people receiving SGAs. Another RCT (up to 600mg/day) shows attenuated olanzapine-induced weight gain. Sedation, diarrhoea and cognitive impairment are the most common problems. Not recommended.

References

1. Pillinger T, et al. Comparative effects of 18 antipsychotics on metabolic function in patients with schizophrenia, predictors of metabolic dysregulation, and association with psychopathology: a systematic review and network meta-analysis. *Lancet Psychiatry* 2020; 7:64–77.

2. Bak M, et al. Almost all antipsychotics result in weight gain: a meta-analysis. *PLoS One* 2014; 9:e94112.

3. Stamoula E, et al. Weight gain, gender, and antipsychotics: a disproportionality analysis of the FDA Adverse Event Reporting System database (FAERS). *Expert Opin Drug Saf* 2024; 23:239–245.

4. Marder SR, et al. Physical health monitoring of patients with schizophrenia. *Am J Psychiatry* 2004; 161:1334–1349.

5. Cooper SJ, et al. BAP guidelines on the management of weight gain, metabolic disturbances and cardiovascular risk associated with psychosis and antipsychotic drug treatment. *J Psychopharmacol* 2016; 30:717–748.

6. Galletly C, et al. Royal Australian and New Zealand College of Psychiatrists clinical practice guidelines for the management of schizophrenia and related disorders. *Aust N Z J Psychiatry* 2016; 50:410–472.

7. American Diabetes Association, et al. Consensus development conference on antipsychotic drugs and obesity and diabetes. *Diabetes Care* 2004; 27:596–601.

8. Vandenberghe F, et al. Importance of early weight changes to predict long-term weight gain during psychotropic drug treatment. *J Clin Psychiatry* 2015; 76:e1417–1423.

9. Lipkovich I, et al. Early evaluation of patient risk for substantial weight gain during olanzapine treatment for schizophrenia, schizophreniform, or schizoaffective disorder. *BMC Psychiatry* 2008; 8:78.

10. Fitzgerald I, et al. Predicting antipsychotic-induced weight gain in first episode psychosis: a field-wide systematic review and meta-analysis of non-genetic prognostic factors. *Eur Psychiatry* 2023; 66:e42.

11. National Institute for Health and Care Excellence. Psychosis and schizophrenia in adults. Quality standard [QS80]. 2015 (last accessed February 2024); https://www.nice.org.uk/guidance/qs80.

12. Mitchell AJ, et al. Guideline concordant monitoring of metabolic risk in people treated with antipsychotic medication: systematic review and meta-analysis of screening practices. *Psychol Med* 2012; 42:125–147.

13. Barnes TR, et al. Screening for the metabolic side effects of antipsychotic medication: findings of a 6-year quality improvement programme in the UK. *BMJ Open* 2015; 5:e007633.

14. Crawford MJ, et al. Assessment and treatment of physical health problems among people with schizophrenia: national cross-sectional study. *Br J Psychiatry* 2014; 205:473–477.

15. Hammoudeh S, et al. Risk factors of metabolic syndrome among patients receiving antipsychotics: a retrospective study. *Community Ment Health J* 2020; 56:760–770.

16. Ward T, et al. Who is responsible for metabolic screening for mental health clients taking antipsychotic medications? *Int J Ment Health Nurs* 2018; 27:196–203.

17. Bruins J, et al. The effects of lifestyle interventions on (long-term) weight management, cardiometabolic risk and depressive symptoms in people with psychotic disorders: a meta-analysis. *PLoS One* 2014; 9:e112276.

18. Mizuno Y, et al. Pharmacological strategies to counteract antipsychotic-induced weight gain and metabolic adverse effects in schizophrenia: a systematic review and meta-analysis. *Schizophr Bull* 2014; 40:1385–1403.

19. Stroup TS, et al. A randomized trial examining the effectiveness of switching from olanzapine, quetiapine, or risperidone to aripiprazole to reduce metabolic risk: comparison of antipsychotics for metabolic problems (CAMP). *Am J Psychiatry* 2011; 168:947–956.

20. Mukundan A, et al. Antipsychotic switching for people with schizophrenia who have neuroleptic-induced weight or metabolic problems. *Cochrane Database Syst Rev* 2010; (12):CD006629.

21. Montes JM, et al. Improvement in antipsychotic-related metabolic disturbances in patients with schizophrenia switched to ziprasidone. *Prog Neuropsychopharmacol Biol Psychiatry* 2007; 31:383–388.

22. Wu H, et al. Antipsychotic-induced weight gain: dose-response meta-analysis of randomized controlled trials. *Schizophr Bull* 2022; 48:643–654.

23. Akinola PS, et al. Antipsychotic-induced metabolic syndrome: a review. *Metab Syndr Relat Disord* 2023; 21:294–305.

24. Galling B, et al. Antipsychotic augmentation vs. monotherapy in schizophrenia: systematic review, meta-analysis and meta-regression analysis. *World Psychiatry* 2017; 16:77–89.

25. de Kuijper G, et al. Effects of controlled discontinuation of long-term used antipsychotics on weight and metabolic parameters in individuals with intellectual disability. *J Clin Psychopharmacol* 2013; 33:520–524.

26. Chen EY, et al. Maintenance treatment with quetiapine versus discontinuation after one year of treatment in patients with remitted first episode psychosis: randomised controlled trial. *BMJ* 2010; 341:c4024.

27. Speyer H, et al. Reversibility of antipsychotic-induced weight gain: a systematic review and meta-analysis. *Front Endocrinol (Lausanne)* 2021; 12:577919.

28. Werneke U, et al. Behavioural management of antipsychotic-induced weight gain: a review. *Acta Psychiatr Scand* 2003; 108:252–259.

29. Caemmerer J, et al. Acute and maintenance effects of non-pharmacologic interventions for antipsychotic associated weight gain and metabolic abnormalities: a meta-analytic comparison of randomized controlled trials. *Schizophr Res* 2012; 140:159–168.

30. Rice J, et al. Integrative management of metabolic syndrome in youth prescribed second-generation antipsychotics. *Med Sci (Basel)* 2020; 8:34.

31. Vancampfort D, et al. The impact of pharmacological and non-pharmacological interventions to improve physical health outcomes in people with schizophrenia: a meta-review of meta-analyses of randomized controlled trials. *World Psychiatry* 2019; 18:53–66.

32. Naslund JA, et al. Lifestyle interventions for weight loss among overweight and obese adults with serious mental illness: a systematic review and meta-analysis. *Gen Hosp Psychiatry* 2017; 47:83–102.

33. Mohanty K, et al. Effectiveness of lifestyle intervention on prevention/management of antipsychotic-induced weight gain among persons with severe mental illness: a systematic review and meta-analysis. *J Health Psychol* 2024; **29**:690–706.

34. Lee K, et al. Antipsychotic-induced weight gain: exploring the role of psychiatrists in managing patients' physical health – challenges, current options and direction for future care. *BJPsych Bull* 2024; **48**:24–29.

35. Manu P, et al. Weight gain and obesity in schizophrenia: epidemiology, pathobiology, and management. *Acta Psychiatr Scand* 2015; **132**:97–108.

36. Kucukgoncu S, et al. Alpha-lipoic acid (ALA) as a supplementation for weight loss: results from a meta-analysis of randomized controlled trials. *Obes Rev* 2017; **18**:594–601.

37. Kim E, et al. A preliminary investigation of alpha-lipoic acid treatment of antipsychotic drug-induced weight gain in patients with schizophrenia. *J Clin Psychopharmacol* 2008; **28**:138–146.

38. Ratliff JC, et al. An open-label pilot trial of alpha-lipoic acid for weight loss in patients with schizophrenia without diabetes. *Clin Schizophr Relat Psychoses* 2015; **8**:196–200.

39. Praharaj SK, et al. Amantadine for olanzapine-induced weight gain: a systematic review and meta-analysis of randomized placebo-controlled trials. *Ther Adv Psychopharmacol* 2012; **2**:151–156.

40. Zheng W, et al. Amantadine for antipsychotic-related weight gain: meta-analysis of randomized placebo-controlled trials. *J Clin Psychopharmacol* 2017; **37**:341–346.

41. Zheng W, et al. Efficacy and safety of adjunctive aripiprazole in schizophrenia: meta-analysis of randomized controlled trials. *J Clin Psychopharmacol* 2016; **36**:628–636.

42. Barak N, et al. A randomized, double-blind, placebo-controlled pilot study of betahistine to counteract olanzapine-associated weight gain. *J Clin Psychopharmacol* 2016; **36**:253–256.

43. Lian J, et al. Ameliorating antipsychotic-induced weight gain by betahistine: mechanisms and clinical implications. *Pharmacol Res* 2016; **106**:51–63.

44. Gadde KM, et al. Bupropion for weight loss: an investigation of efficacy and tolerability in overweight and obese women. *Obes Res* 2001; **9**:544–551.

45. Jain AK, et al. Bupropion SR vs. placebo for weight loss in obese patients with depressive symptoms. *Obes Res* 2002; **10**:1049–1056.

46. Tsoi DT, et al. Interventions for smoking cessation and reduction in individuals with schizophrenia. *Cochrane Database Syst Rev* 2013; 2:CD007253.

47. Weizman S, et al. A double-blind, placebo-controlled trial of bupropion add-on to olanzapine or risperidone in overweight individuals with schizophrenia. *J Clin Psychopharmacol* 2021; **41**:629–631.

48. Greig SL, et al. Naltrexone ER/bupropion ER: a review in obesity management. *Drugs* 2015; **75**:1269–1280.

49. Hinze-Selch D, et al. Effect of coadministration of clozapine and fluvoxamine versus clozapine monotherapy on blood cell counts, plasma levels of cytokines and body weight. *Psychopharmacology (Berl)* 2000; **149**:163–169.

50. Lu ML, et al. Effects of adjunctive fluvoxamine on metabolic parameters and psychopathology in clozapine-treated patients with schizophrenia: a 12-week, randomized, double-blind, placebo-controlled study. *Schizophr Res* 2017; **193**:126–133.

51. Lu ML, et al. Adjunctive fluvoxamine inhibits clozapine-related weight gain and metabolic disturbances. *J Clin Psychiatry* 2004; **65**:766–771.

52. Larsen JR, et al. Effect of liraglutide treatment on prediabetes and overweight or obesity in clozapine- or olanzapine-treated patients with schizophrenia spectrum disorder: a randomized clinical trial. *JAMA Psychiatry* 2017; **74**:719–728.

53. Mayfield K, et al. Glucagon-like peptide-1 agonists combating clozapine-associated obesity and diabetes. *J Psychopharmacol* 2016; **30**:227–236.

54. Lee K, et al. A systematic review of licensed weight-loss medications in treating antipsychotic-induced weight gain and obesity in schizophrenia and psychosis. *Gen Hosp Psychiatry* 2022; **78**:58–67.

55. Siskind D, et al. Treatment of clozapine-associated obesity and diabetes with exenatide (CODEX) in adults with schizophrenia: a randomised controlled trial. *Diabetes Obes Metab* 2017; **20**:1050–1055.

56. Ishoy PL, et al. Effect of GLP-1 receptor agonist treatment on body weight in obese antipsychotic-treated patients with schizophrenia: a randomized, placebo-controlled trial. *Diabetes Obes Metab* 2017; **19**:162–171.

57. Agahi M, et al. Effect of melatonin in reducing second-generation antipsychotic metabolic effects: a double blind controlled clinical trial. *Diabetes Metab Syndr* 2017; **12**:9–15.

58. Wang HR, et al. The role of melatonin and melatonin agonists in counteracting antipsychotic-induced metabolic side effects: a systematic review. *Int Clin Psychopharmacol* 2016; **31**:301–306.

59. Porfirio MC, et al. Can melatonin prevent or improve metabolic side effects during antipsychotic treatments? *Neuropsychiatr Dis Treat* 2017; **13**:2167–2174.

60. Zheng W, et al. Metformin for weight gain and metabolic abnormalities associated with antipsychotic treatment: meta-analysis of randomized placebo-controlled trials. *J Clin Psychopharmacol* 2015; **35**:499–509.

61. Wang C, et al. Outcomes and safety of concomitant topiramate or metformin for antipsychotics-induced obesity: a randomized-controlled trial. *Ann Gen Psychiatry* 2020; **19**:68.

62. Agarwal SM, et al. Pharmacological interventions for prevention of weight gain in people with schizophrenia. *Cochrane Database Syst Rev* 2022; **10**:CD013337.

63. Stogios N, et al. Metformin for the prevention of clozapine-induced weight gain: a retrospective naturalistic cohort study. *Acta Psychiatr Scand* 2022; **146**:190–200.

64. Anagnostou E, et al. Metformin for treatment of overweight induced by atypical antipsychotic medication in young people with autism spectrum disorder: a randomized clinical trial. *JAMA Psychiatry* 2016; **73**:928–937.

65. Handen BL, et al. A randomized, placebo-controlled trial of metformin for the treatment of overweight induced by antipsychotic medication in young people with autism spectrum disorder: open-label extension. *J Am Acad Child Adolesc Psychiatry* 2017; **56**:849-856.e6.
66. Chapman LE, et al. Association between metformin and vitamin B12 deficiency in patients with type 2 diabetes: a systematic review and meta-analysis. *Diabetes Metab* 2016; **42**:316–327.
67. Henderson DC, et al. Effects of modafinil on weight, glucose and lipid metabolism in clozapine-treated patients with schizophrenia. *Schizophr Res* 2011; **130**:53–56.
68. Roerig JL, et al. An exploration of the effect of modafinil on olanzapine associated weight gain in normal human subjects. *Biol Psychiatry* 2009; **65**:607–613.
69. Taveira TH, et al. The effect of naltrexone on body fat mass in olanzapine-treated schizophrenic or schizoaffective patients: a randomized double-blind placebo-controlled pilot study. *J Psychopharmacol* 2014; **28**:395–400.
70. Tek C, et al. A randomized, double-blind, placebo-controlled pilot study of naltrexone to counteract antipsychotic-associated weight gain: proof of concept. *J Clin Psychopharmacol* 2014; **34**:608–612.
71. Sjostrom L, et al. Randomised placebo-controlled trial of orlistat for weight loss and prevention of weight regain in obese patients. European Multicentre Orlistat Study Group. *Lancet* 1998; **352**:167–172.
72. Hilger E, et al. The effect of orlistat on plasma levels of psychotropic drugs in patients with long-term psychopharmacotherapy. *J Clin Psychopharmacol* 2002; **22**:68–70.
73. Pavlovic ZM. Orlistat in the treatment of clozapine-induced hyperglycemia and weight gain. *Eur Psychiatry* 2005; **20**:520.
74. Carpenter LL, et al. A case series describing orlistat use in patients on psychotropic medications. *Med Health R I* 2004; **87**:375–377.
75. Joffe G, et al. Orlistat in clozapine- or olanzapine-treated patients with overweight or obesity: a 16-week randomized, double-blind, placebo-controlled trial. *J Clin Psychiatry* 2008; **69**:706–711.
76. Tchoukhine E, et al. Orlistat in clozapine- or olanzapine-treated patients with overweight or obesity: a 16-week open-label extension phase and both phases of a randomized controlled trial. *J Clin Psychiatry* 2011; **72**:326–330.
77. Chukhin E, et al. In a randomized placebo-controlled add-on study orlistat significantly reduced clozapine-induced constipation. *Int Clin Psychopharmacol* 2013; **28**:67–70.
78. Amrami-Weizman A, et al. The effect of reboxetine co-administration with olanzapine on metabolic and endocrine profile in schizophrenia patients. *Psychopharmacology (Berl)* 2013; **230**:23–27.
79. Gao J, et al. Samidorphan for the treatment of weight gain associated with olanzapine in patients with schizophrenia and bipolar disorder. *Expert Rev Clin Pharmacol* 2022; **15**:1011–1016.
80. Laguado SA, et al. Opioid antagonists to prevent olanzapine-induced weight gain: a systematic review. *Ment Health Clin* 2022; **12**:254–262.
81. Meyer JM, et al. Olanzapine/samidorphan combination consistently mitigates weight gain across various subgroups of patients. *CNS Spectr* 2023; **28**:478–481.
82. Grywińska WB, et al. Combining samidorphan with olanzapine to mitigate weight gain as a side effect in schizophrenia treatment. *Postep Psychiatr Neurol* 2023; **32**:128–137.
83. Peng Z, et al. Effects of combined therapy of olanzapine and samidorphan on safety and metabolic parameters in schizophrenia patients: a meta-analysis. *Neuropsychiatr Dis Treat* 2023; **19**:2295–2308.
84. Kahn RS, et al. Olanzapine/samidorphan in young adults with schizophrenia, schizophreniform disorder, or bipolar I disorder who are early in their illness: results of the randomized, controlled ENLIGHTEN-Early study. *J Clin Psychiatry* 2023; **84**:22m14674.
85. Correll CU, et al. Reduction in multiple cardiometabolic risk factors with combined olanzapine/samidorphan compared with olanzapine: post hoc analyses from a 24-week phase 3 study. *Schizophr Bull* 2023; **49**:454–463.
86. Prasad F, et al. Semaglutide for the treatment of antipsychotic-associated weight gain in patients not responding to metformin: a case series. *Ther Adv Psychopharmacol* 2023; **13**:20451253231165169.
87. Stogios N, et al. Antipsychotic-induced weight gain in severe mental illness: risk factors and special considerations. *Curr Psychiatry Rep* 2023; **25**:707–721.
88. Correll CU, et al. Efficacy for psychopathology and body weight and safety of topiramate-antipsychotic cotreatment in patients with schizophrenia spectrum disorders: results from a meta-analysis of randomized controlled trials. *J Clin Psychiatry* 2016; **77**:e746–e756.
89. Zheng W, et al. Efficacy and safety of adjunctive topiramate for schizophrenia: a meta-analysis of randomized controlled trials. *Acta Psychiatr Scand* 2016; **134**:385–398.
90. Buoli M, et al. The use of zonisamide for the treatment of psychiatric disorders: a systematic review. *Clin Neuropharmacol* 2017; **40**:85–92.

Neuroleptic malignant syndrome

NMS occurs as a rare but potentially serious or even fatal adverse effect of antipsychotics and other dopamine antagonists (Table 1.33).[1,2] It is an acute disorder of thermoregulation and neuromotor control, characterised by muscular rigidity, hyperthermia, altered consciousness and autonomic dysfunction, although there is considerable heterogeneity in the clinical presentation.[1,3–5] In many cases, the presentation is atypical, lacking key signs and symptoms such as hyperthermia and muscle rigidity.[6–8] Asymptomatic rises in plasma creatine kinase (CK) seem to be fairly common and so CK cannot be used as a diagnostic marker of NMS.[9]

Table 1.33 Neuroleptic malignant syndrome.

Signs and symptoms[10–13] (presentation varies considerably)[14]	Fever, diaphoresis, muscle rigidity, confusion, fluctuating level of consciousness, labile or high BP, tachycardia
	Elevated CK, often >1000 units/L,[2,15] leukocytosis, altered LFTs
Risk factors[12,13,16–21]	High-potency FGAs, recent or rapid dose increase, rapid dose reduction, abrupt withdrawal of anticholinergic agents, antipsychotic polypharmacy
	Psychosis, organic brain disease, alcoholism, Parkinson's disease, hyperthyroidism, psychomotor agitation, cognitive impairment
	Male gender, younger age
	Agitation, dehydration
Treatments[10,12,22–25] (note that guideline recommendations for NMS vary widely and are based on limited evidence)[26]	**In the psychiatric unit:** withdraw antipsychotic medication, monitor temperature, pulse, BP. Consider benzodiazepines if not already prescribed – IM lorazepam has been used.[27]
	In the medical/emergency unit: rehydration, bromocriptine + dantrolene, sedation with benzodiazepines, artificial ventilation if required
	L-dopa, apomorphine and carbamazepine have also been used, among many other drugs. ECT may be effective for NMS, even after pharmacotherapy has failed.[28–30]
Restarting antipsychotics[12,22,31,32]	Antipsychotic treatment will be required in most instances and rechallenge is associated with acceptable risk
	Stop antipsychotic medication for at least 5 days, preferably longer. Allow time for symptoms and signs of NMS to resolve completely
	Begin with very small dose and increase very slowly with close monitoring of temperature, pulse and blood pressure. CK monitoring may be used but is controversial.[13,33] Close monitoring of physical and biochemical parameters is effective in reducing progression to 'full-blown' NMS.[34,35]
	Consider using an antipsychotic medication structurally unrelated to that previously associated with NMS or a drug with low dopamine affinity (quetiapine or clozapine). Aripiprazole may also be considered[36] but it has a long plasma half-life and has been linked to an increased risk of NMS.[17]
	Avoid depot/LAI antipsychotic preparations (of any kind) and high-potency FGAs

CK, creatine kinase; FGA, first-generation antipsychotic.

Risk factors for developing NMS include being male, dehydration, exhaustion and confusion/agitation.[4,37] Although NMS has commonly been reported to occur at standard doses of antipsychotics, there is some evidence that higher dosage or combined antipsychotic medications may also be risk factors.[2] Young adult males seem to be particularly at risk, while the condition is more likely to be lethal in older people.[4,16,38,39] Other predictors of mortality with NMS are the presence of respiratory difficulties, the severity of hyperthermia, and failing to stop antipsychotic medication.[39]

The incidence and mortality rate of NMS are difficult to establish and probably vary as medication regimens change and recognition of NMS waxes and wanes. The incidence of NMS has been estimated at 0.02–0.03%, with a mortality rate of 5.6%.[25] However, data from a drug safety programme from 1993 to 2015 yielded an overall incidence of 0.16%,[10] while a similar study, covering the period 2004 to 2017, reported an incidence of 0.11%.[40] High-potency FGAs seem to be associated with the greatest incidence, while SGAs and low-potency FGAs seem to have a lower incidence.[3,10,17]

Most available antipsychotic medications have been reported to be associated with NMS,[41–45] including more recently introduced SGAs such as lurasidone,[46] ziprasidone,[47,48] iloperidone,[49] aripiprazole,[6,50,52] paliperidone[53] (including paliperidone palmitate),[54] asenapine[55] and risperidone injection.[56] Mortality is probably lower with SGAs than with FGAs,[3,57–59] although the clinical picture is essentially similar[58] except that rigidity and fever may be less common.[3,58] In 2020, NMS had yet to be associated with pimavanserin, cariprazine, brexpiprazole or lumateperone,[60] and we could find no reports of NMS being linked to these drugs in mid-2024.

NMS is also sometimes seen with other medications, such as antidepressants,[61–64] valproate,[65,66] phenytoin[31] and lithium.[67,68] The co-prescription of SSRIs[69] or cholinesterase inhibitors[70,71] with antipsychotic medication may increase the risk of NMS. NMS-type syndromes induced by combinations of SGA and SSRI medications may share their symptoms and pathogenesis with the serotonin syndrome.[72,73] Benzodiazepines are a recommended treatment for NMS,[26] but an association between their use and NMS has been reported, possibly confounded by diagnosis or explained by the occurrence of NMS-like symptoms during benzodiazepine withdrawal.[17,18,74] NMS is also occasionally seen in people given non-psychotropic dopamine antagonists such as metoclopramide[75] and prochlorperazine.[76,77]

References

1. Caroff SN, et al. Neuroleptic malignant syndrome. *Med Clin North Am* 1993; 77:185–202.

2. Tse L, et al. Neuroleptic malignant syndrome: a review from a clinically oriented perspective. *Curr Neuropharmacol* 2015; 13:395–406.

3. Belvederi Murri M, et al. Second-generation antipsychotics and neuroleptic malignant syndrome: systematic review and case report analysis. *Drugs R D* 2015; 15:45–62.

4. Ware MR, et al. Neuroleptic malignant syndrome: diagnosis and management. *Prim Care Companion CNS Disord* 2018; 20:17r02185.

5. Tan CM, et al. Neuroleptic malignant syndrome. *CMAJ* 2023; 195:E1481.

6. Rodriguez OP, et al. A case report of neuroleptic malignant syndrome without fever in a patient given aripiprazole. *J Okla State Med Assoc* 2006; 99:435–438.

7. Singhai K, et al. Atypical neuroleptic malignant syndrome: a systematic review of case reports. *Gen Hosp Psychiatry* 2019; 60:12–19.

8. Szota AM, et al. Atypical neuroleptic malignant syndrome: case reports and diagnostic challenges. *J Psychoactive Drugs* 2022; 54:284–293.

9. Meltzer HY, et al. Marked elevations of serum creatine kinase activity associated with antipsychotic drug treatment. *Neuropsychopharmacology* 1996; 15:395–405.

10. Schneider M, et al. Neuroleptic malignant syndrome: evaluation of drug safety data from the AMSP program during 1993–2015. *Eur Arch Psychiatry Clin Neurosci* 2020; 270:23–33.

11. Gurrera RJ. Sympathoadrenal hyperactivity and the etiology of neuroleptic malignant syndrome. *Am J Psychiatry* 1999; 156:169–180.

12. Levenson JL. Neuroleptic malignant syndrome. *Am J Psychiatry* 1985; 142:1137–1145.

13. Hermesh H, et al. High serum creatinine kinase level: possible risk factor for neuroleptic malignant syndrome. *J Clin Psychopharmacol* 2002; 22:252–256.

14. Picard LS, et al. Atypical neuroleptic malignant syndrome: diagnostic controversies and considerations. *Pharmacotherapy* 2008; 28:530–535.

15. Gurrera RJ, et al. An international consensus study of neuroleptic malignant syndrome diagnostic criteria using the Delphi method. *J Clin Psychiatry* 2011; 72:1222–1228.

16. Gurrera RJ. A systematic review of sex and age factors in neuroleptic malignant syndrome diagnosis frequency. *Acta Psychiatr Scand* 2017; 135:398–408.

17. Su YP, et al. Retrospective chart review on exposure to psychotropic medications associated with neuroleptic malignant syndrome. *Acta Psychiatr Scand* 2014; 130:52–60.

18. Nielsen RE, et al. Neuroleptic malignant syndrome—an 11-year longitudinal case-control study. *Can J Psychiatry* 2012; 57:512–518.

19. Viejo LF, et al. Risk factors in neuroleptic malignant syndrome: a case–control study. *Acta Psychiatr Scand* 2003; 107:45–49.

20. Spivak B, et al. Neuroleptic malignant syndrome during abrupt reduction of neuroleptic treatment. *Acta Psychiatr Scand* 1990; 81:168–169.

21. Spivak B, et al. Neuroleptic malignant syndrome associated with abrupt withdrawal of anticholinergic agents. *Int Clin Psychopharmacol* 1996; 11:207–209.

22. Olmsted TR. Neuroleptic malignant syndrome: guidelines for treatment and reinstitution of neuroleptics. *South Med J* 1988; 81:888–891.

23. Lattanzi L, et al. Subcutaneous apomorphine for neuroleptic malignant syndrome. *Am J Psychiatry* 2006; 163:1450–1451.

24. Kuhlwilm L, et al. The neuroleptic malignant syndrome—a systematic case series analysis focusing on therapy regimes and outcome. *Acta Psychiatr Scand* 2020; 142:233–241.

25. Pileggi DJ, et al. Neuroleptic malignant syndrome. *Ann Pharmacother* 2016; 50:973–981.

26. Schönfeldt-Lecuona C, et al. Treatment of the neuroleptic malignant syndrome in international therapy guidelines: a comparative analysis. *Pharmacopsychiatry* 2020; 53:51–59.

27. Francis A, et al. Is lorazepam a treatment for neuroleptic malignant syndrome? *CNS Spectr* 2000; 5:54–57.

28. Morcos N, et al. Electroconvulsive therapy for neuroleptic malignant syndrome: a case series. *J ECT* 2019; 35:225–230.

29. Aki Ö E, et al. A severe neuroleptic malignant syndrome treated with daily electroconvulsive therapy: a case report. *Turk Psikiyatri Derg* 2022; 33:139–142.

30. Katzell L, et al. Rapid symptom control in neuroleptic malignant syndrome with electroconvulsive therapy: a case report. *Front Psychiatry* 2023; 14:1143407.

31. Shin HW, et al. Neuroleptic malignant syndrome induced by phenytoin in a patient with drug-induced Parkinsonism. *Neurol Sci* 2014; 35:1641–1643.

32. Wells AJ, et al. Neuroleptic rechallenge after neuroleptic malignant syndrome: case report and literature review. *Drug Intell Clin Pharm* 1988; 22:475–480.

33. Klein JP, et al. Massive creatine kinase elevations with quetiapine: report of two cases. *Pharmacopsychiatry* 2006; 39:39–40.

34. Shiloh R, et al. Precautionary measures reduce risk of definite neuroleptic malignant syndrome in newly typical neuroleptic-treated schizophrenia inpatients. *Int Clin Psychopharmacol* 2003; 18:147–149.

35. Hatch CD, et al. Failed challenge with quetiapine after neuroleptic malignant syndrome with conventional antipsychotics. *Pharmacotherapy* 2001; 21:1003–1006.

36. Trutia A, et al. Neuroleptic rechallenge with aripiprazole in a patient with previously documented neuroleptic malignant syndrome. *J Psychiatry Pract* 2008; 14:398–402.

37. Keck PE, Jr., et al. Risk factors for neuroleptic malignant syndrome: a case–control study. *Arch Gen Psychiatry* 1989; 46:914–918.

38. Isik AT, et al. Neuroleptic malignant syndrome in patients with dementia: experiences of a single memory clinic. *Clin Neuropharmacol* 2023; 46:209–213.

39. Guinart D, et al. A systematic review and pooled, patient-level analysis of predictors of mortality in neuroleptic malignant syndrome. *Acta Psychiatr Scand* 2021; 144:329–341.

40. Lao KSJ, et al. Antipsychotics and risk of neuroleptic malignant syndrome: a population-based cohort and case-crossover study. *CNS Drugs* 2020; 34:1165–1175.

41. Sierra-Biddle D, et al. Neuropletic malignant syndrome and olanzapine. *J Clin Psychopharmacol* 2000; 20:704–705.

42. Hasan S, et al. Novel antipsychotics and the neuroleptic malignant syndrome: a review and critique. *Am J Psychiatry* 1998; 155:1113–1116.

43. Tsai JH, et al. Zotepine-induced catatonia as a precursor in the progression to neuroleptic malignant syndrome. *Pharmacotherapy* 2005; 25:1156–1159.

44. Gortney JS, et al. Neuroleptic malignant syndrome secondary to quetiapine. *Ann Pharmacother* 2009; 43:785–791.

45. Saraiva R, et al. Quetiapine-induced neuroleptic malignant syndrome. *Prim Care Companion CNS Disord* 2023; 25:22cr03332.

46. Pàmpols-Pérez S, et al. Neuroleptic malignant syndrome associated with lurasidone: a case report. *J Clin Psychopharmacol* 2023; 43:548–549.

47. Leibold J, et al. Neuroleptic malignant syndrome associated with ziprasidone in an adolescent. *Clin Ther* 2004; 26:1105–1108.

48. Borovicka MC, et al. Ziprasidone- and lithium-induced neuroleptic malignant syndrome. *Ann Pharmacother* 2006; 40:139–142.

49. Guanci N, et al. Atypical neuroleptic malignant syndrome associated with iloperidone administration. *Psychosomatics* 2012; 53:603–605.

50. Spalding S, et al. Aripiprazole and atypical neuroleptic malignant syndrome. *J Am Acad Child Adolesc Psychiatry* 2004; 43:1457–1458.

51. Chakraborty N, et al. Aripiprazole and neuroleptic malignant syndrome. *Int Clin Psychopharmacol* 2004; 19:351–353.

52. Srephichit S, et al. Neuroleptic malignant syndrome and aripiprazole in an antipsychotic-naive patient. *J Clin Psychopharmacol* 2006; **26**:94–95.

53. Duggal HS. Possible neuroleptic malignant syndrome associated with paliperidone. *J Neuropsychiatry Clin Neurosci* 2007; **19**:477–478.

54. Langley-DeGroot M, et al. Atypical neuroleptic malignant syndrome associated with paliperidone long-acting injection: a case report. *J Clin Psychopharmacol* 2016; **36**:277–279.

55. Singh N, et al. Neuroleptic malignant syndrome after exposure to asenapine: a case report. *Prim Care Companion J Clin Psychiatry* 2010; **12**:e1.

56. Mall GD, et al. Catatonia and mild neuroleptic malignant syndrome after initiation of long-acting injectable risperidone: case report. *J Clin Psychopharmacol* 2008; **28**:572–573.

57. Ananth J, et al. Neuroleptic malignant syndrome and atypical antipsychotic drugs. *J Clin Psychiatry* 2004; **65**:464–470.

58. Trollor JN, et al. Comparison of neuroleptic malignant syndrome induced by first- and second-generation antipsychotics. *Br J Psychiatry* 2012; **201**:52–56.

59. Nakamura M, et al. Mortality of neuroleptic malignant syndrome induced by typical and atypical antipsychotic drugs: a propensity-matched analysis from the Japanese Diagnosis Procedure Combination database. *J Clin Psychiatry* 2012; **73**:427–430.

60. Orsolini L, et al. Up-to-date expert opinion on the safety of recently developed antipsychotics. *Expert Opinion on Drug Safety* 2020; **19**:981–998.

61. Kontaxakis VP, et al. Neuroleptic malignant syndrome after addition of paroxetine to olanzapine. *J Clin Psychopharmacol* 2003; **23**:671–672.

62. Young C. A case of neuroleptic malignant syndrome and serotonin disturbance. *J Clin Psychopharmacol* 1997; **17**:65–66.

63. June R, et al. Neuroleptic malignant syndrome associated with nortriptyline. *Am J Emerg Med* 1999; **17**:736–737.

64. Lu TC, et al. Neuroleptic malignant syndrome after the use of venlafaxine in a patient with generalized anxiety disorder. *J Formos Med Assoc* 2006; **105**:90–93.

65. Verma R, et al. An atypical case of neuroleptic malignant syndrome precipitated by valproate. *BMJ Case Rep* 2014; **2014**:bcr2013202578.

66. Menon V, et al. Atypical neuroleptic malignant syndrome in a young male precipitated by oral sodium valproate. *Aust N Z J Psychiatry* 2016; **50**:1208–1209.

67. Gill J, et al. Acute lithium intoxication and neuroleptic malignant syndrome. *Pharmacotherapy* 2003; **23**:811–815.

68. Ramadas S, et al. Neuroleptic malignant syndrome with low dose lithium, without concomitant antipsychotics. *Indian J Psychol Med* 2023; **45**:92–94.

69. Stevens DL. Association between selective serotonin-reuptake inhibitors, second-generation antipsychotics, and neuroleptic malignant syndrome. *Ann Pharmacother* 2008; **42**:1290–1297.

70. Stevens DL, et al. Olanzapine-associated neuroleptic malignant syndrome in a patient receiving concomitant rivastigmine therapy. *Pharmacotherapy* 2008; **28**:403–405.

71. Warwick TC, et al. Neuroleptic malignant syndrome variant in a patient receiving donepezil and olanzapine. *Nat Clin Pract Neurol* 2008; **4**:170–174.

72. Odagaki Y. Atypical neuroleptic malignant syndrome or serotonin toxicity associated with atypical antipsychotics? *Curr Drug Saf* 2009; **4**:84–93.

73. Maktabi L, et al. Serotonin syndrome and neuroleptic malignant syndrome: a case report of intersecting symptomatology. *Ment Health Clin* 2024; **14**:23–27.

74. Kishimoto S, et al. Postoperative neuroleptic malignant syndrome-like symptoms improved with intravenous diazepam: a case report. *J Anesth* 2013; **27**:768–770.

75. Wittmann O, et al. Neuroleptic malignant syndrome associated with metoclopramide use in a boy: case report and review of the literature. *Am J Ther* 2016; **23**:e1246–e1249.

76. Pesola GR, et al. Prochlorperazine-induced neuroleptic malignant syndrome. *J Emerg Med* 1996; **14**:727–729.

77. Tee ZJ. A rare case of prochlorperazine-induced neuroleptic malignant syndrome. *Am J Emerg Med* 2024; **81**:160.e1–160.e2.

Catatonia

Catatonia is a neuropsychiatric disorder that presents with a wide range of signs and symptoms, covering focal and generalised motor activity, speech, affect, complex behaviour and autonomic function.[1] A comprehensive meta-analysis of international data from 74 studies, conducted between 1935 and 2017 and involving 107,304 individuals, found an overall pooled, mean prevalence of catatonia of just over 9% in patients diagnosed with a range of psychiatric and medical conditions.[2]

Three main catatonia subtypes are recognised: a **retarded** or **stuporous** form with decreased psychomotor behaviour; an **excited** form, characterised by agitation, combativeness, impulsivity and apparently purposeless overactivity; and **malignant catatonia**, a life-threatening state that presents as catatonia with clinically significant autonomic abnormalities, including raised blood pressure and body temperature, and change in heart rate and respiratory rate.[1,3–5]

The retarded form tends to present as stupor – the key features include mutism, rigidity, marked psychomotor retardation, negativism, posturing, waxy flexibility and catalepsy. While historically associated with schizophrenia, stupor is also seen in other psychiatric conditions such as depression and, less commonly, mania,[6–11] alcohol[12] or benzodiazepine withdrawal,[13] and conversion disorder.[6,7,14–20] If psychiatric stupor is left untreated, physical health complications are unavoidable and develop rapidly. Prompt treatment is crucial to prevent serious complications such as dehydration, venous thrombosis, pulmonary embolism, pneumonia and, ultimately, death.[21]

A catatonic syndrome is most commonly associated with psychiatric conditions such as bipolar disorder, schizophrenia and major depressive disorder,[1,2] but may also be seen in patients with postpartum psychosis,[22–24] post-traumatic stress disorder,[25,26] developmental disorders such as autism spectrum disorder, neurodegenerative conditions,[27,28] and a range of underlying medical conditions, including:

- subarachnoid haemorrhages
- basal ganglia disorders
- non-convulsive status epilepticus
- locked-in and akinetic mutism states
- endocrine and metabolic disorders (e.g. Wilson's)[29]
- Prader–Willi syndrome
- antiphospholipid syndrome[30]
- autoimmune encephalitis, such as anti-NMDAR encephalitis[1,31–33]
- systemic lupus erythematosus[34,35]
- infections (especially CNS infections)
- dementia
- drug withdrawal and toxic drug states (e.g. after abrupt withdrawal of clozapine and withdrawal of zolpidem, benzodiazepines[36] and many non-psychotropic medications, including medicines used in oncology).

Treatment

The treatment of stupor in the context of catatonia is somewhat dependent on its cause but should usually include benzodiazepines. Benzodiazepine monotherapy is the treatment of choice for stupor occurring in the context of affective and conversion disorders.[8,9,37] It is postulated that benzodiazepines may act by increasing gamma-aminobutyric acid (GABA)ergic transmission or reducing levels of brain-derived neurotropic factor.[38]

There is most clinical experience with lorazepam.[32,39] Many patients will respond to standard doses (up to 4mg/day) but repeated and higher doses (between 8 and 24mg per day) may be needed.[40] One small, observational study of patients with catatonic stupor in the context of a mood disorder[8] (either major depressive disorder or bipolar I disorder) used a lorazepam–diazepam treatment protocol and reported a response in 10 of the 12 patients with intramuscular lorazepam 2–4mg. In another study, which followed a very similar protocol, relief of symptoms was achieved in 18 of 21 patients with catatonia caused by general medical conditions or substance misuse.[41] Where benzodiazepines are effective, onset effect is rapid. A test dose of zolpidem (10mg) may predict response to benzodiazepines[42] and frequent dosing of zolpidem may provide effective treatment.[43,44] IV lorazepam has also been used to predict response.[45]

Catatonia in schizophrenia may be somewhat less likely to respond to benzodiazepines alone, with a response in 40–50%[46] of cases. A double-blind, placebo-controlled, crossover trial with lorazepam up to 6mg/day demonstrated no effect on chronic catatonic symptoms in patients with established schizophrenia,[47] similar to the poor effect of lorazepam seen in a non-randomised trial.[48] A Cochrane review[49] searched for RCTs in which people with schizophrenia or other similar severe mental illness had received benzodiazepines or another relevant treatment for catatonia. Only one study was eligible, which involved 17 participants treated with lorazepam or oxazepam; there was no clear difference in effect. The authors noted that no data were available for benzodiazepines compared with either placebo or standard care.

A further complication in schizophrenia is that of differential diagnosis, which includes EPSEs and the NMS. Debate continues regarding the similarities and differences between catatonic stupor in psychosis and NMS.[50–53] Malignant catatonia[5] may not be distinguishable from NMS, either clinically or by laboratory testing, which has prompted the view that NMS may be a variant form of malignant catatonia.[54] However, NMS can probably be ruled out in the absence of any prior or recent administration of a dopamine antagonist.

The vast majority of evidence published recently and over previous decades suggests that prompt ECT remains the most successful treatment for catatonia.[39,45,48,55–71] ECT-responsive catatonia has been recognised in the context of NMS, delirious mania, autism spectrum disorder and limbic encephalitis.[53,72] While it has been suggested that response to ECT may be lower in patients with schizophrenia (or in those who have been treated with antipsychotic medication) than in patients with mood disorders,[73] ECT is still considered the treatment of choice for catatonic schizophrenia that has failed to respond to an adequate trial of benzodiazepines.[1,74] In malignant catatonia, every effort should be made to maximise the effect of ECT by using liberal stimulus dosing to induce well-generalised seizures.[75] Physical health needs should be prioritised, with inpatient medical care being provided, when necessary, especially for those showing autonomic instability and those for whom dietary intake cannot be managed in psychiatric care. A 2024 systematic review[76] of studies of 'non-invasive brain stimulation' techniques for catatonia reinforced ECT as an effective treatment and suggested that it may be considered as first-line therapy in certain cases, but also identified rTMS and tDCS as promising treatments, although high-quality RCTs are required to establish efficacy.[76,77]

The use of antipsychotic medication should be carefully considered. Some authors recommend that such treatment should be avoided altogether in patients with catatonia, although there are reports of successful treatment of catatonia with clozapine,[78] as well as other SGAs, such as olanzapine, aripiprazole, risperidone and ziprasidone[1,79–85] (particularly in cases of catatonic schizophrenia).[86] There are also case reports of combination treatment with antipsychotic and benzodiazepine medication proving effective when each has failed individually.[87,88]

When considering the use of antipsychotic medication, account should be taken of the patient's history, their psychiatric diagnosis and previous response to antipsychotic treatment. If stupor develops in a patient on antipsychotic medication, any treatment with antipsychotic medication should be avoided if there are any signs or symptoms of NMS. Where NMS can be ruled out and stupor occurs in the context of non-adherence to antipsychotic treatment, early re-establishment of antipsychotic medication is recommended, with consideration of adjunctive benzodiazepines. This may be particularly relevant when catatonic symptoms have occurred following discontinuation of clozapine.[36,89] Catatonia has also been reported after withdrawal of long-term benzodiazepine treatment.[36]

When physical health conditions, as in the examples listed earlier this section, are associated with a catatonia-like clinical picture, treatment of the underlying medical condition (e.g. lupus)[90] is warranted.

A treatment algorithm for catatonic stupor[91] is provided in Figure 1.4. The 2023 British Association for Psychopharmacology consensus guideline for the management of catatonia[1] includes a more detailed referenced algorithm for the management of the condition. Medications other than benzodiazepines reported as treatments for catatonia/stupor are listed in Table 1.34.

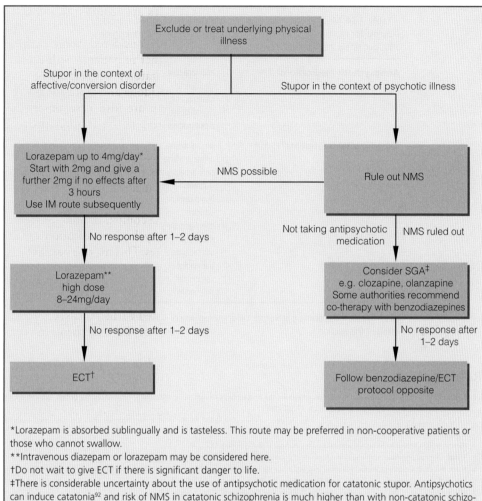

Figure 1.4 Algorithm for treating catatonic stupor.[91]

*Lorazepam is absorbed sublingually and is tasteless. This route may be preferred in non-cooperative patients or those who cannot swallow.

**Intravenous diazepam or lorazepam may be considered here.

†Do not wait to give ECT if there is significant danger to life.

‡There is considerable uncertainty about the use of antipsychotic medication for catatonic stupor. Antipsychotics can induce catatonia[92] and risk of NMS in catatonic schizophrenia is much higher than with non-catatonic schizo-phrenia.[93] An alternative approach is to use antipsychotic medication either once catatonia has resolved or when benzodiazepines or ECT have failed and there is clear evidence of a psychotic illness.[91]

Table 1.34 Medications other than benzodiazepines reported as treatments for catatonia/stupor (listed in alphabetical order – no ranking or judgement is implied by the order).

Antipsychotic medications[1,78–84,94–97]	aripiprazole
	clozapine
	olanzapine
	risperidone
	ziprasidone
Experimental treatments *[9,10,43,44,64,98–103]	amantadine
	amitriptyline
	carbamazepine
	fluoxetine
	fluvoxamine
	lithium
	memantine
	methylphenidate
	mirtazapine
	tramadol
	valproate
	zolpidem

* Always read the primary literature before using any of the medications listed in this section.

References

1. Rogers JP, et al. Evidence-based consensus guidelines for the management of catatonia: recommendations from the British Association for Psychopharmacology. *J Psychopharmacol* 2023; 37:327–369.
2. Solmi M, et al. Prevalence of catatonia and its moderators in clinical samples: results from a meta-analysis and meta-regression analysis. *Schizophr Bull* 2018; 44:1133–1150.
3. Morrison JR. Catatonia. Retarded and excited types. *Arch Gen Psychiatry* 1973; 28:39–41.
4. Walther S, et al. Structure and neural mechanisms of catatonia. *Lancet Psychiatry* 2019; 6:610–619.
5. Mann SC, et al. Catatonia, malignant catatonia, and neuroleptic malignant syndrome. *Current Psychiatry Reviews* 2013; 9:111–119.
6. Takacs R, et al. Catatonia in affective disorders. *Current Psychiatry Reviews* 2013; 9:101–105.
7. Mangas MCC, et al. P-167: catatonia in bipolar disorder. *Eur Psychiatry* 2012; 27 Suppl 1:1.
8. Huang YC, et al. Rapid relief of catatonia in mood disorder by lorazepam and diazepam. *Biomed J* 2013; 36:35–39.
9. Vasudev K, et al. What works for delirious catatonic mania? *BMJ Case Rep* 2010; 2010:bcr0220102713.
10. Neuhut R, et al. Resolution of catatonia after treatment with stimulant medication in a patient with bipolar disorder. *Psychosomatics* 2012; 53:482–484.
11. Ghaffarinejad AR, et al. Periodic catatonia: challenging diagnosis for psychiatrists. *Neurosciences (Riyadh)* 2012; 17:156–158.
12. Oldham MA, et al. Alcohol and sedative-hypnotic withdrawal catatonia: two case reports, systematic literature review, and suggestion of a potential relationship with alcohol withdrawal delirium. *Psychosomatics* 2016; 57:246–255.
13. Banerjee D. Etizolam withdrawal catatonia: the first case report. *Asian J Psychiatr* 2018; 37:32–33.
14. Fink M. Rediscovering catatonia: the biography of a treatable syndrome. *Acta Psychiatr Scand Suppl* 2013; (441):1–47.
15. Bartolommei N, et al. Catatonia: a critical review and therapeutic recommendation. *J Psychopathol* 2012; 18:234–246.
16. Lee J. Dissociative catatonia: dissociative-catatonic reactions, clinical presentations and responses to benzodiazepines. *Aust N Z J Psychiatry* 2011; 45:A42.
17. Suzuki K, et al. Hysteria presenting as a prodrome to catatonic stupor in a depressive patient resolved with electroconvulsive therapy. *J ECT* 2006; 22:276.
18. Alwaki A, et al. Catatonia: an elusive diagnosis. *Neurology* 2013; 80 Suppl 1:P05.127.
19. Dhadphale M. Eye gaze diagnostic sign in hysterical stupor. *Lancet* 1980; 2:374–375.
20. Gomez J. Hysterical stupor and death. *Br J Psychiatry* 1980; 136:105–106.
21. Petrides G, et al. Synergism of lorazepam and electroconvulsive therapy in the treatment of catatonia. *Biol Psychiatry* 1997; 42:375–381.
22. Nahar A, et al. Catatonia among women with postpartum psychosis in a mother–baby inpatient psychiatry unit. *Gen Hosp Psychiatry* 2017; 45:40–43.
23. Csihi L, et al. Catatonia during pregnancy and the postpartum period. *Schizophr Res* 2024; 263:257–264.
24. Delvi A, et al. Catatonia in the peripartum: a cohort study using electronic health records. *Schizophr Res* 2024; 263:252–256.

25. Biles TR, et al. Should catatonia be conceptualized as a pathological response to trauma? *J Nerv Ment Dis* 2021; **209**:320–323.

26. Bonomo N, et al. Rapid resolution of catatonia secondary to post traumatic stress disorder with secondary psychotic features through scheduled zolpidem tartrate. *BMC Psychiatry* 2023; **23**:258.

27. Mazzone L, et al. Catatonia in patients with autism: prevalence and management. *CNS Drugs* 2014; **28**:205–215.

28. Dhossche DM, et al. Catatonia in psychiatric illnesses. In: Fatemi SH, Clayton PJ, eds. *The Medical Basis of Psychiatry*. Totowa, NJ: Humana Press; 2008:471–486.

29. Shetageri VN, et al. Case report: catatonia as a presenting symptom of Wilsons disease. *Indian J Psychiatry* 2011; **53** Suppl 5:S93–S94.

30. Cardinal RN, et al. Psychosis and catatonia as a first presentation of antiphospholipid syndrome. *Br J Psychiatry* 2009; **195**:272.

31. Rogers JP, et al. Catatonia and the immune system: a review. *Lancet Psychiatry* 2019; **6**:620–630.

32. Edinoff AN, et al. Catatonia: clinical overview of the diagnosis, treatment, and clinical challenges. *Neurol Int* 2021; **13**:570–586.

33. Wadi L, et al. Electroconvulsive therapy for catatonia in anti-NMDA receptor encephalitis: a case series. *J Neuroimmunol* 2024; **386**:578271.

34. Pustilnik S, et al. Catatonia as the presenting symptom in systemic lupus erythematosus. *J Psychiatr Pract* 2011; **17**:217–221.

35. Sundaram TG, et al. Catatonia in systemic lupus erythematosus: case based review. *Rheumatol Int* 2022; **42**:1461–1476.

36. Lander M, et al. Review of withdrawal catatonia: what does this reveal about clozapine? *Transl Psychiatry* 2018; **8**:139.

37. Sienaert P, et al. Adult catatonia: etiopathogenesis, diagnosis and treatment. *Neuropsychiatry* 2013; **3**:391–399.

38. Huang TL, et al. Lorazepam reduces the serum brain-derived neurotrophic factor level in schizophrenia patients with catatonia. *Prog Neuropsychopharmacol Biol Psychiatry* 2009; **33**:158–159.

39. Sienaert P, et al. A clinical review of the treatment of catatonia. *Front Psychiatry* 2014; **5**:181.

40. Fink M, et al. Neuroleptic malignant syndrome is malignant catatonia, warranting treatments efficacious for catatonia. *Prog Neuropsychopharmacol Biol Psychiatry* 2006; **30**:1182–1183.

41. Lin CC, et al. The lorazepam and diazepam protocol for catatonia due to general medical condition and substance in liaison psychiatry. *PLoS One* 2017; **12**:e0170452.

42. Javelot H, et al. Zolpidem test and catatonia. *J Clin Pharm Ther* 2015; **40**:699–701.

43. Bastiampillai T, et al. Treatment refractory chronic catatonia responsive to zolpidem challenge. *Aust N Z J Psychiatry* 2016; **50**:98.

44. Peglow S, et al. Treatment of catatonia with zolpidem. *J Neuropsychiatry Clin Neurosci* 2013; **25**:E13.

45. Bush G, et al. Catatonia. II. Treatment with lorazepam and electroconvulsive therapy. *Acta Psychiatr Scand* 1996; **93**:137–143.

46. Rosebush PI, et al. Catatonia: re-awakening to a forgotten disorder. *Mov Disord* 1999; **14**:395–397.

47. Ungvari GS, et al. Lorazepam for chronic catatonia: a randomized, double-blind, placebo-controlled cross-over study. *Psychopharmacology (Berl)* 1999; **142**:393–398.

48. Dutt A, et al. Phenomenology and treatment of catatonia: a descriptive study from north India. *Indian J Psychiatry* 2011; **53**:36–40.

49. Zaman H, et al. Benzodiazepines for catatonia in people with schizophrenia or other serious mental illnesses. *Cochrane Database Syst Rev* 2019; **8**:CD006570.

50. Luchini F, et al. Catatonia and neuroleptic malignant syndrome: two disorders on a same spectrum? Four case reports. *J Nerv Ment Dis* 2013; **201**:36–42.

51. Mishima T, et al. [Diazepam-responsive malignant catatonia in a patient with an initial clinical diagnosis of neuroleptic malignant syndrome: a case report]. *Brain Nerve* 2011; **63**:503–507.

52. Rodriguez S, et al. Neuroleptic malignant syndrome or catatonia? A case report. *J Crit Care Med (Targu Mures)* 2020; **6**:190–193.

53. Fink M. Expanding the catatonia tent: recognizing electroconvulsive therapy responsive syndromes. *J ECT* 2021; **37**:77–79.

54. Taylor MA, et al. Catatonia in psychiatric classification: a home of its own. *Am J Psychiatry* 2003; **160**:1233–1241.

55. Cristancho P, et al. Successful use of right unilateral ECT for catatonia: a case series. *J ECT* 2014; **30**:69–72.

56. Philbin D, et al. Catatonic schizophrenia: therapeutic challenges and potentially a new role for electroconvulsive therapy? *BMJ Case Rep* 2013; **2013**:bcr2013009153.

57. Takebayashi M. [Electroconvulsive therapy in schizophrenia]. *Nihon Rinsho* 2013; **71**:694–700.

58. Oviedo G, et al. Trends in the administration of electroconvulsive therapy for schizophrenia in Colombia: descriptive study and literature review. *Eur Arch Psychiatry Clin Neurosci* 2013; **263** Suppl 1:S98.

59. Pompili M, et al. Indications for electroconvulsive treatment in schizophrenia: a systematic review. *Schizophr Res* 2013; **146**:1–9.

60. Ogando Portilla N, et al. Electroconvulsive therapy as an effective treatment in neuroleptic malignant syndrome: purposely a case. *Eur Psychiatry* 2013; **28** Suppl 1:1.

61. Unal A, et al. Effective treatment of catatonia by combination of benzodiazepine and electroconvulsive therapy. *J ECT* 2013; **29**:206–209.

62. Kaliora SC, et al. The practice of electroconvulsive therapy in Greece. *J ECT* 2013; **29**:219–224.

63. Girardi P, et al. Life-saving electroconvulsive therapy in a patient with near-lethal catatonia. *Riv Psichiatr* 2012; **47**:535–537.

64. Kumar V, et al. Electroconvulsive therapy in pregnancy. *Indian J Psychiatry* 2011; **53** Suppl 5:S100–S101.

65. Weiss M, et al. Treatment of catatonia with electroconvulsive therapy in adolescents. *J Child Adolesc Psychopharmacol* 2012; **22**:96–100.

66. Bauer J, et al. Should the term catatonia be explicitly included in the ICD-10 description of acute transient psychotic disorder F23.0? *Nord J Psychiatry* 2012; **66**:68–69.

67. Mohammadbeigi H, et al. Electroconvulsive therapy in single manic episodes: a case series. *Afr J Psychiatry* 2011; **14**:56–59.

68. Dragasek J. [Utilisation of electroconvulsive therapy in treatment of depression disorders]. *Psychiatrie* 2011; **15**:1211–1219.

69. Luchini F, et al. Electroconvulsive therapy in catatonic patients: efficacy and predictors of response. *World J Psychiatry* 2015; **5**:182–192.

70. Lloyd JR, et al. Electroconvulsive therapy for patients with catatonia: current perspectives. *Neuropsychiatr Dis Treat* 2020; **16**:2191–2208.

71. Breit S, et al. The effect of electroconvulsive therapy on specific catatonia symptoms and predictors of late response. *Pharmacopsychiatry* 2024; **57**:13–20.

72. Sajith SG, et al. Response to electroconvulsive therapy in patients with autism spectrum disorder and intractable challenging behaviors associated with symptoms of catatonia. *J ECT* 2017; 33:63–67.

73. van Waarde JA, et al. Electroconvulsive therapy for catatonia: treatment characteristics and outcomes in 27 patients. *J ECT* 2010; 26:248–252.

74. Jain A, et al. *Catatonic Schizophrenia.* StatPearls. Treasure Island (FL): StatPearls Publishing LLC; 2020.

75. Kellner CH, et al. Electroconvulsive therapy for catatonia. *Am J Psychiatry* 2010; 167:1127–1128.

76. Xiao H, et al. Non-invasive brain stimulation for treating catatonia: a systematic review. *Front Psychiatry* 2023; 14:1135583.

77. Hansbauer M, et al. rTMS and tDCS for the treatment of catatonia: a systematic review. *Schizophr Res* 2020; 222:73–78.

78. Saini A, et al. Clozapine as a treatment for catatonia: a systematic review. *Schizophr Res* 2024; 263:275–281.

79. Van Den EF, et al. The use of atypical antipsychotics in the treatment of catatonia. *Eur Psychiatry* 2005; 20:422–429.

80. Caroff SN, et al. Movement disorders associated with atypical antipsychotic drugs. *J Clin Psychiatry* 2002; 63 Suppl 4:12–19.

81. Guzman CS, et al. Treatment of periodic catatonia with atypical antipsychotic, olanzapine. *Psychiatry Clin Neurosci* 2008; 62:482.

82. Babington PW, et al. Treatment of catatonia with olanzapine and amantadine. *Psychosomatics* 2007; 48:534–536.

83. Bastiampillai T, et al. Catatonia resolution and aripiprazole. *Aust N Z J Psychiatry* 2008; 42:907.

84. Strawn JR, et al. Successful treatment of catatonia with aripiprazole in an adolescent with psychosis. *J Child Adolesc Psychopharmacol* 2007; 17:733–735.

85. Kufert Y, et al. Catatonic symptoms successfully treated with olanzapine in an adolescent with schizophrenia. *J Child Adolesc Psychopharmacol* 2021; 31:327–330.

86. Gazdag G, et al. Diagnosing and treating catatonia: an update. *Curr Psychiatr Rev* 2013; 9:130–135.

87. Spiegel DR, et al. A case of schizophrenia with catatonia resistant to lorazepam and olanzapine monotherapy but responsive to combination treatment: is it time to consider using select second-generation antipsychotics earlier in the treatment algorithm for this patient type? *Clin Neuropharmacol* 2019; 42:57–59.

88. Cevher Binici N, et al. Response of catatonia to amisulpride and lorazepam in an adolescent with schizophenia. *J Child Adolesc Psychopharmacol* 2018; 28:151–152.

89. Bilbily J, et al. Catatonia secondary to sudden clozapine withdrawal: a case with three repeated episodes and a literature review. *Case Rep Psychiatry* 2017; 2017:2402731.

90. Grover S, et al. Catatonia in systemic lupus erythematosus: a case report and review of literature. *Lupus* 2013; 22:634–638.

91. Rosebush PI, et al. Catatonia and its treatment. *Schizophr Bull* 2010; 36:239–242.

92. Caroff SN, et al. Movement disorders induced by antipsychotic drugs: implications of the CATIE schizophrenia trial. *Neurol Clin* 2011; 29:127–148, viii.

93. Funayama M, et al. Catatonic stupor in schizophrenic disorders and subsequent medical complications and mortality. *Psychosom Med* 2018; 80:370–376.

94. Voros V, et al. [Use of aripiprazole in the treatment of catatonia]. *Neuropsychopharmacol Hung* 2010; 12:373–376.

95. Yoshimura B, et al. Is quetiapine suitable for treatment of acute schizophrenia with catatonic stupor? A case series of 39 patients. *Neuropsychiatr Dis Treat* 2013; 9:1565–1571.

96. Todorova K. Olanzapine in the treatment of catatonic stupor - two case reports and discussion. *Eur Neuropsychopharmacol* 2012; 22 Suppl 2:S326.

97. Prakash O, et al. Catatonia and mania in patient with AIDS: treatment with lorazepam and risperidone. *Gen Hosp Psychiatry* 2012; 34:321–326.

98. Daniels J. Catatonia: clinical aspects and neurobiological correlates. *J Neuropsychiatry Clin Neurosci* 2009; 21:371–380.

99. Obregon DF, et al. Memantine and catatonia: a case report and literature review. *J Psychiatr Pract* 2011; 17:292–299.

100. Hervey WM, et al. Treatment of catatonia with amantadine. *Clin Neuropharmacol* 2012; 35:86–87.

101. Consoli A, et al. Lorazepam, fluoxetine and packing therapy in an adolescent with pervasive developmental disorder and catatonia. *J Physiol Paris* 2010; 104:309–314.

102. Lewis AL, et al. Malignant catatonia in a patient with bipolar disorder, B12 deficiency, and neuroleptic malignant syndrome: one cause or three? *J Psychiatr Pract* 2009; 15:415–422.

103. Padhy SK, et al. The catatonia conundrum: controversies and contradictions. *Asian J Psychiatr* 2014; 7:6–9.

ECG changes – QT prolongation

Introduction

Many psychotropic drugs are associated with ECG changes and some are causally linked to serious ventricular arrhythmia and sudden cardiac death. Specifically, some antipsychotics block cardiac potassium channels and are linked to prolongation of the cardiac QT interval, a risk factor for the ventricular arrhythmia TdP, which is sometimes fatal.[1]

Case–control studies have suggested that the use of most antipsychotics is associated with an increase in the rate of sudden cardiac death.[2-8] This risk is probably a result of the arrhythmogenic potential of antipsychotics,[9,10] although schizophrenia itself may be associated with QT prolongation,[11] QT interval is longer in patients with schizophrenia than in controls (e.g. 418ms vs 393ms in one study)[12] and in one study prolonged QTc was identified in 7.6% of psychiatric in-patients who had an ECG.[13] A more recent systematic review[14] suggested that 4% of people with schizophrenia and receiving an antipsychotic had a prolonged QTc.

Antipsychotic-related risk is probably dose-related and, although the absolute risk is low, it is substantially higher than, say, the risk of fatal agranulocytosis with clozapine.[9] One report of cases gathered by a national database put the risk of TdP at between 0 and 19.2 cases per 100,000 patient years, depending on the individual antipsychotic and age of patients.[15] The effect of antipsychotic polypharmacy on QT is somewhat uncertain,[16] but the extent of QT prolongation is probably a function of overall dose.[17]

ECG monitoring of drug-induced changes in mental health settings is complicated by a number of factors. Psychiatrists may have limited expertise in ECG interpretation, for example, and still less expertise in manually measuring QT intervals. Even cardiologists show an inter-rater reliability in QT measurement of up to 20ms.[18] Self-reading, computerised ECG devices are now widely available and compensate for some lack of expertise, but different models use different algorithms and different correction formulae.[19] ECG machines may not be as readily available as they are in general medicine. Also, there may be insufficient time for ECG determination in many areas (e.g. out-patients). Lastly, ECG determination may be difficult to perform in acutely disturbed, physically uncooperative patients.

ECG monitoring is nonetheless essential for all patients prescribed antipsychotics. An estimate of QTc interval should be made on admission to in-patient units (in the UK this is recommended in the NICE schizophrenia guideline)[20] and yearly thereafter.

QT prolongation

- The cardiac QT interval (usually cited as QTc – QT corrected for heart rate) is a useful but imprecise indicator of risk of TdP and of increased cardiac mortality.[21] Different correction factors and methods may give markedly different values.[22] The most widely used formula is Bazett's. This tends to overestimate QT length, especially when heart rate is increased.[23]
- The QT interval broadly reflects the duration of cardiac repolarisation. Lengthening of repolarisation duration induces heterogeneity of electrical phasing in different ventricular structures (a phenomenon known as dispersion), which in turn allows the emergence of early after-depolarisations, which may provoke ventricular extrasystole and TdP. Measures have been developed (QT dispersion ratio, dispersion transmural repolarisation time) which may better predict arrhythmia.[12]

- There is some controversy over the exact association between QTc and risk of arrhythmia. Very limited evidence suggests that risk is exponentially related to the extent of prolongation beyond normal limits (440ms for men; 470ms for women), although there are well-known exceptions which appear to disprove this theory[24] (some drugs prolong QT without increasing dispersion). Rather stronger evidence links QTc values over 500ms to a clearly increased risk of arrhythmia.[25] QT intervals of >650ms may be more likely than not to induce torsades.[26] Overall, despite some uncertainties, QTc determination remains an important measure in estimating risk of arrhythmia and sudden death.
- Individual components of the QT interval may have particular importance. The time from the start of the T wave to T-wave peak has been shown to be an important aspect of QT prolongation associated with sudden cardiac deaths;[27] T-wave peak to end interval may also be predictive of arrhythmia.[12]
- QTc measurements and evaluation are complicated by:
  - difficulty in determining the end of the T wave, particularly where U waves are present (this applies to both manual and self-reading ECG machines)[25]
  - normal physiological variation in QTc interval: QT varies with gender, time of day, food intake, alcohol intake, menstrual cycle, ECG lead, etc.[22,24]
  - variation in the extent of drug-induced prolongation of QTc because of changes in plasma levels. QTc prolongation is most prominent at peak drug plasma levels and least obvious at trough levels.[22,24]

Other ECG changes

Other reported antipsychotic-induced changes include atrial fibrillation, giant P waves, T-wave changes and heart block.[24]

Quantifying risk

Drugs are categorised here according to data available on their effects on the cardiac QTc interval as reported, mostly using Bazett's correction formula (Table 1.35). 'No-effect' drugs are those with which QTc prolongation has not been reported either at therapeutic doses or in overdose. 'Low-effect' drugs are those for which severe QTc prolongation has been reported only following overdose or where only small average increases (<10ms) have been observed at clinical doses. 'Moderate-effect' drugs are those which have been observed to prolong QTc by >10ms on average when given at normal clinical doses or where ECG monitoring is officially recommended in some circumstances. 'High-effect' drugs are those for which there is extensive average QTc prolongation (usually >20ms at normal clinical doses).

As outlined above, effect on QTc may not necessarily equate directly to risk of TdP or sudden death,[28] although this is often assumed.[29] (A good example here is ziprasidone – a drug with a moderate effect on QTc but with minimal evidence of cardiac toxicity.[30]) Also, categorisation is inevitably approximate given the problems associated with QTc measurements. Lastly, keep in mind that differences in the effects of different antipsychotics on the QT interval rarely reach statistical significance even in meta-analyses.[31]

Outside these guidelines, readers are directed to the RISQ-PATH study,[32] which provides a scoring system for the prediction of QT prolongation (to above normal ranges) in any patient. RISQ-PATH has a 98% negative predictive value, so allowing a reduction in monitoring in low-risk patients. The RISQ-PATH method uses CredibleMeds categorisation for drug effects on QT – this, too, is recommended.[33]

Table 1.35 Antipsychotics – effect on QTc.[12,22,24,34–59]

Effect on QTc	Drug
No effect	Brexpiprazole Cariprazine Lurasidone Lumateperone*
Low effect	Aripiprazole** Asenapine Clozapine Flupentixol Fluphenazine Perphenazine Prochlorperazine Olanzapine† Paliperidone Risperidone Sulpiride Zuclopenthixol
Moderate effect	Amisulpride‡ Chlorpromazine Haloperidol Iloperidone Levomepromazine Melperone Pimavanserin Quetiapine Ziprasidone
High effect	Pimozide Sertindole
Unknown effect	Loxapine Pipotiazine Trifluoperazine

* Limited clinical experience (association with QT prolongation may emerge).
** One case of TdP reported,[60] two cases of QT prolongation[61,62] and an association with TdP found in database studies.[63,64] Healthy volunteer data suggest aripiprazole causes QTc prolongation of around 8ms.[65] Aripiprazole may increase QT dispersion.[66] Low-dose aripiprazole has no effect on QT when added to another antipsychotic.[67]
† Isolated cases of QTc prolongation[38,68] and has effects on cardiac ion channel, IKr.[69] Other data suggest no effect on QTC.[24,36,37,70]
‡ TdP common in overdose,[26,71] strong association with TdP in clinical doses.[63]

Aripiprazole remains in the low-effect group having previously been firmly placed in 'no effect'. Data are rather contradictory, with most studies showing a decrease in QTc associated with aripiprazole use,[51] even in children and adolescents.[72] However, later data[60,61,63,65,73] cast doubt on assumptions of cardiac safety. Nonetheless, a 2020 paper analysing reports of events in >400,000 in-patients over 20 years found aripiprazole had the lowest rate of cardiac events (0.06%) of all antipsychotics.[74]

Lurasidone remains in the 'no-effect' group,[51] although one study mentioned in the US labelling[75] reports a QT lengthening of 7.5ms in people receiving 120mg (111mg) a day. Those receiving 600mg (555mg) daily showed a lower change (+4.6ms). These findings are in some contrast with those from studies in patients which uniformly suggest no or minimal effect.[76–78] This disparity is probably explained by the use of different correction factors and by random change, as often seen in placebo-treated patients[78] and as suggested by the apparent lack of dose-related effect. One case of QTc >500ms has been reported with lurasidone in which lurasidone was judged the 'probable' cause.[79]

Brexpiprazole remains in the 'no-effect' group although one study of 16 patients found an increase in QTc (Hodges' formula) of 10.1ms and an important increase in dispersion transmural repolarisation time.[12] All other data suggest no effect.

Other risk factors

A number of physiological, pathological and genetic[80] factors are associated with an increased risk of QT changes and of arrhythmia (Table 1.36) and many non-psychotropic drugs are linked to QT prolongation (Table 1.37).[25] These additional risk factors seem almost always to be present in cases of antipsychotic-induced TdP.[81]

Table 1.36 Physiological risk factors for QTc prolongation and arrhythmia.

Cardiac	Long QT syndrome
	Bradycardia
	Ischaemic heart disease
	Myocarditis
	Myocardial infarction
	Left ventricular hypertrophy
Metabolic	Hypokalaemia
	Hypomagnesaemia
	Hypocalcaemia
Others	Extreme physical exertion
	Stress or shock
	Anorexia nervosa
	Extremes of age – children and elderly may be more susceptible to QT changes
	Female gender

Note: Hypokalaemia-related QTc prolongation is more commonly observed in acute psychotic admissions.[82] There are a number of physical and genetic factors (related to cardiac potassium channels or CYP enzyme function),[80] which may not be discovered on routine examination but which probably predispose patients to arrhythmia.[83,84]

Table 1.37 Non-psychotropics associated with QT prolongation (see Crediblemeds.org for latest information; this is not a complete list).

Antibiotics	Erythromycin
	Clarithromycin
	Ampicillin
	Co-trimoxazole
	Pentamidine
	(Some 4 quinolones affect QTc – see manufacturers' literature)
Antimalarials	Chloroquine
	Mefloquine
	Quinine
Antiarrhythmics	Quinidine
	Disopyramide
	Procainamide
	Sotalol
	Amiodarone
	Bretylium
Others	Amantadine
	Cyclosporin
	Diphenhydramine
	Hydroxyzine
	Methadone
	Nicardipine
	Tamoxifen

Note: β_2 agonists and sympathomimetics may provoke TdP in patients with prolonged QTc.

ECG monitoring

Measure QTc in all patients prescribed antipsychotics:

- on admission
- if previous abnormality or known additional risk factor, at annual physical health check.

Consider measuring QTc within a week of achieving a therapeutic dose of a newly prescribed antipsychotic that is associated with a moderate or high risk of QTc prolongation or of newly prescribed combined antipsychotics. Management of QT prolongation in patients receiving antipsychotic drugs is detailed in Table 1.38.

Metabolic inhibition

The effect of drugs on the QTc interval is usually plasma level dependent. Drug interactions are therefore important, especially when metabolic inhibition results in increased plasma levels of the drug affecting QTc. Commonly used metabolic inhibitors include fluvoxamine, fluoxetine, paroxetine and valproate.

Table 1.38 Management of QT prolongation in patients receiving antipsychotic drugs.

QTc	Action	Refer to cardiologist
<440ms (men) or <470ms (women)	None unless abnormal T-wave morphology	Consider if in doubt
>440ms (men) or >470ms (women) but <500ms	Consider reducing dose or switching to drug of lower effect; repeat ECG	Consider
>500ms	Repeat ECG. Stop suspected causative drug(s) and switch to drug of lower effect.	Immediately
Abnormal T-wave morphology	Review treatment. Consider reducing dose or switching to drug of lower effect.	Immediately

Other cardiovascular risk factors

The risk of drug-induced arrhythmia and sudden cardiac death with psychotropics is an important consideration. With respect to cardiovascular disease, note that other risk factors such as smoking, obesity and impaired glucose tolerance present a much greater risk to patient morbidity and mortality than the uncertain outcome of QT changes. See the relevant sections for discussion of these problems.

Summary

- In the absence of conclusive data, assume that all antipsychotics are linked to sudden cardiac death.
- Prescribe the lowest dose possible and avoid polypharmacy/metabolic interactions.
- Perform ECG on admission and, if previous abnormality or additional risk factor, at yearly check-up.
- Consider measuring QTc within a week of achieving a therapeutic dose of a moderate/high-risk antipsychotic.

References

1. Sicouri S, et al. Mechanisms underlying the actions of antidepressant and antipsychotic drugs that cause sudden cardiac arrest. *Arrhythm Electrophysiol Rev* 2018; **7**:199–209.
2. Reilly JG, et al. Thioridazine and sudden unexplained death in psychiatric in-patients. *Br J Psychiatry* 2002; **180**:515–522.
3. Murray-Thomas T, et al. Risk of mortality (including sudden cardiac death) and major cardiovascular events in atypical and typical antipsychotic users: a study with the general practice research database. *Cardiovasc Psychiatry Neurol* 2013; **2013**:247486.
4. Ray WA, et al. Antipsychotics and the risk of sudden cardiac death. *Arch Gen Psychiatry* 2001; **58**:1161–1167.
5. Hennessy S, et al. Cardiac arrest and ventricular arrhythmia in patients taking antipsychotic drugs: cohort study using administrative data. *BMJ* 2002; **325**:1070.
6. Straus SM, et al. Antipsychotics and the risk of sudden cardiac death. *Arch Intern Med* 2004; **164**:1293–1297.
7. Liperoti R, et al. Conventional and atypical antipsychotics and the risk of hospitalization for ventricular arrhythmias or cardiac arrest. *Arch Intern Med* 2005; **165**:696–701.
8. Ray WA, et al. Atypical antipsychotic drugs and the risk of sudden cardiac death. *N Engl J Med* 2009; **360**:225–235.
9. Schneeweiss S, et al. Antipsychotic agents and sudden cardiac death: how should we manage the risk? *N Engl J Med* 2009; **360**:294–296.
10. Nakagawa S, et al. Antipsychotics and risk of first-time hospitalization for myocardial infarction: a population-based case–control study. *J Intern Med* 2006; **260**:451–458.
11. Fujii K, et al. QT is longer in drug-free patients with schizophrenia compared with age-matched healthy subjects. *PLoS One* 2014; **9**:e98555.

CHAPTER 1

12. Okayasu H, et al. Effects of antipsychotics on arrhythmogenic parameters in schizophrenia patients: beyond corrected QT interval. *Neuropsychiatr Dis Treat* 2021; 17:239–249.

13. Ansermot N, et al. Prevalence of ECG abnormalities and risk factors for QTc interval prolongation in hospitalized psychiatric patients. *Ther Adv Psychopharmacol* 2019; 9:2045125319891386.

14. Du W, et al. QTc prolongation in patients with schizophrenia taking antipsychotics: prevalence and risk factors. *J Psychopharmacol* 2023; 37:971–981.

15. Danielsson B, et al. Drug use and torsades de pointes cardiac arrhythmias in Sweden: a nationwide register-based cohort study. *BMJ Open* 2020; 10:e034560.

16. Takeuchi H, et al. Antipsychotic polypharmacy and corrected QT interval: a systematic review. *Can J Psychiatry* 2015; 60:215–222.

17. Barbui C, et al. Antipsychotic dose mediates the association between polypharmacy and corrected QT interval. *PLoS One* 2016; 11:e0148212.

18. Goldenberg I, et al. QT interval: how to measure it and what is 'normal'. *J Cardiovasc Electrophysiol* 2006; 17:333–336.

19. Nielsen J, et al. Assessing QT interval prolongation and its associated risks with antipsychotics. *CNS Drugs* 2011; 25:473–490.

20. National Institute for Health and Care Excellence. Psychosis and schizophrenia in adults: prevention and management. Clinical guideline [CG178]. 2014 (last checked November 2024); https://www.nice.org.uk/guidance/cg178.

21. Malik M, et al. Evaluation of drug-induced QT interval prolongation: implications for drug approval and labelling. *Drug Saf* 2001; 24:323–351.

22. Haddad PM, et al. Antipsychotic-related QTc prolongation, torsade de pointes and sudden death. *Drugs* 2002; 62:1649–1671.

23. Andric T, et al. Estimation of cardiac QTc intervals in people prescribed antipsychotics: a comparison of correction factors. *Ther Adv Psychopharmacol* 2022; 12:20451253221104947.

24. Taylor DM. Antipsychotics and QT prolongation. *Acta Psychiatr Scand* 2003; 107:85–95.

25. Botstein P. Is QT interval prolongation harmful? A regulatory perspective. *Am J Cardiol* 1993; 72:50B–52B.

26. Joy JP, et al. Prediction of torsade de pointes from the QT interval: analysis of a case series of amisulpride overdoses. *Clin Pharmacol Ther* 2011; 90:243–245.

27. O'Neal WT, et al. Association between QT-interval components and sudden cardiac death: the ARIC study (Atherosclerosis Risk in Communities). *Circ Arrhythm Electrophysiol* 2017; 10:e005485.

28. Witchel HJ, et al. Psychotropic drugs, cardiac arrhythmia, and sudden death. *J Clin Psychopharmacol* 2003; 23:58–77.

29. Melo L, et al. An updated safety review of the relationship between atypical antipsychotic drugs, the QTc interval and torsades de pointe As: implications for clinical use. *Expert Opin Drug Saf* 2024; 23:1127–1134.

30. Strom BL, et al. Comparative mortality associated with ziprasidone and olanzapine in real-world use among 18,154 patients with schizophrenia: the ziprasidone observational study of cardiac outcomes (ZODIAC). *Am J Psychiatry* 2011; 168:193–201.

31. Chung AK, et al. Effects on prolongation of Bazett's corrected QT interval of seven second-generation antipsychotics in the treatment of schizophrenia: a meta-analysis. *J Psychopharmacol* 2011; 25:646–666.

32. Vandael E, et al. Development of a risk score for QTc-prolongation: the RISQ-PATH study. *Int J Clin Pharm* 2017; 39:424–432.

33. CredibleMeds®. Tucson, AZ: CredibleMeds; 2024; https://www.crediblemeds.org.

34. Hui WK, et al. Melperone: electrophysiologic and antiarrhythmic activity in humans. *J Cardiovasc Pharmacol* 1990; 15:144–149.

35. Glassman AH, et al. Antipsychotic drugs: prolonged QTc interval, torsade de pointes, and sudden death. *Am J Psychiatry* 2001; 158:1774–1782.

36. Harrigan EP, et al. A randomized evaluation of the effects of six antipsychotic agents on QTc, in the absence and presence of metabolic inhibition. *J Clin Psychopharmacol* 2004; 24:62–69.

37. Lindborg SR, et al. Effects of intramuscular olanzapine vs. haloperidol and placebo on QTc intervals in acutely agitated patients. *Psychiatry Res* 2003; 119:113–123.

38. Dineen S, et al. QTc prolongation and high-dose olanzapine [Letter]. *Psychosomatics* 2003; 44:174–175.

39. Gupta S, et al. Quetiapine and QTc issues: a case report [Letter]. *J Clin Psychiatry* 2003; 64:612–613.

40. Su KP, et al. A pilot cross-over design study on QTc interval prolongation associated with sulpiride and haloperidol. *Schizophr Res* 2003; 59:93–94.

41. Stollberger C, et al. Antipsychotic drugs and QT prolongation. *Int Clin Psychopharmacol* 2005; 20:243–251.

42. Ward DI. Two cases of amisulpride overdose: a cause for prolonged QT syndrome. *Emerg Med Australas* 2005; 17:274–276.

43. Vieweg WV, et al. Torsade de pointes in a patient with complex medical and psychiatric conditions receiving low-dose quetiapine. *Acta Psychiatr Scand* 2005; 112:318–322.

44. Huang BH, et al. Sulpiride induced torsade de pointes. *Int J Cardiol* 2007; 118:e100–e102.

45. Kane JM, et al. Long-term efficacy and safety of iloperidone: results from 3 clinical trials for the treatment of schizophrenia. *J Clin Psychopharmacol* 2008; 28:S29–S35.

46. Kim MD, et al. Blockade of HERG human K+ channel and IKr of guinea pig cardiomyocytes by prochlorperazine. *Eur J Pharmacol* 2006; 544:82–90.

47. Meltzer H, et al. Efficacy and tolerability of oral paliperidone extended-release tablets in the treatment of acute schizophrenia: pooled data from three 6-week placebo-controlled studies. *J Clin Psychiatry* 2006; 69:817–829.

48. Chapel S, et al. Exposure-response analysis in patients with schizophrenia to assess the effect of asenapine on QTc prolongation. *J Clin Pharmacol* 2009; 49:1297–1308.

49. Ozeki Y, et al. QTc prolongation and antipsychotic medications in a sample of 1017 patients with schizophrenia. *Prog Neuropsychopharmacol Biol Psychiatry* 2010; 34:401–405.

50. Girardin FR, et al. Drug-induced long QT in adult psychiatric inpatients: the 5-year cross-sectional ECG Screening Outcome in Psychiatry study. *Am J Psychiatry* 2013; 170:1468–1476.

51. Leucht S, et al. Comparative efficacy and tolerability of 15 antipsychotic drugs in schizophrenia: a multiple-treatments meta-analysis. *Lancet* 2013; **382**:951–962.
52. Hong HK, et al. Block of hERG K+ channel and prolongation of action potential duration by fluphenazine at submicromolar concentration. *Eur J Pharmacol* 2013; **702**:165–173.
53. Vieweg WV, et al. Risperidone, QTc interval prolongation, and torsade de pointes: a systematic review of case reports. *Psychopharmacology (Berl)* 2013; **228**:515–524.
54. Suzuki Y, et al. QT prolongation of the antipsychotic risperidone is predominantly related to its 9-hydroxy metabolite paliperidone. *Hum Psychopharmacol* 2012; **27**:39–42.
55. Polcwiartek C, et al. The cardiac safety of aripiprazole treatment in patients at high risk for torsade: a systematic review with a meta-analytic approach. *Psychopharmacology (Berl)* 2015; **232**:3297–3308.
56. Citrome L. Cariprazine in schizophrenia: clinical efficacy, tolerability, and place in therapy. *Adv Ther* 2013; **30**:114–126.
57. Das S, et al. Brexpiprazole: so far so good. *Ther Adv Psychopharmacol* 2016; **6**:39–54.
58. Meyer JM, et al. Lurasidone: a new drug in development for schizophrenia. *Expert Opin Investig Drugs* 2009; **18**:1715–1726.
59. Kim K, et al. Clozapine blood concentration predicts corrected QT-interval prolongation in patients with psychoses. *J Clin Psychopharmacol* 2022; **42**:536–543.
60. Nelson S, et al. Torsades de pointes after administration of low-dose aripiprazole. *Ann Pharmacother* 2013; **47**:e11.
61. Hategan A, et al. Aripiprazole-associated QTc prolongation in a geriatric patient. *J Clin Psychopharmacol* 2014; **34**:766–768.
62. Suzuki Y, et al. Dose-dependent increase in the QTc interval in aripiprazole treatment after risperidone. *Prog Neuropsychopharmacol Biol Psychiatry* 2011; **35**:643–644.
63. Raschi E, et al. The contribution of national spontaneous reporting systems to detect signals of torsadogenicity: issues emerging from the ARITMO Project. *Drug Saf* 2016; **39**:59–64.
64. He L, et al. Characteristics and spectrum of cardiotoxicity induced by various antipsychotics: a real-world study from 2015 to 2020 based on FAERS. *Front Pharmacol* 2021; **12**:815151.
65. Belmonte C, et al. Evaluation of the relationship between pharmacokinetics and the safety of aripiprazole and its cardiovascular effects in healthy volunteers. *J Clin Psychopharmacol* 2016; **36**:608–614.
66. Germano E, et al. ECG parameters in children and adolescents treated with aripiprazole and risperidone. *Prog Neuropsychopharmacol Biol Psychiatry* 2014; **51**:23–27.
67. Pilunthanakul T, et al. The impact of adjunctive aripiprazole on QT interval: A 12-week open label study in patients on olanzapine, clozapine or risperidone. *Hum Psychopharmacol* 2023; **38**:e2863.
68. Su KP, et al. Olanzapine-induced QTc prolongation in a patient with Wolff–Parkinson–White syndrome. *Schizophr Res* 2004; **66**:191–192.
69. Morissette P, et al. Olanzapine prolongs cardiac repolarization by blocking the rapid component of the delayed rectifier potassium current. *J Psychopharmacol* 2007; **21**:735–741.
70. Bar KJ, et al. Influence of olanzapine on QT variability and complexity measures of heart rate in patients with schizophrenia. *J Clin Psychopharmacol* 2008; **28**:694–698.
71. Berling I, et al. Prolonged QT risk assessment in antipsychotic overdose using the QT nomogram. *Ann Emerg Med* 2015; **66**:154–164.
72. Jensen KG, et al. Corrected QT changes during antipsychotic treatment of children and adolescents: a systematic review and meta-analysis of clinical trials. *J Am Acad Child Adolesc Psychiatry* 2015; **54**:25–36.
73. Karz AJ, et al. Effects of aripiprazole on the QTc: a case report. *J Clin Psychiatry* 2015; **76**:1648–1649.
74. Friedrich ME, et al. Cardiovascular adverse reactions during antipsychotic treatment: results of AMSP, a drug surveillance program between 1993 and 2013. *Int J Neuropsychopharmacol* 2020; **23**:67–75.
75. Sunovion Pharmaceuticals Inc. Highlights of Prescribing Information: LATUDA (lurasidone hydrochloride) tablets for oral use. 2022 (last checked December 2024); http://www.latuda.com/LatudaPrescribingInformation.pdf.
76. Potkin SG, et al. Double-blind comparison of the safety and efficacy of lurasidone and ziprasidone in clinically stable outpatients with schizophrenia or schizoaffective disorder. *Schizophr Res* 2011; **132**:101–107.
77. Nakamura M, et al. Lurasidone in the treatment of acute schizophrenia: a double-blind, placebo-controlled trial. *J Clin Psychiatry* 2009; **70**:829–836.
78. Meltzer HY, et al. Lurasidone in the treatment of schizophrenia: a randomized, double-blind, placebo- and olanzapine-controlled study. *Am J Psychiatry* 2011; **168**:957–967.
79. Naguy A, et al. Possible lurasidone-associated dose-dependent QTc prolongation in first-episode psychosis. *Psychopharmacol Bull* 2022; **52**:68–71.
80. Vaiman EE, et al. Genetic biomarkers of antipsychotic-induced prolongation of the QT interval in patients with schizophrenia. *Int J Mol Sci* 2022; **23**:15786.
81. Hasnain M, et al. Quetiapine, QTc interval prolongation, and torsade de pointes: a review of case reports. *Ther Adv Psychopharmacol* 2014; **4**:130–138.
82. Hatta K, et al. Prolonged QT interval in acute psychotic patients. *Psychiatry Res* 2000; **94**:279–285.
83. Priori SG, et al. Low penetrance in the long-QT syndrome: clinical impact. *Circulation* 1999; **99**:529–533.
84. Frassati D, et al. Hidden cardiac lesions and psychotropic drugs as a possible cause of sudden death in psychiatric patients: a report of 14 cases and review of the literature. *Can J Psychiatry* 2004; **49**:100–105.

Effects of antipsychotic medications on plasma lipids

Morbidity and mortality from cardiovascular disease are higher in people with schizophrenia than in the general population.[1-3] Dyslipidaemia is an established risk factor for cardiovascular disease, together with obesity, hypertension, smoking, diabetes and sedentary lifestyle. Specifically, reduced high-density lipoprotein (HDL) cholesterol and raised triglyceride levels are included in the definition of the metabolic syndrome.[4] The majority of patients with schizophrenia have several of these cardiometabolic risk factors and can be considered at 'high risk' of developing cardiovascular disease. Dyslipidaemia is treatable and intervention is known to reduce morbidity and mortality.[5] Aggressive treatment is particularly important in people with diabetes, the prevalence of which is increased two- to three-fold over population norms in people with schizophrenia (see section on diabetes and impaired glucose tolerance).

Effect of antipsychotic medications on lipids

Antipsychotic medications show a marked variation in their effects on total cholesterol, low-density lipoprotein (LDL) cholesterol, HDL cholesterol and triglycerides.[6,7] Regarding FGAs, phenothiazines are known to be associated with increases in triglycerides and LDL cholesterol and decreases in HDL[8] cholesterol, but the magnitude of these effects is poorly quantified.[9] Haloperidol seems to have minimal effect on lipid profiles.[8] Although there are relatively more data pertaining to some SGAs, they are derived from a variety of sources and are reported in different ways, making it difficult to compare such medications directly. While cholesterol levels can rise, the most profound effect of antipsychotic medications seems to be on triglycerides. Raised triglycerides are, in general, associated with obesity and diabetes. From the available data, clozapine and olanzapine[6,10] would seem to have the greatest propensity to increase lipids, while quetiapine and risperidone have a moderate propensity.[11,12] Aripiprazole, lurasidone and ziprasidone appear to have minimal adverse effect on blood lipids[6,10,13-18] and may even modestly reverse dyslipidaemias associated with previous antipsychotics.[17,19,20] For cariprazine and brexpiprazole, the effects on plasma lipids would also appear to be relatively limited.[6,21-24] Iloperidone causes some weight gain but may not have an equivalent impact on cholesterol or triglycerides.[6,25,26] Early RCT data suggest that lumateperone is not associated with any significant effects on plasma cholesterol or triglycerides in the short term, compared with placebo.[27]

Olanzapine

In people with schizophrenia, olanzapine has a relatively high propensity to induce dyslipidaemia,[6,7] which is characterised by elevated levels of plasma triglyceride, total cholesterol and LDL cholesterol and can occur in the first 4 weeks of treatment.[28] Triglyceride levels have been shown to increase by 40% over the short (12 weeks) and medium (16 months) term.[29,30] Levels may continue to rise for up to a year.[31] Up to two-thirds of patients treated with olanzapine have raised triglycerides[32] and just under 10% may develop severe hypertriglyceridaemia.[33] While weight gain with olanzapine is generally associated with increases in both cholesterol[30,34] and triglycerides,[33] severe hypertriglyceridaemia can occur independently of weight gain.[33] In one study, patients treated with olanzapine or risperidone gained a similar amount of weight, but with olanzapine, serum triglyceride levels increased by four times as much (105mg/dL) as for risperidone (32 mg/dL).[35] Quetiapine[36] seems to have more modest effects than olanzapine, although the data are conflicting.[37]

A case–control study conducted in the UK found that patients with schizophrenia who were treated with olanzapine were five times more likely to develop hyperlipidaemia than those with no antipsychotic exposure and three times more likely to develop hyperlipidaemia than patients receiving FGAs.[38] Risperidone treatment was not associated with an increased likelihood of hyperlipidaemia compared with no antipsychotic exposure or treatment with an FGA.

Clozapine

Clozapine also has a relatively high propensity to induce dyslipidaemia.[6,7] Mean triglyceride levels have been shown to double and cholesterol levels to increase by at least 10% after 5 years of treatment with clozapine.[39] Patients treated with clozapine have triglyceride levels that are almost double those of patients who are treated with FGA medications.[40,41] Cholesterol levels are also increased.[10]

Particular care should be taken before prescribing clozapine or olanzapine for patients who are obese, diabetic or known to have pre-existing hyperlipidaemia.[42]

Screening and monitoring

In patients with schizophrenia treated with antipsychotic medication, the monitoring of plasma lipids by mental health services and in primary care is generally insufficient,[43–47] falling short of recommended practice.[48,49] All patients should have their lipids measured at baseline, 3 months after starting treatment with a new antipsychotic medication and then annually. Those prescribed clozapine and olanzapine should ideally have their serum lipids measured every 3 months for the first year of treatment, and then annually.

Clinically significant changes in cholesterol are unlikely over the short term but triglycerides can increase dramatically.[50] In practice, dyslipidaemia is widespread in patients on long-term antipsychotic treatment irrespective of the medication prescribed or of diagnosis.[51–53]

Severe hypertriglyceridaemia (fasting level of >5mmol/L) is a risk factor for pancreatitis. Note that antipsychotic-induced dyslipidaemia can occur independent of weight gain.[54]

Clinical management of dyslipidaemia

Patients with raised cholesterol may benefit from dietary advice, lifestyle changes and/ or treatment with statins.[49,55] Statins seem to be effective in this patient group, although pharmacokinetic and pharmacodynamic interactions are possible.[56,57] The outline of a systematic approach to the diagnosis and management of hypercholesterolaemia is available,[58] based on NICE guidance in the UK.[59] Further, risk tables and treatment guidelines can be found in the BNF. Evidence supports the treatment of cholesterol concentrations as low as 4mmol/L in high-risk patients[60] and this is the highest level recommended by NICE for secondary prevention of cardiovascular events.[61] NICE makes no recommendations on target levels for primary prevention but recent advice promotes the use of statins for anyone with a >10% 10-year risk of cardiovascular disease.[61] Coronary heart disease and stroke risk can be reduced by a third by reducing cholesterol to as low as 3.5mmol/L. When triglycerides alone are raised, diets low in saturated fats and the taking of fish oil and fibrates are effective treatments,[31,62,63] although there is no proof that mortality is reduced. Such patients should be screened for impaired glucose tolerance and diabetes.

If moderate to severe hyperlipidaemia develops during antipsychotic treatment, a switch to another antipsychotic medication less likely to cause this problem should be considered in the first instance. Although not recommended as a strategy in patients with treatment-resistant illness, clozapine-induced hypertriglyceridaemia has been shown to reverse after a switch to risperidone.[64] This may hold true with other switching regimens but data are scarce.[65] Aripiprazole and other D2 partial agonists seem to be the treatments of choice in those with prior antipsychotic-induced dyslipidaemia (lumateperone and ziprasidone are options outside the UK).[20,66] There is evidence to suggest that adjunctive aripiprazole may have beneficial effects on measures of plasma cholesterol and triglycerides when combined with clozapine or olanzapine[19,49,67] and that metformin added to antipsychotic medication may improve total cholesterol and triglyceride levels[49,68] (see Buzea et al. 2022[57] and the 'BAP guidelines on the management of weight gain, metabolic disturbances and cardiovascular risk associated with psychosis and antipsychotic drug treatment'[49] for discussion of the potential risks and benefits of these two strategies).

Summary of monitoring

Medication	Suggested monitoring schedule
Clozapine	Fasting lipids at baseline then every 3 months for a year, then annually
Olanzapine	
Other antipsychotic medications	Fasting lipids at baseline, 3 months, and then annually[66]

References

1. Brown S, et al. Causes of the excess mortality of schizophrenia. *Br J Psychiatry* 2000; **177**:212–217.
2. Correll CU, et al. Prevalence, incidence and mortality from cardiovascular disease in patients with pooled and specific severe mental illness: a large-scale meta-analysis of 3,211,768 patients and 113,383,368 controls. *World Psychiatry* 2017; **16**:163–180.
3. Lemogne C, et al. Management of cardiovascular health in people with severe mental disorders. *Curr Cardiol Rep* 2021; **23**:7.
4. Alberti KG, et al. The metabolic syndrome: a new worldwide definition. *Lancet* 2005; **366**:1059–1062.
5. Durrington P. Dyslipidaemia. *Lancet* 2003; **362**:717–731.
6. Pillinger T, et al. Comparative effects of 18 antipsychotics on metabolic function in patients with schizophrenia, predictors of metabolic dysregulation, and association with psychopathology: a systematic review and network meta-analysis. *Lancet Psychiatry* 2020; **7**:64–77.
7. Burschinski A, et al. Metabolic side effects in persons with schizophrenia during mid- to long-term treatment with antipsychotics: a network meta-analysis of randomized controlled trials. *World Psychiatry* 2023; **22**:116–128.
8. Sasaki J, et al. Lipids and apolipoproteins in patients treated with major tranquilizers. *Clin Pharmacol Ther* 1985; **37**:684–687.
9. Henkin Y, et al. Secondary dyslipidemia: inadvertent effects of drugs in clinical practice. *JAMA* 1992; **267**:961–968.
10. Chaggar PS, et al. Effect of antipsychotic medications on glucose and lipid levels. *J Clin Pharmacol* 2011; **51**:631–638.
11. Smith RC, et al. Effects of olanzapine and risperidone on lipid metabolism in chronic schizophrenic patients with long-term antipsychotic treatment: a randomized five month study. *Schizophr Res* 2010; **120**:204–209.

CHAPTER 1

12. Perez-Iglesias R, et al. Glucose and lipid disturbances after 1 year of antipsychotic treatment in a drug-naive population. *Schizophr Res* 2009; **107**:115–121.
13. Olfson M, et al. Hyperlipidemia following treatment with antipsychotic medications. *Am J Psychiatry* 2006; **163**:1821–1825.
14. L'Italien GJ, et al. Comparison of metabolic syndrome incidence among schizophrenia patients treated with aripiprazole versus olanzapine or placebo. *J Clin Psychiatry* 2007; **68**:1510–1516.
15. Fenton WS, et al. Medication-induced weight gain and dyslipidemia in patients with schizophrenia. *Am J Psychiatry* 2006; **163**:1697–1704.
16. Meyer JM, et al. Change in metabolic syndrome parameters with antipsychotic treatment in the CATIE schizophrenia trial: prospective data from phase 1. *Schizophr Res* 2008; **101**:273–286.
17. Potkin SG, et al. Double-blind comparison of the safety and efficacy of lurasidone and ziprasidone in clinically stable outpatients with schizophrenia or schizoaffective disorder. *Schizophr Res* 2011; **132**:101–107.
18. Correll CU, et al. Long-term safety and effectiveness of lurasidone in schizophrenia: a 22-month, open-label extension study. *CNS Spectr* 2016; **21**:393–402.
19. Fleischhacker WW, et al. Effects of adjunctive treatment with aripiprazole on body weight and clinical efficacy in schizophrenia patients treated with clozapine: a randomized, double-blind, placebo-controlled trial. *Int J Neuropsychopharmacol* 2010; **13**:1115–1125.
20. Chen Y, et al. Comparative effectiveness of switching antipsychotic drug treatment to aripiprazole or ziprasidone for improving metabolic profile and atherogenic dyslipidemia: a 12-month, prospective, open-label study. *J Psychopharmacol* 2012; **26**:1201–1210.
21. Lao KS, et al. Tolerability and safety profile of cariprazine in treating psychotic disorders, bipolar disorder and major depressive disorder: a systematic review with meta-analysis of randomized controlled trials. *CNS Drugs* 2016; **30**:1043–1054.
22. Earley W, et al. Tolerability of cariprazine in the treatment of acute bipolar I mania: a pooled post hoc analysis of 3 phase II/III studies. *J Affect Disord* 2017; **215**:205–212.
23. McEvoy J, et al. Brexpiprazole for the treatment of schizophrenia: a review of this novel serotonin-dopamine activity modulator. *Clin Schizophr Relat Psychoses* 2016; **9**:177–186.
24. Correll CU, et al. Efficacy and safety of brexpiprazole for the treatment of acute schizophrenia: a 6-week randomized, double-blind, placebo-controlled trial. *Am J Psychiatry* 2015; **172**:870–880.
25. Citrome L. Iloperidone: chemistry, pharmacodynamics, pharmacokinetics and metabolism, clinical efficacy, safety and tolerability, regulatory affairs, and an opinion. *Expert Opin Drug Metab Toxicol* 2010; **6**:1551–1564.
26. Cutler AJ, et al. Long-term safety and tolerability of iloperidone: results from a 25-week, open-label extension trial. *CNS Spectr* 2013; **18**:43–54.
27. Correll CU, et al. Efficacy and safety of lumateperone for treatment of schizophrenia: a randomized clinical trial. *JAMA Psychiatry* 2020; **77**:349–358.
28. Li R, et al. Effects of olanzapine treatment on lipid profiles in patients with schizophrenia: a systematic review and meta-analysis. *Sci Rep* 2020; **10**:17028.
29. Sheitman BB, et al. Olanzapine-induced elevation of plasma triglyceride levels. *Am J Psychiatry* 1999; **156**:1471–1472.
30. Osser DN, et al. Olanzapine increases weight and serum triglyceride levels. *J Clin Psychiatry* 1999; **60**:767–770.
31. Meyer JM. Effects of atypical antipsychotics on weight and serum lipid levels. *J Clin Psychiatry* 2001; **62** Suppl 27:27–34.
32. Melkersson KI, et al. Elevated levels of insulin, leptin, and blood lipids in olanzapine-treated patients with schizophrenia or related psychoses. *J Clin Psychiatry* 2000; **61**:742–749.
33. Meyer JM. Novel antipsychotics and severe hyperlipidemia. *J Clin Psychopharmacol* 2001; **21**:369–374.
34. Kinon BJ, et al. Long-term olanzapine treatment: weight change and weight-related health factors in schizophrenia. *J Clin Psychiatry* 2001; **62**:92–100.
35. Meyer JM. A retrospective comparison of weight, lipid, and glucose changes between risperidone- and olanzapine-treated inpatients: metabolic outcomes after 1 year. *J Clin Psychiatry* 2002; **63**:425–433.
36. Atmaca M, et al. Serum leptin and triglyceride levels in patients on treatment with atypical antipsychotics. *J Clin Psychiatry* 2003; **64**:598–604.
37. de Leon J, et al. A clinical study of the association of antipsychotics with hyperlipidemia. *Schizophr Res* 2007; **92**:95–102.
38. Koro CE, et al. An assessment of the independent effects of olanzapine and risperidone exposure on the risk of hyperlipidemia in schizophrenic patients. *Arch Gen Psychiatry* 2002; **59**:1021–1026.
39. Henderson DC, et al. Clozapine, diabetes mellitus, weight gain, and lipid abnormalities: a five-year naturalistic study. *Am J Psychiatry* 2000; **157**:975–981.
40. Ghaeli P, et al. Serum triglyceride levels in patients treated with clozapine. *Am J Health Syst Pharm* 1996; **53**:2079–2081.
41. Spivak B, et al. Diminished suicidal and aggressive behavior, high plasma norepinephrine levels, and serum triglyceride levels in chronic neuroleptic-resistant schizophrenic patients maintained on clozapine. *Clin Neuropharmacol* 1998; **21**:245–250.
42. Baptista T, et al. Novel antipsychotics and severe hyperlipidemia: comments on the Meyer paper. *J Clin Psychopharmacol* 2002; **22**:536–537.
43. Barnes TR, et al. Screening for the metabolic side effects of antipsychotic medication: findings of a 6-year quality improvement programme in the UK. *BMJ Open* 2015; **5**:e007633.
44. Fond G, et al. How can we improve the care of patients with schizophrenia in the real-world? A population-based cohort study of 456,003 patients. *Mol Psychiatry* 2023; **28**:5328–5336.
45. Ali RA, et al. Guideline adherence for cardiometabolic monitoring of patients prescribed antipsychotic medications in primary care: a retrospective observational study. *Int J Clin Pharm* 2023; **45**:1241–1251.

46. Mitchell AJ, et al. Guideline concordant monitoring of metabolic risk in people treated with antipsychotic medication: systematic review and meta-analysis of screening practices. *Psychol Med* 2012; **42**:125–147.

47. Al-Awad FA, et al. Adherence to the monitoring of metabolic syndrome in patients receiving antipsychotics in outpatient clinics in Saudi Arabia. *J Family Community Med* 2024; **31**:42–47.

48. National Institute for Health and Care Excellence. Psychosis and schizophrenia in adults: prevention and management. Clinical guideline [CG178]. 2014 (last checked February 2024); https://www.nice.org.uk/guidance/cg178.

49. Cooper SJ, et al. BAP guidelines on the management of weight gain, metabolic disturbances and cardiovascular risk associated with psychosis and antipsychotic drug treatment. *J Psychopharmacol* 2016; **30**:717–748.

50. Meyer JM, et al. The effects of antipsychotic therapy on serum lipids: a comprehensive review. *Schizophr Res* 2004; **70**:1–17.

51. Paton C, et al. Obesity, dyslipidaemias and smoking in an inpatient population treated with antipsychotic drugs. *Acta Psychiatr Scand* 2004; **110**:299–305.

52. De Hert M, et al. The METEOR study of diabetes and other metabolic disorders in patients with schizophrenia treated with antipsychotic drugs. I. Methodology. *Int J Methods Psychiatr Res* 2010; **19**:195–210.

53. Jin H, et al. Comparison of longer-term safety and effectiveness of 4 atypical antipsychotics in patients over age 40: a trial using equipoise-stratified randomization. *J Clin Psychiatry* 2013; **74**:10–18.

54. Birkenaes AB, et al. Dyslipidemia independent of body mass in antipsychotic-treated patients under real-life conditions. *J Clin Psychopharmacol* 2008; **28**:132–137.

55. Ojala K, et al. Statins are effective in treating dyslipidemia among psychiatric patients using second-generation antipsychotic agents. *J Psychopharmacol* 2008; **22**:33–38.

56. Tse L, et al. Pharmacological treatment of antipsychotic-induced dyslipidemia and hypertension. *Int Clin Psychopharmacol* 2014; **29**:125–137.

57. Buzea CA, et al. Drug-drug interactions involving combinations of antipsychotic agents with antidiabetic, lipid-lowering, and weight loss drugs. *Expert Opin Drug Metab Toxicol* 2022; **18**:729–744.

58. Ryan A, et al. Dyslipidaemia and cardiovascular risk. *BMJ* 2018; **360**:k835.

59. Rabar S, et al. Lipid modification and cardiovascular risk assessment for the primary and secondary prevention of cardiovascular disease: summary of updated NICE guidance. *BMJ* 2014; **349**:g4356.

60. Group HPSC. MRC/BHF Heart Protection Study of cholesterol lowering with simvastatin in 20,536 high-risk individuals: a randomised placebo-controlled trial. *Lancet* 2002; **360**:7–22.

61. National Institute for Health and Care Excellence. Cardiovascular disease: risk assessment and reduction, including lipid modification. NICE guideline [NG238]. 2023 (last accessed February 2024); https://www.nice.org.uk/guidance/ng238.

62. Caniato RN, et al. Effect of omega-3 fatty acids on the lipid profile of patients taking clozapine. *Aust N Z J Psychiatry* 2006; **40**:691–697.

63. Freeman MP, et al. Omega-3 fatty acids for atypical antipsychotic-associated hypertriglyceridemia. *Ann Clin Psychiatry* 2015; **27**:197–202.

64. Ghaeli P, et al. Elevated serum triglycerides with clozapine resolved with risperidone in four patients. *Pharmacotherapy* 1999; **19**:1099–1101.

65. Weiden PJ. Switching antipsychotics as a treatment strategy for antipsychotic-induced weight gain and dyslipidemia. *J Clin Psychiatry* 2007; **68** Suppl 4:34–39.

66. Newcomer JW, et al. A multicenter, randomized, double-blind study of the effects of aripiprazole in overweight subjects with schizophrenia or schizoaffective disorder switched from olanzapine. *J Clin Psychiatry* 2008; **69**:1046–1056.

67. Henderson DC, et al. Aripiprazole added to overweight and obese olanzapine-treated schizophrenia patients. *J Clin Psychopharmacol* 2009; **29**:165–169.

68. Jiang WL, et al. Adjunctive metformin for antipsychotic-induced dyslipidemia: a meta-analysis of randomized, double-blind, placebo-controlled trials. *Transl Psychiatry* 2020; **10**:117.

Diabetes and impaired glucose tolerance

Schizophrenia

Schizophrenia is associated with relatively high rates of insulin resistance and type 2 diabetes[1,2] – an observation that predates the discovery and widespread use of antipsychotic medication.[3-5] Lifestyle interventions (healthy diet, losing weight, regular physical activity) are effective in preventing diabetes[6,7] and should be considered for all people with a diagnosis of schizophrenia.

Antipsychotic medications

The data relating to diabetes and the use of antipsychotic medication are numerous but less than perfect.[8-12] The main problem is that while incidence and prevalence studies assume full or uniform screening for diabetes, this is unlikely to be occurring in clinical practice.[13] Many studies do not account for other factors affecting the risk of developing diabetes.[14] Small differences between medications are therefore difficult to substantiate but may, in any case, be ultimately unimportant: risk is probably increased for all those with schizophrenia receiving any antipsychotic medication. This risk is fairly strongly linked to increased diabetes-related mortality.[11]

The mechanisms involved in the development of antipsychotic-related diabetes are unclear, but may include $5HT_{2A}/5HT_{2C}$ antagonism, increased plasma lipids, weight gain and leptin resistance.[15] Pancreatic insulin secretion is controlled by dopamine[16] and this may explain why so many antipsychotics cause impaired glucose tolerance.[17] Insulin resistance may occur in the absence of weight gain.[18]

First-generation antipsychotic medications

Phenothiazine derivatives have long been associated with impaired glucose tolerance and diabetes.[19] Diabetes prevalence was reported to have substantially increased following the introduction and widespread use of FGA medications.[20] The prevalence of impaired glucose tolerance seems to be higher with the aliphatic phenothiazines than with fluphenazine or haloperidol.[21] Hyperglycaemia has also been reported with other FGAs, such as loxapine,[22] and other data confirm an association with haloperidol.[23] Some studies have suggested that FGAs are no different from SGAs in their propensity to cause diabetes,[24,25] whereas others suggest a modest but statistically significant excess incidence of diabetes with SGAs.[26]

Second-generation antipsychotic medications

Clozapine

Clozapine is strongly linked to hyperglycaemia, impaired glucose tolerance and diabetic ketoacidosis.[27] The risk of diabetes appears to be higher with clozapine than with other SGAs or FGAs, especially in younger patients,[28-31] although this is not a consistent finding.[32,33]

As many as a third of patients on continuing treatment with clozapine might develop diabetes after 5 years.[34] Many cases of diabetes occur in the first 6 months of treatment, some within a month,[35] and some only after many years.[33] Death from ketoacidosis has also been reported.[35] Diabetes associated with clozapine is not necessarily linked to obesity or to family history of diabetes,[27,36] although these factors greatly increase the risk of developing diabetes on this medication.[37]

Clozapine appears to increase plasma levels of insulin in a clozapine level-dependent fashion.[38,39] It has been shown to be more likely than FGAs to increase plasma glucose and insulin following oral glucose challenge.[40] Testing for diabetes is essential, given the high prevalence of the condition in people receiving clozapine.[41,42]

Olanzapine

As with clozapine, olanzapine has been strongly linked to impaired glucose tolerance, diabetes and diabetic ketoacidosis.[43] Olanzapine and clozapine appear to directly induce insulin resistance.[44,45] Risk of diabetes has also been reported to be higher with olanzapine than with FGA drugs,[46] again with a particular risk in younger patients.[29] The time course of development of diabetes has not been established, but impaired glucose tolerance seems to occur even in the absence of obesity and family history of diabetes.[27,36] Olanzapine is probably more diabetogenic than risperidone.[47–51] Olanzapine is also associated with plasma levels of glucose and insulin higher than those seen with FGAs (after oral glucose load).[40,52]

Risperidone

Risperidone has been linked, mainly in case reports, to impaired glucose tolerance,[53] diabetes[54] and ketoacidosis.[55] The number of reports of such adverse effects is substantially smaller than with either clozapine or olanzapine.[56] At least one study has suggested that changes in fasting glucose are significantly less common with risperidone than with olanzapine,[47] but other studies have detected no difference.[57]

Risperidone seems no more likely than FGA drugs to be associated with diabetes,[29,46,48] although there may be an increased risk in patients under 40 years of age.[29] Risperidone has, however, been observed to adversely affect fasting glucose and plasma glucose (following glucose challenge) compared with the levels seen in healthy volunteers (but not compared with patients taking FGAs).[40]

Quetiapine

Like risperidone, quetiapine has been linked to cases of new-onset diabetes and ketoacidosis,[58–60] and associated with an increased risk of diabetes.[61,62] Two studies showed quetiapine to be equal to olanzapine in the incidence of diabetes.[57,63] The risk with quetiapine may be dose related, with daily doses of 400mg or more being clearly linked to changes in HbA_{1C}.[64]

Other SGAs

Amisulpride appears not to elevate plasma glucose,[65] although there is one reported case of ketoacidosis occurring in a patient given the closely related medication sulpiride.[66] Data for **aripiprazole**[67–70] and **ziprasidone**[71,72] suggest that neither drug alters glucose homeostasis. Aripiprazole may even reverse diabetes caused by other drugs[73] (although ketoacidosis has been reported with aripiprazole).[74–76] Further, studies have not found amisulpride or aripiprazole to be associated with a significantly greater risk of diabetes.[61,77,78] So, these three drugs (amisulpride, aripiprazole and ziprasidone) are recommended for those with a history of, or predisposition to, diabetes mellitus or as an alternative to other antipsychotic medications known to be diabetogenic.

Data suggest that neither **lurasidone**[79,80] nor **asenapine**[81,82] has any effect on glucose homeostasis. Likewise, early data on **brexpiprazole**[83,84] and **cariprazine**[85–87] suggest minimal effects on glucose tolerance. Thus, for patients developing prediabetes or diabetes who are being treated with clozapine, olanzapine or quetiapine, switching to antipsychotic medications with a lower cardiometabolic risk, such as aripiprazole, brexpiprazole, cariprazine, lurasidone or ziprasidone, has been recommended.[88] **Lumateperone** appears to have no effect on glucose parameters[89] but clinical experience is limited.

Predicting antipsychotic-related diabetes

The risk of diabetes is increased to a much greater extent in younger adults than in the elderly[90,91] (for whom antipsychotic medication may show no increased risk).[92] Patients with first-episode schizophrenia seem particularly prone to the development of diabetes with a variety of antipsychotic medications.[93–95] During treatment, rapid weight gain and a rise in plasma triglycerides seem to be predictive of the development of diabetes.[96,97] Monitoring of abnormal glucose metabolism is particularly warranted in those with obesity or hypertriglyceridaemia.[42]

Monitoring

Diabetes is a growing problem in western society and has a strong association with obesity, (older) age, (lower) educational achievement and certain ethnic groups.[98,99] Diabetes markedly increases cardiovascular mortality, largely as a consequence of atherosclerosis.[100] Likewise, the use of antipsychotic medication also increases cardiovascular mortality.[101–103] Intervention to reduce plasma glucose levels and minimise other risk factors (obesity, hypercholesterolaemia) is therefore essential.[104]

There is no clear consensus on diabetes monitoring practice for those receiving antipsychotic medication,[105] and the recommendations in formal guidelines vary considerably.[106] Given the previous known parlous state of testing for diabetes in the UK[13,107–109] and elsewhere,[110] arguments over precisely which tests are done and when seem to miss the point. There is an overwhelming need to improve monitoring by any means and so any tests for diabetes are supported – urine glucose and random plasma glucose included.

Ideally, though, all patients should have oral glucose tolerance tests (OGTT) performed as this is the most sensitive method of detection.[111,112] Fasting plasma glucose (FPG) tests are less sensitive but recommended.[113] Any abnormality in FPG should provoke an OGTT. Fasting tests are often difficult to obtain in acutely ill, disorganised patients, so measurement of random plasma glucose or glycated haemoglobin (HbA_{1c}) may also be used (fasting not required). HbA_{1C} is recognised as a useful tool in detecting and monitoring diabetes.[7] In the UK, NICE[114] recommendations for monitoring people with a psychotic disorder, treated with antipsychotic medication, include the measurement of plasma glucose or HbA_{1C} 3 months after starting treatment and then annually (Table 1.39).

Table 1.39 Recommended monitoring for diabetes in patients receiving antipsychotic drugs.

Treatment stage	Recommended monitoring	
	Ideally	Minimum
At baseline	OGTT or FPG. HbA$_{1C}$ if fasting not possible.	UG, RPG
Continuing	All antipsychotic medications: OGTT or FPG + HbA$_{1C}$ at 4–6 months then every 12 months	UG or RPG every 12 months, with symptom monitoring
	For clozapine and olanzapine or if other risk factors present: OGTT or FPG after 1 month, then every 4–6 months	
	HbA$_{1C}$ is a suitable test for monitoring. But note that this test is not suitable for detecting short-term change.	

FPG, fasting plasma glucose; HbA$_{1C}$, glycated haemoglobin; OGTT, oral glucose tolerance tests; RPG, random plasma glucose; UG, urine glucose.

Frequency of monitoring should be determined by physical factors (e.g. weight gain) and known risk factors (e.g. family history of diabetes, lipid abnormalities, smoking status). In addition, all patients should be asked to look out for and report signs and symptoms of diabetes (fatigue, candida infection, thirst polyuria).

Treatment of antipsychotic-related diabetes

Switching to an antipsychotic medication with a lower cardiometabolic risk is often effective in reversing changes in glucose tolerance. In this respect, the most compelling evidence is for switching to aripiprazole,[115,116] but also to ziprasidone[116] and lurasidone.[80,117] Standard antidiabetic treatments are otherwise recommended.[88] Pioglitazone[118] may have particular benefit, but note the hepatotoxic potential of this drug. GLP-1 agonists such as liraglutide, exenatide and semaglutide are increasingly used.[119–121]

Summary: antipsychotic medications – risk of diabetes and impaired glucose tolerance

High risk	Clozapine, olanzapine
Moderate risk	Phenothiazines, quetiapine, risperidone
Low risk	High-potency FGAs (e.g. haloperidol)
Minimal risk	Aripiprazole, amisulpride, asenapine, brexpiprazole, cariprazine, lumateperone, lurasidone, ziprasidone

References

1. Schimmelbusch WH, et al. The positive correlation between insulin resistance and duration of hospitalization in untreated schizophrenia. *Br J Psychiatry* 1971; **118**:429–436.
2. Waitzkin L. A survey for unknown diabetics in a mental hospital. I. Men under age fifty. *Diabetes* 1966; **15**:97–104.
3. Kasanin J. The blood sugar curve in mental disease. II. The schizophrenia (dementia praecox) groups. *Arch Neurol Psychiatry* 1926; **16**:414–419.
4. Braceland FJ, et al. Delayed action of insulin in schizophrenia. *Am J Psychiatry* 1945; **102**:108–110.
5. Kohen D. Diabetes mellitus and schizophrenia: historical perspective. *Br J Psychiatry Suppl* 2004; **47**:S64–S66.
6. Glechner A, et al. Effects of lifestyle changes on adults with prediabetes: a systematic review and meta-analysis. *Prim Care Diabetes* 2018; **12**:393–408.
7. National Institute for Health and Care Excellence. Type 2 diabetes in adults: management. NICE guideline [NG28]; 2015 (last updated June 2022, last checked March 2024); https://www.nice.org.uk/guidance/ng28.
8. Haddad PM. Antipsychotics and diabetes: review of non-prospective data. *Br J Psychiatry Suppl* 2004; **47**:S80–S86.
9. Bushe C, et al. Association between atypical antipsychotic agents and type 2 diabetes: review of prospective clinical data. *Br J Psychiatry* 2004; **184**:S87–S93.
10. Hirigo AT, et al. The magnitude of undiagnosed diabetes and hypertension among adult psychiatric patients receiving antipsychotic treatment. *Diabetol Metab Syndr* 2020; **12**:79.
11. Poulos J, et al. Antipsychotics and the risk of diabetes and death among adults with serious mental illnesses. *Psychol Med* 2023; **53**:7677–7684.
12. Lindekilde N, et al. Risk of developing type 2 diabetes in individuals with a psychiatric disorder: a nationwide register-based cohort study. *Diabetes Care* 2022; **45**:724–733.
13. Taylor D, et al. Testing for diabetes in hospitalised patients prescribed antipsychotic drugs. *Br J Psychiatry* 2004; **185**:152–156.
14. Gianfrancesco F, et al. The influence of study design on the results of pharmacoepidemiologic studies of diabetes risk with antipsychotic therapy. *Ann Clin Psychiatry* 2006; **18**:9–17.
15. Buchholz S, et al. Atypical antipsychotic-induced diabetes mellitus: an update on epidemiology and postulated mechanisms. *Intern Med J* 2008; **38**:602–606.
16. Farino ZJ, et al. New roles for dopamine D2 and D3 receptors in pancreatic beta cell insulin secretion. *Mol Psychiatry* 2020; **25**:2070–2085.
17. Wei H, et al. Dopamine D2 receptor signaling modulates pancreatic beta cell circadian rhythms. *Psychoneuroendocrinology* 2020; **113**:104551.
18. Teff KL, et al. Antipsychotic-induced insulin resistance and postprandial hormonal dysregulation independent of weight gain or psychiatric disease. *Diabetes* 2013; **62**:3232–3240.
19. Arneson GA. Phenothiazine derivatives and glucose metabolism. *J Neuropsychiatr* 1964; **5**:181.
20. Lindenmayer JP, et al. Hyperglycemia associated with the use of atypical antipsychotics. *J Clin Psychiatry* 2001; **62** Suppl 23:30–38.
21. Keskiner A, et al. Psychotropic drugs, diabetes and chronic mental patients. *Psychosomatics* 1973; **14**:176–181.
22. Tollefson G, et al. Nonketotic hyperglycemia associated with loxapine and amoxapine: case report. *J Clin Psychiatry* 1983; **44**:347–348.
23. Lindenmayer JP, et al. Changes in glucose and cholesterol levels in patients with schizophrenia treated with typical or atypical antipsychotics. *Am J Psychiatry* 2003; **160**:290–296.
24. Carlson C, et al. Diabetes mellitus and antipsychotic treatment in the United Kingdom. *Eur Neuropsychopharmacol* 2006; **16**:366–375.
25. Ostbye T, et al. Atypical antipsychotic drugs and diabetes mellitus in a large outpatient population: a retrospective cohort study. *Pharmacoepidemiol Drug Saf* 2005; **14**:407–415.
26. Smith M, et al. First- v. second-generation antipsychotics and risk for diabetes in schizophrenia: systematic review and meta-analysis. *Br J Psychiatry* 2008; **192**:406–411.
27. Mir S, et al. Atypical antipsychotics and hyperglycaemia. *Int Clin Psychopharmacol* 2001; **16**:63–74.
28. Lund BC, et al. Clozapine use in patients with schizophrenia and the risk of diabetes, hyperlipidemia, and hypertension: a claims-based approach. *Arch Gen Psychiatry* 2001; **58**:1172–1176.
29. Sernyak MJ, et al. Association of diabetes mellitus with use of atypical neuroleptics in the treatment of schizophrenia. *Am J Psychiatry* 2002; **159**:561–566.
30. Gianfrancesco FD, et al. Differential effects of risperidone, olanzapine, clozapine, and conventional antipsychotics on type 2 diabetes: findings from a large health plan database. *J Clin Psychiatry* 2002; **63**:920–930.
31. Guo JJ, et al. Risk of diabetes mellitus associated with atypical antipsychotic use among patients with bipolar disorder: a retrospective, population-based, case-control study. *J Clin Psychiatry* 2006; **67**:1055–1061.
32. Wang PS, et al. Clozapine use and risk of diabetes mellitus. *J Clin Psychopharmacol* 2002; **22**:236–243.
33. Sumiyoshi T, et al. A comparison of incidence of diabetes mellitus between atypical antipsychotic drugs: a survey for clozapine, risperidone, olanzapine, and quetiapine [Letter]. *J Clin Psychopharmacol* 2004; **24**:345–348.
34. Henderson DC, et al. Clozapine, diabetes mellitus, weight gain, and lipid abnormalities: a five-year naturalistic study. *Am J Psychiatry* 2000; **157**:975–981.
35. Koller E, et al. Clozapine-associated diabetes. *Am J Med* 2001; **111**:716–723.
36. Sumiyoshi T, et al. The effect of hypertension and obesity on the development of diabetes mellitus in patients treated with atypical antipsychotic drugs [Letter]. *J Clin Psychopharmacol* 2004; **24**:452–454.

37. Zhang R, et al. The prevalence and clinical-demographic correlates of diabetes mellitus in chronic schizophrenic patients receiving clozapine. *Hum Psychopharmacol* 2011; **26**:392–396.

38. Melkersson KI, et al. Different influences of classical antipsychotics and clozapine on glucose-insulin homeostasis in patients with schizophrenia or related psychoses. *J Clin Psychiatry* 1999; **60**:783–791.

39. Melkersson K. Clozapine and olanzapine, but not conventional antipsychotics, increase insulin release in vitro. *Eur Neuropsychopharmacol* 2004; **14**:115–119.

40. Newcomer JW, et al. Abnormalities in glucose regulation during antipsychotic treatment of schizophrenia. *Arch Gen Psychiatry* 2002; **59**:337–345.

41. Lamberti JS, et al. Diabetes mellitus among outpatients receiving clozapine: prevalence and clinical-demographic correlates. *J Clin Psychiatry* 2005; **66**:900–906.

42. Miyakoshi T, et al. Risk factors for abnormal glucose metabolism during antipsychotic treatment: a prospective cohort study. *J Psychiatr Res* 2023; **168**:149–156.

43. Wirshing DA, et al. Novel antipsychotics and new onset diabetes. *Biol Psychiatry* 1998; **44**:778–783.

44. Engl J, et al. Olanzapine impairs glycogen synthesis and insulin signaling in L6 skeletal muscle cells. *Mol Psychiatry* 2005; **10**:1089–1096.

45. Vestri HS, et al. Atypical antipsychotic drugs directly impair insulin action in adipocytes: effects on glucose transport, lipogenesis, and antilipolysis. *Neuropsychopharmacology* 2007; **32**:765–772.

46. Koro CE, et al. Assessment of independent effect of olanzapine and risperidone on risk of diabetes among patients with schizophrenia: population based nested case-control study. *BMJ* 2002; **325**:243.

47. Meyer JM. A retrospective comparison of weight, lipid, and glucose changes between risperidone- and olanzapine-treated inpatients: metabolic outcomes after 1 year. *J Clin Psychiatry* 2002; **63**:425–433.

48. Gianfrancesco F, et al. Antipsychotic-induced type 2 diabetes: evidence from a large health plan database. *J Clin Psychopharmacol* 2003; **23**:328–335.

49. Leslie DL, et al. Incidence of newly diagnosed diabetes attributable to atypical antipsychotic medications. *Am J Psychiatry* 2004; **161**:1709–1711.

50. Duncan E, et al. Relative risk of glucose elevation during antipsychotic exposure in a Veterans Administration population. *Int Clin Psychopharmacol* 2007; **22**:1–11.

51. Meyer JM, et al. Change in metabolic syndrome parameters with antipsychotic treatment in the CATIE schizophrenia trial: prospective data from phase 1. *Schizophr Res* 2008; **101**:273–286.

52. Ebenbichler CF, et al. Olanzapine induces insulin resistance: results from a prospective study. *J Clin Psychiatry* 2003; **64**:1436–1439.

53. Mallya A, et al. Resolution of hyperglycemia on risperidone discontinuation: a case report. *J Clin Psychiatry* 2002; **63**:453–454.

54. Wirshing DA, et al. Risperidone-associated new-onset diabetes. *Biol Psychiatry* 2001; **50**:148–149.

55. Croarkin PE, et al. Diabetic ketoacidosis associated with risperidone treatment? *Psychosomatics* 2000; **41**:369–370.

56. Koller EA, et al. Risperidone-associated diabetes mellitus: a pharmacovigilance study. *Pharmacotherapy* 2003; **23**:735–744.

57. Lambert BL, et al. Diabetes risk associated with use of olanzapine, quetiapine, and risperidone in Veterans Health Administration patients with schizophrenia. *Am J Epidemiol* 2006; **164**:672–681.

58. Henderson DC. Atypical antipsychotic-induced diabetes mellitus: how strong is the evidence? *CNS Drugs* 2002; **16**:77–89.

59. Koller EA, et al. A survey of reports of quetiapine-associated hyperglycemia and diabetes mellitus. *J Clin Psychiatry* 2004; **65**:857–863.

60. Nanasawa H, et al. Development of diabetes mellitus associated with quetiapine: a case series. *Medicine (Baltimore)* 2017; **96**:e5900.

61. Ulcickas Yood M, et al. Association between second-generation antipsychotics and newly diagnosed treated diabetes mellitus: does the effect differ by dose? *BMC Psychiatry* 2011; **11**:197.

62. Correll CU, et al. Cardiovascular and cerebrovascular risk factors and events associated with second-generation antipsychotic compared to antidepressant use in a non-elderly adult sample: results from a claims-based inception cohort study. *World Psychiatry* 2015; **14**:56–63.

63. Bushe C, et al. Comparison of metabolic and prolactin variables from a six-month randomised trial of olanzapine and quetiapine in schizophrenia. *J Psychopharmacol* 2010; **24**:1001–1009.

64. Guo Z, et al. A real-world data analysis of dose effect of second-generation antipsychotic therapy on hemoglobin A1C level. *Prog Neuropsychopharmacol Biol Psychiatry* 2011; **35**:1326–1332.

65. Vanelle JM, et al. A double-blind randomised comparative trial of amisulpride versus olanzapine for 2 months in the treatment of subjects with schizophrenia and comorbid depression. *Eur Psychiatry* 2006; **21**:523–530.

66. Toprak O, et al. New-onset type II diabetes mellitus, hyperosmolar non-ketotic coma, rhabdomyolysis and acute renal failure in a patient treated with sulpiride. *Nephrol Dial Transplant* 2005; **20**:662–663.

67. Keck PE, Jr., et al. Aripiprazole: a partial dopamine D2 receptor agonist antipsychotic. *Expert Opin Invest Drugs* 2003; **12**:655–662.

68. Pigott TA, et al. Aripiprazole for the prevention of relapse in stabilized patients with chronic schizophrenia: a placebo-controlled 26-week study. *J Clin Psychiatry* 2003; **64**:1048–1056.

69. van WR, et al. Major changes in glucose metabolism, including new-onset diabetes, within 3 months after initiation of or switch to atypical antipsychotic medication in patients with schizophrenia and schizoaffective disorder. *J Clin Psychiatry* 2008; **69**:472–479.

70. Baker RA, et al. Atypical antipsychotic drugs and diabetes mellitus in the US Food and Drug Administration Adverse Event Database: a systematic Bayesian signal detection analysis. *Psychopharmacol Bull* 2009; **42**:11–31.

71. Simpson GM, et al. Randomized, controlled, double-blind multicenter comparison of the efficacy and tolerability of ziprasidone and olanzapine in acutely ill inpatients with schizophrenia or schizoaffective disorder. *Am J Psychiatry* 2004; **161**:1837–1847.

72. Sacher J, et al. Effects of olanzapine and ziprasidone on glucose tolerance in healthy volunteers. *Neuropsychopharmacology* 2008; **33**:1633–1641.

73. De Hert M, et al. A case series: evaluation of the metabolic safety of aripiprazole. *Schizophr Bull* 2007; **33**:823–830.

74. Church CO, et al. Diabetic ketoacidosis associated with aripiprazole. *Diabet Med* 2005; **22**:1440–1443.

75. Reddymasu S, et al. Elevated lipase and diabetic ketoacidosis associated with aripiprazole. *J Pancreas* 2006; **7**:303–305.

76. Campanella LM, et al. Severe hyperglycemic hyperosmolar nonketotic coma in a nondiabetic patient receiving aripiprazole. *Ann Emerg Med* 2009; **53**:264–266.

77. Kessing LV, et al. Treatment with antipsychotics and the risk of diabetes in clinical practice. *Br J Psychiatry* 2010; **197**:266–271.

78. Vancampfort D, et al. Diabetes mellitus in people with schizophrenia, bipolar disorder and major depressive disorder: a systematic review and large scale meta-analysis. *World Psychiatry* 2016; **15**:166–174.

79. McEvoy JP, et al. Effectiveness of lurasidone in patients with schizophrenia or schizoaffective disorder switched from other antipsychotics: a randomized, 6-week, open-label study. *J Clin Psychiatry*, 2013; **74**:170–179.

80. Stahl SM, et al. Effectiveness of lurasidone for patients with schizophrenia following 6 weeks of acute treatment with lurasidone, olanzapine, or placebo: a 6-month, open-label, extension study. *J Clin Psychiatry* 2013; **74**:507–515.

81. McIntyre RS, et al. Asenapine for long-term treatment of bipolar disorder: a double-blind 40-week extension study. *J Affect Disord* 2010; **126**:358–365.

82. McIntyre RS, et al. Asenapine versus olanzapine in acute mania: a double-blind extension study. *Bipolar Disord* 2009; **11**:815–826.

83. Garnock-Jones KP. Brexpiprazole: a review in schizophrenia. *CNS Drugs* 2016; **30**:335–342.

84. Newcomer JW, et al. Changes in metabolic parameters and body weight in patients with major depressive disorder treated with adjunctive brexpiprazole: pooled analysis of phase 3 clinical studies. *J Clin Psychiatry* 2019; **80**:18m12680.

85. Lao KS, et al. Tolerability and safety profile of cariprazine in treating psychotic disorders, bipolar disorder and major depressive disorder: a systematic review with meta-analysis of randomized controlled trials. *CNS Drugs* 2016; **30**:1043–1054.

86. Earley W, et al. Tolerability of cariprazine in the treatment of acute bipolar I mania: a pooled post hoc analysis of 3 phase II/III studies. *J Affect Disord* 2017; **215**:205–212.

87. Barabássy Á, et al. Safety and tolerability of cariprazine in patients with schizophrenia: a pooled analysis of eight phase II/III studies. *Neuropsychiatr Dis Treat* 2021; **17**:957–970.

88. Cernea S, et al. Pharmacological management of glucose dysregulation in patients treated with second-generation antipsychotics. *Drugs* 2020; **80**:1763–1781.

89. Correll CU, et al. Efficacy and safety of lumateperone for treatment of schizophrenia: a randomized clinical trial. *JAMA Psychiatry* 2020; **77**:349–358.

90. Hammerman A, et al. Antipsychotics and diabetes: an age-related association. *Ann Pharmacother* 2008; **42**:1316–1322.

91. Galling B, et al. Type 2 diabetes mellitus in youth exposed to antipsychotics: a systematic review and meta-analysis. *JAMA Psychiatry* 2016; **73**:247–259.

92. Albert SG, et al. Atypical antipsychotics and the risk of diabetes in an elderly population in long-term care: a retrospective nursing home chart review study. *J Am Med Dir Assoc* 2009; **10**:115–119.

93. De Hert M, et al. Typical and atypical antipsychotics differentially affect long-term incidence rates of the metabolic syndrome in first-episode patients with schizophrenia: a retrospective chart review. *Schizophr Res* 2008; **101**:295–303.

94. Saddichha S, et al. Metabolic syndrome in first episode schizophrenia: a randomized double-blind controlled, short-term prospective study. *Schizophr Res* 2008; **101**:266–272.

95. Saddichha S, et al. Diabetes and schizophrenia – effect of disease or drug? Results from a randomized, double-blind, controlled prospective study in first-episode schizophrenia. *Acta Psychiatr Scand* 2008; **117**:342–347.

96. Reaven GM, et al. In search of moderators and mediators of hyperglycemia with atypical antipsychotic treatment. *J Psychiatr Res* 2009; **43**:997–1002.

97. Heald AH, et al. Changes in metabolic parameters in patients with severe mental illness over a 10-year period: a retrospective cohort study. *Aust N Z J Psychiatry* 2017; **51**:75–82.

98. Mokdad AH, et al. The continuing increase of diabetes in the US. *Diabetes Care* 2001; **24**:412.

99. Mokdad AH, et al. Diabetes trends in the US: 1990–1998. *Diabetes Care* 2000; **23**:1278–1283.

100. Beckman JA, et al. Diabetes and atherosclerosis: epidemiology, pathophysiology, and management. *JAMA* 2002; **287**:2570–2581.

101. Henderson DC, et al. Clozapine, diabetes mellitus, hyperlipidemia, and cardiovascular risks and mortality: results of a 10-year naturalistic study. *J Clin Psychiatry* 2005; **66**:1116–1121.

102. Lamberti JS, et al. Prevalence of the metabolic syndrome among patients receiving clozapine. *Am J Psychiatry* 2006; **163**:1273–1276.

103. Goff DC, et al. A comparison of ten-year cardiac risk estimates in schizophrenia patients from the CATIE study and matched controls. *Schizophr Res* 2005; **80**:45–53.

104. Haupt DW, et al. Hyperglycemia and antipsychotic medications. *J Clin Psychiatry* 2001; **62** Suppl 27:15–26.

105. Cohn TA, et al. Metabolic monitoring for patients treated with antipsychotic medications. *Can J Psychiatry* 2006; **51**:492–501.

106. De Hert M, et al. Guidelines for screening and monitoring of cardiometabolic risk in schizophrenia: systematic evaluation. *Br J Psychiatry* 2011; **199**:99–105.

107. Barnes TR, et al. Screening for the metabolic syndrome in community psychiatric patients prescribed antipsychotics: a quality improvement programme. *Acta Psychiatr Scand* 2008; **118**:26–33.

108. Barnes TR, et al. Screening for the metabolic side effects of antipsychotic medication: findings of a 6-year quality improvement programme in the UK. *BMJ Open* 2015; **5**:e007633.

109. Crawford MJ, et al. Assessment and treatment of physical health problems among people with schizophrenia: national cross-sectional study. *Br J Psychiatry* 2014; **205**:473–477.

110. Morrato EH, et al. Metabolic screening after the ADA's consensus statement on antipsychotic drugs and diabetes. *Diabetes Care* 2009; **32**:1037–1042.

111. De Hert M, et al. Oral glucose tolerance tests in treated patients with schizophrenia. Data to support an adaptation of the proposed guidelines for monitoring of patients on second generation antipsychotics? *Eur Psychiatry* 2006; **21**:224–226.

112. Pillinger T, et al. Impaired glucose homeostasis in first-episode schizophrenia: a systematic review and meta-analysis. *JAMA Psychiatry* 2017; **74**:261–269.

113. Marder SR, et al. Physical health monitoring of patients with schizophrenia. *Am J Psychiatry* 2004; **161**:1334–1349.

114. National Institute for Health and Care Excellence. Prescribing information: monitoring. Psychosis and schizophrenia: what monitoring is required? (Last revised October 2024; last checked January 2025); https://cks.nice.org.uk/topics/psychosis-schizophrenia/prescribing-information.

115. Stroup TS, et al. Effects of switching from olanzapine, quetiapine, and risperidone to aripiprazole on 10-year coronary heart disease risk and metabolic syndrome status: results from a randomized controlled trial. *Schizophr Res* 2013; **146**:190–195.

116. Chen Y, et al. Comparative effectiveness of switching antipsychotic drug treatment to aripiprazole or ziprasidone for improving metabolic profile and atherogenic dyslipidemia: a 12-month, prospective, open-label study. *J Psychopharmacol* 2012; **26**:1201–1210.

117. Wang YH, et al. Lurasidone successfully reversed clozapine-induced type 2 diabetes mellitus and hypertriglyceridemia in a patient with schizophrenia. *Am J Ther* 2023; **30**:e490–e491.

118. Smith RC, et al. Effects of pioglitazone on metabolic abnormalities, psychopathology, and cognitive function in schizophrenic patients treated with antipsychotic medication: a randomized double-blind study. *Schizophr Res* 2013; **143**:18–24.

119. Larsen JR, et al. Effect of liraglutide treatment on prediabetes and overweight or obesity in clozapine- or olanzapine-treated patients with schizophrenia spectrum disorder: a randomized clinical trial. *JAMA Psychiatry* 2017; **74**:719–728.

120. Patoulias D, et al. Effect of glucagon-like peptide-1 receptor agonists on cardio-metabolic risk factors among obese/overweight individuals treated with antipsychotic drug classes: an updated systematic review and meta-analysis of randomized controlled trials. *Biomedicines* 2023; **11**:669.

121. Noda K, et al. Semaglutide is effective in type 2 diabetes and obesity with schizophrenia. *Diabetol Int* 2022; **13**:693–697.

Blood pressure changes with antipsychotics

Orthostatic hypotension

Orthostatic hypotension (postural hypotension) is one of the most common cardiovascular adverse effects of antipsychotics and some antidepressants. Orthostatic hypotension generally presents acutely, during the initial dose titration period, but it can also be a chronic problem.[1] Symptoms include dizziness, light-headedness, asthenia, headache and visual disturbance. Patients may not be able to communicate the severity of these symptoms effectively and subjective reports of postural dizziness correlate only weakly with the magnitude of measured postural hypotension.[2]

Blood pressure monitoring is recommended in suspected cases to confirm orthostatic hypotension (usually defined as a ≥20mmHg fall in systolic blood pressure and/or a ≥10mmHg fall in diastolic blood pressure within 3 minutes of standing).[3] Orthostatic hypotension impairs quality of life and is associated with an increased risk of falls, cardiovascular disease, depression and death.[3] Risk factors are shown in Table 1.40.

Slow dose titration is a commonly used and often effective strategy to avoid or minimise orthostatic hypotension. However, in some cases orthostasis may be a dose-limiting side effect, preventing optimal treatment. Potential management strategies are shown in Table 1.41.

Table 1.40 Risk factors for orthostatic hypotension.[2]

Treatment factors	▪ IM administration route (peak levels higher and achieved more rapidly) ▪ Rapid dose increases ▪ Antipsychotic polypharmacy ▪ Drug interactions (e.g. tricyclic antidepressants, antihypertensive drugs – particularly alpha blockers, beta blockers and diuretics, although the number of antihypertensive drugs prescribed may be more predictive than the class)[3]
Patient factors	▪ Old age (young patients may have sinus tachycardia with minimal change in blood pressure) ▪ Disease states associated with autonomic dysfunction (e.g. Parkinson's disease) ▪ Dehydration ▪ Cardiovascular disease

Table 1.41 Management of antipsychotic-induced orthostatic hypotension.[2,4]

Minimise the risk of treatment	▪ Limit initial doses and titrate slowly according to tolerability (most people develop a tolerance to the hypotensive effect) ▪ Consider a temporary dose reduction if hypotension develops ▪ Reduce peak plasma levels by using smaller and more frequent dosing or by using modified-release preparations
Non-pharmacological therapies	▪ Advice to patients (e.g. sitting on the edge of the bed for several minutes before attempting to stand in the morning and slowly rising from a seated position) ▪ Abdominal binders and compression stockings can be used ▪ Increasing fluid intake to 1.25–2.5L/day is advisable for all patients who are not fluid restricted

(Continued)

Table 1.41 *(Continued)*	
Pharmacological therapies for patients with a compelling indication for treatment where alternatives are not suitable (e.g. clozapine) and management strategies have failed	■ Sodium chloride supplementation may help antidepressant-induced orthostatic hypotension ■ Fludrocortisone has been used to treat clozapine-induced orthostatic hypotension where other measures have failed (electrolyte and blood pressure monitoring essential). Long-term use is not recommended.[4] ■ Midodrine, an α1 receptor agonist, has been used in one small case series (including one patient on clozapine) to reduce symptom severity.[4] Of note, midodrine has been linked to acute dystonia when used alongside antipsychotics.[5] A review suggests that midodrine should be considered second line in clozapine-induced orthostatic hypotension or where fludrocortisone is contraindicated or poorly tolerated.[4] ■ Other sympathomimetic drugs have also been used to treat orthostatic hypotension, although for most there is an absence of evidence in the treatment of psychotropic-related cases. Etilefrine has shown benefit in psychotropic-induced hypotension but cannot be recommended owing to unfavourable risk–benefit profile.[4]

Antipsychotics with a high affinity for postsynaptic α_1-adrenergic receptors are most frequently implicated in postural hypotension. Among the SGAs, the reported incidence is highest with clozapine (24%), quetiapine (27%) and iloperidone (19.5%) and lowest with lurasidone (<2%) and asenapine (<2%).[2] There are limited quantitative data for FGAs,[6] but low-potency phenothiazines (e.g. chlorpromazine) are considered most likely to cause orthostatic hypotension.[7] All reported frequencies are somewhat dependent on titration schedules used. Please see the section on relative adverse effects – a rough guide in this chapter for a summary of the relative incidence and severity of hypotension with antipsychotics.

Hypertension

There are two ways in which antipsychotic drugs may be associated with the development or worsening of hypertension:

- **Slow steady rise in blood pressure over time.** This may be linked to weight gain. Being overweight increases the risk of developing hypertension. The magnitude of the effect has been modelled using the Framingham data: for every 30 people who gain 4kg, one will develop hypertension over the next 10 years.[8] Note that this is a very modest weight gain. The majority of patients treated with some antipsychotics gain more than this, increasing further the risk of developing hypertension (see section on antipsychotic-induced weight gain in this chapter).
- **Unpredictable rapid sharp increase in blood pressure on starting a new drug or increasing the dose.** Increases in blood pressure occur shortly after starting, ranging from within hours of the first dose to a month.

The mechanism for the rapid increase in blood pressure (i.e. that independent of obesity) is uncertain, so the risk of hypertension cannot be predicted from antipsychotic pharmacology. One review of the literature suggested a possible mechanism related to dopamine receptor antagonism.[9] All five dopamine receptor subtypes (D_{1-5}) are known to be involved in renal sodium excretion and blood pressure regulation.[9] Antipsychotics vary in their affinity for these dopamine receptor subtypes, and the relative importance of each receptor subtype is unclear. Other suggested mechanisms include α_2 antagonism leading to prolonged noradrenaline release, hypertension through renal potassium loss, and sodium and fluid retention, possibly owing to D_4 receptor antagonism.[10]

Some antipsychotics are more commonly implicated than others, although individual patient factors are also likely to be important. Most case reports involve clozapine,[11,12] with some clearly describing normal blood pressure before clozapine was introduced, a sharp rise during treatment and return to normal when clozapine was discontinued or doses were decreased.[12] Blood pressure has also been reported to rise again on rechallenge and increased urinary catecholamines mimicking phaeochromocytoma have been noted in some cases. Clozapine can usually be continued with antihypertensive drugs.[12] Case reports also implicate aripiprazole,[13–16] sulpiride,[17,18] risperidone,[19] quetiapine[20] and ziprasidone.[21] Olanzapine has been linked to water retention and hypertension in a pregnant woman[22] and intracranial hypertension in an adolescent.[23]

Data available through the UK Medicines and Healthcare products Regulatory Authority yellow card system indicate that clozapine is the antipsychotic drug most associated with hypertension. There are substantially fewer reports with aripiprazole, olanzapine, quetiapine and risperidone.[24] The timing of the onset of hypertension in these reports with respect to antipsychotic initiation is unknown.

In long-term treatment, hypertension is seen in around 30–40% of patients regardless of antipsychotic prescribed.[25] A cross-sectional study found an increased risk of hypertension only for perphenazine,[26] a finding not readily explained by its pharmacology.

No antipsychotic is contraindicated in essential hypertension, but extreme care is needed when clozapine is prescribed. Concomitant treatment with SSRIs may increase risk of hypertension, possibly via inhibition of the metabolism of the co-prescribed antipsychotic.[20] It is also theoretically possible that α_2 antagonism may be at least partially responsible for clozapine-induced tachycardia and nausea.[27]

Treatment of antipsychotic-associated hypertension should follow standard protocols. Switching to alternative antipsychotics with a lower cardiometabolic risk should be considered where possible. There is specific evidence for the efficacy of valsartan and telmisartan in antipsychotic-related hypertension.[28]

References

1. Silver H, et al. Postural hypotension in chronically medicated schizophrenics. *J Clin Psychiatry* 1990; 51:459–462.
2. Gugger JJ. Antipsychotic pharmacotherapy and orthostatic hypotension: identification and management. *CNS Drugs* 2011; 25:659–671.
3. Gilani A, et al. Postural hypotension. *BMJ* 2021; 373:n922.
4. Tanzer TD, et al. Treatment strategies for clozapine-induced hypotension: a systematic review. *Ther Adv Psychopharmacol* 2022; 12:20451253221092931.
5. Stroup TS, et al. Management of common adverse effects of antipsychotic medications. *World Psychiatry* 2018; 17:341–356.
6. Bhanu C, et al. Drug-induced orthostatic hypotension: a systematic review and meta-analysis of randomised controlled trials. *PLoS Med* 2021; 18:e1003821.
7. Li XQ, et al. Antipsychotics cardiotoxicity: what's known and what's next. *World J Psychiatry* 2021; 11:736–753.
8. Fontaine KR, et al. Estimating the consequences of anti-psychotic induced weight gain on health and mortality rate. *Psychiatry Res* 2001; 101:277–288.
9. Gonsai NH, et al. Effects of dopamine receptor antagonist antipsychotic therapy on blood pressure. *J Clin Pharm Ther* 2018; 43:1–7.

10. Deepak MB, et al. Clozapine induced hypertension and its association with autonomic dysfunction. *Psychopharmacol Bull* 2021; **51**:122–127.

11. Yuen JWY, et al. Clozapine-induced cardiovascular side effects and autonomic dysfunction: a systematic review. *Front Neurosci* 2018; **12**:203.

12. Grover S, et al. Clozapine-induced hypertension: a case report and review of literature. *Ind Psychiatry J* 2017; **26**:103–105.

13. Hsiao YL, et al. Aripiprazole augmentation induced hypertension in major depressive disorder: a case report. *Prog Neuropsychopharmacol Biol Psychiatry* 2011; **35**:305–306.

14. Yasui-Furukori N, et al. Worsened hypertension control induced by aripiprazole. *Neuropsychiatr Dis Treat* 2013; **9**:505–507.

15. Seven H, et al. Aripiprazole-induced asymptomatic hypertension: a case report. *Psychopharmacol Bull* 2017; **47**:53–56.

16. Alves BB, et al. Use of atypical antipsychotics and risk of hypertension: a case report and review literature. *SAGE Open Med Case Rep* 2019; **7**:2050313x19841825.

17. Mayer RD, et al. Acute hypertensive episode induced by sulpiride: a case report. *Hum Psychopharmacol* 1989; **4**:149–150.

18. Corvol P, et al. Hypertensive episodes initiated by sulpiride (Dogmatil). *Ann Med Interne (Paris)* 1973; **124**:647–649.

19. Thomson SR, et al. Risperidone induced hypertension in a young female: a case report. *Advanced Science Letters* 2017; **23**:1980–1982.

20. Coulter D. Atypical antipsychotics may cause hypertension. *Prescriber Update* 2003; **24**:4.

21. Villanueva N, et al. Probable association between ziprasidone and worsening hypertension. *Pharmacotherapy* 2006; **26**:1352–1357.

22. Izsak J, et al. Case report: olanzapine-associated water retention, high blood pressure, and subsequent preterm preeclampsia. *Front Psychiatry* 2023; **14**:1301348.

23. Naguy A, et al. Probable olanzapine-related idiopathic intracranial hypertension in an adolescent with first-episode psychosis. *Psychopharmacol Bull* 2023; **53**:69–72.

24. Medicines and Healthcare products Regulatory Agency. Drug Analysis Profiles (iDAPs). 2024; https://www.gov.uk/drug-analysis-prints.

25. Kelly AC, et al. A naturalistic comparison of the long-term metabolic adverse effects of clozapine versus other antipsychotics for patients with psychotic illnesses. *J Clin Psychopharmacol* 2014; **34**:441–445.

26. Boden R, et al. A comparison of cardiovascular risk factors for ten antipsychotic drugs in clinical practice. *Neuropsychiatr Dis Treat* 2013; **9**:371–377.

27. Pandharipande P, et al. Alpha-2 agonists: can they modify the outcomes in the postanesthesia care unit? *Curr Drug Targets* 2005; **6**:749–754.

28. Tse L, et al. Pharmacological treatment of antipsychotic-induced dyslipidemia and hypertension. *Int Clin Psychopharmacol* 2014; **29**:125–137.

CHAPTER 1

Antipsychotic-associated hyponatraemia

Hyponatraemia can occur in the context of:

- **Water intoxication,** where water consumption exceeds the maximal renal clearance capacity. Serum and urine osmolality are low. Cross-sectional studies of chronically ill, hospitalised, psychiatric patients have found the prevalence of water intoxication to be 6–17%.[1,2] A longitudinal study found that 10% of severely ill patients with a diagnosis of schizophrenia had episodic hyponatraemia secondary to fluid overload.[3] The primary aetiology is poorly understood. It may be driven, at least in part, by an extreme compensatory response to the anticholinergic adverse effects of some antipsychotic drugs.[4] An alternative theory is that post-synaptic dopamine receptor antagonism results in receptor supersensitivity, increased presynaptic dopamine release, and elevated dopamine in the hypothalamus, driving thirst and polydipsia.[5] The fact that many reported cases occur in patients with long illness histories and treatment with antipsychotics with high D_2 receptor affinity (and that clozapine can improve polydipsia independent of improvement in psychosis) appears to support this suggestion.[5]

- **Drug-induced syndrome of inappropriate antidiuretic hormone (SIADH),** where the kidney retains an excessive quantity of solute-free water. Serum osmolality is low and urine osmolality relatively high. The prevalence of SIADH may be as high as 11% in acutely ill psychiatric patients.[6] Risk factors for antidepressant-induced SIADH (increasing age, female gender, medical comorbidity and polypharmacy) seem to be less relevant to the population of patients treated with antipsychotic drugs.[7] SIADH usually develops in the first few weeks of treatment with the offending drug[8] but can appear at a later time.[8] Case reports/series[7,9–30] implicate various phenothiazines, haloperidol, pimozide, risperidone, paliperidone, quetiapine, olanzapine, aripiprazole, cariprazine and clozapine. Systematic review[31] and case–control studies[32,33] suggest a clear increase in risk of hyponatraemia with antipsychotics. One large Swedish study found a stronger association for first-generation antipsychotics than for SGAs.[33] Analysis of pharmacovigilance reports appears to support this.[34] Another review[35] confirmed that drug-induced hyponatraemia is associated with concentrated urine and suggested that antipsychotic treatment was five times more likely than water intoxication to be the cause of hyponatraemia. Overall prevalence of antipsychotic-induced hyponatraemia has been estimated at 0.004%[36] and 26.1%.[37] It is assumed that the true figure is somewhere between these two widely different extremes. Desmopressin, when used for clozapine-induced enuresis, can also result in hyponatraemia.[38] Other drugs, including antidepressants and anticonvulsants (especially carbamazepine),[39] valbenazine[40] and many drugs for physical health conditions (diuretics, angiotensin-converting-enzyme [ACE] inhibitors, angiotensin II receptor blockers, proton pump inhibitors), have also been implicated.[41] The risk of hyponatraemia is probably additive with concomitant prescriptions.[42–44]

- Severe **hyperlipidaemia** and/or **hyperglycaemia** lead to secondary increases in plasma volume and 'pseudohyponatraemia'.[4] Both are more common in people treated with antipsychotic drugs than in the general population and should be excluded as causes.

Mild to moderate hyponatraemia presents as confusion, nausea, headache and lethargy. As the plasma sodium falls, these symptoms become increasingly severe, and seizures and coma can develop.

Monitoring of plasma sodium is desirable for all those receiving antipsychotics, particularly if several risk factors for hyponatraemia are present. A risk-scoring algorithm has been proposed.[45] Signs of confusion or lethargy should provoke thorough diagnostic analysis, including plasma sodium determination and urine osmolality (Table 1.42).

Tolvaptan,[46] a so-called vaptan (non-peptide arginine-vasopressin antagonist, also known as aquaretics because they induce a highly hypotonic diuresis),[47] shows promise in the treatment of hyponatraemia of various aetiologies, including that caused by drug-related SIADH and psychogenic polydipsia.[48]

Table 1.42 Treatment of hyponatraemia associated with antipsychotic treatment.[4,6]

Cause of hyponatraemia	Antipsychotic drugs implicated	Treatment
Water intoxication (serum and urine osmolality low)	Only very speculative evidence to support drugs as a cause. Core part of illness in a minority of patients (e.g. psychotic polydipsia)	■ **Fluid restriction** with careful monitoring of serum sodium, particularly diurnal variation (Na drops as the day progresses). Refer urgently to specialist medical care if Na <125 mmol/L. Note that over-rapid correction of sodium levels can cause irreversible osmotic demyelination syndrome.[49] ■ Consider treatment with **clozapine**, which has been shown to increase plasma osmolality into the normal range and increase urine osmolality.[50,51] These effects are consistent with reduced fluid intake but are not clearly related to improvements in mental state.[52] ■ There are both[7] positive and negative reports for olanzapine[53] and risperidone[54] and one positive case report for quetiapine.[55] Compared with clozapine, the evidence base is weak. ■ There is no evidence that either reducing or increasing the dose of an antipsychotic results in improvements in serum sodium in water-intoxicated patients[56] although reducing the number and dose of antipsychotics prescribed may decrease dopamine receptor supersensitivity and drug adverse effects[5] ■ **Demeclocyline** may be used[57,58] and it is included in some practice guidelines for psychogenic polydipsia.[59] However, it exerts its effect by interfering with alcohol dehydrogenase and increasing water excretion, which is already at capacity in these patients. Any rationale for its use in the absence of SIADH is therefore debatable (and some cases in the literature may have been complicated by undiagnosed SIADH).[60] A single small RCT showed no benefit.[61] ■ Many other drugs have been used (naloxone, enalapril, clonidine, naltrexone, acetazolamide, captopril, propranolol, losartan, carbamazepine, fluoxetine, bupropion, trazodone, mianserin) but data are limited.[62] Successful use of the carbonic anhydrase inhibitor acetazolamide has also been reported.[63,64]

(Continued)

Table 1.42 *(Continued)*

Cause of hyponatraemia	Antipsychotic drugs implicated	Treatment
SIADH (serum osmolality low; urine osmolality relatively high)	All antipsychotic drugs	■ If mild, **fluid restriction** with careful monitoring of serum sodium. Refer urgently to specialist medical care if Na <125mmol/L. ■ **Dose reduction** of the antipsychotic has been suggested[45] but evidence to support this strategy is lacking ■ **Switching to a different antipsychotic drug**. There are insufficient data available to guide choice. Be aware that cross-sensitivity may occur (the individual may be predisposed overall and the choice of drug unimportant). ■ Consider **demeclocycline** (see formal prescribing information for details) ■ Lithium may be effective[7] but is a potentially toxic drug (and hyponatraemia predisposes to lithium toxicity)

References

1. de Leon J, et al. Polydipsia and water intoxication in psychiatric patients: a review of the epidemiological literature. *Biol Psychiatry* 1994; 35:408–419.
2. Patel JK. Polydipsia, hyponatremia, and water intoxication among psychiatric patients. *Hosp Community Psychiatry* 1994; 45:1073–1074.
3. de Leon J. Polydipsia: a study in a long-term psychiatric unit. *Eur Arch Psychiatry Clin Neurosci* 2003; 253:37–39.
4. Siegel AJ, et al. Primary and drug-induced disorders of water homeostasis in psychiatric patients: principles of diagnosis and management. *Harv Rev Psychiatry* 1998; 6:190–200.
5. Kirino S, et al. Relationship between polydipsia and antipsychotics: a systematic review of clinical studies and case reports. *Prog Neuropsychopharmacol Biol Psychiatry* 2020; 96:109756.
6. Siegler EL, et al. Risk factors for the development of hyponatremia in psychiatric inpatients. *Arch Intern Med* 1995; 155:953–957.
7. Madhusoodanan S, et al. Hyponatraemia associated with psychotropic medications: a review of the literature and spontaneous reports. *Adverse Drug React Toxicol Rev* 2002; 21:17–29.
8. Takeda K, et al. Analysis of the frequency and onset time of hyponatremia/syndrome of inappropriate antidiuretic hormone induced by antidepressants or antipsychotics. *Ann Pharmacother* 2022; 56:303–308.
9. Bachu K, et al. Aripiprazole-induced syndrome of inappropriate antidiuretic hormone secretion (SIADH). *Am J Ther* 2006; 13:370–372.
10. Dudeja SJ, et al. Olanzapine induced hyponatraemia. *Ulster Med J* 2010; 79:104–105.
11. Yam FK, et al. Syndrome of inappropriate antidiuretic hormone associated with aripiprazole. *Am J Health Syst Pharm* 2013; 70:2110–2114.
12. Kaur J, et al. Paliperidone inducing concomitantly syndrome of inappropriate antidiuretic hormone, neuroleptic malignant syndrome, and rhabdomyolysis. *Case Rep Crit Care* 2016; 2016:2587963.
13. Lin MW, et al. Aripiprazole-related hyponatremia and consequent valproic acid-related hyperammonemia in one patient. *Aust N Z J Psychiatry* 2017; 51:296–297.
14. Koufakis T. Quetiapine-induced syndrome of inappropriate secretion of antidiuretic hormone. *Case Rep Psychiatry* 2016; 2016:4803132.
15. Chen LC, et al. Polydipsia, hyponatremia and rhabdomyolysis in schizophrenia: a case report. *World J Psychiatry* 2014; 4:150–152.
16. Bakhla AK, et al. A suspected case of olanzapine induced hyponatremia. *Indian J Pharmacol* 2014; 46:441–442.
17. Kane JM, et al. Efficacy and safety of cariprazine in acute exacerbation of schizophrenia: results from an international, phase III clinical trial. *J Clin Psychopharmacol* 2015; 35:367–373.
18. Tibrewal P, et al. Paliperidone-induced hyponatremia. *Prim Care Companion CNS Disord* 2017; 19:16l02088.
19. McNally MA, et al. Olanzapine-induced hyponatremia presenting with seizure requiring intensive care unit admission. *Cureus* 2020; 12:e8212.
20. Sachdeva A, et al. Hyponatremia with olanzapine: a suspected association. *Shanghai Arch Psychiatry* 2017; 29:177–179.
21. Kumar PNS, et al. Hyponatremia secondary to SIADH in a schizophrenic patient treated with Quetiapine. *Asian J Psychiatr* 2018; 35:89–90.
22. Mazhar F, et al. Paliperidone-associated hyponatremia: report of a fatal case with analysis of cases reported in the literature and to the US Food and Drug Administration Adverse Event Reporting System. *J Clin Psychopharmacol* 2020; 40:202–205.
23. Chowdhury W, et al. Management of persistent hyponatremia induced by long-acting injectable risperidone therapy. *Cureus* 2018; 10:e2657.
24. Anil SS, et al. A case report of rapid-onset hyponatremia induced by low-dose olanzapine. *J Family Med Prim Care* 2017; 6:878–880.
25. Kang SG, et al. Addendum: low-dose quetiapine-induced syndrome of inappropriate antidiuretic hormone in a patient with traumatic brain syndrome. *Clin Psychopharmacol Neurosci* 2021; 19:179.
26. Aruachán S, et al. Hyponatraemia associated with the use of quetiapine: case report. *Rev Colomb Psiquiatr* 2020; 49:297–300.

27. Zhu X, et al. Rhabdomyolysis and elevated liver enzymes after rapid correction of hyponatremia due to pneumonia and concurrent use of aripiprazole: a case report. *Aust N Z J Psychiatry* 2018; **52**:206.

28. Mc Donald D, et al. Extreme hyponatraemia due to primary polydipsia and quetiapine-induced SIAD. *Endocrinol Diabetes Metab Case Rep* 2021; **2021**:21-0028.

29. Younes N, et al. Olanzapine induced hyponatremia and rhabdomyolysis. *Clin Case Rep* 2023; **11**:e5951.

30. Soenarti S, et al. Chlorpromazine-induced severe hyponatremia in 66 years old patient. *Acta Med Indones* 2023; **55**:444–448.

31. Meulendijks D, et al. Antipsychotic-induced hyponatraemia: a systematic review of the published evidence. *Drug Saf* 2010; **33**:101–114.

32. Mannesse CK, et al. Hyponatraemia as an adverse drug reaction of antipsychotic drugs: a case-control study in VigiBase. *Drug Saf* 2010; **33**:569–578.

33. Falhammar H, et al. Antipsychotics and severe hyponatraemia: a Swedish population-based case–control study. *Eur J Intern Med* 2019; **60**:71–77.

34. Mazhar F, et al. Hyponatremia following antipsychotic treatment: in silico pharmacodynamics analysis of spontaneous reports from the US Food and Drug Administration Adverse Event Reporting System Database and an updated systematic review. *Int J Neuropsychopharmacol* 2021; **24**:477–489.

35. Atsariyasing W, et al. A systematic review of the ability of urine concentration to distinguish antipsychotic- from psychosis-induced hyponatremia. *Psychiatry Res* 2014; **217**:129–133.

36. Letmaier M, et al. Hyponatraemia during psychopharmacological treatment: results of a drug surveillance programme. *Int J Neuropsychopharmacol* 2012; **15**:739–748.

37. Serrano A, et al. Safety of long-term clozapine administration. Frequency of cardiomyopathy and hyponatraemia: two cross-sectional, naturalistic studies. *Aust N Z J Psychiatry* 2014; **48**:183–192.

38. Sarma S, et al. Severe hyponatraemia associated with desmopressin nasal spray to treat clozapine-induced nocturnal enuresis. *Aust N Z J Psychiatry* 2005; **39**:949.

39. Yang HJ, et al. Antipsychotic use is a risk factor for hyponatremia in patients with schizophrenia: a 15-year follow-up study. *Psychopharmacology* 2017; **234**:869–876.

40. Adelakun AA, et al. Severe syndrome of inappropriate antidiuretic hormone secretion (SIADH) following the initiation of valbenazine for tardive dyskinesia: a case report. *Cureus* 2024; **16**:e58493.

41. Shepshelovich D, et al. Medication-induced SIADH: distribution and characterization according to medication class. *Br J Clin Pharmacol* 2017; **83**:1801–1807.

42. Yamamoto Y, et al. Prevalence and risk factors for hyponatremia in adult epilepsy patients: large-scale cross-sectional cohort study. *Seizure* 2019; **73**:26–30.

43. Fabrazzo M, et al. The unmasking of hidden severe hyponatremia after long-term combination therapy in exacerbated bipolar patients: a case series. *Int Clin Psychopharmacol* 2019; **34**:206–210.

44. Seifert J, et al. Psychotropic drug-induced hyponatremia: results from a drug surveillance program—an update. *J Neural Transm (Vienna)* 2021; **128**:1249–1264.

45. Pinkhasov A, et al. Management of SIADH-related hyponatremia due to psychotropic medications – an expert consensus from the Association of Medicine and Psychiatry. *J Psychosom Res* 2021; **151**:110654.

46. Josiassen RC, et al. Tolvaptan: a new tool for the effective treatment of hyponatremia in psychotic disorders. *Expert Opin Pharmacother* 2010; **11**:637–648.

47. Decaux G, et al. Non-peptide arginine-vasopressin antagonists: the vaptans. *Lancet* 2008; **371**:1624–1632.

48. Bhatia MS, et al. Psychogenic polydipsia – management challenges. *Shanghai Arch Psychiatry* 2017; **29**:180–183.

49. Zaidi AN. Rhabdomyolysis after correction of hyponatremia in psychogenic polydipsia possibly complicated by ziprasidone. *Ann Pharmacother* 2005; **39**:1726–1731.

50. Canuso CM, et al. Clozapine restores water balance in schizophrenic patients with polydipsia-hyponatremia syndrome. *J Neuropsychiatry Clin Neurosci* 1999; **11**:86–90.

51. Fujimoto M, et al. Clozapine improved the syndrome of inappropriate antidiuretic hormone secretion in a patient with treatment-resistant schizophrenia. *Psychiatry Clin Neurosci* 2016; **70**:469.

52. Spears NM, et al. Clozapine treatment in polydipsia and intermittent hyponatremia. *J Clin Psychiatry* 1996; **57**:123–128.

53. Littrell KH, et al. Effects of olanzapine on polydipsia and intermittent hyponatremia. *J Clin Psychiatry* 1997; **58**:549.

54. Kawai N, et al. Risperidone failed to improve polydipsia-hyponatremia of the schizophrenic patients. *Psychiatry Clin Neurosci* 2002; **56**:107–110.

55. Montgomery JH, et al. Adjunctive quetiapine treatment of the polydipsia, intermittent hyponatremia, and psychosis syndrome: a case report. *J Clin Psychiatry* 2003; **64**:339–341.

56. Canuso CM, et al. Does minimizing neuroleptic dosage influence hyponatremia? *Psychiatry Res* 1996; **63**:227–229.

57. Nixon RA, et al. Demeclocycline in the prophylaxis of self-induced water intoxication. *Am J Psychiatry* 1982; **139**:828–830.

58. Vieweg WV, et al. The use of demeclocycline in the treatment of patients with psychosis, intermittent hyponatremia, and polydipsia (PIP syndrome). *Psychiatr Q* 1988; **59**:62–68.

59. Srinivasan S, et al. Psychogenic polydipsia. 2022 (last updated April 2024, last checked May 2024); https://bestpractice.bmj.com/topics/en-gb/865.

60. Walter-Ryan WG. Water intoxication, demeclocycline, and antidiuretic hormone. *Am J Psychiatry* 1983; **140**:815.

61. Alexander RC, et al. A double blind, placebo-controlled trial of demeclocycline treatment of polydipsia-hyponatremia in chronically psychotic patients. *Biol Psychiatry* 1991; **30**:417–420.

62. Havens TH, et al. Non-antipsychotic pharmacotherapy of psychogenic polydipsia: a systematic review. *J Psychosom Res* 2021; **152**:110674.

63. Ahmed SE, et al. Acetazolamide: treatment of psychogenic polydipsia. *Cureus* 2017; **9**:e1553.

64. Takagi S, et al. Treatment of psychogenic polydipsia with acetazolamide: a report of 5 cases. *Clin Neuropharmacol* 2011; **34**:5–7.

Hyperprolactinaemia

Dopamine inhibits prolactin release and so dopamine antagonists can be expected to increase prolactin plasma levels. The degree of prolactin elevation is probably dose-related,[1] and for most antipsychotic medications the threshold activity (D_2 occupancy) for increased prolactin is very close to that of therapeutic efficacy.[2] Genetic differences may also play a part.[3] Table 1.43 groups individual antipsychotics according to their effect on prolactin concentrations.

Table 1.43 Effects of antipsychotic medication on prolactin concentration.[4-12]

Effect	Risk	Drug
Prolactin-sparing	Prolactin increase very rare	Aripiprazole Asenapine Brexpiprazole Cariprazine Clozapine Iloperidone Lumateperone Pimavanserin Quetiapine Xanomeline
Prolactin-elevating	Low risk, minor changes only	Lurasidone Olanzapine Ziprasidone
Prolactin-elevating	High risk; major changes	Amisulpride Paliperidone Risperidone Sulpiride First-generation antipsychotics

Hyperprolactinaemia is often superficially asymptomatic (that is, the patient does not spontaneously report problems) and there is some evidence that hyperprolactinaemia does not affect subjective quality of life.[13] Nonetheless, persistent elevation of plasma prolactin is associated with suppression of the hypothalamic–pituitary–gonadal axis.[14] Symptoms of this include sexual dysfunction[15] (but note that other pharmacological activities also give rise to sexual dysfunction),[16] menstrual disturbances,[4,17] breast growth and galactorrhoea,[17] and may include delusions of pregnancy.[18] Long-term adverse consequences are reductions in bone mineral density[19,20] and a possible increase in the risk of breast cancer.[21]

Prolactin can also be raised because of stress, pregnancy and lactation, seizures, renal impairment and other medical conditions,[7,22,23] including prolactinoma. When measuring prolactin, the sample should be taken early in the morning and stress during venepuncture should be minimised.[23]

Contraindications

Prolactin-elevating drugs with high risk should, if possible, be avoided in the following patient groups:

- Patients under 25 years of age (i.e. before peak bone mass).
- Patients with osteoporosis.
- Patients with a history of hormone-dependent breast cancer.
- Young women.

Management

Treatment of hyperprolactinaemia depends more on symptoms and long-term risk than on the reported plasma prolactin level.

Below, we suggest an algorithm for managing antipsychotic-induced hyperprolactinaemia (Figure 1.5). If treatment of hyperprolactinaemia is required, switching to an antipsychotic with a lower liability for prolactin elevation is usually the first choice, although switching always carries a risk of destabilising the illness and of relapse.[24] An alternative is to add aripiprazole to existing treatment.[25] Aripiprazole lowers prolactin levels in a dose-dependent manner: 3mg/day is effective but 6mg/day more so. Higher doses appear unnecessary.[26] Other strategies to reduce long-term risk to bone mineral density should also be discussed (e.g. stopping smoking, increasing weight-bearing exercise and ensuring adequate calcium and vitamin D3 intake).[19,27]

For patients who need to remain on a prolactin-elevating antipsychotic medication and who cannot tolerate aripiprazole, dopamine agonists can be effective.[28-30] Amantadine, cabergoline and bromocriptine have all been used, but each has, theoretically at least, the potential to worsen psychosis (although this has not been reported in trials). High-dose vitamin B6 (600mg/day) seems to be effective in reducing antipsychotic-induced hyperprolactinaemia and is well tolerated.[31] A herbal remedy – Peony–Glycyrrhiza Decoction – has also been shown to improve prolactin-related symptoms,[32,33] but the data are limited. A reduction in prolactin levels was also achieved by taking high daily doses (2.5–3g) of metformin[34] in a study of women with diabetes on antipsychotic medication. A 2022 network meta-analysis of all the above treatments confirmed the efficacy of aripiprazole 5mg a day and of vitamin B6 600mg/day in patients whose baseline prolactin exceeded 50ng/mL.[35] Two other meta-analyses concluded that adjunctive aripiprazole was the most effective treatment.[36,37]

Summary of management

First-choice adjunct treatment	Aripiprazole 5mg/day
Second-choice adjunct	Vitamin B6 600mg/day
Third-choice adjunct (in no particular order)	DA agonists – cabergoline, bromocriptine, amantadine Peony–Glycyrrhiza Decoction Metformin 2.5–3g/day

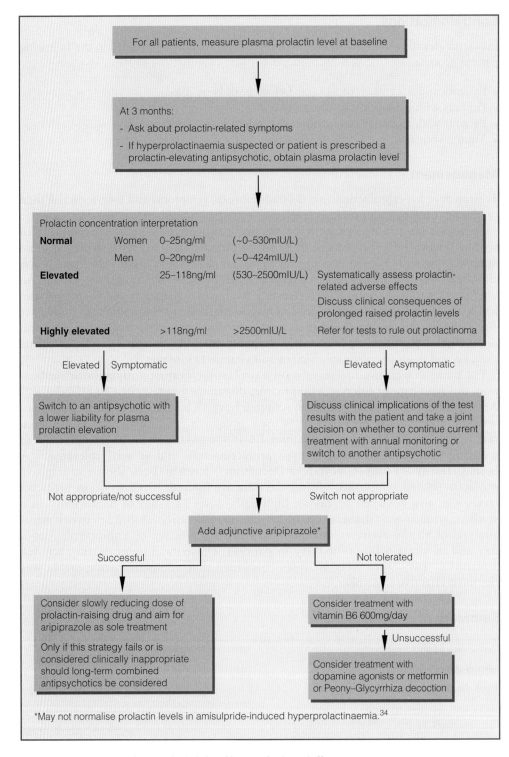

Figure 1.5 Management of antipsychotic-induced hyperprolactinaemia.[38]

References

1. Suzuki Y, et al. Differences in plasma prolactin levels in patients with schizophrenia treated on monotherapy with five second-generation antipsychotics. *Schizophr Res* 2013; **145**:116–119.

2. Tsuboi T, et al. Hyperprolactinemia and estimated dopamine D2 receptor occupancy in patients with schizophrenia: analysis of the CATIE data. *Prog Neuropsychopharmacol Biol Psychiatry* 2013; **45**:178–182.

3. Young RM, et al. Prolactin levels in antipsychotic treatment of patients with schizophrenia carrying the DRD2*A1 allele. *Br J Psychiatry* 2004; **185**:147–151.

4. Haddad PM, et al. Antipsychotic-induced hyperprolactinaemia: mechanisms, clinical features and management. *Drugs* 2004; **64**:2291–2314.

5. Holt RI, et al. Antipsychotics and hyperprolactinaemia: mechanisms, consequences and management. *Clin Endocrinol (Oxf)* 2011; **74**:141–147.

6. Leucht S, et al. Comparative efficacy and tolerability of 15 antipsychotic drugs in schizophrenia: a multiple-treatments meta-analysis. *Lancet* 2013; **382**:951–962.

7. Peuskens J, et al. The effects of novel and newly approved antipsychotics on serum prolactin levels: a comprehensive review. *CNS Drugs* 2014; **28**:421–453.

8. Citrome L. Cariprazine: chemistry, pharmacodynamics, pharmacokinetics, and metabolism, clinical efficacy, safety, and tolerability. *Expert Opin Drug Metab Toxicol* 2013; **9**:193–206.

9. Marder SR, et al. Brexpiprazole in patients with schizophrenia: overview of short- and long-term phase 3 controlled studies. *Acta Neuropsychiatr* 2017; **29**:278–290.

10. Vanover KE, et al. Dopamine D(2) receptor occupancy of lumateperone (ITI-007): a positron emission tomography study in patients with schizophrenia. *Neuropsychopharmacology* 2019; **44**:598–605.

11. Yunusa I, et al. Pimavanserin: a novel antipsychotic with potentials to address an unmet need of older adults with dementia-related psychosis. *Front Pharmacol* 2020; **11**:87.

12. Correll CU, et al. Safety and tolerability of KarXT (xanomeline-trospium) in a phase 2, randomized, double-blind, placebo-controlled study in patients with schizophrenia. *Schizophrenia (Heidelb)* 2022; **8**:109.

13. Kaneda Y. The impact of prolactin elevation with antipsychotic medications on subjective quality of life in patients with schizophrenia. *Clin Neuropharmacol* 2003; **26**:182–184.

14. Smith S, et al. The effects of antipsychotic-induced hyperprolactinaemia on the hypothalamic-pituitary-gonadal axis. *J Clin Psychopharmacol* 2002; **22**:109–114.

15. De Hert M, et al. Second-generation and newly approved antipsychotics, serum prolactin levels and sexual dysfunctions: a critical literature review. *Expert Opin Drug Saf* 2014; **13**:605–624.

16. Baldwin D, et al. Sexual side-effects of antidepressant and antipsychotic drugs. *Adv Psychiatr Treat* 2003; **9**:202–210.

17. Wieck A, et al. Antipsychotic-induced hyperprolactinaemia in women: pathophysiology, severity and consequences. Selective literature review. *Br J Psychiatry* 2003; **182**:199–204.

18. Ali JA, et al. Delusions of pregnancy associated with increased prolactin concentrations produced by antipsychotic treatment. *Int J Neuropsychopharmacol* 2003; **6**:111–115.

19. De Hert M, et al. Relationship between antipsychotic medication, serum prolactin levels and osteoporosis/osteoporotic fractures in patients with schizophrenia: a critical literature review. *Expert Opin Drug Saf* 2016; **15**:809–823.

20. Tseng PT, et al. Bone mineral density in schizophrenia: an update of current meta-analysis and literature review under guideline of PRISMA. *Medicine (Baltimore)* 2015; **94**:e1967.

21. De Hert M, et al. Relationship between prolactin, breast cancer risk, and antipsychotics in patients with schizophrenia: a critical review. *Acta Psychiatr Scand* 2016; **133**:5–22.

22. Holt RI. Medical causes and consequences of hyperprolactinaemia: a context for psychiatrists. *J Psychopharmacol* 2008; **22**:28–37.

23. Melmed S, et al. Diagnosis and treatment of hyperprolactinemia: an Endocrine Society clinical practice guideline. *J Clin Endocrinol Metab* 2011; **96**:273–288.

24. Montejo AL, et al. Multidisciplinary consensus on the therapeutic recommendations for iatrogenic hyperprolactinemia secondary to antipsychotics. *Front Neuroendocrinol* 2017; **45**:25–34.

25. Sá Esteves P, et al. Low doses of adjunctive aripiprazole as treatment for antipsychotic-induced hyperprolactinemia: a literature review. *Eur Psychiatry* 2015; **30** Suppl 1:393.

26. Yasui-Furukori N, et al. Dose-dependent effects of adjunctive treatment with aripiprazole on hyperprolactinemia induced by risperidone in female patients with schizophrenia. *J Clin Psychopharmacol* 2010; **30**:596–599.

27. Meaney AM, et al. Bone mineral density changes over a year in young females with schizophrenia: relationship to medication and endocrine variables. *Schizophr Res* 2007; **93**:136–143.

28. Hamner MB, et al. Hyperprolactinaemia in antipsychotic-treated patients: guidelines for avoidance and management. *CNS Drugs* 1998; **10**:209–222.

29. Duncan D, et al. Treatment of psychotropic-induced hyperprolactinaemia. *Psychiatr Bull* 1995; **19**:755–757.

30. Cavallaro R, et al. Cabergoline treatment of risperidone-induced hyperprolactinemia: a pilot study. *J Clin Psychiatry* 2004; **65**:187–190.

31. Zhuo C, et al. Safety and efficacy of high-dose vitamin B6 as an adjunctive treatment for antipsychotic-induced hyperprolactinemia in male patients with treatment-resistant schizophrenia. *Front Psychiatry* 2021; **12**:681418.

32. Yuan HN, et al. A randomized, crossover comparison of herbal medicine and bromocriptine against risperidone-induced hyperprolactinemia in patients with schizophrenia. *J Clin Psychopharmacol* 2008; **28**:264–370.

33. Man SC, et al. Peony–glycyrrhiza decoction for antipsychotic-related hyperprolactinemia in women with schizophrenia: a randomized controlled trial. *J Clin Psychopharmacol* 2016; **36**:572–579.
34. Krysiak R, et al. The effect of metformin on prolactin levels in patients with drug-induced hyperprolactinemia. *Eur J Intern Med* 2016; **30**:94–98.
35. Lu Z, et al. Pharmacological treatment strategies for antipsychotic-induced hyperprolactinemia: a systematic review and network meta-analysis. *Transl Psychiatry* 2022; **12**:267.
36. Zhang L, et al. Efficacy and safety of adjunctive aripiprazole, metformin, and paeoniae-glycyrrhiza decoction for antipsychotic-induced hyperprolactinemia: a network meta-analysis of randomized controlled trials. *Front Psychiatry* 2021; **12**:728204.
37. Jiang Q, et al. Treatment of antipsychotic-induced hyperprolactinemia: an umbrella review of systematic reviews and meta-analyses. *Front Psychiatry* 2024; **15**:1337274.
38. Walters J, et al. Clinical questions and uncertainty: prolactin measurement in patients with schizophrenia and bipolar disorder. *J Psychopharmacol* 2008; **22**:82–89.
39. Chen CK, et al. Differential add-on effects of aripiprazole in resolving hyperprolactinemia induced by risperidone in comparison to benzamide antipsychotics. *Prog Neuropsychopharmacol Biol Psychiatry* 2010; **34**:1495–1499.

Sexual dysfunction and antipsychotics

A 2023 meta-analysis found the global prevalence of sexual dysfunction in people with schizophrenia to be 56% in men and 60% in women.[1] Problems are not always reported by patients. In one study of patients with psychosis, 37% spontaneously reported sexual problems but 46% were found to be experiencing difficulties when directly questioned.[2]

Baseline sexual functioning should be determined if possible (questionnaires may be useful) because sexual function can affect both quality of life[3] and compliance with medication (sexual dysfunction is one of the major causes of treatment dropout).[4,5] Complaints of sexual dysfunction may also indicate progression or inadequate treatment of underlying medical or psychiatric conditions.[6,7] Sexual problems may also be caused by drug treatment and are associated with early discontinuation of antipsychotics.[8] Intervention may greatly improve quality of life.[9]

The human sexual response

There are four phases of the human sexual response, as detailed in Table 1.44.[10-12]

Effects of psychosis

Sexual dysfunction is a well-established phenomenon in first-episode schizophrenia.[13,14] Up to 82% of men and 96% of women report problems, with associated reductions in quality of life.[3] Antipsychotic adverse effects are not solely responsible, because prevalence is also high (17–70%) in patients who are unmedicated.[15] Men complain of reduced desire,[16] inability to achieve an erection and premature ejaculation,[1] whereas women complain of lowered libido and orgasm dysfunction.[1] Women with psychosis also have reduced fertility.[17]

Table 1.44 The human sexual response.

Desire	■ Related to testosterone levels in men
	■ Possibly increased by dopamine and decreased by prolactin
	■ Psychosocial context and conditioning significantly affect desire
Arousal	■ Influenced by testosterone in men and oestrogen in women
	■ Other potential mechanisms include central dopamine stimulation, modulation of the cholinergic/adrenergic balance, peripheral α1 agonism and nitric oxide pathways
	■ Physical pathology such as hypertension or diabetes can have a significant effect
Orgasm	■ May be related to oxytocin
	■ Inhibition of orgasm may be caused by an increase in serotonin activity and raised prolactin, as well as α1 blockade
Resolution	■ Occurs passively after orgasm

Note: Many other hormones and neurotransmitters may interact in a complex way at each phase.

People with psychosis are less able to develop good psychosexual relationships and, for some, treatment with an antipsychotic can improve sexual functioning via an improvement in psychotic symptoms.[18] Assessment of sexual functioning can clearly be difficult in someone who is psychotic. The Arizona Sexual Experience Scale may be useful in this respect.[19]

Effects of antipsychotic drugs

Sexual dysfunction is an adverse effect of most antipsychotics. Individual susceptibility varies and effects are usually reversible. Psychosis, physical illness and drugs other than antipsychotics can also contribute to sexual dysfunction. Many studies do not control for these factors, making the prevalence of sexual dysfunction with different antipsychotics difficult to compare.[20]

Antipsychotics decrease dopaminergic transmission, which in itself can decrease libido but may also increase prolactin levels via negative feedback. Hyperprolactinaemia is a key factor in sexual dysfunction[21,22] but may only explain 40% of the sexual dysfunction that is associated with antipsychotic medication.[23] Hyperprolactinaemia can also cause amenorrhoea and infertility[24] in women, and breast enlargement and galactorrhoea in both men and women.[25] The overall propensity of an antipsychotic to cause sexual dysfunction is a function of the facility to raise prolactin (i.e. risperidone > haloperidol > olanzapine > quetiapine > aripiprazole).[6,20,26] Aripiprazole is relatively free of sexual adverse effects when used as monotherapy[27] and may improve symptoms in combination with another antipsychotic.[28,29] The same is probably true for brexpiprazole, and cariprazine is a theoretically appropriate alternative.[30]

Anticholinergic effects of drugs can cause disorders of arousal[31] and concomitant anticholinergics may thus contribute to sexual dysfunction.[32] Drugs that block peripheral α_1 receptors cause particular problems with erection and ejaculation in men.[9] Antipsychotic-induced sedation and weight gain may reduce sexual desire.[33] Table 1.45 gives details of the nature and frequency of sexual adverse effects caused by antipsychotics.

Table 1.45 Sexual adverse effects of antipsychotics.

Drug	Type of problem
Aripiprazole	▪ No effect on prolactin or α_1 receptors. No reported adverse effects on sexual function. Improves sexual function in those switched from other antipsychotics[27,29,34–36] and when added as an adjunct.[37] Case reports of aripiprazole-induced hypersexuality have been published.[38,39]
Asenapine	▪ Does not appear to significantly affect prolactin levels[40] ▪ No reported cases of sexual dysfunction
Brexpiprazole	▪ Similar mechanism of action to aripiprazole (5-HT$_{1A}$ agonist, 5-HT$_{2A}$ antagonist and partial D$_2$ agonist) ▪ Causes negligible increases in prolactin[41] ▪ No problems with sexual dysfunction reported in clinical trials[42]

(Continued)

CHAPTER 1

Table 1.45 (*Continued*)

Drug	Type of problem
Cariprazine	▪ Similar mechanism of action to aripiprazole (5-HT$_{1A}$ agonist, 5-HT$_{2A}$ antagonist and partial D$_2$ agonist) ▪ Not associated with hyperprolactinaemia[43] ▪ Very low rates of sexual dysfunction reported in clinical trials[44]
Clozapine	▪ Significant α1 adrenergic blockade and anticholinergic effects.[45] No effect on prolactin.[46] ▪ Probably fewer problems than with typical antipsychotics[47]
Haloperidol	▪ Similar problems to phenothiazines[48] but anticholinergic effects reduced[49] ▪ Prevalence of sexual dysfunction up to 70%[50]
Lurasidone	▪ Does not appear to affect prolactin levels[51] ▪ No reported cases of sexual dysfunction[52]
Olanzapine	▪ Possibly less sexual dysfunction than drugs such as haloperidol owing to relative lack of prolactin-related effects[48] ▪ Priapism reported rarely[53,54] ▪ Prevalence of sexual dysfunction >50%[50]
Paliperidone	▪ Similar prolactin elevations to risperidone ▪ One small study[55] and one case report[56] showing reduction in sexual dysfunction following switching to paliperidone depot from risperidone oral or depot
Phenothiazines (e.g. chlorpromazine)	▪ Hyperprolactinaemia and anticholinergic effects. May cause delayed orgasm at lower doses followed by normal orgasm but without ejaculation at higher doses.[57] ▪ Priapism has been reported with thioridazine and chlorpromazine (probably due to α1 blockade)[49,58,59]
Quetiapine	▪ No effect on prolactin[60] ▪ Possibly associated with low risk of sexual dysfunction,[61–64] but studies are conflicting[65,66]
Risperidone	▪ Potent elevator of serum prolactin ▪ Less anticholinergic than some other antipsychotics (olanzapine, quetiapine) ▪ Specific peripheral α1 adrenergic blockade leads to a moderately high reported incidence of ejaculatory problems such as retrograde ejaculation[67,68] ▪ Priapism reported rarely[33] ▪ Prevalence of sexual dysfunction 60–70%[50]
Sulpiride/amisulpride	▪ Potent elevators of serum prolactin[69] but note that sulpiride was not associated with greater sexual dysfunction than SGAs in CUtLASS-1[18]
Thioxanthenes (e.g. flupentixol)	▪ Arousal problems and anorgasmia[70]
Lumateperone	▪ Does not appear to affect prolactin[71] ▪ No sexual adverse effects reported in clinical trials[72]
Pimavanserin	▪ Does not bind to dopamine receptors,[73] so has no effect on prolactin ▪ May improve sexual function in patients with depression[74]
Iloperidone	▪ Does not usually affect prolactin[75] ▪ Some reports of sexual dysfunction in adverse event reporting databases,[76] case reports of retrograde ejaculation[77]

CUtLASS-1, Cost Utility of the Latest Antipsychotic Drugs in Schizophrenia Study; SGA, second-generation antipsychotic.

Treatment of sexual dysfunction

Before attempting to treat sexual dysfunction, a thorough assessment is essential to determine the most likely cause. A large meta-analysis of 72 studies from 33 different countries found that for patients with schizophrenia spectrum disorders, concurrent antidepressant and mood stabiliser prescriptions were associated with *lower* rates of erection and ejaculation disorders.[1] This suggests that treating a comorbid depression or mood disorder is an important strategy to improve sexual health. Assuming that psychiatric comorbidity or physical pathology (diabetes, hypertension, cardiovascular disease, etc.) has been excluded or treated (e.g. obesity),[78] the following principles apply when considering the prescribing of antipsychotics:

- Spontaneous remission may occasionally occur[33] but may take 6 months to become apparent, if at all,[30] and may be more likely related to a reduction in severity of illness, rather than tolerance to the antipsychotic itself.
- When symptoms persist, the most obvious first step is to decrease the dose (although a correlation between dose and all types of sexual dysfunction has not been conclusively demonstrated)[79] or discontinue the offending drug, where appropriate.
- The next step is to switch to a different drug that is less likely to cause the specific sexual problem experienced (Table 1.46). Another option is to add 5–10mg aripiprazole – this can normalise prolactin and improve sexual function.[37,80]
- If this fails or is not practicable, 'antidote' drugs can be tried: for example, cyproheptadine (a $5HT_2$ antagonist at doses of 4–16mg/day) has been used to treat SSRI-induced sexual dysfunction but sedation is a common adverse effect. There is some evidence that mirtazapine (also a $5HT_2$ antagonist as well as an α_2 antagonist) may relieve orgasmic dysfunction in patients treated with FGAs.[81] Amantadine, bupropion, buspirone, bethanechol and yohimbine have all been used with varying degrees of success but have several adverse effects and interactions with other drugs. Given that hyperprolactinaemia contributes to sexual dysfunction, selegiline, which enhances dopamine activity, has been investigated but was not effective.[82] Testosterone patches have been shown to increase libido in women, although breast cancer risk may be significantly increased.[83,84]

Table 1.46 lists remedial treatments for psychotropic-induced sexual dysfunction.

Table 1.46 Remedial treatments for psychotropic-induced sexual dysfunction.

Drug	Pharmacology	Potential treatment for	Adverse effects
Alprostadil[12,85]	Prostaglandin	Erectile dysfunction	Pain, fibrosis, hypotension, priapism
Amantadine[85,86,87]	Dopamine agonist	Prolactin-induced reduction in desire and arousal (dopamine increases libido and facilitates ejaculation)	Return of psychotic symptoms, GI effects, nervousness, insomnia, rash
Bethanechol[88]	Cholinergic or cholinergic potentiation of adrenergic neurotransmission	Anticholinergic-induced arousal problems and anorgasmia (from TCAs, antipsychotics, etc.)	Nausea and vomiting, colic, bradycardia, blurred vision, sweating
Bromocriptine[9]	Dopamine agonist	Prolactin-induced reduction in desire and arousal	Return of psychotic symptoms, GI effects
Bupropion[89,90]	Noradrenaline and dopamine reuptake inhibitor	SSRI-induced sexual dysfunction	Concentration problems, reduced sleep, tremor
Buspirone[91]	$5HT_{1a}$ partial agonist	SSRI-induced sexual dysfunction, particularly decreased libido and anorgasmia	Nausea, dizziness, headache
Cyproheptadine[85,91,92]	$5HT_2$ antagonist	Sexual dysfunction caused by increased serotonin transmission (e.g. SSRIs), particularly anorgasmia	Sedation and fatigue. Reversal of the therapeutic effect of antidepressants.
Flibanserin (licensed in USA)[93]	$5HT_{1A}$ agonist, $5HT_{2A}$ antagonist, dopamine antagonist	Lack or loss of sexual desire in premenopausal women. Appears to be safe in women taking antidepressants.[94]	Hypotension, syncope, sedation, dizziness, nausea, dry mouth
Sildenafil,[12,95–98] **tadalafil,**[99] **lodenafil,**[100] **vardenafil**[101]	Phosphodiesterase inhibitors	Erectile dysfunction of any aetiology. Anorgasmia in women. Effective even when prolactin raised.	Mild headaches, dizziness, nasal congestion
Yohimbine[12,85,102–104]	Central and peripheral α_2 adrenoceptor antagonist	SSRI-induced sexual dysfunction, particularly erectile dysfunction, decreased libido and anorgasmia	Anxiety, nausea, fine tremor, increased blood pressure, sweating, fatigue
Pimavanserin[74]	Inverse agonist at $5HT_{2A}$ and $5HT_{2C}$	Sexual dysfunction in depression with inadequate response to antidepressants. Improvement in sexual function independent of effect on depression unconfirmed.	Peripheral oedema, nausea, confusion
Bremelanotide[105]	Melanocortin receptor agonist	Hypoactive sexual desire in premenopausal women. No published data on use in patients with psychiatric diagnoses.	Flushing, nausea, headache

Note: The use of the drugs listed above should ideally be under the care or supervision of a specialist in sexual dysfunction.
GI, gastrointestinal; TCA, tricyclic antidepressant.

The evidence base supporting the use of 'antidotes' is often poor and specific to particular drug-induced problems.[33,106] The generalisability of results from positive trials is limited by small sample sizes, short trial durations and lack of controlling for confounding factors (age, concurrent medication, antipsychotic switches for reasons other than baseline sexual dysfunction).[106] Comparison of data between studies is further complicated by the use of varying assessment tools to measure outcomes.[107]

Drugs such as sildenafil (Viagra) or alprostadil (Caverject) are effective only in the treatment of erectile dysfunction (they have no effect on libido or central arousal). Psychological approaches used by sexual dysfunction clinics may be difficult for clients with mental health problems to engage in.[9]

References

1. Korchia T, et al. Sexual dysfunction in schizophrenia: a systematic review and meta-analysis. *JAMA Psychiatry* 2023; **80**:1110–1120.
2. Montejo AL, et al. Frequency of sexual dysfunction in patients with a psychotic disorder receiving antipsychotics. *J Sex Med* 2010; 7:3404–3413.
3. Olfson M, et al. Male sexual dysfunction and quality of life in schizophrenia. *J Clin Psychiatry* 2005; **66**:331–338.
4. Montejo AL, et al. Incidence of sexual dysfunction associated with antidepressant agents: a prospective multicenter study of 1022 outpatients. Spanish Working Group for the Study of Psychotropic-Related Sexual Dysfunction. *J Clin Psychiatry* 2001; 62 Suppl 3:10–21.
5. Souaiby L, et al. Sexual dysfunction in patients with schizophrenia and schizoaffective disorder and its association with adherence to antipsychotic medication. *J Ment Health* 2020; **29**:623–630.
6. Baggaley M. Sexual dysfunction in schizophrenia: focus on recent evidence. *Hum Psychopharmacol* 2008; **23**:201–209.
7. Ucok A, et al. Sexual dysfunction in patients with schizophrenia on antipsychotic medication. *Eur Psychiatry* 2007; **22**:328–333.
8. Patel R, et al. Oral and long-acting injectable antipsychotic discontinuation and relationship to side effects in people with first episode psychosis: a longitudinal analysis of electronic health record data. *Ther Adv Psychopharmacol* 2023; **13**:20451253231211575.
9. Segraves RT. Effects of psychotropic drugs on human erection and ejaculation. *Arch Gen Psychiatry* 1989; **46**:275–284.
10. Pollack MH, et al. Genitourinary and sexual adverse effects of psychotropic medication. *Int J Psychiatry Med* 1992; **22**:305–327.
11. Stahl SM. The psychopharmacology of sex, part 1: neurotransmitters and the 3 phases of the human sexual response. *J Clin Psychiatry* 2001; **62**:80–81.
12. Garcia-Reboll L, et al. Drugs for the treatment of impotence. *Drugs Aging* 1997; **11**:140–151.
13. Bitter I, et al. Antipsychotic treatment and sexual functioning in first-time neuroleptic-treated schizophrenic patients. *Int Clin Psychopharmacol* 2005; **20**:19–21.
14. Dembler-Stamm T, et al. Sexual dysfunction in unmedicated patients with schizophrenia and in healthy controls. *Pharmacopsychiatry* 2018; **51**:251–256.
15. Vargas-Cáceres S, et al. The impact of psychosis on sexual functioning: a systematic review. *J Sex Med* 2021; **18**:457–466.
16. Macdonald S, et al. Nithsdale Schizophrenia Surveys 24: sexual dysfunction. Case-control study. *Br J Psychiatry* 2003; **182**:50–56.
17. Howard LM, et al. The general fertility rate in women with psychotic disorders. *Am J Psychiatry* 2002; **159**:991–997.
18. Peluso MJ, et al. Non-neurological and metabolic side effects in the Cost Utility of the Latest Antipsychotics in Schizophrenia Randomised Controlled Trial (CUtLASS-1). *Schizophr Res* 2013; **144**:80–86.
19. Byerly MJ, et al. An empirical evaluation of the Arizona sexual experience scale and a simple one-item screening test for assessing antipsychotic-related sexual dysfunction in outpatients with schizophrenia and schizoaffective disorder. *Schizophr Res* 2006; **81**:311–316.
20. Serretti A, et al. A meta-analysis of sexual dysfunction in psychiatric patients taking antipsychotics. *Int Clin Psychopharmacol* 2011; **26**:130–140.
21. Zhang Y, et al. Prolactin and thyroid stimulating hormone (TSH) levels and sexual dysfunction in patients with schizophrenia treated with conventional antipsychotic medication: a cross-sectional study. *Med Sci Monit* 2018; **24**:9136–9143.
22. Martínez-Giner G, et al. Sexual dysfunction in people treated with long-acting injectable antipsychotics in monotherapy or polypharmacy: a naturalistic study. *Int J Ment Health Nurs* 2022; **31**:576–590.
23. Nunes LV, et al. Strategies for the treatment of antipsychotic-induced sexual dysfunction and/or hyperprolactinemia among patients of the schizophrenia spectrum: a review. *J Sex Marital Ther* 2012; **38**:281–301.
24. Edinoff AN, et al. Hyperprolactinemia, clinical considerations, and infertility in women on antipsychotic medications. *Psychopharmacol Bull* 2021; **51**:131–148.
25. Adverse effects of the atypical antipsychotics. Collaborative Working Group on Clinical Trial Evaluations. *J Clin Psychiatry* 1998; 59 Suppl 12:17–22.
26. Knegtering H, et al. Are sexual side effects of prolactin-raising antipsychotics reducible to serum prolactin? *Psychoneuroendocrinology* 2008; **33**:711–717.
27. Hanssens L, et al. The effect of antipsychotic medication on sexual function and serum prolactin levels in community-treated schizophrenic patients: results from the Schizophrenia Trial of Aripiprazole (STAR) study (NCT00237913). *BMC Psychiatry* 2008; **8**:95.
28. Mir A, et al. Change in sexual dysfunction with aripiprazole: a switching or add-on study. *J Psychopharm* 2008; **22**:244–253.

29. Byerly MJ, et al. Effects of aripiprazole on prolactin levels in subjects with schizophrenia during cross-titration with risperidone or olanzapine: analysis of a randomized, open-label study. *Schizophr Res* 2009; **107**:218–222.

30. Montejo AL, et al. Management strategies for antipsychotic-related sexual dysfunction: a clinical approach. *J Clin Med* 2021; **10**:308.

31. Aldridge SA. Drug-induced sexual dysfunction. *Clin Pharm* 1982; **1**:141–147.

32. Fond G, et al. Sexual dysfunctions are associated with major depression, chronic inflammation and anticholinergic consumption in the real-world schizophrenia FACE-SZ national cohort. *Prog Neuropsychopharmacol Biol Psychiatry* 2019; **94**:109654.

33. Baldwin D, et al. Sexual side-effects of antidepressant and antipsychotic drugs. *Adv Psychiatr Treat* 2003; **9**:202–210.

34. Rykmans V, et al. P0106: A comparision of switching strategies from risperidone to aripiprazole in patients with schizophrenia with insufficient efficacy/tolerability on risperidone (cn138-169). *Eur Psychiatry* 2008; **23** Suppl 2:S111.

35. Potkin SG, et al. Reduced sexual dysfunction with aripiprazole once-monthly versus paliperidone palmitate: results from QUALIFY. *Int Clin Psychopharmacol* 2017; **32**:147–154.

36. Kelly DL, et al. Analysis of prolactin and sexual side effects in patients with schizophrenia who switched from paliperidone palmitate to aripiprazole lauroxil. *Psychiatry Res* 2021; **302**:114030.

37. Kelly DL, et al. Adjunct aripiprazole reduces prolactin and prolactin-related adverse effects in premenopausal women with psychosis: results from the DAAMSEL clinical trial. *J Clin Psychopharmacol* 2018; **38**:317–326.

38. Chen CY, et al. Improvement of serum prolactin and sexual function after switching to aripiprazole from risperidone in schizophrenia: a case series. *Psychiatry Clin Neurosci* 2011; **65**:95–97.

39. Vrignaud L, et al. [Hypersexuality associated with aripiprazole: a new case and review of the literature]. *Therapie* 2014; **69**:525–527.

40. Ajmal A, et al. Psychotropic-induced hyperprolactinemia: a clinical review. *Psychosomatics* 2014; **55**:29–36.

41. Kane JM, et al. A multicenter, randomized, double-blind, controlled phase 3 trial of fixed-dose brexpiprazole for the treatment of adults with acute schizophrenia. *Schizophr Res* 2015; **164**:127–135.

42. Citrome L. Brexpiprazole for schizophrenia and as adjunct for major depressive disorder: a systematic review of the efficacy and safety profile for this newly approved antipsychotic – what is the number needed to treat, number needed to harm and likelihood to be helped or harmed? *Int J Clin Pract* 2015; **69**:978–997.

43. Nasrallah HA, et al. The safety and tolerability of cariprazine in long-term treatment of schizophrenia: a post hoc pooled analysis. *BMC Psychiatry* 2017; **17**:305.

44. Barabássy Á, et al. Safety and tolerability of cariprazine in patients with schizophrenia: a pooled analysis of eight phase II/III studies. *Neuropsychiatr Dis Treat* 2021; **17**:957–970.

45. Coward DM. General pharmacology of clozapine. *Br J Psychiatry Suppl* 1992; **160**:5–11.

46. Meltzer HY, et al. Effect of clozapine on human serum prolactin levels. *Am J Psychiatry* 1979; **136**:1550–1555.

47. Aizenberg D, et al. Comparison of sexual dysfunction in male schizophrenic patients maintained on treatment with classical antipsychotics versus clozapine. *J Clin Psychiatry* 2001; **62**:541–544.

48. Crawford AM, et al. The acute and long-term effect of olanzapine compared with placebo and haloperidol on serum prolactin concentrations. *Schizophr Res* 1997; **26**:41–54.

49. Mitchell JE, et al. Antipsychotic drug therapy and sexual dysfunction in men. *Am J Psychiatry* 1982; **139**:633–637.

50. Serretti A, et al. Sexual side effects of pharmacological treatment of psychiatric diseases. *Clin Pharmacol Ther* 2011; **89**:142–147.

51. Citrome L, et al. Long-term safety and tolerability of lurasidone in schizophrenia: a 12-month, double-blind, active-controlled study. *Int Clin Psychopharmacol* 2012; **27**:165–176.

52. Clayton AH, et al. Safety of flibanserin in women treated with antidepressants: a randomized, placebo-controlled study. *J Sex Med* 2018; **15**:43–51.

53. Dossenbach M, et al. Effects of atypical and typical antipsychotic treatments on sexual function in patients with schizophrenia: 12-month results from the Intercontinental Schizophrenia Outpatient Health Outcomes (IC-SOHO) study. *Eur Psychiatry* 2006; **21**:251–258.

54. Aurobindo Pharma - Milpharm Ltd. Summary of Product Characteristics. Olanzapine 10 mg tablets 2023 (last checked May 2024); http://www.medicines.org.uk/emc/medicine/27661/SPC/Olanzapine++10+mg+tablets/.

55. Montalvo I, et al. Changes in prolactin levels and sexual function in young psychotic patients after switching from long-acting injectable risperidone to paliperidone palmitate. *Int Clin Psychopharmacol* 2013; **28**:46–49.

56. Shiloh R, et al. Risperidone-induced retrograde ejaculation. *Am J Psychiatry* 2001; **158**:650.

57. Smith S. Effects of antipsychotics on sexual and endocrine function in women: implications for clinical practice. *J Clin Psychopharmacol* 2003; **23**(3 Suppl 1):S27–S32.

58. Loh C, et al. Risperidone-induced retrograde ejaculation: case report and review of the literature. *Int Clin Psychopharmacol* 2004; **19**:111–112.

59. Thompson JW, Jr., et al. Psychotropic medication and priapism: a comprehensive review. *J Clin Psychiatry* 1990; **51**:430–433.

60. Peuskens J, et al. A comparison of quetiapine and chlorpromazine in the treatment of schizophrenia. *Acta Psychiatr Scand* 1997; **96**:265–273.

61. Bobes J, et al. Frequency of sexual dysfunction and other reproductive side-effects in patients with schizophrenia treated with risperidone, olanzapine, quetiapine, or haloperidol: the results of the EIRE study. *J Sex Marital Ther* 2003; **29**:125–147.

62. Byerly MJ, et al. An open-label trial of quetiapine for antipsychotic-induced sexual dysfunction. *J Sex Marital Ther* 2004; **30**:325–332.

63. Knegtering R, et al. A randomized open-label study of the impact of quetiapine versus risperidone on sexual functioning. *J Clin Psychopharmacol* 2004; **24**:56–61.

64. Montejo Gonzalez AL, et al. A 6-month prospective observational study on the effects of quetiapine on sexual functioning. *J Clin Psychopharmacol* 2005; **25**:533–538.

65. Atmaca M, et al. A new atypical antipsychotic: quetiapine-induced sexual dysfunctions. *Int J Impot Res* 2005; **17**:201–203.

66. Kelly DL, et al. A randomized double-blind 12-week study of quetiapine, risperidone or fluphenazine on sexual functioning in people with schizophrenia. *Psychoneuroendocrinology* 2006; **31**:340–346.

67. Tran PV, et al. Double-blind comparison of olanzapine versus risperidone in the treatment of schizophrenia and other psychotic disorders. *J Clin Psychopharmacol* 1997; **17**:407–418.

68. Raja M. Risperidone-induced absence of ejaculation. *Int Clin Psychopharmacol* 1999; **14**:317–319.

69. Smith SM, et al. Sexual dysfunction in patients taking conventional antipsychotic medication. *Br J Psychiatry* 2002; **181**:49–55.

70. Aizenberg D, et al. Sexual dysfunction in male schizophrenic patients. *J Clin Psychiatry* 1995; **56**:137–141.

71. Correll CU, et al. Safety and tolerability of lumateperone 42 mg: an open-label antipsychotic switch study in outpatients with stable schizophrenia. *Schizophr Res* 2021; **228**:198–205.

72. Correll CU, et al. Efficacy and safety of lumateperone for treatment of schizophrenia: a randomized clinical trial. *JAMA Psychiatry* 2020; **77**:349–358.

73. Cruz MP. Pimavanserin (Nuplazid): a treatment for hallucinations and delusions associated with Parkinson's disease. *P T* 2017; **42**:368–371.

74. Freeman MP, et al. Improvement of sexual functioning during treatment of MDD with adjunctive pimavanserin: a secondary analysis. *Depress Anxiety* 2020; **37**:485–495.

75. Peuskens J, et al. The effects of novel and newly approved antipsychotics on serum prolactin levels: a comprehensive review. *CNS Drugs* 2014; **28**:421–453.

76. Subeesh V, et al. Novel adverse events of iloperidone: a disproportionality analysis in US Food and Drug Administration Adverse Event Reporting System (FAERS) Database. *Curr Drug Saf* 2019; **14**:21–26.

77. Freeman SA. Iloperidone-induced retrograde ejaculation. *Int Clin Psychopharmacol* 2013; **28**:156.

78. Theleritis C, et al. Sexual dysfunction and central obesity in patients with first episode psychosis. *Eur Psychiatry* 2017; **42**:1–7.

79. Yoshida K, et al. Dose-dependent effects of antipsychotics on efficacy and adverse effects in schizophrenia. *Behav Brain Res* 2021; **402**:113098.

80. Besag FMC, et al. Is adjunct aripiprazole effective in treating hyperprolactinemia induced by psychotropic medication? A narrative review. *CNS Drugs* 2021; **35**:507–526.

81. Terevnikov V, et al. Add-on mirtazapine improves orgasmic functioning in patients with schizophrenia treated with first-generation antipsychotics. *Nord J Psychiatry* 2017; **71**:77–80.

82. Kodesh A, et al. Selegiline in the treatment of sexual dysfunction in schizophrenic patients maintained on neuroleptics: a pilot study. *Clin Neuropharmacol* 2003; **26**:193–195.

83. Davis SR, et al. Testosterone for low libido in postmenopausal women not taking estrogen. *N Engl J Med* 2008; **359**:2005–2017.

84. Schover LR. Androgen therapy for loss of desire in women: is the benefit worth the breast cancer risk? *Fertil Steril* 2008; **90**:129–140.

85. Baldwin DS, et al. Effects of antidepressant drugs on sexual function. *Int J Psychiatry Clin Pract* 1997; **1**:47–58.

86. Krzystanek M, et al. Amantadine in the treatment of sexual inactivity in schizophrenia patients taking atypical antipsychotics: the pilot case series study. *Pharmaceuticals (Basel)* 2021; **14**:947.

87. Valevski A, et al. Effect of amantadine on sexual dysfunction in neuroleptic-treated male schizophrenic patients. *Clin Neuropharmacol* 1998; **21**:355–357.

88. Gross MD. Reversal by bethanechol of sexual dysfunction caused by anticholinergic antidepressants. *Am J Psychiatry* 1982; **139**:1193–1194.

89. Masand PS, et al. Sustained-release bupropion for selective serotonin reuptake inhibitor-induced sexual dysfunction: a randomized, double-blind, placebo-controlled, parallel-group study. *Am J Psychiatry* 2001; **158**:805–807.

90. Rezaei O, et al. The effect of bupropion on sexual function in patients with Schizophrenia: a randomized clinical trial. *Eur J Psychiatry* 2017; **32**:11–15.

91. Rothschild AJ. Sexual side effects of antidepressants. *J Clin Psychiatry* 2000; **61** Suppl 11:28–36.

92. Lauerma H. Successful treatment of citalopram-induced anorgasmia by cyproheptadine. *Acta Psychiatr Scand* 1996; **93**:69–70.

93. IBM Watson Health. IBM Micromedex Solutions. 2024; https://www.ibm.com/watson-health/about/micromedex.

94. Clayton AH, et al. Effect of lurasidone on sexual function in major depressive disorder patients with subthreshold hypomanic symptoms (mixed features): results from a placebo-controlled trial. *J Clin Psychiatry* 2018; **79**:18m12132.

95. Nurnberg HG, et al. Sildenafil for women patients with antidepressant-induced sexual dysfunction. *Psychiatr Serv* 1999; **50**:1076–1078.

96. Salerian AJ, et al. Sildenafil for psychotropic-induced sexual dysfunction in 31 women and 61 men. *J Sex Marital Ther* 2000; **26**:133–140.

97. Gopalakrishnan R, et al. Sildenafil in the treatment of antipsychotic-induced erectile dysfunction: a randomized, double-blind, placebo-controlled, flexible-dose, two-way crossover trial. *Am J Psychiatry* 2006; **163**:494–499.

98. Mazzilli R, et al. Erectile dysfunction in patients taking psychotropic drugs and treated with phosphodiesterase-5 inhibitors. *Arch Ital Urol Androl* 2018; **90**:44–48.

99. de Boer MK, et al. Efficacy of tadalafil on erectile dysfunction in male patients using antipsychotics: a double-blind, placebo-controlled, crossover pilot study. *J Clin Psychopharmacol* 2014; **34**:380–382.

100. Nunes LV, et al. Adjunctive treatment with lodenafil carbonate for erectile dysfunction in outpatients with schizophrenia and spectrum: a randomized, double-blind, crossover, placebo-controlled trial. *J Sex Med* 2013; **10**:1136–1145.

101. Mitsonis CI, et al. Vardenafil in the treatment of erectile dysfunction in outpatients with chronic schizophrenia: a flexible-dose, open-label study. *J Clin Psychiatry* 2008; **69**:206–212.

102. Jacobsen FM. Fluoxetine-induced sexual dysfunction and an open trial of yohimbine. *J Clin Psychiatry* 1992; **53**:119–122.

103. Michelson D, et al. Mirtazapine, yohimbine or olanzapine augmentation therapy for serotonin reuptake-associated female sexual dysfunction: a randomized, placebo controlled trial. *J Psychiatr Res* 2002; **36**:147–152.

104. Woodrum ST, et al. Management of SSRI-induced sexual dysfunction. *Ann Pharmacother* 1998; **32**:1209–1215.

105. Kingsberg SA, et al. Bremelanotide for the treatment of hypoactive sexual desire disorder: two randomized phase 3 trials. *Obstet Gynecol* 2019; **134**:899–908.

106. Allen K, et al. Management of antipsychotic-related sexual dysfunction: systematic review. *J Sex Med* 2019; **16**:1978–1987.

107. Basson R, et al. Women's sexual dysfunction associated with psychiatric disorders and their treatment. *Womens Health* 2018; **14**:1745506518762664.

CHAPTER 1

Pneumonia

Background

A 2018 meta-analysis of 14 observational studies ($n = 206,899$) reported that antipsychotic use was associated with a near doubling of pneumonia incidence compared with no use.[1] This same analysis found no difference in incidence of pneumonia between FGAs and SGAs and no increase in fatality rate. A later analysis of spontaneous reporting to the US FDA uncovered relatively greater incidence of pneumonia in people prescribed clozapine, olanzapine and antipsychotic polypharmacy (compared with haloperidol).[2] In 2024, a 20-year observational study ($n = 61,889$) in Finland found increased risk of hospitalisation with pneumonia in people prescribed antipsychotic monotherapy compared with no antipsychotic use.[3]

There is some dispute over the causal association between antipsychotic use and risk of pneumonia. One study looked at the incidence of pneumonia in over 8,000 people before and after starting various antipsychotics and found no change overall (or for any individual antipsychotic).[4] Another analysis, a case–control study, found that duration of antipsychotic use was just one of three factors linked to increased risk of pneumonia (the others being severity of illness and comorbidity index).[5] Schizophrenia itself seems to afford a higher risk of complications (e.g. admission to intensive care) in people diagnosed with pneumonia,[6] although neither diagnosis nor age appears to modify the effect of antipsychotic use on pneumonia.[7] Risk of antipsychotic-associated pneumonia is increased in patients with Alzheimer's disease and those without.[8] Factors associated with antipsychotic-induced pneumonia are listed in Table 1.47.

Table 1.47 Factors associated with antipsychotic-induced pneumonia.

Treatment factors	■ Antipsychotics with high anticholinergic effects (e.g. clozapine and olanzapine)[3,9]
	■ High antipsychotic doses[10]
	■ Antipsychotic polypharmacy*[11–13]
	■ Concomitant benzodiazepines[14,15]
	■ Concomitant mood stabilisers**
Patient factors	■ Decreased CYP2C19 and CYP1A2 activity[16]
	■ Smoking[17]
	■ Obesity[17]
	■ Diagnosis of schizophrenia (especially TRS)[17]

* Not found in one study.[3]
** Lithium seems to have a protective effect.

The risk of pneumonia seems to be most pronounced in people prescribed antipsychotics with high anticholinergic effects (notably clozapine and high-dose olanzapine or quetiapine) and is probably dose dependent.[3,9] Among antipsychotics, clozapine is most often associated with pneumonia, with an estimated incidence of up to 30%[16] (although TRS itself increases risk of pneumonia by two-thirds).[18] In two studies, clozapine re-exposure was associated with a greater risk for recurrent pneumonia than the risk of baseline pneumonia with initial clozapine treatment.[16,19] Aripiprazole (and probably other dopamine partial agonists) seem to have a lower risk of pneumonia than pure dopamine antagonists.[9] Another study found amisulpride (a dopamine antagonist with minimal anticholinergic activity) is not linked to pneumonia.[11]

Mechanisms

Although studies rarely distinguish between the various forms of pneumonia, cases of antipsychotic-induced aspiration, infective (viral and bacterial) and hypersensitivity pneumonia have been documented.[16] The mechanism by which antipsychotics increase the risk of such pneumonia is not known but is probably multifactorial. Proposed mechanisms are outlined in Box 1.2.

Box 1.2 Proposed mechanisms for antipsychotic-induced pneumonia

- Sedation
- Dystonia or dyskinesia
- Dry mouth
- General poor physical health
- Reduced immune response*
- Clozapine-specific: hypersalivation, constipation

* Clozapine is associated with antibody deficiency and greater use of antibiotics. This increased risk of infection is not related to neutrophil counts.[20]

An increased risk of pneumonia should probably be assumed for all patients taking any antipsychotic (but especially clozapine)[21] for any period. All patients should be very carefully monitored for signs of chest infection and effective treatment started promptly. Consideration should be given to using COVID-19, influenza and pneumococcal vaccines, although there is no direct evidence to support benefit for pneumonia prevention in this specific group of patients. Those patients prescribed clozapine should be proactively monitored and treated for hypersalivation. Pneumonia is likely to increase clozapine levels (see section on clozapine: common adverse effects in this chapter) so close monitoring is required. Slower-than-usual clozapine titration may prevent cases of hypersensitivity pneumonia.[14] Extra vigilance is required when re-exposing to patients with history of clozapine-induced pneumonia who are taking clozapine. With all cases, early referral to general medical services should be considered where there is any doubt about the severity or type of chest infection.

Summary

- Assume that the use of all antipsychotics increases the risk of pneumonia, but especially clozapine and high-dose olanzapine or quetiapine.
- Concomitant benzodiazepine use should be avoided, where possible.
- Monitor all patients for signs of chest infection and treat promptly.
- Offer vaccination against COVID-19, influenza and pneumococcus to all high-risk patients.

References

1. Dzahini O, et al. Antipsychotic drug use and pneumonia: systematic review and meta-analysis. *J Psychopharmacol* 2018; 32:1167–1181.
2. Cepaityte D, et al. Exploring a safety signal of antipsychotic-associated pneumonia: a pharmacovigilance–pharmacodynamic study. *Schizophr Bull* 2020; 47:672–681.
3. Luykx JJ, et al. Pneumonia risk, antipsychotic dosing, and anticholinergic burden in schizophrenia. *JAMA Psychiatry* 2024; 81:967–975.
4. Rohde C, et al. Antipsychotic medication exposure, clozapine, and pneumonia: results from a self-controlled study. *Acta Psychiatr Scand* 2020; 142:78–86.
5. Chan HY, et al. Is antipsychotic treatment associated with risk of pneumonia in people with serious mental illness? The roles of severity of psychiatric symptoms and global functioning. *J Clin Psychopharmacol* 2019; 39:434–440.
6. Chen YH, et al. Poor clinical outcomes among pneumonia patients with schizophrenia. *Schizophr Bull* 2011; 37:1088–1094.
7. Nose M, et al. Antipsychotic drug exposure and risk of pneumonia: a systematic review and meta-analysis of observational studies. *Pharmacoepidemiol Drug Saf* 2015; 24:812–820.
8. Tolppanen AM, et al. Antipsychotic use and risk of hospitalization or death due to pneumonia in persons with and those without Alzheimer disease. *Chest* 2016; 150:1233–1241.
9. Cepaityte D, et al. Exploring a safety signal of antipsychotic-associated pneumonia: a pharmacovigilance-pharmacodynamic study. *Schizophr Bull* 2021; 47:672–681.
10. Chen YH, et al. Analysis of risk factors for hospital-acquired pneumonia in schizophrenia. *Front Psychiatry* 2024; 15:1414332.
11. Kuo CJ, et al. Second-generation antipsychotic medications and risk of pneumonia in schizophrenia. *Schizophr Bull* 2013; 39:648–657.
12. Yang SY, et al. Antipsychotic drugs, mood stabilizers, and risk of pneumonia in bipolar disorder: a nationwide case-control study. *J Clin Psychiatry* 2013; 74:e79–e86.
13. Trifiro G, et al. Association of community-acquired pneumonia with antipsychotic drug use in elderly patients: a nested case-control study. *Ann Intern Med* 2010; 152:418–440.
14. Kang N, et al. Association between initial clozapine titration and pneumonia risk among patients with schizophrenia in a Korean tertiary hospital. *Schizophr Res* 2024; 268:107–113.
15. Cheng SY, et al. Benzodiazepines and risk of pneumonia in schizophrenia: a nationwide case-control study. *Psychopharmacology (Berl)* 2018; 235:3329–3338.
16. Partanen JJ, et al. High burden of ileus and pneumonia in clozapine-treated individuals with schizophrenia: a Finnish 25-year follow-up register study. *Am J Psychiatry* 2024; 181:879–892.
17. Schoretsanitis G, et al. An update on the complex relationship between clozapine and pneumonia. *Expert Rev Clin Pharmacol* 2021; 14:145–149.
18. Villasante-Tezanos AG, et al. Pneumonia risk: approximately one-third is due to clozapine and two-thirds is due to treatment-resistant schizophrenia. *Acta Psychiatr Scand* 2020; 142:66–67.
19. Hung GC, et al. Antipsychotic reexposure and recurrent pneumonia in schizophrenia: a nested case-control study. *J Clin Psychiatry* 2016; 77:60–66.
20. Mace S, et al. Incident infection during the first year of treatment: a comparison of clozapine and paliperidone palmitate long-acting injection. *J Psychopharmacol* 2022; 36:232–237.
21. de Leon J, et al. Pneumonia may be more frequent and have more fatal outcomes with clozapine than with other second-generation antipsychotics. *World Psychiatry* 2020; 19:120–121.

Switching antipsychotics

Table 1.48 gives a summary of recommendations for switching antipsychotic medications because of poor tolerability.

Table 1.48 Switching antipsychotic medications because of poor tolerability – a summary of recommendations.

Adverse effect	Suggested medications	Alternative medications
Acute EPS[1–8] (dystonia, parkinsonism, bradykinesia)	Aripiprazole Brexpiprazole Cariprazine Olanzapine Quetiapine	Clozapine Lurasidone Ziprasidone
Akathisia[2,9,10]	Olanzapine Quetiapine	Clozapine Brexpiprazole
Dyslipidaemia[7,8,11–16]	Amisulpride Aripiprazole* Lurasidone Ziprasidone	Asenapine Brexpiprazole Cariprazine
Impaired glucose tolerance[7,8,15,17–21]	Amisulpride Aripiprazole* Lurasidone Ziprasidone	Brexpiprazole Cariprazine Haloperidol
Hyperprolactinaemia[7,8,15,22–29]	Aripiprazole* Brexpiprazole Cariprazine Lurasidone Quetiapine	Clozapine Olanzapine Ziprasidone
Postural hypotension[8,15,30]	Amisulpride Aripiprazole Brexpiprazole Cariprazine Lurasidone	Haloperidol Sulpiride Trifluoperazine
QT prolongation[27,31–38]	Brexpiprazole Cariprazine Lurasidone Paliperidone	Low-dose monotherapy of any drug not formally contraindicated in QT prolongation (with ECG monitoring)
Sedation[7,8,27]	Amisulpride Aripiprazole Brexpiprazole Cariprazine Risperidone Sulpiride	Haloperidol Trifuoperazine Ziprasidone
Sexual dysfunction[8,29,39–46]	Aripiprazole Brexpiprazole Cariprazine Lurasidone Quetiapine	Clozapine

(Continued)

Table 1.48 (*Continued*)

Adverse effect	Suggested medications	Alternative medications
Tardive dyskinesia[47–53]	Clozapine	Aripiprazole Olanzapine Quetiapine
Weight gain[16,36,38,54–65]	Amisulpride Aripiprazole* Brexpiprazole Cariprazine Lurasidone Ziprasidone	Asenapine Haloperidol Trifluoperazine

* There is evidence that both switching to and co-prescription of aripiprazole can be associated with reductions in body weight and plasma prolactin levels, better lipid profiles and a decrease in plasma glucose levels.[66–69]

Lumateperone and pimavanserin are not listed in the table because of their limited availability. Both drugs cause few or no EPSEs or akathisa, have no effect on prolactin or blood pressure and cause minimal weight gain and metabolic disturbance.[70,71] Pimvanserin prolongs QT,[72] whereas lumateperone seems to have no effect on the ECG.[73] To see the relative effect of all antipsychotics on these parameters, please see the Psymatik Treatment Optimizer.[74]

References

1. Stanniland C, et al. Tolerability of atypical antipsychotics. *Drug Saf* 2000; **22**:195–214.
2. Tarsy D, et al. Effects of newer antipsychotics on extrapyramidal function. *CNS Drugs* 2002; **16**:23–45.
3. Caroff SN, et al. Movement disorders associated with atypical antipsychotic drugs. *J Clin Psychiatry* 2002; 63 Suppl 4:12–19.
4. Lemmens P, et al. A combined analysis of double-blind studies with risperidone vs. placebo and other antipsychotic agents: factors associated with extrapyramidal symptoms. *Acta Psychiatr Scand* 1999; **99**:160–170.
5. Taylor DM. Aripiprazole: a review of its pharmacology and clinical use. *Int J Clin Pract* 2003; **57**:49–54.
6. Meltzer HY, et al. Lurasidone in the treatment of schizophrenia: a randomized, double-blind, placebo- and olanzapine-controlled study. *Am J Psychiatry* 2011; **168**:957–967.
7. Garnock-Jones KP. Cariprazine: a review in schizophrenia. *CNS Drugs* 2017; **31**:513–525.
8. Garnock-Jones KP. Brexpiprazole: a review in schizophrenia. *CNS Drugs* 2016; **30**:335–342.
9. Buckley PF. Efficacy of quetiapine for the treatment of schizophrenia: a combined analysis of three placebo-controlled trials. *Curr Med Res Opin* 2004; **20**:1357–1363.
10. Pringsheim T, et al. The assessment and treatment of antipsychotic-induced akathisia. *Can J Psychiatry* 2018; **63**:719–729.
11. Rettenbacher MA, et al. Early changes of plasma lipids during treatment with atypical antipsychotics. *Int Clin Psychopharmacol* 2006; **21**:369–372.
12. Ball MP, et al. Clozapine-induced hyperlipidemia resolved after switch to aripiprazole therapy. *Ann Pharmacother* 2005; **39**:1570–1572.
13. Chrzanowski WK, et al. Effectiveness of long-term aripiprazole therapy in patients with acutely relapsing or chronic, stable schizophrenia: a 52-week, open-label comparison with olanzapine. *Psychopharmacology (Berl)* 2006; **189**:259–266.
14. De Hert M, et al. A case series: evaluation of the metabolic safety of aripiprazole. *Schizophr Bull* 2007; **33**:823–830.
15. Citrome L, et al. Long-term safety and tolerability of lurasidone in schizophrenia: a 12-month, double-blind, active-controlled study. *Int Clin Psychopharmacol* 2012; **27**:165–176.
16. Kemp DE, et al. Weight change and metabolic effects of asenapine in patients with schizophrenia and bipolar disorder. *J Clin Psychiatry* 2014; **75**:238–245.
17. Haddad PM. Antipsychotics and diabetes: review of non-prospective data. *Br J Psychiatry Suppl* 2004; **47**:S80–S86.
18. Berry S, et al. Improvement of insulin indices after switch from olanzapine to risperidone. *Eur Neuropsychopharmacol* 2002; **12**:316.
19. Gianfrancesco FD, et al. Differential effects of risperidone, olanzapine, clozapine, and conventional antipsychotics on type 2 diabetes: findings from a large health plan database. *J Clin Psychiatry* 2002; **63**:920–930.
20. Mir S, et al. Atypical antipsychotics and hyperglycaemia. *Int Clin Psychopharmacol* 2001; **16**:63–74.

21. Cernea S, et al. Pharmacological management of glucose dysregulation in patients treated with second-generation antipsychotics. *Drugs* 2020; **80**:1763–1781.

22. Turrone P, et al. Elevation of prolactin levels by atypical antipsychotics. *Am J Psychiatry* 2002; **159**:133–135.

23. David SR, et al. The effects of olanzapine, risperidone, and haloperidol on plasma prolactin levels in patients with schizophrenia. *Clin Ther* 2000; **22**:1085–1096.

24. Hamner MB, et al. Hyperprolactinaemia in antipsychotic-treated patients: guidelines for avoidance and management. *CNS Drugs* 1998; **10**:209–222.

25. Trives MZ, et al. Effect of the addition of aripiprazole on hyperprolactinemia associated with risperidone long-acting injection. *J Clin Psychopharmacol* 2013; **33**:538–541.

26. Suzuki Y, et al. Differences in plasma prolactin levels in patients with schizophrenia treated on monotherapy with five second-generation antipsychotics. *Schizophr Res* 2013; **145**:116–119.

27. Leucht S, et al. Comparative efficacy and tolerability of 15 antipsychotic drugs in schizophrenia: a multiple-treatments meta-analysis. *Lancet* 2013; **382**:951–962.

28. Keks N, et al. Comparative tolerability of dopamine D2/3 receptor partial agonists for schizophrenia. *CNS Drugs* 2020; **34**:473–507.

29. Kelly DL, et al. Analysis of prolactin and sexual side effects in patients with schizophrenia who switched from paliperidone palmitate to aripiprazole lauroxil. *Psychiatry Res* 2021; **302**:114030.

30. Citrome L. Cariprazine: chemistry, pharmacodynamics, pharmacokinetics, and metabolism, clinical efficacy, safety, and tolerability. *Expert Opin Drug Metab Toxicol* 2013; **9**:193–206.

31. Glassman AH, et al. Antipsychotic drugs: prolonged QTc interval, torsade de pointes, and sudden death. *Am J Psychiatry* 2001; **158**:1774–1782.

32. Taylor D. Antipsychotics and QT prolongation. *Acta Psychiatr Scand* 2003; **107**:85–95.

33. Titier K, et al. Atypical antipsychotics: from potassium channels to torsade de pointes and sudden death. *Drug Saf* 2005; **28**:35–51.

34. Ray WA, et al. Atypical antipsychotic drugs and the risk of sudden cardiac death. *N Engl J Med* 2009; **360**:225–235.

35. Loebel A, et al. Efficacy and safety of lurasidone 80 mg/day and 160 mg/day in the treatment of schizophrenia: a randomized, double-blind, placebo- and active-controlled trial. *Schizophr Res* 2013; **145**:101–109.

36. Das S, et al. Brexpiprazole: so far so good. *Ther Adv Psychopharmacol* 2016; **6**:39–54.

37. Citrome L. Cariprazine for the treatment of schizophrenia: a review of this dopamine D3-preferring D3/D2 receptor partial agonist. *Clin Schizophr Relat Psychoses* 2016; **10**:109–119.

38. Huhn M, et al. Comparative efficacy and tolerability of 32 oral antipsychotics for the acute treatment of adults with multi-episode schizophrenia: a systematic review and network meta-analysis. *Lancet* 2019; **394**:939–951.

39. Byerly MJ, et al. An open-label trial of quetiapine for antipsychotic-induced sexual dysfunction. *J Sex Marital Ther* 2004; **30**:325–332.

40. Byerly MJ, et al. Sexual dysfunction associated with second-generation antipsychotics in outpatients with schizophrenia or schizoaffective disorder: an empirical evaluation of olanzapine, risperidone, and quetiapine. *Schizophr Res* 2006; **86**:244–250.

41. Montejo Gonzalez AL, et al. A 6-month prospective observational study on the effects of quetiapine on sexual functioning. *J Clin Psychopharmacol* 2005; **25**:533–538.

42. Dossenbach M, et al. Effects of atypical and typical antipsychotic treatments on sexual function in patients with schizophrenia: 12-month results from the Intercontinental Schizophrenia Outpatient Health Outcomes (IC-SOHO) study. *Eur Psychiatry* 2006; **21**:251–258.

43. Kerwin R, et al. A multicentre, randomized, naturalistic, open-label study between aripiprazole and standard of care in the management of community-treated schizophrenic patients Schizophrenia Trial of Aripiprazole: (STAR) study. *Eur Psychiatry* 2007; **22**:433–443.

44. Hanssens L, et al. The effect of antipsychotic medication on sexual function and serum prolactin levels in community-treated schizophrenic patients: results from the Schizophrenia Trial of Aripiprazole (STAR) study (NCT00237913). *BMC Psychiatry* 2008; **8**:95.

45. Loebel A, et al. Effectiveness of lurasidone vs. quetiapine XR for relapse prevention in schizophrenia: a 12-month, double-blind, noninferiority study. *Schizophr Res* 2013; **147**:95–102.

46. Silva C, et al. Managing antipsychotic-related sexual dysfunction in patients with schizophrenia. *Expert Rev Neurother* 2023; **23**:1147–1155.

47. Lieberman J, et al. Clozapine pharmacology and tardive dyskinesia. *Psychopharmacology (Berl)* 1989; **99** Suppl 1:S54–S59.

48. O'Brien J, et al. Marked improvement in tardive dyskinesia following treatment with olanzapine in an elderly subject. *Br J Psychiatry* 1998; **172**:186.

49. Sacchetti E, et al. Quetiapine, clozapine, and olanzapine in the treatment of tardive dyskinesia induced by first-generation antipsychotics: a 124-week case report. *Int Clin Psychopharmacol* 2003; **18**:357–359.

50. Witschy JK, et al. Improvement in tardive dyskinesia with aripiprazole use. *Can J Psychiatry* 2005; **50**:188.

51. Ricciardi L, et al. Treatment recommendations for tardive dyskinesia. *Can J Psychiatry* 2019; **64**:388–399.

52. Lee D, et al. Long-term response to clozapine and its clinical correlates in the treatment of tardive movement syndromes: a naturalistic observational study in patients with psychotic disorders. *J Clin Psychopharmacol* 2019; **39**:591–596.

53. Takeuchi H, et al. Pathophysiology, prognosis and treatment of tardive dyskinesia. *Ther Adv Psychopharmacol* 2022; **12**:20451253221117313.

54. Taylor DM, et al. Atypical antipsychotics and weight gain: a systematic review. *Acta Psychiatr Scand* 2000; **101**:416–432.

55. Allison D, et al. Antipsychotic-induced weight gain: a comprehensive research synthesis. *Am J Psychiatry* 1999; **156**:1686–1696.

56. Brecher M, et al. The long term effect of quetiapine (Seroquel™) monotherapy on weight in patients with schizophrenia. *Int J Psychiatry Clin Pract* 2000; **4**:287–291.

57. Casey DE, et al. Switching patients to aripiprazole from other antipsychotic agents: a multicenter randomized study. *Psychopharmacology (Berl)* 2003; **166**:391–399.

58. Newcomer JW, et al. A multicenter, randomized, double-blind study of the effects of aripiprazole in overweight subjects with schizophrenia or schizoaffective disorder switched from olanzapine. *J Clin Psychiatry* 2008; **69**:1046–1056.

59. McEvoy JP, et al. Effectiveness of lurasidone in patients with schizophrenia or schizoaffective disorder switched from other antipsychotics: a randomized, 6-week, open-label study. *J Clin Psychiatry* 2013; **74**:170–179.

60. McEvoy JP, et al. Effectiveness of paliperidone palmitate vs haloperidol decanoate for maintenance treatment of schizophrenia: a randomized clinical trial. *JAMA* 2014; **311**:1978–1987.

61. Nasrallah HA, et al. The safety and tolerability of cariprazine in long-term treatment of schizophrenia: a post hoc pooled analysis. *BMC Psychiatry* 2017; **17**:305.

62. Speyer H, et al. Reversibility of antipsychotic-induced weight gain: a systematic review and meta-analysis. *Front Endocrinol (Lausanne)* 2021; **12**:577919.

63. Siskind D, et al. Does switching antipsychotics ameliorate weight gain in patients with severe mental illness? A systematic review and meta-analysis. *Schizophr Bull* 2021; **47**:948–958.

64. Miura I, et al. Lurasidone for the treatment of schizophrenia: design, development, and place in therapy. *Drug Des Devel Ther* 2023; **17**:3023–3031.

65. Pillinger T, et al. Comparative effects of 18 antipsychotics on metabolic function in patients with schizophrenia, predictors of metabolic dysregulation, and association with psychopathology: a systematic review and network meta-analysis. *Lancet Psychiatry* 2020; **7**:64–77.

66. Shim JC, et al. Adjunctive treatment with a dopamine partial agonist, aripiprazole, for antipsychotic-induced hyperprolactinemia: a placebo-controlled trial. *Am J Psychiatry* 2007; **164**:1404–1410.

67. Fleischhacker WW, et al. Weight change on aripiprazole-clozapine combination in schizophrenic patients with weight gain and suboptimal response on clozapine: 16-week double-blind study. *Eur Psychiatry* 2008; **23** Suppl 2:S114–S115.

68. Henderson DC, et al. Aripiprazole added to overweight and obese olanzapine-treated schizophrenia patients. *J Clin Psychopharmacol* 2009; **29**:165–169.

69. Preda A, et al. A safety evaluation of aripiprazole in the treatment of schizophrenia. *Expert Opin Drug Saf* 2020; **19**:1529–1538.

70. Correll CU, et al. Safety and tolerability of lumateperone 42mg: an open-label antipsychotic switch study in outpatients with stable schizophrenia. *Schizophr Res* 2021; **228**:198–205.

71. Mathis MV, et al. The US Food and Drug Administration's perspective on the new antipsychotic pimavanserin. *J Clin Psychiatry* 2017; **78**:e668–e673.

72. Cruz MP. Pimavanserin (Nuplazid): a treatment for hallucinations and delusions associated with Parkinson's disease. *P T* 2017; **42**:368–371.

73. Greenwood J, et al. Lumateperone: a novel antipsychotic for schizophrenia. *Ann Pharmacother* 2021; **55**:98–104.

74. Pillinger T, et al. Antidepressant and antipsychotic side-effects and personalised prescribing: a systematic review and digital tool development. *Lancet Psychiatry* 2023; **10**:860–876.

Venous thromboembolism

Evidence of an association

Antipsychotic treatment was first linked to an increased risk of thromboembolism in 1965.[1] Over a 10-year observation period, 3.1% of 1,590 patients developed thromboembolism, of whom 9 (0.6%) died. However, the use of antipsychotic medication is a proxy for severe and enduring mental illness and so observed associations with antipsychotics may at least partly reflect inherent pathological processes in the conditions for which they are prescribed. To some extent, the relative contributions to the risk of thromboembolism of antipsychotic treatment and the conditions they treat remain to be clearly defined.

In a case–control study of nearly 30,000 patients,[2] risk of thromboembolism was greatly increased overall in people prescribed antipsychotics (odds ratio [OR] 7.1). The increased risk was driven by low-potency phenothiazines (thioridazine, chlorpromazine; OR 24.1) and was seen chiefly in the first few weeks of treatment. Absolute risk of VTE was low – it was seen in only 0.14% of patients (about 1 in every 714 people). A secondary analysis suggested no association with diagnosis, apparently ruling out an association with schizophrenia itself.

A later meta-analysis of seven case–control studies[3] confirmed an increased risk of thromboembolism with low-potency FGAs (OR 2.91) and suggested lower but significantly increased risks with all types of antipsychotics. Later, a meta-analysis of 17 studies[4] reported a small increased risk of thromboembolism with antipsychotics as a whole (OR 1.54) and with FGAs (OR 1.74) and SGAs (OR 2.07) as individual groups. Risk of thromboembolism clearly decreased with age. The authors suggested that the best that could be said was that antipsychotics probably increased the risk by about 50% but that residual confounding could not be discounted (i.e. other factors may have accounted for the effect seen).

Since this time, several more case–control studies have confirmed both the slightly increased risk of thromboembolism and the small risk overall.[5–7] One study reported a risk for older people taking antipsychotics as 43 per 10,000 patient years.[7] Other noteworthy findings were a substantially increased association with thromboembolism for prochlorperazine – a drug not always (or even often) prescribed for psychotic disorders[5] – and an increased risk linked to antipsychotic dosage (risk was quadrupled in high-dose patients).[6] An association with prochlorperazine prescribing had previously been suggested by a UK study.[8] These findings add weight to the theory that antipsychotic medication (and not only the conditions it treats) is responsible for the increased hazard of thromboembolism.

The highest risk of pathological blood clotting may be in the first 3 months or so of treatment.[9,10] Several meta-analyses have been published in recent years. The findings of two studies are presented in Table 1.49.

Table 1.49 Findings of meta-analyses of the risk of pathological blood clotting.

Reference	Number of studies included	Relative risk vs no use			Comments
		FGAs (OR)	SGAs (OR)	All anti-psychotics (OR)	
Di et al, 2021[9]	22	1.83 VTE/PE	1.75 VTE	1.53 VTE	Highest risk in younger patients (<60 years). Low-potency FGAs highest risk.
			3.79 PE	3.69 PE	
			2.06 VTE/PE	1.60 VTE/PE	
Liu et al, 2021[10]	28	1.47 VTE/PE	1.62 VTE/PE	1.55 VTE	New users of antipsychotics had higher risk than continuing patients. Risk slightly elevated with higher doses vs low doses. Similar effect sizes for FGA vs SGA.
				3.68 PE	
				2.01 VTE/PE	

FGA, first-generation antipsychotic; OR, odds ratio; PE, pulmonary embolism; SGA, second-generation antipsychotic; VTE, venous thromboembolism.

Mechanisms

Several mechanisms have been suggested to explain the association between antipsychotics and thromboembolism. These proposed mechanisms are outlined in Box 1.3.

Box 1.3 Proposed mechanisms for antipsychotic-associated venous thromboembolism[11–15]

Sedation*
Obesity*
Hyperprolactinaemia*
Elevated phospholipid antibodies
Elevated platelet aggregation**
Elevated plasma homocysteine
Elevated tissue plasminogen activator
Elevated platelet count

---

* Some evidence that these factors are not the mechanism for antipsychotic-induced thromboembolism.[16]
** In vitro data suggest radically different effects on platelet aggregation for different antipsychotics.[12]

Outcomes

Increased risk of thromboembolism is reflected in numerous published reports of elevated incidence of pulmonary embolism,[17] stroke[18] and myocardial infarction.[19] A 2022 study suggested that antipsychotics increase the risk of fatal thromboembolism (OR 6.68),[17] although, again, the absolute risk remains low.

Summary

Antipsychotics are almost certainly associated with a small but important increased risk of venous thromboembolism and associated hazards of pulmonary embolism, stroke and myocardial infarction. Risk appears to be greatest during the early part of treatment and in younger people and is probably dose-related.

Practice points

- Monitor closely all patients (but especially younger patients) starting antipsychotic treatment for signs of venous thromboembolism:
  - calf pain or swelling
  - sudden breathing difficulties
  - signs of myocardial infarction (chest pain, nausea, etc.)
  - signs of stroke (sudden unilateral weakness, etc.).
- Use the lowest therapeutic dose.
- Encourage good hydration and physical mobility.

References

1. Häfner H, et al. Thromboembolic complications in neuroleptic treatment. *Compr Psychiatry* 1965; 6:25–34.
2. Zornberg GL, et al. Antipsychotic drug use and risk of first-time idiopathic venous thromboembolism: a case-control study. *Lancet* 2000; 356:1219–1223.
3. Zhang R, et al. Antipsychotics and venous thromboembolism risk: a meta-analysis. *Pharmacopsychiatry* 2011; 44:183–188.
4. Barbui C, et al. Antipsychotic drug exposure and risk of venous thromboembolism: a systematic review and meta-analysis of observational studies. *Drug Saf* 2014; 37:79–90.
5. Ishiguro C, et al. Antipsychotic drugs and risk of idiopathic venous thromboembolism: a nested case–control study using the CPRD. *Pharmacoepidemiol Drug Saf* 2014; 23:1168–1175.
6. Wang MT, et al. Use of antipsychotics and risk of venous thromboembolism in postmenopausal women: a population-based nested case–control study. *Thromb Haemost* 2016; 115:1209–1219.
7. Letmaier M, et al. Venous thromboembolism during treatment with antipsychotics: results of a drug surveillance programme. *World J Biol Psychiatry* 2018; 19:175–186.
8. Parker C, et al. Antipsychotic drugs and risk of venous thromboembolism: nested case–control study. *BMJ* 2010; 341:c4245.
9. Di X, et al. Antipsychotic use and risk of venous thromboembolism: a meta-analysis. *Psychiatry Res* 2021; 296:113691.
10. Liu Y, et al. Current antipsychotic agent use and risk of venous thromboembolism and pulmonary embolism: a systematic review and meta-analysis of observational studies. *Ther Adv Psychopharmacol* 2021; 11:2045125320982720.
11. Hagg S, et al. Risk of venous thromboembolism due to antipsychotic drug therapy. *Expert Opin Drug Saf* 2009; 8:537–547.
12. Dietrich-Muszalska A, et al. The first- and second-generation antipsychotic drugs affect ADP-induced platelet aggregation. *World J Biol Psychiatry* 2010; 11:268–275.
13. Tromeur C, et al. Antipsychotic drugs and venous thromboembolism. *Thromb Res* 2012; 130 Suppl 1:S29–S31.
14. Zheng C, et al. Hypercoagulable state in patients with schizophrenia: different effects of acute and chronic antipsychotic medications. *Ther Adv Psychopharmacol* 2023; 13:20451253231200257.
15. Zhang Y, et al. New role of platelets in schizophrenia: predicting drug response. *Gen Psychiatr* 2024; 37:e101347.
16. Ferraris A, et al. Antipsychotic use among adult outpatients and venous thromboembolic disease: a retrospective cohort study. *J Clin Psychopharmacol* 2017; 37:405–411.
17. Manoubi SA, et al. Fatal pulmonary embolism in patients on antipsychotics: case series, systematic review and meta-analysis. *Asian J Psychiatr* 2022; 73:103105.
18. Zivkovic S, et al. Antipsychotic drug use and risk of stroke and myocardial infarction: a systematic review and meta-analysis. *BMC Psychiatry* 2019; 19:189.
19. Papola D, et al. Antipsychotic use and risk of life-threatening medical events: umbrella review of observational studies. *Acta Psychiatr Scand* 2019; 140:227–243.

REFRACTORY SCHIZOPHRENIA AND CLOZAPINE

Clozapine initiation schedules

Clozapine dosing regimen

Many of the adverse effects of clozapine are dose dependent and linked to speed of titration. Adverse effects tend to be more common and severe at the beginning of treatment. Titration is required to allow tolerance to develop to the pharmacological effects of clozapine. The degree to which tolerance ultimately develops is evidenced by the fact that standard maintenance doses would be fatal in a clozapine-naïve person.[1]

To minimise adverse effects and maximise the chances of successful titration, it is clearly important to start treatment at a low dose and to increase dosage slowly. There are many different opinions on exactly how slowly clozapine should be titrated.

Titration schedules should certainly be individualised. This is something everyone agrees on. There are, however, competing imperatives: the need to establish an effective dose quickly, the need to allow time for the patient to gain tolerance to adverse effects, the need to minimise the risk of myocarditis and the need to account for very different rates of clozapine metabolism.

The aim of dose titration is to attain a minimum therapeutic plasma concentration of approximately 350mcg/L over the course of about 3 weeks. The average dose at which this plasma concentration is achieved varies according to sex, smoking status and genetic variability in cytochrome enzyme activity, such as lower CYP1A2 activity for people of Asian or Native American heritage.[2] Achieving a therapeutic concentration over a period of 2–3 weeks will require very different titration schedules for people with different metabolic capacities.

A dose that will achieve a plasma concentration of 350mcg/L for an individual patient can be estimated by extrapolation of concentrations reported for different populations. This method groups patients according to sex and smoking status to produce predictive models.[3-5] Results are summarised in Table 1.50.

Table 1.50 Clozapine dose (in mg/day) with the highest likelihood of providing a plasma concentration of 350mcg/L, estimated by extrapolation of concentrations reported for different populations.

| Patient group | Rostami-Hodjegan[3] (ethnicity not described) | Schoretsanitis[4] (White Europeans) | Reeves[5] | | |
			Asian	White	Afro-Caribbean
Female non-smoker	265	236	175	225	250
Female smoker	435	357	25	300	325
Male non-smoker	325	256	225	275	300
Male smoker	525	368	250	375	400

Alternatively, an attempt can be made to include other factors into the predictive models, such as cytochrome enzyme metaboliser status, ancestry and concurrent medication to predict target dose and corresponding titration schedule.[2,6] The most accurate dose prediction is given by a genetic test that incorporates gene variant activity scores into a mathematical algorithm.[7] Results from this test can be used to select a titration schedule from the four provided here by choosing the schedule with the calculated target dose closest to the final dose in the schedule.

Clozapine should normally be started at a dose of 6.25mg – this is effectively a test dose for everyone. On subsequent days, the dose can be increased according to the selected schedule, provided the patient is tolerating clozapine. A flexible approach should be taken, altering schedules in response to adverse effects if needed (e.g. pausing titration, returning temporarily to a dose that was previously tolerated, or slowing the speed and/or reducing the magnitude of dose increases). Wherever possible, plasma concentration testing should be used in conjunction with adverse effect monitoring to inform dosing. Monitoring blood levels can help ensure that titration does not overshoot the target blood level. Use of point of care testing (delivering results within minutes) means this is possible without interrupting the dose regimen.[8,9] If results cannot be obtained rapidly then levels should be checked when titration is complete or if adverse effects cause problems during titration. The dose should be divided (usually into two daily doses) and, if sedation is a problem, the larger portion of the dose can be given at night.

The following tables outline four different starting regimens for clozapine. These are based on over 30 years' clinical experience and the published protocols described above. The concept behind the schedules is that every patient reaches, over 20 days, the lowest dose estimated to give a therapeutic blood concentration. The schedules should ensure that the rate of increase in clozapine plasma concentration is approximately the same for all people. This is important to note: the rate of *dose* increase may be very different in these schedules, but the rate of increase in *blood concentration* is the same. The reason we have moved away from providing a single titration schedule is because a single schedule has the opposite effect: the rate of change of plasma level will be vastly different for people with different metabolic capacities.

More rapid increases than those suggested here have been used, as has an extremely slow titration (the 'Laitman protocol' allows dose increases of only 25mg per week). Slower titration may be necessary where sedation or other dose-related side effects are severe, in the elderly, the very young, those who are physically compromised or those who have poorly tolerated other antipsychotics.

The target dose for patients with Asian ancestry should be around 65–75% of that given below. For older patients (>70 years), the target dose is around 50% of that given in the tables.

Faster titrations

The titration schedules listed here are aimed at maximising the likelihood of a successful titration – the aim is to establish the patient on a well-tolerated and therapeutic dose of clozapine. Faster titrations can be used and have been widely used in the past. The main risk with faster titrations, assuming the patient tolerates such a regimen, is myocarditis (see section on clozapine: serious cardiovascular adverse effects in this chapter). If tolerability is not assumed, the main risk is titration failure resulting from the patient's inability or unwillingness to tolerate rapid titration.

Female non-smoker – target dose 225mg/day.

Day	Morning dose (mg)	Evening dose (mg)	Total daily dose (mg)
1	–	6.25	6.25
2	–	6.25	6.25
3	6.25	6.25	12.5
4	6.25	12.5	18.75
5	12.5	12.5	25
6	12.5	12.5	25
7	25	25	50
8	25	25	50
9	25	50	75
10	25	50	75
11	50	50	100
12	50	50	100
13	50	75	125
14	50	75	125
15	75	75	150
16	75	75	150
17	75	100	175
18	75	100	175
19	100	100	200
20	100	100	225

Female smoker – target dose 300mg/day.

Day	Morning dose (mg)	Evening dose (mg)	Total daily dose (mg)
1	–	6.25	6.25
2	6.25	6.25	12.5
3	12.5	12.5	25
4	12.5	12.5	25
5	25	25	50
6	25	25	50
7	25	50	75
8	25	50	75
9	50	50	100
10	50	50	100
11	50	75	125

Day	Morning dose (mg)	Evening dose (mg)	Total daily dose (mg)
12	50	75	125
13	75	75	150
14	75	75	150
15	75	100	175
16	100	100	200
17	100	125	225
18	125	125	250
19	125	150	275
20	150	150	300

Male non-smoker – target dose 250mg/day.

Day	Morning dose (mg)	Evening dose (mg)	Total daily dose (mg)
1	–	6.25	6.25
2	–	6.25	6.25
3	6.25	6.25	12.5
4	6.25	12.5	18.75
5	12.5	12.5	25
6	12.5	12.5	25
7	25	25	50
8	25	25	50
9	25	50	75
10	25	50	75
11	50	50	100
12	50	50	100
13	50	75	125
14	50	75	125
15	75	75	150
16	75	75	150
17	75	100	175
18	100	100	200
19	100	125	225
20	125	125	250

Male smoker – target dose 375mg/day.

Day	Morning dose (mg)	Evening dose (mg)	Total daily dose (mg)
1	–	6.25	6.25
2	6.25	6.25	12.5
3	12.5	12.5	25
4	12.5	25	37.5
5	25	25	50
6	25	25	50
7	25	50	75
8	25	50	75
9	50	50	100
10	50	75	125
11	75	75	150
12	75	100	175
13	100	100	200
14	100	125	225
15	125	125	250
16	125	150	275
17	150	150	300
18	150	175	325
19	175	175	350
20	175	200	375

References

1. Stanworth D, et al. Clozapine: a dangerous drug in a clozapine-naive subject. *Forensic Sci Int* 2011; **214**:e23–e25.
2. Ruan CJ, et al. Is there a future for CYP1A2 pharmacogenetics in the optimal dosing of clozapine? *Pharmacogenomics* 2020; **21**:369–373.
3. Rostami-Hodjegan A, et al. Influence of dose, cigarette smoking, age, sex, and metabolic activity on plasma clozapine concentrations: a predictive model and nomograms to aid clozapine dose adjustment and to assess compliance in individual patients. *J Clin Psychopharmacol* 2004; **24**:70–78.
4. Schoretsanitis G, et al. European whites may need lower minimum therapeutic clozapine doses than those customarily proposed. *J Clin Psychopharmacol* 2021; **41**:140–147.
5. Reeves S, et al. A population pharmacokinetic model to guide clozapine dose selection, based on age, sex, ethnicity, body weight and smoking status. *Br J Clin Pharmacol* 2024; **90**:135–145.
6. de Leon J, et al. An international adult guideline for making clozapine titration safer by using six ancestry-based personalized dosing titrations, CRP, and clozapine levels. *Pharmacopsychiatry* 2022; **55**:73–86.
7. Taylor D, et al. Predicting clozapine dose required to achieve a therapeutic plasma concentration: a comparison of a population algorithm and three algorithms based on gene variant models. *J Psychopharmacol* 2023; **37**:1030–1039.
8. Atkins M, et al. Haematological point of care testing for clozapine monitoring. *J Psychiatr Res* 2023; **157**:66–71.
9. Atkins M, et al. Acceptability of point of care testing for antipsychotic medication levels in schizophrenia. *Psychiatry Research Communications* 2022; **2**:100070.

Intramuscular clozapine

Intramuscular clozapine is a short-term intervention for patients with a treatment-refractory psychotic disorder who refuse oral medication. It is always used with a view to converting to oral clozapine once treatment is established.[1] IM clozapine has also been used for patients who are unable to take oral medication because of physical illness.[2] Although evidence is relatively limited, observational data indicate that initiating treatment with IM clozapine does not adversely affect long-term adherence to oral treatment.[1,3] IM clozapine is similar to oral clozapine in respect to short-term safety and tolerability.[4,5] The IM preparation is unlicensed in the UK and many other countries, so adequate precautions should be taken and patient or carer consent obtained.

General recommendations for prescribing intramuscular clozapine in adults are summarised in Table 1.51.

Table 1.51 General recommendations for prescribing intramuscular clozapine.

Strength	25mg/mL
Maximum dose*	100mg (4mL) per site
Oral equivalent dose	The oral bioavailability of clozapine is about half that of the IM injection (e.g. 50mg IM injection daily = 100mg tablets/oral solution daily)
Site of administration†	The manufacturer states deep intramuscular gluteal injection
Maximum treatment length‡	Before administering each injection, the patient should be offered oral clozapine. Clozapine injection should be used for the shortest duration possible (maximum 2 weeks consecutively).
Dosing frequency	To minimise the number of injections, once daily dosing is preferred
Monitoring	After each administration, patients should be observed every 15 minutes for the first 2 hours to check for excess sedation. Routine clozapine monitoring also applies.

*For doses >100mg, the dose may be divided and administered into two sites.
†Case series data report administration via lateral thigh or deltoid – note that the injection is painful[3] and the maximum volume for the deltoid route is 2mL (50mg).
‡Case series data report use of intramuscular clozapine for up to 96 days.[3,4] Injection site reactions become common with longer-term treatment.
Note: Simultaneous injection of IM clozapine and parenteral benzodiazepines has not been studied. If IM benzodiapines are required leave at least **1 hour** between administration of IM clozapine and IM benzodiapines.

References

1. Casetta C, et al. A retrospective study of intramuscular clozapine prescription for treatment initiation and maintenance in treatment-resistant psychosis. *Br J Psychiatry* 2020; **217**:506–513.
2. Gee S, et al. Intramuscular clozapine in the acute medical hospital: experiences from a liaison psychiatry team. *SAGE Open Med Case Rep* 2021; 9:2050313x211004796.
3. Henry R, et al. Evaluation of the effectiveness and acceptability of intramuscular clozapine injection: illustrative case series. *BJPsych Bull* 2020:1–5.
4. Schulte PF, et al. Compulsory treatment with clozapine: a retrospective long-term cohort study. *Int J Law Psychiatry* 2007; 30:539-545.
5. Gee S, et al. Alternative routes of administration of clozapine. *CNS Drugs* 2022; 36:105–111.

Optimising clozapine treatment

Using clozapine alone

Target dose (dose is best adjusted according to patient tolerability and plasma level)	■ Average dose in UK is around 450mg/day[1] ■ Response usually seen in the range 150–900mg/day[2] ■ Lower doses required in the elderly, females, people of Asian or Native American heritage, non-smokers, and those prescribed certain enzyme inhibitors[3,4] ■ Genetic testing of CYP enzymes accurately predicts therapeutic dose[5]
Plasma levels	■ Most studies indicate that threshold for response is in the range 350–420mcg/L.[6,7] Threshold in some may be as high as 500mcg/L.[8] One study suggests a minority of patients only respond at levels between 500 and 1000mcg/L.[9] ■ In male smokers who cannot achieve therapeutic plasma levels, metabolic inhibitors (fluvoxamine[10,11] or cimetidine,[12] for example) can be co-prescribed, but extreme caution is required[13] ■ Importance of norclozapine levels not established. Clozapine/norclozapine ratio is not a reliable indicator of partial adherence nor of clozapine metabolism.[14]

Clozapine augmentation

Clozapine augmentation has become common practice because inadequate response to clozapine on its own is a frequent clinical event. The evidence base supporting augmentation strategies is fairly large but, despite more than 50 reviews and meta-analyses on the subject, it remains insufficient to allow the development of any algorithm or schedule of treatment options.[15] In practice, the result of clozapine augmentation is often disappointing and substantial changes in symptom severity are rarely observed. This clinical impression is supported by the equivocal results of many studies, which suggest a small effect size at best.

Network meta-analyses examining pharmacological augmentation options often draw conclusions based on only a few studies of dubious merit and may come to different conclusions.[16–19] That mirtazapine augmentation has the largest effect size (and the addition of memantine, the second largest) is something most recent systematic reviews agree on[17–19] although, with both strategies, the supporting evidence was, at best, weak. Meta-analyses of antipsychotic augmentation of clozapine suggest either no effect,[20] a small effect in long-term studies,[21] a very small effect overall[22] or small effects in specific symptom domains.[23] Few high-quality studies in this area exist – when only large, high-quality studies are included, most meta-analyses report no benefit to pharmacological augmentation.[24] This is consistent with imaging studies – investigations into dopaminergic activity in refractory schizophrenia suggest there is no overproduction of dopamine.[25,26] Dopamine antagonists are thus unlikely to be effective.

All augmentation attempts should be carefully monitored and, if no clear benefit is forthcoming, abandoned after 3–6 months. The addition of another drug to clozapine treatment might be expected to worsen overall adverse effect burden, so continuing ineffective treatment is only likely to be detrimental. In some cases, however, the addition of an augmenting agent may reduce the severity of some adverse effects (e.g. weight gain, dyslipidaemia – see below) or allow a reduction in clozapine dose. The addition of aripiprazole to clozapine may be particularly effective in reversing metabolic effects.[27,28] International consensus guidelines recommend (after optimising plasma levels) tailoring augmentation agent choice to residual symptoms, and adding amisulpride or aripiprazole for positive symptoms, antidepressants for negative symptoms, and mood stabilisers for suicidal ideation or aggression.[24] Recent data on cariprazine suggest particular benefit on negative symptoms unresponsive to clozapine.[29-32]

Table 1.52 shows suggested treatment options (in alphabetical order) where 3–6 months of optimised clozapine alone at maximum tolerated dose has provided unsatisfactory benefit.

Table 1.52 Suggested options for augmenting clozapine.

Option	Comment
Add amisulpride[33-40] (400–800mg/day)	Some evidence and experience suggest that amisulpride augmentation may be worthwhile. Five small RCTs (not all positive), the largest of which showed some benefit to positive symptoms and cognition, two of which found an increased adverse-effect burden, including cardiac adverse effects.[41,42] May allow clozapine dose reduction.[43]
Add antipsychotic long-acting injection[15,44-48]	Case series and observational studies suggest benefits to residual symptoms as well as number and length of hospitalisations. Appears to be well tolerated. Does not protect against relapse if clozapine is not taken.
Add aripiprazole[27,49-52] (15–30mg/day)	Very limited evidence of therapeutic benefit, although a meta-analysis suggests some effect.[53] Reduces weight and LDL cholesterol.[53] LAI has been used.[54,55]
Add cariprazine[56]	Three small case series and one pilot study suggest benefit, particularly for negative symptoms.[29-32] Two case reports of worsening psychosis.[57]
Add haloperidol[51,58,59] (2–3mg/day)	Modest evidence of benefit
Add lamotrigine[60-62] (25–300mg/day)	May be useful in partial or non-responders. May reduce alcohol consumption.[63] Several equivocal reports.[64-66] Some meta-analyses suggest moderate effect size[67] but this is largely influenced by two outlying studies.[68]
Add lurasidone[32,69]	One case series, one retrospective chart review and a case report. Appears to be well tolerated.
Add omega-3 triglycerides[70,71] (2–3g EPA daily)	Modest, and somewhat contested, evidence to support efficacy in non- or partial responders to antipsychotics, including clozapine
Add risperidone[72,73] (2–6mg/day)	Supported by an RCT but there are also two negative RCTs, each with minuscule response rates.[74,75] Small number of reports of increases in clozapine plasma levels. LAI also an option.[55,76] Paliperidone LAI has also been used.[48,55]
Add sodium valproate[68,77] (400–800mg/day)	Pooled effects from five Chinese RCTs[68] suggest improvement in positive symptoms, although studies are mostly of poor quality. Cochrane suggests benefit of adding valproate to antipsychotics in general, especially for excitement and aggression.[78]
Add sulpiride[79] (400mg/day)	May be useful in partial or non-responders. Supported by a single randomised trial in English and three in Chinese.[80] Overall effect modest.
Add topiramate[81-85] (50–300mg/day)	Two positive RCTs, two negative. Can worsen psychosis in some.[61,86] Two meta-analyses including hitherto unknown Chinese data[68,87] suggested robust effect on positive and negative symptoms, substantial weight loss but often with psychomotor slowing and attention difficulties.
Add ziprasidone[88-91] (80–160mg/day)	Supported by three RCTs.[91,92] Associated with QTc prolongation. Rarely used.

Note: consider the use of mood stabilisers and/or antidepressants especially where mood disturbance is thought to contribute to symptoms.[93-95]
EPA, eicosapentaenoic acid; LAI, long-acting injection; LDL, low-density lipoprotein.

Other options include adding pimozide, olanzapine or sertindole. None is recommended: pimozide and sertindole have important cardiac toxicity and the addition of olanzapine is poorly supported[96] and likely to exacerbate metabolic adverse effects. Studies of pimozide[97,98] and sertindole[99] have shown no effect. One small RCT supports the use of Ginkgo biloba[100] and another two support the use of memantine.[101,102] Another study suggests possible benefit of augmentation with acetyl-L-carnitine[103] and a case study reports good outcome with thyroxine.[104] A single RCT describes successful use of sodium benzoate.[105] Minocycline is probably not effective.[77,106] Glycine may be effective for positive symptoms, but studies are of poor quality.[107] A small case series (*n* = 6) found benefit from adding pimavanserin.[108] N-acetylcysteine is probably of no benefit.[109–111]

References

1. Taylor D, et al. A prescription survey of the use of atypical antipsychotics for hospital inpatients in the United Kingdom. *Int J Psychiatry Clin Pract* 2000; 4:41–46.

2. Murphy B, et al. Maintenance doses for clozapine. *Psychiatr Bull* 1998; 22:12–14.

3. Taylor D. Pharmacokinetic interactions involving clozapine. *Br J Psychiatry* 1997; 171:109–112.

4. Lane HY, et al. Effects of gender and age on plasma levels of clozapine and its metabolites: analyzed by critical statistics. *J Clin Psychiatry* 1999; 60:36–40.

5. Taylor D, et al. Predicting clozapine dose required to achieve a therapeutic plasma concentration: a comparison of a population algorithm and three algorithms based on gene variant models. *J Psychopharmacol* 2023; 37:1030–1039.

6. Taylor D, et al. The use of clozapine plasma levels in optimising therapy. *Psychiatr Bull* 1995; 19:753–755.

7. Spina E, et al. Relationship between plasma concentrations of clozapine and norclozapine and therapeutic response in patients with schizophrenia resistant to conventional neuroleptics. *Psychopharmacology* 2000; 148:83–89.

8. Perry PJ. Therapeutic drug monitoring of antipsychotics. *Psychopharmacol Bull* 2001; 35:19–29.

9. Kronig MH, et al. Plasma clozapine levels and clinical response for treatment-refractory schizophrenic patients. *Am J Psychiatry* 1995; 152:179–182.

10. Polcwiartek C, et al. The clinical potentials of adjunctive fluvoxamine to clozapine treatment: a systematic review. *Psychopharmacology (Berl)* 2016; 233:741–750.

11. Leising J, et al. High-dose fluvoxamine augmentation to clozapine in treatment-resistant psychosis. *J Clin Psychopharmacol* 2021; 41:186–190.

12. Watras M, et al. A therapeutic interaction between cimetidine and clozapine: case study and review of the literature. *Ther Adv Psychopharmacol* 2013; 3:294–297.

13. Gee S, et al. Optimising treatment of schizophrenia: the role of adjunctive fluvoxamine. *Psychopharmacology (Berl)* 2016; 233:739–740.

14. Schoretsanitis G, et al. A comprehensive review of the clinical utility of and a combined analysis of the clozapine/norclozapine ratio in therapeutic drug monitoring for adult patients. *Expert Rev Clin Pharmacol* 2019; 12:603–621.

15. Chakrabarti S. Clozapine resistant schizophrenia: newer avenues of management. *World J Psychiatry* 2021; 11:429–448.

16. Etchecopar-Etchart D, et al. Comprehensive evaluation of 45 augmentation drugs for schizophrenia: a network meta-analysis. *EClinicalMedicine* 2024; 69:102473.

17. Mishra A, et al. Augmentation strategies for partial or non-responders to clozapine in patients with schizophrenia: A Bayesian network meta-analysis of randomized controlled trials. *Clin Psychopharmacol Neurosci* 2024; 22:232–252.

18. Grover S, et al. Augmentation strategies for clozapine resistance: a systematic review and meta-analysis. *Acta Neuropsychiatr* 2023; 35:65–75.

19. Yeh TC, et al. Pharmacological and nonpharmacological augmentation treatments for clozapine-resistant schizophrenia: a systematic review and network meta-analysis with normalized entropy assessment. *Asian J Psychiatr* 2023; 79:103375.

20. Barbui C, et al. Does the addition of a second antipsychotic drug improve clozapine treatment? *Schizophr Bull* 2009; 35:458–468.

21. Paton C, et al. Augmentation with a second antipsychotic in patients with schizophrenia who partially respond to clozapine: a meta-analysis. *J Clin Psychopharmacol* 2007; 27:198–204.

22. Taylor D, et al. Augmentation of clozapine with a second antipsychotic: a meta analysis. *Acta Psychiatr Scand* 2012; 125:15–24.

23. Bartoli F, et al. Adjunctive second-generation antipsychotics for specific symptom domains of schizophrenia resistant to clozapine: a meta-analysis. *J Psychiatr Res* 2019; 108:24–33.

24. Wagner E, et al. Clozapine combination and augmentation strategies in patients with schizophrenia: recommendations from an international expert survey among the Treatment Response and Resistance in Psychosis (TRRIP) working group. *Schizophr Bull* 2020; 46:1459–1470.

25. Demjaha A, et al. Dopamine synthesis capacity in patients with treatment-resistant schizophrenia. *Am J Psychiatry* 2012; 169:1203–1210.

26. Demjaha A, et al. Antipsychotic treatment resistance in schizophrenia associated with elevated glutamate levels but normal dopamine function. *Biol Psychiatry* 2014; 75:e11–e13.

27. Fleischhacker WW, et al. Effects of adjunctive treatment with aripiprazole on body weight and clinical efficacy in schizophrenia patients treated with clozapine: a randomized, double-blind, placebo-controlled trial. *Int J Neuropsychopharmacol* 2010; 13:1115–1125.

28. Correll CU, et al. Selective effects of individual antipsychotic cotreatments on cardiometabolic and hormonal risk status: results from a systematic review and meta-analysis. *Schizophr Bull* 2013; 39 Suppl 1:S29–S30.

29. Oloyede E, et al. Clozapine augmentation with cariprazine for negative symptoms: a case series and literature review. *Ther Adv Psychopharmacol* 2022; **12**:20451253211066642.

30. Berardis D, et al. Cariprazine add-on in inadequate clozapine response: a report on two cases. *Clin Psychopharmacol Neurosci* 2021; **19**:174–178.

31. Pappa S, et al. Efficacy and safety of cariprazine augmentation in patients treated with clozapine: a pilot study. *Ther Adv Psychopharmacol* 2022; **12**:20451253221132087.

32. Siwek M, et al. Cariprazine augmentation of clozapine in schizophrenia—a retrospective chart review. *Front Pharmacol* 2024; **14**:1321112.

33. Matthiasson P, et al. Relationship between dopamine D2 receptor occupancy and clinical response in amisulpride augmentation of clozapine non-response. *J Psychopharmacol* 2001; **15**:S41.

34. Munro J, et al. Amisulpride augmentation of clozapine: an open non-randomized study in patients with schizophrenia partially responsive to clozapine. *Acta Psychiatr Scand* 2004; **110**:292–298.

35. Zink M, et al. Combination of clozapine and amisulpride in treatment-resistant schizophrenia: case reports and review of the literature. *Pharmacopsychiatry* 2004; **37**:26–31.

36. Ziegenbein M, et al. Augmentation of clozapine with amisulpride in patients with treatment-resistant schizophrenia: an open clinical study. *German J Psychiatry* 2006; **9**:17–21.

37. Kampf P, et al. Augmentation of clozapine with amisulpride: a promising therapeutic approach to refractory schizophrenic symptoms. *Pharmacopsychiatry* 2005; **38**:39–40.

38. Assion HJ, et al. Amisulpride augmentation in patients with schizophrenia partially responsive or unresponsive to clozapine: a randomized, double-blind, placebo-controlled trial. *Pharmacopsychiatry* 2008; **41**:24–28.

39. Poonia S, et al. Amisulpride augmentation of clozapine in clozapine-resistant schizophrenia: a case series. *Can J Hosp Pharm* 2022; **75**:234–238.

40. Zhu MH, et al. Amisulpride augmentation therapy improves cognitive performance and psychopathology in clozapine-resistant treatment-refractory schizophrenia: a 12-week randomized, double-blind, placebo-controlled trial. *Mil Med Res* 2022; **9**:59.

41. Barnes TR, et al. Amisulpride augmentation in clozapine-unresponsive schizophrenia (AMICUS): a double-blind, placebo-controlled, randomised trial of clinical effectiveness and cost-effectiveness. *Health Technol Assess* 2017; **21**:1–56.

42. Barnes TRE, et al. Amisulpride augmentation of clozapine for treatment-refractory schizophrenia: a double-blind, placebo-controlled trial. *Ther Adv Psychopharmacol* 2018; **8**:185–197.

43. Croissant B, et al. Reduction of side effects by combining clozapine with amisulpride: case report and short review of clozapine-induced hypersalivation – a case report. *Pharmacopsychiatry* 2005; **38**:38–39.

44. Oloyede E, et al. Clozapine augmentation with long-acting antipsychotic injections: a case series and systematic review. *Acta Psychiatr Scand* 2023; **148**:538–552.

45. Joo SW, et al. Comparative effectiveness of antipsychotic monotherapy and polypharmacy in schizophrenia patients with clozapine treatment: a nationwide, health insurance data-based study. *Eur Neuropsychopharmacol* 2022; **59**:36–44.

46. Nováková M, et al. Potential impact on mental health in patients with treatment-resistant schizophrenia: clozapine augmentation with long-acting parenteral antipsychotics: a case series. *Ceska Slov Farm* 2024; **72**:277–287.

47. Mukherjee H, et al. Predictors of functioning and clinical outcomes in inpatient with schizophrenia on clozapine augmented with antipsychotics. *Australas Psychiatry* 2022; **30**:100–104.

48. Bioque M, et al. Clozapine and paliperidone palmitate antipsychotic combination in treatment-resistant schizophrenia and other psychotic disorders: a retrospective 6-month mirror-image study. *Eur Psychiatry* 2020; **63**:e71.

49. Chang JS, et al. Aripiprazole augmentation in clozapine-treated patients with refractory schizophrenia: an 8-week, randomized, double-blind, placebo-controlled trial. *J Clin Psychiatry* 2008; **69**:720–731.

50. Muscatello MR, et al. Effect of aripiprazole augmentation of clozapine in schizophrenia: a double-blind, placebo-controlled study. *Schizophr Res* 2011; **127**:93–99.

51. Cipriani A, et al. Aripiprazole versus haloperidol in combination with clozapine for treatment-resistant schizophrenia: a 12-month, randomized, naturalistic trial. *J Clin Psychopharmacol* 2013; **33**:533–537.

52. Tiihonen J, et al. Association of antipsychotic polypharmacy vs monotherapy with psychiatric rehospitalization among adults with schizophrenia. *JAMA Psychiatry* 2019; **76**:499–507.

53. Srisurapanont M, et al. Efficacy and safety of aripiprazole augmentation of clozapine in schizophrenia: a systematic review and meta-analysis of randomized-controlled trials. *J Psychiatr Res* 2015; **62**:38–47.

54. Balcioglu YH, et al. One plus one sometimes equals more than two: long-acting injectable aripiprazole adjunction in clozapine-resistant schizophrenia. *Clin Neuropharmacol* 2020; **43**:166–168.

55. Grimminck R, et al. Combination of clozapine with long-acting injectable antipsychotics in treatment-resistant schizophrenia: preliminary evidence from health care utilization indices. *Prim Care Companion CNS Disord* 2020; **22**:19m02560.

56. Karoline RD, et al. Cariprazine augmentation in a patient with clozapine-resistant schizophrenia. *Ind Psychiatry J* 2023; **32**:S279–S280.

57. Weise J, et al. Add-on cariprazine in patients with long-term clozapine treatment and treatment resistant schizophrenia: two cases of psychotic deterioration and Pisa syndrome. *Clin Psychopharmacol Neurosci* 2022; **20**:398–401.

58. Rajarethinam R, et al. Augmentation of clozapine partial responders with conventional antipsychotics. *Schizophr Res* 2003; **60**:97–98.

59. Barbui C, et al. Aripiprazole versus haloperidol in combination with clozapine for treatment-resistant schizophrenia in routine clinical care: a randomized, controlled trial. *J Clin Psychopharmacol* 2011; **31**:266–273.

60. Dursun SM, et al. Clozapine plus lamotrigine in treatment-resistant schizophrenia. *Arch Gen Psychiatry* 1999; **56**:950.

61. Dursun SM, et al. Augmenting antipsychotic treatment with lamotrigine or topiramate in patients with treatment-resistant schizophrenia: a naturalistic case-series outcome study. *J Psychopharmacol* 2001; **15**:297–301.

62. Tiihonen J, et al. Lamotrigine in treatment-resistant schizophrenia: a randomized placebo-controlled crossover trial. *Biol Psychiatry* 2003; **54**:1241–1248.

63. Kalyoncu A, et al. Use of lamotrigine to augment clozapine in patients with resistant schizophrenia and comorbid alcohol dependence: a potent anti-craving effect? *J Psychopharmacol* 2005; **19**:301–305.

64. Goff DC, et al. Lamotrigine as add-on therapy in schizophrenia: results of 2 placebo-controlled trials. *J Clin Psychopharmacol* 2007; **27**:582–589.

65. Heck AH, et al. Addition of lamotrigine to clozapine in inpatients with chronic psychosis. *J Clin Psychiatry* 2005; **66**:1333.

66. Vayisoglu S, et al. Lamotrigine augmentation in patients with schizophrenia who show partial response to clozapine treatment. *Schizophr Res* 2013; **143**:207–214.

67. Tiihonen J, et al. The efficacy of lamotrigine in clozapine-resistant schizophrenia: a systematic review and meta-analysis. *Schizophr Res* 2009; **109**:10–14.

68. Zheng W, et al. Clozapine augmentation with antiepileptic drugs for treatment-resistant schizophrenia: a meta-analysis of randomized controlled trials. *J Clin Psychiatry* 2017; **78**:e498–e505.

69. Olivola M, et al. Lurasidone augmentation of clozapine in refractory schizophrenia: a case series. *J Clin Psychopharmacol* 2023; **43**:157–160.

70. Peet M, et al. Double-blind placebo controlled trial of N-3 polyunsaturated fatty acids as an adjunct to neuroleptics. *Schizophr Res* 1998; **29**:160–161.

71. Puri BK, et al. Sustained remission of positive and negative symptoms of schizophrenia following treatment with eicosapentaenoic acid. *Arch Gen Psychiatry* 1998; **55**:188–189.

72. Josiassen RC, et al. Clozapine augmented with risperidone in the treatment of schizophrenia: a randomized, double-blind, placebo-controlled trial. *Am J Psychiatry* 2005; **162**:130–136.

73. Raskin S, et al. Clozapine and risperidone: combination/augmentation treatment of refractory schizophrenia: a preliminary observation. *Acta Psychiatr Scand* 2000; **101**:334–336.

74. Anil Yagcioglu AE, et al. A double-blind controlled study of adjunctive treatment with risperidone in schizophrenic patients partially responsive to clozapine: efficacy and safety. *J Clin Psychiatry* 2005; **66**:63–72.

75. Honer WG, et al. Clozapine alone versus clozapine and risperidone with refractory schizophrenia. *N Engl J Med* 2006; **354**:472–482.

76. Se HK, et al. The combined use of risperidone long-acting injection and clozapine in patients with schizophrenia non-adherent to clozapine: a case series. *J Psychopharmacol* 2010; **24**:981–986.

77. Siskind DJ, et al. Augmentation strategies for clozapine refractory schizophrenia: a systematic review and meta-analysis. *Aust N Z J Psychiatry* 2018; **52**:751–767.

78. Wang Y, et al. Valproate for schizophrenia. *Cochrane Database Syst Rev* 2016; **11**:CD004028.

79. Shiloh R, et al. Sulpiride augmentation in people with schizophrenia partially responsive to clozapine. A double-blind, placebo-controlled study. *Br J Psychiatry* 1997; **171**:569–573.

80. Wang J, et al. Sulpiride augmentation for schizophrenia. *Schizophr Bull* 2010; **36**:229–230.

81. Tiihonen J, et al. Topiramate add-on in treatment-resistant schizophrenia: a randomized, double-blind, placebo-controlled, crossover trial. *J Clin Psychiatry* 2005; **66**:1012–1015.

82. Afshar H, et al. Topiramate add-on treatment in schizophrenia: a randomised, double-blind, placebo-controlled clinical trial. *J Psychopharmacol* 2009; **23**:157–162.

83. Muscatello MR, et al. Topiramate augmentation of clozapine in schizophrenia: a double-blind, placebo-controlled study. *J Psychopharmacol* 2011; **25**:667–674.

84. Hahn MK, et al. Topiramate augmentation in clozapine-treated patients with schizophrenia: clinical and metabolic effects. *J Clin Psychopharmacol* 2010; **30**:706–710.

85. Behdani F, et al. Effect of topiramate augmentation in chronic schizophrenia: a placebo-controlled trial. *Arch Iran Med* 2011; **14**:270–275.

86. Millson RC, et al. Topiramate for refractory schizophrenia. *Am J Psychiatry* 2002; **159**:675.

87. Zheng W, et al. Efficacy and safety of adjunctive topiramate for schizophrenia: a meta-analysis of randomized controlled trials. *Acta Psychiatr Scand* 2016; **134**:385–398.

88. Zink M, et al. Combination of ziprasidone and clozapine in treatment-resistant schizophrenia. *Hum Psychopharmacol* 2004; **19**:271–273.

89. Ziegenbein M, et al. Clozapine and ziprasidone: a useful combination in patients with treatment-resistant schizophrenia. *J Neuropsychiatry Clin Neurosci* 2006; **18**:246–247.

90. Ziegenbein M, et al. Combination of clozapine and ziprasidone in treatment-resistant schizophrenia: an open clinical study. *Clin Neuropharmacol* 2005; **28**:220–224.

91. Zink M, et al. Efficacy and tolerability of ziprasidone versus risperidone as augmentation in patients partially responsive to clozapine: a randomised controlled clinical trial. *J Psychopharmacol* 2009; **23**:305–314.

92. Muscatello MR, et al. Augmentation of clozapine with ziprasidone in refractory schizophrenia: a double-blind, placebo-controlled study. *J Clin Psychopharmacol* 2014; **34**:129–133.

93. Citrome L. Schizophrenia and valproate. *Psychopharmacol Bull* 2003; 37 Suppl 2:74–88.

94. Tranulis C, et al. Somatic augmentation strategies in clozapine resistance: what facts? *Clin Neuropharmacol* 2006; **29**:34–44.

95. Suzuki T, et al. Augmentation of atypical antipsychotics with valproic acid. An open-label study for most difficult patients with schizophrenia. *Hum Psychopharmacol* 2009; **24**:628–638.

96. Gupta S, et al. Olanzapine augmentation of clozapine. *Ann Clin Psychiatry* 1998; **10**:113–115.

97. Friedman JI, et al. Pimozide augmentation of clozapine inpatients with schizophrenia and schizoaffective disorder unresponsive to clozapine monotherapy. *Neuropsychopharmacology* 2011; **36**:1289–1295.

98. Gunduz-Bruce H, et al. Efficacy of pimozide augmentation for clozapine partial responders with schizophrenia. *Schizophr Res* 2013; **143**:344–347.

99. Nielsen J, et al. Augmenting clozapine with sertindole: a double-blind, randomized, placebo-controlled study. *J Clin Psychopharmacol* 2012; **32**:173–178.

100. Doruk A, et al. A placebo-controlled study of extract of ginkgo biloba added to clozapine in patients with treatment-resistant schizophrenia. *Int Clin Psychopharmacol* 2008; **23**:223–227.

101. de Lucena D, et al. Improvement of negative and positive symptoms in treatment-refractory schizophrenia: a double-blind, randomized, placebo-controlled trial with memantine as add-on therapy to clozapine. *J Clin Psychiatry* 2009; **70**:1416–1423.

102. Veerman SR, et al. Adjunctive memantine in clozapine-treated refractory schizophrenia: an open-label 1-year extension study. *Psychol Med* 2017; **47**:363–375.

103. Bruno A, et al. Acetyl-L-carnitine augmentation of clozapine in partial-responder schizophrenia: a 12-week, open-label uncontrolled preliminary study. *Clin Neuropharmacol* 2016; **39**:277–280.

104. Seddigh R, et al. Levothyroxine augmentation in clozapine resistant schizophrenia: a case report and review. *Case Rep Psychiatry* 2015; **2015**:678040.

105. Lin CH, et al. Sodium benzoate, a D-amino acid oxidase inhibitor, added to clozapine for the treatment of schizophrenia: a randomized, double-blind, placebo-controlled trial. *Biol Psychiatry* 2018; **84**:422–432.

106. Kelly DL, et al. Adjunctive minocycline in clozapine-treated schizophrenia patients with persistent symptoms. *J Clin Psychopharmacol* 2015; **35**:374–381.

107. Correll CU, et al. Efficacy of 42 pharmacologic cotreatment strategies added to antipsychotic monotherapy in schizophrenia: systematic overview and quality appraisal of the meta-analytic evidence. *JAMA Psychiatry* 2017; **74**:675–684.

108. Nasrallah HA, et al. Successful treatment of clozapine-nonresponsive refractory hallucinations and delusions with pimavanserin, a serotonin 5HT-2A receptor inverse agonist. *Schizophr Res* 2019; **208**:217–220.

109. Yolland CO, et al. Meta-analysis of randomised controlled trials with N-acetylcysteine in the treatment of schizophrenia. *Aust N Z J Psychiatry* 2020; **54**:453–466.

110. Neill E, et al. N-acetylcysteine (NAC) in schizophrenia resistant to clozapine: a double-blind, randomized, placebo-controlled trial targeting negative symptoms. *Schizophr Bull* 2022; **48**:1263–1272.

111. Andrade C. Antipsychotic augmentation with N-acetylcysteine for patients with schizophrenia. *J Clin Psychiatry* 2022; **83**:22f14664.

Alternatives to clozapine

Clozapine has the strongest evidence for efficacy for schizophrenia that has proved refractory to adequate trials of standard antipsychotic medication. About three-quarters of these patients are treatment resistant from the onset of illness.[1] Where treatment resistance has been established, clozapine treatment should not be delayed or withheld.[2,3] The practice of using successive antipsychotic medications (or the latest) instead of clozapine is widespread but not supported by any research. Where clozapine cannot be used because of toxicity or patient refusal or unwillingness to comply with the mandatory monitoring tests, other drugs or drug combinations may be tried (Table 1.53). In practice, outcome is usually disappointing and long-term data on efficacy and safety are generally lacking.

Available data do not allow any distinction between treatment regimens to be drawn, particularly choice of antipsychotic medication,[4,5] but it seems wise to use single drugs before trying polypharmacy options. Olanzapine is perhaps the most often used antipsychotic monotherapy, usually in doses above the licensed range. If this fails, then the addition of a second antipsychotic (amisulpride, for example) is a possible next step, although the risk–benefit balance of combined antipsychotic medication regimens remains unclear.[6] In people who have stopped clozapine, clozapine reintroduction and olanzapine are the only effective treatments.[7] Among unconventional agents, minocycline and ondansetron have the advantage of low toxicity and good tolerability. With advances in the understanding of the neurobiology of TRS, non-dopaminergic treatments are an area of active research. Glutamatergic drugs such as evenamide[8] (although bitopertin is inactive),[9] $5HT_{2A}$ inverse agonists,[10] trace amine-associated receptor 1 (TAAR1) agonists and muscarinic receptor agonists such as xanomeline may hold some promise.[11]

Many of the treatments listed in Table 1.53 are somewhat experimental and some of the compounds difficult to obtain (e.g. glycine, D-serine, sarcosine, etc.). Before using any of the regimens outlined, readers should consult the primary literature cited. Particular care should be taken to inform patients where prescribing is off-label and to ensure that they understand the potential adverse effects of the more experimental treatments.

Table 1.53 Alternatives to clozapine (treatments are listed in alphabetical order – no preference is implied by position in table).

Treatment	Comments
Allopurinol 300–600mg/day (+ antipsychotic)[12–15]	Increases adenosinergic transmission, which may reduce effects of dopamine. Three positive RCTs.[12,13,15]
Amisulpride[16] (up to 1200mg/day)	Single, small open study
Antipsychotic polypharmacy	Various antipsychotics in combination have been used. Data are limited, mainly in the form of case reports, open and naturalistic studies. RCTs show no advantage for polypharmacy over monotherapy.[17]
Aripiprazole[18,19] (15–30mg/day)	Single RCT indicating moderate effect in patients resistant to risperidone or olanzapine (+ others). Higher doses (60mg/day) have been used.[20]

Table 1.53 (*Continued*)

Treatment	Comments
Asenapine (+ antipsychotic)[21]	A post-hoc analysis of a phase III extension study showed that add-on asenapine may be beneficial in some patients with TRS
Blonanserin (+ antipsychotic)[22]	Atypical antipsychotic licensed in Japan and Korea. A retrospective cohort study involving 69 patients showed improved PANSS scores with add-on blonanserin[23]
Cariprazine (+ antipsychotic)[24–26]	Case reports of successful use of cariprazine as monotherapy or as add-on
CBT[27]	Non-drug therapies should always be considered[28]
Deep brain stimulation	Effectiveness of nucleus accumbens and subgenual anterior cingulate cortex targeted deep brain stimulation demonstrated in 4 of 7 patients with TRS[29]
D–Alanine 100mg/kg/day (+ antipsychotic)[30]	Glycine (NMDA) agonist. One positive RCT.
D–Serine 30mg/kg/day (+ olanzapine)[31]	Glycine (NMDA) agonist. One positive RCT.
D–Serine up to 3g as monotherapy[32]	Improved negative symptoms in one RCT, but inferior to high-dose olanzapine for treatment of positive symptoms
ECT[33]	Open studies suggest moderate effect, as does a retrospective study.[34] Often reserved for last-line treatment in practice but can be successful in the short[35] and long[36] term. A 2024 RCT was negative.[37]
Estradiol 100–200mcg transdermal/day (+ antipsychotic)[38]	Oestrogens may be psychoprotective and/or antipsychotic in women of child-bearing age especially on positive symptoms, at higher doses.[39] Contraindications include being post-menopausal, history of VTE, stroke, breast cancer, migraine with aura. Unopposed estradiol increases risk of endometrial hyperplasia and malignancy – consult an endocrinologist. Evidence in men is lacking.
Famotidine 100mg bd + antipsychotic[40]	H_2 antagonist. One short (4-week) RCT suggested some benefit in overall PANSS and CGI scale scores.
Ginkgo biloba (+ antipsychotic)[41]	A systematic review of studies published in China showed improvements in total and negative symptoms
Lurasidone up to 240mg/day[42] (+ vortioxetine)	One RCT comparing standard with high-dose lurasidone produced comparable improvements in TRS when given up to 24 weeks.[43] Appears to be well tolerated. The addition of vortioxetine to lurasidone was effective in a small case series.[44]
Memantine 20mg/day (+ antipsychotic)[45–47]	Memantine is an NMDA antagonist. Two RCTs. The larger of the two (*n* = 138) was negative. In the smaller (*n* = 21), memantine improved positive and negative symptoms when added to clozapine. In another study in non-refractory schizophrenia, memantine improved negative symptoms when added to risperidone.
Minocycline 200mg/day (+ antipsychotic)[48,49]	May be anti-inflammatory and neuroprotective. One open study (*n* = 22) and one RCT (*n* = 54) suggest good effect on negative and cognitive symptoms. Also, one RCT (*n* = 52) of augmentation of clozapine showed improvement in some symptoms.[50] RCT evidence of neuroprotective effect in early psychosis.[51]
Mirtazapine 30mg/day (+ antipsychotic)[52–54]	Two RCTs, one negative,[53] one positive.[52] Effect seems to be mainly on positive symptoms.
N–acetylcysteine 2g/day (+ antipsychotic)[40]	One RCT suggests small benefits in negative symptoms and rates of akathisia. Another RCT showed benefits in chronic schizophrenia.[55] Case study of successful use of 600mg/day.[56] A large RCT failed to show any benefit when added to clozapine.[57]

(Continued)

Table 1.53 (Continued)

Treatment	Comments
Olanzapine[58-63] 5–25mg/day	Supported by some well-conducted trials but clinical experience disappointing. Some patients show moderate response.
Olanzapine 30–60mg/day	High-dose olanzapine is more effective than other non-clozapine antipsychotics.[64] High-dose olanzapine is not atypical[65] and can be poorly tolerated[66] with gross metabolic changes.[67]
Olanzapine + glycine[68] (0.8g/kg/day)	Small, double-blind crossover trial suggests clinically relevant improvement in negative symptoms
Olanzapine + lamotrigine[66,69] (up to 400mg/day)	Reports contradictory and rather unconvincing. Reasonable theoretical basis for adding lamotrigine which is usually well tolerated.
Ondansetron 8mg/day (+ antipsychotic)	A systematic review of RCTs showed improvements in negative symptoms and general psychopathology. Effect on cognition inconclusive.[70]
Paliperidone LAI	Improvement in endocrine and hepatic parameters and lower antipsychotic exposure in a small number of patients switched from clozapine to paliperidone 3-monthly. No data on clinical outcomes.[71]
Pimavanserin (+ antipsychotics)	Clinical improvement with pimavanserin alone or as adjunct to clozapine or other antipsychotics in 10 patients, 6 of whom had failed to respond to clozapine[72]
Propentofylline + risperidone[73] (900mg + 6mg/day)	One RCT suggests some activity against positive symptoms
Quetiapine[74-77]	Very limited evidence and clinical experience not encouraging. High doses (>1200mg/day) have been used but are no more effective.[78]
Raloxifene 60–120mg/day (+ antipsychotic)[39]	Selective oestrogen receptor modulator. May offer benefits of estradiol without long-term risks, but sexual dysfunction and weight gain may occur.[39] Data in non-treatment resistance are rather conflicting, with two overlapping positive trials[79,80] and one negative trial.[81] One positive RCT in refractory psychosis in women.[82] Evidence in men is lacking.
Riluzole 100mg/day + risperidone up to 6mg/day[83]	Glutamate modulating agent. One RCT demonstrated improvement in negative symptoms.
Risperidone[84-86] 4–8mg/day	Doubtful efficacy in true TRS but some supporting evidence. May also be tried in combination with glycine[68] or lamotrigine[60] or indeed with other SGAs.[87]
Risperidone LAI 50/100mg 2/52[88]	One RCT showing good response for both doses in refractory schizophrenia. Plasma levels for 100mg dose similar to 6–8mg/day oral risperidone.
Ritanserin + risperidone (12mg + 6mg/day)	$5HT_{2A/2C}$ antagonist. One RCT suggests small effect on negative symptoms.
Sarcosine (2g/day)[89,90] (+ antipsychotic)	Enhances glycine action. Supported by two RCTs. Benefits may be in patients with non-TRS.[91]
Sertindole[92] (12–24mg/day)	One large RCT (conducted in 1996–68 but published in 2011) suggested good effect and equivalence to risperidone. Around half of subjects responded. Another RCT[93] showed no effect at all when added to clozapine. Little experience in practice.
Topiramate (300mg/day) (+ antipsychotic)[94]	Small effect shown in single RCT. Induces weight loss. Cognitive adverse effects likely. Teratogenic.

(Continued)

Table 1.53 (*Continued*)

Treatment	Comments
Transcranial magnetic stimulation[95,96]	Conflicting results
Ursodeoxycholic acid[97]	Single case reports
Valproate[98]	Doubtful effect but may be useful where there is a clear affective component
Yokukansan (+ antipsychotic)[99]	Japanese herbal medicine, partial agonist at D_2 and $5HT_{1A}$, antagonist at $5HT_{2A}$ and glutamate receptors. Potential small benefit in excitement/hostility symptoms. Another 12-week double-blind placebo-controlled RCT showed modest symptomatic improvement.[100]
Ziprasidone 80–160mg/day[101–103]	Two good RCTs. One[103] suggests superior efficacy to chlorpromazine in refractory schizophrenia, the other[101] suggests equivalence to clozapine in subjects with treatment intolerance/resistance. Disappointing results in practice. Supratherapeutic doses offer no advantage.[104]
Zotepine 300mg/day+[105]	One study showed that some patients do not deteriorate when switched from clozapine to zotepine

CGI, Clinical Global Impression; LAI, long-acting injection; NMDA, N-methyl-D-aspartate; PANSS, Positive and Negative Syndrome Scale; TRS, treatment-resistant schizophrenia; VTE, venous thromboembolism.

Summary of alternatives to clozapine

Table 1.54 provides a summary of alternatives to clozapine in refractory schizophrenia.

Table 1.54 Summary of alternatives to clozapine in refractory schizophrenia.

Treatment	Examples	Comments	Strength of evidence
Monotherapy using non-clozapine antipsychotics in standard or high doses	Aripiprazole 15–30mg daily Olanzapine 25–60mg daily	Evidence of efficacy for any antipsychotic other than clozapine in refractory schizophrenia is controversial. Some data suggest efficacy for olanzapine above licensed doses but at the risk of metabolic adverse effects.	Weak +
Non-clozapine antipsychotic polypharmacy	Amisulpride + olanzapine, quetiapine + amisulpride, aripiprazole + olanzapine, and various other combinations	Polypharmacy is common in clinical practice. Evidence from controlled studies limited but open studies and real-world data suggest some effectiveness. Burden of adverse effects is increased.	Weak +
Anti-inflammatory agents as adjuncts to antipsychotics	N-acetylcysteine, NSAIDs, minocycline, oestrogens, aspirin, omega-3 fatty acids	A heterogeneous group of medicinal agents with inflammatory properties have been tried as adjuncts. Possible benefits in negative and cognitive symptoms but sample sizes have been small.	Very weak ±
NMDA receptor modulators as adjuncts	Memantine, glycine, D-serine and sarcosine	Rarely used in clinical practice. May have some benefit in negative symptoms.	Very weak ±

(Continued)

Table 1.54 *(Continued)*

Treatment	Examples	Comments	Strength of evidence
Physical treatments	ECT, rTMS, tDCS, DBS	Best evidence for ECT as adjunct to clozapine. Others still largely experimental.	Modest ++
Adjunctive antidepressants	Mirtazapine, vortioxetine, SSRIs	Limited data available suggest small benefits in negative and cognitive symptoms.	Weak +
Adjunctive anticonvulsants	Lamotrigine, topiramate, sodium valproate, carbamazepine	Data difficult to interpret	Weak +
Psychological therapies	CBT	Conflicting findings, effects small.	Very weak ±

CBT, cognitive behavioural therapy; DBS, deep brain stimulation; NSAIDs, non-steroidal anti-inflammatory drugs; rTMS, repetitive transcranial magnetic stimulation; tDCS, transcranial direct current stimulation.

References

1. Millgate E, et al. Neuropsychological differences between treatment-resistant and treatment-responsive schizophrenia: a meta-analysis. *Psychol Med* 2022; **52**:1–13.
2. Yoshimura B, et al. The critical treatment window of clozapine in treatment-resistant schizophrenia: secondary analysis of an observational study. *Psychiatry Res* 2017; **250**:65–70.
3. Shah P, et al. The impact of delay in clozapine initiation on treatment outcomes in patients with treatment-resistant schizophrenia: a systematic review. *Psychiatry Res* 2018; **268**:114–122.
4. Molins C, et al. Response to antipsychotic drugs in treatment-resistant schizophrenia: conclusions based on systematic review. *Schizophr Res* 2016; **178**:64–67.
5. Samara MT, et al. Efficacy, acceptability, and tolerability of antipsychotics in treatment-resistant schizophrenia: a network meta-analysis. *JAMA Psychiatry* 2016; **73**:199–210.
6. Galling B, et al. Antipsychotic augmentation vs. monotherapy in schizophrenia: systematic review, meta-analysis and meta-regression analysis. *World Psychiatry* 2017; **16**:77–89.
7. Luykx JJ, et al. In the aftermath of clozapine discontinuation: comparative effectiveness and safety of antipsychotics in patients with schizophrenia who discontinue clozapine. *Br J Psychiatry* 2020; **217**:498–505.
8. Anand R, et al. Phase 2 results indicate evenamide, a selective modulator of glutamate release, is associated with clinically important long-term efficacy when added to an antipsychotic in patients with treatment-resistant schizophrenia. *Int J Neuropsychopharmacol* 2023; **26**:523–528.
9. Bugarski-Kirola D, et al. Efficacy and safety of adjunctive bitopertin versus placebo in patients with suboptimally controlled symptoms of schizophrenia treated with antipsychotics: results from three phase 3, randomised, double-blind, parallel-group, placebo-controlled, multicentre studies in the SearchLyte clinical trial programme. *Lancet Psychiatry* 2016; **3**:1115–1128.
10. Garay RP, et al. Potential serotonergic agents for the treatment of schizophrenia. *Expert Opin Investig Drugs* 2016; **25**:159–170.
11. de Bartolomeis A, et al. Update on novel antipsychotics and pharmacological strategies for treatment-resistant schizophrenia. *Expert Opin Pharmacother* 2022; **23**:2035–2052.
12. Akhondzadeh S, et al. Beneficial antipsychotic effects of allopurinol as add-on therapy for schizophrenia: a double blind, randomized and placebo controlled trial. *Prog Neuropsychopharmacol Biol Psychiatry* 2005; **29**:253–259.
13. Brunstein MG, et al. A clinical trial of adjuvant allopurinol therapy for moderately refractory schizophrenia. *J Clin Psychiatry* 2005; **66**:213–219.
14. Buie LW, et al. Allopurinol as adjuvant therapy in poorly responsive or treatment refractory schizophrenia. *Ann Pharmacother* 2006; **40**:2200–2204.
15. Dickerson FB, et al. A double-blind trial of adjunctive allopurinol for schizophrenia. *Schizophr Res* 2009; **109**:66–69.
16. Kontaxakis VP, et al. Switching to amisulpride monotherapy for treatment-resistant schizophrenia. *Eur Psychiatry* 2006; **21**:214–217.
17. Lochmann van Bennekom MWH, et al. Efficacy and tolerability of antipsychotic polypharmacy for schizophrenia spectrum disorders: a systematic review and meta-analysis of individual patient data. *Schizophr Res* 2024; **272**:1–11.
18. Kane JM, et al. Aripiprazole for treatment-resistant schizophrenia: results of a multicenter, randomized, double-blind, comparison study versus perphenazine. *J Clin Psychiatry* 2007; **68**:213–223.
19. Hsu WY, et al. Aripiprazole in treatment-refractory schizophrenia. *J Psychiatr Pract* 2009; **15**:221–226.

20. Crossman AM, et al. Tolerability of high-dose aripiprazole in treatment-refractory schizophrenic patients. *J Clin Psychiatry* 2006; **67**:1158–1159.

21. Kishi T, et al. Asenapine add-on treatment for schizophrenia adults who received antipsychotics: a 52-week, open-label study. *Psychiatry Clin Neurosci* 2023; **77**:365–366.

22. Tachibana M, et al. Effectiveness of blonanserin for patients with drug treatment-resistant schizophrenia and dopamine supersensitivity: a retrospective analysis. *Asian J Psychiatr* 2016; **24**:28–32.

23. Tang S, et al. Efficacy of add-on blonanserin in treatment-resistant schizophrenia therapy: a retrospective cohort study. *Asian J Psychiatr* 2024; **91**:103867.

24. Aubel T. Cariprazine: patients with treatment-resistant schizophrenia. *Neuropsychiatr Dis Treat* 2021; **17**:2327–2332.

25. Montgomery A, et al. Cariprazine: an alternative treatment for clozapine-resistant schizophrenia? *Clin Psychopharmacol Neurosci* 2023; **21**:202–206.

26. Boydstun C, et al. Cariprazine: an augmentation strategy for treatment-resistant schizophrenia with pro-cognitive and anti-hostility effects. *Int Clin Psychopharmacol* 2023; **38**:361–366.

27. Valmaggia LR, et al. Cognitive-behavioural therapy for refractory psychotic symptoms of schizophrenia resistant to atypical antipsychotic medication: randomised controlled trial. *Br J Psychiatry* 2005; **186**:324–330.

28. Polese D, et al. Treatment-resistant to antipsychotics: a resistance to everything? Psychotherapy in treatment-resistant schizophrenia and nonaffective psychosis: a 25-year systematic review and exploratory meta-analysis. *Front Psychiatry* 2019; **10**:210.

29. Corripio I, et al. Deep brain stimulation in treatment resistant schizophrenia: a pilot randomized cross-over clinical trial. *EBioMedicine* 2020; **51**:102568.

30. Tsai GE, et al. D-alanine added to antipsychotics for the treatment of schizophrenia. *Biol Psychiatry* 2006; **59**:230–234.

31. Heresco-Levy U, et al. D-serine efficacy as add-on pharmacotherapy to risperidone and olanzapine for treatment-refractory schizophrenia. *Biol Psychiatry* 2005; **57**:577–585.

32. Ermilov M, et al. A pilot double-blind comparison of d-serine and high-dose olanzapine in treatment-resistant patients with schizophrenia. *Schizophr Res* 2013; **150**:604–605.

33. Zheng W, et al. Electroconvulsive therapy added to non-clozapine antipsychotic medication for treatment resistant schizophrenia: meta-analysis of randomized controlled trials. *PLoS One* 2016; **11**:e0156510.

34. Grover S, et al. Effectiveness of electroconvulsive therapy in patients with treatment resistant schizophrenia: a retrospective study. *Psychiatry Res* 2017; **249**:349–353.

35. Chanpattana W, et al. Electroconvulsive therapy in treatment-resistant schizophrenia: prediction of response and the nature of symptomatic improvement. *J ECT* 2010; **26**:289–298.

36. Ravanic DB, et al. Long-term efficacy of electroconvulsive therapy combined with different antipsychotic drugs in previously resistant schizophrenia. *Psychiatr Danub* 2009; **21**:179–186.

37. Melzer-Ribeiro DL, et al. Randomized, double-blind, sham-controlled trial to evaluate the efficacy and tolerability of electroconvulsive therapy in patients with clozapine-resistant schizophrenia. *Schizophr Res* 2024; **268**:252–260.

38. Kulkarni J, et al. Estradiol for treatment-resistant schizophrenia: a large-scale randomized-controlled trial in women of child-bearing age. *Mol Psychiatry* 2015; **20**:695–702.

39. Li Z, et al. Estradiol and raloxifene as adjunctive treatment for women with schizophrenia: a meta-analysis of randomized, double-blind, placebo-controlled trials. *Acta Psychiatr Scand* 2023; **147**:360–372.

40. Meskanen K, et al. A randomized clinical trial of histamine 2 receptor antagonism in treatment-resistant schizophrenia. *J Clin Psychopharmacol* 2013; **33**:472–478.

41. Chen X, et al. Efficacy and safety of extract of Ginkgo biloba as an adjunct therapy in chronic schizophrenia: a systematic review of randomized, double-blind, placebo-controlled studies with meta-analysis. *Psychiatry Res* 2015; **228**:121–127.

42. Meltzer H, et al. W162 lurasidone is an effective treatment for treatment resistant schizophrenia. *Neuropsychopharmacology* 2015; **40** Suppl 1:S546.

43. Meltzer HY, et al. Lurasidone improves psychopathology and cognition in treatment-resistant schizophrenia. *J Clin Psychopharmacol* 2020; **40**:240–249.

44. Lowe P, et al. When the drugs don't work: treatment-resistant schizophrenia, serotonin and serendipity. *Ther Adv Psychopharmacol* 2018; **8**:63–70.

45. Lieberman JA, et al. A randomized, placebo-controlled study of memantine as adjunctive treatment in patients with schizophrenia. *Neuropsychopharmacology* 2009; **34**:1322–1329.

46. de Lucena D, et al. Improvement of negative and positive symptoms in treatment-refractory schizophrenia: a double-blind, randomized, placebo-controlled trial with memantine as add-on therapy to clozapine. *J Clin Psychiatry* 2009; **70**:1416–1423.

47. Rezaei F, et al. Memantine add-on to risperidone for treatment of negative symptoms in patients with stable schizophrenia: randomized, double-blind, placebo-controlled study. *J Clin Psychopharmacol* 2013; **33**:336–342.

48. Levkovitz Y, et al. A double-blind, randomized study of minocycline for the treatment of negative and cognitive symptoms in early-phase schizophrenia. *J Clin Psychiatry* 2010; **71**:138–149.

49. Miyaoka T, et al. Minocycline as adjunctive therapy for schizophrenia: an open-label study. *Clin Neuropharmacol* 2008; **31**:287–292.

50. Kelly DL, et al. Adjunctive minocycline in clozapine-treated schizophrenia patients with persistent symptoms. *J Clin Psychopharmacol* 2015; **35**:374–381.

51. Chaudhry IB, et al. Minocycline benefits negative symptoms in early schizophrenia: a randomised double-blind placebo-controlled clinical trial in patients on standard treatment. *J Psychopharmacol* 2012; **26**:1185–1193.

52. Joffe G, et al. Add-on mirtazapine enhances antipsychotic effect of first generation antipsychotics in schizophrenia: a double-blind, randomized, placebo-controlled trial. *Schizophr Res* 2009; **108**:245–251.

53. Berk M, et al. Mirtazapine add-on therapy in the treatment of schizophrenia with atypical antipsychotics: a double-blind, randomised, placebo-controlled clinical trial. *Hum Psychopharmacol* 2009; 24:233–238.

54. Delle CR, et al. Add-on mirtazapine enhances effects on cognition in schizophrenic patients under stabilized treatment with clozapine. *Exp Clin Psychopharmacol* 2007; 15:563–568.

55. Sepehrmanesh Z, et al. Therapeutic effect of adjunctive N-acetyl cysteine (NAC) on symptoms of chronic schizophrenia: a double-blind, randomized clinical trial. *Prog Neuropsychopharmacol Biol Psychiatry* 2017; 82:289–296.

56. Bulut M, et al. Beneficial effects of N-acetylcysteine in treatment resistant schizophrenia. *World J Biol Psychiatry* 2009; 10:626–628.

57. Neill E, et al. N-acetylcysteine (NAC) in schizophrenia resistant to clozapine: a double-blind, randomized, placebo-controlled trial targeting negative symptoms. *Schizophr Bull* 2022; 48:1263–1272.

58. Breier A, et al. Comparative efficacy of olanzapine and haloperidol for patients with treatment-resistant schizophrenia. *Biol Psychiatry* 1999; 45:403–411.

59. Conley RR, et al. Olanzapine compared with chlorpromazine in treatment-resistant schizophrenia. *Am J Psychiatry* 1998; 155:914–920.

60. Sanders RD, et al. An open trial of olanzapine in patients with treatment-refractory psychoses. *J Clin Psychopharmacol* 1999; 19:62–66.

61. Taylor D, et al. Olanzapine in practice: a prospective naturalistic study. *Psychiatr Bull* 1999; 23:178–180.

62. Bitter I, et al. Olanzapine versus clozapine in treatment-resistant or treatment-intolerant schizophrenia. *Prog Neuropsychopharmacol Biol Psychiatry* 2004; 28:173–180.

63. Tollefson GD, et al. Double-blind comparison of olanzapine versus clozapine in schizophrenic patients clinically eligible for treatment with clozapine. *Biol Psychiatry* 2001; 49:52–63.

64. Gannon L, et al. High-dose olanzapine in treatment-resistant schizophrenia: a systematic review. *Ther Adv Psychopharmacol* 2023; 13:20451253231168788.

65. Bronson BD, et al. Adverse effects of high-dose olanzapine in treatment-refractory schizophrenia. *J Clin Psychopharmacol* 2000; 20:382–384.

66. Kelly DL, et al. Adverse effects and laboratory parameters of high-dose olanzapine vs. clozapine in treatment-resistant schizophrenia. *Ann Clin Psychiatry* 2003; 15:181–186.

67. Meltzer HY, et al. A randomized, double-blind comparison of clozapine and high-dose olanzapine in treatment-resistant patients with schizophrenia. *J Clin Psychiatry* 2008; 69:274–285.

68. Heresco-Levy U, et al. High-dose glycine added to olanzapine and risperidone for the treatment of schizophrenia. *Biol Psychiatry* 2004; 55:165–171.

69. Dursun SM, et al. Augmenting antipsychotic treatment with lamotrigine or topiramate in patients with treatment-resistant schizophrenia: a naturalistic case-series outcome study. *J Psychopharmacol* 2001; 15:297–301.

70. Zheng W, et al. Adjunctive ondansetron for schizophrenia: a systematic review and meta-analysis of randomized controlled trials. *J Psychiatr Res* 2019; 113:27–33.

71. Martínez-Andrés JA, et al. Switching from clozapine to paliperidone palmitate-3-monthly improved obesity, hyperglycemia and dyslipidemia lowering antipsychotic dose equivalents in a treatment-resistant schizophrenia cohort. *Int Clin Psychopharmacol* 2020; 35:163–169.

72. Nasrallah HA, et al. Successful treatment of clozapine-nonresponsive refractory hallucinations and delusions with pimavanserin, a serotonin 5HT-2A receptor inverse agonist. *Schizophr Res* 2019; 208:217–220.

73. Salimi S, et al. A placebo controlled study of the propentofylline added to risperidone in chronic schizophrenia. *Prog Neuropsychopharmacol Biol Psychiatry* 2008; 32:726–732.

74. Reznik I, et al. Long-term efficacy and safety of quetiapine in treatment-refractory schizophrenia: a case report. *Int J Psychiatry Clin Pract* 2000; 4:77–80.

75. De Nayer A, et al. Efficacy and tolerability of quetiapine in patients with schizophrenia switched from other antipsychotics. *Int J Psychiatry Clin Pract* 2003; 7:59–66.

76. Larmo I, et al. Efficacy and tolerability of quetiapine in patients with schizophrenia who switched from haloperidol, olanzapine or risperidone. *Hum Psychopharmacol* 2005; 20:573–581.

77. Boggs DL, et al. Quetiapine at high doses for the treatment of refractory schizophrenia. *Schizophr Res* 2008; 101:347–348.

78. Lindenmayer JP, et al. A randomized, double-blind, parallel-group, fixed-dose, clinical trial of quetiapine at 600 versus 1200 mg/d for patients with treatment-resistant schizophrenia or schizoaffective disorder. *J Clin Psychopharmacol* 2011; 31:160–168.

79. Usall J, et al. Raloxifene as an adjunctive treatment for postmenopausal women with schizophrenia: a 24-week double-blind, randomized, parallel, placebo-controlled trial. *Schizophr Bull* 2016; 42:309–317.

80. Usall J, et al. Raloxifene as an adjunctive treatment for postmenopausal women with schizophrenia: a double-blind, randomized, placebo-controlled trial. *J Clin Psychiatry* 2011; 72:1552–1557.

81. Weiser M, et al. Raloxifene plus antipsychotics versus placebo plus antipsychotics in severely ill decompensated postmenopausal women with schizophrenia or schizoaffective disorder: a randomized controlled trial. *J Clin Psychiatry* 2017; 78:e758–e765.

82. Kulkarni J, et al. Effect of adjunctive raloxifene therapy on severity of refractory schizophrenia in women: a randomized clinical trial. *JAMA Psychiatry* 2016; 73:947–954.

83. Farokhnia M, et al. A double-blind, placebo controlled, randomized trial of riluzole as an adjunct to risperidone for treatment of negative symptoms in patients with chronic schizophrenia. *Psychopharmacology (Berl)* 2014; 231:533–542.

84. Breier AF, et al. Clozapine and risperidone in chronic schizophrenia: effects on symptoms, parkinsonian side effects, and neuroendocrine response. *Am J Psychiatry* 1999; 156:294–298.

85. Bondolfi G, et al. Risperidone versus clozapine in treatment-resistant chronic schizophrenia: a randomized double-blind study. The Risperidone Study Group. *Am J Psychiatry* 1998; 155:499–504.

86. Conley RR, et al. Risperidone, quetiapine, and fluphenazine in the treatment of patients with therapy-refractory schizophrenia. *Clin Neuropharmacol* 2005; **28**:163–168.

87. Lerner V, et al. Combination of 'atypical' antipsychotic medication in the management of treatment-resistant schizophrenia and schizoaffective disorder. *Prog Neuropsychopharmacol Biol Psychiatry* 2004; **28**:89–98.

88. Meltzer HY, et al. A six month randomized controlled trial of long acting injectable risperidone 50 and 100mg in treatment resistant schizophrenia. *Schizophr Res* 2014; **154**:14–22.

89. Lane HY, et al. Sarcosine or D-serine add-on treatment for acute exacerbation of schizophrenia: a randomized, double-blind, placebo-controlled study. *Arch Gen Psychiatry* 2005; **62**:1196–1204.

90. Tsai G, et al. Glycine transporter I inhibitor, N-methylglycine (sarcosine), added to antipsychotics for the treatment of schizophrenia. *Biol Psychiatry* 2004; **55**:452–456.

91. Marchi M, et al. Sarcosine as an add-on treatment to antipsychotic medication for people with schizophrenia: a systematic review and meta-analysis of randomized controlled trials. *Expert Opin Drug Metab Toxicol* 2021; **17**:483–493.

92. Kane JM, et al. A double-blind, randomized study comparing the efficacy and safety of sertindole and risperidone in patients with treatment-resistant schizophrenia. *J Clin Psychiatry* 2011; **72**:194–204.

93. Nielsen J, et al. Augmenting clozapine with sertindole: a double-blind, randomized, placebo-controlled study. *J Clin Psychopharmacol* 2012; **32**:173–178.

94. Tiihonen J, et al. Topiramate add-on in treatment-resistant schizophrenia: a randomized, double-blind, placebo-controlled, crossover trial. *J Clin Psychiatry* 2005; **66**:1012–1015.

95. Lorentzen R, et al. The efficacy of transcranial magnetic stimulation (TMS) for negative symptoms in schizophrenia: a systematic review and meta-analysis. *Schizophrenia (Heidelb)* 2022; **8**:35.

96. Guttesen LL, et al. Repetitive transcranial magnetic stimulation and transcranial direct current stimulation for auditory hallucinations in schizophrenia: systematic review and meta-analysis. *J Psychiatr Res* 2021; **143**:163–175.

97. Khosravi M. Ursodeoxycholic acid augmentation in treatment-refractory schizophrenia: a case report. *J Med Case Rep* 2020; **14**:137.

98. Basan A, et al. Valproate as an adjunct to antipsychotics for schizophrenia: a systematic review of randomized trials. *Schizophr Res* 2004; **70**:33–37.

99. Miyaoka T, et al. Efficacy and safety of yokukansan in treatment-resistant schizophrenia: a randomized, multicenter, double-blind, placebo-controlled trial. *Evid Based Complement Alternat Med* 2015; **2015**:201592.

100. Horiguchi J, et al. A multicenter, double-blind, randomized, controlled study of patients with treatment-resistant schizophrenia treated with yokukansan for 12 weeks. *PCN Rep* 2023; **2**:e155.

101. Sacchetti E, et al. Ziprasidone vs clozapine in schizophrenia patients refractory to multiple antipsychotic treatments: the MOZART study. *Schizophr Res* 2009; **110**:80–89.

102. Loebel AD, et al. Ziprasidone in treatment-resistant schizophrenia: a 52-week, open-label continuation study. *J Clin Psychiatry* 2007; **68**:1333–1338.

103. Kane JM, et al. Efficacy and tolerability of ziprasidone in patients with treatment-resistant schizophrenia. *Int Clin Psychopharmacol* 2006; **21**:21–28.

104. Goff DC, et al. High-dose oral ziprasidone versus conventional dosing in schizophrenia patients with residual symptoms: the ZEBRAS study. *J Clin Psychopharmacol* 2013; **33**:485–490.

105. Lin CC, et al. Switching from clozapine to zotepine in patients with schizophrenia: a 12-week prospective, randomized, rater blind, and parallel study. *J Clin Psychopharmacol* 2013; **33**:211–214.

Restarting clozapine after a break in treatment

Interruptions in clozapine treatment are commonplace.[1] Patients prescribed clozapine should be advised to contact their prescriber if they stop taking the medication. This is partly because, if clozapine treatment is stopped abruptly, there is a need to monitor for symptoms of cholinergic rebound, such as nausea, vomiting, diarrhoea, sweating and headache,[2,3] as well as the possible emergence of dystonias, dyskinesias and catatonic symptoms.[4–7] If the last dose of clozapine was more than 48 hours ago, it should be re-introduced using a suitable dosage titration schedule.[8]

Depending on the time since clozapine was last taken, it may be feasible to re-titrate the dose to a therapeutic level more rapidly than is recommended for initial treatment. While there is some evidence to suggest that faster titrations may be safe in those patients naïve to clozapine[2] as well as those re-starting it,[3] there is the risk that such schedules could lead to drug discontinuation because of adverse effects. The risk of myocarditis, pneumonia, agranulocytosis and seizures, as well as the occurrence of adverse effects such as tachycardia and orthostatic hypotension, are probably reduced with slower initial titration schedules,[8,9] and the same may apply to restarting. More cautious dosage titration will be appropriate for certain patients, such as those who are elderly, people with Parkinson's disease and outpatients starting clozapine who are uncertain about the potential benefits of the medication.[10–12] Furthermore, there is some evidence that tolerance to the effects of clozapine is lost after only a few weeks,[13,14] so people who have missed clozapine treatment for more than a week should probably restart clozapine as if it were being initiated for the first time.

Restarting clozapine after gaps of various lengths should take account of the need to regain antipsychotic activity with clozapine while ensuring safety during titration. Examples of slow, fast and ultra-fast titration schedules are available[15] but it is probably best to individualise titration according to patient tolerability. A key element is flexibility: the dosage schedule prescribed for a patient will depend upon how previous dosages within the schedule are tolerated. In broad terms, this means starting with 12.5mg and increasing to 25mg for the next dose if the initial dose caused no adverse effects, such as sedation, increased heart rate or lowered blood pressure. If the 25mg dose is well tolerated then 50mg can be given for the next dose, and so on. In other words, the dose is doubled each time until the target daily dosage is reached (which is likely to be the dose the patient was taking before the break in medication).

Twice daily dosing allows for a faster rate of titration than once daily dosing. Some centres use three times daily dosing, which allows for even quicker titration but may increase the risk of adverse effects caused by accumulation. For example, if a patient were to receive 12.5mg, 25mg and 50mg doses of clozapine on the first day of re-titration, then each successive dose would be added to what remains of previous doses. Thus, the effect of the 50mg dose in this schedule would be greater than a single (i.e. stat) dose of 50mg. The same phenomenon occurs with twice daily dosing, but with 12 hours between doses the contribution of the prior dose is more limited.

Where a given dose in the titration schedule is not tolerated, the next dose should usually be delayed and not increased (or possibly decreased). Therefore, it is usually better to prescribe a series of single 'stat' doses, one at a time, rather than write up a complete schedule of doses that may then have to be changed.

References

1. John AP, et al. Rates and reasons for clozapine treatment interruptions: impact of the frequency of hematologic monitoring and cardiac adverse events. *J Clin Psychopharmacol* 2023; **43**:233–238.

2. Shiovitz TM, et al. Cholinergic rebound and rapid onset psychosis following abrupt clozapine withdrawal. *Schizophr Bull* 1996; **22**:591–595.

3. Galova A, et al. A case report of cholinergic rebound syndrome following abrupt low-dose clozapine discontinuation in a patient with type I bipolar affective disorder. *BMC Psychiatry* 2019; **19**:73.

4. Ahmed S, et al. Clozapine withdrawal-emergent dystonias and dyskinesias: a case series. *J Clin Psychiatry* 1998; **59**:472–477.

5. Shrivastava M, et al. Relapse of tardive dyskinesia due to reduction in clozapine dose. *Indian J Pharmacol* 2009; **41**:201–202.

6. Boazak M, et al. Catatonia due to clozapine withdrawal: a case report and literature review. *Psychosomatics* 2019; **60**:421–427.

7. Lander M, et al. Review of withdrawal catatonia: what does this reveal about clozapine? *Transl Psychiatry* 2018; **8**:139.

8. Flanagan RJ, et al. Clozapine in the treatment of refractory schizophrenia: a practical guide for healthcare professionals. *Br Med Bull* 2020; **135**:73–89.

9. de Leon J, et al. An international adult guideline for making clozapine titration safer by using six ancestry-based personalized dosing titrations, CRP, and clozapine levels. *Pharmacopsychiatry* 2022; **55**:73–86.

10. Gee SH, et al. Patient attitudes to clozapine initiation. *Int Clin Psychopharmacol* 2017; **32**:337–342.

11. Schulte PF, et al. Comment on 'effectiveness and safety of rapid clozapine titration in schizophrenia'. *Acta Psychiatr Scand* 2014; **130**:69–70.

12. Correll CU, et al. A guideline and checklist for initiating and managing clozapine treatment in patients with treatment-resistant schizophrenia. *CNS Drugs* 2022; **36**:659–679.

13. National Association of Boards of Pharmacy (NABP). ISMP: Restarting clozapine too rapidly can cause severe cardiovascular effects. 2022 (last accessed February 2025); https://nabp.pharmacy/news/blog/regulatory_news/ismp-restarting-clozapine-too-rapidly-can-cause-severe-cardiovascular-effects.

14. Shastay A. Caution when restarting clozapine. *Home Healthc Now* 2022; **40**:54–55.

15. Rubio JM, et al. How and when to use clozapine. *Acta Psychiatr Scand* 2020; **141**:178–189.

Initiation of clozapine in the community

While in-patient initiation remains the main method of starting clozapine, community initiation is fairly common in many countries. The likelihood of successful titration is similar for both methods (about 60%),[1] indicating that any risks associated with reduced monitoring frequency are offset by the relatively slower initiation schedules employed in the community.

Relative contraindications to community initiation

- History of uncontrolled seizures, significant cardiac disease, unstable diabetes, paralytic ileus, significant blood dyscrasia, neuroleptic malignant syndrome or other disorder that increases the risk of serious adverse effects (initiation with close monitoring in hospital may still be possible).
- Previous severe adverse effects on titration of clozapine or other antipsychotics.
- Unreliable or chaotic lifestyle that may affect adherence to the medication or the monitoring regimen.
- Significant abuse of alcohol or other drugs likely to increase the risk of adverse effects (e.g. cocaine).

Essential criteria for suitability for community initiation

- Is the patient likely to be adherent with oral medication and to monitoring requirements or is there support for these?
- Has the patient understood the need for regular physical monitoring and blood tests?
- Has the patient understood the possible adverse effects and what to do about them (particularly the rare but serious ones)?
- Is the patient readily contactable (e.g. in the event of a result that needs follow-up)?
- Is it possible for the patient to be seen weekly or more often during the early titration phase?
- Is the patient able to collect medication every week or can medication be delivered to their home?
- Is the patient likely to be able to seek help out-of-hours if they experience potentially serious adverse effects (e.g. indicators of myocarditis or infection such as fever, malaise, chest pain)?
- Has the patient understood what needs to be done in the event of an abnormal blood test (e.g. daily monitoring of FBC until normalisation in the case of a RED result)?

Initial work-up

To screen for risk factors and provide a baseline:

- Physical examination, FBC (see below), liver function tests, urea and electrolytes, lipids, glucose/HbA_{1c}. Also, C-reactive protein (CRP), CK, troponin, beta-natriuretic peptide (BEN; as baseline for further tests).
- ECG: particularly to screen for evidence of past myocardial infarction or ventricular abnormality.

- Echocardiogram if clinically indicated.
- Consider work-up for BEN where baseline neutrophil counts are low (see section on clozapine, neutropenia and lithium in this chapter). Genetic testing for BEN is also available (see section on clozapine: genetic testing for clozapine treatment in this chapter).

Mandatory blood monitoring and registration

- Register with the relevant monitoring service.
- Perform baseline blood tests (white cell and differential counts) before starting clozapine.
- Further blood testing continues weekly for the first 18 weeks and then every 2 weeks for the remainder of the year. After that, the blood monitoring is usually done monthly.
- Inform the patient's GP.

Dosing

Starting clozapine in the community requires a slow and flexible titration schedule. Prior antipsychotics should be slowly discontinued during the titration phase (depots can usually be stopped at the start of titration). Clozapine can, of course, cause marked postural hypotension. The initial monitoring is partly aimed at detecting and managing this, partly at ensuring sedative effects are manageable.

There are two approaches to giving the first dose of clozapine in the community. One is to give the first dose in the morning in clinic and then monitor the patient for postural hypotension for at least 1 hour. If the dose is well tolerated, the patient is then allowed home with a dose to take before going to bed. The second approach involves giving the patient the first dose to take immediately before bed, thereby avoiding the need for close physical monitoring immediately after administration. All initiations should take place early in the week (e.g. on a Monday) so that adequate staffing and monitoring are assured. Unless there are significant concerns regarding tolerability (e.g. postural hypotension), the 1-hour monitoring for morning doses in clinic can be omitted.

Previous guidelines[2,3] recommended physical observations on 5 days/week during weeks one and two of community clozapine initiations, followed by 3 days/week for weeks three and four. A 2023 study showed that this frequency can be reduced when using a slower titration schedule.[4] Example titration schedules for these two protocols are shown in Table 1.55. These dose increase schedules are examples and may need to be adjusted based on tolerability and target dose. Additional reviews may be necessary to manage adverse effects. The low-frequency monitoring (on the left of the table) is suitable for most patients and even lower frequency of monitoring may be feasible in some patients (e.g. re-titration of clozapine where the patient tolerated it well previously). The standard monitoring frequency is recommended for patients who may be more sensitive to adverse effects (e.g. female non-smokers) or who may struggle to adhere to frequent dose adjustments. The two protocols do not differ in the frequency of physical monitoring after week four (i.e. both reduce to once a week). As with in-patient initiation, estimating the target dose for each individual patient is recommended before starting clozapine. This gives some idea of the likely duration of the titration schedule. Genetic testing appears to be the most accurate method of predicting an effective dose.[5]

Table 1.55 Suggested titration regimens for initiation of clozapine in the community.

Day	Low-frequency monitoring	Morning dose (mg)	Evening dose (mg)	Standard-frequency monitoring	Morning dose (mg)	Evening dose (mg)	Approximate percentage dose of previous antipsychotic
1	Mon #*	0	6.25	Mon #*	6.25	6.25	100
2	Tue	0	12.5	Tue #	6.25	12.5	
3	Wed #	6.25	12.5	Wed #	12.5	12.5	
4	Thu	6.25	25	Thu #	12.5	25	
5	Fri #	12.5	25	Fri #	25	25	
6	Sat	12.5	25	Sat	25	25	
7	Sun	12.5	37.5	Sun	25	50	
8	Mon #*	25	37.5	Mon #*	25	50	75
9	Tue	25	50	Tue #	50	50	
10	Wed #	25	62.5	Wed #	50	50	
11	Thu	25	75	Thu #	50	75	
12	Fri #	37.5	75	Fri #	50	75	
13	Sat	37.5	75	Sat	75	75	
14	Sun	37.5	87.5	Sun	75	75	
15	Mon #*	50	87.5	Mon #*	75	100	50
16	Tue	50	100	Tue	75	100	
17	Wed	50	125	Wed #	75	125	
18	Thu #	50	125	Thu	75	125	
19	Fri	50	125	Fri #	75	150	
20	Sat	50	125	Sat	75	150	
21	Sun	50	150	Sun	75	150	
22	Mon #*	50	150	Mon #*	75	175	25
23	Tue	50	150	Tue	75	175	
24	Wed	50	150	Wed	75	200	
25	Thu #	75	150	Thu #	75	200	
26	Fri	75	150	Fri	75	225	
27	Sat	75	150	Sat	75	225	
28	Sun	75	175	Sun	75	225	
29	Further increments should be 25–50mg/day (generally 25mg/day) until target dose is reached (use plasma levels). Beware of sudden increase in plasma levels due to saturation of first-pass metabolism (watch for increase in sedation/other adverse effects).						0

Face-to-face assessments including physical observations (sitting and standing blood pressure, heart rate, oxygen saturation, temperature and respiratory rate), adverse effect and mental state review, actively manage adverse effects (e.g. behavioural advice, slow clozapine titration or reduce dose of other antipsychotic, start adjunctive treatments – see sections on clozapine adverse effects in this chapter).

* Full blood count; also consider C-reactive protein, CK, troponin, beta-natriuretic peptide.

Adverse effects

Sedation, hypersalivation and hypotension are common at the start of treatment. These effects can usually be managed (see section on clozapine: common adverse effects in this chapter) but require particular attention in community titration. Consider regular systematic assessment of adverse effects using a recognised scale such as the GASS for Clozapine.

The formal carer (usually the community psychiatric nurse) should inform the prescriber if:

- temperature rises above 38°C (this is very common and is not a good reason, on its own, for stopping clozapine)
- pulse is >100bpm (also common and not, on its own, a reason for stopping, but may sometimes be linked to myocarditis)
- postural drop of >30mmHg
- patient is clearly over-sedated
- any signs of constipation (initiate laxatives early)
- flu-like symptoms (malaise, fatigue, etc.)
- chest pain, dyspnoea, tachypnoea
- any other adverse effect that is intolerable
- changes in smoking habit.

The patient should be reviewed at least once a week for the first month to assess mental and physical state.

Recommended additional monitoring

Baseline	1 month	3 months	4–6 months	12 months
Weight/BMI/waist	Weight/BMI/weight	Weight/BMI/waist	Weight/BMI/waist	Weight/BMI/waist
Plasma glucose and lipids	Plasma glucose and lipids		Plasma glucose and lipids	Plasma glucose and lipids
LFTs			LFTs	

Monitor CRP, CK, troponin weekly in the first four weeks of treatment or if temperature is above 38°C (see section on clozapine and myocarditis). CK, B-natriuretic peptide and echocardiogram should be used to confirm or rule out myocarditis if CRP and troponin are raised above thresholds.[6]

Switching from other antipsychotics

- The switching regimen will be largely dependent on the patient's mental state.
- Consider potential additive adverse effects of antipsychotics (e.g. hypotension, sedation, effect on QTc interval).
- Consider drug interactions (e.g. some SSRIs may increase clozapine levels).
- Other antipsychotics and clozapine may be cross-tapered with varying degrees of caution. ECG monitoring is prudent when clozapine is co-prescribed with other drugs known to affect QT interval. (Pimozide and ziprasidone should be stopped before clozapine is started.)

Serious cardiac adverse effects

See section on clozapine: serious cardiovascular adverse effects in this chapter. Patients should be closely observed for signs or symptoms of myocarditis, particularly during the first month,[7] and advised to inform staff if they experience cardiac symptoms and to seek out-of-hours review if necessary. These symptoms include persistent tachycardia (although commonly benign), palpitations, shortness of breath, fever, arrhythmia, symptoms mimicking myocardial infarction, chest pain, unusually low blood pressure and other unexplained symptoms of heart failure. Myocarditis risk is probably lower when using the slow titrations used in the community.[8]

References

1. Butler E, et al. Real-world clinical and cost-effectiveness of community clozapine initiation: mirror cohort study. *Br J Psychiatry* 2022; **221**:740–747.
2. Beck K, et al. The practical management of refractory schizophrenia—the Maudsley Treatment REview and Assessment Team service approach. *Acta Psychiatr Scand* 2014; **130**:427–438.
3. Taylor DM, et al. *The Maudsley Prescribing Guidelines in Psychiatry*, 14th edn. Oxford: Wiley-Blackwell; 2021.
4. Mizuno Y, et al. Low-frequency monitoring for community clozapine initiations: a comparative study relative to standard frequency assessments. *J Psychopharm* 2023; **37**:627–629.
5. Taylor D, et al. Predicting clozapine dose required to achieve a therapeutic plasma concentration: a comparison of a population algorithm and three algorithms based on gene variant models. *J Psychopharmacol* 2023; **37**:1030–1039.
6. Clark SR, et al. Dotting the I's and crossing the T's: a South Australian perspective on variability in troponin thresholds for myocarditis risk in clozapine treatment. *Schizophr Res* 2023; **268**:114–117.
7. Correll CU, et al. A guideline and checklist for initiating and managing clozapine treatment in patients with treatment-resistant schizophrenia. *CNS Drugs* 2022; **36**:659–679.
8. de Leon J, et al. Escaping the long shadow cast by agranulocytosis: reflections on clozapine pharmacovigilance focused on the United Kingdom. *J Clin Psychopharmacol* 2023; **43**:239–245.

CLOZAPINE ADVERSE EFFECTS

Clozapine: common adverse effects

This section provides a summary of management of the common adverse effects of clozapine.

Adverse effect	Time course	Action
Constipation	First 4 months are the highest risk.[1] Usually persists and so requires continuous monitoring and treatment.	Advise patients of the risks before starting, screen regularly, ensure adequate fibre, fluid and exercise. Consider early or even prophylactic laxatives. Stimulant laxatives (senna or bisacodyl) are first-line treatments, with emollients (docusate) and/or osmotics (macrogols).[2] Bulk-forming laxatives should be avoided. Stop other medicines that may be contributing and reduce clozapine dose if possible. Effective treatment or prevention of constipation is essential, as death may result.[3,4] See section on clozapine-induced gastrointestinal hypomotility in this chapter.
Fever[5]	First 4 weeks[6]	Clozapine induces inflammatory response (increased CRP, interleukin-6 and eosinophils).[7–9] Give paracetamol but check FBC for neutropenia. Reduce rate of dose titration.[10] Concurrent valproate or quetiapine may increase risk.[11] This fever is not usually related to blood dyscrasias[12] but beware myocarditis, NMS, pneumonia and other rarer types of inflammatory organ damage (see section on clozapine: uncommon or unusual adverse effects in this chapter).
Gastro-esophageal reflux disease[13,14]	Any time	Proton pump inhibitors often prescribed but some are CYP1A2 inducers and possibly increase risk of neutropenia and agranulocytosis.[15,16] Reasons for GERD association unclear – clozapine is an H_2 antagonist.[17]
Hypersalivation	First few months. Usually persists but sometimes wears off. Often very troublesome at night.	Reduce dose if possible.[18] Many options available[19] (see section on clozapine-induced hypersalivation in this chapter). Systemic anticholinergic drugs worsen constipation and cognition and so should not be used first line.
Hypertension[20]	First 4 weeks, sometimes longer	Monitor closely and increase dose as slowly as is necessary. Hypotensive therapy is sometimes necessary.[21]
Hypotension	First 4 weeks	Advise patient to stand up in stages. Reduce dose or slow down rate of increase. Ensure fluid intake of >2L daily.[22] If severe, consider fludrocortisone 0.05–0.3mg daily first line (monitor fluid intake, potassium and sodium) or midodrine 2.5–5mg three times a day (maximum 30mg/day).[23] Other options include moclobemide and Bovril® in combination or etilefrine.[23]
Myoclonus[24–27]	During dose titration or plasma level increases	May precede full tonic-clonic seizure. May present as knee-buckling.[28] Reduce dose. Antiseizure drugs may help and will reduce the likelihood of progression to seizures. Valproate is first choice but has limited utility. Referral to neurology specialist is advised.
Nausea	First 6 weeks	May give anti-emetic. Avoid prochlorperazine if previous EPS. Avoid domperidone if underlying cardiac risk or QTc prolongation. Ondansetron is a good choice, but it may worsen constipation. Metoclopramide may help with hypersalivation. Nausea and vomiting can be the only presenting symptoms of myocarditis.[29]

(Continued)

(Continued)

Adverse effect	Time course	Action
Nocturnal enuresis	May occur at any time	Try reducing the dose or manipulating dose schedule to avoid periods of deep sedation. Avoid fluids before bedtime. Consider scheduled night-time toileting. May resolve spontaneously,[30] but may persist for months or years.[31] Seems to affect 1 in 5 people on clozapine.[32] Try aripiprazole (10–15mg daily) or desmopressin (10mcg/mL nasal spray into each nostril at night, or 200–400mcg orally at night).[33] Monitoring for hyponatraemia is essential. Other options include oxybutynin, trihexyphenidyl, imipramine, amitriptyline and verapamil.[33]
Pneumonia[34,35]	Usually early in treatment, but may be any time	May result from saliva aspiration (this may be why pneumonia appears to be dose related),[36,37] and very rarely from constipation.[38] Pneumonia is a common cause of death in people on clozapine.[39] Infections in general may be more common in those on clozapine[40] and use of antibiotics is also increased.[41] Obesity,[34] anticholinergic burden[35] and treatment-resistant schizophrenia itself may also contribute to risk.[34] Respiratory infections may give rise to elevated clozapine levels.[42,43–45] This may be an artefact: smoking usually ceases during an infection and inflammation itself causes a reduction in CYP1A2 activity.[46,47] Clozapine is often successfully continued after the pneumonia has resolved, but recurrence may be more likely.[48–50]
Sedation	First few months. May persist, but usually wears off to some extent.	Give smaller dose in the morning. Give evening dose earlier if morning waking is troublesome. Once daily dosing in the evening seems effective and well tolerated.[51,52] Case reports of successful use of psychostimulants (methylphenidate[53]) and betahistine.[54] Modafinil does not appear to be effective.[55] Aripiprazole may help.[56]
Seizures[57]	May occur at any time[58]	Related to dose, plasma level and rapid dose escalation.[25] There is no step-change in risk at a particular dose or level. Consider prophylactic, topiramate, lamotrigine, gabapentin or valproate* if there are risk factors for seizures and or plasma level is high (≥600mcg/L). Some suggest risk of seizures below 1300mcg/L is not enough to support primary prophylaxis.[59] After a seizure: withhold clozapine for one day; restart at half previous dose; give antiseizure medication.**
Tachycardia	First 4 weeks, but usually persists	Very common in early stages of treatment but usually benign. May be dose-related.[60] Tachycardia, if persistent at rest and associated with fever, hypotension or chest pain, may indicate myocarditis or pericarditis (see section on clozapine: serious cardiovascular adverse effects in this chapter). Referral to a cardiologist is advised. Benign sinus tachycardia can be treated with bisoprolol[61] or atenolol,[62] although evidence base is poor.[63,64] Ivabradine may be used if hypotension or contraindications limit the use of beta blockers.[65] Prolonged tachycardia can itself precipitate cardiomyopathy[66] or other cardiovascular consequences.[22]
Weight gain	Usually during the first year of treatment, but may continue	Dietary counselling is essential. Advice may be more effective if given before weight gain occurs. Weight gain is common and often profound (4.5kg in the first 10 weeks).[67] Many treatments available (see section on treatment of antipsychotic-induced weight gain in this chapter).

* Usual dose is 1000–2000mg/day. Plasma levels may be useful as a rough guide to dosing – aim for 50–100mg/L. Use of modified-release preparation (Epilim Chrono) may aid compliance: can be given once daily and may be better tolerated.

** Lamotrigine may be helpful if poor response to clozapine or continued negative symptoms; topiramate if weight loss required (but beware cognitive adverse effects); gabapentin if other anticonvulsants are poorly tolerated.[25] Valproate should be avoided in most cases because of the risks of neurodevelopmental disorders and birth defects if valproate is taken during pregnancy or prior to conception (in the case of men). EEG abnormalities are common in those on clozapine.[68,69] CRP, C-reactive protein; EPS, extrapyramidal symptoms; GERD, gastro-esophageal reflux disease.

References

1. Palmer SE, et al. Life-threatening clozapine-induced gastrointestinal hypomotility: an analysis of 102 cases. *J Clin Psychiatry* 2008; **69**:759–768.

2. Taylor D, et al. *The Maudsley Practice Guidelines for Physical Health Conditions in Psychiatry*. Chichester: Wiley-Blackwell; 2021.

3. Handley SA, et al. Clozapine-induced gastrointestinal hypomotility: presenting features and outcomes, UK pharmacovigilance reports, 1992–2017. *Br J Psychiatry* 2022; **220**:355–363.

4. Partanen JJ, et al. High burden of ileus and pneumonia in clozapine-treated individuals with schizophrenia: a Finnish 25-year follow-up register study. *Am J Psychiatry* 2024; **181**:879–892.

5. Verdoux H, et al. Clinical determinants of fever in clozapine users and implications for treatment management: a narrative review. *Schizophr Res* 2019; **211**:1–9.

6. Martins PLB, et al. Immunoinflammatory and oxidative alterations in subjects with schizophrenia under clozapine: a meta-analysis. *Eur Neuropsychopharmacol* 2023; **73**:82–95.

7. Hung YP, et al. Role of cytokine changes in clozapine-induced fever: a cohort prospective study. *Psychiatry Clin Neurosci* 2017; **71**:395–402.

8. Kohen I, et al. Increases in C-reactive protein may predict recurrence of clozapine-induced fever. *Ann Pharmacother* 2009; **43**:143–146.

9. Kluge M, et al. Effects of clozapine and olanzapine on cytokine systems are closely linked to weight gain and drug-induced fever. *Psychoneuroendocrinology* 2009; **34**:118–128.

10. Chung JP, et al. The incidence and characteristics of clozapine- induced fever in a local psychiatric unit in Hong Kong. *Can J Psychiatry* 2008; **53**:857–862.

11. Kikuchi Y, et al. Effects of titration speed, gender, obesity and concomitant medications on the risk and onset time of clozapine-associated fever among Japanese patients with schizophrenia: retrospective review of charts from 21 hospitals. *Br J Psychiatry* 2024; **6**:1–7.

12. Tham JC, et al. Clozapine-induced fevers and 1-year clozapine discontinuation rate. *J Clin Psychiatry* 2002; **63**:880–884.

13. Taylor D, et al. Use of antacid medication in patients receiving clozapine: a comparison with other second-generation antipsychotics. *J Clin Psychopharmacol* 2010; **30**:460–461.

14. Van Veggel M, et al. Clozapine and gastro-oesophageal reflux disease (GORD): an investigation of temporal association. *Acta Psychiatr Scand* 2013; **127**:69–77.

15. Wicinski M, et al. Potential mechanisms of hematological adverse drug reactions in patients receiving clozapine in combination with proton pump inhibitors. *J Psychiatr Pract* 2017; **23**:114–120.

16. Shuman MD, et al. Exploring the potential effect of polypharmacy on the hematologic profiles of clozapine patients. *J Psychiatr Pract* 2014; **20**:50–58.

17. Humbert-Claude M, et al. Involvement of histamine receptors in the atypical antipsychotic profile of clozapine: a reassessment in vitro and in vivo. *Psychopharmacology (Berl)* 2011; **220**:225–241.

18. Schorctsanitis G, et al. Elevated clozapine concentrations in clozapine-treated patients with hypersalivation. *Clin Pharmacokinet* 2021; **60**:329–335.

19. Fornaro M, et al. Pharmacological interventions for antipsychotic-related sialorrhea: a systematic review and network meta-analysis of randomized trials. *Mol Psychiatry* 2023; **28**:3648–3660.

20. Gonsai NH, et al. Effects of dopamine receptor antagonist antipsychotic therapy on blood pressure. *J Clin Pharm Ther* 2017; **43**:1–7.

21. Henderson DC, et al. Clozapine and hypertension: a chart review of 82 patients. *J Clin Psychiatry* 2004; **65**:686–689.

22. Ronaldson KJ. Cardiovascular disease in clozapine-treated patients: evidence, mechanisms and management. *CNS Drugs* 2017; **31**:777–795.

23. Tanzer TD, et al. Treatment strategies for clozapine-induced hypotension: a systematic review. *Ther Adv Psychopharmacol* 2022; **12**:20451253221092931.

24. Osborne IJ, et al. Clozapine-induced myoclonus: a case report and review of the literature. *Ther Adv Psychopharmacol* 2015; **5**:351–356.

25. Varma S, et al. Clozapine-related EEG changes and seizures: dose and plasma-level relationships. *Ther Adv Psychopharmacol* 2011; **1**:47–66.

26. Praharaj SK, et al. Clozapine-induced myoclonus: a case study and brief review. *Prog Neuropsychopharmacol Biol Psychiatry* 2010; **34**:242–243.

27. Sajatovic M, et al. Clozapine-induced myoclonus and generalized seizures. *Biol Psychiatry* 1996; **39**:367–370.

28. Sahib Din J, et al. Knee buckling as an atypical adverse effect of clozapine: a case report. *Cureus* 2024; **16**:e55865.

29. van der Horst MZ, et al. Isolated nausea and vomiting as the cardinal presenting symptoms of clozapine-induced myocarditis: a case report. *BMC Psychiatry* 2020; **20**:568.

30. Warner JP, et al. Clozapine and urinary incontinence. *Int Clin Psychopharmacol* 1994; **9**:207–209.

31. Jeong SH, et al. A 2-year prospective follow-up study of lower urinary tract symptoms in patients treated with clozapine. *J Clin Psychopharmacol* 2008; **28**:618–624.

32. Harrison-Woolrych M, et al. Nocturnal enuresis in patients taking clozapine, risperidone, olanzapine and quetiapine: comparative cohort study. *Br J Psychiatry* 2011; **199**:140–144.

33. Tanzer T, et al. Treatment strategies for clozapine-induced nocturnal enuresis and urinary incontinence: a systematic review. *CNS Spectr* 2023; **28**:133–144.

34. Schoretsanitis G, et al. An update on the complex relationship between clozapine and pneumonia. *Expert Rev Clin Pharmacol* 2021; **14**:145–149.

35. Luykx JJ, et al. Pneumonia risk, antipsychotic dosing, and anticholinergic burden in schizophrenia. *JAMA Psychiatry* 2024; **81**:967–975.

36. Trigoboff E, et al. Sialorrhea and aspiration pneumonia: a case study. *Innov Clin Neurosci* 2013; **10**:20–27.

37. Kuo CJ, et al. Second-generation antipsychotic medications and risk of pneumonia in schizophrenia. *Schizophr Bull* 2013; **39**:648–657.

38. Galappathie N, et al. Clozapine-associated pneumonia and respiratory arrest secondary to severe constipation. *Med Sci Law* 2014; **54**:105–109.

39. Taylor DM, et al. Reasons for discontinuing clozapine: matched, case-control comparison with risperidone long-acting injection. *Br J Psychiatry* 2009; **194**:165–167.

40. Landry P, et al. Increased use of antibiotics in clozapine-treated patients. *Int Clin Psychopharmacol* 2003; **18**:297–298.

41. Nielsen J, et al. Increased use of antibiotics in patients treated with clozapine. *Eur Neuropsychopharmacol* 2009; **19**:483–486.

42. Raaska K, et al. Bacterial pneumonia can increase serum concentration of clozapine. *Eur J Clin Pharmacol* 2002; **58**:321–322.

43. de Leon J, et al. Serious respiratory infections can increase clozapine levels and contribute to side effects: a case report. *Prog Neuropsychopharmacol Biol Psychiatry* 2003; **27**:1059–1063.

44. Ruan CJ, et al. Pneumonia can cause clozapine intoxication: a case report. *Psychosomatics* 2017; **58**:652–656.

45. Leung JG, et al. Necrotizing pneumonia in the setting of elevated clozapine levels. *J Clin Psychopharmacol* 2016; **36**:176–178.

46. de Leon J, et al. A rational use of clozapine based on adverse drug reactions, pharmacokinetics, and clinical pharmacopsychology. *Psychother Psychosom* 2020; **89**:200–214.

47. Clark SR, et al. Elevated clozapine levels associated with infection: a systematic review. *Schizophr Res* 2018; **192**:50–56.

48. Hung GC, et al. Antipsychotic reexposure and recurrent pneumonia in schizophrenia: a nested case-control study. *J Clin Psychiatry* 2016; **77**:60–66.

49. Galappathie N, et al. Clozapine re-trial in a patient with repeated life threatening pneumonias. *Acta Biomed* 2014; **85**:175–179.

50. Schmidinger S, et al. Pulmonary embolism and aspiration pneumonia after reexposure to clozapine: pulmonary adverse effects of clozapine. *J Clin Psychopharmacol* 2014; **34**:385–387.

51. Tsukahara M, et al. Impact of clozapine once-daily versus multiple-daily dosing regimen on relapse in patients with treatment-resistant schizophrenia: a 1-year retrospective cohort study. *Psychopharmacology* 2025; **242**:161–171.

52. Sathienluckana T, et al. Comparison of the effectiveness and safety of clozapine between once-daily and divided dosing regimen in patients with treatment-resistant schizophrenia. *Ann Pharmacother* 2024; **58**:598–604.

53. Sarfati D, et al. Methylphenidate as treatment for clozapine-induced sedation in patients with treatment-resistant schizophrenia. *Clin Schizophr Relat Psychoses* 2018; doi: 10.3371/CSRP.SALA.061518.

54. Poyurovsky M, et al. Beneficial effect of betahistine, a structural analog of histamine, in clozapine-related sedation. *Clin Neuropharmacol* 2019; **42**:145.

55. Freudenreich O, et al. Modafinil for clozapine-treated schizophrenia patients: a double-blind, placebo-controlled pilot trial. *J Clin Psychiatry* 2009; **70**:1674–1680.

56. Fernandez-Egea E, et al. The effect of clozapine on self-reported duration of sleep and its interaction with 23 other medications: a 5-year naturalistic study. *J Clin Psychopharmacol* 2021; **41**:534–539.

57. Grover S, et al. Association of clozapine with seizures: a brief report involving 222 patients prescribed clozapine. *East Asian Arch Psychiatry* 2015; **25**:73–78.

58. Pacia SV, et al. Clozapine-related seizures: experience with 5,629 patients. *Neurology* 1994; **44**:2247–2249.

59. Caetano D. Use of anticonvulsants as prophylaxis for seizures in patients on clozapine. *Australas Psychiatry* 2014; **22**:78–83.

60. Nilsson BM, et al. Tachycardia in patients treated with clozapine versus antipsychotic long-acting injections. *Int Clin Psychopharmacol* 2017; **32**:219–224.

61. Nilsson BM, et al. Persistent tachycardia in clozapine treated patients: a 24-hour ambulatory electrocardiogram study. *Schizophr Res* 2018; **199**:403–406.

62. Stryjer R, et al. Beta-adrenergic antagonists for the treatment of clozapine-induced sinus tachycardia: a retrospective study. *Clin Neuropharmacol* 2009; **32**:290–292.

63. Lally J, et al. Pharmacological interventions for clozapine-induced sinus tachycardia. *Cochrane Database Syst Rev* 2016; (6):CD011566.

64. Yuen JWY, et al. Clozapine-induced cardiovascular side effects and autonomic dysfunction: a systematic review. *Front Neurosci* 2018; **12**:203.

65. Lally J, et al. Ivabradine, a novel treatment for clozapine-induced sinus tachycardia: a case series. *Ther Adv Psychopharmacol* 2014; **4**:117–122.

66. Shinbane JS, et al. Tachycardia-induced cardiomyopathy: a review of animal models and clinical studies. *J Am Coll Cardiol* 1997; **29**:709–715.

67. Allison D, et al. Antipsychotic-induced weight gain: a comprehensive research synthesis. *Am J Psychiatry* 1999; **156**:1686–1696.

68. Centorrino F, et al. EEG abnormalities during treatment with typical and atypical antipsychotics. *Am J Psychiatry* 2002; **159**:109–115.

69. Jackson A, et al. EEG changes in patients on antipsychotic therapy: a systematic review. *Epilepsy Behav* 2019; **95**:1–9.

Clozapine: uncommon or unusual adverse effects

Adverse effect	Time course	Comment
Agranulocytosis (delayed)[1–4]	Usually first 3 months but may occur at any time	Occasional reports of apparent clozapine-related blood dyscrasia even after 1 year of treatment. Some suggest risk may be elevated for up to 9 years.[5] It is very likely that clozapine is not the causative agent in most, if not all late cases[6,7] (see section on clozapine: serious haematological adverse effects in this chapter).
Colitis/gastrointestinal necrosis[8–15]	Usually within the first month but may be any time[16]	Growing body of case reports. Any severe or chronic diarrhoea should prompt specialist referral as there is a substantial risk of death. Use of drugs with anticholinergic effects probably increases risk of colitis and necrosis.[17]
Delirium[18–20]	Any time	Reported rates vary (0.1–10%)[18,21,22] but rarely seen in practice if dose is titrated slowly and plasma level determinations are used. Older age and medical comorbidity increase the risk of delirium. Ensure common causes of delirium are treated. Cholinergic rebound resulting from abrupt cessation of clozapine can cause delirium.
Eosinophilia[23–25]	First week,[26,27] but can be any time	Reasonably common but significance unclear. Eosinophilia may predict neutropenia but this is disputed. Usually benign but investigate for signs of inflammatory organ damage[28] (myocarditis,[29] interstitial nephritis,[27,30] interstitial lung disease, hepatitis, pancreatitis).[31] May be associated with colitis and related symptoms.[15,32] DRESS syndrome described in case reports.[33,34] Successful rechallenge is possible.[35] Concomitant antidepressants may increase risk.[36,37]
Heat stroke[38,39]	Any time	Two cases reported, both occurred during a heatwave. May be mistaken for NMS (CK was elevated in both cases).
Hepatic failure/enzyme abnormalities[40–46]	First few months	Benign changes in LFTs are common (up to 50% of patients) but worth monitoring because of the very small risk of fulminant hepatic failure.[47] Rash may be associated with clozapine-related hepatitis[48] (see section on hepatic impairment in Chapter 8).
Hypothermia[49]	Any time	A few case reports and events in pharmacovigilance databases. Can be fatal.
Interstitial nephritis[50,51]	Usually first 3 weeks, possibly up to 3 months[27]	A handful of reports implicating clozapine. Probably immune mediated. May occur after only a few doses. Symptoms include fever, tachycardia, nausea, vomiting, diarrhoea, raised creatinine, urinary difficulties and eosinophilia. The classic nephritis-associated rash may not be present.[27] There are no published cases of successful rechallenge.[27]
Interstitial lung disease	Usually first few months, possibly later in treatment	Six case reports.[52] May be caused by aspiration or an immune reaction. Symptoms are non-specific: shortness of breath, fever, cough, fatigue. Pneumonitis has also been reported.[53]
Knee-buckling[54,55]	Usually at the start of treatment	Several cases reported. May be mistaken for postural hypotension.
Ocular effects[56]	Any time	Single case report of ocular pigmentation,[57] five of periorbital oedema.[58] Clozapine may cause dry eye syndrome.[59]

(Continued)

(Continued)

Adverse effect	Time course	Comment
Pancreatitis[60–69]	Usually first 6 weeks, possibly later in treatment[70]	Several reports of asymptomatic and symptomatic pancreatitis. Symptoms include fever, abdominal pain and distension, nausea and vomiting, raised CRP and raised lipase and/or amylase. Concomitant valproate may increase the risk.[27] The majority of attempts to rechallenge fail[63,71–74] but one successful case is reported.[75]
Parotid gland swelling[76–80]	Usually first few weeks, but may occur later[81]	Several case reports. Unclear mechanism, possibly immunological or thickening of saliva leading to calcium precipitation. Can be recurrent. May resolve spontaneously.[82] Terazosin in combination with benztropine may be helpful.
Pericarditis and pericardial effusion[69,83–90]	Any time	Several reports in the literature. Symptoms include fatigue, chest pain, dyspnoea, orthostatic hypotension and tachycardia, but may be asymptomatic.[91] Signs include raised inflammatory markers (specifically trop I) and pro-BNP levels.[91] Use echocardiogram to confirm/rule out effusion. Successful rechallenge possible.[92–94]
Stuttering[95,96]	Any time	Case reports only. Check plasma levels, consider dose reduction and/or antiseizure drugs – may be a warning sign for impending generalised seizures.[97]
Thrombocytopenia[98–101]	First 3 months	Few data but apparently fairly common (incidence over 1 year of 3[102]–8%[103]). Probably transient and clinically unimportant, but persistent in some cases[104,105] and recurrent on rechallenge in others.[106,107] Thrombocytosis also reported.[108]
Skin reactions[109]	Any time	Presence of skin diseases in general is higher in those with schizophrenia.[110] Four reports of vasculitis[111–114] in which patients developed confluent erythematous rash on lower limbs. One report of Stevens–Johnson syndrome,[115] two of pityriasis rosea,[116,117] one of a papular rash,[118] one of exanthematic pustulosis,[119] one of cholinergic urticaria[120] and two of Sweet's syndrome,[121] one fatal.[122] Rash is often reported in DRESS syndrome.[123]
Thromboembolism[124–126]	Any time[127]	Weight increase and sedation may contribute to risk. Mechanism may be increased platelet aggregation via $5HT_{2A}$ receptor activation.[128] Clozapine increases risk of pulmonary thromboembolism by 28 times compared with the general population.[129] The risk may be dose related[130] but cases are reported across the dose range.[131,132] Consider prophylactic antithrombotic treatment where additional risk factors are present (surgery, immobility). Continuation of therapy after embolism may be possible[133] but consult haematologist as without prophylactic antithrombotic treatment recurrence is likely[134,135] and may be fatal.[131,136]
Polyserositis	Usually first few weeks, but can occur at any time	Case reports describe a wide variety of symptoms related to inflammatory processes, including flu-like symptoms, fever, eosinophilia, diarrhoea, shortness of breath, tachycardia, thoracic pain.[137] Other inflammatory conditions may be present (hepatitis, pancreatitis, dermatosis). Suggested to be either IgE-mediated hypersensitivity or an immunomodulatory effect.[138] All reported cases have resolved on discontinuation of clozapine.[138]

CK, creatine kinase; CRP, C-reactive protein; DRESS, drug rash with eosinophilia and systemic symptoms; IgE, immunoglobulin E; NMS, neuroleptic malignant syndrome; pro-BNP, pro-brain natriuretic peptide.

References

1. Thompson A, et al. Late onset neutropenia with clozapine. *Can J Psychiatry* 2004; **49**:647–648.

2. Bhanji NH, et al. Late-onset agranulocytosis in a patient with schizophrenia after 17 months of clozapine treatment. *J Clin Psychopharmacol* 2003; **23**:522–523.

3. Sedky K, et al. Clozapine-induced agranulocytosis after 11 years of treatment [Letter]. *Am J Psychiatry* 2005; **162**:814.

4. de Araujo CF, et al. Delayed-onset severe neutropenia associated with clozapine with successful rechallenge at lower dose. *J Clin Psychopharmacol* 2021; **41**:77–79.

5. Kang BJ, et al. Long-term patient monitoring for clozapine-induced agranulocytosis and neutropenia in Korea: when is it safe to discontinue CPMS? *Hum Psychopharmacol* 2006; **21**:387–391.

6. Panesar N, et al. Late onset neutropenia with clozapine. *Aust N Z J Psychiatry* 2011; **45**:684.

7. Tourian L, et al. Late-onset agranulocytosis in a patient treated with clozapine and lamotrigine. *J Clin Psychopharmacol* 2011; **31**:665–667.

8. Hawe R, et al. Response to clozapine-induced microscopic colitis: a case report and review of the literature. *J Clin Psychopharmacol* 2008; **28**:454–455.

9. Shah V, et al. Clozapine-induced ischaemic colitis. *BMJ CaseRep* 2013; **2013**:bcr2012007933.

10. Linsley KR, et al. Clozapine-associated colitis: case report and review of the literature. *J Clin Psychopharmacol* 2012; **32**:564–566.

11. Baptista T. A fatal case of ischemic colitis during clozapine administration. *Rev Bras Psiquiatr* 2014; **36**:358.

12. Rodriguez-Sosa JT, et al. Apropos of a case: relationship of ischemic colitis with clozapine. *Actas Esp Psiquiatr* 2014; **42**:325–326.

13. Osterman MT, et al. Clozapine-induced acute gastrointestinal necrosis: a case report. *J Med Case Rep* 2017; **11**:270.

14. Holz K, et al. Clozapine associated with microscopic colitis in the setting of biopsy-proven celiac disease. *J Clin Psychopharmacol* 2018; **38**:150–152.

15. Rask SM, et al. Clozapine-related diarrhea and colitis: report of 4 cases. *J Clin Psychopharmacol* 2020; **40**:293–296.

16. Verdoux H, et al. Clinical determinants of fever in clozapine users and implications for treatment management: a narrative review. *Schizophr Res* 2019; **211**:1–9.

17. Peyriere H, et al. Antipsychotics-induced ischaemic colitis and gastrointestinal necrosis: a review of the French pharmacovigilance database. *Pharmacoepidemiol Drug Saf* 2009; **18**:948–955.

18. Centorrino F, et al. Delirium during clozapine treatment: incidence and associated risk factors. *Pharmacopsychiatry* 2003; **36**:156–160.

19. Shankar BR. Clozapine-induced delirium. *J Neuropsychiatry Clin Neurosci* 2008; **20**:239–240.

20. Khanra S, et al. An unusual case of delirium after restarting clozapine. *Clin Psychopharmacol Neurosci* 2016; **14**:107–108.

21. Gaertner HJ, et al. Side effects of clozapine. *Psychopharmacology (Berl)* 1989; 99 Suppl:S97–S100.

22. Friedrich ME, et al. Incidence of drug-induced delirium during treatment with antidepressants or antipsychotics: a drug surveillance report of German-speaking countries between 1993 and 2016. *Int J Neuropsychopharmacol* 2022; **25**:556–566.

23. Hummer M, et al. Does eosinophilia predict clozapine induced neutropenia? *Psychopharmacology* 1996; **124**:201–204.

24. Ames D, et al. Predictive value of eosinophilia for neutropenia during clozapine treatment. *J Clin Psychiatry* 1996; **57**:579–581.

25. Wysokinski A, et al. Rapidly developing and self-limiting eosinophilia associated with clozapine. *Psychiatry Clin Neurosci* 2015; **69**:122.

26. Aneja J, et al. Eosinophilia induced by clozapine: a report of two cases and review of the literature. *J Family Med Prim Care* 2015; **4**:127–129.

27. Lally J, et al. Hepatitis, interstitial nephritis, and pancreatitis in association with clozapine treatment: a systematic review of case series and reports. *J Clin Psychopharmacol* 2018; **38**:520–527.

28. Marchel D, et al. Multiorgan eosinophilic infiltration after initiation of clozapine therapy: a case report. *BMC Res Notes* 2017; **10**:316.

29. Chatterton R. Eosinophilia after commencement of clozapine treatment. *Aust N Z J Psychiatry* 1997; **31**:874–876.

30. Chan SY, et al. Clozapine-induced acute interstitial nephritis. *Hong Kong Med J* 2015; **21**:372–374.

31. Lally J, et al. Rechallenge following clozapine-associated eosinophilia: a case report and literature review. *J Clin Psychopharmacol* 2019; **39**:504–506.

32. Karmacharya R, et al. Clozapine-induced eosinophilic colitis [Letter]. *Am J Psychiatry* 2005; **162**:1386–1387.

33. de Filippis R, et al. Antipsychotic-related DRESS syndrome: analysis of individual case safety reports of the WHO Pharmacovigilance Database. *Drug Saf* 2024; **47**:745–757.

34. de Filippis R, et al. Unravelling cases of clozapine-related drug reaction with eosinophilia and systemic symptoms (DRESS) in patients reported otherwise: a systematic review. *J Psychopharmacol* 2021; **35**:1062–1073.

35. McArdle PA, et al. Successful rechallenge with clozapine after treatment associated eosinophilia. *Australas Psychiatry* 2016; **24**:365–367.

36. Fabrazzo M, et al. Clozapine versus other antipsychotics during the first 18 weeks of treatment: a retrospective study on risk factor increase of blood dyscrasias. *Psychiatry Res* 2017; **256**:275–282.

37. Sanader B, et al. Clozapine-induced DRESS syndrome: a case series from the AMSP Multicenter Drug Safety Surveillance Project. *Pharmacopsychiatry* 2019; **52**:156–159.

38. Kerwin RW, et al. Heat stroke in schizophrenia during clozapine treatment: rapid recognition and management. *J Psychopharmacol* 2004; **18**:121–123.

39. Hoffmann MS, et al. Heat stroke during long-term clozapine treatment: should we be concerned about hot weather? *Trends Psychiatry Psychother* 2016; **38**:56–59.

40. Erdogan A, et al. Management of marked liver enzyme increase during clozapine treatment: a case report and review of the literature. *Int J Psychiatry Med* 2004; **34**:83–89.

41. Macfarlane B, et al. Fatal acute fulminant liver failure due to clozapine: a case report and review of clozapine-induced hepatotoxicity. *Gastroenterology* 1997; **112**:1707–1709.

42. Chang A, et al. Clozapine-induced fatal fulminant hepatic failure: a case report. *Can J Gastroenterol* 2009; **23**:376–378.

43. Chaplin AC, et al. Re: Recent case report of clozapine-induced acute hepatic failure. *Can J Gastroenterol* 2010; **24**:739–740.

44. Wu Chou AI, et al. Hepatotoxicity induced by clozapine: a case report and review of literature. *Neuropsychiatr Dis Treat* 2014; **10**:1585–1587.

45. Kane JP, et al. Clozapine-induced liver injury and pleural effusion. *Ment Illn* 2014; **6**:5403.

46. Douros A, et al. Drug-induced liver injury: results from the hospital-based Berlin Case–Control Surveillance Study. *Br J Clin Pharmacol* 2015; **79**:988–999.

47. Tucker P. Liver toxicity with clozapine. *Aust N Z J Psychiatry* 2013; **47**:975–976.

48. Fong SY, et al. Clozapine-induced toxic hepatitis with skin rash. *J Psychopharmacol* 2005; **19**:107.

49. Burk BG, et al. A case report of acute hypothermia during initial inpatient clozapine titration with review of current literature on clozapine-induced temperature dysregulations. *BMC Psychiatry* 2020; **20**:290.

50. McLoughlin C, et al. Clozapine-induced interstitial nephritis in a patient with schizoaffective disorder in the forensic setting: a case report and review of the literature. *Ir J Psychol Med* 2022; **39**:106–111.

51. Vantipalli P, et al. Acute interstitial nephritis induced by clozapine. *J Med Cases* 2022; **13**:322–329.

52. Can KC, et al. A very rare adverse effect of clozapine, clozapine-induced interstitial lung disease: case report and literature review. *Noro Psikiyatr Ars* 2019; **56**:313–315.

53. Torrico T, et al. Clozapine-induced pneumonitis: a case report. *Front Psychiatry* 2020; **11**:572102.

54. Sahib Din J, et al. Knee buckling as an atypical adverse effect of clozapine: a case report. *Cureus* 2024; **16**:e55865.

55. Uzun Ö, et al. Knee buckling (negative myoclonus) associated with clozapine: reports on 3 cases. *Clin Neuropharmacol* 2020; **43**:26–27.

56. Mu C, et al. Characteristics of eye disorders induced by atypical antipsychotics: a real-world study from 2016 to 2022 based on Food and Drug Administration Adverse Event Reporting System. *Front Psychiatry* 2024; **15**:1322939.

57. Borovik AM, et al. Ocular pigmentation associated with clozapine. *Med J Aust* 2009; **190**:210–211.

58. Huttlin EA, et al. Periorbital edema associated with clozapine and gabapentins: a case report. *J Clin Psychopharmacol* 2020; **40**:198–199.

59. Ceylan E, et al. The ocular surface side effects of an anti-psychotic drug, clozapine. *Cutan Ocul Toxicol* 2016; **35**:62–66.

60. Bergemann N, et al. Asymptomatic pancreatitis associated with clozapine. *Pharmacopsychiatry* 1999; **32**:78–80.

61. Raja M, et al. A case of clozapine-associated pancreatitis. *Open Neuropsychopharmacol J* 2011; **4**:5–7.

62. Bayard JM, et al. Case report: acute pancreatitis induced by Clozapine. *Acta Gastroenterol Belg* 2005; **68**:92–94.

63. Sani G, et al. Development of asymptomatic pancreatitis with paradoxically high serum clozapine levels in a patient with schizophrenia and the CYP1A2*1F/1F genotype. *J Clin Psychopharmacol* 2010; **30**:737–739.

64. Wehmeier PM, et al. Pancreatitis followed by pericardial effusion in an adolescent treated with clozapine. *J Clin Psychopharmacol* 2003; **23**:102–103.

65. Garlipp P, et al. The development of a clinical syndrome of asymptomatic pancreatitis and eosinophilia after treatment with clozapine in schizophrenia: implications for clinical care, recognition and management. *J Psychopharmacol* 2002; **16**:399–400.

66. Gatto EM, et al. Clozapine and pancreatitis. *Clin Neuropharmacol* 1998; **21**:203.

67. Martin A. Acute pancreatitis associated with clozapine use. *Am J Psychiatry* 1992; **149**:714.

68. Yildiz MI, et al. All in one: clozapine-associated acute pancreatitis with multiple organ involvement. *J Clin Psychopharmacol* 2021; **41**:214–216.

69. de Filippis R, et al. Clozapine-associated pericarditis and pancreatitis in children and adolescents: a systematic literature review and pharmacovigilance study using the VigiBase database. *Schizophr Res* 2024; **268**:118–130.

70. Cerulli TR. Clozapine-associated pancreatitis. *Harv Rev Psychiatry* 1999; **7**:61–63.

71. Huang YJ, et al. Recurrent pancreatitis without eosinophilia on clozapine rechallenge. *Prog Neuropsychopharmacol Biol Psychiatry* 2009; **33**:1561–1562.

72. Chengappa KN, et al. Recurrent pancreatitis on clozapine re-challenge. *J Psychopharmacol* 1995; **9**:381–382.

73. Frankenburg FR, et al. Eosinophilia, clozapine, and pancreatitis. *Lancet* 1992; **340**:251.

74. Ratcliff K, et al. Clozapine rechallenge with recurrent pancreatitis. *Prim Care Companion CNS Disord* 2022; **24**:22cr03237.

75. DeRemer CE, et al. Clozapine drug-induced pancreatitis of intermediate latency of onset confirmed by de-challenge and re-challenge. *Int J Clin Pharmacol Ther* 2019; **57**:37–40.

76. Immadisetty V, et al. A successful treatment strategy for clozapine-induced parotid swelling: a clinical case and systematic review. *Ther Adv Psychopharmacol* 2012; **2**:235–239.

77. Gouzien C, et al. [Clozapine-induced parotitis: a case study]. *Encephale* 2014; **40**:81–85.

78. Saguem BN, et al. Eosinophilia and parotitis occurring early in clozapine treatment. *Int J Clin Pharm* 2015; **37**:992–995.

79. Vohra A. Clozapine-induced recurrent and transient parotid gland swelling. *Afr J Psychiatry (Johannesbg)* 2013; **16**:236, 238.

80. Kathirvel N, et al. Recurrent transient parotid gland swelling with clozapine therapy. *Ir J Psychol Med* 2014; **25**:69–70.

81. Brodkin ES, et al. Treatment of clozapine-induced parotid gland swelling. *Am J Psychiatry* 1996; **153**:445.

82. Vasile JS, et al. Clozapine and the development of salivary gland swelling: a case study. *J Clin Psychiatry* 1995; **56**:511–513.

83. Bhatti MA, et al. Clozapine-induced pericarditis, pericardial tamponade, polyserositis, and rash. *J Clin Psychiatry* 2005; **66**:1490–1491.

84. Boot E, et al. Pericardial and bilateral pleural effusion associated with clozapine treatment. *Eur Psychiatry* 2004; **19**:65.

85. Murko A, et al. Clozapine and pericarditis with pericardial effusion. *Am J Psychiatry* 2002; **159**:494.

86. Imon Paul MD, et al. Clozapine induced pericarditis: an overlooked adverse effect. *Clin Schizophr Relat Psychoses* 2014; **8**:133–134.

87. Bath AS, et al. Pericardial effusion: rare adverse effect of clozapine. *Cureus* 2019; **11**:e4890.

88. Johal HK, et al. Clozapine-induced pericarditis: an ethical dilemma. *BMJ Case Rep* 2019; **12**:e229872.

89. Sahyouni C, et al. Clozapine induced pericarditis: a case report. *Psychiatry Res* 2021; **305**:114250.

90. Gilbreth N, et al. Clozapine-induced pericardial effusion presenting with persistent tachycardia. *Case Rep Med* 2021; **2021**:5523562.

91. Prisco V, et al. Brain natriuretic peptide as a biomarker of asymptomatic clozapine-related heart dysfunction: a criterion for a more cautious administration. *Clin Schizophr Relat Psychoses* 2016; **12**:185–188.

92. Crews MP, et al. Clozapine rechallenge following clozapine-induced pericarditis. *J Clin Psychiatry* 2010; **71**:959–961.

93. Sarathy K, et al. A successful re-trial after clozapine myopericarditis. *J R Coll Physicians Edinb* 2017; **47**:146–147.

94. Boscutti A, et al. Successful clozapine rechallenge after myopericarditis: a case report. *Int Clin Psychopharmacol* 2022; **37**:179–181.

95. Nikvarz N, et al. Drug-induced stuttering: a comprehensive literature review. *World J Psychiatry* 2022; **12**:236–263.

96. Trenque T, et al. Drug induced stuttering: pharmacovigilance data. *Expert Opin Drug Saf* 2021; **20**:373–378.

97. Duggal HS, et al. Clozapine-induced stuttering and seizures. *Am J Psychiatry* 2002; **159**:315.

98. Jagadheesan K, et al. Clozapine-induced thrombocytopenia: a pilot study. *Hong Kong J Psychiatry* 2003; **13**:12–15.

99. Mihaljevic-Peles A, et al. Thrombocytopenia associated with clozapine and fluphenazine. *Nord J Psychiatry* 2001; **55**:449–450.

100. Rudolf J, et al. Clozapine-induced agranulocytosis and thrombopenia in a patient with dopaminergic psychosis. *J Neural Transm (Vienna)* 1997; **104**:1305–1311.

101. Assion HJ, et al. Lymphocytopenia and thrombocytopenia during treatment with risperidone or clozapine. *Pharmacopsychiatry* 1996; **29**:227–228.

102. Lee J, et al. The effect of clozapine on hematological indices: a 1-year follow-up study. *J Clin Psychopharmacol* 2015; **35**:510–516.

103. Grover S, et al. Haematological side effects associated with clozapine: a retrospective study from India. *Asian J Psychiatr* 2020; **48**:101906.

104. Kate N, et al. Clozapine associated thrombocytopenia. *J Pharmacol Pharmacother* 2013; **4**:149–151.

105. Gonzales MF, et al. Evidence for immune etiology in clozapine-induced thrombocytopenia of 40 months' duration: a case report. *CNS Spectr* 2000; **5**:17–18.

106. Hauseux PA, et al. Clozapine rechallenge after thrombocytopenia: a case report. *Schizophr Res* 2020; **222**:477–479.

107. Thapaliya S, et al. Effective and safe use of intramuscular clozapine in a patient presenting with catatonia and thrombocytopenia. *BMJ Case Rep* 2024; **17**:e260197.

108. Hampson ME. Clozapine-induced thrombocytosis. *Br J Psychiatry* 2000; **176**:400.

109. Warnock JK, et al. Adverse cutaneous reactions to antipsychotics. *Am J Clin Dermatol* 2002; **3**:629–636.

110. Wu BY, et al. Prevalence and associated factors of comorbid skin diseases in patients with schizophrenia: a clinical survey and national health database study. *Gen Hosp Psychiatry* 2014; **36**:415–421.

111. Voulgari C, et al. Clozapine-induced late agranulocytosis and severe neutropenia complicated with streptococcus pneumonia, venous thromboembolism, and allergic vasculitis in treatment-resistant female psychosis. *Case Rep Med* 2015; **2015**:703218.

112. Penaskovic K, et al. Clozapine-induced allergic vasculitis [Letter]. *Am J Psychiatry* 2005; **162**:1543–1542.

113. Mukherjee S, et al. Leukocytoclastic vasculitis secondary to clozapine. *Indian J Psychiatry* 2019; **61**:94–96.

114. Fujimoto S, et al. Clozapine-induced antineutrophil cytoplasmic antibody-associated vasculitis: a case report. *Mod Rheumatol Case Rep* 2020; **4**:70–73.

115. Wu MK, et al. The severe complication of Stevens–Johnson syndrome induced by long-term clozapine treatment in a male schizophrenia patient: a case report. *Neuropsychiatr Dis Treat* 2015; **11**:1039–1041.

116. Lai YW, et al. Pityriasis rosea-like eruption associated with clozapine: a case report. *Gen Hosp Psychiatry* 2012; **34**:703.e5–e7.

117. Bhatia MS, et al. Clozapine induced pityriasiform eruption. *Indian J Dermatol* 1997; **42**:245–246.

118. Stanislav SW, et al. Papular rash and bilateral pleural effusion associated with clozapine. *Ann Pharmacother* 1999; **33**:1008–1009.

119. Bosonnet S, et al. [Acute generalized exanthematic pustulosis after intake of clozapine (leponex). First case]. *Ann Dermatol Venereol* 1997; **124**:547–548.

120. El Ouni Amami N, et al. Clozapine-induced cholinergic urticaria: a case report. *Ther Adv Psychopharmacol* 2024; **14**:20451253241241056.

121. Bunting A, et al. Clozapine and Sweet's syndrome: case report. *BJPsych Open* 2023; **9**:e166.

122. Kleinen JM, et al. [Clozapine-induced agranulocytosis and Sweet's syndrome in a 74-year-old female patient: a case study]. *Tijdschr Psychiatr* 2008; **50**:119–123.

123. de Filippis R, et al. Clozapine-related drug reaction with eosinophilia and systemic symptoms (DRESS) syndrome: a systematic review. *Expert Rev Clin Pharmacol* 2020; **13**:875–883.

124. Chate S, et al. Pulmonary thromboembolism associated with clozapine. *J Neuropsychiatry Clin Neurosci* 2013; **25**:E3–E6.

125. Yang TY, et al. Massive pulmonary embolism in a young patient on clozapine therapy. *J Emerg Med* 2004; **27**:27–29.

126. Huang J, et al. Association between antipsychotics and pulmonary embolism: a pharmacovigilance analysis. *Expert Opin Drug Saf* 2024; doi: 10.1080/14740338.2024.2396390.

127. Gami RK, et al. Pulmonary embolism and clozapine use: a case report and literature review. *Psychosomatics* 2017; **58**:203–208.

128. Hagg S, et al. Risk of venous thromboembolism due to antipsychotic drug therapy. *Expert Opin Drug Saf* 2009; **8**:537–547.

129. De Fazio P, et al. Rare and very rare adverse effects of clozapine. *Neuropsychiatr Dis Treat* 2015; **11**:1995–2003.

130. Sarvaiya N, et al. Clozapine-associated pulmonary embolism: a high-mortality, dose-independent and early-onset adverse effect. *Am J Ther* 2018; **25**:e434–e438.

131. Pallares Vela E, et al. Clozapine-related thromboembolic events. *Cureus* 2021; **13**:e16883.

132. Robbins-Welty GA, et al. Pulmonary embolism during a retrial of low-dose clozapine. *Clin Psychopharmacol Neurosci* 2022; **20**:578–580.

133. Goh JG, et al. A case report of clozapine continuation after pulmonary embolism in the context of other risk factors for thromboembolism. *Aust N Z J Psychiatry* 2016; **50**:1205–1206.

134. Munoli RN, et al. Clozapine-induced recurrent pulmonary thromboembolism. *J Neuropsychiatry Clin Neurosci* 2013; **25**:E50–E51.

135. Selten JP, et al. Clozapine and venous thromboembolism: further evidence. *J Clin Psychiatry* 2003; **64**:609.

136. Manoubi SA, et al. Fatal pulmonary embolism in patients on antipsychotics: case series, systematic review and meta-analysis. *Asian J Psychiatr* 2022; **73**:103105.

137. Mouaffak F, et al. Clozapine-induced serositis: review of its clinical features, pathophysiology and management strategies. *Clin Neuropharmacol* 2009; **32**:219–223.

138. Bonnet U, et al. Late-onset polyserositis emerging during long-term clozapine treatment and persisting after clozapine discontinuation: is clozapine really innocent? *J Clin Psychopharmacol* 2022; **42**:106–107.

Clozapine: serious haematological adverse effects

Agranulocytosis

Clozapine is a somewhat toxic drug. Despite this, clozapine reduces overall mortality in schizophrenia,[1] in part owing to a reduction in the rate of suicide.[2-4] Non-clozapine antipsychotics also reduce natural-cause mortality,[5] possibly because of improved adherence to cardiometabolic medication.[6] Clozapine is more effective than any other antipsychotic in this regard.[6]

Clozapine can cause serious, life-threatening adverse effects, of which **agranulocytosis** is the best known, and which is seen in 0.4% of patients.[7] The incidence of death related to agranulocytosis following clozapine prescription is 0.013%, with a case fatality rate for agranulocytosis of 2.1%.[8] Risk is clearly well managed by the approved clozapine monitoring systems. The incidence of severe neutropenia declines to negligible levels after the first year of treatment.[8]

Successful rechallenge after neutropenia occurring during clozapine treatment may be possible,[9] but rechallenge should not be attempted after confirmed clozapine-related agranulocytosis.[10] Most neutropenia occurring in the context of clozapine treatment is coincidental to the use of clozapine.[11] Distinguishing between benign, clinically insignificant neutropenia and clozapine-related life-threatening agranulocytosis (CRLTA) is vital. CRLTA is usually characterised by a continuous and rapid neutrophil count decline to zero, or near zero, mostly within the first 18 weeks of clozapine treatment. A prolonged nadir and delayed recovery (range 4–16 days) follow[12] unless GCSF is given. Non-CRLTA episodes are more often brief, show a non-continuous and/or slow decline in neutrophils, or have an obvious cause that is not clozapine.[12,13] However, if clozapine is withdrawn very early, the typical catastrophic fall in neutrophil counts may not develop.[13] Distinguishing between non-clozapine-related neutropenia and CRLTA is difficult, but cases can usually reliably be classified as non-CRLTA, possible CRLTA and definite CRLTA.

The mandatory threshold-based method of detecting agranulocytosis has a very low specificity for CRLTA – the system creates a huge number of false positives. Pattern-based criteria based on the above factors are more specific without loss of sensitivity.[14] Misdiagnosing benign neutropenia as CRLTA has resulted in many thousands of patients being denied access to clozapine.[11] The most common reason for misdiagnosis is the failure to detect BEN.[15]

Summary

- Overall mortality is lower for those on clozapine than in schizophrenia as a whole.
- Risk of fatal agranulocytosis is less than 1 in 8,000 during standard monitoring.
- Real clozapine-related agranulocytosis usually follows a distinctive, catastrophic pattern.
- Pattern-based criteria are more specific for clozapine-related agranulocytosis than standard threshold-based monitoring.

CHAPTER 1

References

1. Vermeulen JM, et al. Clozapine and long-term mortality risk in patients with schizophrenia: a systematic review and meta-analysis of studies lasting 1.1–12.5 years. *Schizophr Bull* 2019; **45**:315–329.

2. Walker AM, et al. Mortality in current and former users of clozapine. *Epidemiology* 1997; **8**:671–677.

3. van der Zalm Y, et al. Clozapine and mortality: a comparison with other antipsychotics in a nationwide Danish cohort study. *Acta Psychiatr Scand* 2021; **143**:216–226.

4. Munro J, et al. Active monitoring of 12760 clozapine recipients in the UK and Ireland. *Br J Psychiatry* 1999; **175**:576–580.

5. Correll CU, et al. Mortality in people with schizophrenia: a systematic review and meta-analysis of relative risk and aggravating or attenuating factors. *World Psychiatry* 2022; **21**:248–271.

6. Solmi M, et al. Antipsychotics use is associated with greater adherence to cardiometabolic medications in patients with schizophrenia: results from a nationwide, within-subject design study. *Schizophr Bull* 2022; **48**:166–175.

7. Li XH, et al. The prevalence of agranulocytosis and related death in clozapine-treated patients: a comprehensive meta-analysis of observational studies. *Psychol Med* 2020; **50**:583–594.

8. Myles N, et al. Meta-analysis examining the epidemiology of clozapine-associated neutropenia. *Acta Psychiatr Scand* 2018; **138**:101–109.

9. Prokopez CR, et al. Clozapine rechallenge after neutropenia or leucopenia. *J Clin Psychopharmacol* 2016; **36**:377–380.

10. Manu P, et al. Clozapine rechallenge after major adverse effects: clinical guidelines based on 259 cases. *Am J Ther* 2018; **25**:e218–e223.

11. Oloyede E, et al. There is life after the UK Clozapine Central Non-Rechallenge Database. *Schizophr Bull* 2021; **47**:1088–1098.

12. Taylor D, et al. Distinctive pattern of neutrophil count change in clozapine-associated, life-threatening agranulocytosis. *Schizophrenia (Heidelb)* 2022; **8**:21.

13. Taylor D, et al. Severe neutropenia unrelated to clozapine in patients receiving clozapine. *J Psychopharmacol* 2024; **38**:624–635.

14. Oloyede E, et al. Identifying clinically relevant agranulocytosis in people registered on the UK clozapine Central Non-Rechallenge Database: retrospective cohort study. *Br J Psychiatry* 2024; **225**:484–491.

15. Oloyede E, et al. Benign ethnic neutropenia: an analysis of prevalence, timing and identification accuracy in two large inner-city NHS hospitals. *BMC Psychiatry* 2021; **21**:502.

Clozapine: serious cardiovascular adverse effects

Thromboembolism

Over 30 years ago a possible association between clozapine and thromboembolism was first suggested.[1,2] Later, data from Sweden[3] suggested the risk of thromboembolism was 1 in 2,000 to 1 in 6,000 patients treated.

Thromboembolism may be related to clozapine's effects on antiphospholipid antibodies[4] and platelet aggregation.[5] It seems most likely to occur in the first 6 months of treatment[6] but can occur at any time. The risk may be independent of dose,[6] but some studies suggest a correlation with higher doses.[7] Other antipsychotics are also strongly linked to thromboembolism,[8] although clozapine may present the highest risk.[7,9]

With all drugs, the causes of thromboembolism are probably multifactorial.[10] Sedation may lead to a reduction in movement and consequent venous stasis. Obesity, hyperprolactinaemia and smoking are additional independent risk factors for thromboembolism.[11,12] Encouraging exercise and ensuring good hydration are essential precautionary measures.[13]

Myocarditis

Clozapine is associated with **myocarditis** and **cardiomyopathy**. Myocarditis is a hypersensitivity response to clozapine, resulting in inflammation of the myocardium. Some debate surrounds the prevalence of myocarditis, with several Australian studies reporting an incidence of 3%[14-16] and one finding a rate of 9.8%.[17] Studies conducted outside Australia[18-20] have suggested an incidence of 1% or less. The reason for such variation is unclear but it may be that a lack of robust monitoring leads to missed diagnoses in those countries reporting lower incidences.[21] Geography, environment and higher starting doses may also play a role.[17,22] A 2020 meta-analysis suggested an event rate of less than 1% – 7/1,000 patients.[23]

Myocarditis is potentially fatal (case fatality rate of 12.7%)[23] and is most likely to occur in the first 6–8 weeks of starting clozapine treatment (median 3 weeks),[24] but may occur at any time.

Despite uncertainty over incidence, all patients should be closely monitored for signs and symptoms of myocarditis especially in the first few months of treatment.[25] Symptoms include hypotension, tachycardia, fever, flu-like symptoms, fatigue, dyspnoea (with increased respiratory rate) and chest pain.[26] Signs include ECG changes (ST depression), enlarged heart on radiography/echo and eosinophilia. Many of these symptoms occur in patients on clozapine not developing myocarditis[27] and, conversely, their absence does not rule out myocarditis.[28,29] Nonetheless, signs of heart failure should provoke immediate cessation of clozapine and referral to a cardiologist.

Rechallenge has been successfully completed[29-36] (the use of beta blockers, ACE inhibitors and mineralocorticoid receptor antagonists may help)[37-39] but recurrence is also possible.[29,40-43] Published cases suggest a success rate of 62%.[44] Use of echocardiography, measurement of CRP and troponin are obviously absolutely essential in cases of rechallenge.[45-47] Effective treatment of comorbid metabolic syndrome and diabetes may also help.[23] Most cases of successful rechallenge employ a very slow rate of titration.[44] One proposed schedule is to limit dose increases to 6.25mg increments every

4 days until a daily dose of 75mg is reached.[22] Dose increases (of 6.25mg) can then be made every 3 days after this point, and every 2 days after reaching a daily dose of 150mg.

Autopsy findings suggest that fatal myocarditis can occur in the absence of clear cardiac symptoms, although tachycardia and fever are usually present.[48] A monitoring programme which is said to detect 100% of symptomatic cases of myocarditis[49] using measurement of troponin I or T and CRP has been developed (Table 1.56). The additional measuring of NT-proBNP (an indicator of cardiac failure) and continuing cardiac and blood marker monitoring for 8 weeks have also been suggested[50] (5-8% of cases occur in the second month of treatment,[50,51] almost all of these in weeks four to six).[52] Echocardiography at baseline, 6 months and yearly thereafter is routine practice in Australia, although the benefit of this monitoring in the absence of other symptoms has been questioned.[53] Baseline echocardiography may at least be useful to establish a comparator if concerns arise later, especially in those with known cardiac disease, structural abnormalities or other cardiac risk factors.[54] The absence of resources to provide monitoring beyond routine blood tests (including CRP and troponin) and ECG should not be a barrier to prescribing for most patients.[20]

Factors that may increase the risk of developing myocarditis include rapid titration, concurrent use of sodium valproate[55] and older age (31% increased risk for each additional decade).[56] Other psychotropics, including lithium, risperidone, haloperidol, chlorpromazine and fluphenazine, have also been associated with myocarditis.[57] It is probably preferable to avoid concomitant use of other medicines that may contribute to the risk, but this may be practically difficult. Any pre-existing cardiac disorder, previous cardiac event, use of illicit drugs[15] or family history of cardiac disease should provoke extra caution.

Cardiomyopathy

Cardiomyopathy is usually diagnosed from echocardiography to establish left ventricular dilatation (resulting in a reduced ejection fraction) and/or hypertrophy. It may develop following myocarditis (if clozapine is not stopped), but other causative factors may include persistent tachycardia, obesity, diabetes and previous personal or familial cardiac events.[21] Long-term clozapine seems to induce cardiac myocyte autophagy and structural remodelling of the heart.[58] Most incidence data originate from Australia and range from 0.02 to 5%.[16,59] Meta-analysis suggests an event rate of 6 per 1,000 patients, with a case fatality rate of 7.8%.[23] Cardiomyopathy occurs later in treatment than myocarditis (median 9 months)[24] but, as with myocarditis, it may occur at any time. Cardiomyopathy should be suspected in any patient showing signs of heart failure, which should provoke immediate cessation of clozapine and referral. Presentation of cardiomyopathy varies somewhat[60,61] and is often asymptomatic in the early stages,[16] so any reported symptoms of palpitations, chest pain, syncope, sweating, decreased exercise capacity or breathing difficulties should be closely investigated. Successful rechallenge with rigorous cardiac monitoring (including ECHO) and instigation of disease-modifying cardiac medications may be possible,[39,62–66] including in cases of pre-existing cardiomyopathy or heart failure (as opposed to clozapine-induced cardiomyopathy).

Despite an overall reduction in mortality, younger patients may have an increased risk of sudden death,[67] perhaps because of clozapine-induced ECG changes.[68] There may, of course, be similar problems with other antipsychotics.[57,69,70]

Table 1.56 Suggested monitoring for myocarditis.[22,49,71,72]

Baseline*	Pulse, BP, temperature, respiratory rate
	FBC
	CRP
	Troponin
	Echocardiography (if available)
	ECG
Daily, if possible	Pulse, BP, temperature, respiratory rate
	Ask about: chest pain, fever, cough, shortness of breath, exercise capacity
On days 7, 14, 21, and 28	CRP
	Troponin
	FBC
	ECG if possible
If CRP >100mg/L or troponin > twice upper limit of normal	Stop clozapine; repeat echo
	NT-proBNP
If fever + tachycardia* + raised CRP or troponin (but not as above)	Daily CRP and troponin measures
	NT-proBNP

*Tachycardia is not a good indicator of myocarditis – almost all cases have tachycardia, but tachycardia is very common in people who do not have myocarditis.[52]

CRP, C-reactive protein; NT-proBNP, N-terminal pro b-type brain natriuretic peptide.

References

1. Paciullo CA. Evaluating the association between clozapine and venous thromboembolism. *Am J Health Syst Pharm* 2008; **65**:1825–1829.
2. Walker AM, et al. Mortality in current and former users of clozapine. *Epidemiology* 1997; **8**:671–677.
3. Hagg S, et al. Association of venous thromboembolism and clozapine. *Lancet* 2000; **355**:1155–1156.
4. Davis S, et al. Antiphospholipid antibodies associated with clozapine treatment. *Am J Hematol* 1994; **46**:166–167.
5. Axelsson S, et al. In vitro effects of antipsychotics on human platelet adhesion and aggregation and plasma coagulation. *Clin Exp Pharmacol Physiol* 2007; **34**:775–780.
6. Sarvaiya N, et al. Clozapine-associated pulmonary embolism: a high-mortality, dose-independent and early-onset adverse effect. *Am J Ther* 2018; **25**:e434–e438.
7. Allenet B, et al. Antipsychotic drugs and risk of pulmonary embolism. *Pharmacoepidemiol Drug Saf* 2012; **21**:42–48.
8. Huang J, et al. Association between antipsychotics and pulmonary embolism: a pharmacovigilance analysis. *Expert Opin Drug Saf* 2024; doi: 10.1080/14740338.2024.2396390.
9. Dai L, et al. The association and influencing factors between antipsychotics exposure and the risk of VTE and PE: a systematic review and meta-analysis. *Curr Drug Targets* 2020; **21**:930–942.
10. Lacut K. Association between antipsychotic drugs, antidepressant drugs, and venous thromboembolism. *Clin Adv Hematol Oncol* 2008; **6**:887–890.
11. Masopust J, et al. Risk of venous thromboembolism during treatment with antipsychotic agents. *Psychiatry Clin Neurosci* 2012; **66**:541–552.
12. Jonsson AK, et al. Venous thromboembolism in recipients of antipsychotics: incidence, mechanisms and management. *CNS Drugs* 2012; **26**:649–662.
13. Maly R, et al. Assessment of risk of venous thromboembolism and its possible prevention in psychiatric patients. *Psychiatry Clin Neurosci* 2008; **62**:3–8.
14. Ronaldson KJ. Cardiovascular disease in clozapine-treated patients: evidence, mechanisms and management. *CNS Drugs* 2017; **31**:777–795.
15. Khan AA, et al. Clozapine and incidence of myocarditis and sudden death: long term Australian experience. *Int J Cardiol* 2017; **238**:136–139.
16. Youssef DL, et al. Incidence and risk factors for clozapine-induced myocarditis and cardiomyopathy at a regional mental health service in Australia. *Australas Psychiatry* 2016; **24**:176–180.
17. Tirupati S, et al. High rates of myocarditis with clozapine in the Hunter region of Australia. *Schizophr Res* 2024; **264**:543–548.
18. Cohen D, et al. Beyond white blood cell monitoring: screening in the initial phase of clozapine therapy. *J Clin Psychiatry* 2012; **73**:1307–1312.
19. Kilian JG, et al. Myocarditis and cardiomyopathy associated with clozapine. *Lancet* 1999; **354**:1841–1845.
20. Freudenreich O. Clozapine-induced myocarditis: prescribe safely but do prescribe. *Acta Psychiatr Scand* 2015; **132**:240–241.
21. Ronaldson KJ, et al. Clozapine-induced myocarditis, a widely overlooked adverse reaction. *Acta Psychiatr Scand* 2015; **132**:231–240.
22. Qubad M, et al. When, why and how to re-challenge clozapine in schizophrenia following myocarditis. *CNS Drugs* 2024; **38**:671–696.
23. Siskind D, et al. Systematic review and meta-analysis of rates of clozapine-associated myocarditis and cardiomyopathy. *Aust N Z J Psychiatry* 2020; **54**:467–481.
24. La Grenade L, et al. Myocarditis and cardiomyopathy associated with clozapine use in the United States [Letter]. *N Engl J Med* 2001; **345**:224–225.
25. Marder SR, et al. Physical health monitoring of patients with schizophrenia. *Am J Psychiatry* 2004; **161**:1334–1349.
26. Annamraju S, et al. Early recognition of clozapine-induced myocarditis. *J Clin Psychopharmacol* 2007; **27**:479–483.
27. Wehmeier PM, et al. Chart review for potential features of myocarditis, pericarditis, and cardiomyopathy in children and adolescents treated with clozapine. *J Child Adolesc Psychopharmacol* 2004; **14**:267–271.
28. McNeil JJ, et al. Clozapine-induced myocarditis: characterisation using case-control design. *Eur Heart J* 2013; **34** Suppl 1:688.
29. Richardson N, et al. Clozapine-induced myocarditis and patient outcomes after drug rechallenge following myocarditis: a systematic case review. *Psychiatry Res* 2021; **305**:114247.
30. Reinders J, et al. Clozapine-related myocarditis and cardiomyopathy in an Australian metropolitan psychiatric service. *Aust N Z J Psychiatry* 2004; **38**:915–922.
31. Manu P, et al. Clozapine rechallenge after major adverse effects: clinical guidelines based on 259 cases. *Am J Ther* 2018; **25**:e218–e223.
32. Bellissima BL, et al. A systematic review of clozapine-induced myocarditis. *Int J Cardiol* 2018; **259**:122–129.
33. Nguyen B, et al. Successful clozapine re-challenge following myocarditis. *Australas Psychiatry* 2017; **25**:385–386.
34. Otsuka Y, et al. Clozapine-induced myocarditis: follow-up for 3.5 years after successful retrial. *J Gen Fam Med* 2019; **20**:114–117.
35. Noël MC, et al. Clozapine-related myocarditis and rechallenge: a case series and clinical review. *J Clin Psychopharmacol* 2019; **39**:380–385.
36. Hosseini SA, et al. Successful clozapine re-challenge after suspected clozapine-induced myocarditis. *Am J Case Rep* 2020; **21**:e926507.
37. Rostagno C, et al. Beta-blocker and angiotensin-converting enzyme inhibitor may limit certain cardiac adverse effects of clozapine. *Gen Hosp Psychiatry* 2008; **30**:280–283.
38. Floreani J, et al. Successful re-challenge with clozapine following development of clozapine-induced cardiomyopathy. *Aust N Z J Psychiatry* 2008; **42**:747–748.
39. Patel RK, et al. Clozapine and cardiotoxicity: a guide for psychiatrists written by cardiologists. *Psychiatry Res* 2019; **282**:112491.

40. Roh S, et al. Cardiomyopathy associated with clozapine. *Exp Clin Psychopharmacol* 2006; **14**:94–98.

41. Masopust J, et al. Repeated occurrence of clozapine-induced myocarditis in a patient with schizoaffective disorder and comorbid Parkinson's disease. *Neuro Endocrinol Lett* 2009; **30**:19–21.

42. Ronaldson KJ, et al. Observations from 8 cases of clozapine rechallenge after development of myocarditis. *J Clin Psychiatry* 2012; **73**:252–254.

43. Nielsen J, et al. Termination of clozapine treatment due to medical reasons: when is it warranted and how can it be avoided? 2013; **74**: 603–613; quiz 613.

44. Holden J, et al. Successful rechallenge after clozapine-associated myocarditis. *BMJ Case Rep* 2022; **15**:e248909.

45. Hassan I, et al. Monitoring in clozapine rechallenge after myocarditis. *Australas Psychiatry* 2011; **19**:370–371.

46. Bray A, et al. Successful clozapine rechallenge after acute myocarditis. *Aust N Z J Psychiatry* 2011; **45**:90.

47. Rosenfeld AJ, et al. Successful clozapine retrial after suspected myocarditis. *Am J Psychiatry* 2010; **167**:350–351.

48. Ronaldson KJ, et al. Clinical course and analysis of ten fatal cases of clozapine-induced myocarditis and comparison with 66 surviving cases. *Schizophr Res* 2011; **128**:161–165.

49. Ronaldson KJ, et al. A new monitoring protocol for clozapine-induced myocarditis based on an analysis of 75 cases and 94 controls. *Aust N Z J Psychiatry* 2011; **45**:458–465.

50. Griffin JM, et al. Clozapine-associated myocarditis: a protocol for monitoring upon clozapine initiation and recommendations for how to conduct a clozapine rechallenge. *J Clin Psychopharmacol* 2021; **41**:180–185.

51. De Las Cuevas C, et al. Clozapine-associated myocarditis in the World Health Organization's pharmacovigilance database: focus on reports from various countries. *Rev Psiquiatr Salud Ment (Engl Ed)* 2022; **15**:238–250.

52. Segev A, et al. Clozapine-induced myocarditis: electronic health register analysis of incidence, timing, clinical markers and diagnostic accuracy. *Br J Psychiatry* 2021; **219**:644–651.

53. Robinson G, et al. Echocardiography and clozapine: is current clinical practice inhibiting use of a potentially life-transforming therapy? *Aust Fam Physician* 2017; **46**:169–170.

54. Knoph KN, et al. Clozapine-induced cardiomyopathy and myocarditis monitoring: a systematic review. *Schizophr Res* 2018; **199**:17–30.

55. Vickers M, et al. Risk factors for clozapine-induced myocarditis and cardiomyopathy: a systematic review and meta-analysis. *Acta Psychiatr Scand* 2022; **145**:442–455.

56. Ronaldson KJ, et al. Rapid clozapine dose titration and concomitant sodium valproate increase the risk of myocarditis with clozapine: a case-control study. *Schizophr Res* 2012; **141**:173–178.

57. Coulter DM, et al. Antipsychotic drugs and heart muscle disorder in international pharmacovigilance: data mining study. *BMJ* 2001; **322**:1207–1209.

58. Zhang S, et al. Exploration of clozapine-induced cardiomyopathy and its mechanism. *Cardiovasc Toxicol* 2024; **24**:1192–1203.

59. Curto M, et al. Systematic review of clozapine cardiotoxicity. *Curr Psychiatry Rep* 2016; **18**:68.

60. Pastor CA, et al. Masked clozapine-induced cardiomyopathy. *J Am Board Fam Med* 2008; **21**:70–74.

61. Sagar R, et al. Clozapine-induced cardiomyopathy presenting as panic attacks. *J Psychiatr Pract* 2008; **14**:182–185.

62. Nederlof M, et al. Clozapine re-exposure after dilated cardiomyopathy. *BMJ Case Rep* 2017; **2017**:bcr2017219652.

63. Alawami M, et al. A systematic review of clozapine induced cardiomyopathy. *Int J Cardiol* 2014; **176**:315–320.

64. Williams F, et al. Continuing clozapine treatment after a diagnosis of cardiomyopathy. *Ir J Psychol Med* 2021; **38**:227–231.

65. Grover S, et al. Safe use of clozapine in a patient with treatment resistant schizophrenia with co-morbid dilated cardiomyopathy: a case report. *Asian J Psychiatr* 2022; **68**:102971.

66. Whiskey E, et al. Resolution without discontinuation: heart failure during clozapine treatment. *Ther Adv Psychopharmacol* 2020; **10**:2045125320924786.

67. Modai I, et al. Sudden death in patients receiving clozapine treatment: a preliminary investigation. *J Clin Psychopharmacol* 2000; **20**:325–327.

68. Kang UG, et al. Electrocardiographic abnormalities in patients treated with clozapine. *J Clin Psychiatry* 2000; **61**:441–446.

69. Thomassen R, et al. Antipsychotic drugs and venous thromboembolism [Letter]. *Lancet* 2000; **356**:252.

70. Hagg S, et al. Antipsychotic-induced venous thromboembolism: a review of the evidence. *CNS Drugs* 2002; **16**:765–776.

71. Ronaldson KJ, et al. Diagnostic characteristics of clozapine-induced myocarditis identified by an analysis of 38 cases and 47 controls. *J Clin Psychiatry* 2010; **71**:976–981.

72. Yuen JWY, et al. Clozapine-induced cardiovascular side effects and autonomic dysfunction: a systematic review. *Front Neurosci* 2018; **12**:203.

Clozapine-induced hypersalivation

Clozapine is well known to be causally associated with hypersalivation (sialorrhoea):[1] excess salivary pooling in the mouth and drooling, particularly at night. Hypersalivation is dose-[2] and plasma concentration-related[3] but some degree of excess salvation may be seen in the vast majority of patients.[4] Clinical observation suggests that hypersalivation reduces in severity somewhat over time (usually several months) but normally persists to some extent.

Clozapine-induced hypersalivation is socially embarrassing and discomfiting, has a negative impact on quality of life[4] and is often a reason for patients stopping clozapine treatment.[5] Further, hypersalivation has been implicated as a contributory factor in the development of aspiration pneumonia and so is potentially life-threatening.[6–10] Effective treatment is a matter of some urgency.

The pharmacological basis of clozapine-related hypersalivation remains unclear.[11] Suggested mechanisms include muscarinic M_4 agonism, adrenergic α_2 antagonism, and inhibition of the swallowing reflex.[12,13] The last of these is supported by trials which suggest that saliva production is not increased in patients treated with clozapine,[14,15] although at least one study has observed marked increases in salivary flow in the first 3 weeks of treatment.[16]

Whatever the mechanism, medications that reduce saliva production might be expected to diminish the severity of clozapine-induced sialorrhoea. However, there are no medications licensed for this condition and many of the relevant published studies have limitations that preclude any confident treatment recommendations.[17] A 2023 network analysis of RCTs testing a range of pharmacological interventions for clozapine-induced sialorrhoea in adults[18] yielded 'low confidence' findings of efficacy, ranking metoclopramide highest, and decreasing through cyproheptadine, sulpiride, propantheline, diphenhydramine, benzhexol, doxepin, amisulpride, chlorpheniramine, to amitriptyline and atropine. Overall, the evidence, such as it is, seems to favour antimuscarinic agents, such as propantheline and diphenhydramine.[19,20] Use of antimuscarinic agents should take account of the risk of compounding clozapine's liability for serious, potentially life-threatening, gastrointestinal hypomotility.[21,22] Topical antimuscarinic treatment might be preferred. Several topical agents have been shown to be effective and a small RCT of sofpironium bromide gel in 2023 produced encouraging results.[23] In 2024, another small RCT[24] found topical atropine to be more effective than amitriptyline and ipratropium bromide nasal spray. Metoclopramide and other benzamide compounds are probably second-line treatments.[25]

Table 1.57 describes pharmacological treatments that have been examined. Non-drug treatments may be used if appropriate – these include chewing gum during the day, elevating pillows and placing a towel on the pillow to prevent soaking.[11] Nonetheless, problematic hypersalivation should not be considered an inevitable consequence of clozapine use and strenuous efforts should be made to minimise its severity.

Table 1.57 Clozapine-related hypersalivation – summary.

Treatment	Comments
Amisulpride 100–400mg/day[20,26,27]	Supported by a positive RCT compared with placebo, one other in which it was compared with moclobemide and numerous case studies.[28–32] May allow dose reduction of clozapine.
Amitriptyline 25–100 mg/day[33–36]	Limited literature support. Adverse effects may be troublesome. Worsens constipation.
Atropine given sublingually[37–41] or as solution (1mg/10mL) used as a mouthwash	Limited literature support and the benefit–risk balance is uncertain, although case reports suggest that it may be a relatively effective and tolerable treatment for some patients in clinical practice[41,42] and a 2024 RCT yielded positive findings.[24] But one meta-analysis[18] failed to find atropine superior to placebo for nocturnal sialorrhoea. Problems with administration have been reported.[43]
Benzhexol (trihexyphenidyl) 5–15mg/day[44]	Small, open study suggests useful activity. Used in some centres but may impair cognitive function. Lower doses (2mg) may be effective.[45]
Benztropine 2mg/day + terazosin 2mg/day[46]	Combination shown to be better than either drug alone. Terazosin is an α_1 antagonist so may cause hypotension.
Botulinum toxin[47–50] (Botox) bilateral parotid gland injections (150IU into each gland)	Effective in treating sialorrhoea associated with neurological disorders. Six cases of successful treatment of clozapine-related hypersalivation in the literature. Widely used in some US centres. Slow onset of effect. Some botulinum preparations are formally licensed for chronic sialorrhoea caused by neurological conditions in adults.
Bupropion 100–150mg/day[51]	Single case report. May lower seizure threshold.
Chlorphenamine[20]	Antihistamine and relatively weak antimuscarinic. One high-quality study.
Clonidine 0.1–0.2mg patch weekly or 0.1mg orally at night[52,53]	α_2 partial agonist. Limited literature support. May exacerbate psychosis, depression and cause hypotension.
Diphenhydramine[19,20]	Antihistamine and potent antimuscarinic. Few high-quality studies.
Glycopyrrolate 0.5–4mg bd[54–59]	One RCT showed glycopyrrolate to be more effective than biperiden without worsening cognitive function while another found significant clinical improvement of 'nocturnal sialorrhoea' with 2mg a day, compared with placebo. May worsen constipation.
Guanfacine 1mg/day[60]	α_2 agonist. Single case report. May cause hypotension.
Hyoscine 0.3mg tablet sucked or chewed up to three times daily or 1.5mg/72 hr patch[61–64]	Hyoscine hydrobromide is a peripheral and central anticholinergic that is commonly prescribed for clozapine-induced hypersalivation,[59] but in the UK is an unlicensed use.[65] There is one double-blind RCT.[53] May cause cognitive impairment, drowsiness and worsen constipation.
Ipratropium nasal spray (0.03% or 0.06%) given sublingually up to two sprays three times a day of the 0.06% or intranasally, one spray into each nostril daily of the 0.03%[66,67]	Limited literature support. The only placebo-controlled RCT conducted was negative.[68]
Lofexidine 0.2 mg twice daily[69]	α_2 agonist. Very few data. May exacerbate psychosis, depression and cause hypotension.

(Continued)

Table 1.57 (Continued)

Treatment	Comments
Metoclopramide Starting dose of 10mg/day[20,70,71]	Double-blind, RCT trial found metoclopramide was associated with a significant reduction in nocturnal hypersalivation and drooling. Described as an 'effective and tolerated' treatment in cases in clinical practice.[72]
Moclobemide 150–300mg/day[45]	Effective in 9 of 14 patients treated in one open study. Appears to be as effective as amisulpride (see above).
N–acetylcysteine[73]	An antioxidant that also modulates glutamatergic, neurotrophic and inflammatory pathways. Small case series reported with significant decrease in sialorrhea.
Oxybutynin 5mg up to twice daily[74]	Single case report
Pirenzepine 50–150mg/day[75–77]	Selective M_1, M_4 antagonist. Extensive clinical experience suggests efficacy in some but only randomised trial suggested no effect. Still widely used. Does not have a UK or US licence for any indication. May cause constipation.
Propantheline 7.5mg at night[19,20]	Peripheral anticholinergic. No central effects. Meta-analyses of relevant trials have found that propantheline outperforms placebo for the treatment of antipsychotic-induced sialorrhoea.[18–20] May worsen constipation.
Quetiapine[51]	May reduce hypersalivation by allowing lower doses of clozapine to be used
Sofpironium bromide 5% gel[23]	A small RCT reported a 40% reduction in saliva flow at 4 weeks. Very limited availability – Japan only.
Sulpiride 150–300mg/day[20,78–80]	Supported by one, small positive RCT and a Cochrane review of clozapine augmentation with sulpiride (at higher sulpiride doses). May allow dose reduction of clozapine.

References

1. Man WH, et al. Reporting patterns of sialorrhea comparing users of clozapine to users of other antipsychotics: a disproportionality analysis using VigiBase. *J Clin Psychopharmacol* 2020; 40:283–286.
2. Subramanian S, et al. Clozapine dose for schizophrenia. *Cochrane Database Syst Rev* 2017; 6:CD009555.
3. Schoretsanitis G, et al. Elevated clozapine concentrations in clozapine-treated patients with hypersalivation. *Clin Pharmacokinet* 2021; 60:329–335.
4. Sanagustin D, et al. Prevalence of clozapine-induced sialorrhea and its effect on quality of life. *Psychopharmacology (Berl)* 2023; 240:203–211.
5. Grover S, et al. Patient and caregivers perspective about clozapine: a systematic review. *Schizophr Res* 2024; 268:223–232.
6. Hinkes R, et al. Aspiration pneumonia possibly secondary to clozapine-induced sialorrhea. *J Clin Psychopharmacol* 1996; 16:462–463.
7. Saenger RC, et al. Aspiration pneumonia due to clozapine-induced sialorrhea. *Clin Schizophr Relat Psychoses* 2016; 9:170–172.
8. Gurrera RJ, et al. Aspiration pneumonia: an underappreciated risk of clozapine treatment. *J Clin Psychopharmacol* 2016; 36:174–176.
9. Kaplan J, et al. Clozapine-associated aspiration pneumonia: case series and review of the literature. *Psychosomatics* 2017; 58:199–203.
10. Cicala G, et al. A comprehensive review of swallowing difficulties and dysphagia associated with antipsychotics in adults. *Expert Rev Clin Pharmacol* 2019; 12:219–234.
11. Praharaj SK, et al. Clozapine-induced sialorrhea: pathophysiology and management strategies. *Psychopharmacology (Berl)* 2006; 185:265–273.
12. Davydov L, et al. Clozapine-induced hypersalivation. *Ann Pharmacother* 2000; 34:662–665.
13. Rogers DP, et al. Therapeutic options in the treatment of clozapine-induced sialorrhea. *Pharmacotherapy* 2000; 20:1092–1095.
14. Rabinowitz T, et al. The effect of clozapine on saliva flow rate: a pilot study. *Biol Psychiatry* 1996; 40:1132–1134.
15. Ben Aryeh H, et al. Salivary flow-rate and composition in schizophrenic patients on clozapine: subjective reports and laboratory data. *Biol Psychiatry* 1996; 39:946–949.
16. Praharaj SK, et al. Salivary flow rate in patients with schizophrenia on clozapine. *Clin Neuropharmacol* 2010; 33:176–178.
17. Sockalingam S, et al. Review: insufficient evidence to guide use of drugs for clozapine induced hypersalivation. *Evid Based Ment Health* 2009; 12:12.

18. Fornaro M, et al. Pharmacological interventions for antipsychotic-related sialorrhea: a systematic review and network meta-analysis of randomized trials. *Mol Psychiatry* 2023; **28**:3648–3660.

19. Syed R, et al. Pharmacological interventions for clozapine-induced hypersalivation. *Cochrane Database Syst Rev* 2008; (3):CD005579.

20. Chen SY, et al. Treatment strategies for clozapine-induced sialorrhea: a systematic review and meta-analysis. *CNS Drugs* 2019; **33**:225–238.

21. Palmer SE, et al. Life-threatening clozapine-induced gastrointestinal hypomotility: an analysis of 102 cases. *J Clin Psychiatry* 2008; **69**:759–768.

22. West S, et al. Clozapine induced gastrointestinal hypomotility: a potentially life threatening adverse event: a review of the literature. *Gen Hosp Psychiatry* 2017; **46**:32–37.

23. Amano Y, et al. Efficacy of sofpironium bromide gel on clozapine-induced hypersalivation in patients with treatment-resistant schizophrenia: double-blind, controlled crossover study. *BJPsych Open* 2023; **9**:e14.

24. Mohammad-Gholizad F, et al. Evaluation and comparison of the effectiveness of atropine eye drops, ipratropium bromide nasal spray, and amitriptyline tablet in the management of clozapine-associated sialorrhea in patients with refractory schizophrenia: a randomized clinical trial. *J Clin Psychopharmacol* 2024; **44**:9–15.

25. Miodownik C, et al. Treatment of clozapine-associated sialorrhea: the role of benzamide derivatives. *J Clin Psychopharmacol* 2023; **43**:171–177.

26. Kreinin A, et al. Amisulpride treatment of clozapine-induced hypersalivation in schizophrenia patients: a randomized, double-blind, placebo-controlled cross-over study. *Int Clin Psychopharmacol* 2006; **21**:99–103.

27. Kreinin A, et al. Amisulpride versus moclobemide in treatment of clozapine-induced hypersalivation. *World J Biol Psychiatry* 2010; **12**:620–626.

28. Praharaj SK, et al. Amisulpride treatment for clozapine-induced sialorrhea. *J Clin Psychopharmacol* 2009; **29**:189–190.

29. Aggarwal A, et al. Amisulpride for clozapine induced sialorrhea. *Psychopharmacol Bull* 2009; **42**:69–71.

30. Croissant B, et al. Reduction of side effects by combining clozapine with amisulpride: case report and short review of clozapine-induced hypersalivation—a case report. *Pharmacopsychiatry* 2005; **38**:38–39.

31. Praharaj SK, et al. Amisulpride improved debilitating clozapine-induced sialorrhea. *Am J Ther* 2011; **18**:e84–e85.

32. Kulkarni RR. Low-dose amisulpride for debilitating clozapine-induced sialorrhea: case series and review of literature. *Indian J Psychol Med* 2015; **37**:446–448.

33. Copp P, et al. Amitriptyline in clozapine-induced sialorrhoea. *Br J Psychiatry* 1991; **159**:166.

34. Praharaj SK, et al. Amitriptyline for clozapine-induced nocturnal enuresis and sialorrhoea. *Br J Clin Pharmacol* 2007; **63**:128–129.

35. Sinha S, et al. Very low dose amitriptyline for clozapine-associated sialorrhea. *Curr Drug Saf* 2016; **11**:262–263.

36. Cereda G, et al. Amitriptyline for clozapine-induced hypersalivation: a case series. *Schizophr Res* 2022; **243**:110–111.

37. Antonello C, et al. Clozapine and sialorrhea: a new intervention for this bothersome and potentially dangerous side effect. *J Psychiatry Neurosci* 1999; **24**:250.

38. Mustafa FA, et al. Sublingual atropine for the treatment of severe and hyoscine-resistant clozapine-induced sialorrhea. *Afr J Psychiatry* 2013; **16**:242.

39. Matos Santana TE, et al. Sublingual atropine in the treatment of clozapine-induced sialorrhea. *Schizophr Res* 2017; **182**:144–145.

40. Mubaslat O, et al. The effect of sublingual atropine sulfate on clozapine-induced hypersalivation: a multicentre, randomised placebo-controlled trial. *Psychopharmacology (Berl)* 2020; **237**:2905–2915.

41. Van der Poorten T, et al. The sublingual use of atropine in the treatment of clozapine-induced sialorrhea: a systematic review. *Clin Case Rep* 2019; **7**:2108–2113.

42. Mutlu E, et al. A systematic chart review of pharmacological interventions in patients with clozapine-induced hypersalivation. *Schizophr Res* 2024; **268**:138–144.

43. Leung JG, et al. Potential problems surrounding the use of sublingually administered ophthalmic atropine for sialorrhea. *Schizophr Res* 2017; **185**:202–203.

44. Spivak B, et al. Trihexyphenidyl treatment of clozapine-induced hypersalivation. *Int Clin Psychopharmacol* 1997; **12**:213–215.

45. Praharaj SK, et al. Complete resolution of clozapine-induced sialorrhea with low dose trihexyphenidyl. *Psychopharmacol Bull* 2010; **43**:73–75.

46. Reinstein M, et al. Comparative efficacy and tolerability of benzatropine and terazosin in the treatment of hypersalivation secondary to clozapine. *Clin Drug Investig* 1999; **17**:97–102.

47. Kahl KG, et al. Botulinum toxin as an effective treatment of clozapine-induced hypersalivation. *Psychopharmacology (Berl)* 2004; **173**:229–230.

48. Steinlechner S, et al. Botulinum toxin B as an effective and safe treatment for neuroleptic-induced sialorrhea. *Psychopharmacology (Berl)* 2010; **207**:593–597.

49. Kahl KG, et al. [Pharmacological strategies for clozapine-induced hypersalivation: treatment with botulinum toxin B in one patient and review of the literature]. *Nervenarzt* 2005; **76**:205–208.

50. Verma R, et al. Botulinum toxin: a novel therapy for clozapine-induced sialorrhoea. *Psychopharmacology (Berl)* 2018; **235**:369–371.

51. Stern RG, et al. Clozapine-induced sialorrhea alleviated by bupropion: a case report. *Prog Neuropsychopharmacol Biol Psychiatry* 2009; **33**:1578–1580.

52. Grabowski J. Clonidine treatment of clozapine-induced hypersalivation. *J Clin Psychopharmacol* 1992; **12**:69–70.

53. Praharaj SK, et al. Is clonidine useful for treatment of clozapine-induced sialorrhea? *J Psychopharmacol* 2005; **19**:426–428.

54. Duggal HS. Glycopyrrolate for clozapine-induced sialorrhea. *Prog Neuropsychopharmacol Biol Psychiatry* 2007; **31**:1546–1547.

55. Robb AS, et al. Glycopyrrolate for treatment of clozapine-induced sialorrhea in three adolescents. *J Child Adolesc Psychopharmacol* 2008; **18**:99–107.

56. Liang CS, et al. Comparison of the efficacy and impact on cognition of glycopyrrolate and biperiden for clozapine-induced sialorrhea in schizophrenic patients: a randomized, double-blind, crossover study. *Schizophr Res* 2010; **119**:138–144.

57. Man WH, et al. The effect of glycopyrrolate on nocturnal sialorrhea in patients using clozapine: a randomized, crossover, double-blind, placebo-controlled trial. *J Clin Psychopharmacol* 2017; **37**:155–161.

58. Praharaj SK, et al. Low-dose glycopyrrolate for clozapine-associated sialorrhea. *J Clin Psychopharmacol* 2014; **34**:392.

59. Qurashi I, et al. Glycopyrrolate in comparison to hyoscine hydrobromide and placebo in the treatment of hypersalivation induced by clozapine (GOTHIC1): a feasibility study. *Pilot Feasibility Stud* 2019; **5**:79.

60. Webber MA, et al. Guanfacine treatment of clozapine-induced sialorrhea. *J Clin Psychopharmacol* 2004; **24**:675–676.

61. McKane JP, et al. Hyoscine patches in clozapine-induced hypersalivation. *Psychiatr Bull* 2001; **25**:277.

62. Gaftanyuk O, et al. Scolpolamine patch for clozapine-induced sialorrhea. *Psychiatr Serv* 2004; **55**:318.

63. Segev A, et al. Hyoscine for clozapine-induced hypersalivation: a double-blind, randomized, placebo-controlled cross-over trial. *Int Clin Psychopharmacol* 2019; **34**:101–107.

64. Takeuchi I, et al. Effect of scopolamine butylbromide on clozapine-induced hypersalivation in schizophrenic patients: a case series. *Clin Psychopharmacol Neurosci* 2015; **13**:109–112.

65. British National Formulary JFC. Hyoscine hydrobromide – unlicensed use. 2023 (last accessed December 2023); https://bnf.nice.org.uk/drugs/hyoscine-hydrobromide/#unlicensed-use.

66. Calderon J, et al. Potential use of ipatropium bromide for the treatment of clozapine-induced hypersalivation: a preliminary report. *Int Clin Psychopharmacol* 2000; **15**:49–52.

67. Freudenreich O, et al. Clozapine-induced sialorrhea treated with sublingual ipratropium spray: a case series. *J Clin Psychopharmacol* 2004; **24**:98–100.

68. Sockalingam S, et al. Treatment of clozapine-induced hypersalivation with ipratropium bromide: a randomized, double-blind, placebo-controlled crossover study. *J Clin Psychiatry* 2009; **70**:1114–1119.

69. Corrigan FM, et al. Clozapine-induced hypersalivation and the alpha 2 adrenoceptor. *Br J Psychiatry* 1995; **167**:412.

70. Kreinin A, et al. Double-blind, randomized, placebo-controlled trial of metoclopramide for hypersalivation associated with clozapine. *J Clin Psychopharmacol* 2016; **36**:200–205.

71. Hallahan B. Metoclopramide may be effective for clozapine-induced hypersalivation. *Evid Based Ment Health* 2016; **19**:124.

72. Livermore C, et al. A retrospective case notes review of the effectiveness and tolerability of metoclopramide in the treatment of clozapine-induced hypersalivation (CIH). *BMC Psychiatry* 2022; **22**:277.

73. Uzun Ö, et al. Effect of N-acetylcysteine on clozapine-induced sialorrhea in schizophrenic patients: a case series. *Int Clin Psychopharmacol* 2020; **35**:229–231.

74. Leung JG, et al. Immediate-release oxybutynin for the treatment of clozapine-induced sialorrhea. *Ann Pharmacother* 2011; **45**:e45.

75. Fritze J, et al. Pirenzepine for clozapine-induced hypersalivation. *Lancet* 1995; **346**:1034.

76. Bai YM, et al. Therapeutic effect of pirenzepine for clozapine-induced hypersalivation: a randomized, double-blind, placebo-controlled, crossover study. *J Clin Psychopharmacol* 2001; **21**:608–611.

77. Schneider B, et al. Reduction of clozapine-induced hypersalivation by pirenzepine is safe. *Pharmacopsychiatry* 2004; **37**:43–45.

78. Kreinin A, et al. Sulpiride addition for the treatment of clozapine-induced hypersalivation: preliminary study. *Isr J Psychiatry Relat Sci* 2005; **42**:61–63.

79. Wang J, et al. Sulpiride augmentation for schizophrenia. *Cochrane Database Syst Rev* 2010; (1):CD008125.

80. Prljača E, et al. Clozapine-induced hypersalivation treated with sulpiride: is it a solution? *Psychiatr Danub* 2021; **33**:1230–1232.

Clozapine-induced gastrointestinal hypomotility

Constipation is a common adverse effect of clozapine treatment with a prevalence of more than 30%, three times that seen with other antipsychotics.[1] The mechanism of action is not completely understood but is thought to be a combination of the drug's anticholinergic[2,3] and antihistaminergic properties,[4] which are further complicated by antagonism at 5-HT$_3$ receptors.[2,3,5] In addition, clozapine-induced sedation can result in a sedentary lifestyle,[4] which is itself a risk factor for constipation. Clozapine causes constipation by slowing transit time through the gut. Mean transit times are four times longer than normal and 80% of patients taking clozapine show reduced transit time.[6]

Clozapine-induced GI hypomotility (CIGH) is a much greater risk to life than clozapine-related agranulocytosis.[4] When constipation is severe, the case fatality rate is around 20–30%.[4,7–9] One long-term study[10] found an incidence of 37/10,000 cases of severe hypomotility and 7/10,000 constipation-related deaths. Case fatality was 18%. Enhanced monitoring and effective treatment of CIGH are clearly needed to reduce the likelihood of constipation-related fatality.

A GI history and abdominal examination are recommended prior to starting treatment and, if the patient is constipated, clozapine should not be initiated until this has resolved.[8] CIGH is most severe during the first 4 months of treatment,[8] but may occur at any time. Adopting the Rome III criteria[11] at routine FBCs might be a successful strategy to combat preventable deaths due to CIGH, but even this does not guarantee identification of hypomotility.[12] A study that examined the diagnostic accuracy of constipation screening found self-reporting to have a sensitivity of just 18%. Adding the Rome criteria improved this to 50%, but this means half of cases were still missed.[13]

Opinions differ on the relationship between clozapine dose and constipation, and between clozapine plasma level and constipation.[8,14,15] However, most studies report that deaths that have occurred as a result of CIGH have higher than average daily doses.[8,9,16] Older age, male sex and higher daily doses have been proposed as possible risk factors for death based on case series review[16] and pharmacovigilance database studies (Box 1.4).[9]

Box 1.4 Risk factors for developing clozapine-induced constipation[8,17–20]

- Increasing age
- Female sex
- Anticholinergic medication
- Higher clozapine dose/plasma concentration
- Hypercalcaemia
- GI disease
- Obesity
- Diaphoresis
- Low-fibre diet
- Poor bowel habit
- Dehydration (exacerbated by hypersalivation)
- Diabetes
- Hypothyroidism
- Parkinson's disease
- Multiple sclerosis

Prevention and simple management of CIGH

A slow clozapine titration may reduce the risk of developing constipation, with dose increments not exceeding 25mg/day or 100mg/week.[21] Increasing dietary fibre intake to at least 20–25g/day can increase stool weight but can decrease gut transit time[20,22] (fibre decreases or increases transit time depending on the initial transit time).[23] If fibre intake is increased it is important that adequate fluid intake (1.5–2L/day) is also maintained to avoid intestinal obstruction.[8,20,24] Daily food and fluid charts would be ideal to monitor fibre and fluid intake, especially during the titration phase of clozapine. Regular exercise (150 minutes/week)[25] in addition to a high-fibre diet and increased fluid intake also assists in the prevention of CIGH.[26,27]

Active monitoring of patients, including direct questioning, is essential. Patients often do not self-report even life-threatening constipation.[8] Use of stool charts daily for the first 4 weeks and weekly or monthly thereafter is recommended. If there is a change from usual baseline bowel habit or fewer than three bowel movements a week,[11] an abdominal examination is indicated.[8] Where this excludes intestinal obstruction, both a stimulant and stool-softening laxative should be started, as suggested by the Porirua protocol[28] (for example senna 15mg at night and docusate 100mg three times daily).[8,28,29] Bulk-forming laxatives are not usually effective in slow-transit constipation[2,30] and therefore should be avoided. There is some evidence that lactulose and polyethylene glycol (for example Movicol®) are effective[2,31] and could be considered in addition to the stimulant and softener combination.[28] Most people with CIGH will need a stimulant laxative such as senna or bisacodyl, or both. These should not be withheld on the basis that long-term use of stimulants is usually proscribed. In addition to laxative treatment, a review of the anticholinergic burden of other prescribed medicines should be undertaken. Consideration may be made of reducing the clozapine dose, but this step alone cannot be considered treatment of CIGH – use of laxatives is still essential.

Choice of laxative should also be guided by the patient's previous response to certain agents in association with consideration of the required speed of action. Lactulose takes up to 72 hours of regular use to work,[32] so is of no use for urgent treatment. Stimulant laxatives are usually the fastest acting (6–10 hours). Laxative doses should be increased every 24 hours until resolution of symptoms (usual maximum daily dose of senna is 30mg, bisacodyl 20mg and docusate 500mg). Glycerin or bisacodyl suppositories can be used and are usually effective within 30 minutes but there are no data on their use in CIGH. In fact, published data supporting laxative choice for antipsychotic-related constipation are sparse and of poor quality.[12]

Management of suspected acute CIGH

Up to 30% of patients on long-term clozapine will suffer severe GI hypomotility unless preventative steps are taken.[33] Signs and symptoms that warrant immediate medical attention are abdominal pain, distension, vomiting, overflow diarrhoea, absent bowel sounds, acute abdomen, feculent vomitus and symptoms of sepsis.[7,8,21,34–38] There have been case reports of fatalities occurring only hours after first symptoms present,[39] and this emphasises the urgency for prompt assessment and management (including cessation of clozapine). There should therefore be a low threshold for referral to emergency medical services when conservative management fails or constipation is severe and acute.[8,40]

Clozapine rechallenge following severe constipation

Some patients have been successfully rechallenged following severe cases of CIGH, but this process does not come without risk. Prophylactic measures should be used for those with a history of CIGH or who are deemed high risk of developing CIGH. Minimise the use of other constipating drugs and ensure other modifiable risk factors are addressed (fibre and fluid intake, exercise). Conventional laxatives should be started in regular and adequate doses to prevent constipation from developing. A number of more experimental options are available. Prescribers must familiarise themselves with the literature (at the very least by reading the SPC) before using any of these treatments and involvement of gastrointestinal specialists is encouraged.

Orlistat, a drug used to aid weight loss, is also known to have a laxative effect, particularly when a high-fat diet is consumed. It was reported as being successfully used for three patients with severe constipation associated with opioid use (hypomotility-induced constipation).[41] A small, randomised placebo controlled study of orlistat for clozapine-induced constipation found a favourable difference at study endpoint (week 16) for the prevalence of constipation, diarrhoea and normal stools for orlistat compared with placebo,[42] although 47 of the 54 participants required conventional laxatives. Orlistat is known to reduce the absorption of some drugs from the GI tract. It is therefore important to monitor plasma clozapine levels if starting treatment with orlistat.

Bethanechol, a cholinergic agonist, was effective at 30mg/day in reducing the amount of laxatives and enemas required to maintain regular bowel movements for a patient diagnosed with clozapine-related CIGH.[43] Another case report described use in a patient with a gastrostomy, where up to 200mg/day bethanechol was given to reduce dilation of the bowel.[44] Bethanechol should only ever be initiated after other options have failed and in consultation with a gastroenterologist.[43]

Prucalopride is a $5HT_4$ agonist which increases gut motility and is licensed for chronic constipation where laxatives have failed to provide adequate relief. Case reports of successful use for clozapine-induced constipation have been described,[45,46] and superior efficacy to lactulose for this indication was demonstrated in an open-label study.[47]

Linaclotide (licensed in the UK for constipation in irritable bowel syndrome) and **plecanatide** (available in the USA for chronic idiopathic constipation) are oral guanylate cyclase C agonists. Neither has any published data to date supporting use in antipsychotic-induced constipation, beyond a single case report for linaclotide.[44]

Key message

- Prevent clozapine-related constipation by aggressive use of stimulant laxatives.

References

1. Shirazi A, et al. Prevalence and predictors of clozapine-associated constipation: a systematic review and meta-analysis. *Int J Mol Sci* 2016; 17:863.

2. Hibbard KR, et al. Fatalities associated with clozapine-related constipation and bowel obstruction: a literature review and two case reports. *Psychosomatics* 2009; 50:416–419.

3. Rege S, et al. Life-threatening constipation associated with clozapine. *Australas Psychiatry* 2008; 16:216–219.

4. De Hert M, et al. Second-generation antipsychotics and constipation: a review of the literature. *Eur Psychiatry* 2011; 26:34–44.

5. Meltzer HY, et al. Effects of antipsychotic drugs on serotonin receptors. *Pharmacol Rev* 1991; 43:587–604.

6. Every-Palmer S, et al. Clozapine-treated patients have marked gastrointestinal hypomotility, the probable basis of life-threatening gastrointestinal complications: a cross sectional study. *EBioMedicine* 2016; 5:125–134.

7. Cohen D, et al. Beyond white blood cell monitoring: screening in the initial phase of clozapine therapy. *J Clin Psychiatry* 2012; 73:1307–1312.

8. Palmer SE, et al. Life-threatening clozapine-induced gastrointestinal hypomotility: an analysis of 102 cases. *J Clin Psychiatry* 2008; 69:759–768.

9. Handley SA, et al. Clozapine-induced gastrointestinal hypomotility: presenting features and outcomes, UK pharmacovigilance reports, 1992–2017. *Br J Psychiatry* 2022; 220:355–363.

10. Every-Palmer S, et al. Clozapine-induced gastrointestinal hypomotility: a 22-year bi-national pharmacovigilance study of serious or fatal 'slow gut' reactions, and comparison with international drug safety advice. *CNS Drugs* 2017; 31:699–709.

11. Rome Foundation. Rome IV Disorders and Criteria. 2021 (last accessed October 2024). https://theromefoundation.org.

12. Every-Palmer S, et al. Pharmacological treatment for antipsychotic-related constipation. *Cochrane Database Syst Rev* 2017; 1:CD011128.

13. Every-Palmer S, et al. Constipation screening in people taking clozapine: a diagnostic accuracy study. *Schizophr Res* 2020; 220:179–186.

14. Chengappa KN, et al. Anticholinergic differences among patients receiving standard clinical doses of olanzapine or clozapine. *J Clin Psychopharmacol* 2000; 20:311–316.

15. Vella-Brincat J, et al. Clozapine-induced gastrointestinal hypomotility. *Australas Psychiatry* 2011; 19:450–451.

16. West S, et al. Clozapine induced gastrointestinal hypomotility: a potentially life threatening adverse event: a review of the literature. *Gen Hosp Psychiatry* 2017; 46:32–37.

17. Nielsen J, et al. Termination of clozapine treatment due to medical reasons: when is it warranted and how can it be avoided? *J Clin Psychiatry* 2013; 74:603–613; quiz 613.

18. Nielsen J, et al. Risk factors for ileus in patients with schizophrenia. *Schizophr Bull* 2012; 38:592–598.

19. Longmore M, et al. *Oxford Handbook of Clinical Medicine*. Oxford: Oxford University Press; 2010.

20. ZTAS. Zaponex Fact Sheet – Constipation. 2023 (last accessed February 2025); https://www.ztas.com/PDF/FS_Constipation_jan2023.pdf.

21. Hayes G, et al. Clozapine-induced constipation. *Am J Psychiatry* 1995; 152:298.

22. Muller-Lissner SA. Effect of wheat bran on weight of stool and gastrointestinal transit time: a meta analysis. *Br Med J* 1988; 296:615–617.

23. Harvey RF, et al. Effects of increased dietary fibre on intestinal transit. *Lancet* 1973; 1:1278–1280.

24. National Prescribing Centre. The management of constipation. *Med Rec Bulletin* 2011; 21:1–8.

25. NHS. Exercise. Physical activity guidelines for adults aged 19 to 64. 2024 (last accessed October 2024); https://www.nhs.uk/live-well/exercise.

26. Fitzsimons J, et al. A review of clozapine safety. *Expert Opin Drug Saf* 2005; 4:731–744.

27. Young CR, et al. Management of the adverse effects of clozapine. *Schizophr Bull* 1998; 24:381–390.

28. Every-Palmer S, et al. The Porirua protocol in the treatment of clozapine-induced gastrointestinal hypomotility and constipation: a pre- and post-treatment study. *CNS Drugs* 2017; 31:75–85.

29. Swegle JM, et al. Management of common opioid-induced adverse effects. *Am Fam Physician* 2006; 74:1347–1354.

30. Voderholzer WA, et al. Clinical response to dietary fiber treatment of chronic constipation. *Am J Gastroenterol* 1997; 92:95–98.

31. Brandt LJ, et al. Systematic review on the management of chronic constipation in North America. *Am J Gastroenterol* 2005; 100 Suppl 1:S5–S21.

32. Esteve Pharmaceuticals (formerly Intrapharm Laboratories). Summary of Product Characteristics. Lactulose 10g / 15ml oral solution sachets. 2023 (last accessed October 2024); https://www.medicines.org.uk/emc/medicine/25597.

33. Partanen JJ, et al. High burden of ileus and pneumonia in clozapine-treated individuals with schizophrenia: a Finnish 25-year follow-up register study. *Am J Psychiatry* 2024; 181:879–892.

34. Leong QM, et al. Necrotising colitis related to clozapine? A rare but life threatening side effect. *World J Emerg Surg* 2007; 2:21.

35. Townsend G, et al. Case report: rapidly fatal bowel ischaemia on clozapine treatment. *BMC Psychiatry* 2006; 6:43.

36. Karmacharya R, et al. Clozapine-induced eosinophilic colitis. *Am J Psychiatry* 2005; 162:1386–1387.

37. Erickson B, et al. Clozapine-associated postoperative ileus: case report and review of the literature. *Arch Gen Psychiatry* 1995; 52:508–509.

38. Schwartz BJ, et al. A case report of clozapine-induced gastric outlet obstruction. *Am J Psychiatry* 1993; 150:1563.

39. Drew L, et al. Clozapine and constipation: a serious issue. *Aust N Z J Psychiatry* 1997; 31:149.

40. Ikai S, et al. Reintroduction of clozapine after perforation of the large intestine: a case report and review of the literature. *Ann Pharmacother* 2013; 47:e31.

41. Guarino AH. Treatment of intractable constipation with orlistat: a report of three cases. *Pain Med* 2005; 6:327–328.

42. Chukhin E, et al. In a randomized placebo-controlled add-on study orlistat significantly reduced clozapine-induced constipation. *Int Clin Psychopharmacol* 2013; 28:67–70.

43. Poetter CE, et al. Treatment of clozapine-induced constipation with bethanechol. *J Clin Psychopharmacol* 2013; 33:713–714.

44. Tomulescu S, et al. Managing recurrent clozapine-induced constipation in a patient with resistant schizophrenia. *Case Rep Psychiatry* 2021; 2021:9649334.

45. Thomas N, et al. Prucalopride in clozapine-induced constipation. *Aust N Z J Psychiatry* 2018; 52:804.

46. Hui KO. Prucalopride for the treatment of clozapine induced constipation: a case report. *Juniper Online J Case Stud* 2018; 6:555683.

47. Damodaran I, et al. An open-label, head to head comparison study between prucalopride and lactulose for clozapine induced constipation in patients with treatment resistant schizophrenia. *Healthcare (Basel)* 2020; 8:533.

Clozapine, neutropenia and lithium

Mild neutropenia

Around 3.8% of patients treated with clozapine develop neutropenia.[1] Most of these cases are unrelated to clozapine treatment, and clozapine in fact may not cause neutropenia per se.[2] The risk of neutropenia ($<1.5\times10^9$/L) in patients treated with clozapine is broadly similar to the cross-sectional prevalence of neutropenia in otherwise healthy individuals (0.4–4.5% depending on ethnicity).[3] Indeed, a meta-analysis comparing the risk of neutropenia between clozapine and other antipsychotics found that clozapine did not have a stronger association with neutropenia than other antipsychotic medications.[4]

Most people developing mild neutropenia will not develop severe neutropenia or agranulocytosis. Risk factors for neutropenia include being Afro-Caribbean, younger age and having a low baseline white cell count (WCC).[5] The vast majority of patients who stop clozapine because they have developed neutropenia can be successfully rechallenged.[6] Adopting the US monitoring criteria would eliminate the requirement to discontinue clozapine treatment in cases of mild neutropenia (absolute neutrophil count [ANC] between 1 and 1.5×10^9/L).

Confusion arises because of the various possible reasons for a low neutrophil count in people taking clozapine. A single low count might just be a coincidental finding of no clinical relevance, as is common with all drugs. Several low counts (consecutive or intermittent) might be seen in people with BEN (see below) or as a result of clozapine-associated bone marrow suppression (especially if consecutive and progressively falling). Full-blown agranulocytosis can probably always be interpreted as being the result of severe bone marrow suppression caused by clozapine.

Severe neutropenia or agranulocytosis

The risk of agranulocytosis during clozapine treatment is 1 in 250 (0.4%),[7] lower than previously thought, and risk of death resulting from this is 0.05% – a rare event. Most cases of agranulocytosis develop within the first 18 weeks of treatment. Thereafter, the risk diminishes steeply.[8] The mechanism of clozapine-induced agranulocytosis is not fully understood but is thought to be immune mediated, given the significant association with certain human leucocyte antigen variants.[9]

Identifying with certainty whether an episode of severe neutropenia is clozapine-related may be difficult. However, the pattern of neutrophil count change is important. A single episode of a below-threshold ANC $<0.5\times10^9$/L may be unrelated to clozapine but would normally promptly lead to treatment cessation. In patients without BEN, agranulocytosis is generally preceded by normal neutrophil counts, which are then followed by a precipitous fall in neutrophils (usually over a week or less) and a prolonged period of counts near to zero (assuming that it has not been treated).[10] Neutrophil counts that do not follow this characteristic pattern are difficult to interpret.

The Netherlands Clozapine Collaboration Group[11] considers the risk of agranulocytosis so low that a mentally competent patient may stop routine haematological monitoring after 6 months of treatment. The group still nevertheless recommends low-frequency testing (for example four times a year if routine monitoring is stopped).

Risk factors for agranulocytosis include increasing age and Asian race.[5] Unlike neutropenia, risk of agranulocytosis appears to be higher in people of European ancestry than in those of African descent.[12] Some patients may be genetically predisposed[13] (see section on clozapine: genetic testing for clozapine treatment in this chapter). Although the timescale and individual risk factors for the development of agranulocytosis are different from those associated with neutropenia/coincidental low neutrophil counts, it is difficult to be certain in any given patient that neutropenia is not a precursor to agranulocytosis. However, it is notable that only 30% of confirmed cases of agranulocytosis pass through a neutropenia phase during the precipitous fall in counts.[12]

Haematological monitoring is mandatory to mitigate haematological risk. However, worldwide, there are marked variations in the recommendations for monitoring frequency and the threshold for clozapine cessation,[14] reflecting, perhaps, the weak evidence on which they are based. In 2015, the US FDA introduced changes to the clozapine monitoring system making only the ANC mandatory and effectively lowering the threshold for cessation of clozapine treatment.[15] It is recommended that treatment with clozapine be stopped when neutrophils fall below 1000/mm[16] (compared with UK recommendations for cessation if ANC <1500/mm).[16]

There is evidence that clozapine is grossly under-used worldwide, with very wide variation in prescribing frequency from one country to another.[17] This may be explained at least in part by the stringent blood monitoring requirements. The worldwide outbreak of COVID-19 in 2020 prompted a re-evaluation of clozapine haematological monitoring, with a group proposing a reduction from monthly to 3-monthly for patients who have received clozapine for more than 1 year without a history of neutropenia.[18] Implementation of the extended 3-monthly monitoring found no difference in the rates of severe neutropenia compared with monthly monitoring.[19] In addition to this, when considering that the development of true agranulocytosis occurs over 10 days or less, the value of monthly monitoring is clearly questionable, especially in patients for whom the overall risk of agranulocytosis is near to zero.

Benign ethnic neutropenia

BEN is a widely recognised hereditary condition in which the neutrophil count is relatively low – there is a left shift in the normal distribution of counts. People of African or Middle Eastern descent have a high prevalence. BEN is characterised by low WCC, which may frequently fall below the lower limit of normal. This pattern may be observed before, during and after the use of clozapine and very probably accounts for a proportion of observed or apparent clozapine-associated neutropenias and treatment cessation. Many countries allow registration of BEN status whereby different (lower) limits are set for neutrophil counts in these patients. While true clozapine-induced neutropenia can occur in the context of BEN, evidence suggests that BEN does not pose an increased risk of dyscrasias during clozapine treatment.[20,21] The use of genetic testing to identify BEN may be useful in reducing the risk of unnecessary termination of treatment and is strongly recommended for all patients starting clozapine, regardless of ethnicity.[22,23]

Concurrent medications

Different classes of medicines associated with haematological adverse effects are co-prescribed with clozapine. These include other antipsychotics, anticonvulsants such as sodium valproate and carbamazepine, antibacterials and GI agents such as proton-pump inhibitors. Many patients develop neutropenia on clozapine but not all are clozapine-related or even pathological. The possible contributory role of these agents should always be considered and these drugs discontinued if clozapine rechallenge is attempted.[24]

Management options

Before treatment initiation, it is important to evaluate baseline haematological values. All patients should be genetically tested for BEN.[25]

In those already taking clozapine, there are three distinct patient groups: those with normal neutrophil counts, those with neutropenia unrelated to clozapine, and those with clozapine-related agranulocytosis. Here, we discuss options for the middle group – those with mild neutropenia unrelated to clozapine. The use of iatrogenic agents to elevate WCC in patients with clear prior clozapine-induced severe neutropenia or agranulocytosis (i.e. there is certainty that clozapine was the cause) is not recommended. Lithium or other medicines should only be used to elevate WCC where it is strongly felt that prior neutropenic episodes were unrelated to clozapine. Patients who have had a previous episode of agranulocytosis that is attributable to clozapine should not be rechallenged either with or without lithium.

Lithium

Lithium increases the neutrophil count and total WCC both acutely and chronically. The magnitude of this effect is poorly quantified, but a mean neutrophil count of 11.9×10^9/L has been reported in patients treated with lithium, and a mean rise in neutrophil count of 2×10^9/L was seen in patients treated with clozapine after the addition of lithium. This effect does not seem to be clearly dose-related, although a minimum lithium serum level of at least 0.4mmol/L may be required. The mechanism is not completely understood.[26]

Lithium has been used to increase the WCC in patients who have developed neutropenia while taking clozapine, allowing clozapine treatment to continue. Several case reports in adults[27–31] and in children[32,33] have been published. Almost all patients had plasma lithium levels of >0.6mmol/L. In a case series (n = 25) of patients who had stopped clozapine because of an apparent blood dyscrasia and were rechallenged in the presence of lithium, only one developed a subsequent dyscrasia.[34]

If considering lithium, discuss with the medical adviser at the relevant monitoring service to determine the optimum pharmacological strategy for the particular patient. Increased risk of neurological adverse effects such as myoclonus, ataxia and seizures should be considered when using the combination.[35] Where there are valid concerns regarding neurotoxic effect, it may be prudent to use clozapine alone (off-licence) with US monitoring criteria (Figure 1.6).[36]

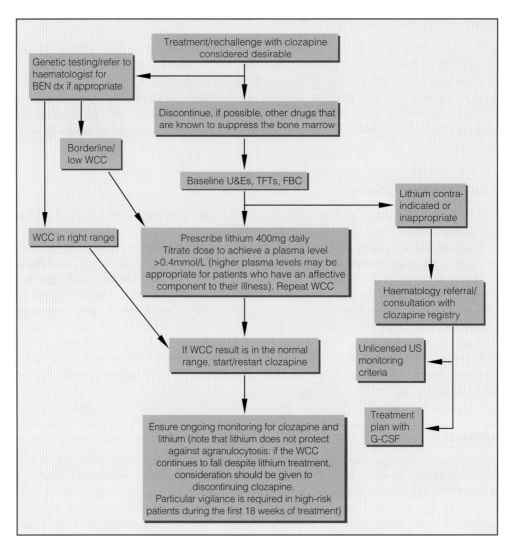

Figure 1.6 The use of lithium with clozapine.

Lithium does not protect against true clozapine-induced agranulocytosis. One case of fatal agranulocytosis has occurred with this combination[25] and a second case of agranulocytosis has been reported with the combination with subsequent resistant to treatment with granulocyte colony-stimulating factor (G-CSF).[37]

Granulocyte colony-stimulating factor

The use of G-CSF to facilitate uninterrupted clozapine therapy in patients with previous neutropenia is a strategy that is attracting increasing interest but is somewhat controversial. In one study, clozapine was successfully rechallenged using G-CSF in 76% of patients for an average follow-up period of 1.9 years.[38] As well as the commonly reported adverse effects of bone pain[39] and neutrophil dysplasia,[40] the administration of

G-CSF in the face of a low or declining neutrophil count may mask an impending neutropenia or agranulocytosis, leading to dire consequences. The long-term safety of G-CSF has not been determined but bone density and spleen size should probably be monitored.

'When required' G-CSF, to be administered if neutrophils drop below a defined threshold, may allow rechallenge with clozapine of patients in whom lithium is insufficient to prevent 'dipping' of WCC below the normal range. Again, this strategy risks masking a severe neutropenia/agranulocytosis. It is also likely to be practically difficult to manage outside a specialist unit, as frequent blood testing (twice to three times a week) is required, as well as immediate access to medical review and the G-CSF itself.

Consultation with a haematologist and discussion with the medical adviser at the clozapine monitoring service are essential before considering the use of G-CSF. A patient's individual clinical circumstances should be considered. In particular, patients should be considered to be very high risk for rechallenge with clozapine if the first episode of dyscrasia fulfilled any of the following criteria, all of which suggest that the low counts are clozapine-related:

- inconsistent with previous WCCs (i.e. not part of a pattern of repeated low WCCs)
- occurred within the first 18 weeks of treatment
- severe (neutrophils $<0.5\times10^9$/L) or
- prolonged.

While G-CSF has been reported as allowing successful rechallenge with clozapine in some people with previous episodes of clozapine-induced neutropenia,[41] the available evidence should exclude this course of action for someone with a true clozapine-related agranulocytosis.[42]

Lithium is indicated in the management of patients with:

- low initial WCC ($<4\times10^9$/L) or neutrophils ($< 2.5\times10^9$/L)
- leucopenia (WCC $<3\times10^9$/L) or neutropenia (neutrophils $<1.5\times10^9$/L) thought to be linked to benign ethnic neutropenia. Such patients may be of African or Middle Eastern descent, have no history of susceptibility to infection and have morphologically normal white blood cells[3]
- recurrent 'amber' results during clozapine treatment
- a 'red' result probably unrelated to clozapine.

References

1. Myles N, et al. Meta-analysis examining the epidemiology of clozapine-associated neutropenia. *Acta Psychiatr Scand* 2018; **138**:101–109.

2. Johannsen CF, et al. Clozapine- and non-clozapine-associated neutropenia in patients with schizophrenia: a retrospective cohort study. *Ther Adv Psychopharmacol* 2022; **12**:20451253211072341.

3. Hsieh MM, et al. Prevalence of neutropenia in the U.S. population: age, sex, smoking status, and ethnic differences. *Ann Intern Med* 2007; **146**:486–492.

4. Myles N, et al. A meta-analysis of controlled studies comparing the association between clozapine and other antipsychotic medications and the development of neutropenia. *Aust N Z J Psychiatry* 2019; **53**:403–412.

5. Munro J, et al. Active monitoring of 12760 clozapine recipients in the UK and Ireland. *Br J Psychiatry* 1999; **175**:576–580.

6. Oloyede E, et al. Relaxation of the criteria for entry to the UK Clozapine Central Non-Rechallenge Database: a modelling study. *Lancet Psychiatry* 2022; **9**:636–644.

7. Li XH, et al. The prevalence of agranulocytosis and related death in clozapine-treated patients: a comprehensive meta-analysis of observational studies. *Psychol Med* 2020; **50**:583–594.

8. Northwood K, et al. Evaluating the epidemiology of clozapine-associated neutropenia among people on clozapine across Australia and Aotearoa New Zealand: a retrospective cohort study. *Lancet Psychiatry* 2024; **11**:27–35.

9. Islam F, et al. Pharmacogenomics of clozapine-induced agranulocytosis: a systematic review and meta-analysis. *Pharmacogenomics J* 2022; **22**:230–240.

10. Taylor D, et al. Distinctive pattern of neutrophil count change in clozapine-associated, life-threatening agranulocytosis. *Schizophrenia (Heidelb)* 2022; **8**:21.

11. Netherlands Clozapine Collaboration Group. Guideline for the use of Clozapine version 05-02-2013. 2013 (last accessed February 2025); https://www.clozapinepluswerkgroep.nl/wp-content/uploads/2013/07/Guideline-for-the-use-of-Clozapine-2013.pdf.

12. Oloyede E, et al. Identifying clinically relevant agranulocytosis in people registered on the UK clozapine Central Non-Rechallenge Database: retrospective cohort study. *Br J Psychiatry* 2024; **225**:484–491.

13. Dettling M, et al. Further evidence of human leukocyte antigen-encoded susceptibility to clozapine-induced agranulocytosis independent of ancestry. *Pharmacogenetics* 2001; **11**:135–141.

14. Nielsen J, et al. Worldwide differences in regulations of clozapine use. *CNS Drugs* 2016; **30**:149–161.

15. FDA. FDA Drug Safety Communication: FDA modifies monitoring for neutropenia associated with schizophrenia medicine clozapine; approves new shared REMS program for all clozapine medicines. 2016 (last accessed November 2024); https://www.fda.gov/Drugs/DrugSafety/ucm461853.htm.

16. Dunk LR, et al. Rechallenge with clozapine following leucopenia or neutropenia during previous therapy. *Br J Psychiatry* 2006; **188**:255–263.

17. Bachmann CJ, et al. International trends in clozapine use: a study in 17 countries. *Acta Psychiatr Scand* 2017; **136**:37–51.

18. Siskind D, et al. Consensus statement on the use of clozapine during the COVID-19 pandemic. *J Psychiatry Neurosci* 2020; **45**:222–223.

19. Oloyede E, et al. Clinical impact of reducing the frequency of clozapine monitoring: controlled mirror-image cohort study. *Br J Psychiatry* 2023; **223**:382–388.

20. Manu P, et al. Benign ethnic neutropenia and clozapine use: a systematic review of the evidence and treatment recommendations. *J Clin Psychiatry* 2016; **77**:e909–e916.

21. Richardson CM, et al. Evaluation of the safety of clozapine use in patients with benign neutropenia. *J Clin Psychiatry* 2016; **77**:e1454–e1459.

22. Aziri H, et al. Genetic identification of undiagnosed benign ethnic neutropenia in patients receiving clozapine treatment. *Br J Psychiatry* 2024; doi: 10.1192/bjp.2024.236.

23. Borinstein SC, et al. Frequency of benign neutropenia among black versus white individuals undergoing a bone marrow assessment. *J Cell Mol Med* 2022; **26**:3628–3635.

24. Shuman MD, et al. Exploring the potential effect of polypharmacy on the hematologic profiles of clozapine patients. *J Psychiatr Pract* 2014; **20**:50–58.

25. Whiskey E, et al. The importance of the recognition of benign ethnic neutropenia in black patients during treatment with clozapine: case reports and database study. *J Psychopharmacol* 2011; **25**:842–845.

26. Paton C, et al. Managing clozapine-induced neutropenia with lithium. *Psychiatr Bull* 2005; **29**:186–188.

27. Adityanjee A. Modification of clozapine-induced leukopenia and neutropenia with lithium carbonate. *Am J Psychiatry* 1995; **152**:648–649.

28. Silverstone PH. Prevention of clozapine-induced neutropenia by pretreatment with lithium. *J Clin Psychopharmacol* 1998; **18**:86–88.

29. Boshes RA, et al. Initiation of clozapine therapy in a patient with preexisting leukopenia: a discussion of the rationale of current treatment options. *Ann Clin Psychiatry* 2001; **13**:233–237.

30. Papetti F, et al. Treatment of clozapine-induced granulocytopenia with lithium (two observations). *Encephale* 2004; **30**:578–582.

31. Kutscher EC, et al. Clozapine-induced leukopenia successfully treated with lithium. *Am J Health Syst Pharm* 2007; **64**:2027–2031.

32. Sporn A, et al. Clozapine-induced neutropenia in children: management with lithium carbonate. *J Child Adolesc Psychopharmacol* 2003; **13**:401–404.

33. Mattai A, et al. Adjunctive use of lithium carbonate for the management of neutropenia in clozapine-treated children. *Hum Psychopharmacol* 2009; **24**:584–589.

34. Kanaan RA, et al. Lithium and clozapine rechallenge: a restrospective case analysis. *J Clin Psychiatry* 2006; **67**:756–760.

35. Verdoux H, et al. Risks and benefits of clozapine and lithium co-prescribing: a systematic review and expert recommendations. *Schizophr Res* 2024; **268**:233–242.

36. Silva E, et al. Understanding clozapine-related blood dyscrasias. Developments, genetics, ethnicity and disparity: it's a CIN. *BJPsych Bull* 2024:1–6.

37. Valevski A, et al. Clozapine–lithium combined treatment and agranulocytosis. *Int Clin Psychopharmacol* 1993; **8**:63–65.

38. Corbeil O, et al. Clozapine rechallenge or continuation despite neutropenia or agranulocytosis using colony-stimulating factor: a systematic review. *J Psychopharmacol* 2023; **37**:370–377.

39. Puhalla S, et al. Hematopoietic growth factors: personalization of risks and benefits. *Mol Oncol* 2012; **6**:237–241.

40. Bain BJ, et al. Neutrophil dysplasia induced by granulocyte colony-stimulating factor. *Am J Hematol* 2010; **85**:354.

41. Myles N, et al. Use of granulocyte-colony stimulating factor to prevent recurrent clozapine-induced neutropenia on drug rechallenge: a systematic review of the literature and clinical recommendations. *Aust N Z J Psychiatry* 2017:4867417720516.

42. Lally J, et al. The use of granulocyte colony-stimulating factor in clozapine rechallenge: a systematic review. *J Clin Psychopharmacol* 2017; **37**:600–604.

Clozapine and chemotherapy

The use of clozapine with agents that cause neutropenia is formally contraindicated. Most chemotherapy treatments cause significant bone marrow suppression. When the white blood cell count drops below 3.0×10^9/L clozapine is usually discontinued. This is an important safety precaution outlined in the formal licence/labelling. For many regimens it can be predicted that chemotherapy will reduce the white blood cell (WBC) count below this level, irrespective of the use of clozapine.

The use of chemotherapy may be more likely in people taking clozapine because of its association with malignancy.[1,2] Ideally, clozapine should be discontinued before chemotherapy starts. However, this will place most patients at high risk of relapse or at least significant deterioration of their psychotic illness, which may then affect their capacity to consent to chemotherapy. This poses a therapeutic dilemma in patients prescribed clozapine and requiring chemotherapy. In practice, most patients do continue on clozapine treatment during chemotherapy.

Liaison with regulatory bodies is essential in ensuring continuity of clozapine treatment for patients who are also receiving chemotherapy. Severe clozapine-induced neutropenia is very rare in people taking clozapine for longer than a year, while neutropenia is a known adverse effect of many chemotherapy regimens. Chemotherapy has a predictable effect on neutrophil counts, both in terms of magnitude of effect and the timing, so knowledge of these factors should help determine the cause of any neutropenia that develops.

There are a number of case reports supporting continuing clozapine during chemotherapy,[3–18] but interpretation of this literature should take account of possible publication bias.[3] Before initiating chemotherapy for a patient receiving clozapine, it is essential to put in place a treatment plan that is agreed with all relevant healthcare staff involved and, of course, the patient and family members/carers. This will include the oncologist/physician, psychiatrist, haematologist, pharmacist and the clozapine monitoring service. Plans should be made in advance for the action that should be taken when the WBC count drops below the normally accepted minimum. This plan should cover the frequency of haematological monitoring, increased vigilance regarding the clinical consequences of neutropenia/agranulocytosis, if and when clozapine should be stopped, and the place of medication such as lithium and G-CSF[19,20] to try and support the maintenance of normal neutrophil counts.

In the UK, the clozapine monitoring service will normally ask the psychiatrist to sign an 'unlicensed use' form and will request additional blood monitoring. Complications appear to be rare but there is one case report of neutropenia persisting for 6 months after doxorubicin, radiotherapy and clozapine.[6] G-CSF has been used to treat agranulocytosis associated with chemotherapy and clozapine in combination.[7,8,21] As discussed above, the risks of life-threatening blood dyscrasia are probably lowest in those who have received clozapine for longer than a year, in whom a clozapine-induced severe neutropenia would be highly unusual.

Summary

- If possible, clozapine should be discontinued before starting chemotherapy but, for almost all people, the risk–benefit analysis will be judged to be in favour of continuing clozapine.

- The likelihood of relapse or deterioration of the psychotic illness must be considered before discontinuing clozapine.
- Consideration should be given to the possibility that, if the patient's mental state deteriorates, they may retract their consent for chemotherapy.
- When clozapine treatment is continued during chemotherapy, a collaborative approach is strongly recommended, involving an oncologist, a psychiatrist, a haematologist, a pharmacist, the patient and their relatives/carers and the relevant clozapine monitoring service.

References

1. Chrétien B, et al. Haematologic malignancies associated with clozapine v. all other antipsychotic agents: a pharmacovigilance study in VigiBase(®). *Psychol Med* 2021; 51:1459–1466.
2. Tiihonen J, et al. Long-term treatment with clozapine and other antipsychotic drugs and the risk of haematological malignancies in people with schizophrenia: a nationwide case-control and cohort study in Finland. *Lancet Psychiatry* 2022; 9:353–362.
3. Cunningham NT, et al. Continuation of clozapine during chemotherapy: a case report and review of literature. *Psychosomatics* 2014; 55:673–679.
4. Bareggi C, et al. Clozapine and full-dose concomitant chemoradiation therapy in a schizophrenic patient with nasopharyngeal cancer. *Tumori* 2002; 88:59–60.
5. Hundertmark J, et al. Reintroduction of clozapine after diagnosis of lymphoma. *Br J Psychiatry* 2001; 178:576.
6. Rosenstock J. Clozapine therapy during cancer treatment. *Am J Psychiatry* 2004; 161:175.
7. Lee SY, et al. Combined antitumor chemotherapy in a refractory schizophrenic receiving clozapine. *J Korean Neuropsychiatr Assoc* 2000; 39:234–239.
8. Usta NG, et al. Clozapine treatment of refractory schizophrenia during essential chemotherapy: a case study and mini review of a clinical dilemma. *Ther Adv Psychopharmacol* 2014; 4:276–281.
9. Rosenberg I, et al. Restarting clozapine treatment during ablation chemotherapy and stem cell transplant for Hodgkin's lymphoma. *Am J Psychiatry* 2007; 164:1438–1439.
10. Goulet K, et al. Case report: clozapine given in the context of chemotherapy for lung cancer. *Psychooncology* 2008; 17:512–516.
11. Frieri T, et al. Maintaining clozapine treatment during chemotherapy for non-Hodgkin's lymphoma. *Prog Neuropsychopharmacol Biol Psychiatry* 2008; 32:1611–1612.
12. Sankaranarayanan A, et al. Clozapine, cancer chemotherapy and neutropenia: dilemmas in management. *Psychiatr Danub* 2013; 25:419–422.
13. De Berardis D, et al. Safety and efficacy of combined clozapine-azathioprine treatment in a case of resistant schizophrenia associated with Behcet's disease: a 2-year follow-up. *Gen Hosp Psychiatry* 2013; 35:213–211.
14. Deodhar JK, et al. Clozapine and cancer treatment: adding to the experience and evidence. *Indian J Psychiatry* 2014; 56:191–193.
15. Monga V, et al. Clozapine and concomitant chemotherapy in a patient with schizophrenia and new onset esophageal cancer. *Psychooncology* 2015; 24:971–972.
16. Overbeeke MR, et al. Successful clozapine continuation during chemotherapy for the treatment of malignancy: a case report. *Int J Clin Pharm* 2016; 38:199–202.
17. Campbell G, et al. Clozapine and chemotherapy: a dangerous couple or a necessary partnership? *Drug Ther Bull* 2022; 60:29–31.
18. Wright T, et al. Should clozapine be discontinued in a patient receiving chemotherapy? *Current Psychiatry* 2022; 21:44–49.
19. Whiskey E, et al. Restarting clozapine after neutropenia: evaluating the possibilities and practicalities. *CNS Drugs* 2007; 21:25–35.
20. Silva E, et al. Clozapine rechallenge and initiation despite neutropenia- a practical, step-by-step guide. *BMC Psychiatry* 2020; 20:279.
21. Kolli V, et al. Treating chemotherapy induced agranulocytosis with granulocyte colony-stimulating factors in a patient on clozapine. *Psychooncology* 2013; 22:1674–1675.

Genetic testing for clozapine treatment

A great number of studies have sought to detect genetic predictors of clozapine outcomes, both therapeutic and adverse. Generally, only small effects have been uncovered and clinical utility is limited unless genetic variant effects are mathematically combined. Sensitivity (the likelihood of accurately predicting a specific outcome) is usually low but specificity (the likelihood of correctly excluding that outcome) is often very high. Numerical values for these categories can be combined with population incidence data to generate positive predictive value (PPV – the % of people who will experience the outcome when predicted) and negative predictive value (NPV – the % of people who will not experience that outcome when it is not predicted). This concept is applicable to genetic variants linked to agranulocytosis. The presence of a candidate variant (see PPV below) should provoke caution and perhaps more frequent testing. The absence of a candidate variant (see NPV) may give some reassurance about the likelihood of agranulocytosis, especially if the NPV is >99.6% (that is, 100 minus 0.4%, the risk of agranulocytosis in the wider population).

Response

Three variants have been reliably shown to predict therapeutic outcome with clozapine:[1]

HTR2A rs6313C   CC carriers less likely to respond than <u>T carriers</u>
CC 146/272 response, CT/TT 366/596 response (54% vs 62%)

HTR2A rs6314   <u>C allele</u> more likely to respond than T allele
C allele response 685/1,215, T allele 55/127 (56% vs 43%)

HTR3A rs1062613   C allele less likely to respond than <u>T allele</u>
C allele response 528/841, T allele 134/185 (63% vs 72%)

Mathematical modelling of these three variants can generate an overall percentage chance of response with confidence intervals. Other variants may be linked to response.

Agranulocytosis

Several genetic variants are reliably associated with altered risk of agranulocytosis. Some variants are found only in certain ethnic groups.

HLA-DQB1   Sequence variant 6672G>C (REC 21G) confers 1,175% higher risk of agranulocytosis than general population.

         Sensitivity 21.5%, specificity 98.4%.[2] PPV 5.1%, NPV 99.7%.

         In people of European ancestry, sensitivity is 53.7% and this variant confers a 10-fold greater risk of agranulocytosis.[3]

HLA-DQB1   DQB1*0502 allele is associated with agranulocytosis in 5 of 7 studies (e.g. Dettling and colleagues,[4] Yunis and colleagues[5]). Effect size variable.

HLA-B*59:01	Presence of allele highly predictive of agranulocytosis but is rare in East Asian populations and almost absent in people of European descent.
	Sensitivity 31.8%, specificity 95.3%.[6] PPV 6.4%, NPV 99.3%.
HLA DQB1/HLA-B	Single amino acid changes HLA DQB1 126Q and HLA-B 158T associated with increased risk of agranulocytosis. Overall, 39 of 95 cases had one or both alleles; 175 of 206 controls had neither allele.
	Sensitivity 41.0%, specificity 85.0%[7,8] (36% and 89% figures given elsewhere).[9] PPV/NPV not given but can be calculated.
HLA-DRB1	DRB1*04:02 confers a six-fold higher risk of agranulocytosis. NPV is 99.3%.[10]

The HLA-DQB1 variants and the HLA-B variants are in linkage disequilibrium[9] and are likely to convey the same association signal. Variants in linkage disequilibrium are inherited together.

Benign ethnic neutropenia

ACKR1 rs2814778	CC genotype at rs2814778 (Duffy Null Status) is considered to be the cause of BEN.[11]

All patients starting clozapine should undergo genetic testing for BEN.[12]

Metabolism

Clozapine is largely metabolised by CYP1A2 and, to a lesser extent in most people, CYP3A4/5. Despite early reports, CYP2D6 plays almost no role in the metabolism of clozapine.[13] Metabolic rate is usually classified as poor (PM), intermediate (IM) or extensive (EM) and each is associated with a particular genetic variant. Genetic analysis can therefore allow an estimate of the target dose of clozapine for an individual. This is the most accurate method of predicting clozapine dose.[14]

Cytochrome p4501A2	PM/IM/EM status as normally defined by analysis of e.g. CYP1A2*1F/1C/1A/1K.[15]
Cytochrome p4503A4	PM/IM/EM status. CYP3A4 is usually a minor route of clozapine metabolism but metaboliser status affects blood concentration.[16]
Cytochrome p4503A5	PM/IM/EM status. CYP3A5 PM status associated with elevated clozapine blood levels.[17]

Other non-CYP genetic associations have also been demonstrated.

NFIB rs28379954 *T>C* CT carriers have much lower blood concentrations than TT carriers in both smokers and non-smokers.[18]

Also, the **rs2472297** genotype independently predicts clozapine plasma levels.[19] Levels are highest in C/C carriers and lowest in T/T carriers (C/T somewhere in between).

Genetic analysis of CYP function can identify the cause of low clozapine blood concentrations and allow selection of appropriate enzyme inhibitors.[20]

Other adverse effects

Genetic predictors of myocarditis[21] and weight gain[22] have also been found, but associations are probably too weak to allow clinical application.[15]

References

1. Gressier F, et al. Pharmacogenetics of clozapine response and induced weight gain: a comprehensive review and meta-analysis. *Eur Neuropsychopharmacol* 2016; **26**:163–185.
2. Athanasiou MC, et al. Candidate gene analysis identifies a polymorphism in HLA-DQB1 associated with clozapine-induced agranulocytosis. *J Clin Psychiatry* 2011; **72**:458–463.
3. Konte B, et al. HLA-DQB1 6672G>C (rs113332494) is associated with clozapine-induced neutropenia and agranulocytosis in individuals of European ancestry. *Transl Psychiatry* 2021; **11**:214.
4. Dettling M, et al. Genetic determinants of clozapine-induced agranulocytosis: recent results of HLA subtyping in a non-Jewish Caucasian sample. *Arch Gen Psychiatry* 2001; **58**:93–94.
5. Yunis JJ, et al. HLA associations in clozapine-induced agranulocytosis. *Blood* 1995; **86**:1177–1183.
6. Saito T, et al. Pharmacogenomic study of clozapine-induced agranulocytosis/granulocytopenia in a Japanese population. *Biol Psychiatry* 2016; **80**:636–642.
7. Girardin FR, et al. Cost-effectiveness of HLA-DQB1/HLA-B pharmacogenetic-guided treatment and blood monitoring in US patients taking clozapine. *Pharmacogenomics J* 2019; **19**:211–218.
8. Goldstein JI, et al. Clozapine-induced agranulocytosis is associated with rare HLA-DQB1 and HLA-B alleles. *Nat Commun* 2014; **5**:4757.
9. Legge SE, et al. Genetics of clozapine-associated neutropenia: recent advances, challenges and future perspective. *Pharmacogenomics* 2019; **20**:279–290.
10. Islam F, et al. Pharmacogenomics of clozapine-induced agranulocytosis: a systematic review and meta-analysis. *Pharmacogenomics J* 2022; **22**:230–240.
11. Charles BA, et al. Analyses of genome wide association data, cytokines, and gene expression in African-Americans with benign ethnic neutropenia. *PLoS One* 2018; **13**:e0194400.
12. Aziri H, et al. Genetic identification of undiagnosed benign ethnic neutropenia in patients receiving clozapine treatment. *Br J Psychiatry* 2024; doi: 10.1192/bjp.2024.236.
13. Olesen OV, et al. Contributions of five human cytochrome P450 isoforms to the N-demethylation of clozapine in vitro at low and high concentrations. *J Clin Pharmacol* 2001; **41**:823–832.
14. Taylor D, et al. Predicting clozapine dose required to achieve a therapeutic plasma concentration: a comparison of a population algorithm and three algorithms based on gene variant models. *J Psychopharmacol* 2023; **37**:1030–1039.
15. Thorn CF, et al. PharmGKB summary: clozapine pathway, pharmacokinetics. *Pharmacogenet Genomics* 2018; **28**:214–222.
16. Tóth K, et al. Potential role of patients' CYP3A-status in clozapine pharmacokinetics. *Int J Neuropsychopharmacol* 2017; **20**:529–537.
17. John AP, et al. Unusually high serum levels of clozapine associated with genetic polymorphism of CYP3A enzymes. *Asian J Psychiatr* 2020; **10**:21283.
18. Smith RL, et al. Identification of a novel polymorphism associated with reduced clozapine concentration in schizophrenia patients: a genome-wide association study adjusting for smoking habits. *Transl Psychiatry* 2020; **10**:198.
19. Pardiñas AF, et al. Pharmacogenomic variants and drug interactions identified through the genetic analysis of clozapine metabolism. *Am J Psychiatry* 2019; **176**:477–486.
20. Okon-Rocha E, et al. Genetic analysis of clozapine metabolism in a patient with subtherapeutic clozapine plasma concentrations: the importance of CYP3A5: a case report. *J Clin Psychopharmacol* 2022; **42**:604–606.
21. Lacaze P, et al. Genetic associations with clozapine-induced myocarditis in patients with schizophrenia. *Transl Psychiatry* 2020; **10**:37.
22. Li N, et al. Progress in genetic polymorphisms related to lipid disturbances induced by atypical antipsychotic drugs. *Front Pharmacol* 2020; **10**:1669.

Bipolar disorder

Lithium

Mechanism of action

Lithium is implicated in a wide range of biological processes, with a multiplicity of effects. Consequently it has proven very difficult to ascertain the key mechanism(s) of action of lithium in regulating mood and behaviour. For example, there is some older evidence that people with bipolar illness have higher intracellular concentrations of sodium and calcium than controls and that lithium can reduce these. Interestingly, calcium-related genes have been implicated by genetic studies in bipolar disorder.[1] *GSK3* (glycogen synthase kinase 3), *CREB* (cAMP response element-binding protein) and Na^+/K^+ adenosine triphosphatase (ATPase) related mechanisms may be important for lithium's effects.[2] Lithium may have neuroprotective effects that preserve the function of neurons and neuronal circuits.[3] Lithium also promotes neurogenesis in the hippocampus, which is important for learning, memory and stress responses.[4] A meta-analysis suggests lithium may prevent transition to dementia[5] and lithium appears to be more effective than aducanumab in preventing cognitive decline.[6] However, the largest study to date showed no beneficial effect on risk of neurocognitive disorders.[7] Both reversible and irreversible neurotoxicity related to lithium are recognised adverse effects.[8,9] Lithium is present in low levels in the environment (e.g. in drinking water sources) and environmental lithium concentration has been reported to be inversely related to suicide and dementia at a population level.[10,11]

Clinical indications

Acute treatment of mania

Lithium is effective for the treatment of mania, at a plasma level of 0.8–1.0mmol/L.[12] If a faster onset of action is needed an adjunctive or single-agent antipsychotic with an evidence base for treating mania is recommended.[12] It can be difficult to achieve

The Maudsley® Prescribing Guidelines in Psychiatry, Fifteenth Edition. David M. Taylor, Thomas R. E. Barnes and Allan H. Young.

therapeutic plasma lithium levels rapidly and monitoring may be problematic if the patient is uncooperative. Treatment may be most successful in those without psychotic symptoms or evidence of rapid cycling.[13]

Treatment of acute mania in patients already on long-term lithium

The 2016 British Association for Psychopharmacology guidelines[12] suggest that in the event of relapse, an urgent plasma lithium level should be obtained to indicate the level of compliance with lithium therapy and inform possible dose adjustment. If lithium level measurement indicates non-compliance, the reason should be ascertained. If the lithium level is confirmed to be optimal, but the control of mania is inadequate, then adding a dopamine antagonist, dopamine partial agonist or valproate (given the conditions with regard to reproductive potential) is recommended.[12]

Bipolar depression

Lithium is widely used in bipolar depression but evidence supporting robust efficacy for acute episodes is somewhat unconvincing.[14,15] Evidence for prevention of depressive episodes is more compelling.

Maintenance treatment of bipolar disorder

Aim for the highest tolerable lithium plasma level in the range of 0.6–0.8mmol/L[12,16] with the option to reduce it to 0.4–0.6mmol/L in case of good response but poor tolerance, or to increase it to 0.8–1.0mmol/L in case of insufficient response and good tolerance. The aim of treatment is complete remission and prevention of both manic and depressive episodes.[17] Lithium is the best-performing mood stabiliser for bipolar disorder in practice with a prophylactic effectiveness similar to long-acting antipsychotics.[18] In 2024, it remains the gold standard treatment for bipolar disorder.[19]

Augmentation of antidepressants in unipolar depression

Approximately 30–50% of patients fail to respond to trials of first- or second-line antidepressants and outcomes from treatment-resistant depression are poor.[20] Evidence-based guidelines for treating depressive disorders with antidepressants[21] suggest that either lithium or quetiapine is the agent of first choice for augmenting the existing antidepressant and that lithium augmentation is most effective at a lithium plasma level of 0.6–1.0mmol/L. Recent meta-analyses suggest robust efficacy for lithium, alongside quetiapine, D_2 partial agonists and ketamine.[22,23] One meta-analysis suggested lithium to be most effective.[24] Clinical predictors associated with a better outcome in lithium augmentation for treatment-resistant depression included more severe depressive symptomatology, psychomotor retardation, significant weight loss, a family history of major depression or a personal experience of more than three episodes.[25] Of course, compliance with lithium augmentation should also be added to this list. Lithium is widely underused in resistant depression.[26]

Prophylaxis of unipolar depression

Lithium is significantly superior to antidepressants in preventing relapses that require hospitalisation, with a relative risk of 0.34.[27] Lithium prophylaxis is indicated in unipolar depression (i) if a patient has suffered two depressive episodes in 5 years; (ii) after one episode if the episode is severe and there is a strong suicide risk; (iii) with indefinite treatment if there is adherence and adverse events are not problematic, particularly if a bipolar background is suspected.[28]

Other uses of lithium

Lithium is also used to treat aggressive and self-mutilating behaviour and studies have confirmed benefits[29] to both prevent and treat steroid-induced psychosis[30] and to raise the white blood cell count in patients receiving clozapine.[31]

Lithium and suicide

It is estimated that 15% of people with bipolar disorder eventually take their own life.[32] A meta-analysis of clinical trials concluded that lithium reduced the risk of both attempted and completed suicide by 80% in patients with bipolar illness,[33] and large database studies have shown that lithium-treated patients are less likely to complete suicide than patients treated with other mood-stabilising drugs.[34]

In patients with unipolar depression, lithium also seems to protect against suicide although the mechanism of this protective effect is unknown.[33] As noted, environmental lithium has been reported to be inversely related to suicide at a population level.[10,35]

Plasma levels

The minimum effective plasma level for prophylaxis of mood disorder episodes is probably 0.4mmol/L, with the optimal concentration being in the range 0.6–0.8mmol/L.[36] Levels above 0.75mmol/L offer additional protection only against manic symptoms[37] so the target range for prophylaxis is effectively 0.6–0.8mmol/L.[16,38] Changes in plasma levels in either direction seem to worsen the risk of relapse.[37] The optimal plasma level range in patients who have unipolar depression is less clear.[39] Taking account of evidence from clinical trials, naturalistic studies and lithium in drinking water, studies seem to suggest that various benefits of lithium begin at a low concentration and increase over a narrow range up to 1.0mmol/L. Low-dose lithium regimens are under investigation but not yet clinically recommended.[40]

Children and adolescents may require higher plasma levels than adults to ensure that an adequate concentration of lithium is present in the central nervous system (CNS).[41]

Lithium is rapidly absorbed from the gastrointestinal tract but has a long distribution phase. Blood samples for plasma lithium level estimations should be taken 10–14 (ideally 12) hours post-dose in patients who are prescribed a single daily dose of a prolonged-release preparation at bedtime.[12]

Formulations

There is no clinically significant difference in the pharmacokinetics of the two most widely prescribed brands of lithium in the UK: Priadel and Camcolit. In other countries, standard lithium carbonate tablets are often given twice or three times daily.

The amount of elemental lithium varies by salt used.

- Lithium carbonate 400mg tablets each contain 10.8mmol lithium.
- Lithium citrate liquid is available in two strengths:
  - 5.4mmol/5mL (equivalent to 200mg lithium carbonate).
  - 10.8mmol/5mL (equivalent to 400mg lithium carbonate).

Lack of clarity over which liquid preparation is intended when prescribing can lead to the patient receiving a sub-therapeutic or toxic dose. Liquid preparations need to be given 12-hourly.

Adverse effects

Most adverse effects are dose- and plasma level-related. These include mild gastrointestinal upset, fine tremor, polyuria and polydipsia. Polyuria may occur more frequently with twice daily dosing.[42,43] Propranolol can be useful in lithium-induced tremor. Some skin conditions such as psoriasis and acne can be aggravated by lithium therapy. Lithium can also cause a metallic taste in the mouth, ankle oedema and weight gain.

Lithium can cause a reduction in urinary concentrating capacity – nephrogenic diabetes insipidus – hence the occurrence of thirst and polyuria. This effect is usually reversible in the short to medium term, but renal effects may be irreversible after long-term treatment (>15 years).[44] Lithium treatment can also lead to a reduction in the glomerular filtration rate (GFR) although the magnitude of the risk is uncertain.[44] Lithium levels of >0.8mmol/L are associated with a higher risk of renal toxicity and prolonged lithium treatment of course requires regular monitoring of kidney function.[45] Hypertension and a diagnosis of bipolar disorder worsen the risk of lithium-related chronic kidney disease.[46]

In the longer term, lithium increases the risk of hypothyroidism;[47] in middle-aged women the risk may be up to 20%.[48] A case has been made for testing thyroid autoantibodies in this group before starting lithium (to better estimate risk) and for performing thyroid function tests (TFTs) more frequently in the first year of treatment.[49] Hypothyroidism is readily treated with thyroxine. TFTs usually return to normal when lithium is discontinued. Lithium also more rarely causes hyperthyroidism.[50]

Hyperparathyroidism causes hypercalcaemia in about 4% of patients[51] and calcium levels should be monitored in patients on long-term treatment.[50,52] Clinical consequences of chronically increased serum calcium include renal stones, osteoporosis, dyspepsia, hypertension and renal impairment.

Lithium toxicity

Toxic effects reliably occur at levels >1.5mmol/L and usually consist of gastrointestinal symptoms (increasing anorexia, nausea and diarrhoea) and CNS effects (muscle weakness, drowsiness, confusion, ataxia, coarse tremor and muscle twitching).[53]

Above 2mmol/L, increased disorientation and seizures usually occur, which can progress to coma and ultimately death. In the presence of more severe symptoms, osmotic or forced alkaline diuresis should be used in a medical facility. Above 3mmol/L, peritoneal or haemodialysis is often used. These plasma levels are only a guide and individuals vary in their susceptibility to symptoms of toxicity. Neurotoxicity at normal plasma levels has also been described, as brain lithium levels may not be reflected by concentration in the plasma.[54,55]

Most risk factors for toxicity involve changes in sodium levels or in the way the body handles sodium, for example low salt diets, dehydration, drug interactions (see later Table 2.2) and some uncommon physical illnesses such as Addison's disease.

Information relating to the symptoms of toxicity and the common risk factors (especially drug interactions) should always be given to patients when treatment with lithium is initiated.[56] This information should be repeated at appropriate intervals to make sure that it is clearly understood.

Pre-treatment tests

Before prescribing lithium, renal, thyroid and cardiac function should be checked. As a minimum, the estimated GFR (eGFR),[57] urea and electrolytes (U&Es) and TFTs should be checked. A baseline calcium level is also helpful. An electrocardiogram (ECG) is also recommended in patients who have risk factors for, or existing, cardiovascular disease. A baseline measure of weight is also desirable.

Lithium is a putative human teratogen. Women of child-bearing age should be advised to use a reliable form of contraception. See the section on psychotropics and pregnancy (Chapter 7).

On-treatment monitoring[12,58]

Plasma lithium, eGFR, U&Es and TFTs should be checked every 6 months. More frequent tests may be required in those who are prescribed interacting drugs, who are elderly or who have established chronic kidney disease. Weight (or body mass index [BMI]) should also be monitored. Lithium monitoring in clinical practice in the UK is known to be suboptimal[59] although there has been a modest improvement over time.[60] The use of automated reminder systems has been shown to improve monitoring rates.[61]

Discontinuation

Intermittent treatment with lithium may worsen the natural course of bipolar illness. A much greater than expected incidence of manic relapse is seen in the first few months after abruptly discontinuing lithium,[62] even in patients who have been symptom-free for as long as 5 years.[63] Lithium treatment should not be started unless there is a clear intention to continue it for several years and where compliance can be reasonably assured.[64] This advice has obvious implications for initiating lithium treatment against a patient's will (or in a patient known to be non-compliant with medication) during a period of acute illness.

The risk of relapse is probably reduced by decreasing the dose gradually over a period of at least a month[65] and avoiding decremental plasma level reductions of >0.2mmol/L.[37]

In contrast with these recommendations, a naturalistic study found that, in patients who had been in remission for at least 2 years and had discontinued lithium very slowly, the recurrence rate was at least three times greater than in patients who continued lithium and that significant survival differences persisted for many years. Patients maintained on high lithium levels before discontinuation were particularly prone to relapse.[66]

One large US study based on prescription records found that half of those prescribed lithium took almost all of their prescribed doses, a quarter took between 50% and 80% and the remaining quarter took less than 50%. A third of patients took lithium for less than 6 months in total.[67] A large audit found that 1 in 10 patients prescribed long-term lithium treatment had a plasma level below the therapeutic range.[68] It is clear that suboptimal adherence limits the effectiveness of lithium in clinical practice. One database study suggested the extent to which lithium was taken was directly related to the risk of suicide (more prescriptions were associated with lower suicide rate).[69] Less convincing data support the emergence of depressive symptoms in bipolar patients after lithium discontinuation.[62] There are few data relating to patients with unipolar depression.

Table 2.1 summarises the prescribing and monitoring of lithium.

Table 2.1 Lithium: prescribing and monitoring.

Indications	Mania, hypomania, prophylaxis of bipolar affective disorder and recurrent depression. Reduces aggression and suicidality.
Pre-lithium work-up	Estimated glomerular filtration rate (eGFR) and thyroid function tests (TFTs). ECG recommended in patients who have risk factors for, or existing, cardiovascular disease. Baseline measure of weight desirable. U&Es (including calcium).
Prescribing	Start at 400mg at night (200mg in the elderly). Plasma level after 7 days, then 7 days after every dose change until the desired level is reached (0.4mmol/L may be effective in unipolar depression, 0.6–1.0mmol/L in bipolar illness, slightly higher levels in this range in difficult to treat mania). Blood should be taken 12 hours after the last dose. Take care when prescribing liquid preparations to clearly specify the strength required.
Monitoring	Plasma lithium every 6 months (more frequent monitoring is necessary in those prescribed interacting drugs, the elderly and those with established renal impairment or other relevant physical illness). eGFR, U&Es and TFTs every 6 months. Weight (or body mass index) should also be monitored.
Stopping	Reduce slowly over at least 1 month and preferably 3 months. Avoid reductions in plasma levels of >0.2mmol/L at a time (see section on discontinuation).

Interactions with other drugs[70–72]

Because of lithium's relatively narrow therapeutic index, pharmacokinetic interactions with other drugs can precipitate lithium toxicity. Most clinically significant interactions are largely with drugs that alter renal sodium handling. Rarely, neurotoxicity results from co-prescribing lithium and antipsychotics.[73,74]

ACE inhibitors

Angiotensin-converting enzyme (ACE) inhibitors can (i) reduce thirst, which can lead to mild dehydration; and (ii) increase renal sodium loss leading to increased sodium reabsorption by the kidney, resulting in an increase in lithium plasma levels. The magnitude of this effect is variable, from no increase to a fourfold increase. The full effect can take several weeks to develop. The risk seems to be increased in patients with heart failure, dehydration and renal impairment (presumably because of changes in fluid balance/handling). In the elderly, ACE inhibitors increase sevenfold the risk of hospitalisation due to lithium toxicity. ACE inhibitors can also precipitate renal failure so, if co-prescribed with lithium, more frequent monitoring of eGFR and plasma lithium is required.

The following drugs are ACE inhibitors: captopril, cilazapril, enalapril, fosinopril, imidapril, lisinopril, moexipril, perindopril, quinapril, ramipril and trandolapril.

Care is also required with the **angiotensin II receptor antagonists** candesartan, eprosartan, irbesartan, losartan, olmesartan, telmisartan and valsartan.

Diuretics

Diuretics can reduce the renal clearance of lithium, the magnitude of this effect being greater with thiazide than with loop diuretics. Lithium levels usually rise within 10 days of a **thiazide diuretic** being prescribed; the magnitude of the rise is unpredictable and can vary from an increase of 25% to 400%.

The following drugs are thiazide (or related) diuretics: bendroflumethiazide, chlortalidone, cyclopenthiazide, indapamide, metolazone and xipamide.

Although there are case reports of lithium toxicity induced by **loop diuretics**, many patients receive this combination of drugs without apparent problems. The risk of an interaction seems to be greatest in the first month after the loop diuretic has been prescribed and additional lithium plasma level monitoring during this time is recommended if these drugs are co-prescribed. Loop diuretics can increase sodium loss and subsequent reabsorption by the kidney. Patients taking loop diuretics may also have been advised to restrict their salt intake; this may contribute to the risk of lithium toxicity in these individuals.

The following drugs are loop diuretics: bumetanide, furosemide and torasemide.

Non-steroidal anti-inflammatory drugs

Non-steroidal anti-inflammatory drugs (NSAIDs) inhibit the synthesis of renal prostaglandins, thereby reducing renal blood flow and possibly increasing renal reabsorption of sodium and therefore lithium. The magnitude of the rise in lithium concentration is unpredictable for any given patient; case reports vary from increases of around 10% to over 400%. The onset of effect also seems to be variable, from a few days to several months. Risk appears to be increased in those patients who have impaired renal function, renal artery stenosis or heart failure and who are dehydrated or on a low salt diet. There are a number of case reports of an interaction between lithium and COX-2 inhibitors. NSAIDs do not appear to diminish the therapeutic effects of lithium,[75] as has previously been reported.

NSAIDs (or COX-2 inhibitors) can be very carefully combined with lithium, but they should be prescribed regularly, not intermittently, and more frequent plasma lithium monitoring is essential. Some NSAIDs can be purchased without a prescription, so it is particularly important that patients are aware of the potential for interaction.

The following drugs are NSAIDs or COX-2 inhibitors: aceclofenac, acemetacin, celecoxib, dexibuprofen, dexketoprofen, diclofenac, diflunisal, etodolac, etoricoxib, fenbufen, fenoprofen, flurbiprofen, ibuprofen, indometacin, ketoprofen, lumiracoxib, mefenamic acid, meloxicam, nabumetone, naproxen, piroxicam, sulindac, tenoxicam and tiaprofenic acid.

Carbamazepine

There are rare reports of neurotoxicity when carbamazepine is combined with lithium. Most reports are old and in the context of treatment involving high plasma lithium levels. It is of note though that carbamazepine can cause hyponatraemia, which may in turn lead to lithium retention and toxicity. Similarly, rare reports of CNS toxicity implicate **selective serotonin reuptake inhibitors** (SSRIs), another group of drugs that can cause hyponatraemia.

Table 2.2 summarises drugs that may clinically interact with lithium.

Table 2.2 Lithium: clinically relevant drug interactions.

Drug group	Magnitude of effect	Timescale of effect	Additional information
ACE inhibitors	Unpredictable Up to fourfold increases in [Li]	Develops over several weeks	Sevenfold increased risk of hospitalisation for lithium toxicity in the elderly Angiotensin II receptor antagonists may be associated with similar risk
Thiazide diuretics	Unpredictable Up to fourfold increases in [Li]	Usually apparent in first 10 days	Loop diuretics are safer Any effect will be apparent in the first month
NSAIDs	Unpredictable From 10% to over fourfold increases in [Li]	Variable; few days to several months	NSAIDs are widely used on a when necessary basis Can be bought without a prescription

ACE, angiotensin-converting enzyme; [Li], lithium concentration; NSAIDs, non-steroidal anti-inflammatory drugs.

References

1. Bray NJ, et al. The genetics of neuropsychiatric disorders. *Brain Neurosci Adv* 2019; 2:2398212818799271.
2. Bortolozzi A, et al. New advances in the pharmacology and toxicology of lithium: a neurobiologically oriented overview. *Pharmacol Rev* 2024; 76:323–357.
3. Jope RS, et al. Lithium to the rescue. *Cerebrum* 2016; 2016:cer-02-16.
4. Hanson ND, et al. Lithium, but not fluoxetine or the corticotropin-releasing factor receptor 1 receptor antagonist R121919, increases cell proliferation in the adult dentate gyrus. *J Pharmacol Exp Ther* 2011; 337:180–186.
5. Matsunaga S, et al. Lithium as a treatment for Alzheimer's disease: a systematic review and meta-analysis. *J Alzheimers Dis* 2015; 48:403–410.
6. Terao I, et al. Comparative efficacy of lithium and aducanumab for cognitive decline in patients with mild cognitive impairment or Alzheimer's disease: a systematic review and network meta-analysis. *Ageing Res Rev* 2022; 81:101709.
7. Huang Q, et al. Lithium exposure and risk of major neurocognitive disorders: a systematic review and meta-analysis. *J Clin Psychopharmacol* 2024; 44:418–423.
8. Netto I, et al. Reversible lithium neurotoxicity: review of the literature. *Prim Care Companion CNS Disord* 2012; 14:PCC.11r01197.
9. Adityanjee, et al. The syndrome of irreversible lithium-effectuated neurotoxicity. *Clin Neuropharmacol* 2005; 28:38–49.
10. Memon A, et al. Association between naturally occurring lithium in drinking water and suicide rates: systematic review and meta-analysis of ecological studies. *Br J Psychiatry* 2020; 217:667–678.
11. Kessing LV, et al. Association of lithium in drinking water with the incidence of dementia. *JAMA Psychiatry* 2017; 74:1005–1010.
12. Goodwin GM, et al. Evidence-based guidelines for treating bipolar disorder: revised third edition recommendations from the British Association for Psychopharmacology. *J Psychopharmacol* 2016; 30:495–553.
13. Hui TP, et al. A systematic review and meta-analysis of clinical predictors of lithium response in bipolar disorder. *Acta Psychiatr Scand* 2019; 140:94–115.

CHAPTER 2

14. Bahji A, et al. Comparative efficacy and tolerability of pharmacological treatments for the treatment of acute bipolar depression: a systematic review and network meta-analysis. *J Affect Disord* 2020; **269**:154–184.

15. Taylor DM, et al. Comparative efficacy and acceptability of drug treatments for bipolar depression: a multiple-treatments meta-analysis. *Acta Psychiatr Scand* 2014; **130**:452–469.

16. Nolen WA, et al. What is the optimal serum level for lithium in the maintenance treatment of bipolar disorder? A systematic review and recommendations from the ISBD/IGSLI Task Force on treatment with lithium. *Bipolar Disord* 2019; **21**:394–409.

17. Severus E, et al. Lithium for prevention of mood episodes in bipolar disorders: systematic review and meta-analysis. *Int J Bipolar Disord* 2014; **2**:15.

18. Lähteenvuo M, et al. Real-world effectiveness of pharmacological treatments for bipolar disorder: register-based national cohort study. *Br J Psychiatry* 2023; **223**:456–464.

19. Airainer M, et al. Lithium, the gold standard drug for bipolar disorder: analysis of current clinical studies. *Naunyn Schmiedebergs Arch Pharmacol* 2024; **397**:9723–9743.

20. Dunner DL, et al. Prospective, long-term, multicenter study of the naturalistic outcomes of patients with treatment-resistant depression. *J Clin Psychiatry* 2006; **67**:688–695.

21. Cleare A, et al. Evidence-based guidelines for treating depressive disorders with antidepressants: a revision of the 2008 British Association for Psychopharmacology guidelines. *J Psychopharmacol* 2015; **29**:459–525.

22. Scott F, et al. Systematic review and meta-analysis of augmentation and combination treatments for early-stage treatment-resistant depression. *J Psychopharmacol* 2023; **37**:268–278.

23. Nuñez NA, et al. Augmentation strategies for treatment resistant major depression: a systematic review and network meta-analysis. *J Affect Disord* 2022; **302**:385–400.

24. Vázquez GH, et al. Efficacy and tolerability of combination treatments for major depression: antidepressants plus second-generation antipsychotics vs. esketamine vs. lithium. *J Psychopharmacol* 2021; **35**:890–900.

25. Bauer M, et al. Role of lithium augmentation in the management of major depressive disorder. *CNS Drugs* 2014; **28**:331–342.

26. Ercis M, et al. When and how to use lithium augmentation for treating major depressive disorder. *J Clin Psychiatry* 2023; **84**:23ac14813.

27. Cipriani A, et al. Lithium versus antidepressants in the long-term treatment of unipolar affective disorder. *Cochrane Database Syst Rev* 2006; **4**:CD003492.

28. Abou-Saleh MT, et al. Lithium in the episode and suicide prophylaxis and in augmenting strategies in patients with unipolar depression. *Int J Bipolar Disord* 2017; **5**:11.

29. Correll CU, et al. Biological treatment of acute agitation or aggression with schizophrenia or bipolar disorder in the inpatient setting. *Ann Clin Psychiatry* 2017; **29**:92–107.

30. Sirois F. Steroid psychosis: a review. *Gen Hosp Psychiatry* 2003; **25**:27–33.

31. Aydin M, et al. Continuing clozapine treatment with lithium in schizophrenic patients with neutropenia or leukopenia: brief review of literature with case reports. *Ther Adv Psychopharmacol* 2016; **6**:33–38.

32. Harris EC, et al. Excess mortality of mental disorder. *Br J Psychiatry* 1998; **173**:11–53.

33. Cipriani A, et al. Lithium in the prevention of suicide in mood disorders: updated systematic review and meta-analysis. *BMJ* 2013; **346**:f3646.

34. Hayes JF, et al. Self-harm, unintentional injury, and suicide in bipolar disorder during maintenance mood stabilizer treatment: a UK population-based electronic health records study. *JAMA Psychiatry* 2016; **73**:630–637.

35. Fadaei A. An investigation into the association between suicide mortality rate and lithium levels in potable water: a review study. *Int Clin Psychopharmacol* 2023; **38**:73–80.

36. Nolen WA, et al. The association of the effect of lithium in the maintenance treatment of bipolar disorder with lithium plasma levels: a post hoc analysis of a double-blind study comparing switching to lithium or placebo in patients who responded to quetiapine (Trial 144). *Bipolar Disord* 2013; **15**:100–109.

37. Severus WE, et al. What is the optimal serum lithium level in the long-term treatment of bipolar disorder—a review? *Bipolar Disord* 2008; **10**:231–237.

38. Manchia M, et al. Lithium and its effects: does dose matter? *Int J Bipolar Disord* 2024; **12**:23.

39. Young AH. Lithium for long-term treatment of unipolar depression. *Lancet Psychiatry* 2017; **4**:511–512.

40. Strawbridge R, et al. Lithium: how low can you go? *Int J Bipolar Disord* 2024; **12**:4.

41. Moore CM, et al. Brain-to-serum lithium ratio and age: an in vivo magnetic resonance spectroscopy study. *Am J Psychiatry* 2002; **159**:1240–1242.

42. Bowen RC, et al. Less frequent lithium administration and lower urine volume. *Am J Psychiatry* 1991; **148**:189–192.

43. Ljubicic D, et al. Lithium treatments: single and multiple daily dosing. *Can J Psychiatry* 2008; **53**:323–331.

44. Gong R, et al. What we need to know about the effect of lithium on the kidney. *Am J Physiol Renal Physiol* 2016; **311**:F1168–F1171.

45. Aiff H, et al. Effects of 10 to 30 years of lithium treatment on kidney function. *J Psychopharmacol* 2015; **29**:608–614.

46. Parsaik AK, et al. Effects of long-term lithium therapy on kidney functioning in mood disorders: a population-based historical cohort study. *Bipolar Disord* 2024; doi: 10.1111/bdi.13501.

47. Frye MA, et al. Depressive relapse during lithium treatment associated with increased serum thyroid-stimulating hormone: results from two placebo-controlled bipolar I maintenance studies. *Acta Psychiatr Scand* 2009; **120**:10–13.

48. Johnston AM, et al. Lithium-associated clinical hypothyroidism. Prevalence and risk factors. *Br J Psychiatry* 1999; **175**:336–339.

49. Livingstone C, et al. Lithium: a review of its metabolic adverse effects. *J Psychopharmacol* 2006; **20**:347–355.

50. McKnight RF, et al. Lithium toxicity profile: a systematic review and meta-analysis. *Lancet* 2012; **379**:721–728.

51. Vandermeulen L, et al. Lithium-associated hypercalcemia and hyperparathyroidism: a systematic review and meta-analysis. *World J Biol Psychiatry* 2024; **25**:417–429.

52. Czarnywojtek A, et al. Effect of lithium carbonate on the function of the thyroid gland: mechanism of action and clinical implications. *J Physiol Pharmacol* 2020; **71**:191–199.

53. Ott M, et al. Lithium intoxication: incidence, clinical course and renal function – a population-based retrospective cohort study. *J Psychopharmacol* 2016; **30**:1008–1019.

54. Bell AJ, et al. Lithium neurotoxicity at normal therapeutic levels. *Br J Psychiatry* 1993; **162**:689–692.

55. Smith FE, et al. 3D ⁷Li magnetic resonance imaging of brain lithium distribution in bipolar disorder. *Mol Psychiatry* 2018; **23**:2184–2191.

56. Gerrett D, et al. Prescribing and monitoring lithium therapy: summary of a safety report from the National Patient Safety Agency. *BMJ* 2010; **341**:c6258.

57. Morriss R, et al. Lithium and eGFR: a new routinely available tool for the prevention of chronic kidney disease. *Br J Psychiatry* 2008; **193**:93–95.

58. National Institute for Health and Care Excellence. Bipolar disorder: assessment and management. Clinical guideline [CG185]. 2014 (last updated December 2023, last accessed October 2024); https://www.nice.org.uk/guidance/cg185.

59. Collins N, et al. Standards of lithium monitoring in mental health trusts in the UK. *BMC Psychiatry* 2010; **10**:80.

60. Paton C, et al. Monitoring lithium therapy: the impact of a quality improvement programme in the UK. *Bipolar Disord* 2013; **15**:865–875.

61. Kirkham E, et al. Impact of active monitoring on lithium management in Norfolk. *Ther Adv Psychopharmacol* 2013; **3**:260–265.

62. Cavanagh J, et al. Relapse into mania or depression following lithium discontinuation: a 7-year follow-up. *Acta Psychiatr Scand* 2004; **109**:91–95.

63. Yazici O, et al. Controlled lithium discontinuation in bipolar patients with good response to long-term lithium prophylaxis. *J Affect Disord* 2004; **80**:269–271.

64. Goodwin GM. Recurrence of mania after lithium withdrawal. Implications for the use of lithium in the treatment of bipolar affective disorder. *Br J Psychiatry* 1994; **164**:149–152.

65. Baldessarini RJ, et al. Effects of the rate of discontinuing lithium maintenance treatment in bipolar disorders. *J Clin Psychiatry* 1996; **57**:441–448.

66. Biel MG, et al. Continuation versus discontinuation of lithium in recurrent bipolar illness: a naturalistic study. *Bipolar Disord* 2007; **9**:435–442.

67. Sajatovic M, et al. Treatment adherence with lithium and anticonvulsant medications among patients with bipolar disorder. *Psychiatr Serv* 2007; **58**:855–863.

68. Paton C, et al. Lithium in bipolar and other affective disorders: prescribing practice in the UK. *J Psychopharmacol* 2010; **24**:1739–1746.

69. Kessing LV, et al. Suicide risk in patients treated with lithium. *Arch Gen Psychiatry* 2005; **62**:860–866.

70. Pharmaceutical Press. Medicines Complete 2024; https://www.pharmaceuticalpress.com/services/medicinescomplete/.

71. Juurlink DN, et al. Drug-induced lithium toxicity in the elderly: a population-based study. *J Am Geriatr Soc* 2004; **52**:794–798.

72. Finley PR. Drug interactions with lithium: an update. *Clin Pharmacokinet* 2016; **55**:925–941.

73. Netto I, et al. Lithium neurotoxicity due to second-generation antipsychotics combined with lithium: a systematic review. *Prim Care Companion CNS Disord* 2019; **21**:17r02225.

74. Konieczny K, et al. The syndrome of irreversible lithium-effectuated neurotoxicity: a scoping review. *Alpha Psychiatry* 2024; **25**:190–205.

75. Kohler-Forsberg O, et al. Nonsteroidal anti-inflammatory drugs (NSAIDs) and paracetamol do not affect 6-month mood-stabilizing treatment outcome among 482 patients with bipolar disorder. *Depress Anxiety* 2017; **34**:281–290.

Valproate

Mechanism of action[1]

Valproate is a simple branched-chain fatty acid. Its mechanism of action is complex and not fully understood. Valproate inhibits the catabolism of gamma-aminobutyric acid (GABA), reduces the turnover of arachidonic acid, activates the extracellular signal-regulated kinase (ERK) pathway and thus alters synaptic plasticity, interferes with intracellular signalling, promotes brain-derived neurotrophic factor (BDNF) expression and reduces levels of protein kinase C. Research has focused on the ability of valproate to alter the expression of various genes that are involved in transcription regulation, cytoskeletal modifications and ion homeostasis. Other mechanisms that have been proposed include depletion of inositol and indirect effects on non-GABA pathways through the inhibition of voltage-gated sodium channels.

There is a growing literature relating to the potential use of valproate as an adjunctive treatment in several types of cancer,[2] a property which may also confer some effects on neuroplasticity.[3]

Formulations

Valproate is available in the UK in three forms: sodium valproate and valproic acid (licensed for the treatment of epilepsy) and semi-sodium valproate (licensed for the treatment of acute mania). Both semi-sodium and sodium valproate are metabolised to valproic acid, which is responsible for the pharmacological activity of all three preparations.[4] Clinical studies of the treatment of affective disorders variably use sodium valproate, semi-sodium valproate, 'valproate' or valproic acid. The great majority have used semi-sodium valproate.

It is unclear if there is any difference in efficacy between valproic acid, valproate semi-sodium and sodium valproate. One large US quasi-experimental study found that in-patients who initially received the semi-sodium preparation had a hospital stay that was a third longer than patients who initially received valproic acid.[5] One clear difference is that controlled-release sodium valproate (Epilim Chrono[6]) can be administered as a once daily dose whereas other sodium and semi-sodium valproate preparations require at least twice daily administration. Overall, there are probably no important differences between different valproate forms,[7] except for the small differences in bioavailability related to valproate content.

Indications

Randomised controlled trials (RCTs) have shown valproate to be effective in the treatment of **mania**,[8,9] with a response rate of 50% and a number needed to treat (NNT) of 2–4,[10] although large negative studies do exist.[11] One RCT found lithium to be more effective overall than valproate[9] but a large (n = 300) randomised open trial of 12 weeks' duration found lithium and valproate to be equally effective in the treatment of acute mania.[12] Valproate may be effective in patients who have failed to respond to lithium.[13] It may be less effective than olanzapine, both as monotherapy[14] *and* as an adjunctive treatment to lithium[12] in acute mania. One network meta-analysis reported that valproate was less effective but better tolerated than lithium.[15] Overall, data relating to efficacy in mania are less convincing for valproate than for lithium and a range of antipsychotics.[16,17]

A meta-analysis of four small RCTs concluded that valproate is effective in **bipolar depression** with a small to medium effect size.[18] A 2020 meta-analysis placed divalproex fifth out of 21 treatments for bipolar depression.[19] Valproate has limited utility in **rapid-cycling bipolar disorder**.[20]

Although open-label studies suggest that valproate is effective in the **prophylaxis** of bipolar affective disorder,[21] RCT data are limited.[22,23] Bowden et al.[24] found no difference between lithium, valproate and placebo in the primary outcome measure, time to any mood episode, although valproate was superior to lithium and placebo on some secondary outcome measures. In another RCT[22] there was no difference in relapse rates between valproate and olanzapine. A post-hoc analysis of data from this study found that patients with rapid-cycling illness had a better very early response to valproate than to olanzapine but that this advantage was not maintained.[23] Outcomes with respect to manic symptoms for those who did not have a rapid-cycling illness were better at 1 year with olanzapine than with valproate. In a further 20-month RCT of lithium versus valproate in patients with rapid-cycling illness, both the relapse and attrition rates were high, and no difference in efficacy between valproate and lithium was apparent.[25] The independent BALANCE study found lithium to be numerically superior to valproate, and the combination of lithium and valproate statistically superior to valproate alone.[26] Aripiprazole in combination with valproate is superior to valproate alone.[27] Overall, data suggest that adjunctive valproate provides additional protection against relapse.[28]

In the UK, the National Institute for Health and Care Excellence (NICE) recommends valproate as a first-line option for the treatment of acute episodes of mania, in combination with an antidepressant for the treatment of acute episodes of depression, and for prophylaxis,[29] but importantly NOT in women of child-bearing potential.[29,30] A Cochrane review concluded that the evidence supporting the use of valproate as prophylaxis is limited.[31]

Valproate is sometimes used to treat aggressive behaviours of variable aetiology.[32] One RCT (n = 16) failed to detect any advantage for risperidone augmented with valproate over risperidone alone in reducing hostility in patients with schizophrenia.[33] A mirror-image study found that, in patients with schizophrenia or bipolar disorder in a secure setting, valproate decreased agitation.[34]

There is a small positive placebo-controlled RCT of valproate in generalised anxiety disorder.[35] Valproate may also have preventive benefits against COVID-19.[36]

Plasma levels

The pharmacokinetics of valproate are complex, following a three-compartmental model and showing protein-binding saturation. Plasma level monitoring is supposedly of more limited use than with lithium or carbamazepine.[37] There may be a linear association between valproate serum levels and response in acute mania, with serum levels <55mg/L being no more effective than placebo, and levels >94mg/L being associated with the most robust response.[38] Optimal serum levels during the maintenance phase are unknown, but are likely to be at least 50mg/L.[39] Achieving therapeutic plasma levels rapidly using a loading dose regimen is generally well tolerated. Plasma levels can also be used to detect non-compliance or toxicity. Using total valproate concentration (the standard method) is no less useful than free valproate levels in most situations.[40]

Adverse effects

Valproate can cause both gastric irritation and hyperammonaemia,[41] both of which can lead to nausea. Lethargy and confusion can occasionally occur with starting doses above 750mg/day. Weight gain can be significant,[42] particularly when valproate is used in combination with clozapine. Valproate causes dose-related tremor in up to a quarter of patients.[43] In most of these patients, it is intention/postural tremor that is problematic, but a very small proportion develop parkinsonism associated with cognitive decline; these symptoms are reversible when valproate is discontinued.[44]

Hair loss (with curly regrowth)[45] and peripheral oedema can occur, as can thrombocytopenia, leucopenia, red cell hypoplasia and pancreatitis.[46] Valproate can cause hyperandrogenism in women[47] and has been linked with the development of polycystic ovaries although the evidence supporting this association is conflicting. Valproate is a major human teratogen (see Chapter 7). Valproate may also affect male fertility[48] but its teratogenic effect in men is disputed.[49–51] Valproate may very rarely cause fulminant hepatic failure. Young children receiving multiple anticonvulsants are most at risk. Any patient with raised liver function tests (LFTs; common in early treatment[52]) should be evaluated clinically and other markers of hepatic function such as albumin and clotting time should be checked.

Many adverse effects of valproate are dose-related (and often peak plasma level related) and increase sharply in frequency and severity when the plasma concentration is >100mg/L. The once daily modified-release form of sodium valproate does not produce as high peak plasma levels as the conventional formulation, and so may be better tolerated.

Valproate and other antiseizure medications have been associated with an increased risk of suicidal behaviour[53] but this finding is not consistent across studies.[54] Patients with depression[55] or who take another antiseizure medication that increases the risk of developing depression may be a subgroup at greater risk.[56]

Pre-treatment tests

Baseline full blood count (FBC), LFTs and weight or BMI are recommended by NICE in the UK.

On-treatment monitoring

In the UK, NICE recommends that an FBC and LFTs should be repeated after 6 months, and that BMI should be monitored. Valproate summary of product characteristics (SPCs) recommends more frequent LFTs during the first 6 months with albumin and clotting measured if enzyme levels are abnormal. Where there is clear hypalbuminaemia, free valproate levels should be measured.

Discontinuation

It is unknown if abrupt discontinuation of valproate worsens the natural course of bipolar illness in the same manner as lithium. One small naturalistic retrospective study suggested that it might.[57] Until further data are available, if valproate is to be discontinued, it should be done slowly over at least a month, preferably longer. In people with epilepsy, valproate withdrawal is associated with depression, falls and hospital admissions.[58]

Use in women of child-bearing age

Valproate is an established human teratogen. NICE recommends that alternative antiseizure medications are preferred in women with epilepsy[59] and that valproate should not be used to treat bipolar illness in women of child-bearing age.[29] The teratogenic potential of valproate is not widely appreciated and in the past many women of child-bearing age were not advised of the need for contraception or prophylactic folate.[60,61] Valproate may also cause impaired cognitive function in children exposed to valproate in utero.[62] Valproate is now contraindicated in women of child-bearing potential in many countries (see Chapter 7).

Interactions with other drugs

Valproate is highly protein bound and can be displaced by other protein bound drugs such as aspirin, leading to toxicity. Aspirin also inhibits the metabolism of valproate; a dose of at least 300mg aspirin is required.[63] Other, less strongly protein bound drugs such as warfarin can be displaced by valproate, leading to higher free levels and toxicity.

Valproate is hepatically metabolised; drugs that inhibit CYP enzymes can increase valproate levels (e.g. erythromycin, fluoxetine and cimetidine). Valproate can increase the plasma levels of some drugs by inhibition of glucuronidation. Examples include tricyclic antidepressants (TCAs; particularly clomipramine[64]), lamotrigine,[65] quetiapine,[66] warfarin[67] and phenobarbital. Valproate may also significantly lower plasma olanzapine concentrations although the mechanism is unknown.[68]

Pharmacodynamic interactions also occur. The anticonvulsant effect of valproate is antagonised by drugs that lower the seizure threshold (e.g. antipsychotics). Weight gain can be exacerbated by other drugs such as clozapine and olanzapine.

Table 2.3 summarises the prescribing and monitoring of valproate.

Table 2.3 Valproate: prescribing and monitoring.

Indications	Mania, hypomania, bipolar depression and prophylaxis of bipolar affective disorder. May reduce aggression in a range of psychiatric disorders (although data are weak).
Pre-valproate work-up	FBC and LFTs. Baseline measure of weight desirable.
Prescribing	Titrate dose upwards against response and adverse effects. Loading doses can be used and are generally well tolerated. Modified-release sodium valproate (Epilim Chrono⁶) can be given once daily. All other formulations must be administered at least twice daily. Plasma levels can be used to assure adequate dosing and treatment compliance. Blood should be taken immediately before the next dose.
Monitoring	FBC and LFTs if clinically indicated. Weight (or body mass index).
Stopping	Reduce slowly over at least 1 month, preferably longer.

References

1. Rosenberg G. The mechanisms of action of valproate in neuropsychiatric disorders: can we see the forest for the trees? *Cell Mol Life Sci* 2007; **64**:2090–2103.
2. Natale G, et al. Valproate and lithium: old drugs for new pharmacological approaches in brain tumors? *Cancer Lett* 2023; **560**:216125.
3. Gervain J, et al. Valproate reopens critical-period learning of absolute pitch. *Front Syst Neurosci* 2013; 7:1–11.
4. Fisher C, et al. Sodium valproate or valproate semisodium: is there a difference in the treatment of bipolar disorder? *Psychiatric Bulletin* 2003; **27**:446–448.
5. Wassef AA, et al. Lower effectiveness of divalproex versus valproic acid in a prospective, quasi-experimental clinical trial involving 9,260 psychiatric admissions. *Am J Psychiatry* 2005; **162**:330–339.
6. SANOFI. Summary of product characteristics. Epilim Chrono (valproic acid, sodium valproate) 500mg. 2024 (last accessed October 2024); https://www.medicines.org.uk/emc/medicine/6779.
7. Delage C, et al. Valproate, divalproex, valpromide: are the differences in indications justified? *Biomed Pharmacother* 2023; **158**:114051.
8. Bowden CL, et al. Efficacy of divalproex vs lithium and placebo in the treatment of mania. The Depakote Mania Study Group. *JAMA* 1994; **271**:918–924.
9. Freeman TW, et al. A double-blind comparison of valproate and lithium in the treatment of acute mania. *Am J Psychiatry* 1992; **149**:108–111.
10. Nasrallah HA, et al. Carbamazepine and valproate for the treatment of bipolar disorder: a review of the literature. *J Affect Disord* 2006; **95**:69–78.
11. Hirschfeld RM, et al. A randomized, placebo-controlled, multicenter study of divalproex sodium extended-release in the acute treatment of mania. *J Clin Psychiatry* 2010; **71**:426–432.
12. Bowden C, et al. A 12-week, open, randomized trial comparing sodium valproate to lithium in patients with bipolar I disorder suffering from a manic episode. *Int Clin Psychopharmacol* 2008; **23**:254–262.
13. Pope HG, Jr, et al. Valproate in the treatment of acute mania. A placebo-controlled study. *Arch Gen Psychiatry* 1991; **48**:62–68.
14. Novick D, et al. Translation of randomised controlled trial findings into clinical practice: comparison of olanzapine and valproate in the EMBLEM study. *Pharmacopsychiatry* 2009; **42**:145–152.
15. Cipriani A, et al. Comparative efficacy and acceptability of antimanic drugs in acute mania: a multiple-treatments meta-analysis. *Lancet* 2011; **378**:1306–1315.
16. Kishi T, et al. Pharmacological treatment for bipolar mania: a systematic review and network meta-analysis of double-blind randomized controlled trials. *Mol Psychiatry* 2022; **27**:1136–1144.
17. Hsu TW, et al. Variability and efficacy in treatment effects on manic symptoms with lithium, anticonvulsants, and antipsychotics in acute bipolar mania: a systematic review and meta-analysis. *EClinicalMedicine* 2022; **54**:101690.
18. Smith LA, et al. Valproate for the treatment of acute bipolar depression: systematic review and meta-analysis. *J Affect Disord* 2010; **122**:1–9.
19. Bahji A, et al. Comparative efficacy and tolerability of pharmacological treatments for the treatment of acute bipolar depression: a systematic review and network meta-analysis. *J Affect Disord* 2020; **269**:154–184.
20. Strawbridge R, et al. A systematic review and meta-analysis of treatments for rapid cycling bipolar disorder. *Acta Psychiatr Scand* 2022; **146**:290–311.
21. Calabrese JR, et al. Spectrum of efficacy of valproate in 55 patients with rapid-cycling bipolar disorder. *Am J Psychiatry* 1990; **147**:431–434.
22. Tohen M, et al. Olanzapine versus divalproex sodium for the treatment of acute mania and maintenance of remission: a 47-week study. *Am J Psychiatry* 2003; **160**:1263–1271.
23. Suppes T, et al. Rapid versus non-rapid cycling as a predictor of response to olanzapine and divalproex sodium for bipolar mania and maintenance of remission: post hoc analyses of 47-week data. *J Affect Disord* 2005; **89**:69–77.
24. Bowden CL, et al. A randomized, placebo-controlled 12-month trial of divalproex and lithium in treatment of outpatients with bipolar I disorder. Divalproex Maintenance Study Group. *Arch Gen Psychiatry* 2000; **57**:481–489.
25. Calabrese JR, et al. A 20-month, double-blind, maintenance trial of lithium versus divalproex in rapid-cycling bipolar disorder. *Am J Psychiatry* 2005; **162**:2152–2161.
26. Geddes JR, et al. Lithium plus valproate combination therapy versus monotherapy for relapse prevention in bipolar I disorder (BALANCE): a randomised open-label trial. *Lancet* 2010; **375**:385–395.
27. Marcus R, et al. Efficacy of aripiprazole adjunctive to lithium or valproate in the long-term treatment of patients with bipolar I disorder with an inadequate response to lithium or valproate monotherapy: a multicenter, double-blind, randomized study. *Bipolar Disord* 2011; **13**:133–144.
28. Nestsiarovich A, et al. Preventing new episodes of bipolar disorder in adults: systematic review and meta-analysis of randomized controlled trials. *Eur Neuropsychopharmacol* 2022; **54**:75–89.
29. National Institute for Health and Care Excellence. Bipolar disorder: assessment and management. Clinical guideline [CG185]. 2014 (last updated December 2023, last accessed October 2024); https://www.nice.org.uk/guidance/cg185.
30. National Institute for Health and Care Excellence. Antenatal and postnatal mental health: clinical management and service guidance. Clinical guideline [CG192]. 2014 (last updated February 2020, last accessed October 2024); https://www.nice.org.uk/guidance/cg192.
31. Cipriani A, et al. Valproic acid, valproate and divalproex in the maintenance treatment of bipolar disorder. *Cochrane Database Syst Rev* 2013; **10**:CD003196.
32. Lindenmayer JP, et al. Use of sodium valproate in violent and aggressive behaviors: a critical review. *J Clin Psychiatry* 2000; **61**:123–128.

CHAPTER 2

33. Citrome L, et al. Risperidone alone versus risperidone plus valproate in the treatment of patients with schizophrenia and hostility. *Int Clin Psychopharmacol* 2007; **22**:356–362.

34. Gobbi G, et al. Efficacy of topiramate, valproate, and their combination on aggression/agitation behavior in patients with psychosis. *J Clin Psychopharmacol* 2006; **26**:467–473.

35. Aliyev NA, et al. Valproate (depakine-chrono) in the acute treatment of outpatients with generalized anxiety disorder without psychiatric comorbidity: randomized, double-blind placebo-controlled study. *Eur Psychiatry* 2008; **23**:109–114.

36. Watson A, et al. Valproic acid use is associated with diminished risk of contracting COVID-19, and diminished disease severity: epidemiologic and in vitro analysis reveal mechanistic insights. *PLoS One* 2024; **19**:e0307154.

37. Haymond J, et al. Does valproic acid warrant therapeutic drug monitoring in bipolar affective disorder? *Ther Drug Monit* 2010; **32**:19–29.

38. Allen MH, et al. Linear relationship of valproate serum concentration to response and optimal serum levels for acute mania. *Am J Psychiatry* 2006; **163**:272–275.

39. Taylor D, et al. Doses of carbamazepine and valproate in bipolar affective disorder. *Psychiatric Bulletin* 1997; **21**:221–223.

40. Krishna MBN, et al. Total valproate versus free valproate in therapeutic drug monitoring for bipolar disorder: a cross-sectional study. *Asia Pac Psychiatry* 2024; **16**:e12555.

41. Segura-Bruna N, et al. Valproate-induced hyperammonemic encephalopathy. *Acta Neurol Scand* 2006; **114**:1–7.

42. El-Khatib F, et al. Valproate, weight gain and carbohydrate craving: a gender study. *Seizure* 2007; **16**:226–232.

43. Zadikoff C, et al. Movement disorders in patients taking anticonvulsants. *J Neurol Neurosurg Psychiatry* 2007; **78**:147–151.

44. Ristic AJ, et al. The frequency of reversible parkinsonism and cognitive decline associated with valproate treatment: a study of 364 patients with different types of epilepsy. *Epilepsia* 2006; **47**:2183–2185.

45. Praharaj SK, et al. Valproate-associated hair abnormalities: pathophysiology and management strategies. *Hum Psychopharmacol* 2022; **37**:e2814.

46. Gerstner T, et al. Valproic acid-induced pancreatitis: 16 new cases and a review of the literature. *J Gastroenterol* 2007; **42**:39–48.

47. Joffe H, et al. Valproate is associated with new-onset oligoamenorrhea with hyperandrogenism in women with bipolar disorder. *Biol Psychiatry* 2006; **59**:1078–1086.

48. Asghar MA, et al. Understanding the impact of valproate on male fertility: insights from preclinical and clinical meta-analysis. *BMC Pharmacol Toxicol* 2024; **25**:69.

49. Garey JD, et al. Paternal valproate treatment and risk of childhood neurodevelopmental disorders: precautionary regulatory measures are insufficiently substantiated. *Birth Defects Res* 2024; **116**:e2392.

50. Christensen J, et al. Valproate use during spermatogenesis and risk to offspring. *JAMA Netw Open* 2024; **7**:e2414709.

51. Angus-Leppan H, et al. New valproate regulations, informed choice and seizure risk. *J Neurol* 2024; **271**:5671–5686.

52. Bjornsson E. Hepatotoxicity associated with antiepileptic drugs. *Acta Neurol Scand* 2008; **118**:281–290.

53. Patorno E, et al. Anticonvulsant medications and the risk of suicide, attempted suicide, or violent death. *JAMA* 2010; **303**:1401–1409.

54. Gibbons RD, et al. Relationship between antiepileptic drugs and suicide attempts in patients with bipolar disorder. *Arch Gen Psychiatry* 2009; **66**:1354–1360.

55. Arana A, et al. Suicide-related events in patients treated with antiepileptic drugs. *N Engl J Med* 2010; **363**:542–551.

56. Andersohn F, et al. Use of antiepileptic drugs in epilepsy and the risk of self-harm or suicidal behavior. *Neurology* 2010; **75**:335–340.

57. Franks MA, et al. Bouncing back: is the bipolar rebound phenomenon peculiar to lithium? A retrospective naturalistic study. *J Psychopharmacol* 2008; **22**:452–456.

58. Mbizvo GK, et al. Morbidity and mortality risks associated with valproate withdrawal in young adults with epilepsy. *Brain* 2024; **147**:3426–3441.

59. National Institute for Health and Care Excellence. Epilepsies in children, young people and adults. NICE guideline [NG217]. 2022 (last accessed October 2024); https://www.nice.org.uk/guidance/ng217.

60. James L, et al. Informing patients of the teratogenic potential of mood stabilising drugs; a case notes review of the practice of psychiatrists. *J Psychopharmacol* 2007; **21**:815–819.

61. James L, et al. Mood stabilizers and teratogenicity – prescribing practice and awareness amongst practising psychiatrists. *J Mental Health* 2009; **18**:137–143.

62. Meador KJ, et al. Cognitive function at 3 years of age after fetal exposure to antiepileptic drugs. *N Engl J Med* 2009; **360**:1597–1605.

63. Sandson NB, et al. An interaction between aspirin and valproate: the relevance of plasma protein displacement drug-drug interactions. *Am J Psychiatry* 2006; **163**:1891–1896.

64. Fehr C, et al. Increase in serum clomipramine concentrations caused by valproate. *J Clin Psychopharmacol* 2000; **20**:493–494.

65. Morris RG, et al. Clinical study of lamotrigine and valproic acid in patients with epilepsy: using a drug interaction to advantage? *Ther Drug Monit* 2000; **22**:656–660.

66. Aichhorn W, et al. Influence of age, gender, body weight and valproate comedication on quetiapine plasma concentrations. *Int Clin Psychopharmacol* 2006; **21**:81–85.

67. Gunes A, et al. Inhibitory effect of valproic acid on cytochrome P450 2C9 activity in epilepsy patients. *Basic Clin Pharmacol Toxicol* 2007; **100**:383–386.

68. Bergemann N, et al. Valproate lowers plasma concentration of olanzapine. *J Clin Psychopharmacol* 2006; **26**:432–434.

Carbamazepine

Mechanism of action[1]

Carbamazepine blocks voltage-dependent sodium channels, thus inhibiting repetitive neuronal firing. It reduces glutamate release and decreases the turnover of dopamine and noradrenaline. While carbamazepine has a similar molecular structure to TCAs, it is radically different in respect to both therapeutic and adverse effects.

Oxcarbazepine (a structural derivative of carbamazepine), as well as blocking voltage-dependent sodium channels, also increases potassium conductance and modulates high-voltage activated calcium channels. Eslicarbazepine is available in some countries. Like oxcarbazepine it acts as a pro-drug for licarbazepine, the likely active molecule of all three drugs.

Formulations

Carbamazepine is available as a liquid, chewable and immediate-release and controlled-release tablets. Non-modified release formulations generally have to be administered two to three times daily. The controlled-release preparation can be given once or twice daily, and the reduced fluctuation in serum levels usually leads to improved tolerability. This modified-release preparation has a lower bioavailability and an increase in dose of 10–15% may be required.

Indications

Carbamazepine is primarily used as an antiseizure medication. It is also used in the treatment of trigeminal neuralgia and, in the UK and elsewhere, is licensed for the treatment of bipolar illness in patients who do not respond to lithium.

With respect to the treatment of **mania**, two placebo-controlled randomised studies have found the extended-release formulation of carbamazepine to be effective. In both studies, the response rate in the carbamazepine arm was twice that in the placebo arm.[2,3] Carbamazepine was not particularly well tolerated – the incidence of dizziness, somnolence and nausea was high. Another study found carbamazepine alone to be as effective as carbamazepine plus olanzapine.[4] Most formal guidelines do not recommend carbamazepine as a first-line treatment for mania.[5] A Cochrane review concluded that there were insufficient trials of adequate methodological quality of oxcarbazepine in the acute treatment of bipolar disorder to inform its efficacy and acceptability.[6] More recent reviews suggest oxcarbazepine has useful efficacy in mania.[7] Two 2022 network meta-analyses[8,9] confirmed the efficacy and relatively poor tolerability of carbamazepine.

Open studies suggest that carbamazepine monotherapy has some efficacy in **bipolar depression**[10] but evidence supporting other strategies is stronger (see section on treatment of bipolar depression later in this chapter). Carbamazepine may also be useful in **unipolar depression** either alone[11] or as an augmentation strategy.[12]

Carbamazepine is generally considered to be less effective than lithium in the prophylaxis of bipolar illness.[13] A 2009 meta-analysis failed to find a significant difference in efficacy between lithium and carbamazepine, but those who received carbamazepine were more likely to drop out of treatment because of adverse effects.[14] Lithium is considered to be superior to carbamazepine in reducing suicidal behaviour,[15] although data are not consistent[16] and carbamazepine may have anti-suicidal properties.[17] In the UK, NICE considers carbamazepine to be a third-line prophylactic agent[5] and data emerging since this guidance support this positioning.[18] Three small studies suggest the related oxcarbazepine may have some prophylactic efficacy when used in combination with other mood-stabilising drugs.[19–21]

There are data supporting the use of carbamazepine in the management of **alcohol withdrawal** symptoms,[22] although the high initial doses required are often poorly tolerated. A Cochrane review did not consider the evidence strong enough to support the use of carbamazepine for this indication.[23] Carbamazepine has also been used to manage **aggressive behaviour** in patients with schizophrenia;[24] the quality of data is weak and the mode of action unknown. There are a number of case reports and open case series that report on the use of carbamazepine in various psychiatric illnesses such as **panic disorder, borderline personality disorder** and **episodic dyscontrol syndrome.**

Plasma levels

When carbamazepine is used as an antiseizure medication, the therapeutic range is generally considered to be 4–12mg/L, although the supporting evidence is not strong. In patients with affective illness, a dose of at least 600mg/day and a plasma level of at least 7mg/L may be required,[25] although this is not a consistent finding.[4,11,26] Levels above 12mg/L are associated with a higher adverse effect burden.

Carbamazepine blood concentrations vary markedly within the dosage interval. It is therefore important to sample at a point in time where levels are likely to be reproducible for any given individual. The most appropriate way of monitoring is to take a trough level before the first dose of the day. Carbamazepine metabolism is genetically determined and so genetic testing may be helpful before starting carbamazepine.[27]

Carbamazepine is a hepatic enzyme inducer that induces its own metabolism as well as that of other drugs, including some antipsychotics.[28] An initial plasma half-life of around 30 hours is reduced to around 12 hours on chronic dosing. For this reason, plasma levels should be checked 2–4 weeks after starting or after an increase in dose to ensure that the desired level is still being obtained.

Most published clinical trials that demonstrated the efficacy of carbamazepine as a mood stabiliser used doses that are significantly higher (800–1200mg/day) than those commonly prescribed in UK clinical practice.[29]

Adverse effects[1]

The main adverse effects associated with carbamazepine therapy are dizziness, diplopia, drowsiness, ataxia, nausea and headaches. They can sometimes be avoided by starting with a low dose and increasing slowly. Avoiding high peak blood levels by splitting the dose throughout the day or using a controlled-release formulation may also help. Dry mouth, oedema and hyponatraemia are also common. Sexual dysfunction can occur, probably mediated through reduced testosterone levels.[30] Around 3% of patients treated with carbamazepine develop a generalised erythematous rash. Serious exfoliative dermatological reactions can rarely occur and vulnerability is genetically determined.[31] The human lymphocyte antigen (HLA) variant B*15:02 has a sensitivity of around 70%

and a specificity approaching 100% in certain populations.[32] Genetic testing in people from South-East Asia is recommended before carbamazepine is prescribed. Carbamazepine is a known human teratogen (see Chapter 7).

Carbamazepine commonly causes a chronic low white blood cell (WBC) count. One patient in 20,000 develops agranulocytosis and/or aplastic anaemia.[33] Raised alkaline phosphate (ALP) and gamma-glutamyl transferase (GGT) are common (a GGT of 2–3 times normal is rarely a cause for concern[34]). A delayed multiorgan hypersensitivity reaction rarely occurs, mainly manifesting itself as various skin reactions, a low WBC count and abnormal LFTs. Fatalities have been reported.[34,35] There is no clear timescale for these events.

Some antiseizure drugs have been associated with an increased risk of suicidal behaviour. Carbamazepine has not been implicated, either in general[36,37] or more specifically in those with bipolar illness.[38]

Pre-treatment tests

Baseline U&Es, FBC and LFTs are recommended by NICE. A baseline measure of weight is also desirable.

On-treatment monitoring

In the UK, NICE recommends that U&Es, FBC and LFTs should be repeated after 6 months, and that weight (or BMI) should also be monitored.

Discontinuation

It is not known if abrupt discontinuation of carbamazepine worsens the natural course of bipolar illness in the same way that abrupt cessation of lithium does. In one small case series (n = 6), one patient developed depression within a month of discontinuation,[39] while in another small case series (n = 4), three patients had a recurrence of their mood disorder within 3 months.[40] Until further data are available, if carbamazepine is to be discontinued, it should be done slowly (over at least a month).

Use in women of child-bearing age

Carbamazepine is an established human teratogen (see Chapter 7). Women who have mania are likely to be sexually disinhibited. The risk of unplanned pregnancy is likely to be above population norms (where 50% of pregnancies are unplanned). If carbamazepine cannot be avoided, adequate contraception should be ensured (note the interaction between carbamazepine and oral contraceptives outlined in the next section) and prophylactic folate prescribed.

Interactions with other drugs[41–44]

Carbamazepine is a potent inducer of hepatic cytochrome enzymes and is metabolised by CYP3A4. Plasma levels of most **antidepressants**, most **antipsychotics, benzodiazepines, warfarin, zolpidem,** some **cholinesterase inhibitors, methadone, thyroxine, theophylline, oestrogens** and **other steroids** may be reduced by carbamazepine, possibly resulting in treatment failure. Patients requiring contraception should either receive a preparation containing not less than 50mcg oestrogen or use a non-hormonal method. Drugs that inhibit CYP3A4 will increase carbamazepine plasma levels and may precipitate toxicity. Examples include **fluconazole, cimetidine, diltiazem, verapamil, erythromycin** and some **SSRIs**.

Pharmacodynamic interactions also occur. The antiseizure activity of carbamazepine is reduced by drugs that lower the seizure threshold (e.g. antipsychotics and antidepressants); the potential for carbamazepine to cause neutropenia may be increased by other drugs that depress the bone marrow function (e.g. clozapine); and the risk of hyponatraemia may be increased by other drugs that have the potential to deplete sodium (e.g. diuretics). Neurotoxicity has very rarely been reported when carbamazepine is used in combination with lithium.

As carbamazepine is structurally similar to TCAs, in theory it should not be given within 14 days of discontinuing a monoamine oxidase inhibitor (MAOI). There seems to be no clinical basis to this restriction.

Table 2.4 summarises the prescribing and monitoring of carbamazepine.

Table 2.4 Carbamazepine: prescribing and monitoring.

Indications	Mania (not first line), bipolar depression (evidence weak), unipolar depression (evidence weak) and prophylaxis of bipolar disorder (third line after antipsychotics and valproate). Alcohol withdrawal (may be poorly tolerated). Carbamazepine is licensed for the treatment of bipolar illness in patients who do not respond to lithium.
Pre-carbamazepine work-up	U&Es, FBC and LFTs. Baseline measure of weight desirable. HLA genotyping. CYP3A4 genotyping.
Prescribing	Titrate dose upwards against response and adverse effects; start with 100–200mg twice a day and aim for 400mg twice a day (some patients will require higher doses). The modified-release formulation (Tegretol Retard) can be given once to twice daily, is associated with less severe fluctuations in serum levels and is generally better tolerated. Plasma levels can be used to assure adequate dosing and treatment compliance. Blood should be taken immediately before the next dose. Carbamazepine induces its own metabolism. Blood levels should be re-checked 2 weeks after an increase in dose.
Monitoring	U&Es, FBC and LFTs yearly and when clinically indicated. Weight (or body mass index).
Stopping	Reduce slowly over at least 1 month, preferably longer. Hyperbolic tapering has theoretical support.

References

1. Novartis Pharmaceuticals UK Ltd. Summary of product characteristics. Tegretol tablets 100mg, 200mg, 400mg. 2024 (last accessed October 2024); https://www.medicines.org.uk/emc/medicine/1328.
2. Weisler RH, et al. A multicenter, randomized, double-blind, placebo-controlled trial of extended-release carbamazepine capsules as monotherapy for bipolar disorder patients with manic or mixed episodes. *J Clin Psychiatry* 2004; **65**:478–484.
3. Weisler RH, et al. Extended-release carbamazepine capsules as monotherapy for acute mania in bipolar disorder: a multicenter, randomized, double-blind, placebo-controlled trial. *J Clin Psychiatry* 2005; **66**:323–330.
4. Tohen M, et al. Olanzapine plus carbamazepine v. carbamazepine alone in treating manic episodes. *Br J Psychiatry* 2008; **192**:135–143.
5. National Institute for Health and Care Excellence. Bipolar disorder: assessment and management. Clinical guideline [CG185]. 2014 (last updated December 2023, last accessed October 2024); https://www.nice.org.uk/guidance/cg185.
6. Vasudev A, et al. Oxcarbazepine for acute affective episodes in bipolar disorder. *Cochrane Database Syst Rev* 2011; **12**:CD004857.
7. Grunze A, et al. Efficacy of carbamazepine and its derivatives in the treatment of bipolar disorder. *Medicina (Kaunas)* 2021; **57**:433.

8. Kishi T, et al. Pharmacological treatment for bipolar mania: a systematic review and network meta-analysis of double-blind randomized controlled trials. *Mol Psychiatry* 2022; **27**:1136–1144.

9. Hong Y, et al. A cumulative Bayesian network meta-analysis on the comparative efficacy of pharmacotherapies for mania over the last 40 years. *Psychopharmacology (Berl)* 2022; **239**:3367–3375.

10. Dilsaver SC, et al. Treatment of bipolar depression with carbamazepine: results of an open study. *Biol Psychiatry* 1996; **40**:935–937.

11. Zhang ZJ, et al. The effectiveness of carbamazepine in unipolar depression: a double-blind, randomized, placebo-controlled study. *J Affect Disord* 2008; **109**:91–97.

12. Kramlinger KG, et al. The addition of lithium to carbamazepine. Antidepressant efficacy in treatment-resistant depression. *Arch Gen Psychiatry* 1989; **46**:794–800.

13. Nasrallah HA, et al. Carbamazepine and valproate for the treatment of bipolar disorder: a review of the literature. *J Affect Disord* 2006; **95**:69–78.

14. Ceron-Litvoc D, et al. Comparison of carbamazepine and lithium in treatment of bipolar disorder: a systematic review of randomized controlled trials. *Hum Psychopharmacol* 2009; **24**:19–28.

15. Kleindienst N, et al. Differential efficacy of lithium and carbamazepine in the prophylaxis of bipolar disorder: results of the MAP study. *Neuropsychobiology* 2000; **42** Suppl 1:2–10.

16. Yerevanian BI, et al. Bipolar pharmacotherapy and suicidal behavior. Part I: Lithium, divalproex and carbamazepine. *J Affect Disord* 2007; **103**:5–11.

17. Tsai CJ, et al. The rapid suicide protection of mood stabilizers on patients with bipolar disorder: a nationwide observational cohort study in Taiwan. *J Affect Disord* 2016; **196**:71–77.

18. Peselow ED, et al. Prophylactic efficacy of lithium, valproic acid, and carbamazepine in the maintenance phase of bipolar disorder: a naturalistic study. *Int Clin Psychopharmacol* 2016; **31**:218–223.

19. Vieta E, et al. A double-blind, randomized, placebo-controlled prophylaxis trial of oxcarbazepine as adjunctive treatment to lithium in the long-term treatment of bipolar I and II disorder. *Int J Neuropsychopharmacol* 2008; **11**:445–452.

20. Conway CR, et al. An open-label trial of adjunctive oxcarbazepine for bipolar disorder. *J Clin Psychopharmacol* 2006; **26**:95–97.

21. Juruena MF, et al. Bipolar I and II disorder residual symptoms: oxcarbazepine and carbamazepine as add-on treatment to lithium in a double-blind, randomized trial. *Prog Neuropsychopharmacol Biol Psychiatry* 2009; **33**:94–99.

22. Malcolm R, et al. The effects of carbamazepine and lorazepam on single versus multiple previous alcohol withdrawals in an outpatient randomized trial. *J Gen Intern Med* 2002; **17**:349–355.

23. Minozzi S, et al. Anticonvulsants for alcohol withdrawal. *Cochrane Database Syst Rev* 2010; **3**:CD005064.

24. Brieden T, et al. Psychopharmacological treatment of aggression in schizophrenic patients. *Pharmacopsychiatry* 2002; **35**:83–89.

25. Taylor D, et al. Doses of carbamazepine and valproate in bipolar affective disorder. *Psychiatric Bulletin* 1997; **21**:221–223.

26. Simhandl C, et al. The comparative efficacy of carbamazepine low and high serum level and lithium carbonate in the prophylaxis of affective disorders. *J Affect Disord* 1993; **28**:221–231.

27. Riffi R, et al. Pharmacogenetics of carbamazepine: a systematic review on CYP3A4 and CYP3A5 polymorphisms. *CNS Neurol Disord Drug Targets* 2024; **23**:1463–1473.

28. Cohen H, et al. The extent of cytochrome P450 3A induction by antiseizure medications: a systematic review and network meta-analysis. *Epilepsia* 2024; **65**:445–455.

29. Taylor DM, et al. Prescribing and monitoring of carbamazepine and valproate – a case note review. *Psychiatric Bulletin* 2000; **24**:174–177.

30. Lossius MI, et al. Reversible effects of antiepileptic drugs on reproductive endocrine function in men and women with epilepsy – a prospective randomized double-blind withdrawal study. *Epilepsia* 2007; **48**:1875–1882.

31. Hung SI, et al. Genetic susceptibility to carbamazepine-induced cutaneous adverse drug reactions. *Pharmacogenet Genomics* 2006; **16**:297–306.

32. Moutaouakkil Y, et al. Diagnostic utility of human leukocyte antigen B*15:02 screening in severe carbamazepine hypersensitivity syndrome. *Ann Indian Acad Neurol* 2019; **22**:377–383.

33. Kaufman DW, et al. Drugs in the aetiology of agranulocytosis and aplastic anaemia. *Eur J Haematol Suppl* 1996; **60**:23–30.

34. Bjornsson E. Hepatotoxicity associated with antiepileptic drugs. *Acta Neurol Scand* 2008; **118**:281–290.

35. Ganeva M, et al. Carbamazepine-induced drug reaction with eosinophilia and systemic symptoms (DRESS) syndrome: report of four cases and brief review. *Int J Dermatol* 2008; **47**:853–860.

36. Patorno E, et al. Anticonvulsant medications and the risk of suicide, attempted suicide, or violent death. *JAMA* 2010; **303**:1401–1409.

37. Andersohn F, et al. Use of antiepileptic drugs in epilepsy and the risk of self-harm or suicidal behavior. *Neurology* 2010; **75**:335–340.

38. Gibbons RD, et al. Relationship between antiepileptic drugs and suicide attempts in patients with bipolar disorder. *Arch Gen Psychiatry* 2009; **66**:1354–1360.

39. Macritchie KA, et al. Does 'rebound mania' occur after stopping carbamazepine? A pilot study. *J Psychopharmacol* 2000; **14**:266–268.

40. Franks MA, et al. Bouncing back: is the bipolar rebound phenomenon peculiar to lithium? A retrospective naturalistic study. *J Psychopharmacol* 2008; **22**:452–456.

41. Spina E, et al. Clinical significance of pharmacokinetic interactions between antiepileptic and psychotropic drugs. *Epilepsia* 2002; **43** Suppl 2:37–44.

42. Patsalos PN, et al. The importance of drug interactions in epilepsy therapy. *Epilepsia* 2002; **43**:365–385.

43. Crawford P. Interactions between antiepileptic drugs and hormonal contraception. *CNS Drugs* 2002; **16**:263–272.

44. Citrome L, et al. Pharmacokinetics of aripiprazole and concomitant carbamazepine. *J Clin Psychopharmacol* 2007; **27**:279–283.

Antipsychotic drugs in bipolar disorder

Antipsychotic drugs not only have activity that reduces psychotic symptoms,[1] individual antipsychotics variously possess sedative, anxiolytic, anti-manic, mood-stabilising and antidepressant properties. Some antipsychotics (quetiapine and olanzapine) show all of these activities.

Antipsychotics licensed by the US Food and Drug Administration (FDA) for use in bipolar disorder include aripiprazole (mania, mixed episodes, maintenance treatment), asenapine (mania, mixed states), cariprazine and lumateperone (bipolar depression), lurasidone (bipolar depression), olanzapine (mania, mixed episodes, maintenance), olanzapine and fluoxetine (bipolar depression), quetiapine (mania, maintenance, bipolar depression), risperidone (mania, mixed episodes) and ziprasidone (mania, maintenance). Risperidone LAI has been approved for monotherapy or adjunctive maintenance, and aripiprazole depot for monotherapy maintenance treatment. EU labelling is similar except that olanzapine/fluoxetine in combination is not licensed for any indication and no second-generation antipsychotic (SGA) long-acting injection (LAI) has a licence for maintenance.

First-generation antipsychotics

These agents have long been used in mania and several studies support their use in the acute phase of illness, with superiority over placebo and comparable effects to lithium.[2,3] Their effectiveness is enhanced by combination with lithium.[4,5] In the longer-term maintenance treatment of bipolar disorder, first-generation antipsychotics (FGAs) are widely used[6] but modern, robust supporting data are absent.[7] FGAs are relatively more often associated with both depression and tardive dyskinesia in bipolar disorder[7-9] and their use is declining. The higher rate of tardive dyskinesia with FGAs is not in doubt, but the greater risk of depression,[10,11] while less well supported, is certainly worthy of consideration.

Second-generation antipsychotics

Mania

Network meta-analyses indicate superiority of antipsychotics over placebo in mania, with similar activity to so-called mood stabilisers.[12-14] In a 2023 network meta-analysis, efficacy of individual antipsychotics was broadly similar,[15] with a suggestion of superiority of risperidone.

Adjunctive treatment with antipsychotics is more effective than monotherapy with mood stabiliser medication, and augmentation with mood stabiliser medication is more effective than antipsychotic monotherapy. The combination is associated with more adverse effects, especially somnolence.[16] Interpretation of outcomes is made difficult by trials including patients whose mania occurred in the context of failed mood stabiliser treatment. Participants receive either a failed mood stabiliser or a mood stabiliser plus an antipsychotic. The superior effect of the combination is not surprising in this context.

Although the mechanism is difficult to discern, converging evidence suggests anti-manic effects of antipsychotics are related to their effects on the dopamine system.[17,18]

Bipolar depression

In acute treatment of bipolar depression, antipsychotics found to be effective include cariprazine, lumateperone, lurasidone, olanzapine (± fluoxetine) and quetiapine.[14,19,20] In terms of mechanism, this does not appear to be a dopamine-mediated effect as aripiprazole and most dopamine-blocking antipsychotics do not show efficacy in acute bipolar depression.[19] Efficacy is similar among those shown to be effective, although lurasidone may be superior to cariprazine.[21,22]

Maintenance

Compounds that have efficacy in the acute phase of bipolar disorder, whether that be mania or depression, seem to exert effects in maintenance treatment.[23] This is borne out by a network meta-analysis of maintenance treatments in bipolar disorder, in which olanzapine, quetiapine and risperidone LAIs showed effects against relapse.[24] This analysis did not include more recent (positive) trials of aripiprazole (see next section),[24] nor studies of cariprazine[25] which may not be effective as maintenance treatment.

Specific antipsychotics

Aripiprazole

Aripiprazole is effective in acute treatment of mania both alone,[26–28] as an add-on agent[29] and in long-term prophylaxis.[30,31] No difference is seen when directly compared with lithium or haloperidol although one small RCT suggested lithium was more effective in mania.[32] In trials in mania, aripiprazole is associated with nausea and movement disorder (mainly akathisia).[33] Aripiprazole LAI is also effective for prophylaxis in bipolar I disorder with the effect predominantly on prevention of manic episodes.[34]

Asenapine

Asenapine is given by the sublingual route and is effective in mania.[35,36] Efficacy seems to be maintained in the longer term,[37] with RCT evidence showing efficacy in preventing depression and manic episodes in people with bipolar I disorder.[38] Asenapine is less likely to cause weight gain and metabolic disturbance[39] than some other antipsychotics.

Cariprazine

Cariprazine is efficacious for treating mania as well as depression symptoms in people with mania with mixed features[40] and has a low propensity for weight gain.[39]

Clozapine

The earliest observational study of antipsychotics for maintenance treatment in bipolar disorder examined clozapine in people attending a service for resistant mood disorders.[41] There is evidence from at least 15 trials to suggest improvements in treatment-resistant bipolar disorder (TRBD) (where two treatments have failed, despite adequate dose and duration) and in depression, mania, rapid-cycling states and psychotic symptoms.[42] Clozapine is fairly widely used in bipolar disorder, particularly in South-East Asia.[43]

Lurasidone

Lurasidone is licensed by the FDA as monotherapy and adjunctive treatment to lithium and divalproex for acute treatment of bipolar depression, on the basis of RCTs of monotherapy versus placebo,[44] and as an adjunct to lithium or valproate.[45] The main adverse effects include nausea and akathisia, with minimal effects on weight and metabolic parameters.[39]

Olanzapine

Olanzapine is effective in mania.[46,47] As with other FGAs, olanzapine is most effective when used in combination with a mood stabiliser in acute mania and for symptomatic (though not syndromal) relapse prevention,[48,49] although in one study, olanzapine + carbamazepine was no better than carbamazepine alone.[50] Data suggest olanzapine may offer benefits in longer-term treatment.[51,52] It may be more effective than lithium.[53,54] Olanzapine is, of course, associated with significant metabolic effects, including weight gain, effects that are minimised by the use of the olanzapine/samidorphan combination available in some countries.[55,56]

Quetiapine

Data relating to quetiapine[57–59] suggest robust efficacy in all aspects of bipolar disorder including prevention of mania and bipolar depression.[60] It has low propensity for extrapyramidal side effects (EPSEs), though there are significant effects on weight and metabolic parameters.

Risperidone

Risperidone has shown efficacy in mania,[61] particularly in combination with a mood stabiliser.[62,63] Risperidone LAI (as Risperdal Consta) is also effective[64] (note though that the pharmacokinetics of this formulation generally render it an unsuitable choice for the acute treatment of mania). The long-acting version is used as prophylaxis (an unlicensed use in most countries). It is effective as prophylaxis against mania in the longer term.[23] Paliperidone can be assumed to have similar effects, although prospective, controlled data are lacking.[65]

Other antipsychotics

There are few data for amisulpride[66] and rather more for ziprasidone,[67] which is sometimes used for mania in the USA. Iloperidone may be effective in mixed episodes[68] but data are insufficient to support its use. Lumateperone is effective in bipolar depression.[69,70]

References

1. ECNP. Neuroscience-based nomenclature (NbN). 2024; https://www.ecnp.eu/research-innovation/nomenclature.

2. Cipriani A, et al. Comparative efficacy and acceptability of antimanic drugs in acute mania: a multiple-treatments meta-analysis. *Lancet* 2011; **378**:1306–1315.

3. Goodwin GM, et al. Evidence-based guidelines for treating bipolar disorder: revised third edition recommendations from the British Association for Psychopharmacology. *J Psychopharmacol* 2016; **30**:495–553.

4. Chou JC, et al. Acute mania: haloperidol dose and augmentation with lithium or lorazepam. *J Clin Psychopharmacol* 1999; **19**:500–505.

5. Small JG, et al. A placebo-controlled study of lithium combined with neuroleptics in chronic schizophrenic patients. *Am J Psychiatry* 1975; **132**:1315–1317.

6. Soares JC, et al. Adjunctive antipsychotic use in bipolar patients: an open 6-month prospective study following an acute episode. *J Affect Disord* 1999; **56**:1–8.

7. Keck PE, Jr, et al. Anticonvulsants and antipsychotics in the treatment of bipolar disorder. *J Clin Psychiatry* 1998; **59** Suppl 6:74–81.

8. Tohen M, et al. Antipsychotic agents and bipolar disorder. *J Clin Psychiatry* 1998; **59** Suppl 1:38–48.

9. Zarate CA, Jr, et al. Double-blind comparison of the continued use of antipsychotic treatment versus its discontinuation in remitted manic patients. *Am J Psychiatry* 2004; **161**:169–171.

10. Gigante AD, et al. Long-acting injectable antipsychotics for the maintenance treatment of bipolar disorder. *CNS Drugs* 2012; **26**:403–420.

11. Goikolea JM, et al. Lower rate of depressive switch following antimanic treatment with second-generation antipsychotics versus haloperidol. *J Affect Disord* 2013; **144**:191–198.

12. Yildiz A, et al. A network meta-analysis on comparative efficacy and all-cause discontinuation of antimanic treatments in acute bipolar mania. *Psychol Med* 2015; **45**:299–317.

13. Kishi T, et al. Pharmacological treatment for bipolar mania: a systematic review and network meta-analysis of double-blind randomized controlled trials. *Mol Psychiatry* 2022; **27**:1136–1144.

14. Baldessarini RJ, et al. Pharmacological treatment of adult bipolar disorder. *Mol Psychiatry* 2019; **24**:198–217.

15. Yu CL, et al. Comparison of antipsychotic dose equivalents for acute bipolar mania and schizophrenia. *BMJ Ment Health* 2023; **26**:e300546.

16. Ogawa Y, et al. Mood stabilizers and antipsychotics for acute mania: a systematic review and meta-analysis of combination/augmentation therapy versus monotherapy. *CNS Drugs* 2014; **28**:989–1003.

17. Ashok AH, et al. The dopamine hypothesis of bipolar affective disorder: the state of the art and implications for treatment. *Mol Psychiatry* 2017; **22**:666–679.

18. Jauhar S, et al. A test of the transdiagnostic dopamine hypothesis of psychosis using positron emission tomographic imaging in bipolar affective disorder and schizophrenia. *JAMA Psychiatry* 2017; **74**:1206–1213.

19. Taylor DM, et al. Comparative efficacy and acceptability of drug treatments for bipolar depression: a multiple-treatments meta-analysis. *Acta Psychiatr Scand* 2014; **130**:452–469.

20. Yildiz A, et al. Comparative efficacy and tolerability of pharmacological interventions for acute bipolar depression in adults: a systematic review and network meta-analysis. *Lancet Psychiatry* 2023; **10**:693–705.

21. Kadakia A, et al. Efficacy and tolerability of atypical antipsychotics for acute bipolar depression: a network meta-analysis. *BMC Psychiatry* 2021; **21**:249.

22. Martins-Correia J, et al. Cariprazine in the acute treatment of unipolar and bipolar depression: a systematic review and meta-analysis. *J Affect Disord* 2024; **362**:297–307.

23. Taylor MJ. Bipolar treatment efficacy. *Lancet Psychiatry* 2014; **1**:418.

24. Miura T, et al. Comparative efficacy and tolerability of pharmacological treatments in the maintenance treatment of bipolar disorder: a systematic review and network meta-analysis. *Lancet Psychiatry* 2014; **1**:351–359.

25. McIntyre RS, et al. Cariprazine as a maintenance therapy in the prevention of mood episodes in adults with bipolar I disorder. *Bipolar Disord* 2024; **26**:442–453.

26. Sachs G, et al. Aripiprazole in the treatment of acute manic or mixed episodes in patients with bipolar I disorder: a 3-week placebo-controlled study. *J Psychopharmacol* 2006; **20**:536–546.

27. Keck PE, et al. Aripiprazole monotherapy in the treatment of acute bipolar I mania: a randomized, double-blind, placebo- and lithium-controlled study. *J Affect Disord* 2009; **112**:36–49.

28. Young AH, et al. Aripiprazole monotherapy in acute mania: 12-week randomised placebo- and haloperidol-controlled study. *Br J Psychiatry* 2009; **194**:40–48.

29. Vieta E, et al. Efficacy of adjunctive aripiprazole to either valproate or lithium in bipolar mania patients partially nonresponsive to valproate/lithium monotherapy: a placebo-controlled study. *Am J Psychiatry* 2008; **165**:1316–1325.

30. Keck PE, Jr, et al. Aripiprazole monotherapy for maintenance therapy in bipolar I disorder: a 100-week, double-blind study versus placebo. *J Clin Psychiatry* 2007; **68**:1480–1491.

31. Vieta E, et al. Assessment of safety, tolerability and effectiveness of adjunctive aripiprazole to lithium/valproate in bipolar mania: a 46-week, open-label extension following a 6-week double-blind study. *Curr Med Res Opin* 2010; **26**:1485–1496.

32. Shafti SS. Aripiprazole versus lithium in management of acute mania: a randomized clinical trial. *East Asian Arch Psychiatry* 2018; **28**:80–84.

33. Brown R, et al. Aripiprazole alone or in combination for acute mania. *Cochrane Database Syst Rev* 2013; **12**:CD005000.

34. Calabrese JR, et al. Efficacy and safety of aripiprazole once-monthly in the maintenance treatment of bipolar I disorder: a double-blind, placebo-controlled, 52-week randomized withdrawal study. *J Clin Psychiatry* 2017; **78**:324–331.

35. McIntyre RS, et al. Asenapine in the treatment of acute mania in bipolar I disorder: a randomized, double-blind, placebo-controlled trial. *J Affect Disord* 2010; **122**:27–38.

36. McIntyre RS, et al. Asenapine versus olanzapine in acute mania: a double-blind extension study. *Bipolar Disord* 2009; **11**:815–826.

37. McIntyre RS, et al. Asenapine for long-term treatment of bipolar disorder: a double-blind 40-week extension study. *J Affect Disord* 2010; **126**:358–365.

38. Szegedi A, et al. Randomized, double-blind, placebo-controlled trial of asenapine maintenance therapy in adults with an acute manic or mixed episode associated with bipolar I disorder. *Am J Psychiatry* 2018; **175**:71–79.

39. Pillinger T, et al. Comparative effects of 18 antipsychotics on metabolic function in patients with schizophrenia, predictors of metabolic dysregulation, and association with psychopathology: a systematic review and network meta-analysis. *Lancet Psychiatry* 2020; **7**:64–77.

40. McIntyre RS, et al. Cariprazine for the treatment of bipolar mania with mixed features: a post hoc pooled analysis of 3 trials. *J Affect Disord* 2019; **257**:600–606.

41. Zarate CA, Jr, et al. Clozapine in severe mood disorders. *J Clin Psychiatry* 1995; **56**:411–417.

42. Li XB, et al. Clozapine for treatment-resistant bipolar disorder: a systematic review. *Bipolar Disord* 2015; **17**:235–247.

43. Loo LWJ, et al. Clozapine use for bipolar disorder: an Asian Psychotropic Prescription Patterns Consortium Study. *J Clin Psychopharmacol* 2023; **43**:278–282.

44. Loebel A, et al. Lurasidone monotherapy in the treatment of bipolar I depression: a randomized, double-blind, placebo-controlled study. *Am J Psychiatry* 2014; **171**:160–168.

45. Loebel A, et al. Lurasidone as adjunctive therapy with lithium or valproate for the treatment of bipolar I depression: a randomized, double-blind, placebo-controlled study. *Am J Psychiatry* 2014; **171**:169–177.

46. Tohen M, et al. Olanzapine versus placebo in the treatment of acute mania. Olanzapine HGEH Study Group. *Am J Psychiatry* 1999; **156**:702–709.

47. Tohen M, et al. Efficacy of olanzapine in acute bipolar mania: a double-blind, placebo-controlled study. The Olanzipine HGGW Study Group. *Arch Gen Psychiatry* 2000; **57**:841–849.

48. Tohen M, et al. Efficacy of olanzapine in combination with valproate or lithium in the treatment of mania in patients partially nonresponsive to valproate or lithium monotherapy. *Arch Gen Psychiatry* 2002; **59**:62–69.

49. Tohen M, et al. Relapse prevention in bipolar I disorder: 18-month comparison of olanzapine plus mood stabiliser v. mood stabiliser alone. *Br J Psychiatry* 2004; **184**:337–345.

50. Tohen M, et al. Olanzapine plus carbamazepine v. carbamazepine alone in treating manic episodes. *Br J Psychiatry* 2008; **192**:135–143.

51. Sanger TM, et al. Long-term olanzapine therapy in the treatment of bipolar I disorder: an open-label continuation phase study. *J Clin Psychiatry* 2001; **62**:273–281.

52. Vieta E, et al. Olanzapine as long-term adjunctive therapy in treatment-resistant bipolar disorder. *J Clin Psychopharmacol* 2001; **21**:469–473.

53. Tohen M, et al. Olanzapine versus lithium in the maintenance treatment of bipolar disorder: a 12-month, randomized, double-blind, controlled clinical trial. *Am J Psychiatry* 2005; **162**:1281–1290.

54. McKnight RF, et al. Lithium for acute mania. *Cochrane Database Syst Rev* 2019; **6**:CD004048.

55. Corrao MM, et al. Olanzapine/samidorphan: a new combination treatment for schizophrenia and bipolar I disorder intended to reduce weight gain. *CNS Drugs* 2022; **36**:605–616.

56. Faden J, et al. Olanzapine-samidorphan combination tablets for the treatment of schizophrenia and bipolar I disorder – what is it, and will it be used? *Expert Rev Neurother* 2022; **22**:365–376.

57. Ghaemi SN, et al. The use of quetiapine for treatment-resistant bipolar disorder: a case series. *Ann Clin Psychiatry* 1999; **11**:137–140.

58. Sachs G, et al. Quetiapine with lithium or divalproex for the treatment of bipolar mania: a randomized, double-blind, placebo-controlled study. *Bipolar Disord* 2004; **6**:213–223.

59. Altamura AC, et al. Efficacy and tolerability of quetiapine in the treatment of bipolar disorder: preliminary evidence from a 12-month open label study. *J Affect Disord* 2003; **76**:267–271.

60. Young AH, et al. A randomised, placebo-controlled 52-week trial of continued quetiapine treatment in recently depressed patients with bipolar I and bipolar II disorder. *World J Biol Psychiatry* 2014; **15**:96–112.

61. Segal J, et al. Risperidone compared with both lithium and haloperidol in mania: a double-blind randomized controlled trial. *Clin Neuropharmacol* 1998; **21**:176–180.

62. Sachs GS, et al. Combination of a mood stabilizer with risperidone or haloperidol for treatment of acute mania: a double-blind, placebo-controlled comparison of efficacy and safety. *Am J Psychiatry* 2002; **159**:1146–1154.

63. Vieta E, et al. Risperidone in the treatment of mania: efficacy and safety results from a large, multicentre, open study in Spain. *J Affect Disord* 2002; **72**:15–19.

64. Quiroz JA, et al. Risperidone long-acting injectable monotherapy in the maintenance treatment of bipolar I disorder. *Biol Psychiatry* 2010; **68**:156–162.

65. Taylor DM, et al. Paliperidone palmitate: factors predicting continuation with treatment at 2 years. *Eur Neuropsychopharmacol* 2016; **26**:2011–2017.

66. Vieta E, et al. An open-label study of amisulpride in the treatment of mania. *J Clin Psychiatry* 2005; **66**:575–578.

67. Vieta E, et al. Ziprasidone in the treatment of acute mania: a 12-week, placebo-controlled, haloperidol-referenced study. *J Psychopharmacol* 2010; **24**:547–558.

68. Singh V, et al. An open trial of iloperidone for mixed episodes in bipolar disorder. *J Clin Psychopharmacol* 2017; **37**:615–619.

69. McIntyre RS, et al. The efficacy of lumateperone in patients with bipolar depression with mixed features. *J Clin Psychiatry* 2023; **84**:22m14739.

70. Calabrese JR, et al. Efficacy and safety of lumateperone for major depressive episodes associated with bipolar I or bipolar II disorder: a phase 3 randomized placebo-controlled trial. *Am J Psychiatry* 2021; **178**:1098–1106.

CHAPTER 2

CHAPTER 2

Antipsychotic long-acting injections in bipolar disorder

LAIs are widely used in bipolar disorder although none is formally licensed in the UK for this indication (Abilify Maintena is approved by the FDA in the USA). Support for their use is rather limited: there have been dozens of open-label trials or case series published, but few included more than a handful of subjects.[1–3] Retrospective cohort studies, mirror-image studies and population-level studies do, nonetheless, offer some support for the use of LAIs (mainly SGAs) in bipolar maintenance.[1] Mirror-image studies uniformly show a reduction in admissions and bed days when patients are switched from oral medication to LAI formulations of aripiprazole[4–6] and paliperidone,[6,7] although study numbers were small. Prospective open-label studies also support the prophylactic effect of aripiprazole LAI, both monthly and two-monthly.[8,9]

There have also been seven RCTs, only five of which were sufficiently powered to produce interpretable results (the remaining two trials included only 30 subjects in total[10,11]). These five RCTs represent the highest level of evidence for LAIs in bipolar disorder. Their details are set out in Table 2.5.

Few firm conclusions can be drawn from the controlled trials outlined in Table 2.5. Risperidone LAI is clearly effective either as the sole treatment or as an adjunct but provides protection only against manic, hypomanic and mixed-manic episodes and

Table 2.5 Randomised controlled trials (RCTs) of the use of long-acting injections (LAIs) in bipolar affective disorder.

Reference	Number	LAI	Comparator	Duration	Outcome
Ahlfors et al., 1981[12]	33 (19/14)	Flupentixol decanoate	Lithium	18 months	Neither treatment improved main outcome (number of mood episodes)
Macfadden et al., 2009[13]*	124 (65/59)	Risperidone (adjunct)	Placebo (adjunct)	12 months	Risperidone LAI reduced rate of relapse compared with placebo (relative risk 2.3)
Quiroz et al., 2010[14]*	303 (154/149)	Risperidone monotherapy	Placebo monotherapy	24 months	Overall relapse rate was 30% with risperidone, 56% with placebo. Risperidone did not protect against depressive relapse.
Vieta et al., 2012[15]*	398 (132/135/131)	Risperidone monotherapy	Placebo or oral olanzapine monotherapy	18 months	Recurrence of any mood episode: oral olanzapine 23.8%; risperidone LAI 38.9%; placebo 56.4%. Olanzapine and risperidone reduced risk of elevated mood episode but only olanzapine reduced risk of depression.
Calabrese et al., 2017[16]*	266 (133/133)	Aripiprazole monotherapy	Placebo monotherapy	12 months	Relapse to any mood episode 26.5% with aripiprazole; 51.1% with placebo. No clear effect on recurrence of depression. An open follow-on study of this RCT (that also included patients newly prescribed aripiprazole) showed somewhat better levels of protection: 87–98% of participants remained well over 12 months.[17]

*Trial sponsored by manufacturer.

neither decreases nor increases the risk of depressive relapse. Risperidone LAI may be less effective than oral olanzapine. It might be assumed that paliperidone LAI has similar effects to risperidone LAI. Oral paliperidone prevents manic relapse in bipolar disorder,[18] there are a few supportive mirror-image studies[6,7] and case reports describe good outcomes with the LAI form.[19,20] Aripiprazole LAI protects against manic relapse but does not appear to affect risk of depression.

Data for FGAs in bipolar disorder are scarce and generally of low quality (open trials, case series and retrospective analyses). In these studies, FGA LAIs seem to reduce the risk of relapse compared with prior treatments. The largest (open) study[12] (n = 85) suggested flupentixol decanoate (20mg every 2–3 weeks) reduced the risk of elevated mood episodes. Reports describe similar effects for other FGA LAIs. The one RCT conducted with flupentixol LAI[12] showed no effect and no superiority over lithium.

Considering this single RCT and all of the small and uncontrolled observations, there is very little evidence to support the often-repeated lore that flupentixol LAI increases the risk of manic relapse and haloperidol LAI and fluphenazine LAI increase the risk of depressive relapse (or that FGAs provoke depression). It is notable that authors of systematic reviews[21,22] reiterate this view, which seems to be based on solely the observed increase in depressive episodes in the open study conducted by Ahlfors and colleagues.[12] In fact, this increase occurred only in subjects whose lithium treatment had been stopped immediately before the study began. Nonetheless, oral haloperidol, when used for mania, is more likely than oral SGAs to cause a switch to depression[23] so some caution is clearly required.

There are no controlled comparisons of FGA and SGA LAIs.[1–3] A Taiwanese retrospective cohort study[24] reported a higher risk of depressive episode recurrence and a higher likelihood of hospitalisation in those prescribed FGA LAIs (50% were prescribed flupentixol, 25% haloperidol and 25% other drugs) compared with those prescribed risperidone LAI. Of particular note was the substantial rate of treatment discontinuation. At 1 year only 7.2% of those initially prescribed risperidone and 2.2% of those initiated on FGA LAIs remained on the original treatment. Another observational study found both SGA and FGA LAIs to be effective but only when treatment continued for at least 6 months.[25]

Conclusion

- Support for the use of FGA LAIs in bipolar disorder is weak.
- Very limited evidence suggests FGA LAIs may be effective in reducing recurrence of mania/hypomania but they do not prevent recurrence of depression and may increase the risk.
- Risperidone LAI and aripiprazole LAI are robustly associated with a reduced risk of recurrence of episodes of mania/hypomania compared with placebo.
- Risperidone LAI and aripiprazole LAI have no effect on the risk of depressive recurrence.
- There is limited evidence to support the benefit of LAIs over oral antipsychotic treatment in bipolar maintenance.
- As with other conditions, the use of LAIs offers the advantage of transparency in respect to compliance: the LAI injection is either given or it is not.

References

1. Keramatian K, et al. Long-acting injectable second-generation/atypical antipsychotics for the management of bipolar disorder: a systematic review. *CNS Drugs* 2019; 33:431–456.
2. Pacchiarotti I, et al. Long-acting injectable antipsychotics (LAIs) for maintenance treatment of bipolar and schizoaffective disorders: a systematic review. *Eur Neuropsychopharmacol* 2019; 29:457–470.
3. Prajapati AR, et al. Second-generation antipsychotic long-acting injections in bipolar disorder: systematic review and meta-analysis. *Bipolar Disord* 2018; 20:687–696.
4. Goto J, et al. Preventive effect of aripiprazole once monthly on rehospitalization for bipolar disorder: a multicenter 1-year retrospective mirror image study. *Neuropsychopharmacol Rep* 2023; 43:425–433.
5. Woo YS, et al. Preventive effect of aripiprazole once-monthly on relapse into mood episodes in bipolar disorder: a multicenter, one-year, retrospective, mirror image study. *J Affect Disord* 2024; 351:381–386.
6. Yıldızhan E, et al. Effect of long acting injectable antipsychotics on course and hospitalizations in bipolar disorder – a naturalistic mirror image study. *Nord J Psychiatry* 2022; 76:37–43.
7. Caliskan AM, et al. Impact of initiating long-acting injectable paliperidone palmitate on relapse and hospitalization in patients with bipolar I disorder: a mirror image retrospective study. *Asian J Psychiatr* 2020; 54:102457.
8. Harlin M, et al. A randomized, open-label, multiple-dose, parallel-arm, pivotal study to evaluate the safety, tolerability, and pharmacokinetics of aripiprazole 2-month long-acting injectable in adults with schizophrenia or bipolar I disorder. *CNS Drugs* 2023; 37:337–350.
9. McIntyre RS, et al. Safety and efficacy of aripiprazole 2-month ready-to-use 960 mg: secondary analysis of outcomes in adult patients with bipolar I disorder in a randomized, open-label, parallel-arm, pivotal study. *Curr Med Res Opin* 2023; 39:1021–1030.
10. Esparon J, et al. Comparison of the prophylactic action of flupenthixol with placebo in lithium treated manic-depressive patients. *Br J Psychiatry* 1986; 148:723–725.
11. Yatham L, et al. Randomised trial of oral vs. injectable antipsychotics in bipolar disorder. Presented at the 6th International Conference on Bipolar Disorder: 16–18 June 2005, Pittsburgh, PA.
12. Ahlfors UG, et al. Flupenthixol decanoate in recurrent manic-depressive illness. A comparison with lithium. *Acta Psychiatr Scand* 1981; 64:226–237.
13. Macfadden W, et al. A randomized, double-blind, placebo-controlled study of maintenance treatment with adjunctive risperidone long-acting therapy in patients with bipolar I disorder who relapse frequently. *Bipolar Disord* 2009; 11:827–839.
14. Quiroz JA, et al. Risperidone long-acting injectable monotherapy in the maintenance treatment of bipolar I disorder. *Biol Psychiatry* 2010; 68:156–162.
15. Vieta E, et al. A randomized, double-blind, placebo-controlled trial to assess prevention of mood episodes with risperidone long-acting injectable in patients with bipolar I disorder. *Eur Neuropsychopharmacol* 2012; 22:825–835.
16. Calabrese JR, et al. Efficacy and safety of aripiprazole once-monthly in the maintenance treatment of bipolar I disorder: a double-blind, placebo-controlled, 52-week randomized withdrawal study. *J Clin Psychiatry* 2017; 78:324–331.
17. Calabrese JR, et al. Aripiprazole once-monthly as maintenance treatment for bipolar I disorder: a 52-week, multicenter, open-label study. *Int J Bipolar Disord* 2018; 6:14.
18. Berwaerts J, et al. A randomized, placebo- and active-controlled study of paliperidone extended-release as maintenance treatment in patients with bipolar I disorder after an acute manic or mixed episode. *J Affect Disord* 2012; 138:247–258.
19. Buoli M, et al. Paliperidone palmitate depot in the long-term treatment of psychotic bipolar disorder: a case series. *Clin Neuropharmacol* 2015; 38:209–211.
20. Li K, et al. Case report: paliperidone palmitate in the management of bipolar I disorder with non-compliance. *Front Psychiatry* 2020; 11:529672.
21. Bond DJ, et al. Depot antipsychotic medications in bipolar disorder: a review of the literature. *Acta Psychiatr Scand Suppl* 2007; 2007:3–16.
22. Gigante AD, et al. Long-acting injectable antipsychotics for the maintenance treatment of bipolar disorder. *CNS Drugs* 2012; 26:403–420.
23. Goikolea JM, et al. Lower rate of depressive switch following antimanic treatment with second-generation antipsychotics versus haloperidol. *J Affect Disord* 2013; 144:191–198.
24. Wu CS, et al. Comparative effectiveness of long-acting injectable risperidone vs. long-acting injectable first-generation antipsychotics in bipolar disorder. *J Affect Disord* 2016; 197:189–195.
25. Bartoli F, et al. Effect of long-acting injectable antipsychotics on 1-year hospitalization in bipolar disorder: a mirror-image study. *Eur Arch Psychiatry Clin Neurosci* 2023; 273:1579–1586.

Physical monitoring for people with bipolar disorder[1,2]

Test or measurement	Monitoring for all patients		Additional monitoring for specific drugs			
	Initial health check	Annual check-up	Antipsychotics	Lithium	Valproate	Carbamazepine
Thyroid function	Yes	Yes		At start and every 6 months. More often if evidence of change.		
Liver function tests (LFTs)	Yes	Yes			Every 3 months for the first year then annually	Monthly for the first 3 months then annually
Renal function (eGFR)	Yes	Yes		At start and every 6 months. More often if there is evidence of deterioration or the patient starts taking interacting drugs.		
Electrolytes, urea and creatinine (EUC)	Yes	Yes		At start and then every 3–6 months (include serum calcium)		Monthly for the first 3 months then annually
Full blood count (FBC)	Yes	Yes		Only if clinically indicated	Every 3 months for the first year then annually	Monthly for the first 3 months then annually
Blood (plasma) glucose	Yes	Yes, as part of a routine physical health check	At start and then every 4–6 months (and at 1 month if taking olanzapine); more often if evidence of elevated levels			
Lipid profile	Yes	Yes, as part of a routine physical health check	At start and at 3 months; more often initially if evidence of elevated levels			
Blood pressure and pulse	Yes	Yes, as part of a routine physical health check	During dosage titration if antipsychotic prescribed is associated with postural hypotension			

Test					
Prolactin	Children and adolescents only	At start and if symptoms of raised prolactin develop	Raised prolactin unlikely with quetiapine or aripiprazole. Very occasionally seen with olanzapine and asenapine. Very common with risperidone and FGAs.		
ECG	If indicated by cardiovascular disease or risk factors	At start if there are risk factors for or existing cardiovascular disease (or haloperidol is prescribed). If relevant abnormalities are detected, re-check after each dose increase.		At start if risk factors for or existing cardiovascular disease. If relevant abnormalities are detected, re-check after each dose increase.	
Waist circumference and/or body mass index	Yes, as part of a routine physical health check	Monthly for the first 3 months then annually	At start, and then every 6 months	Every 3 months for the first year then annually	At start and when needed if the patient gains weight rapidly
Plasma levels of drug		At least 3–4 days after initiation and 3–4 days after every dose change until levels stable, then **every 3 months** in the first year, then every 6 months for most patients (see NICE[2])	Titrate by effect and tolerability. Do not routinely measure unless there is evidence of lack of effectiveness, poor adherence or toxicity.	Two weeks after initiation and 2 weeks after dose change. Thereafter, do not routinely measure unless there is evidence of lack of effectiveness, poor adherence or toxicity.	

For patients on **lamotrigine**, do an annual health check, but no special monitoring tests are needed although blood levels may indicate if high doses might be considered.

References

1. Ng F, et al. The International Society for Bipolar Disorders (ISBD) consensus guidelines for the safety monitoring of bipolar disorder treatments. *Bipolar Disord* 2009; **11**:559–595.
2. National Institute for Health and Care Excellence. Bipolar disorder: assessment and management. Clinical guideline (CG185); 2014 (last updated December 2023, last accessed October 2024); https://www.nice.org.uk/guidance/cg185.

Treatment of acute mania or hypomania

Drug treatment is the mainstay of therapy for mania and hypomania. Both antipsychotics and mood stabilisers are effective (although the nomenclature here is unhelpful – most, possibly all, antipsychotics are anti-manic and most mood stabilisers reduce psychotic symptoms in mania). Sedative and anxiolytic drugs (e.g. benzodiazepines) may add to the effects of these treatments.

Drug choice is made difficult by the small number of direct comparisons, such that no one individual drug can be recommended over another on efficacy grounds. However, an early network meta-analysis[1] suggested that olanzapine, risperidone, haloperidol and quetiapine had the best combination of efficacy and acceptability. Cochrane reviews suggested olanzapine is more effective than both lithium[2] and valproate[3] when used as monotherapy. Olanzapine may also be more effective than asenapine.[4] A 2024 network meta-analysis concluded that tamoxifen was the most effective individual drug.[5]

The benefit of antipsychotic mood stabiliser combinations (compared with a mood stabiliser alone) is established for those relapsing while on mood stabilisers but less clear for those presenting on no treatment.[6–10] The most common study design is for participants to be randomised to continued mood stabiliser alone (a treatment that allows the emergence of mania) or to the failed mood stabiliser with a (newly introduced)

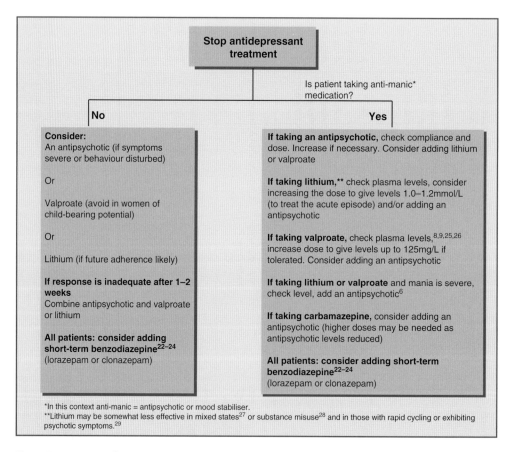

Figure 2.1 Treatment of acute mania or hypomania.[6–21]

antipsychotic. Overall, combination treatment with an antipsychotic and a mood stabiliser is more effective and quicker to act than either individual drug used alone.[5,30] Most formal guidelines recommend drug combinations as the first choice in mania,[31] although single drug treatment may be considered, at least initially, for people presenting on no prior treatment.

Figure 2.1 outlines a treatment strategy for mania and hypomania. These recommendations are based on somewhat dated UK NICE guidelines,[7] British Association for Psychopharmacology (BAP) guidelines[32] and individual references cited in the diagram. Where an antipsychotic is recommended, choose from those licensed for mania/bipolar disorder (i.e. most conventional drugs, aripiprazole, asenapine, olanzapine, risperidone and quetiapine).

Valproate use is now heavily restricted, so lithium is likely to be the mood stabiliser most commonly used, at least in younger men and women. An alternative is carbamazepine, but this, like valproate, is teratogenic. Lamotrigine has no activity in mania[33] and should not be used.

Suggested doses and alternative treatments are outlined in Tables 2.6 and 2.7.

Table 2.6 Mania: suggested drug doses.

Drug	Dose
Mood stabilisers	
Carbamazepine	400mg MR twice daily increasing to 800–1600mg/day.[34,35] Dose may need to be increased after 2 weeks owing to induction of metabolism.
Lithium	400mg/day, increasing every 3–4 days according to plasma levels. At least one study has used 800mg as a starting dose.[36]
Valproate	As **semi-sodium** – 250mg three times daily increasing according to tolerability and plasma levels. Slow-release semi-sodium valproate may also be effective (at 15–30mg/kg)[37] but there is one failed study.[38] As slow-release **sodium valproate** – 500mg/day increasing as above. Higher, 'loading doses' have been used, both oral[39–41] and intravenous.[42–44] The dose is 20–30mg/kg/day.
Antipsychotics	
Aripiprazole	15mg/day increasing up to 30mg/day as required.[45] Doses lower than 15mg may not be effective.[46]
Asenapine	5mg twice daily increasing to 10mg twice daily as required
Cariprazine	3mg/day increasing up to 12mg a day as required[47]
Olanzapine	10mg/day increasing to 15 or 20mg as required
Risperidone	2 or 3mg/day increasing to 6mg/day as required. The use of paliperidone in mania is not well supported.[48]
Quetiapine	**IR** – 100mg/day increasing to 800mg as required. Higher starting doses have been used.[49] **XL** – 300mg/day increasing to 600mg/day on day 2
Haloperidol	5–10mg/day increasing to 15mg if required
Benzodiazepines	
Lorazepam[23,24]	Up to 4mg/day (some centres use higher doses)
Clonzapam[22,24]	Up to 8mg/day

Table 2.7 Mania: other possible treatments.*

Treatment	Comments
Allopurinol (300–600mg/day)	A meta-analysis of five studies of adjunct allopurinol found an effect size of just less than 0.3.[50]
Celecoxib (400mg/day)[51]	Small RCT (n = 46) suggests benefit when used as adjunct to valproate.
Clonidine (450–900mcg/day)[52]	Limited data
Clozapine[53–55]	Established treatment option for refractory mania/bipolar disorder. Rapid titration has been reported.[56]
Endoxifen[57] (4–8mg/day)	RCT evidence of efficacy. Major metabolite of tamoxifen.
Gabapentin[58] (up to 2.4g/day)	Probably only effective by virtue of an anxiolytic effect. Rarely used. Possibly useful as prophylaxis.[59]
Levetiracetam (up to 1500mg/day)	Effective as adjunctive treatment in two RCTs.[60,61] One case of levetiracetam causing mania.[62]
Melatonin (6mg/day)[67]	Preliminary evidence of benefit as an adjunct to standard treatment. One small negative study.[68]
Memantine[63] (10–30mg/day)	Conflicting evidence[64–66]
Oxcarbazepine[69–76] (around 300–3000mg/day)	Probably effective acutely and as prophylaxis although one controlled study (conducted in youths) was negative.[77]
Phenytoin[78] (300–400mg/day)	Rarely used. Limited data. Complex kinetics with narrow therapeutic range.
Ritanserin[79] (10mg/day)	Supported by a single RCT. Well tolerated. May protect against EPSEs.
Tamoxifen[80] (20–140mg/day)	Good evidence for efficacy as adjunct and as monotherapy, with large effect size. May provoke switch to depression.
Topiramate[81] (up to 300mg/day)	Probably not effective. Less effective than lithium.[2]
Tryptophan depletion[82]	Supported by a small RCT.
Ziprasidone[83–85]	Supported by three RCTs. Widely used outside UK.

*Entries are given in alphabetical order; no preference is implied by order in the table. Consult specialist and primary literature before using any treatment listed.
EPSEs, extrapyramidal side effects; RCT, randomised controlled trial.

References

1. Cipriani A, et al. Comparative efficacy and acceptability of antimanic drugs in acute mania: a multiple-treatments meta-analysis. *Lancet* 2011; 378:1306–1315.
2. McKnight RF, et al. Lithium for acute mania. *Cochrane Database Syst Rev* 2019; 6:CD004048.
3. Jochim J, et al. Valproate for acute mania. *Cochrane Database Syst Rev* 2019; 10:CD004052.
4. Mahajan V, et al. Efficacy and safety of asenapine versus olanzapine in combination with divalproex for acute mania: a randomized controlled trial. *J Clin Psychopharmacol* 2019; 39:305–311.
5. Huang W, et al. Comparative efficacy, safety, and tolerability of pharmacotherapies for acute mania in adults: a systematic review and network meta-analysis of randomized controlled trials. *Mol Psychiatry* 2024; doi: 10.1038/s41380-024-02705-3.

6. Smith LA, et al. Acute bipolar mania: a systematic review and meta-analysis of co-therapy vs. monotherapy. *Acta Psychiatr Scand* 2007; **115**:12–20.

7. National Institute for Health and Care Excellence. Bipolar disorder: assessment and management. Clinical guideline [CG185]. 2014 (last updated December 2023, last accessed October 2024); https://www.nice.org.uk/guidance/cg185.

8. Goodwin GM. Evidence-based guidelines for treating bipolar disorder: revised second edition – recommendations from the British Association for Psychopharmacology. *J Psychopharmacol* 2009; **23**:346–388.

9. American Psychiatric Association. Practice guideline for the treatment of patients with bipolar disorder (revision). *Am J Psychiatry* 2002; **159**:1–50.

10. Sachs GS. Decision tree for the treatment of bipolar disorder. *J Clin Psychiatry* 2003; **64** Suppl 8:35–40.

11. Tohen M, et al. A 12-week, double-blind comparison of olanzapine vs haloperidol in the treatment of acute mania. *Arch Gen Psychiatry* 2003; **60**:1218–1226.

12. Baldessarini RJ, et al. Olanzapine versus placebo in acute mania treatment responses in subgroups. *J Clin Psychopharmacol* 2003; **23**:370–376.

13. Sachs G, et al. Quetiapine with lithium or divalproex for the treatment of bipolar mania: a randomized, double-blind, placebo-controlled study. *Bipolar Disord* 2004; **6**:213–223.

14. Yatham LN, et al. Quetiapine versus placebo in combination with lithium or divalproex for the treatment of bipolar mania. *J Clin Psychopharmacol* 2004; **24**:599–606.

15. Yatham LN, et al. Risperidone plus lithium versus risperidone plus valproate in acute and continuation treatment of mania. *Int Clin Psychopharmacol* 2004; **19**:103–109.

16. Bowden CL, et al. Risperidone in combination with mood stabilizers: a 10-week continuation phase study in bipolar I disorder. *J Clin Psychiatry* 2004; **65**:707–714.

17. Hirschfeld RM, et al. Rapid antimanic effect of risperidone monotherapy: a 3-week multicenter, double-blind, placebo-controlled trial. *Am J Psychiatry* 2004; **161**:1057–1065.

18. Bowden CL, et al. A randomized, double-blind, placebo-controlled efficacy and safety study of quetiapine or lithium as monotherapy for mania in bipolar disorder. *J Clin Psychiatry* 2005; **66**:111–121.

19. Khanna S, et al. Risperidone in the treatment of acute mania: double-blind, placebo-controlled study. *Br J Psychiatry* 2005; **187**:229–234.

20. Young RC, et al. GERI-BD: a randomized double-blind controlled trial of lithium and divalproex in the treatment of mania in older patients with bipolar disorder. *Am J Psychiatry* 2017; **174**:1086–1093.

21. Conus P, et al. Olanzapine or chlorpromazine plus lithium in first episode psychotic mania: an 8-week randomised controlled trial. *Eur Psychiatry* 2015; **30**:975–982.

22. Sachs GS, et al. Adjunctive clonazepam for maintenance treatment of bipolar affective disorder. *J Clin Psychopharmacol* 1990; **10**:42–47.

23. Modell JG, et al. Inpatient clinical trial of lorazepam for the management of manic agitation. *J Clin Psychopharmacol* 1985; **5**:109–113.

24. Curtin F, et al. Clonazepam and lorazepam in acute mania: a Bayesian meta-analysis. *J Affect Disord* 2004; **78**:201–208.

25. Taylor D, et al. Doses of carbamazepine and valproate in bipolar affective disorder. *Psychiatric Bulletin* 1997; **21**:221–223.

26. Allen MH, et al. Linear relationship of valproate serum concentration to response and optimal serum levels for acute mania. *Am J Psychiatry* 2006; **163**:272–275.

27. Swann AC, et al. Lithium treatment of mania: clinical characteristics, specificity of symptom change, and outcome. *Psychiatry Res* 1986; **18**:127–141.

28. Goldberg JF, et al. A history of substance abuse complicates remission from acute mania in bipolar disorder. *J Clin Psychiatry* 1999; **60**:733–740.

29. Hui TP, et al. A systematic review and meta-analysis of clinical predictors of lithium response in bipolar disorder. *Acta Psychiatr Scand* 2019; **140**:94–115.

30. Tajika A, et al. Mood stabilizers and antipsychotics for acute mania: systematic review and meta-analysis of augmentation therapy vs monotherapy from the perspective of time to the onset of treatment effects. *Int J Neuropsychopharmacol* 2022; **25**:839–852.

31. Yatham LN, et al. Canadian Network for Mood and Anxiety Treatments (CANMAT) and International Society for Bipolar Disorders (ISBD) 2018 guidelines for the management of patients with bipolar disorder. *Bipolar Disord* 2018; **20**:97–170.

32. Goodwin GM, et al. Evidence-based guidelines for treating bipolar disorder: revised third edition recommendations from the British Association for Psychopharmacology. *J Psychopharmacol* 2016; **30**:495–553.

33. Besag FMC, et al. Efficacy and safety of lamotrigine in the treatment of bipolar disorder across the lifespan: a systematic review. *Ther Adv Psychopharmacol* 2021; **11**:20451253211045870.

34. Weisler RH, et al. A multicenter, randomized, double-blind, placebo-controlled trial of extended-release carbamazepine capsules as monotherapy for bipolar disorder patients with manic or mixed episodes. *J Clin Psychiatry* 2004; **65**:478–484.

35. Weisler RH, et al. Extended-release carbamazepine capsules as monotherapy for acute mania in bipolar disorder: a multicenter, randomized, double-blind, placebo-controlled trial. *J Clin Psychiatry* 2005; **66**:323–330.

36. Bowden CL, et al. Efficacy of valproate versus lithium in mania or mixed mania: a randomized, open 12-week trial. *Int Clin Psychopharmacol* 2010; **25**:60–67.

37. McElroy SL, et al. Randomized, double-blind, placebo-controlled study of divalproex extended release loading monotherapy in ambulatory bipolar spectrum disorder patients with moderate-to-severe hypomania or mild mania. *J Clin Psychiatry* 2010; **71**:557–565.

38. Hirschfeld RM, et al. A randomized, placebo-controlled, multicenter study of divalproex sodium extended-release in the acute treatment of mania. *J Clin Psychiatry* 2010; **71**:426–432.

39. McElroy SL, et al. A randomized comparison of divalproex oral loading versus haloperidol in the initial treatment of acute psychotic mania. *J Clin Psychiatry* 1996; **57**:142–146.

40. Hirschfeld RM, et al. Safety and tolerability of oral loading divalproex sodium in acutely manic bipolar patients. *J Clin Psychiatry* 1999; **60**:815–818.

41. Hirschfeld RM, et al. The safety and early efficacy of oral-loaded divalproex versus standard-titration divalproex, lithium, olanzapine, and placebo in the treatment of acute mania associated with bipolar disorder. *J Clin Psychiatry* 2003; **64**:841–846.

42. Jagadheesan K, et al. Acute antimanic efficacy and safety of intravenous valproate loading therapy: an open-label study. *Neuropsychobiology* 2003; **47**:90–93.

43. Sekhar S, et al. Efficacy of sodium valproate and haloperidol in the management of acute mania: a randomized open-label comparative study. *J Clin Pharmacol* 2010; **50**:688–692.

44. Fontana E, et al. Intravenous valproate in the treatment of acute manic episode in bipolar disorder: a review. *J Affect Disord* 2020; **260**:738–743.

45. Li DJ, et al. Efficacy, safety and tolerability of aripiprazole in bipolar disorder: an updated systematic review and meta-analysis of randomized controlled trials. *Prog Neuropsychopharmacol Biol Psychiatry* 2017; **79**:289–301.

46. Romeo B, et al. Meta-analysis and review of dopamine agonists in acute episodes of mood disorder: efficacy and safety. *J Psychopharmacol* 2018; **32**:385–396.

47. Vieta E, et al. Effect of cariprazine across the symptoms of mania in bipolar I disorder: analyses of pooled data from phase II/III trials. *Eur Neuropsychopharmacol* 2015; **25**:1882–1891.

48. Chang HY, et al. The efficacy and tolerability of paliperidone in mania of bipolar disorder: a preliminary meta-analysis. *Exp Clin Psychopharmacol* 2017; **25**:422–433.

49. Pajonk FG, et al. Rapid dose titration of quetiapine for the treatment of acute schizophrenia and acute mania: a case series. *J Psychopharmacol* 2006; **20**:119–124.

50. Chen AT, et al. Allopurinol augmentation in acute mania: a meta-analysis of placebo-controlled trials. *J Affect Disord* 2018; **226**:245–250.

51. Arabzadeh S, et al. Celecoxib adjunctive therapy for acute bipolar mania: a randomized, double-blind, placebo-controlled trial. *Bipolar Disord* 2015; **17**:606–614.

52. Singal P, et al. Efficacy and safety of clonidine in the treatment of acute mania in bipolar disorder: a systematic review. *Brain Sci* 2023; **13**:547.

53. Mahmood T, et al. Clozapine in the management of bipolar and schizoaffective manic episodes resistant to standard treatment. *Aust NZ J Psychiatry* 1997; **31**:424–426.

54. Green AI, et al. Clozapine in the treatment of refractory psychotic mania. *Am J Psychiatry* 2000; **157**:982–986.

55. Ifteni P, et al. Switching bipolar disorder patients treated with clozapine to another antipsychotic medication: a mirror image study. *Neuropsychiatr Dis Treat* 2017; **13**:201–204.

56. Aksoy Poyraz C, et al. Effectiveness of ultra-rapid dose titration of clozapine for treatment-resistant bipolar mania: case series. *Ther Adv Psychopharmacol* 2015; **5**:237–242.

57. Joseph JT, et al. Efficacy and safety of endoxifen in bipolar disorder: a systematic review. *Hum Psychopharmacol* 2024; **39**:e2899.

58. Ng QX, et al. A systematic review of the clinical use of gabapentin and pregabalin in bipolar disorder. *Pharmaceuticals (Basel)* 2021; **14**:834.

59. Vieta E, et al. A double-blind, randomized, placebo-controlled, prophylaxis study of adjunctive gabapentin for bipolar disorder. *J Clin Psychiatry* 2006; **67**:473–477.

60. Zarezadeh F, et al. Levetiracetam adjunct to quetiapine for the acute manic phase of bipolar disorder: a randomized, double-blind and placebo-controlled clinical trial of efficacy, safety and tolerability. *Int Clin Psychopharmacol* 2022; **37**:46–53.

61. Keshavarzi A, et al. Levetiracetam as an adjunctive treatment for mania: a double-blind, randomized, placebo-controlled trial. *Neuropsychobiology* 2022; **81**:192–203.

62. Park EM, et al. Acute mania associated with levetiracetam treatment. *Psychosomatics* 2014; **55**:98–100.

63. Koukopoulos A, et al. Antimanic and mood-stabilizing effect of memantine as an augmenting agent in treatment-resistant bipolar disorder. *Bipolar Disord* 2010; **12**:348–349.

64. Veronese N, et al. Acetylcholinesterase inhibitors and memantine in bipolar disorder: a systematic review and best evidence synthesis of the efficacy and safety for multiple disease dimensions. *J Affect Disord* 2016; **197**:268–280.

65. Serra G, et al. Three-year, naturalistic, mirror-image assessment of adding memantine to the treatment of 30 treatment-resistant patients with bipolar disorder. *J Clin Psychiatry* 2015; **76**:e91–97.

66. Omranifard V, et al. Evaluation of the effect of memantine supplementation in the treatment of acute phase of mania in bipolar disorder of elderly patients: a double-blind randomized controlled trial. *Adv Biomed Res* 2018; **7**:148.

67. Moghaddam HS, et al. Efficacy of melatonin as an adjunct in the treatment of acute mania: a double-blind and placebo-controlled trial. *Int Clin Psychopharmacol* 2020; **35**:81–88.

68. Quested DJ, et al. Melatonin In Acute Mania Investigation (MIAMI-UK). A randomized controlled trial of add-on melatonin in bipolar disorder. *Bipolar Disord* 2021; **23**:176–185.

69. Benedetti A, et al. Oxcarbazepine as add-on treatment in patients with bipolar manic, mixed or depressive episode. *J Affect Disord* 2004; **79**:273–277.

70. Lande RG. Oxcarbazepine: efficacy, safety, and tolerability in the treatment of mania. *Int J Psychiatry Clin Pract* 2004; **8**:37–40.

71. Ghaemi SN, et al. Oxcarbazepine treatment of bipolar disorder. *J Clin Psychiatry* 2003; **64**:943–945.

72. Pratoomsri W, et al. Oxcarbazepine in the treatment of bipolar disorder: a review. *Can J Psychiatry* 2006; **51**:540–545.

73. Juruena MF, et al. Bipolar I and II disorder residual symptoms: oxcarbazepine and carbamazepine as add-on treatment to lithium in a double-blind, randomized trial. *Prog Neuropsychopharmacol Biol Psychiatry* 2009; **33**:94–99.

74. Suppes T, et al. Comparison of two anticonvulsants in a randomized, single-blind treatment of hypomanic symptoms in patients with bipolar disorder. *Aust NZ J Psychiatry* 2007; **41**:397–402.

75. Vieta E, et al. A double-blind, randomized, placebo-controlled prophylaxis trial of oxcarbazepine as adjunctive treatment to lithium in the long-term treatment of bipolar I and II disorder. *Int J Neuropsychopharmacol* 2008; **11**:445–452.

76. Talaei A, et al. Oxcarbazepine versus sodium valproate in treatment of acute mania: a double-blind randomized clinical trial. *Int Clin Psychopharmacol* 2022; **37**:116–121.

77. Wagner KD, et al. A double-blind, randomized, placebo-controlled trial of oxcarbazepine in the treatment of bipolar disorder in children and adolescents. *Am J Psychiatry* 2006; **163**:1179–1186.

78. Mishory A, et al. Phenytoin as an antimanic anticonvulsant: a controlled study. *Am J Psychiatry* 2000; **157**:463–465.

79. Akhondzadeh S, et al. Ritanserin as an adjunct to lithium and haloperidol for the treatment of medication-naive patients with acute mania: a double blind and placebo controlled trial. *BMC Psychiatry* 2003; **3**:7.

80. Carmassi C, et al. Prescribing tamoxifen in patients with mood disorders: a systematic review of potential antimanic versus depressive effects. *J Clin Psychopharmacol* 2021; **41**:450–460.

81. Pigott K, et al. Topiramate for acute affective episodes in bipolar disorder in adults. *Cochrane Database Syst Rev* 2016; **9**:CD003384.

82. Applebaum J, et al. Rapid tryptophan depletion as a treatment for acute mania: a double-blind, pilot-controlled study. *Bipolar Disord* 2007; **9**:884–887.

83. Keck PE, Jr, et al. Ziprasidone in the treatment of acute bipolar mania: a three-week, placebo-controlled, double-blind, randomized trial. *Am J Psychiatry* 2003; **160**:741–748.

84. Potkin SG, et al. Ziprasidone in acute bipolar mania: a 21-day randomized, double-blind, placebo-controlled replication trial. *J Clin Psychopharmacol* 2005; **25**:301–310.

85. Vieta E, et al. Ziprasidone in the treatment of acute mania: a 12-week, placebo-controlled, haloperidol-referenced study. *J Psychopharmacol* 2010; **24**:547–558.

CHAPTER 2

Rapid-cycling bipolar affective disorder

Rapid-cycling bipolar affective disorder is usually defined as bipolar disorder in which four or more episodes of (hypo-)mania or depression (or four clear switches in polarity) occur in a 12-month period. It is generally considered to be less responsive to drug treatment than non-rapid-cycling bipolar illness[1] and entails considerable depressive morbidity and suicide risk.[2] Bipolar patients with rapid cycling have more depressive morbidity, a higher incidence of anxiety disorders, addiction, bulimia and borderline personality disorder, as well as atypical features during depression and symptoms such as irritability, risky behaviour, impulsivity and agitation. Rapid-cycling patients have poorer overall functioning, more obesity and are treated with a greater number of drugs.[3] Drug doses tend to be somewhat higher in rapid-cycling than in other bipolar patients.[4] Recent electroconvulsive therapy (ECT) treatment is associated with greater risk of rapid cycling.[5]

Table 2.8 outlines a treatment strategy for rapid cycling based on rather limited data and few direct comparisons of drugs.[6] This strategy is broadly in line with the findings of published systematic reviews.[7,8] NICE concluded that there is no evidence to support rapid-cycling illness being managed any differently from that with a more conventional course.[9] There is no formal first choice agent or combination – prescribing depends partly on what treatments have already been used to prevent or treat mood episodes. Lithium is less likely to be effective in rapid cycling than in non-rapid cycling,[10] a finding supported by psychiatrists' experiences.[11]

In practice, response to treatment is sometimes idiosyncratic: individuals may show significant response to a particular drug. Spontaneous or treatment-related remissions occur in around a third of rapid cyclers[12] and rapid cycling may come and go in many patients.[13]

Table 2.8 Recommended treatment strategy fo rapid-cycling bipolar disorder.

Step	Suggested treatment
Step 1	**Withdraw antidepressants** in all patients[10,11] (some controversial evidence supports continuation of SSRIs[12,13])
Step 2	**Evaluate possible precipitants** e.g. alcohol, thyroid dysfunction (including antithyroid antibodies[14]), external stressors[15]
Step 3	**Optimise mood stabiliser treatment**[16–19] (using plasma levels) and **Consider combining mood stabilisers** e.g. lithium + valproate, lithium + lamotrigine, valproate + carbamazepine or go to Step 4
Step 4	**Consider other (usually adjunctive) treatment options** (alphabetical order; preferred treatment options in bold[8]) **Aripiprazole**[20,21] (15–30mg/day) Clozapine[22] (usual doses) ECT[23] Lamotrigine[24–26] (up to 225mg/day) Levetiracetam[27] (up to 2000mg/day) Lurasidone[28,29] (40–120mg/day) Nimodipine[30–32] (180mg/day) **Olanzapine**[33] (usual doses) **Quetiapine**[34–37] (300–600mg/day) Risperidone[38,39] (up to 6mg/day) Thyroxine[40,41] (150–400mcg/day) Topiramate[42] (up to 300mg/day) Transcranial magnetic stimulation (rTMS)[43,44]

The choice of drug is determined by patient factors – there are few comparative efficacy data to guide choice at the time of writing. **Quetiapine** probably has the best supporting data[34–36] but it has similar efficacy to aripiprazole or olanzapine. Supporting data for levetiracetam, nimodipine, thyroxine and topiramate are relatively limited.

Clozapine has a clear role in treatment-resistant bipolar disorder,[45] a definition that might include rapid cycling, in which it shows some acute and long-term efficacy.[22,46]

References

1. Miola A, et al. Prevalence and outcomes of rapid cycling bipolar disorder: mixed method systematic meta-review. *J Psychiatr Res* 2023; **164**:404–415.
2. Coryell W, et al. The long-term course of rapid-cycling bipolar disorder. *Arch Gen Psychiatry* 2003; **60**:914–920.
3. Furio M, et al. Characterization of rapid cycling bipolar patients presenting with major depressive episode within the BRIDGE-II-MIX study. *Bipolar Disord* 2020; **23**:391–399.
4. Yasui-Furukori N, et al. Factors associated with doses of mood stabilizers in real-world outpatients with bipolar disorder. *Clin Psychopharmacol Neurosci* 2020; **18**:599–606.
5. Xu JJ, et al. Sociodemographic, clinical and treatment characteristics of current rapid-cycling bipolar disorder: a multicenter Chinese study. *Int J Bipolar Disord* 2024; **12**:11.
6. Miola A, et al. Current status and treatment of rapid cycling bipolar disorder. *J Clin Psychopharmacol* 2024; **44**:86–88.
7. Strawbridge R, et al. A systematic review and meta-analysis of treatments for rapid cycling bipolar disorder. *Acta Psychiatr Scand* 2022; **146**:290–311.
8. Roosen L, et al. Evidence-based treatment strategies for rapid cycling bipolar disorder, a systematic review. *J Affect Disord* 2022; **311**:69–77.
9. National Institute for Health and Care Excellence. Bipolar disorder: assessment and management. Clinical guideline [CG185]. 2014 (last updated December 2023, last accessed October 2024); https://www.nice.org.uk/guidance/cg185.
10. Hui TP, et al. A systematic review and meta-analysis of clinical predictors of lithium response in bipolar disorder. *Acta Psychiatr Scand* 2019; **140**:94–115.
11. Montlahuc C, et al. Response to lithium in patients with bipolar disorder: what are psychiatrists' experiences and practices compared to literature review? *Pharmacopsychiatry* 2019; **52**:70–77.
12. Koukopoulos A, et al. Duration and stability of the rapid-cycling course: a long-term personal follow-up of 109 patients. *J Affect Disord* 2003; **73**:75–85.
13. Carvalho AF, et al. Rapid cycling in bipolar disorder: a systematic review. *J Clin Psychiatry* 2014; **75**:e578–e586.

14. Wehr TA, et al. Can antidepressants cause mania and worsen the course of affective illness? *Am J Psychiatry* 1987; **144**:1403–1411.

15. El-Mallakh RS, et al. Antidepressants worsen rapid-cycling course in bipolar depression: a STEP-BD randomized clinical trial. *J Affect Disord* 2015; **184**:318–321.

16. Amsterdam JD, et al. Efficacy and mood conversion rate during long-term fluoxetine v. lithium monotherapy in rapid- and non-rapid-cycling bipolar II disorder. *Br J Psychiatry* 2013; **202**:301–306.

17. Amsterdam JD, et al. Effectiveness and mood conversion rate of short-term fluoxetine monotherapy in patients with rapid cycling bipolar II depression versus patients with nonrapid cycling bipolar II depression. *J Clin Psychopharmacol* 2013; **33**:420–424.

18. Gan Z, et al. Rapid cycling bipolar disorder is associated with antithyroid antibodies, instead of thyroid dysfunction. *BMC Psychiatry* 2019; **19**:378.

19. Kupka RW, et al. Rapid and non-rapid cycling bipolar disorder: a meta-analysis of clinical studies. *J Clin Psychiatry* 2003; **64**:1483–1494.

20. Kemp DE, et al. A 6-month, double-blind, maintenance trial of lithium monotherapy versus the combination of lithium and divalproex for rapid-cycling bipolar disorder and co-occurring substance abuse or dependence. *J Clin Psychiatry* 2009; **70**:113–121.

21. Da Rocha FF, et al. Addition of lamotrigine to valproic acid: a successful outcome in a case of rapid-cycling bipolar affective disorder. *Prog Neuropsychopharmacol Biol Psychiatry* 2007; **31**:1548–1549.

22. Woo YS, et al. Lamotrigine added to valproate successfully treated a case of ultra-rapid cycling bipolar disorder. *Psychiatry Clin Neurosci* 2007; **61**:130–131.

23. Zhihan G, et al. Lamotrigine and lithium combination for treatment of rapid cycling bipolar disorder: results from meta-analysis. *Front Psychiatry* 2022; **13**:913051.

24. Suppes T, et al. Efficacy and safety of aripiprazole in subpopulations with acute manic or mixed episodes of bipolar I disorder. *J Affect Disord* 2008; **107**:145–154.

25. Muzina DJ, et al. Aripiprazole monotherapy in patients with rapid-cycling bipolar I disorder: an analysis from a long-term, double-blind, placebo-controlled study. *Int J Clin Pract* 2008; **62**:679–687.

26. Calabrese JR, et al. Clozapine prophylaxis in rapid cycling bipolar disorder. *J Clin Psychopharmacol* 1991; **11**:396–397.

27. Mosolov S, et al. Electroconvulsive therapy (ECT) in bipolar disorder patients with ultra-rapid cycling and unstable mixed states. *Medicina (Kaunas)* 2021; **57**:624.

28. Fatemi SH, et al. Lamotrigine in rapid-cycling bipolar disorder. *J Clin Psychiatry* 1997; **58**:522–527.

29. Calabrese JR, et al. A double-blind, placebo-controlled, prophylaxis study of lamotrigine in rapid-cycling bipolar disorder. Lamictal 614 Study Group. *J Clin Psychiatry* 2000; **61**:841–850.

30. Wang Z, et al. Lamotrigine adjunctive therapy to lithium and divalproex in depressed patients with rapid cycling bipolar disorder and a recent substance use disorder: a 12-week, double-blind, placebo-controlled pilot study. *Psychopharmacol Bull* 2010; **43**:5–21.

31. Braunig P, et al. Levetiracetam in the treatment of rapid cycling bipolar disorder. *J Psychopharmacol* 2003; **17**:239–241.

32. Siwek M, et al. Lurasidone in therapy of treatment-resistant ultra-rapid cycling bipolar disorder: case report. *Clin Psychopharmacol Neurosci* 2021; **19**:568–571.

33. Kato M, et al. The efficacy and safety of lurasidone in bipolar I depression with and without rapid cycling: a pooled post-hoc analysis of two randomized, placebo-controlled trials. *J Affect Disord* 2023; **337**:150–158.

34. Goodnick PJ. Nimodipine treatment of rapid cycling bipolar disorder. *J Clin Psychiatry* 1995; **56**:330.

35. Pazzaglia PJ, et al. Preliminary controlled trial of nimodipine in ultra-rapid cycling affective dysregulation. *Psychiatry Res* 1993; **49**:257–272.

36. Romanov DV, et al. [Nimodipine in treatment of bipolar disorder]. *Zh Nevrol Psikhiatr Im S S Korsakova* 2023; **123**:20–26.

37. Sanger TM, et al. Olanzapine in the acute treatment of bipolar I disorder with a history of rapid cycling. *J Affect Disord* 2003; **73**:155–161.

38. Goldberg JF, et al. Effectiveness of quetiapine in rapid cycling bipolar disorder: a preliminary study. *J Affect Disord* 2008; **105**:305–310.

39. Vieta E, et al. Quetiapine monotherapy in the treatment of patients with bipolar I or II depression and a rapid-cycling disease course: a randomized, double-blind, placebo-controlled study. *Bipolar Disord* 2007; **9**:413–425.

40. Langosch JM, et al. Efficacy of quetiapine monotherapy in rapid-cycling bipolar disorder in comparison with sodium valproate. *J Clin Psychopharmacol* 2008; **28**:555–560.

41. Vieta E, et al. Quetiapine in the treatment of rapid cycling bipolar disorder. *Bipolar Disord* 2002; **4**:335–340.

42. Bobo WV, et al. A randomized open comparison of long-acting injectable risperidone and treatment as usual for prevention of relapse, rehospitalization, and urgent care referral in community-treated patients with rapid cycling bipolar disorder. *Clin Neuropharmacol* 2011; **34**:224–233.

43. Vieta E, et al. Treatment of refractory rapid cycling bipolar disorder with risperidone. *J Clin Psychopharmacol* 1998; **18**:172–174.

44. Extein IL. High doses of levothyroxine for refractory rapid cycling. *Am J Psychiatry* 2000; **157**:1704–1705.

45. Walshaw PD, et al. Adjunctive thyroid hormone treatment in rapid cycling bipolar disorder: a double-blind placebo-controlled trial of levo-thyroxine (L-T_4) and triiodothyronine (T_3). *Bipolar Disord* 2018; **20**:594–603.

46. Chen CK, et al. Combination treatment of clozapine and topiramate in resistant rapid-cycling bipolar disorder. *Clin Neuropharmacol* 2005; **28**:136–138.

47. Zamar AC, et al. A new treatment protocol of combined high-dose levothyroxine and repetitive transcranial magnetic stimulation for the treatment of rapid-cycling bipolar spectrum disorders: a cohort evaluation of 55 patients. *J Clin Med* 2022; **11**:5830.

48. Tao S, et al. Case report: rTMS in combination with aripiprazole and sodium valproate for the maintenance treatment of rapid cycling bipolar disorder. *Front Psychiatry* 2023; **14**:1070046.

49. Delgado A, et al. Clozapine in bipolar disorder: a systematic review and meta-analysis. *J Psychiatr Res* 2020; **125**:21–27.

50. Kılınçel O, et al. The role of clozapine as a mood regulator in the treatment of rapid cycling bipolar affective disorder. *Turk Psikiyatri Derg* 2019; **30**:268–271.

Bipolar depression

Bipolar depression shares the diagnostic criteria for an episode of major depressive disorder, but episodes may differ in severity, time course, liability to recurrence and response to drug treatment. Episodes of bipolar depression are, compared with unipolar depression, more rapid in onset, more frequent, more severe, shorter and more likely to involve delusions and reverse neuro-vegetative symptoms such as hyperphagia and hypersomnia.[1-3] Around 15% of people with bipolar disorder commit suicide,[4] a statistic that reflects the severity and frequency of depressive episodes. Bipolar depression affords greater socioeconomic burden than either mania or unipolar major depression[5] and comprises the majority of symptomatic illness in bipolar affective disorder with respect to time.[6,7]

In the UK, NICE recommends the combination of fluoxetine with olanzapine or quetiapine on its own (assuming an antipsychotic is not already prescribed).[8] Lamotrigine is considered to be second-line treatment. BAP guidelines[9] have lamotrigine as a first-line option, albeit with the caveat that a mood stabiliser or antipsychotic will be needed to protect against mania in the longer term. Lurasidone is also a first-line option in the BAP guidelines.

The 2020 RANZCP guidelines[10] recommend the use of lithium, lamotrigine, valproate, quetiapine, lurasidone and cariprazine either as individual agents or in combinations of two or three different drugs (including the addition of an antidepressant). Olanzapine and carbamazepine are considered second-line drugs. Similar recommendations are made in the more recent (2023) Canadian guidelines.[11] Differences include the relegation of valproate to a second-line treatment and the inclusion of lumateperone (also as a second-line drug). Lurasidone is suggested as a first-line agent but only as an adjunct. Olanzapine plus fluoxetine is second line but olanzapine itself is demoted to third-line use.

Tables 2.9, 2.10 and 2.11 give some broad guidance on treatment options in bipolar depression.

Meta-analysis in bipolar depression

Meta-analytical studies in bipolar depression are constrained by the variety of methods used to assess efficacy. This means that many scientifically robust studies cannot be included in some meta-analyses because their parameters (outcomes, duration, etc.) are not shared with other studies and so cannot be compared with them. Early lithium studies are an important example – their short duration and cross-over design preclude their inclusion in meta-analysis. BAP guidelines are somewhat dismissive (perhaps correctly) of network meta-analyses because outcome is heavily influenced by inclusion criteria and because findings often contradict direct comparisons.[9]

A 2021 network meta-analysis of 18 RCTs found that, looking only at antipsychotic drugs, lurasidone, quetiapine, olanzapine and cariprazine were all effective, with cariprazine having the smallest effect size.[12] A more recent (2024) review[13] of 16 RCTs of FDA-licensed antipsychotics added lumateperone to the list of robustly effective agents. Olanzapine showed the lowest rate of withdrawals from trials and quetiapine was the least well tolerated. The largest network meta-analysis (101 RCTs) was published in 2023.[14] In this, olanzapine plus fluoxetine was the most effective, followed in order by quetiapine, olanzapine alone, lurasidone, lumateperone, cariprazine and lamotrigine (the least effective). Recent meta-analyses of ketamine and esketamine[15,16] have concluded that ketamine formulations are probably effective in bipolar depression but with a low certainty of evidence.

CHAPTER 2

Table 2.9 Established treatments (listed in alphabetical order).

Drug/regimen	Comments
Lamotrigine[1,17–21]	Lamotrigine appears to be effective both as a treatment for bipolar depression and as prophylaxis against further episodes. It does not induce switching or rapid cycling. It is as effective as citalopram and causes less weight gain than lithium. Overall, the effect of lamotrigine is difficult to be clear about, with numerous equivocal trials[22] that perhaps failed to allow for the time taken for full titration of the drug. It may be useful as an adjunct to lithium[23] or as an alternative to it in pregnancy.[24] A later trial[25] suggested robust efficacy when combined with quetiapine. There is a small anti-manic effect of lamotrigine.[26]

Treatment is somewhat complicated by the small risk of rash, which is associated with speed of dose titration. The necessity for titration may limit clinical utility.

A further complication is the question of dose: 50mg/day has efficacy, but 200mg/day is probably better. In the USA, doses of up to 1200mg/day have been used (mean around 250mg/day). Plasma concentrations (only the range for anti-convulsant effects is known) may guide the need for higher doses. |
| Lithium[1,17,27–29] | Lithium is probably effective in treating bipolar depression but supporting data are methodologically questionable.[30] There is some evidence that lithium prevents depressive relapse but its effects on manic relapse are considered more robust. There is fairly strong support for lithium in reducing suicidality in bipolar disorder.[31,32] |
| Lurasidone | Three RCTs show a good effect for lurasidone either alone[33] or as an adjunct to mood stabilisers.[34,35] A further RCT reported good outcome in bipolar depression with sub-syndromal hypomanic symptoms.[36] Pooled analysis suggests response is dose-related.[37] A network meta-analysis suggested lurasidone is more effective than aripiprazole and ziprasidone but not quetiapine or olanzapine.[38] |
| Mood stabiliser + antidepressant[39–45] | Antidepressants are still widely used in bipolar depression, particularly for breakthrough episodes occurring in those on mood stabilisers. They have been assumed to be effective, although there is a risk of cycle acceleration and/or switching. Studies suggest mood stabilisers alone are just as effective as mood stabilisers/antidepressant combination although subanalysis suggested higher doses of antidepressants may be effective.[46–48] Tricyclics and MAOIs are usually best avoided. SSRIs are generally recommended if an antidepressant is to be prescribed. Venlafaxine and bupropion (amfebutamone) have also been used. Venlafaxine may be more likely to induce a switch to mania.[49,50]

Continuing antidepressant treatment after resolution of symptoms may protect against depressive relapse[51,52] although only in the absence of a mood stabiliser.[53] At the time of writing, there is no consensus on whether or not to continue antidepressants long term.[54] The most recent findings suggest that switch rates are no higher with sertraline alone than with lithium + sertraline,[55] but also that there may be no protective effect against depressive episodes.[56]

Some guidelines recommend the use of antidepressants in bipolar II depression[57] and there is evidence that sertraline does not increase switch rates in these patients.[55] |
| Olanzapine ± fluoxetine[17,30,58–61] | This combination (Symbyax®) is more effective than both placebo and olanzapine alone in treating bipolar depression. The dose is 6 and 25mg or 12 and 50mg/day (so presumably 5/20mg and 10/40mg are effective). It may be more effective than lamotrigine. There is reasonable evidence of prophylactic effect. It is recommended as first-line treatment by NICE[8] but not in other guidelines.

Olanzapine alone is effective when compared with placebo[62] but the combination with fluoxetine is more effective. (This is possibly the strongest evidence for a beneficial effect for an antidepressant in bipolar depression.) |

Table 2.9 (*Continued*)

Drug/regimen	Comments
Quetiapine[63–67]	Five large RCTs have demonstrated clear efficacy for doses of 300 and 600mg daily (as monotherapy) in bipolar I and bipolar II depression. A later study in Chinese patients demonstrated the efficacy of 300mg/day[68] in bipolar I depression. It may be superior to both lithium and paroxetine. Quetiapine also prevents relapse into depression and mania[69,70] and so is one of the treatments of choice in bipolar depression. It appears not to be associated with switching to mania.
Valproate[1,17,71–75]	Limited evidence of efficacy as monotherapy but recommended in some guidelines. Several very small RCTs but many are negative; however meta-analyses do support antidepressant efficacy.[74] Probably protects against depressive relapse but database is small. Not recommended because of its teratogenic effects in both men and women.

MAOIs, monoamine oxidase inhibitors; RCT, randomised controlled trial.

Table 2.10 Alternative treatments (refer to primary literature before using).

Drug/regimen	Comments
Antidepressants[76–84]	'Unopposed' antidepressants (i.e. without mood-stabiliser protection) are generally to be avoided in bipolar depression because of the risk of switching and inducing rapid cycling. There is also evidence that they are relatively less effective (perhaps not effective at all) in bipolar depression than in unipolar depression although dose may be critical.[48] Short-term use of fluoxetine, venlafaxine and moclobemide seems reasonably effective and safe even as monotherapy. A meta-analysis suggested a large effect size for tranylcypromine in the absence of any risk of switching.[85] Overall, however, unopposed antidepressant treatment should be avoided, especially in bipolar I disorder.[54]
Cariprazine[86]	One RCT suggests that cariprazine at 1.5mg/day is effective in bipolar I depression. A second, larger study showed 1.5 and 3mg/day to be effective.[87] The most recent study[87] found benefit for 1.5mg/day but not 3mg/day. Usually has lowest efficacy among effective drugs in meta-analyses.
Ketamine[88–91]	An IV dose of 0.5mg/kg is effective in refractory bipolar depression with a very high response rate. Dissociative symptoms are common but brief. Now accepted as standard treatment for refractory bipolar depression.[92,93] IV racemate is possibly more effective than intranasal esketamine.[94] Switching to mania is a potential problem[95] although probably a remote risk.
Pramipexole[96,97]	Two small placebo-controlled trials suggested useful efficacy in bipolar depression. Effective dose averages around 1.7mg/day. Both studies used pramipexole as an adjunct to existing mood-stabiliser treatment. Neither study detected an increased risk of switching to mania/hypomania (a theoretical consideration) but data are insufficient to exclude this possibility. A meta-analysis of studies showed a robust effect on response but not remission.[98]

RCT, randomised controlled trial.

Table 2.11 Other possible treatments (seek specialist advice before using).

Drug/regimen	Comments
Aripiprazole[99–102]	Limited support from open studies as add-on treatment. One RCT was negative. Possibly not effective.[98]
Carbamazepine[1,17,103]	Occasionally recommended but database is poor and effect modest. May have useful activity when added to other mood stabilisers.
Gabapentin[1,104,105]	Open studies suggest modest effect when added to mood stabilisers or antipsychotics. Doses average around 1750mg/day. Anxiolytic effect may account for apparent effect in bipolar depression.
Inositol[106]	Small, randomised, pilot study suggests that 12g/day inositol is effective in bipolar depression.
Mifepristone[107,108]	Some evidence of mood-elevating properties in bipolar depression although this was not replicated in a larger trial. Improved cognitive function in both trials. Dose used was 600mg/day.
Modafinil[109]	Meta-analysis of five studies of modafinil/armodafinil suggests robust benefit on response and remission with good tolerability and no evidence of increased risk of switching. Some evidence of safety from a later study.[110]
Omega-3 fatty acids[111–113]	One positive RCT (1g/2g a day) and one negative (6g a day). The ratio of omega-6 may determine efficacy.[113]

RCT, randomised controlled trial.

Summary of drug choice

The combination of olanzapine + fluoxetine is probably the most effective treatment available for bipolar depression but its use is constrained by the well-known adverse effect profile of olanzapine. SSRIs other than fluoxetine may be effective but should probably be avoided unless clear individual benefit is obvious.[54] Alternative first-line choices are quetiapine, olanzapine, lurasidone, lamotrigine and cariprazine (and lumateperone in North America). These drugs differ substantially in adverse effect profile, tolerability and cost, each of which needs to be considered when prescribing for an individual. Lithium is also effective but supporting evidence is relatively weak. Second-line drugs include ketamine and, increasingly, modafinil. Aripiprazole, risperidone, ziprasidone, tricyclics (with the exception of imipramine) and MAOIs (with the exception of tranylcypromine) are probably not effective and should not be used routinely.[114]

References

1. Malhi GS, et al. Bipolar depression: management options. *CNS Drugs* 2003; **17**:9–25.
2. Perlis RH, et al. Clinical features of bipolar depression versus major depressive disorder in large multicenter trials. *Am J Psychiatry* 2006; **163**:225–231.
3. Mitchell PB, et al. Comparison of depressive episodes in bipolar disorder and in major depressive disorder within bipolar disorder pedigrees. *Br J Psychiatry* 2011; **199**:303–309.
4. Haddad P, et al. Pharmacological management of bipolar depression. *Acta Psychiatr Scand* 2002; **105**:401–403.
5. Hirschfeld RM. Bipolar depression: the real challenge. *Eur Neuropsychopharmacol* 2004; **14** Suppl 2:S83–S88.
6. Judd LL, et al. The long-term natural history of the weekly symptomatic status of bipolar I disorder. *Arch Gen Psychiatry* 2002; **59**:530–537.
7. Judd LL, et al. A prospective investigation of the natural history of the long-term weekly symptomatic status of bipolar II disorder. *Arch Gen Psychiatry* 2003; **60**:261–269.
8. National Institute for Health and Care Excellence. Bipolar disorder: assessment and management. Clinical guideline [CG185]. 2014 (last updated December 2023, last accessed October 2024); https://www.nice.org.uk/guidance/cg185.

9. Goodwin GM, et al. Evidence-based guidelines for treating bipolar disorder: revised third edition recommendations from the British Association for Psychopharmacology. *J Psychopharmacol* 2016; **30**:495–553.

10. Malhi GS, et al. The 2020 Royal Australian and New Zealand College of Psychiatrists clinical practice guidelines for mood disorders. *Aust NZ J Psychiatry* 2021; **55**:7–117.

11. Keramatian K, et al. The CANMAT and ISBD guidelines for the treatment of bipolar disorder: summary and a 2023 update of evidence. *Focus (Am Psychiatr Publ)* 2023; **21**:344–353.

12. Kadakia A, et al. Efficacy and tolerability of atypical antipsychotics for acute bipolar depression: a network meta-analysis. *BMC Psychiatry* 2021; **21**:249.

13. Li S, et al. Efficacy and tolerability of FDA-approved atypical antipsychotics for the treatment of bipolar depression: a systematic review and network meta-analysis. *Eur Psychiatry* 2024; **67**:e29.

14. Yildiz A, et al. Comparative efficacy and tolerability of pharmacological interventions for acute bipolar depression in adults: a systematic review and network meta-analysis. *Lancet Psychiatry* 2023; **10**:693–705.

15. Zhan Z, et al. Comparative efficacy and side-effect profile of ketamine and esketamine in the treatment of unipolar and bipolar depression: protocol for a systematic review and network meta-analysis. *BMJ Open* 2021; **11**:e043457.

16. Rodolico A, et al. Efficacy and safety of ketamine and esketamine for unipolar and bipolar depression: an overview of systematic reviews with meta-analysis. *Front Psychiatry* 2024; **15**:1325399.

17. Yatham LN, et al. Bipolar depression: criteria for treatment selection, definition of refractoriness, and treatment options. *Bipolar Disord* 2003; **5**:85–97.

18. Calabrese JR, et al. A double-blind placebo-controlled study of lamotrigine monotherapy in outpatients with bipolar I depression. Lamictal 602 Study Group. *J Clin Psychiatry* 1999; **60**:79–88.

19. Bowden CL, et al. Lamotrigine in the treatment of bipolar depression. *Eur Neuropsychopharmacol* 1999; **9** Suppl 4:S113–S117.

20. Marangell LB, et al. Lamotrigine treatment of bipolar disorder: data from the first 500 patients in STEP-BD. *Bipolar Disord* 2004; **6**:139–143.

21. Schaffer A, et al. Randomized, double-blind pilot trial comparing lamotrigine versus citalopram for the treatment of bipolar depression. *J Affect Disord* 2006; **96**:95–99.

22. Calabrese JR, et al. Lamotrigine in the acute treatment of bipolar depression: results of five double-blind, placebo-controlled clinical trials. *Bipolar Disord* 2008; **10**:323–333.

23. Van der Loos ML, et al. Efficacy and safety of lamotrigine as add-on treatment to lithium in bipolar depression: a multicenter, double-blind, placebo-controlled trial. *J Clin Psychiatry* 2009; **70**:223–231.

24. Newport DJ, et al. Lamotrigine in bipolar disorder: efficacy during pregnancy. *Bipolar Disord* 2008; **10**:432–436.

25. Geddes JR, et al. Comparative evaluation of quetiapine plus lamotrigine combination versus quetiapine monotherapy (and folic acid versus placebo) in bipolar depression (CEQUEL): a 2 x 2 factorial randomised trial. *Lancet Psychiatry* 2016; **3**:31–39.

26. Goodwin GM, et al. A pooled analysis of 2 placebo-controlled 18-month trials of lamotrigine and lithium maintenance in bipolar I disorder. *J Clin Psychiatry* 2004; **65**:432–441.

27. Geddes JR, et al. Long-term lithium therapy for bipolar disorder: systematic review and meta-analysis of randomized controlled trials. *Am J Psychiatry* 2004; **161**:217–222.

28. Calabrese JR, et al. A placebo-controlled 18-month trial of lamotrigine and lithium maintenance treatment in recently depressed patients with bipolar I disorder. *J Clin Psychiatry* 2003; **64**:1013–1024.

29. Prien RF, et al. Lithium carbonate and imipramine in prevention of affective episodes. A comparison in recurrent affective illness. *Arch Gen Psychiatry* 1973; **29**:420–425.

30. Grunze H, et al. The World Federation of Societies of Biological Psychiatry (WFSBP) guidelines for the biological treatment of bipolar disorders: update 2010 on the treatment of acute bipolar depression. *World J Biol Psychiatry* 2010; **11**:81–109.

31. Goodwin FK, et al. Suicide risk in bipolar disorder during treatment with lithium and divalproex. *JAMA* 2003; **290**:1467–1473.

32. Kessing LV, et al. Suicide risk in patients treated with lithium. *Arch Gen Psychiatry* 2005; **62**:860–866.

33. Loebel A, et al. Lurasidone monotherapy in the treatment of bipolar I depression: a randomized, double-blind, placebo-controlled study. *Am J Psychiatry* 2014; **171**:160–168.

34. Loebel A, et al. Lurasidone as adjunctive therapy with lithium or valproate for the treatment of bipolar I depression: a randomized, double-blind, placebo-controlled study. *Am J Psychiatry* 2014; **171**:169–177.

35. Suppes T, et al. Lurasidone adjunctive with lithium or valproate for bipolar depression: a placebo-controlled trial utilizing prospective and retrospective enrolment cohorts. *J Psychiatr Res* 2016; **78**:86–93.

36. Suppes T, et al. Lurasidone for the treatment of major depressive disorder with mixed features: a randomized, double-blind, placebo-controlled study. *Am J Psychiatry* 2016; **173**:400–407.

37. Chapel S, et al. Lurasidone dose response in bipolar depression: a population dose-response analysis. *Clin Ther* 2016; **38**:4–15.

38. Ostacher M, et al. Lurasidone compared to other atypical antipsychotic monotherapies for bipolar depression: a systematic review and network meta-analysis. *World J Biol Psychiatry* 2018; **19**:586–601.

39. Calabrese JR, et al. International Consensus Group on Bipolar I Depression Treatment Guidelines. *J Clin Psychiatry* 2004; **65**:571–579.

40. Nemeroff CB, et al. Double-blind, placebo-controlled comparison of imipramine and paroxetine in the treatment of bipolar depression. *Am J Psychiatry* 2001; **158**:906–912.

41. Vieta E, et al. A randomized trial comparing paroxetine and venlafaxine in the treatment of bipolar depressed patients taking mood stabilizers. *J Clin Psychiatry* 2002; **63**:508–512.

42. Young LT, et al. Double-blind comparison of addition of a second mood stabilizer versus an antidepressant to an initial mood stabilizer for treatment of patients with bipolar depression. *Am J Psychiatry* 2000; **157**:124–126.

43. Fawcett JA. Lithium combinations in acute and maintenance treatment of unipolar and bipolar depression. *J Clin Psychiatry* 2003; **64** Suppl 5:32–37.

CHAPTER 2

44. Altshuler L, et al. The impact of antidepressant discontinuation versus antidepressant continuation on 1-year risk for relapse of bipolar depression: a retrospective chart review. *J Clin Psychiatry* 2001; **62**:612–616.

45. Erfurth A, et al. Bupropion as add-on strategy in difficult-to-treat bipolar depressive patients. *Neuropsychobiology* 2002; **45** Suppl 1:33–36.

46. Sachs GS, et al. Effectiveness of adjunctive antidepressant treatment for bipolar depression. *N Engl J Med* 2007; **356**:1711–1722.

47. Goldberg JF, et al. Adjunctive antidepressant use and symptomatic recovery among bipolar depressed patients with concomitant manic symptoms: findings from the STEP-BD. *Am J Psychiatry* 2007; **164**:1348–1355.

48. Tada M, et al. Antidepressant dose and treatment response in bipolar depression: reanalysis of the Systematic Treatment Enhancement Program for Bipolar Disorder (STEP-BD) data. *J Psychiatr Res* 2015; **68**:151–156.

49. Post RM, et al. Mood switch in bipolar depression: comparison of adjunctive venlafaxine, bupropion and sertraline. *Br J Psychiatry* 2006; **189**:124–131.

50. Leverich GS, et al. Risk of switch in mood polarity to hypomania or mania in patients with bipolar depression during acute and continuation trials of venlafaxine, sertraline, and bupropion as adjuncts to mood stabilizers. *Am J Psychiatry* 2006; **163**:232–239.

51. Salvi V, et al. The use of antidepressants in bipolar disorder. *J Clin Psychiatry* 2008; **69**:1307–1318.

52. Altshuler LL, et al. Impact of antidepressant continuation after acute positive or partial treatment response for bipolar depression: a blinded, randomized study. *J Clin Psychiatry* 2009; **70**:450–457.

53. Ghaemi SN, et al. Long-term antidepressant treatment in bipolar disorder: meta-analyses of benefits and risks. *Acta Psychiatr Scand* 2008; **118**:347–356.

54. Pacchiarotti I, et al. The International Society for Bipolar Disorders (ISBD) task force report on antidepressant use in bipolar disorders. *Am J Psychiatry* 2013; **170**:1249–1262.

55. Altshuler LL, et al. Switch rates during acute treatment for bipolar II depression with lithium, sertraline, or the two combined: a randomized double-blind comparison. *Am J Psychiatry* 2017; **174**:266–276.

56. Yatham LN, et al. Duration of adjunctive antidepressant maintenance in bipolar I depression. *N Engl J Med* 2023; **389**:430–440.

57. Yatham LN, et al. Canadian Network for Mood and Anxiety Treatments (CANMAT) and International Society for Bipolar Disorders (ISBD) 2018 guidelines for the management of patients with bipolar disorder. *Bipolar Disord* 2018; **20**:97–170.

58. Tohen M, et al. Efficacy of olanzapine and olanzapine-fluoxetine combination in the treatment of bipolar I depression. *Arch Gen Psychiatry* 2003; **60**:1079–1088.

59. Brown EB, et al. A 7-week, randomized, double-blind trial of olanzapine/fluoxetine combination versus lamotrigine in the treatment of bipolar I depression. *J Clin Psychiatry* 2006; **67**:1025–1033.

60. Corya SA, et al. A 24-week open-label extension study of olanzapine-fluoxetine combination and olanzapine monotherapy in the treatment of bipolar depression. *J Clin Psychiatry* 2006; **67**:798–806.

61. Dube S, et al. Onset of antidepressant effect of olanzapine and olanzapine/fluoxetine combination in bipolar depression. *Bipolar Disord* 2007; **9**:618–627.

62. Tohen M, et al. Randomised, double-blind, placebo-controlled study of olanzapine in patients with bipolar I depression. *Br J Psychiatry* 2012; **201**:376–382.

63. Calabrese JR, et al. A randomized, double-blind, placebo-controlled trial of quetiapine in the treatment of bipolar I or II depression. *Am J Psychiatry* 2005; **162**:1351–1360.

64. Thase ME, et al. Efficacy of quetiapine monotherapy in bipolar I and II depression: a double-blind, placebo-controlled study (the BOLDER II study). *J Clin Psychopharmacol* 2006; **26**:600–609.

65. Suppes T, et al. Effectiveness of the extended release formulation of quetiapine as monotherapy for the treatment of acute bipolar depression. *J Affect Disord* 2010; **121**:106–115.

66. Young AH, et al. A double-blind, placebo-controlled study of quetiapine and lithium monotherapy in adults in the acute phase of bipolar depression (EMBOLDEN I). *J Clin Psychiatry* 2010; **71**:150–162.

67. McElroy SL, et al. A double-blind, placebo-controlled study of quetiapine and paroxetine as monotherapy in adults with bipolar depression (EMBOLDEN II). *J Clin Psychiatry* 2010; **71**:163–174.

68. Li H, et al. Efficacy and safety of quetiapine extended release monotherapy in bipolar depression: a multi-center, randomized, double-blind, placebo-controlled trial. *Psychopharmacology (Berl)* 2016; **233**:1289–1297.

69. Vieta E, et al. Efficacy and safety of quetiapine in combination with lithium or divalproex for maintenance of patients with bipolar I disorder (international trial 126). *J Affect Disord* 2008; **109**:251–263.

70. Suppes T, et al. Maintenance treatment for patients with bipolar I disorder: results from a North American study of quetiapine in combination with lithium or divalproex (trial 127). *Am J Psychiatry* 2009; **166**:476–488.

71. Goodwin GM. Evidence-based guidelines for treating bipolar disorder: revised second edition – recommendations from the British Association for Psychopharmacology. *J Psychopharmacol* 2009; **23**:346–388.

72. Davis LL, et al. Divalproex in the treatment of bipolar depression: a placebo-controlled study. *J Affect Disord* 2005; **85**:259–266.

73. Ghaemi SN, et al. Divalproex in the treatment of acute bipolar depression: a preliminary double-blind, randomized, placebo-controlled pilot study. *J Clin Psychiatry* 2007; **68**:1840–1844.

74. Smith LA, et al. Valproate for the treatment of acute bipolar depression: systematic review and meta-analysis. *J Affect Disord* 2010; **122**:1–9.

75. Muzina DJ, et al. Acute efficacy of divalproex sodium versus placebo in mood stabilizer-naive bipolar I or II depression: a double-blind, randomized, placebo-controlled trial. *J Clin Psychiatry* 2011; **72**:813–819.

76. Amsterdam JD, et al. Short-term fluoxetine monotherapy for bipolar type II or bipolar NOS major depression – low manic switch rate. *Bipolar Disord* 2004; **6**:75–81.

77. Amsterdam JD, et al. Efficacy and safety of fluoxetine in treating bipolar II major depressive episode. *J Clin Psychopharmacol* 1998; **18**:435–440.

78. Amsterdam J. Efficacy and safety of venlafaxine in the treatment of bipolar II major depressive episode. *J Clin Psychopharmacol* 1998; **18**:414–417.

79. Amsterdam JD, et al. Venlafaxine monotherapy in women with bipolar II and unipolar major depression. *J Affect Disord* 2000; **59**:225–229.

80. Silverstone T. Moclobemide vs. imipramine in bipolar depression: a multicentre double-blind clinical trial. *Acta Psychiatr Scand* 2001; **104**:104–109.

81. Ghaemi SN, et al. Antidepressant treatment in bipolar versus unipolar depression. *Am J Psychiatry* 2004; **161**:163–165.

82. Post RM, et al. A re-evaluation of the role of antidepressants in the treatment of bipolar depression: data from the Stanley Foundation Bipolar Network. *Bipolar Disord* 2003; **5**:396–406.

83. Amsterdam JD, et al. Comparison of fluoxetine, olanzapine, and combined fluoxetine plus olanzapine initial therapy of bipolar type I and type II major depression – lack of manic induction. *J Affect Disord* 2005; **87**:121–130.

84. Amsterdam JD, et al. Fluoxetine monotherapy of bipolar type II and bipolar NOS major depression: a double-blind, placebo-substitution, continuation study. *Int Clin Psychopharmacol* 2005; **20**:257–264.

85. Heijnen WT, et al. Efficacy of tranylcypromine in bipolar depression: a systematic review. *J Clin Psychopharmacol* 2015; **35**:700–705.

86. Durgam S, et al. An 8-week randomized, double-blind, placebo-controlled evaluation of the safety and efficacy of cariprazine in patients with bipolar I depression. *Am J Psychiatry* 2016; **173**:271–281.

87. Earley W, et al. Cariprazine treatment of bipolar depression: a randomized double-blind placebo-controlled phase 3 study. *Am J Psychiatry* 2019; **176**:439–448.

88. Diazgranados N, et al. A randomized add-on trial of an N-methyl-D-aspartate antagonist in treatment-resistant bipolar depression. *Arch Gen Psychiatry* 2010; **67**:793–802.

89. Shahani R, et al. Ketamine-associated ulcerative cystitis: a new clinical entity. *Urology* 2007; **69**:810–812.

90. Zarate CA, Jr, et al. Replication of ketamine's antidepressant efficacy in bipolar depression: a randomized controlled add-on trial. *Biol Psychiatry* 2012; **71**:939–946.

91. Permoda-Osip A, et al. Single ketamine infusion and neurocognitive performance in bipolar depression. *Pharmacopsychiatry* 2015; **48**:78–79.

92. Jha MK, et al. Psychopharmacology and experimental therapeutics for bipolar depression. *Focus (Am Psychiatr Publ)* 2019; **17**:232–237.

93. Włodarczyk A, et al. Safety and tolerability of ketamine use in treatment-resistant bipolar depression patients with regard to central nervous system symptomatology: literature review and analysis. *Medicina (Kaunas)* 2020; **56**:67.

94. Bahji A, et al. Comparative efficacy of racemic ketamine and esketamine for depression: a systematic review and meta-analysis. *J Affect Disord* 2021; **278**:542–555.

95. Alison McInnes L, et al. Possible affective switch associated with intravenous ketamine treatment in a patient with bipolar I disorder. *Biol Psychiatry* 2016; **79**:e71–e72.

96. Goldberg JF, et al. Preliminary randomized, double-blind, placebo-controlled trial of pramipexole added to mood stabilizers for treatment-resistant bipolar depression. *Am J Psychiatry* 2004; **161**:564–566.

97. Zarate CA, Jr, et al. Pramipexole for bipolar II depression: a placebo-controlled proof of concept study. *Biol Psychiatry* 2004; **56**:54–60.

98. Romeo B, et al. Meta-analysis and review of dopamine agonists in acute episodes of mood disorder: efficacy and safety. *J Psychopharmacol* 2018; **32**:385–396.

99. Ketter TA, et al. Adjunctive aripiprazole in treatment-resistant bipolar depression. *Ann Clin Psychiatry* 2006; **18**:169–172.

100. Mazza M, et al. Beneficial acute antidepressant effects of aripiprazole as an adjunctive treatment or monotherapy in bipolar patients unresponsive to mood stabilizers: results from a 16-week open-label trial. *Expert Opin Pharmacother* 2008; **9**:3145–3149.

101. Sidor MM, et al. Antidepressants for the acute treatment of bipolar depression: a systematic review and meta-analysis. *J Clin Psychiatry* 2011; **72**:156–167.

102. Cruz N, et al. Efficacy of modern antipsychotics in placebo-controlled trials in bipolar depression: a meta-analysis. *Int J Neuropsychopharmacol* 2010; **13**:5–14.

103. Dilsaver SC, et al. Treatment of bipolar depression with carbamazepine: results of an open study. *Biol Psychiatry* 1996; **40**:935–937.

104. Wang PW, et al. Gabapentin augmentation therapy in bipolar depression. *Bipolar Disord* 2002; **4**:296–301.

105. Ashton H, et al. GABA-ergic drugs: exit stage left, enter stage right. *J Psychopharmacol* 2003; **17**:174–178.

106. Chengappa KN, et al. Inositol as an add-on treatment for bipolar depression. *Bipolar Disord* 2000; **2**:47–55.

107. Young AH, et al. Improvements in neurocognitive function and mood following adjunctive treatment with mifepristone (RU-486) in bipolar disorder. *Neuropsychopharmacology* 2004; **29**:1538–1545.

108. Watson S, et al. A randomized trial to examine the effect of mifepristone on neuropsychological performance and mood in patients with bipolar depression. *Biol Psychiatry* 2012; **72**:943–949.

109. Nunez NA, et al. Efficacy and tolerability of adjunctive modafinil/armodafinil in bipolar depression: a meta-analysis of randomized controlled trials. *Bipolar Disord* 2020; **22**:109–120.

110. Lipschitz JM, et al. Modafinil's effects on cognition and sleep quality in affectively-stable patients with bipolar disorder: a pilot study. *Front Psychiatry* 2023; **14**:1246149.

111. Frangou S, et al. Efficacy of ethyl-eicosapentaenoic acid in bipolar depression: randomised double-blind placebo-controlled study. *Br J Psychiatry* 2006; **188**:46–50.

112. Keck PE, Jr, et al. Double-blind, randomized, placebo-controlled trials of ethyl-eicosapentanoate in the treatment of bipolar depression and rapid cycling bipolar disorder. *Biol Psychiatry* 2006; **60**:1020–1022.

113. Zhang M, et al. Assessment of causal relationships between omega-3 and omega-6 polyunsaturated fatty acids in bipolar disorder: a 2-sample bidirectional mendelian randomization study. *Food Funct* 2023; **14**:6200–6211.

114. Taylor DM, et al. Comparative efficacy and acceptability of drug treatments for bipolar depression: a multiple-treatments meta-analysis. *Acta Psychiatr Scand* 2014; **130**:452–469.

CHAPTER 2

Prophylaxis in bipolar disorder

Any successful drug regimen used for an acute episode should be continued as prophylaxis. To a large extent, therefore, the choice of maintenance treatment for individual patients is dictated by the efficacy and tolerability of acute treatment. Possible exceptions include the consideration of withdrawing antipsychotic treatment from a mood-stabiliser combination after an episode of mania (recommended by some authorities[1]) and the withdrawal of antidepressants after the successful treatment of an acute episode of bipolar depression, assuming a mood stabiliser is continued (recommended by most authorities, at least implicitly[2]). Withdrawing antipsychotics from combination regimens with lithium or valproate may worsen the risk of relapse.[3] Residual mood symptoms after an acute episode are a strong predictor of recurrence.[4,5]

In respect to monotherapy, most evidence supports the efficacy of lithium[6,7] in preventing episodes of mania and depression.[8] Carbamazepine is somewhat less effective[6,9] and the long-term efficacy of valproate is uncertain,[7,10–12] although it too may protect against relapse both into depression and mania.[6,13] Lithium has the advantage of a proven anti-suicidal effect[14–16] but perhaps, relative to other mood stabilisers, the disadvantage of a worsened outcome following abrupt discontinuation[17–20] (although the effect of abrupt discontinuation of other drugs may be similar[20]). Early use of lithium might increase the likelihood of efficacy.[21]

The independent BALANCE study found that valproate as monotherapy was relatively less effective than lithium or the combination of lithium and valproate,[11] casting doubt on its use as a first-line single treatment. Also, a large observational study has shown that lithium is much more effective than valproate in preventing relapse to any condition and in preventing rehospitalisation.[22] Given this, valproate's relative contraindication in women of child-bearing age and the fact that valproate is not licensed for prophylaxis, valproate should be considered a second- or third-line treatment.

Conventional antipsychotics have traditionally been used and are perceived to be effective although the objective evidence base is rather weak.[23,24] FGA depots probably protect against mania but may worsen depression[25] (see 'Antipsychotic long-acting injections in bipolar disorder' earlier in this chapter). Evidence supports the efficacy of many SGAs particularly olanzapine,[26,27] quetiapine,[28] aripiprazole[29] and risperidone.[30] Most studies examine combinations with mood stabilisers and there are fewer supportive monotherapy trials, although asenapine, aripiprazole, olanzapine, quetiapine and risperidone monotherapy are all more effective than placebo.

Olanzapine, quetiapine and aripiprazole are licensed for prophylaxis in many countries although only olanzapine and quetiapine offer protection against depression.[7] Asenapine may also be effective,[31] as may ziprasidone.[32] There is some evidence to support maintenance treatment with lurasidone when added to valproate or lithium,[33] but there are only acute data for lumateperone.[34] Cariprazine may be ineffective as maintenance.[35]

All antipsychotic + mood stabiliser combinations were more effective than mood stabilisers alone in a meta-analysis of 41 studies and 9821 participants.[36] Aripiprazole + valproate was numerically the best maintenance treatment (in terms of risk of relapse to any episode) in this analysis. A later meta-analysis of 14 monotherapy studies found that monotherapy with aripiprazole, olanzapine, lurasidone, risperidone or quetiapine was more effective than placebo over 6 months or longer.[37] A 2022 network meta-analysis found the order of effectiveness to be olanzapine (most effective), quetiapine, aripiprazole, risperidone, lurasidone and paliperidone (least effective).[7]

Long-acting aripiprazole has been shown to delay the time to, and reduced the rate of recurrence of, manic episodes and was generally safe and well tolerated.[38] The use of risperidone LAI is well supported by RCTs[39] and naturalistic studies.[40] The prescribing of LAI SGAs is generally encouraged despite some labelling restrictions[41-44] (see 'Antipsychotic long-acting injections in bipolar disorder' earlier in this chapter).

Box 2.1 summarises recommendations from NICE for prescribing in bipolar disorder.

Box 2.1 NICE recommendations[27]

- When planning long-term pharmacological interventions to prevent relapse, take into account drugs that have been effective during episodes of mania or bipolar depression. Discuss with the person whether they prefer to continue this treatment or switch to lithium, and explain that lithium is the most effective long-term treatment for bipolar disorder.
- Offer lithium as a first-line, long-term pharmacological treatment for bipolar disorder and if lithium is insufficiently effective, consider adding valproate. If lithium is poorly tolerated, consider valproate or olanzapine instead, or if it has been effective during an episode of mania or bipolar depression, quetiapine.
- Do not offer valproate to women of child-bearing potential. Ensure adequate contraception in men taking valproate.
- Discuss with the person the possible benefits and risks of each drug for them.

Optimising lithium treatment[45]

For adults with bipolar disorder the standard lithium plasma level should be 0.6–0.8mmol/L with the option to reduce it to 0.4–0.6mmol/L in cases of good response but poor tolerance, or to increase it to 0.8–1.0mmol/L in cases of insufficient response and good tolerance. For children and adolescents no consensus exists, but the majority of the International Society for Bipolar Disorders (ISBD)/International Study Group on Lithium (IGSLI) task force endorsed this same recommendation. For the elderly, a more conservative approach may be adopted, usually aiming for 0.4–0.6mmol/L, with the option to go to, at most, 0.7 or 0.8mmol/L at age 65–79 years, and only to 0.7mmol/L over age 80 years.

Combination treatment

A significant proportion of patients with bipolar illness fail to be treated adequately with a single mood stabiliser,[11] so combinations of mood stabilisers[46,47] or a mood stabiliser and an antipsychotic[47,48] are commonly used.[49] Also, there is evidence that where combination treatments are effective in mania or depression, then continuation with the same combination provides optimal prophylaxis.[28,48] Overall, combination treatments offer better protection against relapse than monotherapy.[7] The use of polypharmacy needs to be balanced against the likely increased adverse effect burden.

Combinations of olanzapine, risperidone, quetiapine or haloperidol with lithium or valproate are recommended by NICE[27] and by BAP guidelines.[6] Alternative antipsychotics (e.g. aripiprazole) are also options in combinations with lithium or valproate, particularly if these have been found to be effective during the treatment of an acute episode of mania or depression.[28,50] Carbamazepine is considered to be third line. Lamotrigine may be useful in bipolar II disorder[27] but seems only to prevent recurrence of depression.[51] Lurasidone may have broadly similar long-term efficacy, both as monotherapy and when combined with a mood stabiliser.[33,52]

Extrapolation of currently available data suggests that lithium plus an SGA is probably the polypharmacy regimen of choice. There are naturalistic data to support combinations of three treatments; in one study[53] the two best treatments were lithium + valproate + quetiapine followed by lithium + valproate + olanzapine.

Monotherapy with antipsychotics can be considered where mood stabilisers are poorly tolerated or where adherence cannot be assured.[54]

A meta-analysis of long-term antidepressant treatment found that continued treatment was more likely to induce a switch to mania than prevent a depressive episode.[55] The STEP-BD study found no significant benefit for continuing (compared with discontinuing) an antidepressant and worse outcomes in those with rapid-cycling illness.[56] A more recent study found that neither escitalopram nor bupropion had any effect on relapse of depression.[57] There is thus essentially no strong support for long-term use of antidepressants in bipolar illness although some bipolar patients may relapse into depression when antidepressants are discontinued.[20]

Box 2.2 and Table 2.12 summarise prophylaxis and maintenance treatment, respectively, in bipolar disorder.

Box 2.2 Summary of prophylaxis in bipolar disorder

First line: lithium monotherapy
Second line: olanzapine, aripiprazole, risperidone or quetiapine in combination with valproate* or lithium
Third line: alternative antipsychotic (lurasidone, asenapine or ziprasidone) or alternative mood stabiliser (carbamazepine or lamotrigine) in combination
Fourth line: antipsychotic with two mood stabilisers

- Always maintain successful acute treatment regimens (e.g. mood stabiliser + antipsychotic) as prophylaxis
- Avoid long-term antidepressants if possible

*Not in women of child-bearing potential.

Table 2.12 Summary of maintenance in bipolar disorder.[7,57]

	Prevents mania	Prevents depression
Monotherapy		
Antipsychotics		
Aripiprazole	Yes	No
Asenapine	Yes	No
Olanzapine	Yes	Yes
Paliperidone	Yes	No
Risperidone	Yes	No
Quetiapine	Yes	Yes
Mood stabilisers (MS)		
Lamotrigine	No	Yes
Lithium	Yes	Yes
Valproate	Yes (?)	Yes
Antidepressants	No	No
Combination treatment		
Antipsychotic + MS	Yes	Yes
Valproate + lamotrigine	Yes (?)	Yes

References

1. Malhi GS, et al. The 2020 Royal Australian and New Zealand College of Psychiatrists Clinical Practice Guidelines for Mood Disorders: bipolar disorder summary. *Bipolar Disord* 2020; 22:805–821.

2. Yatham LN, et al. Canadian Network for Mood and Anxiety Treatments (CANMAT) and International Society for Bipolar Disorders (ISBD) 2018 guidelines for the management of patients with bipolar disorder. *Bipolar Disord* 2018; 20:97–170.

3. Kang MG, et al. Lithium vs valproate in the maintenance treatment of bipolar I disorder: a post-hoc analysis of a randomized double-blind placebo-controlled trial. *Aust NZ J Psychiatry* 2020; 54:298–307.

4. Solomon DA, et al. Longitudinal course of bipolar I disorder: duration of mood episodes. *Arch Gen Psychiatry* 2010; 67:339–347.

5. Perlis RH, et al. Predictors of recurrence in bipolar disorder: primary outcomes from the Systematic Treatment Enhancement Program for Bipolar Disorder (STEP-BD). *Am J Psychiatry* 2006; 163:217–224.

6. Goodwin GM, et al. Evidence-based guidelines for treating bipolar disorder: revised third edition recommendations from the British Association for Psychopharmacology. *J Psychopharmacol* 2016; 30:495–553.

7. Nestsiarovich A, et al. Preventing new episodes of bipolar disorder in adults: systematic review and meta-analysis of randomized controlled trials. *Eur Neuropsychopharmacol* 2022; 54:75–89.

8. Sani G, et al. Treatment of bipolar disorder in a lifetime perspective: is lithium still the best choice? *Clin Drug Investig* 2017; 37:713–727.

9. Hartong EG, et al. Prophylactic efficacy of lithium versus carbamazepine in treatment-naive bipolar patients. *J Clin Psychiatry* 2003; 64:144–151.

10. Cipriani A, et al. Valproic acid, valproate and divalproex in the maintenance treatment of bipolar disorder. *Cochrane Database Syst Rev* 2013; 10:CD003196.

11. Geddes JR, et al. Lithium plus valproate combination therapy versus monotherapy for relapse prevention in bipolar I disorder (BALANCE): a randomised open-label trial. *Lancet* 2010; 375:385–395.

12. Kemp DE, et al. A 6-month, double-blind, maintenance trial of lithium monotherapy versus the combination of lithium and divalproex for rapid-cycling bipolar disorder and co-occurring substance abuse or dependence. *J Clin Psychiatry* 2009; 70:113–121.

13. Smith LA, et al. Effectiveness of mood stabilizers and antipsychotics in the maintenance phase of bipolar disorder: a systematic review of randomized controlled trials. *Bipolar Disord* 2007; 9:394–412.

14. Cipriani A, et al. Lithium in the prevention of suicidal behavior and all-cause mortality in patients with mood disorders: a systematic review of randomized trials. *Am J Psychiatry* 2005; 162:1805–1819.

15. Kessing LV, et al. Suicide risk in patients treated with lithium. *Arch Gen Psychiatry* 2005; 62:860–866.

16. Song J, et al. Suicidal behavior during lithium and valproate treatment: a within-individual 8-year prospective study of 50,000 patients with bipolar disorder. *Am J Psychiatry* 2017; 174:795–802.

17. Mander AJ, et al. Rapid recurrence of mania following abrupt discontinuation of lithium. *Lancet* 1988; 2:15–17.

18. Faedda GL, et al. Outcome after rapid vs gradual discontinuation of lithium treatment in bipolar disorders. *Arch Gen Psychiatry* 1993; 50:448–455.

19. Macritchie KA, et al. Does 'rebound mania' occur after stopping carbamazepine? A pilot study. *J Psychopharmacol* 2000; 14:266–268.

20. Franks MA, et al. Bouncing back: is the bipolar rebound phenomenon peculiar to lithium? A retrospective naturalistic study. *J Psychopharmacol* 2008; 22:452–456.

21. Kessing LV, et al. Starting lithium prophylaxis early v. late in bipolar disorder. *Br J Psychiatry* 2014; 205:214–220.

22. Kessing LV, et al. Valproate v. lithium in the treatment of bipolar disorder in clinical practice: observational nationwide register-based cohort study. *Br J Psychiatry* 2011; 199:57–63.

23. Gao K, et al. Typical and atypical antipsychotics in bipolar depression. *J Clin Psychiatry* 2005; 66:1376–1385.

24. Hellewell JS. A review of the evidence for the use of antipsychotics in the maintenance treatment of bipolar disorders. *J Psychopharmacol* 2006; 20:39–45.

25. Gigante AD, et al. Long-acting injectable antipsychotics for the maintenance treatment of bipolar disorder. *CNS Drugs* 2012; 26:403–420.

26. Tohen M, et al. Olanzapine versus divalproex sodium for the treatment of acute mania and maintenance of remission: a 47-week study. *Am J Psychiatry* 2003; 160:1263–1271.

27. National Institute for Health and Care Excellence. Bipolar disorder: assessment and management. Clinical guideline [CG185]. 2014 (last updated December 2023, last accessed October 2024); https://www.nice.org.uk/guidance/cg185.

28. Vieta E, et al. Efficacy and safety of quetiapine in combination with lithium or divalproex for maintenance of patients with bipolar I disorder (international trial 126). *J Affect Disord* 2008; 109:251–263.

29. McIntyre RS. Aripiprazole for the maintenance treatment of bipolar I disorder: a review. *Clin Ther* 2010; 32 Suppl 1:S32–S38.

30. Ghaemi SN, et al. Long-term risperidone treatment in bipolar disorder: 6-month follow up. *Int Clin Psychopharmacol* 1997; 12:333–338.

31. Szegedi A, et al. Randomized, double-blind, placebo-controlled trial of asenapine maintenance therapy in adults with an acute manic or mixed episode associated with bipolar I disorder. *Am J Psychiatry* 2017; 175:71–79.

32. Bowden CL, et al. Efficacy of valproate versus lithium in mania or mixed mania: a randomized, open 12-week trial. *Int Clin Psychopharmacol* 2010; 25:60–67.

33. Calabrese JR, et al. Lurasidone in combination with lithium or valproate for the maintenance treatment of bipolar I disorder. *Eur Neuropsychopharmacol* 2017; 27:865–876.

34. McIntyre RS, et al. The efficacy of lumateperone in patients with bipolar depression with mixed features. *J Clin Psychiatry* 2023; 84:22m14739.

35. McIntyre RS, et al. Cariprazine as a maintenance therapy in the prevention of mood episodes in adults with bipolar I disorder. *Bipolar Disord* 2024; 26:442–453.

36. Kishi T, et al. Mood stabilizers and/or antipsychotics for bipolar disorder in the maintenance phase: a systematic review and network meta-analysis of randomized controlled trials. *Mol Psychiatry* 2021; 26:4146–4157.

37. Escudero MAG, et al. Second generation antipsychotics monotherapy as maintenance treatment for bipolar disorder: a systematic review of long-term studies. *Psychiatr Q* 2020; 91:1047–1060.

38. Calabrese JR, et al. Efficacy and safety of aripiprazole once-monthly in the maintenance treatment of bipolar I disorder: a double-blind, placebo-controlled, 52-week randomized withdrawal study. *J Clin Psychiatry* 2017; **78**:324–331.

39. Kishi T, et al. Long-acting injectable antipsychotics for prevention of relapse in bipolar disorder: a systematic review and meta-analyses of randomized controlled trials. *Int J Neuropsychopharmacol* 2016; **19**:pyw038.

40. Hsieh MH, et al. Bipolar patients treated with long-acting injectable risperidone in Taiwan: a 1-year mirror-image study using a national claims database. *J Affect Disord* 2017; **218**:327–334.

41. Belge JB, et al. Long-acting second-generation injectable antipsychotics for the maintenance treatment of bipolar disorder: a narrative review. *Expert Opin Pharmacother* 2024; **25**:295–299.

42. Kishi T, et al. A comparison of recurrence rates after discontinuation of second-generation antipsychotic long-acting injectable versus corresponding oral antipsychotic in the maintenance treatment of bipolar disorder: a systematic review. *Psychiatry Res* 2024; **333**:115761.

43. Pacchiarotti I, et al. Long-acting injectable antipsychotics (LAIs) for maintenance treatment of bipolar and schizoaffective disorders: a systematic review. *Eur Neuropsychopharmacol* 2019; **29**:457–470.

44. Yıldızhan E, et al. Effect of long acting injectable antipsychotics on course and hospitalizations in bipolar disorder – a naturalistic mirror image study. *Nord J Psychiatry* 2022; **76**:37–43.

45. Nolen WA, et al. What is the optimal serum level for lithium in the maintenance treatment of bipolar disorder? A systematic review and recommendations from the ISBD/IGSLI Task Force on treatment with lithium. *Bipolar Disord* 2019; **21**:394–409.

46. Freeman MP, et al. Mood stabilizer combinations: a review of safety and efficacy. *Am J Psychiatry* 1998; **155**:12–21.

47. Muzina DJ, et al. Maintenance therapies in bipolar disorder: focus on randomized controlled trials. *Aust NZ J Psychiatry* 2005; **39**:652–661.

48. Tohen M, et al. Relapse prevention in bipolar I disorder: 18-month comparison of olanzapine plus mood stabiliser v. mood stabiliser alone. *Br J Psychiatry* 2004; **184**:337–345.

49. Paton C, et al. Lithium in bipolar and other affective disorders: prescribing practice in the UK. *J Psychopharmacol* 2010; **24**:1739–1746.

50. Marcus R, et al. Efficacy of aripiprazole adjunctive to lithium or valproate in the long-term treatment of patients with bipolar I disorder with an inadequate response to lithium or valproate monotherapy: a multicenter, double-blind, randomized study. *Bipolar Disord* 2011; **13**:133–144.

51. Bowden CL, et al. A placebo-controlled 18-month trial of lamotrigine and lithium maintenance treatment in recently manic or hypomanic patients with bipolar I disorder. *Arch Gen Psychiatry* 2003; **60**:392–400.

52. Pikalov A, et al. Long-term use of lurasidone in patients with bipolar disorder: safety and effectiveness over 2 years of treatment. *Int J Bipolar Disord* 2017; **5**:9.

53. Wingård L, et al. Monotherapy vs. combination therapy for post mania maintenance treatment: a population based cohort study. *Eur Neuropsychopharmacol* 2019; **29**:691–700.

54. Jauhar S, et al. Controversies in bipolar disorder; role of second-generation antipsychotic for maintenance therapy. *Int J Bipolar Disord* 2019; **7**:10.

55. Ghaemi SN, et al. Long-term antidepressant treatment in bipolar disorder: meta-analyses of benefits and risks. *Acta Psychiatr Scand* 2008; **118**:347–356.

56. Ghaemi SN, et al. Antidepressant discontinuation in bipolar depression: a Systematic Treatment Enhancement Program for Bipolar Disorder (STEP-BD) randomized clinical trial of long-term effectiveness and safety. *J Clin Psychiatry* 2010; **71**:372–380.

57. Yatham LN, et al. Duration of adjunctive antidepressant maintenance in bipolar I depression. *N Engl J Med* 2023; **389**:430–440.

Stopping lithium and mood stabilisers

Rationale for stopping

Patients may ask to stop lithium and other mood stabilisers because of the range of adverse effects experienced. In one cohort 54% of patients discontinued lithium, mostly because of tolerability problems, including diarrhoea (13%), tremor (11%), polyuria/polydipsia/diabetes insipidus (9%), creatinine increase (9%) and weight gain (7%).[1] Alternatively, although lithium and mood stabilisers are useful in controlling acute symptoms and in preventing relapse, a clinician may judge that the balance of risks and benefits has shifted over time (e.g. adverse physical effects accumulate, alternative coping strategies developed) such that dose reduction or stopping may be considered. Other patients may be prescribed mood stabilisers for conditions such as personality disorders, for which there is a lack of evidence. Stopping should be done in a manner that minimises the risk of both withdrawal effects and relapse (the two key risks).

Withdrawal effects from lithium and other mood stabilisers

Discontinuation of lithium can cause withdrawal effects, including both physical and psychological symptoms (Table 2.13). These withdrawal effects include mood episodes (depression, but more commonly mania) and are sometimes called 'rebound' effects.[2,3] The risk of relapse in the period following abrupt cessation greatly exceeds the rate of relapse in the untreated disorder.[2] For example, a review of studies of lithium discontinuation in people with bipolar disorder found that the untreated disorder had a mean cycle length (the average time between episodes) of 11.6 months, whereas the time to a new episode following lithium discontinuation was 1.7 months.[2] This represents a sevenfold increase in the rate of relapse and suggests that manic and depressive symptoms that occur following lithium withdrawal are largely because of lithium withdrawal effects rather than because of the untreated disorder. Nonetheless, it is to be expected that the withdrawal of an effective mood stabiliser leads to mood destabilisation simply because of the removal of an effective treatment for the condition. Relapse may sometimes indicate the need for continued treatment. Distinguishing between withdrawal-related rebound and true relapse of the underlying condition is made easier by extending the withdrawal period (so as to help rule out withdrawal effects).

Table 2.13 Withdrawal effects of lithium.[3-5]

Physical effects	Psychological effects
Tremor	Anxiety
Polyuria	Nervousness
Muscular weakness	Irritability
Polydipsia	Alertness
Dryness of mouth	Sleep disturbances
	Elated mood/mania
	Depressed mood

Withdrawal effects are thought to be due to the development of dopaminergic hypersensitivity[6] and changes in neuronal membranes, cell transport function or other neurotransmitter systems during lithium treatment.[7] Other mood stabilisers have also been associated with a withdrawal syndrome.[8]

Evidence for long-term treatment

Although lithium is accepted as the first-line choice for prophylaxis in bipolar disorder,[9] evidence for long-term treatment with lithium and other mood stabilisers is derived from discontinuation studies where patients established on these medications were randomised to either continue or cease treatment.[10,11] In these studies, lithium was sometimes stopped abruptly. As mentioned, rapid stopping of lithium is likely to produce withdrawal effects, which can include precipitating mood episodes.[2] Indeed, in one study abruptly stopping lithium in patients with depression provoked manic episodes in 13%.[12]

There is evidence that abrupt cessation of other mood stabilisers can also precipitate mood episodes.[3] Patients who are discontinued from these medications often demonstrate relapse rates that are greater than in the untreated disorder, suggesting that withdrawal effects may inflate the apparent rate and extent of relapse.[2,13]

Few maintenance studies extend beyond a 2-year follow-up period. Observational studies (over longer periods) have found lithium to be more effective than other mood stabilisers but these studies are somewhat limited by confounding effects.[14]

Duration of tapering

With lithium, rapid discontinuation (1–14 days) has been shown to produce a much greater risk of relapse than gradual tapering over 15–30 days.[15-17] Time to relapse is decreased and the proportion of patients relapsed at study end is greatly increased in the rapid discontinuation group. These robust and reproducible findings support a recommendation that lithium should not be stopped abruptly unless a serious adverse effect occurs, and that withdrawal should take place over at least a month or preferably longer.

There are few studies examining the optimal rate or duration of tapering lithium. However, the finding that 50% of relapses occur in the first 3 months after lithium is stopped but then lessen over time[2] suggests that this period of 3 months might be required for underlying adaptations to lithium to resolve. One study that discontinued lithium over 2–5 months found higher relapse rates in these patients than in those who stayed on lithium.[18] This might conceivably suggest that tapering should be even slower than the 4-week to 3-month period suggested by NICE in the UK.[19]

Long withdrawal schedules are not unusual in different areas of medicine. Antiseizure drugs are tapered over between 1 month and 4 years in non-psychiatric conditions, with relapse rates increased in the first 6 months before converging with patients continuing with the antiseizure drugs.[8]

Pattern of tapering

Lithium, like all pharmacological agents, conforms to the law of mass action and therefore demonstrates a hyperbolic pattern between dose and pharmacological effect.[12] The mode of action of lithium is unknown, however it is known to affect GSK-3. The relationship between the dose of lithium and effect on this target is hyperbolic.[13] As for other psychotropic agents this justifies a hyperbolically reducing dose pattern (in order to produce linearly reducing effects on its target receptors), which may be clinically approximated by a proportionate dose reduction (a reduction by the same proportion each step, so that the size of the reduction becomes smaller and smaller as the total dose gets lower) (Box 2.3).

> **Box 2.3** Suggested slow reduction regimen for lithium
>
> ■ Reduce by 200mg every month until dose is 800mg daily, *then*
> ■ Reduce by 100mg every month until dose is 400mg daily, *then*
> ■ Reduce by 50mg every month until dose is 100mg daily, *then*
> ■ Reduce by 25mg every month until completely stopped

Practice guide to tapering

■ Patients should be told that there is the possibility of withdrawal effects, and that there may be an increased risk of affective relapse from stopping lithium or mood stabilisers more quickly. These effects will be reduced if these medications are reduced in a more gradual fashion.

■ There is no clear evidence on how to taper (or for how long), but following principles from other psychotropic medications, an initial reduction of 10–25% of the current dose should be offered, with withdrawal symptoms (Table 2.13) and symptoms monitored for at least 4 weeks to ensure stability.

■ Further reductions should be titrated against the tolerability of this dose decrease. Reductions should probably be made according to an exponentially reducing pattern, whereby each reduction is calculated as a fixed proportion (e.g. 10% or 25%) of the **most recent** dose (effectively becoming smaller and smaller as the total dose becomes lower) each month, or until stability is assured.

■ For a very few patients the final dose before completely stopping may be very small, because small doses have relatively large effects on target receptors. This may be as small as 1% of therapeutic doses, for example <10mg for lithium. To achieve small doses, liquid preparations (lithium) will be required.

■ As the process of reducing lithium or mood stabilisers might be destabilising it may be wise to pursue other strategies during the tapering period.[20] Ongoing monitoring may be necessary for a number of months after complete cessation to ensure mood stability.

■ If withdrawal symptoms or symptoms of relapse emerge at any point, pausing the reduction, a small increase in dose or returning to a previously effective dose are all possible responses. Difficulty reducing medication does not preclude a further attempt at reduction but might indicate the need for a more gradual reduction regimen.

■ Other modalities for people with bipolar disorder, including family therapy, interpersonal therapy, cognitive behavioural therapy, psychoeducation and social rhythm therapy, may be considered as well as more individualised, idiosyncratic coping strategies.[21–23]

References

1. Öhlund L, et al. Reasons for lithium discontinuation in men and women with bipolar disorder: a retrospective cohort study. *BMC Psychiatry* 2018; 18:37.
2. Suppes T, et al. Risk of recurrence following discontinuation of lithium treatment in bipolar disorder. *Arch Gen Psychiatry* 1991; 48:1082–1088.
3. Franks MA, et al. Bouncing back: is the bipolar rebound phenomenon peculiar to lithium? A retrospective naturalistic study. *J Psychopharmacol* 2008; 22:452–456.
4. Baastrup PC, et al. Prophylactic lithium: double blind discontinuation in manic-depressive and recurrent-depressive disorders. *Lancet* 1970; 2:326–330.

5. Klein E, et al. Discontinuation of lithium treatment in remitted bipolar patients: relationship between clinical outcome and changes in sleep-wake cycles. *J Nerv Ment Dis* 1991; **179**:499–501.

6. Ferrie L, et al. Effect of chronic lithium and withdrawal from chronic lithium on presynaptic dopamine function in the rat. *J Psychopharmacol* 2005; **19**:229–234.

7. Balon R, et al. Lithium discontinuation: withdrawal or relapse? *Compr Psychiatry* 1988; **29**:330–334.

8. Vernachio K, et al. A review of withdraw strategies for discontinuing antiepileptic therapy in epilepsy and pain management. *Pharm Pharmacol Int J* 2015; **3**:232–235.

9. Nolen WA, et al. What is the optimal serum level for lithium in the maintenance treatment of bipolar disorder? A systematic review and recommendations from the ISBD/IGSLI Task Force on treatment with lithium. *Bipolar Disord* 2019; **21**:394–409.

10. Geddes JR, et al. Long-term lithium therapy for bipolar disorder: systematic review and meta-analysis of randomized controlled trials. *Am J Psychiatry* 2004; **161**:217–222.

11. Moncrieff J. Lithium: evidence reconsidered. *Br J Psychiatry* 1997; **171**:113–119.

12. Faedda GL, et al. Lithium discontinuation: uncovering latent bipolar disorder? *Am J Psychiatry* 2001; **158**:1337–1339.

13. Goodwin GM. Recurrence of mania after lithium withdrawal. Implications for the use of lithium in the treatment of bipolar affective disorder. *Br J Psychiatry* 1994; **164**:149–152.

14. Kessing LV, et al. Effectiveness of maintenance therapy of lithium vs other mood stabilizers in monotherapy and in combinations: a systematic review of evidence from observational studies. *Bipolar Disord* 2018; **20**:419–431.

15. Faedda GL, et al. Outcome after rapid vs gradual discontinuation of lithium treatment in bipolar disorders. *Arch Gen Psychiatry* 1993; **50**:448–455.

16. Baldessarini RJ, et al. Illness risk following rapid versus gradual discontinuation of antidepressants. *Am J Psychiatry* 2010; **167**:934–941.

17. Baldessarini RJ, et al. Effects of the rate of discontinuing lithium maintenance treatment in bipolar disorders. *J Clin Psychiatry* 1996; **57**:441–448.

18. Biel MG, et al. Continuation versus discontinuation of lithium in recurrent bipolar illness: a naturalistic study. *Bipolar Disord* 2007; **9**:435–442.

19. National Institute for Health and Care Excellence. Bipolar disorder: assessment and management. Clinical guideline [CG185]. 2014 (last updated December 2023, last checked July 2024); https://www.nice.org.uk/guidance/cg185.

20. Guy. A, et al. *Guidance for Psychological Therapists: Enabling Conversations with Clients Taking or Withdrawing from Prescribed Psychiatric Drugs*. London: APPG for Prescribed Drug Dependence, 2019.

21. Reinares M, et al. Psychosocial interventions in bipolar disorder: what, for whom, and when. *J Affect Disord* 2014; **156**:46–55.

22. Cappleman R, et al. Managing bipolar moods without medication: a qualitative investigation. *J Affect Disord* 2015; **174**:241–249.

23. Miklowitz DJ. Adjunctive psychotherapy for bipolar disorder: state of the evidence. *Am J Psychiatry* 2008; **165**:1408–1419.

Chapter 3

Depression and anxiety disorders

Introduction to depression

Depression (major depressive disorder, MDD) is widely recognised as a major public health problem around the world. The mainstay of treatment is the prescription of antidepressants, although psychological treatments have a place as a first-line alternative to antidepressants in milder and moderate forms of depression.[1] Other methods of treating depression (vagal nerve stimulation [VNS],[2] repetitive transcranial magnetic stimulation [rTMS],[3,4] transcranial direct current stimulation,[3] etc.) are also used but are not widely available.

The basic principles of prescribing are described in Table 3.1, together with a summary of National Institute for Health and Care Excellence (NICE) guidance.

Table 3.1 Basic principles of prescribing in depression.

- Discuss with the patient choice of drug and utility/availability of other, non-pharmacological treatments.
- Discuss with the patient likely outcomes, such as gradual relief from depressive symptoms over several weeks.
- Prescribe a dose of antidepressant (after titration, if necessary) that is likely to be effective.
- Assess the treatment's efficacy within 2–4 weeks of initiation (sooner in young people).
- Monitor treatment adherence and inform the patient about the risk of withdrawal symptoms.
- Monitor for adverse effects.
- For a single episode, continue treatment for at least 6 months after resolution of symptoms. Multiple episodes or high-risk patients may require longer; continuing treatment may reduce the risk of relapse.
- For patients continuing treatment, review treatment every 6 months.
- Withdraw antidepressants very gradually; always inform patients of the risk, duration and nature of discontinuation symptoms.

The Maudsley® Prescribing Guidelines in Psychiatry, Fifteenth Edition. David M. Taylor, Thomas R. E. Barnes and Allan H. Young.
© 2025 David M. Taylor. Published 2025 by John Wiley & Sons Ltd.

Official guidance on the treatment of depression: a summary of the NICE guidelines[1]

- Depression severity is categorised as less severe (includes subthreshold and mild depression) and more severe (includes moderate to severe depression). The severity of depression is determined by the combined influence of factors such as symptom severity, duration and the impact on personal and social functioning.
- Antidepressants are not recommended as a first-line treatment in less severe depression. Other options such as counselling, guided self-help, cognitive behavioural therapy (CBT), behavioural activation, mindfulness, meditation, short-term psychodynamic psychotherapy, interpersonal psychotherapy or exercise are preferred.
- Antidepressants are recommended for the treatment of more severe depression and for dysthymia.
- When an antidepressant is prescribed, a generic selective serotonin reuptake inhibitor (SSRI) is recommended.
- All patients should be informed about the withdrawal (discontinuation) effects of antidepressants and how they can be minimised or avoided.
- For treatment-resistant depression, recommended strategies include implanted VNS, augmentation with lithium or an antipsychotic, or the addition of a second antidepressant (see section in this chapter).
- Patients with a recurrent episode or at high risk should be treated for at least 2 years.
- The use of electroconvulsive therapy (ECT) is supported for severe and treatment-resistant depression if patient prefers it and has responded in the past or when a rapid response is needed.

Nasal esketamine is a licensed treatment for treatment-resistant MDD,[5] but is not yet approved by NICE in the UK. It is widely used elsewhere.

This chapter concentrates on the use of antidepressants and offers advice on drug choice, dosing, switching strategies and sequencing of treatments. The near exclusion of other non-drug treatment modalities does not imply any lack of confidence in their efficacy but simply reflects the need (in a prescribing guideline) to concentrate on medicines-related subjects.

References

1. National Institute for Health and Care Excellence. Depression in adults: treatment and management. NICE guideline [NG222]. 2022 (last updated May 2024, last checked May 2024); https://www.nice.org.uk/guidance/ng222.
2. George MS, et al. Vagus nerve stimulation for the treatment of depression and other neuropsychiatric disorders. *Expert Rev Neurother* 2007; 7:63–74.
3. Hsu CW, et al. Comparing different non-invasive brain stimulation interventions for bipolar depression treatment: a network meta-analysis of randomized controlled trials. *Neurosci Biobehav Rev* 2024; 156:105483.
4. Loo CK, et al. A review of the efficacy of transcranial magnetic stimulation (TMS) treatment for depression, and current and future strategies to optimize efficacy. *J Affect Disord* 2005; 88:255–267.
5. Janssen-Cilag Ltd. Summary of Product Characteristics. Spravato 28 mg nasal spray, solution (esketamine hydrochloride). 2024 (last checked May 2024); https://www.medicines.org.uk/emc/product/10977/smpc.

Antidepressants – general overview

Effectiveness

All antidepressants are more efficacious than placebo in adults with MDD[1] and there is broadly equal benefit from antidepressant treatments for mild, moderate or severe major depression.[2]

Antidepressants are normally recommended as first-line treatment in patients whose depression is of at least moderate severity, with psychological treatments being used for milder forms. Of the moderate to severe patient group, approximately 20% will recover with no treatment at all, 30% will respond to placebo and 50% will respond to antidepressant drug treatment.[3] This gives a number needed to treat (NNT) of 3 for antidepressant over true no-treatment control and an NNT of 5 for antidepressant over placebo. Response in clinical trials is generally defined by a particular percentage reduction in depression rating scale scores (e.g. 50%), a somewhat arbitrary dichotomy. Change measured using individual scale score tends to show a relatively small mean difference between active treatment and placebo (which itself is an effective treatment for depression).

Drug–placebo differences may have diminished over time because of methodological changes.[4] However, it is possible that rating scales obscure the beneficial effects of antidepressants to some extent. Hieronymus and colleagues[5] undertook patient-level post-hoc analyses of 18 industry-sponsored placebo-controlled trials of paroxetine, citalopram, sertraline or fluoxetine, including in total 6,669 adults with major depression. The aim was to assess what the outcome would have been if the single item 'depressed mood' (rated 0–4) had been used as the sole measure of efficacy. While 18 of 32 comparisons (56%) failed to separate active drug from placebo with respect to reduction in total Hamilton Depression Rating Scale (HAM-D) score, only 3 of 32 comparisons (9%) were negative when depressed mood was used as the sole effect parameter (i.e. 91% of trials favoured the antidepressant). It is also noteworthy that even using total scale scores, placebo never performs better than an active treatment – antidepressants are always shown to be better than or the same as placebo, never worse than. This is arguably the most compelling evidence for the efficacy of antidepressants.

As might be expected, network meta-analyses show robust superiority for antidepressants over placebo, with amitriptyline being the most efficacious.[1] In the same study, mirtazapine was ranked as the second most efficacious antidepressant. However, in a post-hoc analysis, the observed superiority of mirtazapine was found to be attributable to its effects on sleep and appetite, and the absence of gastrointestinal (GI) symptoms. In contrast, when it came to improving depressed mood, suicidality and psychic anxiety, SSRIs and venlafaxine demonstrated relatively greater efficacy.[6] In a 2023 network meta-analysis of people with depression and a wide range of chronic medical conditions, antidepressants more effectively reduced depressive symptoms than placebo.[7]

The 2019 PANDA trial results support the prescription of SSRI antidepressants in a wider group of participants than previously thought, including those with mild to moderate symptoms who do not meet diagnostic criteria for depression or generalised anxiety disorder.[8] Antidepressant treatment seems to only modestly improve quality of life and social functioning in individuals with major depression.[9,10]

Onset of action

It is widely believed that antidepressants do not exert their effects for 2–4 weeks, or even longer. This is a myth. All antidepressants show a pattern of response where the rate of improvement is highest during weeks 1 and 2 and lowest during weeks 4 to 6. Early response strongly predicts later remission.[11] Statistical separation from placebo is seen at 2–4 weeks in individual trials (hence the idea of a lag period of no effect) but after only 1 or 2 weeks in (statistically more powerful) meta-analyses.[12,13] Thus, where large numbers of patients are treated and detailed rating scales are used, an antidepressant effect is usually statistically evident at 1 week. In clinical practice using simple observations, an antidepressant effect in an individual is usually seen by 2 weeks.[14] In individuals where no antidepressant effect is evident after 2–3 weeks of treatment, a change in dose or drug should be considered. It is important, however, to be clear about what constitutes 'no effect'. Different patterns of response have been identified,[15] and in some individuals response is slow to emerge. However, in those ultimately responsive to treatment, all will very probably have begun to show at least minor improvement at 3–4 weeks. Thus, those showing no discernible improvement at this time will likely never respond to the prescribed drug at that dose. In contrast, those showing small improvements at 3–4 weeks (i.e. improvement not necessarily meeting criteria for 'response' but observable nonetheless) may go on to respond fully.[16] A meta-analysis[17] has shown that if antidepressant (citalopram, paroxetine or sertraline specifically) trials are examined for effects on depressed mood alone (rather than the total HAM-D score) then both a rapid effect and a dose–response relationship (as already noted) are clearly evident.

Choice of antidepressant and relative adverse effects

Selective serotonin reuptake inhibitors are well tolerated compared with older tricyclic antidepressants (TCAs) and monoamine oxidase inhibitors (MAOIs), and are universally recommended as first-line pharmacological treatment for depression.[18] There is a suggestion from network meta-analyses[1,19] that some individual antidepressants may be more effective overall than others but this has not been consistently demonstrated in head-to-head studies. Adverse effect profiles of antidepressants do differ. For example, paroxetine has been associated with more weight gain and a higher incidence of sexual dysfunction, and sertraline with a higher incidence of diarrhoea than other SSRIs.[20] Dual reuptake inhibitors such as venlafaxine and duloxetine tend to be tolerated less well than SSRIs but better than TCAs. With all drugs there is marked inter-individual variation in tolerability, which is not easily predicted by knowledge of a drug's likely adverse effects. A flexible approach is usually required in finding the right drug for a particular patient. The Psymatik Treatment Optimizer may be helpful.[21]

As well as headache and GI symptoms, SSRIs as a class are associated with a range of other adverse effects including sexual dysfunction (see relevant section in this chapter), hyponatraemia (see section on antidepressant-induced hyponatraemia in this chapter) and GI bleeds (see section on SSRIs and bleeding in this chapter). TCAs have a number of adverse cardiovascular effects (hypotension, tachycardia and QTc prolongation) and are particularly toxic in overdose[22] (see section on overdose in Chapter 13). The now rarely used MAOIs have the potential to interact with tyramine-containing foods to cause hypertensive crisis and much more commonly cause hypotension. All antidepressant drugs can cause discontinuation symptoms, with short half-life drugs probably being most problematic in this respect (see section on stopping antidepressants in this chapter). See following pages for a summary of the clinically relevant adverse effects of available antidepressant drugs.

Drug interactions

Some SSRIs are potent inhibitors of individual or multiple hepatic cytochrome P450 (CYP) pathways and the magnitude of these effects is dose related. Several clinically significant drug interactions can therefore be predicted. For example, fluvoxamine is a potent inhibitor of CYP1A2 which can result in increased theophylline serum levels, fluoxetine is a potent inhibitor of CYP2D6, which can result in increased seizure risk with clozapine, and paroxetine is a potent inhibitor of CYP2D6, which can result in treatment failure with tamoxifen (a pro-drug) leading to increased mortality.[23]

Antidepressants can also cause pharmacodynamic interactions. For example, the cardiotoxicity of TCAs may be exacerbated by drugs such as diuretics, which can cause electrolyte disturbances. A summary of clinically relevant drug interactions with antidepressants can be found later in this chapter.

Potential pharmacokinetic and pharmacodynamic interactions between antidepressants must be considered when switching from one antidepressant to another (see section on switching antidepressants in this chapter).

Suicidality

Antidepressant treatment has been associated with an increased risk of suicidal thoughts and acts, particularly in adolescents and young adults,[24–27] leading to the recommendation that patients should be warned of this potential adverse effect during the early weeks of treatment and know how to seek help if required. Suicide and self-harm rates tend to be higher when antidepressants are started or stopped so the same care over risk assessment should be carried out when treatment is stopped as when it is started.[28] Furthermore, switching antidepressants may be a marker of increased risk of suicidal behaviours in those who initiate antidepressant treatment aged 75 years and over.[29]

All antidepressants have been implicated,[30] including those that are marketed for an indication other than depression (e.g. atomoxetine). Although the relative risk may be elevated above placebo rates in some patient groups, the absolute risk remains very small. The most effective way to treat or prevent suicidal thoughts and acts is to treat depression[31–33] and antidepressant drugs are the most effective treatment currently available.[3,34] For the most part, suicidality is greatly reduced by the use of antidepressants.[35–37] However, those who experience treatment-emergent or worsening suicidal ideation with one antidepressant may be more likely to have a similar experience with subsequent treatments.[38] Some data suggest that an increasing proportion of young women who later committed suicide had been treated with antidepressants in the last few years before and at the time of their suicide.[39] At the time of writing there is no clear consensus on the potential dangers of antidepressants except that young people are most at risk.[40] Ketamine, in its various forms, may have rapidly apparent anti-suicidal effects.[41]

CHAPTER 3

Toxicity in overdose varies both between and within groups of antidepressants[42] (see section on psychotropics in overdose in Chapter 13).

Duration of treatment

Antidepressants relieve the symptoms of depression but do not treat the underlying cause. A reasonable amount of evidence suggests that they should be taken for 6–9 months after recovery from a single episode (presumably to cover the duration of an untreated episode). In those patients who have had several episodes, there is evidence of benefit from maintenance treatment for at least 2 years, but no upper duration of treatment has been identified (see section on antidepressant prophylaxis in this chapter). Beyond 2 years, continued treatment offers some benefits, but many people can safely stop at this point.[43] There are few data on which to base recommendations about the duration of treatment of augmentation regimens. A minority view is that antidepressants worsen outcome in the long term.[44]

Next-step treatments

Approximately one-third of patients do not respond to the first antidepressant that is prescribed. Options in this group include dose escalation, switching to a different drug and several augmentation strategies. A small proportion of non-responders will respond with each treatment change, but effect sizes are modest and there is no clear difference in effectiveness between strategies (see sections on the management of treatment-resistant depression in this chapter).

Use of antidepressants in anxiety spectrum disorders

Antidepressants are first-line treatments in a number of anxiety spectrum disorders (see section on anxiety spectrum disorders in this chapter).

References

1. Cipriani A, et al. Comparative efficacy and acceptability of 21 antidepressant drugs for the acute treatment of adults with major depressive disorder: a systematic review and network meta-analysis. *Lancet* 2018; **391**:1357–1366.
2. Furukawa TA, et al. Initial severity of major depression and efficacy of new generation antidepressants: individual participant data meta–analysis. *Acta Psychiatr Scand* 2018; **137**:450–458.
3. Anderson IM, et al. Evidence-based guidelines for treating depressive disorders with antidepressants: a revision of the 2000 British Association for Psychopharmacology guidelines. *J Psychopharmacol* 2008; **22**:343–396.
4. Khan A, et al. Why has the antidepressant–placebo difference in antidepressant clinical trials diminished over the past three decades? *CNS Neurosci Ther* 2010; **16**:217–226.
5. Hieronymus F, et al. Consistent superiority of selective serotonin reuptake inhibitors over placebo in reducing depressed mood in patients with major depression. *Mol Psychiatry* 2016; **21**:523–530.
6. Hieronymus F, et al. Impact of sedative and appetite-increasing properties on the apparent antidepressant efficacy of mirtazapine, selective serotonin reuptake inhibitors and amitriptyline: an item-based, patient-level meta-analysis. *eClinicalMedicine* 2024; **77**:102904.
7. Köhler-Forsberg O, et al. Efficacy and safety of antidepressants in patients with comorbid depression and medical diseases: an umbrella systematic review and meta–analysis. *JAMA Psychiatry* 2023; **80**:1196–1207.
8. Lewis G, et al. The clinical effectiveness of sertraline in primary care and the role of depression severity and duration (PANDA): a pragmatic, double-blind, placebo-controlled randomised trial. *Lancet Psychiatry* 2019; **6**:903–914.
9. Wiesinger T, et al. Antidepressants and quality of life in patients with major depressive disorder: systematic review and meta-analysis of double-blind, placebo-controlled RCTs. *Acta Psychiatr Scand* 2023; **147**:545–560.
10. Kremer S, et al. Antidepressants and social functioning in patients with major depressive disorder: systematic review and meta–analysis of double–blind, placebo–controlled RCTs. *Psychother Psychosom* 2023; **92**:304–314.

11. Dos Santos Fernandes F, et al. Rapid response to antidepressants and correlation with response and remission after acute treatment. *Journal of Affective Disorders Reports* 2024; **16**:100725.

12. Taylor MJ, et al. Early onset of selective serotonin reuptake inhibitor antidepressant action: systematic review and meta-analysis. *Arch Gen Psychiatry* 2006; **63**:1217–1223.

13. Papakostas GI, et al. A meta-analysis of early sustained response rates between antidepressants and placebo for the treatment of major depressive disorder. *J Clin Psychopharmacol* 2006; **26**:56–60.

14. Szegedi A, et al. Early improvement in the first 2 weeks as a predictor of treatment outcome in patients with major depressive disorder: a meta-analysis including 6562 patients. *J Clin Psychiatry* 2009; **70**:344–353.

15. Uher R, et al. Early and delayed onset of response to antidepressants in individual trajectories of change during treatment of major depression: a secondary analysis of data from the Genome-Based Therapeutic Drugs for Depression (GENDEP) study. *J Clin Psychiatry* 2011; **72**:1478–1484.

16. Posternak MA, et al. Response rates to fluoxetine in subjects who initially show no improvement. *J Clin Psychiatry* 2011; **72**:949–954.

17. Hieronymus F, et al. A mega-analysis of fixed-dose trials reveals dose-dependency and a rapid onset of action for the antidepressant effect of three selective serotonin reuptake inhibitors. *Transl Psychiatry* 2016; **6**:e834.

18. National Institute for Health and Care Excellence. Depression in adults: treatment and management. NICE Guideline [NG222]. 2022 (last reviewed September 2024, last checked November 2024); https://www.nice.org.uk/guidance/ng222.

19. Cipriani A, et al. Comparative efficacy and acceptability of 12 new-generation antidepressants: a multiple-treatments meta-analysis. *Lancet* 2009; **373**:746–758.

20. Gartlehner G, et al. Comparative benefits and harms of second-generation antidepressants: background paper for the American College of Physicians. *Ann Intern Med* 2008; **149**:734–750.

21. Pillinger T, et al. Antidepressant and antipsychotic side-effects and personalised prescribing: a systematic review and digital tool development. *Lancet Psychiatry* 2023; **10**:860–876.

22. Flanagan RJ. Fatal toxicity of drugs used in psychiatry. *Hum Psychopharmacol* 2008; **23** Suppl 1:43–51.

23. Kelly CM, et al. Selective serotonin reuptake inhibitors and breast cancer mortality in women receiving tamoxifen: a population based cohort study. *BMJ* 2010; **340**:c693.

24. Stone M, et al. Risk of suicidality in clinical trials of antidepressants in adults: analysis of proprietary data submitted to US Food and Drug Administration. *BMJ* 2009; **339**:b2880.

25. Carpenter DJ, et al. Meta-analysis of efficacy and treatment-emergent suicidality in adults by psychiatric indication and age subgroup following initiation of paroxetine therapy: a complete set of randomized placebo-controlled trials. *J Clin Psychiatry* 2011; **72**:1503–1514.

26. Barbui C, et al. Selective serotonin reuptake inhibitors and risk of suicide: a systematic review of observational studies. *CMAJ* 2009; **180**:291–297.

27. Umetsu R, et al. Association between selective serotonin reuptake inhibitor therapy and suicidality: analysis of U.S. Food and Drug Administration adverse event reporting system data. *Biol Pharm Bull* 2015; **38**:1689–1699.

28. Coupland C, et al. Antidepressant use and risk of suicide and attempted suicide or self harm in people aged 20 to 64: cohort study using a primary care database. *BMJ* 2015; **350**:h517.

29. Hedna K, et al. Antidepressants and suicidal behaviour in late life: a prospective population-based study of use patterns in new users aged 75 and above. *Eur J Clin Pharmacol* 2018; **74**:201–208.

30. Schneeweiss S, et al. Variation in the risk of suicide attempts and completed suicides by antidepressant agent in adults: a propensity score-adjusted analysis of 9 years' data. *Arch Gen Psychiatry* 2010; **67**:497–506.

31. Isacsson G, et al. The increased use of antidepressants has contributed to the worldwide reduction in suicide rates. *Br J Psychiatry* 2010; **196**:429–433.

32. Gibbons RD, et al. Suicidal thoughts and behavior with antidepressant treatment: reanalysis of the randomized placebo-controlled studies of fluoxetine and venlafaxine. *Arch Gen Psychiatry* 2012; **69**:580–587.

33. Lu CY, et al. Changes in antidepressant use by young people and suicidal behavior after FDA warnings and media coverage: quasi-experimental study. *BMJ* 2014; **348**:g3596.

34. Isacsson G, et al. Antidepressant medication prevents suicide in depression. *Acta Psychiatr Scand* 2010; **122**:454–460.

35. Simon GE, et al. Suicide risk during antidepressant treatment. *Am J Psychiatry* 2006; **163**:41–47.

36. Mulder RT, et al. Antidepressant treatment is associated with a reduction in suicidal ideation and suicide attempts. *Acta Psychiatr Scand* 2008; **118**:116–122.

37. Tondo L, et al. Suicidal status during antidepressant treatment in 789 Sardinian patients with major affective disorder. *Acta Psychiatr Scand* 2008; **118**:106–115.

38. Perlis RH, et al. Do suicidal thoughts or behaviors recur during a second antidepressant treatment trial? *J Clin Psychiatry* 2012; **73**:1439–1442.

39. Larsson J. Antidepressants and suicide among young women in Sweden 1999–2013. *Int J Risk Saf Med* 2017; **29**:101–106.

40. Spielmans GI, et al. Duty to warn: antidepressant black box suicidality warning is empirically justified. *Front Psychiatry* 2020; **11**:18.

41. Chen CC, et al. Acute effects of intravenous sub-anesthetic doses of ketamine and intranasal inhaled esketamine on suicidal ideation: a systematic review and meta-analysis. *Neuropsychiatr Dis Treat* 2023; **19**:587–599.

42. Hawton K, et al. Toxicity of antidepressants: rates of suicide relative to prescribing and non-fatal overdose. *Br J Psychiatry* 2010; **196**:354–358.

43. Lewis G, et al. Maintenance or discontinuation of antidepressants in primary care. *N Engl J Med* 2021; **385**:1257–1267.

44. Fava GA. May antidepressant drugs worsen the conditions they are supposed to treat? The clinical foundations of the oppositional model of tolerance. *Ther Adv Psychopharmacol* 2020; **10**:2045125320970325.

Recognised minimum effective doses of antidepressants

The recommended minimum effective doses of antidepressants are summarised in Table 3.2.

Table 3.2 Recommended minimum effective doses of antidepressants.

Antidepressant	Dose
Tricyclics	Unclear; at least 75–100mg/day[1], possibly 125mg/day[2]
Lofepramine	140mg/day[3]
SSRIs	
Citalopram	20mg/day[4]
Escitalopram	10mg/day[5]
Fluoxetine	20mg/day[6]
Fluvoxamine	50mg/day[7]
Paroxetine	20mg/day[8]
Sertraline	50mg/day[9]
Others	
Agomelatine	25mg/day[10]
Bupropion	150mg/day[11]
Desvenlafaxine	50mg/day[12]
Dextromethorphan plus bupropion	45/105mg/day[13]
Duloxetine	60mg/day[14,15]
Gepirone	20mg/day[16]
Levomilnacipran	40mg/day[17]
Mirtazapine	30mg/day (15mg?[18])
Moclobemide	300mg/day[19]
Reboxetine	8mg/day[20]
Trazodone	150mg/day[21]
Venlafaxine	75mg/day[22]
Vilazodone	20mg/day[17]
Vortioxetine	10mg/day[17]

References

1. Furukawa TA, et al. Meta-analysis of effects and side effects of low dosage tricyclic antidepressants in depression: systematic review. *BMJ* 2002; 325:991.
2. Donoghue J, et al. Suboptimal use of antidepressants in the treatment of depression. *CNS Drugs* 2000; 13:365–368.
3. Lancaster SG, et al. Lofepramine: a review of its pharmacodynamic and pharmacokinetic properties, and therapeutic efficacy in depressive illness. *Drugs* 1989; 37:123–140.
4. Montgomery SA, et al. The optimal dosing regimen for citalopram: a meta-analysis of nine placebo-controlled studies. *Int Clin Psychopharmacol* 1994; 9 Suppl 1:35–40.
5. Burke WJ, et al. Fixed-dose trial of the single isomer SSRI escitalopram in depressed outpatients. *J Clin Psychiatry* 2002; 63:331–336.
6. Altamura AC, et al. The evidence for 20mg a day of fluoxetine as the optimal dose in the treatment of depression. *Br J Psychiatry Suppl* 1988; (3):109–112.
7. Walczak DD, et al. The oral dose–effect relationship for fluvoxamine: a fixed-dose comparison against placebo in depressed outpatients. *Ann Clin Psychiatry* 1996; 8:139–151.
8. Dunner DL, et al. Optimal dose regimen for paroxetine. *J Clin Psychiatry* 1992; 53 Suppl:21–26.
9. Moon CAL, et al. A double-blind comparison of sertraline and clomipramine in the treatment of major depressive disorder and associative anxiety in general practice. *J Psychopharmacol* 1994; 8:171–176.
10. Loo H, et al. Determination of the dose of agomelatine, a melatoninergic agonist and selective 5-HT(2C) antagonist, in the treatment of major depressive disorder: a placebo-controlled dose range study. *Int Clin Psychopharmacol* 2002; 17:239–247.
11. Hewett K, et al. Eight-week, placebo-controlled, double-blind comparison of the antidepressant efficacy and tolerability of bupropion XR and venlafaxine XR. *J Psychopharmacol* 2009; 23:531–538.
12. Kornstein SG, et al. The effect of desvenlafaxine 50 mg/day on a subpopulation of anxious/depressed patients: a pooled analysis of seven randomized, placebo-controlled studies. *Hum Psychopharmacol* 2014; 29:492–501.
13. Iosifescu DV, et al. Efficacy and safety of axs-05 (dextromethorphan-bupropion) in patients with major depressive disorder: a phase 3 randomized clinical trial (GEMINI). *J Clin Psychiatry* 2022; 83:21m14345.
14. Goldstein DJ, et al. Duloxetine in the treatment of depression: a double-blind placebo-controlled comparison with paroxetine. *J Clin Psychopharmacol* 2004; 24:389–399.
15. Detke MJ, et al. Duloxetine, 60 mg once daily, for major depressive disorder: a randomized double-blind placebo-controlled trial. *J Clin Psychiatry* 2002; 63:308–315.
16. Phillips B, et al. Gepirone: A new extended–release oral selective serotonin receptor agonist for major depressive disorder. *J Pharm Technol* 2024; 40:230–235.
17. He H, et al. Efficacy and tolerability of different doses of three new antidepressants for treating major depressive disorder: a PRISMA-compliant meta-analysis. *J Psychiatr Res* 2018; 96:247–259.
18. Furukawa TA, et al. No benefit from flexible titration above minimum licensed dose in prescribing antidepressants for major depression: systematic review. *Acta Psychiatr Scand* 2020; 141:401–409.
19. Priest RG, et al. Moclobemide in the treatment of depression. *Rev Contemp Pharmacother* 1994; 5:35–43.
20. Schatzberg AF. Clinical efficacy of reboxetine in major depression. *J Clin Psychiatry* 2000; 61 Suppl 10:31–38.
21. Brogden RN, et al. Trazodone: a review of its pharmacological properties and therapeutic use in depression and anxiety. *Drugs* 1981; 21:401–429.
22. Feighner JP, et al. Efficacy of once-daily venlafaxine extended release (XR) for symptoms of anxiety in depressed outpatients. *J Affect Disord* 1998; 47:55–62.

CHAPTER 3

Drug treatment of depression

Drugs used in the treatment of depression are summarised in Figure 3.1.

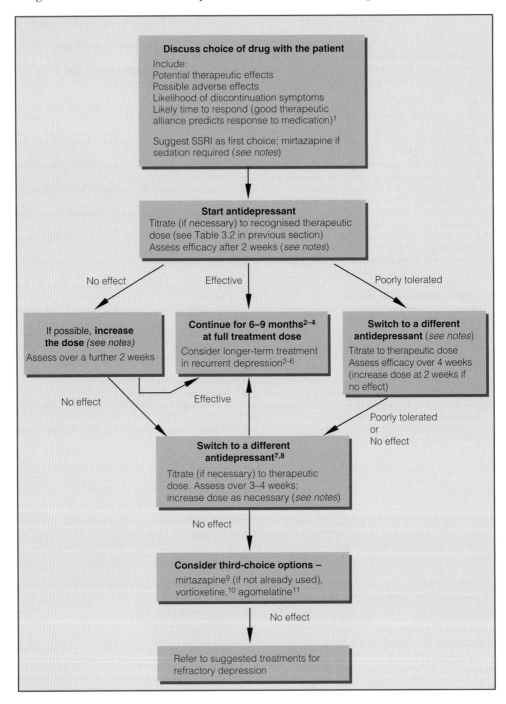

Figure 3.1 Drug treatment for depression.

Notes

- Tools such as the Montgomery–Asberg Depression Rating Scale (MADRS)[12] and the HAM-D[13] are used in trials to assess drug effect. The HAM-D is now somewhat anachronistic and few clinicians are familiar with the MADRS (although it is probably the best scale to measure severity and change). The Patient Health Questionnaire-9[14] is simple to use and is recommended for assessing symptom change in depression (although it better measures frequency rather than severity of symptoms). All rating scales should be treated with caution: someone with an HAM-D score of 30 is not twice as depressed as someone with a score of 15. That is, these scales are not linear and items are not weighted – on most scales insomnia scores more than a suicide attempt.
- Choice of antidepressant is governed largely by patient and clinician preference, but most authorities recommend an SSRI, or mirtazapine where sedation is required. A large network meta-analysis[15] suggested that drugs with effects on both norepinephrine and serotonin uptake are the most effective (five of the top six ranked drugs are dual action) whereas agomelatine and SSRIs have the lowest dropout rates. A 2018 network meta-analysis[16] of newer antidepressants suggested few, if any, clear advantages over older drugs for levomilnacipran, vilazodone and vortioxetine.
- Assessment at 2 weeks has some utility in determining eventual outcome.[17] Only around 30% of those not reaching accepted symptom score threshold for improvement at 2 weeks will ultimately respond. Even fewer people go on to respond if there is no improvement at all or deterioration at 2 weeks.
- Switching between drug classes in cases of poor tolerability is supported by some studies[18] and has a strong theoretical basis. Having said that, in practice, many patients who cannot tolerate one SSRI will readily tolerate another.
- In cases of non-response, there is some evidence that switching within a drug class is effective,[8,19–22] but switching between classes is, in practice, the most common option and is supported by some analyses.[23] The American Psychiatric Association recommends both options.[2] The 2022 NICE guidelines[9] suggest that there is little cogent evidence for switching between antidepressants (an observation in another analysis[24]) and that combining antidepressants or adding a second-generation antipsychotic (SGA) are better-supported options at this stage. The strongest evidence in support of switching after the failure of one treatment is probably for vortioxetine.[10] The most compelling evidence for combination antidepressants is for an SSRI plus mirtazapine.[25]
- There is minimal evidence to recommend increasing the dose of most SSRIs above the minimum therapeutic dose, at least when severity is measured using total rating scale scores.[26] Examining only the mood item on the HAM-D suggests some dose–response relationship for SSRIs.[27] Other evidence suggests that increasing the dose of venlafaxine, escitalopram and tricyclics may be helpful.[3,28] Generally speaking, gains in efficacy afforded by dose increases are small (SSRIs, venlafaxine) or non-existent (e.g. mirtazapine above 30mg/day) while effects on tolerability are reliably and starkly detrimental.[29]
- Switch treatments early (e.g. after 1–2 weeks) if adverse effects are intolerable or if no improvement *at all* is seen after 2–3 weeks. Opinions on when to switch vary somewhat but it is clear that antidepressants have a fairly prompt onset of action[30–32] and that non-response at 2–6 weeks is a good predictor of overall non-response.[33–35] The absence of any improvement *at all* by 2–3 weeks should normally provoke a change

in treatment (British Association for Psychopharmacology guidelines suggest 4 weeks).[3] If there is some improvement at this time, continue and assess for a further 2–3 weeks (see section on general overview of antidepressants in this chapter).

- Our algorithm conveniently dichotomises outcome as response or non-response (effective, not effective). Real-life outcomes include partial response – a positive change that falls short of recovery or remission. In those circumstances there is little evidence to guide practice, but the aim should be to achieve remission by means of dose increase and, if unsuccessful, by changing the antidepressant.

- Adjunctive treatments shown to be effective after the failure of only one antidepressant (early-stage treatment resistance) include (es)ketamine, risperidone, lithium and aripiprazole.[36] Dextromethorphan may improve initial outcomes if added to SSRI treatment.[37]

References

1. Leuchter AF, et al. Role of pill-taking, expectation and therapeutic alliance in the placebo response in clinical trials for major depression. *Br J Psychiatry* 2014; **205**:443–449.

2. American Psychiatric Association. *Practice Guideline for the Treatment of Patients with Major Depressive Disorder*, 3rd edn. Washington, DC: American Psychiatric Association; 2010.

3. Anderson IM, et al. Evidence-based guidelines for treating depressive disorders with antidepressants: a revision of the 2000 British Association for Psychopharmacology guidelines. *J Psychopharmacol* 2008; **22**:343–396.

4. Crismon ML, et al. The Texas Medication Algorithm Project: report of the Texas Consensus Conference Panel on Medication Treatment of Major Depressive Disorder. *J Clin Psychiatry* 1999; **60**:142–156.

5. Kocsis JH, et al. Maintenance therapy for chronic depression: a controlled clinical trial of desipramine. *Arch Gen Psychiatry* 1996; **53**:769–774.

6. Dekker J, et al. The use of antidepressants after recovery from depression. *Eur J Psychiatry* 2000; **14**:207–212.

7. Nelson JC. Treatment of antidepressant nonresponders: augmentation or switch? *J Clin Psychiatry* 1998; **59** Suppl 15:35–41.

8. Joffe RT. Substitution therapy in patients with major depression. *CNS Drugs* 1999; **11**:175–180.

9. National Institute for Health and Care Excellence. Depression in adults: treatment and management. NICE guideline [NG222]. 2022 (last reviewed September 2024, last checked November 2024); https://www.nice.org.uk/guidance/ng222.

10. Montgomery SA, et al. A randomised, double-blind study in adults with major depressive disorder with an inadequate response to a single course of selective serotonin reuptake inhibitor or serotonin-noradrenaline reuptake inhibitor treatment switched to vortioxetine or agomelatine. *Human Psychopharmacol* 2014; **29**:470–482.

11. Sparshatt A, et al. A naturalistic evaluation and audit database of agomelatine: clinical outcome at 12 weeks. *Acta Psychiatr Scand* 2013; **128**:203–211.

12. Montgomery SA, et al. A new depression scale designed to be sensitive to change. *Br J Psychiatry* 1979; **134**:382–389.

13. Hamilton M. Development of a rating scale for primary depressive illness. *Br J Soc Clin Psychol* 1967; **6**:278–296.

14. Kroenke K, et al. The PHQ-9: validity of a brief depression severity measure. *J Gen Intern Med* 2001; **16**:606–613.

15. Cipriani A, et al. Comparative efficacy and acceptability of 21 antidepressant drugs for the acute treatment of adults with major depressive disorder: a systematic review and network meta-analysis. *Lancet* 2018; **391**:1357–1366.

16. Wagner G, et al. Efficacy and safety of levomilnacipran, vilazodone and vortioxetine compared with other second-generation antidepressants for major depressive disorder in adults: a systematic review and network meta-analysis. *J Affect Disord* 2018; **228**:1–12.

17. de Vries YA, et al. Predicting antidepressant response by monitoring early improvement of individual symptoms of depression: individual patient data meta-analysis. *Br J Psychiatry* 2019; **214**:4–10.

18. Köhler-Forsberg O, et al. Efficacy of anti-inflammatory treatment on major depressive disorder or depressive symptoms: meta-analysis of clinical trials. *Acta Psychiatr Scand* 2019; **139**:404–419.

19. Thase ME, et al. Citalopram treatment of fluoxetine nonresponders. *J Clin Psychiatry* 2001; **62**:683–687.

20. Rush AJ, et al. Bupropion-SR, sertraline, or venlafaxine-XR after failure of SSRIs for depression. *N Engl J Med* 2006; **354**:1231–1242.

21. Ruhe HG, et al. Switching antidepressants after a first selective serotonin reuptake inhibitor in major depressive disorder: a systematic review. *J Clin Psychiatry* 2006; **67**:1836–1855.

22. Brent D, et al. Switching to another SSRI or to venlafaxine with or without cognitive behavioral therapy for adolescents with SSRI-resistant depression: the TORDIA randomized controlled trial. *JAMA* 2008; **299**:901–913.

23. Papakostas GI, et al. Treatment of SSRI-resistant depression: a meta-analysis comparing within- versus across-class switches. *Biol Psychiatry* 2008; **63**:699–704.

24. Bschor T, et al. Switching the antidepressant after nonresponse in adults with major depression: a systematic literature search and meta-analysis. *J Clin Psychiatry* 2018; **79**:16r10749.

25. Henssler J, et al. Combining antidepressants vs antidepressant monotherapy for treatment of patients with acute depression: a systematic review and meta-analysis. *JAMA Psychiatry* 2022; **79**:300–312.

26. Adli M, et al. Is dose escalation of antidepressants a rational strategy after a medium-dose treatment has failed? A systematic review. *Eur Arch Psychiatry Clin Neurosci* 2005; **255**:387–400.

27. Hieronymus F, et al. A mega-analysis of fixed-dose trials reveals dose-dependency and a rapid onset of action for the antidepressant effect of three selective serotonin reuptake inhibitors. *Transl Psychiatry* 2016; **6**:e834.

28. Zhou S, et al. Efficacy and dose-response relationships of antidepressants in the acute treatment of major depressive disorders: a systematic review and network meta-analysis. *Chin Med J (Engl)* 2024: doi: 10.1097/CM9.0000000000003138.

29. Furukawa TA, et al. Optimal dose of selective serotonin reuptake inhibitors, venlafaxine, and mirtazapine in major depression: a systematic review and dose–response meta-analysis. *Lancet Psychiatry* 2019; **6**:601–609.

30. Papakostas GI, et al. A meta-analysis of early sustained response rates between antidepressants and placebo for the treatment of major depressive disorder. *J Clin Psychopharmacol* 2006; **26**:56–60.

31. Taylor MJ, et al. Early onset of selective serotonin reuptake inhibitor antidepressant action: systematic review and meta-analysis. *Arch Gen Psychiatry* 2006; **63**:1217–1223.

32. Posternak MA, et al. Is there a delay in the antidepressant effect? A meta-analysis. *J Clin Psychiatry* 2005; **66**:148–158.

33. Szegedi A, et al. Early improvement in the first 2 weeks as a predictor of treatment outcome in patients with major depressive disorder: a meta-analysis including 6562 patients. *J Clin Psychiatry* 2009; **70**:344–353.

34. Baldwin DS, et al. How long should a trial of escitalopram treatment be in patients with major depressive disorder, generalised anxiety disorder or social anxiety disorder? An exploration of the randomised controlled trial database. *Hum Psychopharmacol* 2009; **24**:269–275.

35. Nierenberg AA, et al. Early nonresponse to fluoxetine as a predictor of poor 8-week outcome. *Am J Psychiatry* 1995; **152**:1500–1503.

36. Scott F, et al. Systematic review and meta-analysis of augmentation and combination treatments for early-stage treatment-resistant depression. *J Psychopharmacol* 2023; **37**:268–278.

37. Maji S, et al. Early augmentation therapy with dextromethorphan in mild to moderate major depressive disorder: a group sequential, response adaptive randomized controlled trial. *Psychiatry Res* 2024; **342**:116257.

CHAPTER 3

Management of treatment-resistant depression – commonly used treatments

Resistant depression is difficult to treat successfully and outcomes are often poor,[1-3] especially if evidence-based protocols are not followed.[4] Treatment-resistant depression is not a uniform entity but a complex spectrum of severity which can be graded[5] and in which outcome is closely linked to grading.[6] A significant minority of apparently resistant unipolar depression may in fact be bipolar depression,[7,8] which is often unresponsive to standard antidepressants[9,10] (see section on bipolar depression in Chapter 2). There has been a move to characterise treatment-resistant depression as 'difficult to treat' depression on the basis that the former description implies that depression treatments are normally effective and that non-response is therefore somehow abnormal.[11] Others suggest abandoning treatment-resistant depression as a diagnosis (again proposing 'difficult to treat' depression) because it propels clinicians to try more and more drugs in increasingly complex regimens rather than managing expectations of recovery to a more realistic level.[12]

Management of treatment-resistant depression has been informed by the Sequenced Treatment Alternatives to Relieve Depression (STAR*D) programme. This was a pragmatic effectiveness study, which used remission of symptoms as its main outcome.[13] This study and its various subanalyses have now been somewhat discredited, principally because of high dropout rates after the initial treatment stages.

Other criticisms of the STAR*D programme include the absence of a placebo group, the open nature of treatment and some assessments, the failure to account for patients withdrawing after their first visit, the unexplained use of an a priori secondary measure as the main outcome metric, payments made to subjects, and the observation that 93% of 1,518 patients in remission had relapsed or dropped out of the study at 12 months' follow-up.[14,15] In addition to this, reanalysis of original data collected found the overall remission rate to be 35%, as opposed to the claimed rate of 67%.[16]

Commonly used drugs for refractory depression that are generally well supported by published literature are shown in Table 3.3.

Table 3.3 Commonly used treatments, generally well supported by published literature (no preference implied by order).

Treatment	Advantages	Disadvantages
Add **aripiprazole**[17-23] (2–20mg/day) to antidepressant (brexpiprazole and cariprazine are also effective)[24-26]	■ Good evidence base ■ Usually well tolerated and safe ■ Low doses (2–10mg/day) may be effective ■ Supported by meta-analyses[24,27,28]	■ Akathisia and restlessness common at standard doses (≥10mg/day) ■ Insomnia may be problematic
Add **lithium**[29] Aim for plasma level of 0.4–0.8mmol/L initially, increasing to up to 1.0mmol/L if suboptimal response	■ Well established ■ Well supported in the literature ■ Recommended by NICE[30] ■ Supported by meta-analyses[27,28]	■ Sometimes poorly tolerated at higher plasma levels ■ Potentially toxic ■ Usually needs specialist referral ■ Plasma level monitoring is essential

(Continued)

Table 3.3 (*Continued*)

Treatment	Advantages	Disadvantages
Combine **olanzapine** and **fluoxetine**[31] 6.25–12.5mg + 25–50mg daily (US licensed dose)*	▪ Well researched ▪ Usually well tolerated ▪ Olanzapine + TCA may also be effective[32] ▪ Olanzapine alone may be effective[33,34]	▪ Risk of weight gain ▪ Limited clinical experience outside USA ▪ Most data relate to bipolar depression
Add **quetiapine**[25,26] (150mg or 300mg a day) to SSRI/SNRI	▪ Good evidence base ▪ Usually well tolerated ▪ Plausible explanation for antidepressant effect ▪ Possibly more effective than lithium	▪ Dry mouth, sedation, constipation can be problematic ▪ Weight gain risk in the longer term
SSRI + bupropion[35–40] up to 400mg/day	▪ Well tolerated ▪ May improve sexual adverse effects	▪ Not licensed for depression in the UK
SSRI or **venlafaxine** + **mianserin** (30mg/day) or **mirtazapine**[40,41] (30–45mg/day)	▪ Recommended by NICE ▪ Usually well tolerated ▪ Widely used	▪ Theoretical risk of serotonin syndrome (inform patient) ▪ Risk of blood dyscrasia with mianserin ▪ Weight gain and sedation with mirtazapine ▪ One RCT showed no advantage for mirtazapine added to SSRI/SNRIs[42]

* 5mg + 20mg rising to 10mg + 40mg seems reasonable where combination formulations not available.
TCA, tricyclic antidepressant.

References

1. Dunner DL, et al. Prospective, long-term, multicenter study of the naturalistic outcomes of patients with treatment-resistant depression. *J Clin Psychiatry* 2006; **67**:688–695.
2. Wooderson SC, et al. Prospective evaluation of specialist inpatient treatment for refractory affective disorders. *J Affect Disord* 2011; **131**:92–103.
3. Fekadu A, et al. What happens to patients with treatment-resistant depression? A systematic review of medium to long term outcome studies. *J Affect Disord* 2009; **116**:4–11.
4. Trivedi MH, et al. Clinical results for patients with major depressive disorder in the Texas Medication Algorithm Project. *Arch Gen Psychiatry* 2004; **61**:669–680.
5. Fekadu A, et al. A multidimensional tool to quantify treatment resistance in depression: the Maudsley staging method. *J Clin Psychiatry* 2009; **70**:177–184.
6. Fekadu A, et al. The Maudsley staging method for treatment-resistant depression: prediction of longer-term outcome and persistence of symptoms. *J Clin Psychiatry* 2009; **70**:952–957.
7. Angst J, et al. Toward a re-definition of subthreshold bipolarity: epidemiology and proposed criteria for bipolar-II, minor bipolar disorders and hypomania. *J Affect Disord* 2003; **73**:133–146.
8. Smith DJ, et al. Unrecognised bipolar disorder in primary care patients with depression. *British Journal of Psychiatry* 2011; **199**:49–56.
9. Sidor MM, et al. Antidepressants for the acute treatment of bipolar depression: a systematic review and meta-analysis. *J Clin Psychiatry* 2011; **72**:156–167.
10. Taylor DM, et al. Comparative efficacy and acceptability of drug treatments for bipolar depression: a multiple-treatments meta-analysis. *Acta Psychiatr Scand* 2014; **130**:452–469.
11. Cosgrove L, et al. Reconceptualising treatment-resistant depression as difficult-to-treat depression. *Lancet Psychiatry* 2021; **8**:11–13.
12. Rush AJ, et al. Difficult-to-treat depression: a clinical and research roadmap for when remission is elusive. *Aust N Z J Psychiatry* 2019; **53**:109–118.
13. Trivedi MH, et al. Evaluation of outcomes with citalopram for depression using measurement-based care in STAR*D: implications for clinical practice. *Am J Psychiatry* 2006; **163**:28–40.

14. Pigott HE, et al. Efficacy and effectiveness of antidepressants: current status of research. *Psychother Psychosom* 2010; **79**:267–279.

15. Pigott HE. The STAR*D trial: it is time to reexamine the clinical beliefs that guide the treatment of major depression. *Can J Psychiatry* 2015; **60**:9–13.

16. Pigott HE, et al. What are the treatment remission, response and extent of improvement rates after up to four trials of antidepressant therapies in real-world depressed patients? A reanalysis of the STAR*D study's patient-level data with fidelity to the original research protocol. *BMJ Open* 2023; **13**:e063095.

17. Marcus RN, et al. The efficacy and safety of aripiprazole as adjunctive therapy in major depressive disorder: a second multicenter, randomized, double-blind, placebo-controlled study. *J Clin Psychopharmacol* 2008; **28**:156–165.

18. Hellerstein DJ, et al. Aripiprazole as an adjunctive treatment for refractory unipolar depression. *Prog Neuropsychopharmacol Biol Psychiatry* 2008; **32**:744–750.

19. Simon JS, et al. Aripiprazole augmentation of antidepressants for the treatment of partially responding and nonresponding patients with major depressive disorder. *J Clin Psychiatry* 2005; **66**:1216–1220.

20. Papakostas GI, et al. Aripiprazole augmentation of selective serotonin reuptake inhibitors for treatment-resistant major depressive disorder. *J Clin Psychiatry* 2005; **66**:1326–1330.

21. Berman RM, et al. Aripiprazole augmentation in major depressive disorder: a double-blind, placebo-controlled study in patients with inadequate response to antidepressants. *CNS Spectr* 2009; **14**:197–206.

22. Fava M, et al. A double-blind, placebo-controlled study of aripiprazole adjunctive to antidepressant therapy among depressed outpatients with inadequate response to prior antidepressant therapy (ADAPT-A Study). *Psychother Psychosom* 2012; **81**:87–97.

23. Jon DI, et al. Augmentation of aripiprazole for depressed patients with an inadequate response to antidepressant treatment: a 6-week prospective, open-label, multicenter study. *Clin Neuropharmacol* 2013; **36**:157–161.

24. Nuñez NA, et al. Augmentation strategies for treatment resistant major depression: a systematic review and network meta-analysis. *J Affect Disord* 2022; **302**:385–400.

25. Kishimoto T, et al. Efficacy and safety/tolerability of antipsychotics in the treatment of adult patients with major depressive disorder: a systematic review and meta-analysis. *Psychol Med* 2023; **53**:4064–4082.

26. Yan Y, et al. Efficacy and acceptability of second-generation antipsychotics with antidepressants in unipolar depression augmentation: a systematic review and network meta-analysis. *Psychol Med* 2022; **52**:2224–2231.

27. Strawbridge R, et al. Augmentation therapies for treatment-resistant depression: systematic review and meta-analysis. *Br J Psychiatry* 2019; **214**:42–51.

28. Terao I, et al. Comparative efficacy, tolerability and acceptability of intravenous racemic ketamine with intranasal esketamine, aripiprazole and lithium as augmentative treatments for treatment-resistant unipolar depression: a systematic review and network meta-analysis. *J Affect Disord* 2024; **346**:49–56.

29. Undurraga J, et al. Lithium treatment for unipolar major depressive disorder: systematic review. *J Psychopharmacol* 2019; **33**:167–176.

30. National Institute for Health and Care Excellence. Depression in adults: treatment and management. NICE guideline [NG222]. 2022 (last reviewed September 2024, last checked November 2024); https://www.nice.org.uk/guidance/ng222.

31. Luan S, et al. Efficacy and safety of olanzapine/fluoxetine combination in the treatment of treatment-resistant depression: a meta-analysis of randomized controlled trials. *Neuropsychiatr Dis Treat* 2017; **13**:609–620.

32. Takahashi H, et al. Augmentation with olanzapine in TCA-refractory depression with melancholic features: a consecutive case series. *Hum Psychopharmacol* 2008; **23**:217–220.

33. Corya SA, et al. A randomized, double-blind comparison of olanzapine/fluoxetine combination, olanzapine, fluoxetine, and venlafaxine in treatment-resistant depression. *Depress Anxiety* 2006; **23**:364–372.

34. Thase ME, et al. A randomized, double-blind comparison of olanzapine/fluoxetine combination, olanzapine, and fluoxetine in treatment-resistant major depressive disorder. *J Clin Psychiatry* 2007; **68**:224–236.

35. Trivedi MH, et al. Medication augmentation after the failure of SSRIs for depression. *N Engl J Med* 2006; **354**:1243–1252.

36. Zisook S, et al. Use of bupropion in combination with serotonin reuptake inhibitors. *Biol Psychiatry* 2006; **59**:203–210.

37. Fatemi SH, et al. Venlafaxine and bupropion combination therapy in a case of treatment-resistant depression. *Ann Pharmacother* 1999; **33**:701–703.

38. Lam RW, et al. Citalopram and bupropion-SR: combining versus switching in patients with treatment-resistant depression. *J Clin Psychiatry* 2004; **65**:337–340.

39. Papakostas GI, et al. The combination of duloxetine and bupropion for treatment-resistant major depressive disorder. *Depress Anxiety* 2006; **23**:178–181.

40. Henssler J, et al. Combining antidepressants in acute treatment of depression: a meta-analysis of 38 studies including 4511 patients. *Can J Psychiatry* 2016; **61**:29–43.

41. Ferreri M, et al. Benefits from mianserin augmentation of fluoxetine in patients with major depression non-responders to fluoxetine alone. *Acta Psychiatr Scand* 2001; **103**:66–72.

42. Kessler DS, et al. Mirtazapine added to SSRIs or SNRIs for treatment resistant depression in primary care: phase III randomised placebo controlled trial (MIR). *BMJ* 2018; **363**:k4218.

CHAPTER 3

Management of treatment-resistant depression – other well-supported treatments

Less commonly used treatments for treatment-resistant depression that are generally well supported by published literature are shown in Table 3.4.

Table 3.4 Less commonly used treatments, well supported by published evidence (no preference implied by order).

Treatment	Advantages	Disadvantages
Add **ketamine** (0.5mg/kg IV over 40 minutes)[1] Intranasal **esketamine** (licensed in most countries); dose is 28–84mg[2] (see section on ketamine in this chapter) Oral ketamine (0.5–1.25mg/kg) effective but no licensed products[3]	■ Very rapid response (within hours), including effects on suicidality[4,5] ■ High remission rate[6,7] ■ Some evidence of maintained response if repeated doses given[8] ■ Usually well tolerated at this sub-anaesthetic dose	■ IV needs to be administered in hospital ■ Cognitive effects (confusion, dissociation) and other psychiatric symptoms[9] ■ Associated with transient increases in BP, tachycardia and arrhythmias. Pretreatment ECG required with IV form[10] ■ Adverse effects may have been underestimated[11] ■ Repeated treatment necessary to maintain effect
Add **lamotrigine** (100mg, 200mg and 400mg a day have been used)[12]	■ Reasonably well researched ■ Quite widely used ■ Probably the best tolerated augmentation strategy[13]	■ Slow titration ■ Risk of rash ■ Optimal dosing unclear
ECT[14]	■ Well established ■ Effective ■ Well supported in the literature	■ Necessitates general anaesthetic ■ Needs specialist referral ■ Usually reserved for last-line treatment or if rapid response needed ■ Usually combined with other treatments
Add **tri-iodothyronine** (20–50mcg/day) Higher doses have been safely used[15–21]	■ Usually well tolerated ■ Good literature support[22] ■ May be effective in bipolar depression	■ Clinical and biochemical TFT monitoring required ■ Needs specialist referral ■ Some negative studies ■ No advantage over antidepressant alone in non-refractory illness[23]

TFT, thyroid function test.

CHAPTER 3

CHAPTER 3

References

1. Marcantoni WS, et al. A systematic review and meta-analysis of the efficacy of intravenous ketamine infusion for treatment resistant depression: January 2009 – January 2019. *J Affect Disord* 2020; **277**:831–841.

2. Papakostas GI, et al. Efficacy of esketamine augmentation in major depressive disorder: a meta-analysis. *J Clin Psychiatry* 2020; **81**:19r12889.

3. Meshkat S, et al. Oral ketamine for depression: an updated systematic review. *World J Biol Psychiatry* 2023; **24**:545–557.

4. Wilkinson ST, et al. The effect of a single dose of intravenous ketamine on suicidal ideation: a systematic review and individual participant data meta-analysis. *Am J Psychiatry* 2018; **175**:150–158.

5. Witt K, et al. Ketamine for suicidal ideation in adults with psychiatric disorders: a systematic review and meta-analysis of treatment trials. *Aust N Z J Psychiatry* 2020; **54**:29–45.

6. Alnefeesi Y, et al. Real-world effectiveness of ketamine in treatment-resistant depression: a systematic review and meta-analysis. *J Psychiatr Res* 2022; **151**:693–709.

7. Terao I, et al. Comparative efficacy, tolerability and acceptability of intravenous racemic ketamine with intranasal esketamine, aripiprazole and lithium as augmentative treatments for treatment-resistant unipolar depression: a systematic review and network meta-analysis. *J Affect Disord* 2024; **346**:49–56.

8. Capuzzi E, et al. Long-term efficacy of intranasal esketamine in treatment-resistant major depression: a systematic review. *Int J Mol Sci* 2021; **22**:9338.

9. Beck K, et al. Association of ketamine with psychiatric symptoms and implications for its therapeutic use and for understanding schizophrenia: a systematic review and meta-analysis. *JAMA Netw Open* 2020; **3**:e204693.

10. aan het Rot M, et al. Safety and efficacy of repeated-dose intravenous ketamine for treatment-resistant depression. *Biol Psychiatry* 2010; **67**:139–145.

11. Short B, et al. Side-effects associated with ketamine use in depression: a systematic review. *Lancet Psychiatry* 2018; **5**:65–78.

12. Goh KK, et al. Lamotrigine augmentation in treatment-resistant unipolar depression: a comprehensive meta-analysis of efficacy and safety. *J Psychopharmacol* 2019; **33**:700–713.

13. Papadimitropoulou K, et al. Comparative efficacy and tolerability of pharmacological and somatic interventions in adult patients with treatment-resistant depression: a systematic review and network meta-analysis. *Curr Med Res Opin* 2017; **33**:701–711.

14. Guo Q, et al. Efficacy and safety of eight enhanced therapies for treatment-resistant depression: a systematic review and network meta-analysis of RCTs. *Psychiatry Res* 2024; **339**:116018.

15. Joffe RT, et al. A comparison of triiodothyronine and thyroxine in the potentiation of tricyclic antidepressants. *Psychiatry Res* 1990; **32**:241–251.

16. Anderson IM. Drug treatment of depression: reflections on the evidence. *Adv Psychiatr Treat* 2003; **9**:11–20.

17. Nierenberg AA, et al. A comparison of lithium and T(3) augmentation following two failed medication treatments for depression: a STAR*D report. *Am J Psychiatry* 2006; **163**:1519–1530.

18. Iosifescu DV, et al. An open study of triiodothyronine augmentation of selective serotonin reuptake inhibitors in treatment-resistant major depressive disorder. *J Clin Psychiatry* 2005; **66**:1038–1042.

19. Abraham G, et al. T3 augmentation of SSRI resistant depression. *J Affect Disord* 2006; **91**:211–215.

20. Kelly TF, et al. Long term augmentation with T3 in refractory major depression. *J Affect Disord* 2009; **115**:230–233.

21. Parmentier T, et al. The use of triiodothyronine (T3) in the treatment of bipolar depression: a review of the literature. *J Affect Disord* 2018; **229**:410–414.

22. Nuñez NA, et al. Augmentation strategies for treatment resistant major depression: a systematic review and network meta-analysis. *J Affect Disord* 2022; **302**:385–400.

23. Garlow SJ, et al. The combination of triiodothyronine (T3) and sertraline is not superior to sertraline monotherapy in the treatment of major depressive disorder. *J Psychiatr Res* 2012; **46**:1406–1413.

Treatment-resistant depression – other reported treatments

A very wide range of treatments have been investigated as potential therapy for treatment-resistant depression. Table 3.5 briefly describes strategies that have limited support for their use but may be worth trying in exceptional circumstances. Prescribers should familiarise themselves with the primary literature before using these strategies.

Table 3.5 Other reported treatments (alphabetical order – no preference implied).

Treatment*	Comments
Ayahuasca[1]	Effective but specialist use only
Buprenorphine[2] 0.8–2mg/day?	Reasonable evidence but obvious contraindications
Dexamethasone[3,4] 3–4 mg/day	Limited data
Dextromethorphan + quinidine[5–7] 45/10mg twice a day	Promising novel treatment. NMDA antagonist. Quinidine is needed as CYP2D6 inhibitor to prolong action of dextromethorphan[8]
Folate/methyl folate[9]	Possible benefit
Hyoscine[10,11] (scopolomine) (4mcg/kg IV)	Growing evidence base of prompt and sizeable effect
MAOI and TCA[12–14] e.g. trimipramine and phenelzine	Formerly very widely used, but great care needed
Minocycline 200mg/day	Several positive meta-analyses in both animals[15] and humans.[16,17] Recent failed RCTs.[18,19]
Modafinil[20] 100–400mg/day	See section on stimulants in depression (this chapter)
Naltrexone[21,22] 100mg/day	No studies in non-opiate misusers
Nitrous oxide[23–25]	Short-lived effect
Nortriptyline ± lithium[26–29]	Re-emergent treatment option
Oestrogens[30] (various regimens)	Limited data
Omega–3-triglycerides EPA[31–33]	Many failed trials. Therapeutic dose not defined.
Pindolol[34–39] 5mg three times a day or 7.5mg once daily	Well tolerated, can be initiated in primary care. Data mainly relate to acceleration of response. Refractory data somewhat contradictory.
Pramipexole[40] 0.125–5mg/day	Probably effective
Psilocybin[41] 10/25mg 1 week apart	Effective but specialist use only
Risperidone[42] 0.5–3mg/day to antidepressant	Good RCT support as add-on treatment
S-adenosyl-L-methionine[43–45] 400mg/day IM; 1600mg/day oral	Limited data in treatment-resistant depression. Use weakly supported by a Cochrane review.[46]

(Continued)

CHAPTER 3

Table 3.5 (*Continued*)

Treatment*	Comments
SSRI + buspirone[47,48] Up to 60mg/day	Higher doses required poorly tolerated (dizziness common)
SSRI + TCA[49]	Formerly widely used
Stimulants amfetamine; methylphenidate	Varied outcomes. See section on stimulants in depression in this chapter.
TCA – high dose[50]	Formerly widely used. Cardiac monitoring essential
Testosterone gel[34,51]	Effective in those with low testosterone levels
Tianeptine[52,53] 25–50mg/day	Tiny database. Tianeptine not available in many countries. Potential for misuse.[54]
Tryptophan[55–58] 2–3g three times a day	Long history of successful use
Venlafaxine[59–62] >200mg/day	Nausea and vomiting; discontinuation reactions more common. BP monitoring essential.
Venlafaxine – very high dose (up to 600mg/day)[63]	See above. Cardiac monitoring essential.
Venlafaxine + IV clomipramine[64]	Cardiac monitoring essential
Zinc[65] 25mg Zn+/day	One RCT (*n* = 60) showed good results in refractory depression. A few other small studies.[66]

* Other non-drug treatments are available, including various psychological approaches, rTMS, VNS, deep brain stimulation and psychosurgery. Discussion of these treatments is beyond the scope of this book.
CYP, cytochrome P450; EPA, eicosapentaenoic acid; MAOI, monoamine oxidase inhibitor; NMDA, N-methyl-D-aspartate; TCA, tricyclic antidepressant.

References

1. Gonçalves J, et al. A systematic review on the therapeutic effects of ayahuasca. *Plants (Basel)* 2023; **12**:2573.
2. Stanciu CN, et al. Use of buprenorphine in treatment of refractory depression: a review of current literature. *Asian J Psychiatr* 2017; **26**:94–98.
3. Dinan TG, et al. Dexamethasone augmentation in treatment-resistant depression. *Acta Psychiatr Scand* 1997; **95**:58–61.
4. Bodani M, et al. The use of dexamethasone in elderly patients with antidepressant-resistant depressive illness. *J Psychopharmacol* 1999; **13**:196–197.
5. Murrough JW, et al. Dextromethorphan/quinidine pharmacotherapy in patients with treatment resistant depression: a proof of concept clinical trial. *J Affect Disord* 2017; **218**:277–283.
6. Kelly TF, et al. The utility of the combination of dextromethorphan and quinidine in the treatment of bipolar II and bipolar NOS. *J Affect Disord* 2014; **167**:333–335.
7. Wang PR, et al. An open-label study of adjunctive dextromethorphan/quinidine in treatment-resistant depression. *J Clin Psychopharmacol* 2023; **43**:422–427.
8. Nofziger JL, et al. Evaluation of dextromethorphan with select antidepressant therapy for the treatment of depression in the acute care psychiatric setting. *Ment Health Clin* 2019; **9**:76–81.
9. Maruf AA, et al. Systematic review and meta-analysis of l-methylfolate augmentation in depressive disorders. *Pharmacopsychiatry* 2022; **55**:139–147.
10. Wang X, et al. Group-based symptom trajectory of intramuscular administration of scopolamine augmentation in moderate to severe major depressive disorder: a post-hoc analysis. *Neuropsychiatr Dis Treat* 2023; **19**:1043–1053.
11. Drevets WC, et al. Antidepressant effects of the muscarinic cholinergic receptor antagonist scopolamine: a review. *Biol Psychiatry* 2013; **73**:1156–1163.
12. White K, et al. The combined use of MAOIs and tricyclics. *J Clin Psychiatry* 1984; **45**:67–69.
13. Kennedy N, et al. Treatment and response in refractory depression: results from a specialist affective disorders service. *J Affect Disord* 2004; **81**:49–53.

14. Connolly KR, et al. If at first you don't succeed: a review of the evidence for antidepressant augmentation, combination and switching strategies. *Drugs* 2011; **71**:43–64.

15. Reis DJ, et al. The antidepressant impact of minocycline in rodents: a systematic review and meta-analysis. *Sci Rep* 2019; **9**:261.

16. Zazula R, et al. Minocycline as adjunctive treatment for major depressive disorder: pooled data from two randomized controlled trials. *Aust N Z J Psychiatry* 2020;4867420965697.

17. Strawbridge R, et al. Augmentation therapies for treatment-resistant depression: systematic review and meta-analysis. *Br J Psychiatry* 2019; **214**:42–51.

18. Husain MI, et al. Minocycline and celecoxib as adjunctive treatments for bipolar depression: a multicentre, factorial design randomised controlled trial. *Lancet Psychiatry* 2020; **7**:515–527.

19. Hellmann-Regen J, et al. Effect of minocycline on depressive symptoms in patients with treatment-resistant depression: a randomized clinical trial. *JAMA Netw Open* 2022; **5**:e2230367.

20. Nuñez NA, et al. Augmentation strategies for treatment resistant major depression: a systematic review and network meta-analysis. *J Affect Disord* 2022; **302**:385400.

21. Pettinati HM, et al. A double-blind, placebo-controlled trial combining sertraline and naltrexone for treating co-occurring depression and alcohol dependence. *Am J Psychiatry* 2010; **167**:668–675.

22. Browne CA, et al. Novel targets to treat depression: opioid-based therapeutics. *Harvard Rev Psychiatry* 2020; **28**:40–59.

23. Yan D, et al. Efficacy and safety of nitrous oxide for patients with treatment-resistant depression, a randomized controlled trial. *Psychiatry Res* 2022; **317**:114867.

24. Kim WSH, et al. Proof-of-concept randomized controlled trial of single-session nitrous oxide treatment for refractory bipolar depression: focus on cerebrovascular target engagement. *Bipolar Disord* 2023; **25**:221–232.

25. Nagele P, et al. A phase 2 trial of inhaled nitrous oxide for treatment-resistant major depression. *Sci Transl Med* 2021; **13**:eabe1376.

26. Nierenberg AA, et al. Nortriptyline for treatment-resistant depression. *J Clin Psychiatry* 2003; **64**:35–39.

27. Nierenberg AA, et al. Lithium augmentation of nortriptyline for subjects resistant to multiple antidepressants. *J Clin Psychopharmacol* 2003; **23**:92–95.

28. Fava M, et al. A comparison of mirtazapine and nortriptyline following two consecutive failed medication treatments for depressed outpatients: a STAR*D report. *Am J Psychiatry* 2006; **163**:1161–1172.

29. Shelton RC, et al. Olanzapine/fluoxetine combination for treatment-resistant depression: a controlled study of SSRI and nortriptyline resistance. *J Clin Psychiatry* 2005; **66**:1289–1297.

30. Stahl SM. Basic psychopharmacology of antidepressants, part 2: oestrogen as an adjunct to antidepressant treatment. *J Clin Psychiatry* 1998; 59 Suppl 4:15–24.

31. Liao Y, et al. Efficacy of omega-3 PUFAs in depression: a meta-analysis. *Transl Psychiatry* 2019; **9**:190.

32. Mischoulon D, et al. Omega-3 fatty acids for major depressive disorder with high inflammation: a randomized dose-finding clinical trial. *J Clin Psychiatry* 2022; **83**:21m14074.

33. Wu SK, et al. The efficacy of omega-3 fatty acids as the monotherapy for depression: a randomized, double-blind, placebo-controlled pilot study. *Nutrients* 2024; **16**:3688.

34. Kleeblatt J, et al. Efficacy of off-label augmentation in unipolar depression: a systematic review of the evidence. *Eur Neuropsychopharmacol* 2017; **27**:423–441.

35. McAskill R, et al. Pindolol augmentation of antidepressant therapy. *Br J Psychiatry* 1998; **173**:203–208.

36. Rasanen P, et al. Mitchell B. Balter Award 1998. Pindolol and major affective disorders: a three-year follow-up study of 30,485 patients. *J Clin Psychopharmacol* 1999; **19**:297–302.

37. Perry EB, et al. Pindolol augmentation in depressed patients resistant to selective serotonin reuptake inhibitors: a double-blind, randomized, controlled trial. *J Clin Psychiatry* 2004; **65**:238–243.

38. Sokolski KN, et al. Once-daily high-dose pindolol for SSRI-refractory depression. *Psychiatry Res* 2004; **125**:81–86.

39. Whale R, et al. Pindolol augmentation of serotonin reuptake inhibitors for the treatment of depressive disorder: a systematic review. *J Psychopharmacol* 2010; **24**:513–520.

40. Tundo A, et al. Pramipexole augmentation for treatment-resistant unipolar and bipolar depression in the real world: a systematic review and meta-analysis. *Life (Basel)* 2023; **13**:1043.

41. Metaxa AM, et al. Efficacy of psilocybin for treating symptoms of depression: systematic review and meta-analysis. *BMJ* 2024; **385**:e078084.

42. Kishimoto T, et al. Efficacy and safety/tolerability of antipsychotics in the treatment of adult patients with major depressive disorder: a systematic review and meta-analysis. *Psychol Med* 2023; **53**:4064–4082.

43. Pancheri P, et al. A double-blind, randomized parallel-group, efficacy and safety study of intramuscular S-adenosyl-L-methionine 1,4-butanedisulphonate (SAMe) versus imipramine in patients with major depressive disorder. *Int J Neuropsychopharmacol* 2002; **5**:287–294.

44. Alpert JE, et al. S-adenosyl-L-methionine (SAMe) as an adjunct for resistant major depressive disorder: an open trial following partial or nonresponse to selective serotonin reuptake inhibitors or venlafaxine. *J Clin Psychopharmacol* 2004; **24**:661–664.

45. Sharma A, et al. S-adenosylmethionine (SAMe) for neuropsychiatric disorders: a clinician-oriented review of research. *J Clin Psychiatry* 2017; **78**:e656–e667.

46. Galizia I, et al. S-adenosyl methionine (SAMe) for depression in adults. *Cochrane Database Syst Rev* 2016; **10**:CD011286.

47. Trivedi MH, et al. Medication augmentation after the failure of SSRIs for depression. *N Engl J Med* 2006; **354**:1243–1252.

48. Appelberg BG, et al. Patients with severe depression may benefit from buspirone augmentation of selective serotonin reuptake inhibitors: results from a placebo-controlled, randomized, double-blind, placebo wash-in study. *J Clin Psychiatry* 2001; **62**:448–452.

49. Taylor D. Selective serotonin reuptake inhibitors and tricyclic antidepressants in combination: interactions and therapeutic uses. *Br J Psychiatry* 1995; **167**:575–580.

CHAPTER 3

50. Malhi GS, et al. Management of resistant depression. *Int J Psychiatry Clin Pract* 1997; **1**:269–276.

51. Pope HG, Jr., et al. Testosterone gel supplementation for men with refractory depression: a randomized, placebo-controlled trial. *Am J Psychiatry* 2003; **160**:105–111.

52. Tobe EH, et al. Possible usefulness of tianeptine in treatment-resistant depression. *Int J Psychiatry Clin Pract* 2013; **17**:313–316.

53. Woo YS, et al. Tianeptine combination for partial or non-response to selective serotonin re-uptake inhibitor monotherapy. *Psychiatry Clin Neurosci* 2013; **67**:219–227.

54. Espiridion ED, et al. A case of 'Neptune's fix elixir': the dangerous consequences of unregulated use of tianeptine in over-the-counter products. *Cureus* 2024; **16**:e55120.

55. Angst J, et al. The treatment of depression with L-5-hydroxytryptophan versus imipramine. Results of two open and one double-blind study. *Arch Psychiatr Nervenkr* 1977; **224**:175–186.

56. Alino JJ, et al. 5-Hydroxytryptophan (5-HTP) and a MAOI (nialamide) in the treatment of depressions: a double-blind controlled study. *Int Pharmacopsychiatry* 1976; **11**:8–15.

57. Hale AS, et al. Clomipramine, tryptophan and lithium in combination for resistant endogenous depression: seven case studies. *Br J Psychiatry* 1987; **151**:213–217.

58. Young SN. Use of tryptophan in combination with other antidepressant treatments: a review. *J Psychiatry Neurosci* 1991; **16**:241–246.

59. Poirier MF, et al. Venlafaxine and paroxetine in treatment-resistant depression: double-blind, randomised comparison. *Br J Psychiatry* 1999; **175**:12–16.

60. Nierenberg AA, et al. Venlafaxine for treatment-resistant unipolar depression. *J Clin Psychopharmacol* 1994; **14**:419–423.

61. Smith D, et al. Efficacy and tolerability of venlafaxine compared with selective serotonin reuptake inhibitors and other antidepressants: a meta-analysis. *Br J Psychiatry* 2002; **180**:396–404.

62. Rush AJ, et al. Bupropion-SR, sertraline, or venlafaxine-XR after failure of SSRIs for depression. *N Engl J Med* 2006; **354**:1231–1242.

63. Harrison CL, et al. Tolerability of high-dose venlafaxine in depressed patients. *J Psychopharmacol* 2004; **18**:200–204.

64. Fountoulakis KN, et al. Combined oral venlafaxine and intravenous clomipramine-A: successful temporary response in a patient with extremely refractory depression. *Can J Psychiatry* 2004; **49**:73–74.

65. Siwek M, et al. Zinc supplementation augments efficacy of imipramine in treatment resistant patients: a double blind, placebo-controlled study. *J Affect Disord* 2009; **118**:187–195.

66. Salari S, et al. Zinc sulphate: a reasonable choice for depression management in patients with multiple sclerosis: a randomized, double-blind, placebo-controlled clinical trial. *Pharmacol Rep* 2015; **67**:606–609.

Ketamine

Background

Over the past two decades, ketamine, an uncompetitive N-methyl-D-aspartate (NMDA) receptor antagonist and dissociative anaesthetic, has emerged as a novel and effective rapid-acting antidepressant. In 2000, Berman and colleagues reported findings from a landmark RCT, administering a single subanaesthetic dose of IV ketamine (0.5mg/kg over 40 minutes) to individuals with MDD.[1] Ketamine produced a significant antidepressant effect within hours after the infusion that increased progressively up to 3 days after administration. This finding has since been replicated in several trials in both unipolar and bipolar depression (including treatment-resistant individuals).[2-6] In addition, perinatal or prenatal ketamine and esketamine reduce the risk of postnatal depression by about 50–75%.[7-9] The use of ketamine as anaesthesia may enhance the effect of ECT.[10] Ketamine appears to be broadly as effective as ECT.[11,12]

Ketamine is a racemic mixture composed of equal amounts of the two enantiomers (S)-ketamine and (R)-ketamine (esketamine and arketamine), with esketamine binding more potently to the NMDA receptor. Although racemic ketamine remains an off-label treatment for treatment-resistant depression (TRD), an esketamine nasal spray (Spravato®) is approved for use in TRD (in conjunction with an oral antidepressant) in Europe and the USA. A 2023 trial has shown greater benefit in TRD for augmentation of antidepressants with nasal esketamine than with quetiapine.[13] Interestingly, although benefits were evident for both esketamine and quetiapine immediately, the effects continued to build over 32 weeks. The use of the term 'rapid-acting antidepressant' might be reconsidered in light of these results.

Mechanism

At present, the precise mechanisms of action for the antidepressant effects of ketamine and esketamine are not clear, but it has been proposed these effects are mediated via blockade of NMDA receptors on gamma-aminobutyric acid (GABA)ergic interneurons that normally act to suppress glutamate release from glutamatergic neurons.[14] This disinhibition results in an acute cortical glutamate surge, activation of post-synaptic alpha-amino-3-hydroxy-5-methyl-4-isoxazolepropionic acid (AMPA) receptors, with downstream effects on synaptogenesis and neuroplastic pathways.[14]

Route of administration

The optimal method for administering ketamine for TRD is not fully established. IV ketamine (0.5mg/kg over 40 minutes) is the gold standard for off-label ketamine administration, with the best supporting evidence for efficacy, and may be more effective than intranasal administration.[15,16] Other routes of administration have also been proposed including subcutaneous, intramuscular, oral and sublingual, although further research is needed to qualify the relative efficacy and safety of these routes, as well as the optimal dosing regimen in each case. Each route has its own advantages and challenges in terms of bioavailability, duration of effect, practicality and patient comfort. While no definitive dosing strategy for ketamine has been established across the different routes and doses tested, in Table 3.6 we provide a summary of dosing recommendations, considering available evidence and clinical experience. Novel formulations of oral ketamine are under development.[17]

Adverse effects

Ketamine generally leads to significant dissociative symptoms when given at antidepressant doses.[18] These symptoms include perceptual distortions and can lead to significant anxiety. As a result, it is necessary that any patients administered ketamine should be observed by a trained clinician during dosing and for 1 hour after administration. Although a rare event, ketamine has also been reported to induce laryngospasm and so the observing clinician should be trained in intermediate or advanced life support. When ketamine is given at lower doses by oral or sublingual routes, it is less likely to induce strong dissociative symptoms so, once a test dose has been given under clinical supervision, it may be possible for administration to take place in a non-clinical (home) setting, although patients should be advised not to drive, operate heavy machinery or partake in other high-risk activities for at least 1 hour after administration. In addition, consideration must be given by the prescribing clinician to the risks of diversion and illegal use.

Ketamine can have significant effects on blood pressure and heart rate. Before administration, a physical examination including baseline blood pressure, full blood count, liver function test, thyroid function test plus ECG is recommended. Physical monitoring (blood pressure and heart rate) during and after ketamine administration is also indicated.

In longer-term illicit use, ketamine is associated with urinary pain, epithelial bladder barrier damage, reduced bladder capacity, ureter stenosis and kidney failure.[19] Although this ketamine-induced cystitis is a recognised complication of recreational use of ketamine, its occurrence in therapeutic use of ketamine in depression has so far not been widely reported but remains a concern.[20]

Table 3.6 Dosing recommendations for different routes of ketamine administration and intranasal esketamine in treatment-resistant depression.

Route	Dose	Details	Frequency	Comments
IV[2-6]	■ 0.5mg/kg, increasing up to 1.0mg/kg if no response (limited support for doses higher than 0.5mg/kg[16]) (titrate from 0.25mg/kg in older people)	■ Infuse over 40 minutes	■ Induction phase: once or twice a week ■ Maintenance phase: according to response, weekly then every 2 weeks, or even monthly (consider supplementing with oral/sublingual doses between IV treatments)	■ Must be administered in clinical setting ■ Cognitive effects (confusion, dissociation, etc.) do occasionally occur ■ Associated with transient increase in BP, tachycardia and arrhythmias. Pretreatment ECG required. Monitor BP before and after infusion. ■ Observe during and for 1 hour after infusion

(Continued)

Table 3.6 (*Continued*)

Route	Dose	Details	Frequency	Comments
SC[21,22]	▪ 0.5mg/kg, increasing up to 1.0mg/kg if no response (titrate from 0.25mg/kg in older people)	▪ SC bolus injection to appropriate SC site	▪ As per IV above	▪ As per IV above ▪ May be better tolerated than IV or IM routes[21]
IM[23,24]	▪ 0.5mg/kg, increasing up to 1.0mg/kg if no response (titrate from 0.25mg/kg in older people)	▪ IM bolus injection to appropriate IM site	▪ As per IV above	▪ As per IV above
Oral[25–27]	▪ 0.5–5.0mg/kg depending on dosing strategy	▪ Oral capsules	▪ Regular lower doses: 　▪ 0.5–2.0mg/kg every 1–3 days ▪ Intermittent higher doses to supplement IV/SC/IM treatment: 　▪ 2.0–5.0mg/kg once or twice a week	▪ Can be taken at home ▪ Lower doses show good tolerability, however, antidepressant effects not as rapid as IV/SC/IM ▪ Higher doses may be practical alternative to maintain response to IV/SC/IM treatment. Titrate dose according to response/adverse effects.
Sublingual[27–29]	▪ 0.5–3.0mg/kg depending on dosing strategy	▪ Ketamine solution (held under tongue for 5 minutes and swallowed) ▪ Sublingual ketamine lozenges	▪ Regular lower doses: 　▪ 0.5–1.5mg/kg every 1–3 days 　▪ Limited evidence for very low sublingual dosing (10mg every 2–3 days or weekly)[30] ▪ Intermittent higher doses to supplement IV/SC/IM treatment: 　▪ 1.5–3.0mg/kg once or twice a week	▪ Can be taken at home ▪ Lower doses show good tolerability, however putative antidepressant effects not as rapid as IV/SC/IM ▪ Higher doses may be used as practical alternative to maintain response to IV/SC/IM treatment. Titrate dose according to response/adverse effects.
Intranasal esketamine[31–34]	▪ 56–84mg (28mg in older people)	▪ 28mg in two sprays (1 spray per nostril) ▪ Repeat after 5 minutes, depending on total dose required	▪ Twice weekly, then weekly, then every 2 weeks	▪ Must be administered in clinical setting ▪ Cognitive effects (confusion, dissociation, etc.) do occasionally occur ▪ Associated with transient increase in BP, tachycardia and arrhythmias. Pretreatment ECG recommended. Monitor BP before and after dose. ▪ Observe for approximately 2 hours after dose

CHAPTER 3

References

1. Berman RM, et al. Antidepressant effects of ketamine in depressed patients. *Biol Psychiatry* 2000; **47**:351–354.
2. Zarate CA, Jr., et al. A randomized trial of an N-methyl-D-aspartate antagonist in treatment-resistant major depression. *Arch Gen Psychiatry* 2006; **63**:856–864.
3. Diazgranados N, et al. A randomized add-on trial of an N-methyl-D-aspartate antagonist in treatment-resistant bipolar depression. *Arch Gen Psychiatry* 2010; **67**:793–802.
4. Murrough JW, et al. Antidepressant efficacy of ketamine in treatment-resistant major depression: a two-site randomized controlled trial. *Am J Psychiatry* 2013; **170**:1134–1142.
5. Singh JB, et al. A double-blind, randomized, placebo-controlled, dose-frequency study of intravenous ketamine in patients with treatment-resistant depression. *Am J Psychiatry* 2016; **173**:816–826.
6. Fava M, et al. Double-blind, placebo-controlled, dose-ranging trial of intravenous ketamine as adjunctive therapy in treatment-resistant depression (TRD). *Mol Psychiatry* 2020; **25**:1592–1603.
7. Li S, et al. Effects of ketamine and esketamine on preventing postpartum depression after cesarean delivery: a meta-analysis. *J Affect Disord* 2024; **351**:720–728.
8. Ma S, et al. Association between esketamine interventions and postpartum depression and analgesia following cesarean delivery: a systematic review and meta-analysis. *Am J Obstet Gynecol MFM* 2024; **6**:101241.
9. Wang S, et al. Efficacy of a single low dose of esketamine after childbirth for mothers with symptoms of prenatal depression: randomised clinical trial. *BMJ* 2024; **385**:e078218.
10. Ren L, et al. Comparative efficacy and tolerability of different anesthetics in electroconvulsive therapy for major depressive disorder: a systematic review and network meta-analysis. *J Psychiatr Res* 2024; **171**:116–125.
11. de A Simoes Moreira D, et al. Efficacy and adverse effects of ketamine versus electroconvulsive therapy for major depressive disorder: a systematic review and meta-analysis. *J Affect Disord* 2023; **330**:227–238.
12. Menon V, et al. Ketamine vs electroconvulsive therapy for major depressive episode: a systematic review and meta-analysis. *JAMA Psychiatry* 2023; **80**:639–642.
13. Reif A, et al. Esketamine nasal spray versus quetiapine for treatment-resistant depression. *N Engl J Med* 2023; **389**:1298–1309.
14. Lener MS, et al. Glutamate and gamma-aminobutyric acid systems in the pathophysiology of major depression and antidepressant response to ketamine. *Biol Psychiatry* 2017; **81**:886–897.
15. Terao I, et al. Comparative efficacy, tolerability and acceptability of intravenous racemic ketamine with intranasal esketamine, aripiprazole and lithium as augmentative treatments for treatment-resistant unipolar depression: a systematic review and network meta-analysis. *J Affect Disord* 2024; **346**:49–56.
16. Seshadri A, et al. Efficacy of intravenous ketamine and intranasal esketamine with dose escalation for major depression: a systematic review and meta-analysis. *J Affect Disord* 2024; **356**:379–384.
17. Glue P, et al. Safety and efficacy of extended release ketamine tablets in patients with treatment-resistant depression and anxiety: open label pilot study. *Ther Adv Psychopharmacol* 2020; **10**:2045125320922474.
18. Beck K, et al. Association of ketamine with psychiatric symptoms and implications for its therapeutic use and for understanding schizophrenia: a systematic review and meta-analysis. *JAMA Netw Open* 2020; **3**:e204693.
19. Anderson DJ, et al. Ketamine-induced cystitis: a comprehensive review of the urologic effects of this psychoactive drug. *Health Psychol Res* 2022; **10**:38247.
20. Chang M, et al. Ketamine cystitis following ketamine therapy for treatment-resistant depression - case report. *BMC Psychiatry* 2024; **24**:9.
21. Loo CK, et al. Placebo-controlled pilot trial testing dose titration and intravenous, intramuscular and subcutaneous routes for ketamine in depression. *Acta Psychiatr Scand* 2016; **134**:48–56.
22. George D, et al. Pilot randomized controlled trial of titrated subcutaneous ketamine in older patients with treatment-resistant depression. *Am J Geriatr Psychiatry* 2017; **25**:1199–1209.
23. Glue P, et al. Dose- and exposure-response to ketamine in depression. *Biol Psychiatry* 2011; **70**:e9–e10; author reply e11–e12.
24. Cusin C, et al. Long-term maintenance with intramuscular ketamine for treatment-resistant bipolar II depression. *Am J Psychiatry* 2012; **169**:868–869.
25. Arabzadeh S, et al. Does oral administration of ketamine accelerate response to treatment in major depressive disorder? Results of a double-blind controlled trial. *J Affect Disord* 2018; **235**:236–241.
26. Domany Y, et al. Repeated oral ketamine for out-patient treatment of resistant depression: randomised, double-blind, placebo-controlled, proof-of-concept study. *Br J Psychiatry* 2019; **214**:20–26.
27. Rosenblat JD, et al. Oral ketamine for depression: a systematic review. *J Clin Psychiatry* 2019; **80**:18r12475.
28. Swainson J, et al. Sublingual ketamine: an option for increasing accessibility of ketamine treatments for depression? *J Clin Psychiatry* 2020; **81**:19lr13146.
29. Nguyen L, et al. Off-label use of transmucosal ketamine as a rapid-acting antidepressant: a retrospective chart review. *Neuropsychiatr Dis Treat* 2015; **11**:2667–2673.
30. Lara DR, et al. Antidepressant, mood stabilizing and procognitive effects of very low dose sublingual ketamine in refractory unipolar and bipolar depression. *Int J Neuropsychopharmacol* 2013; **16**:2111–2117.

CHAPTER 3

31. Canuso CM, et al. Efficacy and safety of intranasal esketamine for the rapid reduction of symptoms of depression and suicidality in patients at imminent risk for suicide: results of a double-blind, randomized, placebo-controlled study. *Am J Psychiatry* 2018; **175**:620–630.

32. Daly EJ, et al. Efficacy and safety of intranasal esketamine adjunctive to oral antidepressant therapy in treatment-resistant depression: a randomized clinical trial. *JAMA Psychiatry* 2018; **75**:139–148.

33. Popova V, et al. Efficacy and safety of flexibly dosed esketamine nasal spray combined with a newly initiated oral antidepressant in treatment-resistant depression: a randomized double-blind active-controlled study. *Am J Psychiatry* 2019; **176**:428–438.

34. Daly EJ, et al. Efficacy of esketamine nasal spray plus oral antidepressant treatment for relapse prevention in patients with treatment-resistant depression: a randomized clinical trial. *JAMA Psychiatry* 2019; **76**:893–903.

Psychotic depression

Psychotic depression represents a severe manifestation of depression. It is diagnosed in people experiencing a major depressive illness accompanied by psychotic symptoms such as hallucinations and/or delusions. It can occur in the context of both MDD and bipolar disorder. Psychotic depression has a lifetime prevalence of 1%.[1] However, it is often under-diagnosed and is commonly not adequately identified despite requiring a different treatment approach.[2,3] When compared with non-psychotic depression, psychotic depression is associated with greater illness severity, impairment and episode duration.[4] Once an individual has experienced psychotic symptoms during a depressive episode there is a risk of their recurrence in future episodes.[4,5] Furthermore, long-term outcomes are generally poorer for psychotic than non-psychotic depression.[6–8] Patients with psychotic depression may also have a poorer response to combined pharmacological and psychological treatment than those with non-psychotic depression.[9] People with psychotic depression are much more likely than those with non-psychotic depression to attempt and complete suicide.[8,10]

Acute treatment

While it is important to acknowledge that no treatments have been granted regulatory approval specifically for psychotic depression,[11] there is sufficient evidence to guide treatment decisions. Oliva and colleagues[12] conducted a systematic review and network meta-analysis of pharmacological treatments for psychotic depression in 2024. This network meta-analysis included 14 randomised controlled trials including patients in the acute phase of their illness. It found that, compared with placebo, the combination of an SSRI and an SGA, particularly fluoxetine and olanzapine, resulted in the highest proportion of participants with a treatment response.[12] Overall, this specific combination also showed a good balance between efficacy and tolerability and specifically improved depressive symptom scores compared with placebo.[12] The network meta-analysis concluded that this treatment option is the most appropriate choice in people with psychotic depression.[12]

When different treatment options were compared directly, a combination of antipsychotics and antidepressants was also found to have greater efficacy than monotherapy with either antipsychotic or antidepressant alone.[12] Prior meta-analyses support this outcome, although they were not able to provide specific recommendations on individual drugs because of methodological restrictions.[13,14] UK NICE guidance from 2022, although written some time before the latest network meta-analysis, also advocates this approach.[11,15]

The 2024 network meta-analysis also compared monotherapies and found that TCAs (amoxapine and imipramine) were more efficacious than serotonin–noradrenaline reuptake inhibitors (SNRIs; venlafaxine) and noradrenergic and specific serotonergic reuptake inhibitors (mirtazapine) when overall treatment response was assessed.[12]

It is important to consider that this network meta-analysis only included patients in the acute phase of their illness. Continuation and maintenance studies were excluded. In addition, it only included studies published up to 2013, so drugs used in clinical practice more recently could not be examined.

Ketamine formulations

Many of the more recent studies include ketamine and esketamine, which are increasingly used to treat MDD and bipolar affective disorder,[16] and are possibly efficacious for psychotic depression.[17] Evidence is limited because people with psychotic depression are usually excluded from clinical trials owing to the concern that these drugs may worsen psychotic symptoms, albeit transiently.[17,18] Le et al.[17] reviewed the evidence for the use of ketamine in the treatment of psychotic depression. This comprised two case series, three case reports ($n = 1$), one retrospective chart review ($n = 12$) and one secondary analysis of a randomised controlled trial ($n = 10$). Most patients received ketamine 0.5mg/kg IV (fewer received SC), infused over 40 minutes. The number of treatments was very varied, ranging from one to seven over a number of weeks (approximately 3–8 weeks). The patients in the retrospective chart review were given 30–120mg intranasally at intervals of 3–7 days. A 2023 study[16] examined the effects of add-on ketamine (0.5mg/kg IV twice a week) in 36 patients and found improvements in all domains.

Overall, these lines of evidence indicated that ketamine reduces depressive symptoms and, in a few cases, psychotic symptoms as well. The review did not describe any patients experiencing a worsening of psychotic symptoms. However, all these studies had very small sample sizes. A case series including four patients also provides some limited evidence for the safety and efficacy of esketamine (0.5mg/kg IV or SC) for the treatment of TRD with psychotic features.[19]

ECT

There is a role for ECT in the treatment of psychotic depression, especially where a rapid response is required. Pooled analysis of the two largest sham-controlled ECT trials found a significant improvement in depressive scores with real ECT compared with simulated ECT in patients with depression and delusional features at 4 weeks. However, there was no significant difference between these groups at 6 months.[20] ECT is effective in MDD (see section on ECT and psychotropic drugs in this chapter) and a few studies indicate that ECT may be more efficacious in people with depression with psychotic features.[21–23] ECT may also be more protective against relapse in psychotic depression than in non-psychotic depression.[24,25] One small RCT demonstrated superiority of maintenance ECT plus nortriptyline over nortriptyline alone at 2 years.[26]

Maintenance treatment

Generally, acute treatment should be continued. Evidence from the STOP-PD II (Study of the Pharmacotherapy of Psychotic Depression II) trial suggested that withdrawal of olanzapine from sertraline co-therapy worsens outcomes in the medium term.[27,28] Relapse was more than twice as likely in the sertraline placebo group than in the combination group (55% vs 20%) and almost all the excess risk of relapse occurred in the first 2 months. However, one in five patients in the combined group relapsed over 36 weeks from randomisation into the single drug phase of the study (people were on the combination for much longer than this as all patients in the study started on the combination therapy prior to the 8-week remission phase needed prior to randomisation to monotherapy).[4] The evidence from this study suggests that combined treatment for 4–6 months after remission may be relatively effective at preventing a recurrence in psychotic depression.[4] In the UK, NICE[15] suggests continuing antipsychotic medication for a number of months after remission, but it is not clear how long combination therapy should be continued past this point. This decision could be based on patient preference and adverse effect profile (e.g. weight gain). Options might include slowly tapering the antipsychotic with reintroduction if psychotic symptoms return or switching to an antipsychotic with different adverse effects. Currently there is no evidence to support the best way to do this.

Other treatments

Another potential treatment approach is based on glucocorticoid receptor blocking strategies, since hypothalamic–pituitary–adrenal axis hyperactivity is more common in psychotic depression. A combined analysis of data from five double-blind trials (mifepristone n = 833, placebo n = 627) evaluating the efficacy and safety of 7 days' treatment with mifepristone compared with placebo found that mifepristone reduced psychotic symptoms.[29] Patients with a high mifepristone plasma level ($\geq$1637ng/mL) showed a more significant treatment response.[29]

There is an anecdotal report of the successful use of methylphenidate in a patient who did not respond to robust doses of an antidepressant and antipsychotic combined.[30] Other case reports describe successful outcomes with lamotrigine[31] and a combination of phenelzine, aripiprazole and quetiapine.[32] Minocycline has also shown some effect, albeit in an open study.[33]

Summary

- In the acute phase of psychotic depression, the combination of an antipsychotic and antidepressant is the best treatment option. The strongest evidence is for a combination of olanzapine and fluoxetine.
- Monotherapy is less effective than combined therapy but if this is the best approach for the patient, TCAs are the drugs of choice.
- If using combined therapy, treat with this combination for at least 4–6 months after remission. After this time, consider slowly tapering the antipsychotic but make a decision based on risk (e.g. metabolic syndrome) and potential benefit (e.g. past history of relapse and psychosis).
- ECT is an effective treatment. Consider when a rapid response is required or where other treatments have failed.
- Ketamine formulations may be effective but are not first-line agents.

References

1. Jääskeläinen E, et al. Epidemiology of psychotic depression: systematic review and meta-analysis. *Psychol Med* 2018; 48:905–918.
2. Heslin M, et al. Psychotic major depression: challenges in clinical practice and research. *Br J Psychiatry* 2018; 212:131–133.
3. Rothschild AJ, et al. Missed diagnosis of psychotic depression at 4 academic medical centers. *J Clin Psychiatry* 2008; 69:1293–1296.
4. Coryell WH. Maintenance treatment for psychotic depressive disorders: progress and remaining challenges. *JAMA* 2019; 322:615–617.
5. Tohen M, et al. Two-year outcomes in first-episode psychotic depression the McLean–Harvard First-Episode Project. *J Affect Disord* 2012; 136:1–8.
6. Flint AJ, et al. Two-year outcome of psychotic depression in late life. *Am J Psychiatry* 1998; 155:178–183.

7. Maj M, et al. Phenomenology and prognostic significance of delusions in major depressive disorder: a 10-year prospective follow-up study. *J Clin Psychiatry* 2007; **68**:1411–1417.

8. Paljärvi T, et al. Mortality in psychotic depression: 18-year follow-up study. *Br J Psychiatry* 2023; **222**:37-43.

9. Gaudiano BA, et al. Differential response to combined treatment in patients with psychotic versus nonpsychotic major depression. *J Nerv Ment Dis* 2005; **193**:625–628.

10. Gournellis R, et al. Psychotic (delusional) depression and suicidal attempts: a systematic review and meta-analysis. *Acta Psychiatr Scand* 2018; **137**:18–29.

11. Kendrick T, et al. Management of depression in adults: summary of updated NICE guidance. *BMJ* 2022; **378**:o1557.

12. Oliva V, et al. Pharmacological treatments for psychotic depression: a systematic review and network meta-analysis. *Lancet Psychiatry* 2024; **11**:210–220.

13. Kruizinga J, et al. Pharmacological treatment for psychotic depression. *Cochrane Database Syst Rev* 2021; **12**:CD004044.

14. Farahani A, et al. Are antipsychotics or antidepressants needed for psychotic depression? A systematic review and meta-analysis of trials comparing antidepressant or antipsychotic monotherapy with combination treatment. *J Clin Psychiatry* 2012; **73**:486–496.

15. National Institute for Health and Care Excellence. Depression in adults: treatment and management. NICE guideline [NG222]. 2022 (last updated May 2024, last checked May 2024); https://www.nice.org.uk/guidance/ng222.

16. Gałuszko-Węgielnik M, et al. Central nervous system-related safety and tolerability of add-on ketamine to standard of care treatment in treatment-resistant psychotic depression in patients with major depressive disorder and bipolar disorder. *Front Neurosci* 2023; **17**:1214972.

17. Le TT, et al. Ketamine for psychotic depression: an overview of the glutamatergic system and ketamine's mechanisms associated with antidepressant and psychotomimetic effects. *Psychiatry Res* 2021; **306**:114231.

18. Beck K, et al. Association of ketamine with psychiatric symptoms and implications for its therapeutic use and for understanding schizophrenia: a systematic review and meta-analysis. *JAMA Netw Open* 2020; **3**:e204693.

19. Ajub E, et al. Efficacy of esketamine in the treatment of depression with psychotic features: a case series. *Biol Psychiatry* 2018; **83**:e15–e16.

20. Buchan H, et al. Who benefits from electroconvulsive therapy? Combined results of the Leicester and Northwick Park trials. *Br J Psychiatry* 1992; **160**:355–359.

21. Heijnen W, et al. Influence of age on ECT efficacy in depression and the mediating role of psychomotor retardation and psychotic features. *J Psychiatr Res* 2019; **109**:41–47.

22. Pinna M, et al. Clinical and biological predictors of response to electroconvulsive therapy (ECT): a review. *Neurosci Lett* 2018; **669**:32–42.

23. Spaans HP, et al. Early complete remitters after electroconvulsive therapy: profile and prognosis. *J ECT* 2016; **32**:82–87.

24. Birkenhager TK, et al. One-year outcome of psychotic depression after successful electroconvulsive therapy. *J ECT* 2005; **21**:221–226.

25. Wagenmakers MJ, et al. Psychotic late-life depression less likely to relapse after electroconvulsive therapy. *J Affect Disord* 2020; **276**:984–990.

26. Navarro V, et al. Continuation/maintenance treatment with nortriptyline versus combined nortriptyline and ECT in late-life psychotic depression: a two-year randomized study. *Am J Geriatr Psychiatry* 2008; **16**:498–505.

27. Bingham KS, et al. Stabilization treatment of remitted psychotic depression: the STOP-PD study. *Acta Psychiatr Scand* 2018; **138**:267–273.

28. Flint AJ, et al. Effect of continuing olanzapine vs placebo on relapse among patients with psychotic depression in remission: the STOP-PD II randomized clinical trial. *JAMA* 2019; **322**:622–631.

29. Block T, et al. Mifepristone plasma level and glucocorticoid receptor antagonism associated with response in patients with psychotic depression. *J Clin Psychopharmacol* 2017; **37**:505–511.

30. Huang CC, et al. Adjunctive use of methylphenidate in the treatment of psychotic unipolar depression. *Clin Neuropharmacol* 2008; **31**:245–247.

31. Kajiya T, et al. Effect of lamotrigine in the treatment of bipolar depression with psychotic features: a case report. *Ann Gen Psychiatry* 2017; **16**:31.

32. Meyer JM, et al. Augmentation of phenelzine with aripiprazole and quetiapine in a treatment-resistant patient with psychotic unipolar depression: case report and literature review. *CNS Spectr* 2017; **22**:391–396.

33. Miyaoka T, et al. Minocycline as adjunctive therapy for patients with unipolar psychotic depression: an open-label study. *Prog Neuropsychopharmacol Biol Psychiatry* 2012; **37**:222–226.

CHAPTER 3

Switching antidepressants

General guidelines

When changing from one antidepressant to another, abrupt withdrawal of the first drug should be avoided unless there has been a serious adverse event. Cross-tapering is usually preferred – the dose of the ineffective or poorly tolerated drug is slowly reduced while the new drug is slowly introduced. The time taken to withdraw from the first antidepressant is dependent on the drug, the dose, the duration of prior treatment and the drug to which the patient is being switched.[1]

		Daily dose			
Example		Week 1	Week 2	Week 3	Week 4
Withdrawing **citalopram**	40mg	20mg	10mg	5mg	2.5mg
Introducing **mirtazapine**	Nil	15mg	30mg	30mg	45mg (if required)

- The speed of cross-tapering is best judged by patient tolerability. Extended periods of hyperbolic tapering may be necessary to mitigate withdrawal symptoms when they emerge.[2]
- Cross-tapering is not always possible. The co-administration of some antidepressants, even when cross-tapering, is absolutely contraindicated. In other cases, theoretical risks or lack of experience preclude recommending cross-tapering.
- The switching strategy depends not only on the reason for switching – inadequate or non-response, poor tolerability or adverse effects – but also on the pharmacokinetic and pharmacodynamic properties of the antidepressants involved.[3–5]
- In some cases, cross-tapering may not be necessary. For example, people who have been treated with an antidepressant for less than 3–4 weeks can probably safely stop abruptly and the new antidepressant can be started the next day. Another example is when switching between SSRIs – their effects may be so similar that administration of the second drug is likely to ameliorate withdrawal effects of the first. The use of fluoxetine has been advocated as an abrupt switch treatment to mitigate SSRI discontinuation symptoms[6] (but see below). Abrupt cessation may also, albeit rarely, be acceptable when switching to a drug with a similar, but not identical, mode of action.[7] Thus, in some cases, abruptly stopping one antidepressant and starting another at the usual dose may not only be well tolerated but may also reduce the risk and severity of discontinuation symptoms.
- It is usually advisable to reduce the first antidepressant to the minimum effective dose before directly switching to the minimum effective dose of the second (see section on recognised minimum effective doses of antidepressants in this chapter).

- Stop–start switching is not always successful, particularly when switching to fluoxetine. The probable reason for this is that plasma levels of fluoxetine and its active metabolite take time to build up to steady state – usually 1–2 weeks. So, even when switching from an apparently equivalent dose (say 20mg paroxetine to 20mg fluoxetine) the plasma levels after one 20mg dose[8] of fluoxetine are only 20% of plasma concentration at steady state.[9] Thus, this switch is effectively an 80% reduction in drug activity. Withdrawal reactions are almost inevitable. There is more discussion of this and other relevant issues in the *Maudsley Deprescribing Guidelines*.[10]

- Potential dangers of simultaneously administering two antidepressants include pharmacodynamic interactions (serotonin syndrome, hypotension, drowsiness – depending on the drugs involved) and pharmacokinetic interactions (e.g. elevation of the co-administered antidepressant plasma levels by some SSRIs). In the absence of inhibitory pharmacokinetic interactions, it is best to keep the combined percentage maximum dose below 100% (e.g. 50% maximum dose of one drug + 50% maximum dose of another).

- Agomelatine does not seem to be associated with a discontinuation syndrome,[11] but slow withdrawal when switching is nonetheless recommended. Given agomelatine's mode of action (melatonin agonism; $5HT_{2C}$ antagonism), it is not expected to mitigate discontinuation reactions of other antidepressants. There is no theoretical basis to suggest that pharmacodynamic interactions might occur between agomelatine and other co-administered antidepressants but, in the absence of useful data, caution is advised. Some pharmacokinetic interactions do occur, and agomelatine should not be administered with fluvoxamine or viloxazine.

- Serotonin syndrome can occur with a single serotonergic drug at a therapeutic dose or more commonly in combination of serotonergic drugs or in overdose. Many severe cases of serotonin syndrome involve an MAOI (including moclobemide) plus an SSRI.[12,13] Caution is advised when switching strategies call for the combining of serotonergic drugs.

Serotonin syndrome – symptoms

Increasing severity

Severity	Symptoms
Mild	Insomnia, anxiety, nausea, diarrhoea, hypertension, tachycardia, hyper-reflexia
Moderate	Agitation, myoclonus, tremor, mydriasis, flushing, diaphoresis, low fever (<38.5°C)
Severe	Severe hyperthermia, confusion, rigidity, respiratory failure, coma, death

The advice given in Table 3.7 should be treated with caution and patients should be very carefully monitored when switching.

CHAPTER 3

Table 3.7 Antidepressants – swapping and stopping.*

From \ To	Agomelatine	Bupropion	Clomipramine	Fluoxetine	Fluvoxamine	MAOIs Phenelzine Tranylcypromine Selegiline
Agomelatine[a]		Cross-taper cautiously	Cross-taper cautiously	Cross-taper cautiously	Stop agomelatine then start fluvoxamine	Cross-taper cautiously
Bupropion[b]	Cross-taper cautiously		Cross-taper cautiously with low-dose clomipramine	Cross-taper cautiously	Cross-taper cautiously	Taper and stop then wait for 2 weeks then start MAOIs
Clomipramine	Cross-taper cautiously	Cross-taper cautiously		Taper and stop then start fluoxetine at 10mg/day	Taper and stop then start low-dose fluvoxamine	Taper and stop then wait for 3 weeks then start MAOIs
Fluoxetine[c]	Cross-taper cautiously	Stop fluoxetine then wait for 4–7 days then start bupropion	Stop fluoxetine then wait for 2 weeks then start low-dose clomipramine		Stop fluoxetine then wait for 4–7 days then start fluvoxamine	Stop fluoxetine then wait for 5–6 weeks then start MAOIs
Fluvoxamine[d]	Taper and stop then wait for 4 days	Cross-taper cautiously	Taper and stop then start low-dose clomipramine	Direct switch possible^		Taper and stop then wait for 1 week then start MAOIs
MAOIs Phenelzine Tranylcypromine Selegiline	Cross-taper cautiously	Taper and stop then wait for 2 weeks	Taper and stop then wait for 3 weeks	Taper and stop then wait for 2 weeks	Taper and stop then wait for 2 weeks	Taper and stop then wait for 2 weeks
Moclobemide	Taper and stop then wait for 24 hours	Taper and stop then wait for 24 hours	Taper and stop then wait for 24 hours	Taper and stop then wait for 24 hours	Taper and stop then wait for 24 hours	Taper and stop then wait for 24 hours then start MAOIs
Mirtazapine	Cross-taper cautiously	Cross-taper cautiously	Cross-taper cautiously	Cross-taper cautiously	Cross-taper cautiously	Taper and stop then wait for 2 weeks
Reboxetine[e]	Cross-taper cautiously	Cross-taper cautiously	Cross-taper cautiously	Cross-taper cautiously	Cross-taper cautiously	Taper and stop then wait for 1 week then start MAOIs

Moclobemide	Mirtazapine	Reboxetine	Trazodone	Other SSRIs[f] Vortioxetine	SNRIs Duloxetine Venlafaxine Desvenlafaxine	TCAs (except clomipramine)	Viloxazine
Cross-taper cautiously	Cross-taper cautiously	Cross-taper cautiously	Cross-taper cautiously	Cross-taper cautiously	Cross-taper cautiously	Cross-taper cautiously	Stop agomelatine then start viloxazine
Taper and stop then start moclobemide	Cross-taper cautiously	Cross-taper cautiously	Cross-taper cautiously	Cross-taper cautiously	Cross-taper cautiously	Cross-taper cautiously with low-dose TCA	Cross-taper cautiously
Taper and stop then wait for 1 week then start moclobemide	Cross-taper cautiously	Cross-taper cautiously	Cross-taper cautiously	Taper and stop then start low dose	Taper and stop then start low-dose SNRI	Cross-taper cautiously	Cross-taper cautiously
Stop fluoxetine then wait for 5–6 weeks then start moclobemide	Cross-taper cautiously	Cross-taper cautiously	Cross-taper cautiously	Stop fluoxetine then wait for 4–7 days then start low dose	Stop fluoxetine then wait for 4–7 days then start SNRI	Stop fluoxetine then wait for 4–7 days then start low-dose TCA	Cross-taper cautiously
Taper and stop then wait for 1 week then start moclobemide	Cross-taper cautiously then start mirtazapine at 15mg	Cross-taper cautiously	Cross-taper cautiously	Direct switch possible	Direct switch possible	Cross-taper cautiously with low-dose TCA	Cross-taper cautiously
Taper and stop then wait for 2 weeks then start moclobemide	Taper and stop then wait for 2 weeks	Taper and stop then wait for 2 weeks	Taper and stop then wait for 2 weeks	Taper and stop then wait for 2 weeks	Taper and stop then wait for 2 weeks	Taper and stop then wait for 2 weeks[j]	Taper and stop then wait for 2 weeks
	Taper and stop then wait for 24 hours	Taper and stop then wait for 24 hours	Taper and stop then wait for 24 hours	Taper and stop then wait for 24 hours	Taper and stop then wait for 24 hours	Taper and stop then wait for 24 hours	Taper and stop then wait for 24 hours
Taper and stop then wait for 1 week then start moclobemide		Cross-taper cautiously	Cross-taper cautiously	Cross-taper cautiously	Cross-taper cautiously	Cross-taper cautiously	Cross-taper cautiously
Taper and stop then wait for 1 week then start moclobemide	Cross-taper cautiously			Cross-taper cautiously	Cross-taper cautiously	Cross-taper cautiously	Cross-taper cautiously

(Continued)

Table 3.7 (*Continued*)

From \ To	Agomelatine	Bupropion	Clomipramine	Fluoxetine	Fluvoxamine	MAOIs Phenelzine Tranylcypromine Selegiline
Trazodone	Cross-taper cautiously	Cross-taper cautiously	Cross-taper cautiously with low-dose clomipramine	Cross-taper cautiously	Cross-taper cautiously	Taper and stop then wait for 1 week
Other SSRIs[f] **Vortioxetine**[g]	Cross-taper cautiously	Cross-taper cautiously	Taper and stop then start low-dose clomipramine	Direct switch possible^	Direct switch possible	Taper and stop then wait for 1 week[h]
SNRI Duloxetine[i] **Venlafaxine Desvenlafaxine**	Cross-taper cautiously	Cross-taper cautiously	Taper and stop then start low-dose clomipramine	Direct switch possible^	Direct switch possible	Taper and stop then wait for 1 week
Tricyclics	Cross-taper cautiously	Halve dose and add bupropion and then slow withdrawal	Direct switch possible	Halve dose and add fluoxetine and then slow withdrawal	Cross-taper cautiously	Taper and stop then wait for 2 weeks[j]
Viloxazine[k]	Taper and stop then wait for 48 hours	Cross-taper cautiously	Cross-taper cautiously	Cross-taper cautiously	Cross-taper cautiously	Taper and stop then wait for 2 weeks

Moclobemide	Mirtazapine	Reboxetine	Trazodone	Other SSRIs[f] Vortioxetine	SNRIs Duloxetine Venlafaxine Desvenlafaxine	TCAs (except clomipramine)	Viloxazine
Taper and stop then wait for 1 week then start moclobemide	Cross-taper cautiously	Cross-taper cautiously		Cross-taper cautiously	Cross-taper cautiously	Cross-taper cautiously with low-dose TCA	Cross-taper cautiously
Taper and stop then wait for 1 week then start moclobemide	Cross-taper cautiously	Cross-taper cautiously	Cross-taper cautiously	Direct switch possible	Direct switch possible	Cross-taper cautiously with low-dose TCA	Cross-taper cautiously
Taper and stop then wait for 1 week then start moclobemide	Cross-taper cautiously	Cross-taper cautiously	Cross-taper cautiously	Direct switch possible	Direct switch possible	Cross-taper cautiously with low-dose TCA	Cross-taper cautiously[k]
Taper and stop then wait for 1 week then start moclobemide	Cross-taper cautiously	Cross-taper cautiously	Halve dose and add trazodone and then slow withdrawal	Halve dose and add SSRI and then slow withdrawal	Cross-taper cautiously starting with low-dose SNRI	Direct switch possible	Cross-taper cautiously
Taper and stop then wait for 1 week then start moclobemide	Cross-taper cautiously	Cross-taper cautiously	Cross-taper cautiously	Cross-taper cautiously	Cross-taper cautiously	Cross-taper cautiously	

Notes:

* Advice given in this table is partly derived from manufacturers' information and available published data and partly theoretical. There are several factors that affect individual drug handling and caution is required in every instance. Cross taper cautiously – usually over 2–4 weeks as per example.

ᵃ Agomelatine has no effect on monoamine uptake and no affinity for α, β adrenergic, histaminergic, cholinergic, dopaminergic and benzodiazepine receptors. The potential for interactions between agomelatine and other antidepressants is low and it is not expected to mitigate discontinuation reactions of other antidepressants. Some crossover with other antidepressants might be cautiously attempted when switching from agomelatine, as indicated in the table.

ᵇ Bupropion is licensed for smoking cessation but unlicensed for the treatment of depression in the UK. It is a CYP2D6 inhibitor and particular caution is required when cross-tapering with drugs metabolised by this enzyme.

ᶜ Beware: interactions with fluoxetine may still occur for 5 weeks after stopping fluoxetine because of its metabolite's long half-life.

ᵈ Fluvoxamine is a potent inhibitor of CYP1A2, and to a lesser extent of CYP2C and CYP3A4, and has a high potential for interactions hence extra caution is required.

ᵉ Switching to reboxetine as antidepressant monotherapy is no longer recommended.

ᶠ Citalopram, escitalopram, paroxetine and sertraline.

ᵍ Limited experience with vortioxetine and extra caution is required. Take particular care when switching to or from bupropion and other CYP2D6 inhibitors such as fluoxetine and paroxetine.[14]

ʰ Wait 3 weeks in the case of vortioxetine.[15]

ⁱ Abrupt switch from SSRIs and venlafaxine to duloxetine is possible, starting at 60mg/day.[7]

ʲ Wait 3 weeks in the case of imipramine.

ᵏ Viloxazine is a selective noradrenaline reuptake inhibitor. Now licensed for the treatment of ADHD in the US. Increases in heart rate and diastolic blood pressure have been reported, so caution with SNRIs.

^ Caution when directly switching to fluoxetine. Some overlap (a few days) may be advisable to allow fluoxetine plasma concentration to build up before stopping the first antidepressant. Switching from vortioxetine is a probable exception to this, given its long half-life.

References

1. Horowitz MA, et al. Estimating risk of antidepressant withdrawal from a review of published data. *CNS Drugs* 2023; **37**:143–157.
2. Horowitz MA, et al. Tapering of SSRI treatment to mitigate withdrawal symptoms. *Lancet Psychiatry* 2019; **6**:538–546.
3. Cleare A, et al. Evidence-based guidelines for treating depressive disorders with antidepressants: a revision of the 2008 British Association for Psychopharmacology guidelines. *J Psychopharmacol* 2015; **29**:459–525.
4. Harvey BH, et al. New insights on the antidepressant discontinuation syndrome. *Hum Psychopharmacol* 2014; **29**:503–516.
5. Malhi GS, et al. Royal Australian and New Zealand College of Psychiatrists clinical practice guidelines for mood disorders. *Aust N Z J Psychiatry* 2015; **49**:1087–1206.
6. Benazzi F. Fluoxetine for the treatment of SSRI discontinuation syndrome. *Int J Neuropsychopharmacol* 2008; **11**:725-726.
7. Perahia DG, et al. Switching to duloxetine from selective serotonin reuptake inhibitor antidepressants: a multicenter trial comparing 2 switching techniques. *J Clin Psychiatry* 2008; **69**:95–105.
8. Díaz-Tufinio CA, et al. Pharmacogenetic variants associated with fluoxetine pharmacokinetics from a bioequivalence study in healthy subjects. *Journal of Personalized Medicine* 2023; **13**:1352.
9. el-Yazigi A, et al. Steady-state kinetics of fluoxetine and amitriptyline in patients treated with a combination of these drugs as compared with those treated with amitriptyline alone. *J Clin Pharmacol* 1995; **35**:17–21.
10. Horowitz M, et al. *The Maudsley Deprescribing Guidelines: Antidepressants, Benzodiazepines, Gabapentinoids and Z-drugs*. Oxford: Wiley-Blackwell; 2024.
11. Goodwin GM, et al. Agomelatine prevents relapse in patients with major depressive disorder without evidence of a discontinuation syndrome: a 24-week randomized, double-blind, placebo-controlled trial. *J Clin Psychiatry* 2009; **70**:1128–1137.
12. Buckley NA, et al. Serotonin syndrome. *BMJ* 2014; **348**:g1626.
13. Abadie D, et al. Serotonin syndrome: analysis of cases registered in the French pharmacovigilance database. *J Clin Psychopharmacol* 2015; **35**:382–388.
14. Chen G, et al. Pharmacokinetic drug interactions involving vortioxetine (Lu AA21004), a multimodal antidepressant. *Clin Drug Investig* 2013; **33**:727–736.
15. Citrome L. Vortioxetine for major depressive disorder: a systematic review of the efficacy and safety profile for this newly approved antidepressant: what is the number needed to treat, number needed to harm and likelihood to be helped or harmed? *Int J Clin Pract* 2014; **68**:60–82.

Antidepressant withdrawal symptoms

Signs and symptoms

Antidepressant withdrawal symptoms may be entirely new or similar to some of the original symptoms of the illness for which the medication was originally given. Withdrawal symptoms can be distinguished from a relapse or reoccurrence of the underlying disorder by their rapid onset (days, rather than weeks, or within three to five half-lives of the drug),[1] the rapid response to reintroduction of the antidepressant (generally within hours, certainly within days), and the presence of somatic and psychological symptoms distinct from the original illness (e.g. brain zaps, dizziness, nausea).[2] The wide variety of symptoms reported with SSRIs and related drugs is summarised in Figure 3.2. Symptoms reported with other antidepressants are summarised in Table 3.8.

Incidence and severity

Antidepressant withdrawal/discontinuation symptoms occur in many patients (Box 3.1). Incidence rates from 14 studies that examined antidepressant withdrawal ranged from 27% to 86%, with a weighted average of 56%.[3] Although reported incidence rates vary widely between studies of different drugs and methodologies (9% to 77% for fluoxetine, and from 42% to 100% with paroxetine),[3] symptoms are seen to some extent with all antidepressants, with the possible exception of agomelatine.[1] Two meta-analyses published in 2024 gave strikingly different estimates of withdrawal incidence.[4,5]

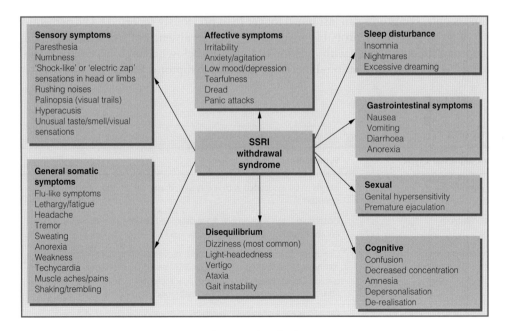

Figure 3.2 Common withdrawal symptoms with SSRIs and similar drugs.

Box 3.1 Factors influencing the incidence and severity of antidepressant withdrawal symptoms

Pharmacological factors:

- Pharmacokinetics
- Drug half-life
- Pharmacodynamics
- Receptor affinities

Treatment factors:

- Duration of treatment
- Dose
- Method of tapering

Patient-specific factors:

- Prior experience and anticipation effects

Other factors:

- Drug half-lives – correlate with the severity and onset of symptoms. Symptoms typically more severe with shorter half-life drugs (e.g. venlafaxine, paroxetine)
- Other pharmacokinetic factors: non-linear pharmacokinetics
- Receptor affinities: higher affinity for the serotonin transporter may confer higher risk of withdrawal symptoms

---

Time course

The onset and severity of symptoms are related to the half-life of the antidepressant. Placebo/nocebo effects and loss of therapeutic efficacy may also be important. Short half-life antidepressants like paroxetine and venlafaxine produce symptoms within a day or two, whereas symptoms with fluoxetine can be delayed by 2–6 weeks.[2] Symptoms can vary in duration, form and intensity and occur in any combination. While they can be mild and self-limiting, there is substantial variation between individuals and, for some people, symptoms can last much longer than previously reported.[6] The perception of symptom severity is probably made worse by the absence of forewarnings. Some symptoms are more likely with individual drugs (see below). Symptoms can be quantified using the Discontinuation–Emergent Signs and Symptoms Scale.[7]

Table 3.8 Symptoms reported with other (non-SSRI) antidepressants.

Antidepressant type	Symptoms
Agomelatine	Seems to be associated with a very low, if any, risk of discontinuation symptoms[1]
Bupropion	Uncommon, but case reports have described anxiety, headache, insomnia, irritability and myalgias;[8,9] single case report of acute dystonia[10]
Monoamine oxidase inhibitors*	Common: agitation, irritability, ataxia, movement disorders, insomnia, somnolence, vivid dreams, cognitive impairment, slowed speech, pressured speech. Occasionally, hallucinations, paranoid delusions. RIMAs: flu-like symptoms reported with moclobemide.[11]
NaSSAs (e.g. mirtazapine)	Panic, anxiety, restlessness, irritability, hypomania, insomnia, dizziness, paraesthesia, nausea, vomiting[10]

(Continued)

Antidepressant type	Symptoms
Serotonin modulators (vortioxetine, vilazodone)	None reported,[10] although these are relatively new antidepressants with less clinical experience. Shared pharmacological actions with other antidepressants (SSRIs) so possibility of withdrawal symptoms cannot be discounted.[10]
TCAs	General somatic and GI distress, sleep disturbances characterised by initial and middle insomnia or excessively vivid and frightening dreams, akathisia or parkinsonism, hypomania or mania, cardiac arrhythmia[10]
Trazodone	Hypomania, anxiety, restless sleep, nightmares, depersonalisation, formication, headache[10]

Table 3.8 *(Continued)*

* Tranylcypromine may have amfetamine-like properties at higher doses[12] and therefore could be associated with a true 'withdrawal syndrome'. Delirium may occur.[13]

NaSSA, noradrenergic and specific serotonergic antidepressant; RIMA, reversible inhibitor of monoamine oxidase A; TCA, tricyclic antidepressant.

Clinical relevance[14,15]

The symptoms of a withdrawal reaction may be mistaken for a relapse of illness or the emergence of a new physical illness,[16] leading to unnecessary investigations or reintroduction of the antidepressant. Symptoms may be severe enough to interfere with daily functioning and those who have experienced discontinuation symptoms may reason (perhaps understandably) that antidepressants are 'addictive' and not wish to accept treatment. There is also evidence of emergent suicidal thoughts on discontinuation with paroxetine.[17]

Who is at risk?[10,14–16,18]

Although anyone can experience discontinuation symptoms, the risk is increased in those prescribed short half-life drugs (e.g. paroxetine, venlafaxine),[7] particularly if they do not take them regularly. Two-thirds of patients prescribed antidepressants skip a few doses from time to time,[19] and many patients stop their antidepressant abruptly.[20] The risk is also increased in those who have been taking antidepressants for 8 weeks or longer,[21] those taking antidepressants at higher doses, those who have developed anxiety symptoms at the start of antidepressant therapy (particularly with SSRIs), those receiving other centrally acting medication (e.g. antihypertensives, antihistamines, antipsychotics), children and adolescents,[7] younger patients,[22] and those who have experienced withdrawal symptoms before.

How to avoid[14–16,18]

Generally, antidepressant therapy should be discontinued gradually.[6] The shorter the half-life of the drug, the more important it is that this rule is followed. The end of the taper may need to be slower, as symptoms may not appear until the reduction in the total daily dosage of the antidepressant is (proportionately) substantial. Patients receiving MAOIs may need to be tapered over a longer period. Tranylcypromine may be particularly difficult to stop.[13] At-risk patients (see above) may need a slower taper. Agomelatine can probably be stopped abruptly without provoking withdrawal symptoms but should be slowly withdrawn as a matter of principle – all psychotropic drugs should be slowly withdrawn where possible.

Many people suffer symptoms despite slow withdrawal and even if they have received adequate education regarding withdrawal symptoms.[7,17] This may be because hyperbolic tapering is not employed (see section on stopping antidepressants in this chapter).

How to treat[14–16,23]

There are few systematic studies in this area. Treatment is pragmatic. If symptoms are mild, reassure the patient that these symptoms are common after discontinuing an antidepressant and will pass in a few days or weeks. If symptoms are severe, reintroduce the original antidepressant (or another with a longer half-life from the same class) and taper gradually while monitoring for symptoms.[6]

Some evidence supports the use of anticholinergic agents in tricyclic withdrawal[24] and fluoxetine for symptoms associated with stopping paroxetine,[25] sertraline,[25] clomipramine[26] or venlafaxine[27] – fluoxetine, with active metabolites, having a much longer plasma half-life, seems to be associated with a lower incidence of discontinuation symptoms than other similar drugs.[7] The use of alternative classes of medications (e.g. short-term symptomatic use of a benzodiazepine) has been suggested for the treatment of anxiety and insomnia.[28]

References

1. Henssler J, et al. Antidepressant withdrawal and rebound phenomena. *Dtsch Arztebl Int* 2019; **116**:355–361.
2. Horowitz MA, et al. Tapering of SSRI treatment to mitigate withdrawal symptoms. *Lancet Psychiatry* 2019; **6**:538–546.
3. Davies J, et al. A systematic review into the incidence, severity and duration of antidepressant withdrawal effects: are guidelines evidence-based? *Addict Behav* 2019; **97**:111–121.
4. Henssler J, et al. Incidence of antidepressant discontinuation symptoms: a systematic review and meta-analysis. *Lancet Psychiatry* 2024; **11**:526–535.
5. Zhang MM, et al. Incidence and risk factors of antidepressant withdrawal symptoms: a meta-analysis and systematic review. *Mol Psychiatry* 2024; doi: 10.1038/s41380-024-02782-4.
6. National Institute for Health and Care Excellence. Depression in adults: treatment and management. NICE guideline [NG222]. 2022 (last reviewed September 2024, last checked November 2024); https://www.nice.org.uk/guidance/ng222.
7. Fava GA, et al. Withdrawal symptoms after selective serotonin reuptake inhibitor discontinuation: a systematic review. *Psychother Psychosom* 2015; **84**:72–81.
8. Berigan TR. Bupropion-associated withdrawal symptoms revisited: a case report. *Prim Care Companion J Clin Psychiatry* 2002; **4**:78.
9. Berigan TR, et al. Bupropion-associated withdrawal symptoms: a case report. *Prim Care Companion J Clin Psychiatry* 1999; **1**:50–51.
10. Cosci F, et al. Acute and persistent withdrawal syndromes following discontinuation of psychotropic medications. *Psychother Psychosom* 2020; **89**:283–306.
11. Curtin F, et al. Moclobemide discontinuation syndrome predominantly presenting with influenza-like symptoms. *J Psychopharmacol* 2002; **16**:271–272.
12. Ricken R, et al. Tranylcypromine in mind (part II): review of clinical pharmacology and meta-analysis of controlled studies in depression. *Eur Neuropsychopharmacol* 2017; **27**:714–731.
13. Gahr M, et al. Withdrawal and discontinuation phenomena associated with tranylcypromine: a systematic review. *Pharmacopsychiatry* 2013; **46**:123–129.
14. Lejoyeux M, et al. Antidepressant withdrawal syndrome: recognition, prevention and management. *CNS Drugs* 1996; **5**:278–292.
15. Haddad PM, et al. Recognising and managing antidepressant discontinuation symptoms. *Adv Psychiatr Treat* 2007; **13**:447–457.
16. Haddad PM. Antidepressant discontinuation syndromes. *Drug Saf* 2001; **24**:183–197.
17. Tint A, et al. The effect of rate of antidepressant tapering on the incidence of discontinuation symptoms: a randomised study. *J Psychopharmacol* 2008; **22**:330–332.
18. Ogle NR, et al. Guidance for the discontinuation or switching of antidepressant therapies in adults. *J Pharm Pract* 2013; **26**:389–396.

19. Meijer WE, et al. Spontaneous lapses in dosing during chronic treatment with selective serotonin reuptake inhibitors. *Br J Psychiatry* 2001; **179**:519–522.

20. van Geffen EC, et al. Discontinuation symptoms in users of selective serotonin reuptake inhibitors in clinical practice: tapering versus abrupt discontinuation. *Eur J Clin Pharmacol* 2005; **61**:303–307.

21. Kramer JC, et al. Withdrawal symptoms following discontinuation of imipramine therapy. *Am J Psychiatry* 1961; **118**:549–550.

22. Read J. How common and severe are six withdrawal effects from, and addiction to, antidepressants? The experiences of a large international sample of patients. *Addict Behav* 2020; **102**:106157.

23. Wilson E, et al. A review of the management of antidepressant discontinuation symptoms. *Ther Adv Psychopharmacol* 2015; **5**:357–368.

24. Dilsaver SC, et al. Antidepressant withdrawal symptoms treated with anticholinergic agents. *Am J Psychiatry* 1983; **140**:249–251.

25. Benazzi F. Re: Selective serotonin reuptake inhibitor discontinuation syndrome: putative mechanisms and prevention strategies. *Can J Psychiatry* 1999; **44**:95–96.

26. Benazzi F. Fluoxetine for clomipramine withdrawal symptoms. *Am J Psychiatry* 1999; **156**:661–662.

27. Giakas WJ, et al. Intractable withdrawal from venlafaxine treated with fluoxetine. *Psychiatr Ann* 1997; **27**:85–93.

28. Fava GA, et al. Understanding and managing withdrawal syndromes after discontinuation of antidepressant drugs. *J Clin Psychiatry* 2019; **80**:19com12794.

CHAPTER 3

Stopping antidepressants

Up to 50% of patients will experience withdrawal symptoms on reducing or stopping an antidepressant,[1,2] but symptoms are less common in shorter-term users.[3] For a small proportion of patients, withdrawal symptoms will be severe[1,3] or will last for months or years.[1,4] Post-acute or protracted withdrawal syndrome (PAWS) is the term used for long-lasting symptoms that last for years and may involve myriad, sometimes debilitating, symptoms.[2,5] Alterations to serotonin and hormonal systems after stopping antidepressants are seen in patients and animals and these changes may persist for months and years after long-term antidepressant exposure.[2]

There are a number of characteristics of antidepressant use that influence the likelihood of withdrawal effects. Patients who have been on antidepressants for longer periods and at higher doses are more likely to have withdrawal effects.[2] Antidepressants with short half-lives and anticholinergic or noradrenergic effects tend to be associated with more severe withdrawal. Venlafaxine, desvenlafaxine, duloxetine and paroxetine are the most often implicated.[2,6] Patients who stop abruptly or rapidly have more withdrawal effects.[7] There are likely to be a range of individual physiological (and psychological) differences, as yet poorly understood, which also determine withdrawal severity.[2]

Withdrawal symptoms include both physical and psychological symptoms, because antidepressants affect a wide variety of bodily systems.[7] Physical symptoms include headache, dizziness, nausea, depersonalisation/derealisation, muscle cramps, brain 'zaps' and akathisia. Psychological symptoms include low mood, anxiety, panic attacks, tearfulness, obsessive thinking, impaired concentration and suicidality. Psychological symptoms can easily be mistaken for a relapse of an underlying condition. Timing of onset, symptoms distinct in nature or severity from the underlying condition and response to reinstatement of the drug can help to distinguish withdrawal effects from relapse.[8] Further details are provided in the *Maudsley Deprescribing Guidelines: Antidepressants, Benzodiazepines, Gabapentinoids and Z-drugs.*[9]

Rate of tapering

There is good evidence that tapering slowly can reduce the likelihood of withdrawal symptoms and also of relapse.[7,10,11] Meta-regression of discontinuation studies found a highly significant lowering of relapse rate with longer tapering.[10] In fact, there was no difference in relapse rate between maintenance treatment and tapering over 6 months.[10]

While tapering over several months reduces the risk of withdrawal symptoms,[7] some patients may take years to withdraw. Clinical experience suggests that long-term users of antidepressants generally take between 3 months and 3 years to withdraw in a tolerable manner.[12] In one study, 40% of patients taking antidepressants for more than 1–2 years were able to taper off successfully in approximately 4 months, suggesting that 60% will need longer than this.[13]

Pattern of tapering

Although reducing by linear amounts (e.g. 50mg, 37.5mg, 25mg, 12.5mg, 0 for sertraline) seems intuitively reasonable (and practical, through splitting tablets), because of the hyperbolic relationship between dose of antidepressant and effect on its principal target, the serotonin receptor (SERT) (following the law of mass action),[14] this is likely to produce increasingly severe withdrawal symptoms (Figure 3.3a).[7] This is consistent with patient reports that reducing at small doses is the most difficult aspect of the process.

It makes more sense to reduce the drug in such a way that it produces a fixed reduction in effect on target receptors at each step: this entails hyperbolic dose reductions (Figure 3.3b). This is most easily approximated by exponential (proportional) reductions of dose – for example, reducing by 10–25% of the *most recent* dose every 2–4 weeks (so that the size of the reductions gets smaller and smaller as the total dose gets lower). The final dose before completely stopping may need to be very small (<1mg) to prevent the reduction to zero being a bigger fall in activity than previously tolerated reductions. This is supported by evidence that tapering down to doses much lower than common therapeutic doses (e.g. 1mg for sertraline) improves the likelihood that people will be able to stop antidepressants,[15,16] and remain off them,[17] as compared with tapering in a 'linear' fashion to minimum therapeutic doses. This approach to tapering is recommended by NICE[18,19] and the Royal College of Psychiatrists.[20]

Further details on how to safely stop antidepressants can be found in the *Maudsley Deprescribing Guidelines: Antidepressants, Benzodiazepines, Gabapentinoids and Z-drugs*, including specific reduction schedules for all licensed antidepressants.[9]

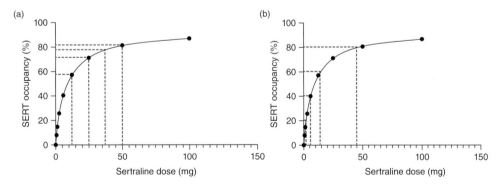

Figure 3.3 (a) Linear reductions of dose cause increasingly large reductions in effect on receptor targets, probably associated with more withdrawal effects. (b) 'Even' reductions of effect at target receptors require hyperbolic dose reductions. The final dose before stopping will need to be very small to minimise the destabilisation caused by this reduction.

Practical application of tapering

Before tapering

All patients should be informed of the risk of withdrawal symptoms on stopping any antidepressant. Some antidepressants, such as paroxetine and SNRIs, are more commonly associated with severe withdrawal symptoms.

Patients should be warned not to stop antidepressants abruptly, because this is the method thought to be most likely to give rise to severe and long-lasting withdrawal symptoms and to an increased risk of relapse.

Although stopping antidepressants can cause some unpleasant symptoms, patients should be told that if they taper gradually and carefully, withdrawal symptoms can be maintained at tolerable levels. As patients may have had negative experiences of too-rapid tapering in the past, reassurance may be required.

It is difficult to predict the exact period required for an individual to taper off antidepressant medication but most patients who have been taking antidepressants long term take between 3 months and 3 years. This may help to set expectations.

Patients' past experiences of stopping should be explored, as they can be informative for predicting what symptoms may arise again on tapering. Careful consideration of past attempts to stop may detect withdrawal symptoms being misdiagnosed as relapse.

Often, patients will require some preparation for antidepressant tapering. This might include arrangements for lightening work or family duties or increased focus on non-pharmacological coping skills (patients have found a wide variety of tools useful, including acceptance, breathing exercises, exercise, hobbies, diary keeping and de-catastrophising).[21,22] Psychological interventions to support tapering demonstrated limited effectiveness, probably because physiological factors predominate, and psychological support, while potentially helpful, is not a substitute for gradual, pharmacologically informed tapering.[13,23]

Both clinicians and patients should be aware that patients can experience negative psychological and physical symptoms during withdrawal that need not indicate that the full dose of the drug is needed (but may indicate that the taper rate needs to be slowed). Familiarity of the patient and the doctor with the wide variety of withdrawal symptoms (Figure 3.3) may help to mitigate unnecessary anxiety when symptoms arise and prevent misdiagnosis of relapse or other physical (such as neurological or psychosomatic conditions) or mental health conditions (such as anxiety, depressive or even psychotic disorders when symptoms are extreme), as often occurs.[24] Patients may require more support during the process, professional or otherwise.[22]

The process of tapering

Patients may be broadly risk-stratified (further details are provided in the *Maudsley Deprescribing Guidelines*):[9]

- For low-risk patients (<6 months of use, low-risk antidepressant, no experience of significant withdrawal symptoms in the past), a test reduction could be made (of 25–50%).
- For high-risk patients (>24 months of use, high-risk antidepressant, past history of severe withdrawal symptoms) a test reduction of 5–10% should be recommended.
- Intermediate-risk patients could reduce by 10–20% of their original dose.

> **Box 3.2** A simplified guide to tapering sertraline according to an exponential pattern
>
> The range of reductions provided is equivalent to about 10–25% dose reductions at each step. Some patients may require smaller reductions and others may tolerate larger reductions at a faster rate.
>
> - Reduce dose by 25–50mg every 2–4 weeks until reaching 50mg per day, then
> - Reduce by 5–10mg every 2–4 weeks until reaching 15mg per day, then
> - Reduce by 1.5–3mg every 2–4 weeks until reaching 6mg per day, then
> - Reduce by 0.5–1mg every 2–4 weeks until reaching 2mg per day, then
> - Reduce by 0.25–0.5mg every 2–4 weeks until completely stopped.
>
> This process normally takes between 3 months and 3 years but in some people can require longer periods.

CHAPTER 3

A cautious initial rate of reduction is prudent. The rate of withdrawal can be sped up if symptoms are tolerable. If severe withdrawal symptoms are precipitated by the first step down, then the process may be set to be a difficult one. The first reduction is perhaps the most important.

Withdrawal symptoms should be monitored for 2–4 weeks for all patients, or until symptoms have resolved. Monitoring may take the form of simple measures of symptoms each day (e.g. out of 10), which may be more convenient than using long standardised measurement such as the Discontinuation–Emergent Signs and Symptoms scale.[25]

Further reductions should be titrated against the tolerability of this experience. If the initial reduction was tolerable and withdrawal symptoms were absent or have resolved by the end of this monitoring period, continue reducing dose by the same *proportion* (worked out on the last dose used; see example regimens in Box 3.2). If symptoms were intolerable, then the taper should proceed at a slower rate. If severe, this may require reinstatement of the previous dose, a period of stabilisation and then a more cautious reduction schedule.

Troubleshooting

If withdrawal symptoms become intolerable at any point, either hold the current dose for longer to allow them to resolve or, if very unpleasant, increase to the last dose at which the symptoms were tolerable and remain there until symptoms resolve. After stabilisation, tapering will need to be more gradual, with reductions made by smaller amounts. Some patients find they cannot reduce at more than 5% of the last dose per month. If a patient experiences distressing withdrawal symptoms, it does not indicate that they cannot stop antidepressants but that they will need to taper more slowly, with smaller reductions than they have been undertaking.

Owing to the long half-life of fluoxetine, withdrawal symptoms can be delayed by weeks, so careful attention should be paid to this. (For reasons that may relate to brain elimination half-lives even shorter-acting antidepressants can present with delayed-onset withdrawal effects.)[26] As the withdrawal period is spread over a longer period, larger reductions of fluoxetine may be relatively tolerable,[7] but fluoxetine cannot be said to be 'self-tapering' for long-term users and so should not be stopped abruptly.

Unfortunately, most current tablet formulations of antidepressants do not permit hyperbolic tapering regimens, so patients will require the use of liquid formulations, as recommended by NICE[18] (or compounded smaller dose formulations, e.g. tapering strips).[15] Off-label options for making up smaller doses also exist, including crushing and suspending tablets, opening up capsules to count or weigh beads or diluting manufacturers' liquid preparations, all of which are permissible according to various pharmaceutical authorities.[27] Again, further details are provided for licensed and off-label options for hyperbolic tapering in the *Maudsley Deprescribing Guidelines: Antidepressants, Benzodiazepines, Gabapentinoids and Z-drugs.*[9]

For many drugs, the final dose before complete stopping will need to be much less than 1mg so that the reduction in effect on target receptors is not greater than the changes previously tolerated.

References

1. Davies J, et al. A systematic review into the incidence, severity and duration of antidepressant withdrawal effects: are guidelines evidence-based? *Addict Behav* 2019; 97:111–121.
2. Horowitz MA, et al. Estimating risk of antidepressant withdrawal from a review of published data. *CNS Drugs* 2023; 37:143-157.
3. Henssler J, et al. Incidence of antidepressant discontinuation symptoms: a systematic review and meta-analysis. *Lancet Psychiatry* 2024; 11:526–535.
4. Stockmann T, et al. SSRI and SNRI withdrawal symptoms reported on an internet forum. *Int J Risk Saf Med* 2018; 29:175–180.
5. Cosci F, et al. Acute and persistent withdrawal syndromes following discontinuation of psychotropic medications. *Psychother Psychosom* 2020; 89:283–306.
6. Gastaldon C, et al. Withdrawal syndrome following discontinuation of 28 antidepressants: pharmacovigilance analysis of 31,688 reports from the WHO Spontaneous Reporting Database. *Drug Saf* 2022; 45:1539–1549.
7. Horowitz MA, et al. Tapering of SSRI treatment to mitigate withdrawal symptoms. *Lancet Psychiatry* 2019; 6:538–546.
8. Horowitz MA, et al. Distinguishing relapse from antidepressant withdrawal: clinical practice and antidepressant discontinuation studies. *B J Psych Advances* 2022; 28:297–311.
9. Horowitz M, et al. *The Maudsley Deprescribing Guidelines: Antidepressants, Benzodiazepines, Gabapentinoids and Z-drugs.* Chichester: Wiley-Blackwell; 2024.
10. Gøtzsche PC, et al. Interventions to help patients withdraw from depression drugs: a systematic review. *Int J Risk Saf Med* 2024; 35:103–116.
11. Baldessarini RJ, et al. Illness risk following rapid versus gradual discontinuation of antidepressants. *Am J Psychiatry* 2010; 167:934–941.
12. Cooper RE, et al. 'Stabilise–reduce, stabilise–reduce': a survey of the common practices of deprescribing services and recommendations for future services. *PLoS One* 2023; 18:e0282988.
13. Kendrick T, et al. Internet and telephone support for discontinuing long-term antidepressants: the REDUCE cluster randomized trial. *JAMA Netw Open* 2024; 7:e2418383.
14. Holford N. Pharmacodynamic principles and the time course of delayed and cumulative drug effects. *Transl Clin Pharmacol* 2018; 26:56–59.
15. Groot PC, et al. How user knowledge of psychotropic drug withdrawal resulted in the development of person-specific tapering medication. *Ther Adv Psychopharmacol* 2020; 10:2045125320932452.
16. Groot PC, et al. Antidepressant tapering strips to help people come off medication more safely. *Psychosis* 2018; 10:142–145.
17. Groot PC, et al. Outcome of antidepressant drug discontinuation with taperingstrips after 1–5 years. *Ther Adv Psychopharmacol* 2020; 10:2045125320954609.
18. National Institute for Health and Care Excellence. Depression in adults: treatment and management. NICE guideline [NG222]. 2022 (last reviewed September 2024, last checked September 2024); https://www.nice.org.uk/guidance/ng222.
19. National Institute for Health and Care Excellence. Medicines associated with dependence or withdrawal symptoms: safe prescribing and withdrawal management for adults [NG215]. 2022 (last checked September 2024); https://www.nice.org.uk/guidance/ng215.
20. Royal College of Psychiatrists. Stopping antidepressants. 2020 (last accessed September 2024); https://www.rcpsych.ac.uk/mental-health/treatments-and-wellbeing/stopping-antidepressants.
21. Inner Compass Initiative. The Withdrawal Project; https://withdrawal.theinnercompass.org.
22. Guy A, et al. *Guidance for Psychological Therapists: Enabling conversations with clients taking or withdrawing from prescribed psychiatric drugs.* London: APPG for Prescribed Drug Dependence; 2019.
23. Scholten WD, et al. The efficacy of a group CBT relapse prevention program for remitted anxiety disorder patients who discontinue antidepressant medication: a randomized controlled trial. *Psychother Psychosom* 2018; 87:240–242.

24. Guy A, et al. The 'patient voice': patients who experience antidepressant withdrawal symptoms are often dismissed, or misdiagnosed with relapse, or a new medical condition. *Ther Adv Psychopharmacol* 2020; **10**:2045125320967183.

25. Rosenbaum JF, et al. Selective serotonin reuptake inhibitor discontinuation syndrome: a randomized clinical trial. *Biol Psychiatry* 1998; **44**:77–87.

26. Sørensen A, et al. The relationship between dose and serotonin transporter occupancy of antidepressants-a systematic review. *Mol Psychiatry* 2022; **27**:192–201.

27. Specialist Pharmacy Service. SSRI suggestions for adults with swallowing difficulties 2021 (last updated July 2024, accessed September 2024); https://www.sps.nhs.uk/articles/selective-serotonin-reuptake-inhibitor-ssri-formulations-suggested-for-adults-with-swallowing-difficulties.

CHAPTER 3

Electroconvulsive therapy and psychotropic drugs

Psychotropics are often continued during ECT. Some agents, such as antidepressants,[1,2] enhance its efficacy.

Table 3.9 summarises the effect of various psychotropics on seizure duration during ECT. There are few well-controlled studies in this area and recommendations should be viewed with this in mind.

The choice of anaesthetic agent may profoundly affect seizure duration[3,4] as well as the severity of post-ictal confusion and ECT efficacy.[5,6] Somewhat against expectation, the use of ketamine or esketamine[7,8] as an anaesthetic does not ultimately improve outcome with ECT,[9] although ketamine may provide short-term improvement of depressive symptoms at the early stages of ECT.[10] Aside from concurrent medication, there are many factors that influence seizure threshold and duration.[11] Caffeine reduces seizure threshold and can be used to enable or prolong seizures in ECT.[12] Flumazenil has similar effects.[13]

ECT frequently causes confusion and disorientation. More rarely, it causes an acute confusional state or delirium. Concurrent lithium may increase the risk of delirium.[2] Agitation may also occur.[14] The use of dexmedetomidine seems to reduce the risk of post-ECT agitation.[15] There have been a few reports of serotonin syndrome when serotonergic medications have been used with ECT.[16–18] Close observation is essential.

Very limited data support the use of thiamine (200mg daily) in reducing post-ECT confusion.[19] Some drugs have been investigated for improving the cognitive adverse effects of ECT.[20] Supporting evidence is of a low (memantine, liothyronine) or a very low quality (acetylcholinesterase inhibitors, piracetam, melatonin).[20] None is recommended.

Paracetamol[21] or ibuprofen may be used to prevent headache;[22] intranasal sumatriptan[23] can be used to treat it.

Table 3.9 Effect of psychotropic drugs on seizure during electroconvulsive therapy.

Drug	Effect on ECT seizure duration	Comments[24–27]
Antipsychotics[2,28–31]	Variable; increased with phenothiazines and clozapine Others; no obvious effect reported	Few published data but widely used. Phenothiazines and clozapine are perhaps most likely to prolong seizures. Some suggest withdrawal before ECT. Safe concurrent use has been reported (particularly with clozapine,[32,33] which is now usually continued).
		ECT and antipsychotics appear generally to be a safe combination. Few data on aripiprazole, quetiapine and ziprasidone, but they also appear to be safe. One case series[24] suggests that antipsychotics increase post-ictal cognitive dysfunction.
Antiseizure medication[2,35,36]	Reduced	If used as a mood stabiliser, continue but be prepared to use higher energy stimulus. Some units omit one or more doses before ECT.
		If used for epilepsy, their effect is to normalise seizure threshold. Interactions are possible. Valproate may prolong the effect of thiopental and carbamazepine may inhibit neuromuscular blockade. A small RCT found no difference between carbamazepine and valproate in seizure duration, seizure threshold and cognition outcomes. Lamotrigine has been associated with shorter seizure duration and reduced remission rates in one cohort study.[37]

Table 3.9 (*Continued*)

Drug	Effect on ECT seizure duration	Comments[24–27]
Barbiturates	Reduced	All barbiturates reduce seizure duration in ECT but are widely used as sedative anaesthetic agents.
		Thiopental and methohexital may be associated with cardiac arrhythmia.
Benzodiazepines[38]	Probably reduced. Mixed evidence and clinical implications unclear.[37–39]	All may raise seizure threshold and so should be avoided where possible. Many are long-acting and may need to be discontinued some days before ECT. Benzodiazepines may also complicate ECT anaesthesia and reduce efficacy of ECT.[37]
		If sedation is required, consider hydroxyzine. If benzodiazepine use is very long term and essential, continue and use higher stimulus, bilaterally.
Bupropion[2]	Possibly increased	Epileptogenic in higher doses so could increase seizure duration. In practice, appears to be well tolerated with ECT.
Duloxetine[40,41]	Not known	One case report suggests duloxetine does not complicate ECT. Another links its use to ventricular tachycardia.
Lithium[2,42,43]	Possibly increased	Conflicting data on lithium and ECT. The combination may be more likely to lead to delirium and confusion. Some authorities suggest discontinuing lithium 48 hours before ECT. In the UK, ECT is often used during lithium therapy but starting with a low stimulus and with very close monitoring. The combination is generally well tolerated. Note that lithium potentiates the effects of non-depolarising neuromuscular blockers such as suxamethonium. Concomitant use of thiopentone or propofol with lithium treatment lowers seizure threshold.[44]
MAOIs[2,45]	Minimal effect	Data relating to ECT very limited but long history of ECT use during MAOI therapy.
		MAOIs probably do not affect seizure duration but interactions with sympathomimetics occasionally used in anaesthesia are possible and may lead to hypertensive crisis. Transdermal selegiline seems safe.[46]
		MAOIs may be continued during ECT but the anaesthetist must be informed. Beware hypotension.
Mirtazapine[47]	Minimal effect; small increase	Apparently safe in ECT and, like other antidepressants, may enhance ECT efficacy. May reduce post-ECT nausea and headache.
SSRIs[1,2,48]	Minimal effect; small increase possible	Generally considered safe to use during ECT. Beware complex pharmacokinetic interactions with anaesthetic agents. Isolated case reports of serotonin syndrome with fluoxetine and paroxetine with ECT.[49,50]
TCAs[51]	Possibly increased	Few data relevant to ECT but many TCAs lower seizure threshold. TCAs are associated with arrhythmia following ECT and should be avoided in elderly patients and those with cardiac disease. In others, it is preferable to continue TCA treatment during ECT. Close monitoring is essential. Beware hypotension and risk of prolonged seizures.
Venlafaxine[52]	Minimal effect at standard doses	Limited data suggest no effect on seizure duration but possibility of increased risk of transient asystole with doses above 300mg/day.[2] Clearly epileptogenic in higher doses. ECG advised.

MAOI, monoamine oxidase inhibitor; TCA, tricyclic antidepressant.

CHAPTER 3

References

1. Pluijms EM, et al. Influence of an adjuvant antidepressant on the efficacy of electroconvulsive therapy: a systematic review and meta-analysis. *Aust N Z J Psychiatry* 2021; **55**:366–380.
2. Janjua AU, et al. The efficacy and safety of concomitant psychotropic medication and electroconvulsive therapy (ECT). *CNS Drugs* 2020; **34**:509–520.
3. Bundy BD, et al. Influence of anesthetic drugs. and concurrent psychiatric medication on seizure adequacy during electroconvulsive therapy. *J Clin Psychiatry* 2010; **71**:775–777.
4. Singh PM, et al. Evaluation of etomidate for seizure duration in electroconvulsive therapy: a systematic review and meta-analysis. *J ECT* 2015; **31**:213–225.
5. Ren L, et al. Comparative efficacy and tolerability of different anesthetics in electroconvulsive therapy for major depressive disorder: a systematic review and network meta-analysis. *J Psychiatr Res* 2024; **171**:116–125.
6. Stripp TK, et al. Anaesthesia for electroconvulsive therapy – new tricks for old drugs: a systematic review. *Acta Neuropsychiatr* 2018; **30**:61–69.
7. Ren L, et al. Clinical efficacy of adjunctive esketamine anesthesia in electroconvulsive therapy for major depressive disorders: a pragmatic, randomized, controlled trial. *Psychiatry Res* 2024; **335**:115843.
8. Zeng QB, et al. Efficacy and safety of esketamine versus propofol in electroconvulsive therapy for treatment-resistant depression: a randomized, double-blind, controlled, non-inferiority trial. *J Affect Disord* 2024; **368**:320–328.
9. McGirr A, et al. Adjunctive ketamine in electroconvulsive therapy: updated systematic review and meta-analysis. *Br J Psychiatry* 2017; **210**:403–407.
10. Zheng W, et al. Adjunctive ketamine and electroconvulsive therapy for major depressive disorder: a meta-analysis of randomized controlled trials. *J Affect Disord* 2019; **250**:123–131.
11. van Waarde JA, et al. Clinical predictors of seizure threshold in electroconvulsive therapy: a prospective study. *Eur Arch Psychiatry Clin Neurosci* 2013; **263**:167–175.
12. Nyhuis P, et al. Augmentation of electroconvulsive therapy with oral caffeine: a retrospective analysis of 40 patients with major depression. *Pharmacopsychiatry* 2024; **57**:30–34.
13. Gistelinck L, et al. Effectiveness and safety of flumazenil augmentation during electroconvulsive therapy. *J ECT* 2024; **40**:e49–e51.
14. Sterina E, et al. Acute and prophylactic management of postictal agitation in electroconvulsive therapy. *J ECT* 2023; **39**:136–140.
15. Feenstra TC, et al. Pharmacological prevention of postictal agitation after electroconvulsive therapy-a systematic review and meta-analysis. *Front Psychiatry* 2023; **14**:1170931.
16. Calderon K, et al. Serotonin toxicity associated with electroconvulsive therapy: a case report. *J Acad Consult Liaison Psychiatry* 2024; S2667-2960(24)00084-3. doi: 10.1016/j.jaclp.2024.08.002.
17. Cheng YC, et al. Serotonin syndrome after electroconvulsive therapy in a patient on trazodone, bupropion, and quetiapine: a case report. *Clin Neuropharmacol* 2015; **38**:112–113.
18. Deuschle M, et al. Electroconvulsive therapy induces transient sensitivity for a serotonin syndrome: a case report. *Pharmacopsychiatry* 2017; **50**:41–42.
19. Linton CR, et al. Using thiamine to reduce post-ECT confusion. *Int J Geriatr Psychiatry* 2002; **17**:189–192.
20. Verdijk J, et al. Pharmacological interventions to diminish cognitive side effects of electroconvulsive therapy: a systematic review and meta-analysis. *Acta Psychiatr Scand* 2022; **145**:343–356.
21. Isuru A, et al. A randomized, double-blind, placebo-controlled trial on the role of preemptive analgesia with acetaminophen [paracetamol] in reducing headache following electroconvulsive therapy [ECT]. *BMC Psychiatry* 2017; **17**:275.
22. Leung M, et al. Pretreatment with ibuprofen to prevent electroconvulsive therapy-induced headache. *J Clin Psychiatry* 2003; **64**:551–553.
23. Markowitz JS, et al. Intranasal sumatriptan in post-ECT headache: results of an open-label trial. *J ECT* 2001; **17**:280–283.
24. Royal College of Psychiatrists. *The ECT Handbook*, 4th edn. London: RCPsych Publications; 2019.
25. Kellner CH, et al. ECT–drug interactions: a review. *Psychopharmacol Bull* 1991; **27**:595–609.
26. Naguib M, et al. Interactions between psychotropics, anaesthetics and electroconvulsive therapy: implications for drug choice and patient management. *CNS Drugs* 2002; **16**:229–247.
27. Maidment I. The interaction between psychiatric medicines and ECT. *Hosp Pharm* 1997; **4**:102–105.
28. Havaki-Kontaxaki BJ, et al. Concurrent administration of clozapine and electroconvulsive therapy in clozapine-resistant schizophrenia. *Clin Neuropharmacol* 2006; **29**:52–56.
29. Nothdurfter C, et al. The influence of concomitant neuroleptic medication on safety, tolerability and clinical effectiveness of electroconvulsive therapy. *World J Biol Psychiatry* 2006; **7**:162–170.
30. Gazdag G, et al. The impact of neuroleptic medication on seizure threshold and duration in electroconvulsive therapy. *Ideggyogy Sz* 2004; **57**:385–390.
31. Oulis P, et al. Corrected QT interval changes during electroconvulsive therapy-antidepressants-atypical antipsychotics coadministration: safety issues. *J ECT* 2011; **27**:e4–e6.
32. Grover S, et al. Combined use of clozapine and ECT: a review. *Acta Neuropsychiatr* 2015; **27**:131–142.
33. Flamarique I, et al. Electroconvulsive therapy and clozapine in adolescents with schizophrenia spectrum disorders: is it a safe and effective combination? *J Clin Psychopharmacol* 2012; **32**:756–766.
34. van Waarde JA, et al. Patient, treatment, and anatomical predictors of outcome in electroconvulsive therapy: a prospective study. *J ECT* 2013; **29**:113–121.
35. Sienaert P, et al. Concurrent use of lamotrigine and electroconvulsive therapy. *J ECT* 2011; **27**:148–152.

36. Jahangard L, et al. Comparing efficacy of ECT with and without concurrent sodium valproate therapy in manic patients. *J ECT* 2012; **28**:118–123.

37. Gillving C, et al. Seizure duration and electroconvulsive therapy in major depressive disorder. *JAMA Netw Open* 2024; 7:e2422738.

38. Tang VM, et al. Should benzodiazepines and anticonvulsants be used during electroconvulsive therapy? A case study and literature review. *J ECT* 2017; 237–242.

39. Chiao S, et al. Psychotropic medication effects on seizure threshold and seizure duration during electroconvulsive therapy stimulus titration. *J ECT* 2020; **36**:115–122.

40. Hanretta AT, et al. Combined use of ECT with duloxetine and olanzapine: a case report. *J ECT* 2006; **22**:139–141.

41. Heinz B, et al. Postictal ventricular tachycardia after electroconvulsive therapy treatment associated with a lithium–duloxetine combination. *J ECT* 2013; **29**:e33–e35.

42. Jha AK, et al. Negative interaction between lithium and electroconvulsive therapy: a case-control study. *Br J Psychiatry* 1996; **168**:241–243.

43. Rucker J, et al. A case of prolonged seizure after ECT in a patient treated with clomipramine, lithium, L-tryptophan, quetiapine, and thyroxine for major depression. *J ECT* 2008; **24**:272–274.

44. Galvez V, et al. Predictors of seizure threshold in right unilateral ultrabrief electroconvulsive therapy: role of concomitant medications and anaesthesia used. *Brain Stimul* 2015; **8**:486–492.

45. Dolenc TJ, et al. Electroconvulsive therapy in patients taking monoamine oxidase inhibitors. *J ECT* 2004; **20**:258–261.

46. Horn PJ, et al. Transdermal selegiline in patients receiving electroconvulsive therapy. *Psychosomatics* 2010; **51**:176–178.

47. Li TC, et al. Mirtazapine relieves post-electroconvulsive therapy headaches and nausea: a case series and review of the literature. *J ECT* 2011; **27**:165–167.

48. Masdrakis VG, et al. The safety of the electroconvulsive therapy-escitalopram combination. *J ECT* 2008; **24**:289–291.

49. Okamoto N, et al. Transient serotonin syndrome by concurrent use of electroconvulsive therapy and selective serotonin reuptake inhibitor: a case report and review of the literature. *Case Rep Psychiatry* 2012; **2012**:215214.

50. Klysner R, et al. Transient serotonin toxicity evoked by combination of electroconvulsive therapy and fluoxetine. *Case Rep Psychiatry* 2014; **2014**:162502.

51. Birkenhager TK, et al. Possible synergy between electroconvulsive therapy and imipramine: a case report. *J Psychiatr Pract* 2016; **22**:478–480.

52. Gonzalez-Pinto A, et al. Efficacy and safety of venlafaxine–ECT combination in treatment-resistant depression. *J Neuropsychiatry Clin Neurosci* 2002; **14**:206–209.

Psychostimulants in depression

Psychostimulants reduce fatigue, promote wakefulness and can be mood elevating. Amfetamines have been used as treatments for depression since the 1930s[1] and more recently modafinil has been evaluated as an adjunct to standard antidepressants. Amfetamines are now rarely used in depression because of their propensity for the development of tolerance and dependence. Prolonged use of high doses is associated with psychosis.[2] Methylphenidate is now more widely used than amfetamines but may have similar shortcomings. Modafinil seems not to induce tolerance, dependence or psychosis but lacks the marked euphoric effects of amfetamines. Armodafinil, the longer-acting isomer of modafinil, is available in some countries.

Psychostimulants differ importantly from standard antidepressants in that their mood-elevating effects are usually seen within a few hours, but their antidepressant action may be short lived. Amfetamines and methylphenidate may thus be useful where a prompt effect is required and where dependence would not be problematic (e.g. in depression associated with terminal illness), although ketamine might also be considered in these cases. Their use might also be justified in severe, prolonged depression unresponsive to standard treatments (e.g. in those considered for psychosurgery). Modafinil might justifiably be used as an adjunct to antidepressants in a wider range of patients and as a specific treatment for hypersomnia and fatigue.[3]

Table 3.10 outlines support (or the absence of it) for the use of psychostimulants in various clinical situations. Generally speaking, data relating to stimulants in depression are rather poor and inconclusive.[4,5] A network meta-analysis[6] concluded that although psychostimulants (particularly methylphenidate) seem to be well tolerated and have some efficacy in depression, the strength of evidence is very low and insufficiently consistent to provide any definitive hierarchy of treatments. Careful consideration should be given to any use of any psychostimulants in depression, since their short- and long-term safety have not been clearly established. Inclusion of individual drugs in Table 3.10 should not in itself be considered a recommendation for their use.

Table 3.10 Stimulants in depression.

Clinical use	Regimens evaluated	Comments	Recommendations
Monotherapy in uncomplicated depression	Modafinil 100–200mg/day[7,8]	Case reports only – efficacy unproven	Standard antidepressants preferred. Avoid psychostimulants as monotherapy in uncomplicated depression.[9]
	Methylphenidate 20–40mg/day[10,11]	Minimal efficacy	
	Dexamfetamine 20mg/day[10]	Minimal efficacy	Meta-analysis found adjunctive therapy but not monotherapy to be associated with clinically significant improvements.[5]

(Continued)

Table 3.10 (Continued)

Clinical use	Regimens evaluated	Comments	Recommendations
Adjunctive therapy to accelerate or improve response	SSRI + methylphenidate 10–20mg/day[12,13]	No clear effect on time to response	Psychostimulants in general not recommended, but modafinil may be useful
	SSRI + modafinil 400mg/day[6]	Improved response over SSRI alone	
	Tricyclic + methylphenidate 5–15mg/day[14]	Single open-label trial suggests faster response	
	SSRI or SNRI + lisdexamfetamine 20–70mg/day[15]	No superiority over placebo	
Adjunctive treatment of depression with fatigue and hypersomnia	SSRI + modafinil 200mg/day[6,16]	Beneficial effect only on hypersomnia. Modafinil may induce suicidal ideation.	Possible effect on fatigue, but weak evidence. An option where fatigue is prominent and otherwise unresponsive.
	SSRI + methylphenidate 10–40mg/day[17]	Clear effect on fatigue in hospice patients	
Adjunctive therapy in treatment-resistant depression	SSRI + modafinil 100–400mg/day[5,6,18–21]	Effect mainly on fatigue and daytime sleepiness. Meta-analysis of 10 trials suggested clinically significant improvement in depressive symptoms.[5]	Data limited. Modafinil may be useful for fatigue[22] and cognition.[23]
	MAOI + dexamfetamine 7.5–40mg/day[24] or lisdexamfetamine 50mg/day[25]	Support from single case series and one case report	Stimulants an option in refractory illness but other options better supported. One naturalistic study suggests methylphenidate may reduce self-harm or suicide attempts.[26]
	Methylphenidate or dexamfetamine +/– antidepressant[27]	Large case series (n = 50) suggests benefit in the majority	
	Lisdexamfetamine 20–70mg/day + antidepressant[5,15,28]	Two meta-analyses found a small, non-significant effect on depressive symptoms compared with placebo	
Adjunctive treatment in bipolar depression[29,30]	Mood stabiliser and/or antidepressants + modafinil 100–200mg/day[31]	Significantly superior to placebo	Possible treatment option where other standard treatments fail. Meta-analysis of trials referenced here found stimulants well tolerated and an overall benefit vs placebo.[32] No evidence of treatment-emergent mania.[29,32–34]
	Mood stabiliser + armodafinil 150–200mg/day[33] (one case report of 1000mg/day[35])	Superior to placebo on some measures	
	Mood stabiliser + methylphenidate 10–40mg/day[36]	Mixed results, mainly positive	
	Mood stabiliser and/or antipsychotic + lisdexamfetamine 20–70mg/day[37]	Greater rates of improvement compared with placebo on patient-rated measures	

CHAPTER 3

(Continued)

Table 3.10 (*Continued*)

Clinical use	Regimens evaluated	Comments	Recommendations
Monotherapy or add-on treatment in late-stage terminal cancer	Methylphenidate 5–30mg/day[38–42]	Case series and open prospective studies	Useful treatment options in those expected to live only for a few weeks
	Dexamfetamine 2.5–20mg/day[43,44]	Beneficial effects seen on mood, fatigue and pain	
	Methylphenidate 20mg/day + mirtazapine 30mg/day[45]	RCT shows benefit for combination from third day of treatment	
	Methylphenidate 20mg/day + SSRI[46]	RCT failed to show benefit for combination	
	Modafinil 200mg/day[47]	Benefit to depression scores only in those also experiencing severe cancer-related fatigue	
Monotherapy or add-on treatment for depression in the elderly	Methylphenidate 1.25–20mg/day[48–50,51]	Use supported by four placebo-controlled studies. Rapid effect observed on mood and activity.	Recommended only where patients fail to tolerate standard antidepressants or where contraindications apply
	Methylphenidate 5–40mg + citalopram 20–60mg/day[52]	Four studies from the same group, two RCTs. Faster rate of response with combination compared with monotherapy with either drug.	Significant increase in heart rate seen in one trial
Monotherapy in post-stroke depression	Methylphenidate 5–40mg/day[53–56]	Variable support but including two placebo-controlled trials.[53,56] Effect on mood evident after a few days.	Standard antidepressants preferred. Further investigation required: stimulants may improve cognition and motor function.
	Modafinil 100mg/day[57]	Single case report	
Monotherapy in depression secondary to medical illness	Methylphenidate 5–20mg/day[58]	Limited data	Psychostimulants not appropriate therapy. Standard antidepressant preferred.
	Dexamfetamine 2.5–30mg/day[59,60]		
Monotherapy in depression and fatigue associated with HIV	Dexamfetamine 2.5–40mg/day[61,62]	Supported by one good, controlled study.[62] Beneficial effect on mood and fatigue.	Possible treatment option where fatigue is not responsive to standard antidepressants
Monotherapy in depression in traumatic brain injury	Methylphenidate 5–20mg/day[63]	Improves depressive symptoms, daytime sleepiness and cognitive function	Appears to outperform antidepressants for this indication, but data are limited to two studies

References

1. Satel SL, et al. Stimulants in the treatment of depression: a critical overview. *J Clin Psychiatry* 1989; **50**:241–249.
2. Warneke L. Psychostimulants in psychiatry. *Can J Psychiatry* 1990; **35**:3–10.
3. Goss AJ, et al. Modafinil augmentation therapy in unipolar and bipolar depression: a systematic review and meta-analysis of randomized controlled trials. *J Clin Psychiatry* 2013; **74**:1101–1107.
4. Candy M, et al. Psychostimulants for depression. *Cochrane Database Syst Rev* 2008; (2):CD006722.
5. McIntyre RS, et al. The efficacy of psychostimulants in major depressive episodes: a systematic review and meta-analysis. *J Clin Psychopharmacol* 2017; **37**:412–418.
6. Bahji A, et al. Comparative efficacy and safety of stimulant-type medications for depression: a systematic review and network meta-analysis. *J Affect Disord* 2021; **292**:416–423.
7. Lundt L. Modafinil treatment in patients with seasonal affective disorder/winter depression: an open-label pilot study. *J Affect Disord* 2004; **81**:173–178.
8. Kaufman KR, et al. Modafinil monotherapy in depression. *Eur Psychiatry* 2002; **17**:167–169.
9. Hegerl U, et al. Why do stimulants not work in typical depression? *Aust N Z J Psychiatry* 2017; **51**:20–22.
10. Little KY. d-Amphetamine versus methylphenidate effects in depressed inpatients. *J Clin Psychiatry* 1993; **54**:349–355.
11. Robin AA, et al. A controlled trial of methylphenidate (ritalin) in the treatment of depressive states. *J Neurol Neurosurg Psychiatry* 1958; **21**:55–57.
12. Lavretsky H, et al. Combined treatment with methylphenidate and citalopram for accelerated response in the elderly: an open trial. *J Clin Psychiatry* 2003; **64**:1410–1414.
13. Postolache TT, et al. Early augmentation of sertraline with methylphenidate. *J Clin Psychiatry* 1999; **60**:123–124.
14. Gwirtsman HE, et al. The antidepressant response to tricyclics in major depressives is accelerated with adjunctive use of methylphenidate. *Psychopharmacol Bull* 1994; **30**:157–164.
15. Giacobbe P, et al. Efficacy and tolerability of lisdexamfetamine as an antidepressant augmentation strategy: a meta-analysis of randomized controlled trials. *J Affect Disord* 2018; **226**:294–300.
16. Fava M, et al. Modafinil augmentation of selective serotonin reuptake inhibitor therapy in MDD partial responders with persistent fatigue and sleepiness. *Ann Clin Psychiatry* 2007; **19**:153–159.
17. Kerr CW, et al. Effects of methylphenidate on fatigue and depression: a randomized, double-blind, placebo-controlled trial. *J Pain Symptom Manage* 2012; **43**:68–77.
18. Rasmussen NA, et al. Modafinil augmentation in depressed patients with partial response to antidepressants: a pilot study on self-reported symptoms covered by the major depression inventory (MDI) and the symptom checklist (SCL-92). *Nord J Psychiatry* 2005; **59**:173–178.
19. DeBattista C, et al. A prospective trial of modafinil as an adjunctive treatment of major depression. *J Clin Psychopharmacol* 2004; **24**:87–90.
20. Markovitz PJ, et al. An open-label trial of modafinil augmentation in patients with partial response to antidepressant therapy. *J Clin Psychopharmacol* 2003; **23**:207–209.
21. Ravindran AV, et al. Osmotic-release oral system methylphenidate augmentation of antidepressant monotherapy in major depressive disorder: results of a double-blind, randomized, placebo-controlled trial. *J Clin Psychiatry* 2008; **69**:87–94.
22. Ghanean H, et al. Fatigue in patients with major depressive disorder: prevalence, burden and pharmacological approaches to management. *CNS Drugs* 2018; **32**:65–74.
23. Vaccarino SR, et al. The potential procognitive effects of modafinil in major depressive disorder: a systematic review. *J Clin Psychiatry* 2019; **80**:19r12767.
24. Fawcett J, et al. CNS stimulant potentiation of monoamine oxidase inhibitors in treatment refractory depression. *J Clin Psychopharmacol* 1991; **11**:127–132.
25. Israel JA. Combining stimulants and monoamine oxidase inhibitors: a reexamination of the literature and a report of a new treatment combination. *Prim Care Companion CNS Disord* 2015; **17**:10.4088/PCC.4015br01836.
26. Rohde C, et al. The use of stimulants in depression: results from a self-controlled register study. *Aust N Z J Psychiatry* 2020; **54**:808–817.
27. Parker G, et al. Do the old psychostimulant drugs have a role in managing treatment-resistant depression? *Acta Psychiatr Scand* 2010; **121**:308–314.
28. Richards C, et al. A randomized, double-blind, placebo-controlled, dose-ranging study of lisdexamfetamine dimesylate augmentation for major depressive disorder in adults with inadequate response to antidepressant therapy. *J Psychopharmacol* 2017; **31**:1190–1203.
29. Szmulewicz AG, et al. Dopaminergic agents in the treatment of bipolar depression: a systematic review and meta-analysis. *Acta Psychiatr Scand* 2017; **135**:527–538.
30. Perugi G, et al. Use of stimulants in bipolar disorder. *Curr Psychiatry Rep* 2017; **19**:7.
31. Frye MA, et al. A placebo-controlled evaluation of adjunctive modafinil in the treatment of bipolar depression. *Am J Psychiatry* 2007; **164**:1242–1249.
32. Tsapakis EM, et al. Adjunctive treatment with psychostimulants and stimulant-like drugs for resistant bipolar depression: a systematic review and meta-analysis. *CNS Spectr* 2020; doi: 10.1017/S109285292000156X.
33. Nunez NA, et al. Efficacy and tolerability of adjunctive modafinil/armodafinil in bipolar depression: a meta-analysis of randomized controlled trials. *Bipolar Disord* 2020; **22**:109–120.
34. Chiorean A, et al. Prescribed psychostimulants and other pro-cognitive medications in bipolar disorder: a systematic review and meta-analysis of recurrence of manic symptoms. *Bipolar Disord* 2024; **26**:418–430.
35. Kwok WY, et al. High-dose armodafinil in treatment-refractory bipolar depression. *Ann Clin Psychiatry* 2023; **35**:195–198.

CHAPTER 3

36. Dell'Osso B, et al. Assessing the roles of stimulants/stimulant-like drugs and dopamine-agonists in the treatment of bipolar depression. *Curr Psychiatry Rep* 2013; **15**:378.

37. McElroy SL, et al. Adjunctive lisdexamfetamine in bipolar depression: a preliminary randomized, placebo-controlled trial. *Int Clin Psychopharmacol* 2015; **30**:6–13.

38. Fernandez F, et al. Methylphenidate for depressive disorders in cancer patients. *Psychosomatics* 1987; **28**:455–461.

39. Macleod AD. Methylphenidate in terminal depression. *J Pain Symptom Manage* 1998; **16**:193–198.

40. Homsi J, et al. Methylphenidate for depression in hospice practice. *Am J Hospice Palliat Care* 2000; **17**:393–398.

41. Sarhill N, et al. Methylphenidate for fatigue in advanced cancer: a prospective open-label pilot study. *Am J Hosp Palliat Care* 2001; **18**:187–192.

42. Homsi J, et al. A phase II study of methylphenidate for depression in advanced cancer. *Am J Hosp Palliat Care* 2001; **18**:403–407.

43. Burns MM, et al. Dextroamphetamine treatment for depression in terminally ill patients. *Psychosomatics* 1994; **35**:80–83.

44. Olin J, et al. Psychostimulants for depression in hospitalized cancer patients. *Psychosomatics* 1996; **37**:57–62.

45. Ng CG, et al. Rapid response to methylphenidate as an add-on therapy to mirtazapine in the treatment of major depressive disorder in terminally ill cancer patients: a four-week, randomized, double-blinded, placebo-controlled study. *Eur Neuropsychopharmacol* 2014; **24**:491–498.

46. Sullivan DR, et al. Randomized, double-blind, placebo-controlled study of methylphenidate for the treatment of depression in SSRI-treated cancer patients receiving palliative care. *Psychooncology* 2017; **26**:1763–1769.

47. Conley CC, et al. Modafinil moderates the relationship between cancer-related fatigue and depression in 541 patients receiving chemotherapy. *J Clin Psychopharmacol* 2016; **36**:82–85.

48. Padala PR, et al. Methylphenidate for apathy in community-dwelling older veterans with mild Alzheimer's disease: a double-blind, randomized, placebo-controlled trial. *Am J Psychiatry* 2018; **175**:159–168.

49. Kaplitz SE. Withdrawn, apathetic geriatric patients responsive to methylphenidate. *J Am Geriatr Soc* 1975; **23**:271–276.

50. Jacobson A. The use of ritalin in psychotherapy of depressions of the aged. *Psychiatr Q* 1958; **32**:474–483.

51. Wallace AE, et al. Double-blind, placebo-controlled trial of methylphenidate in older, depressed, medically ill patients. *Am J Psychiatry* 1995; **152**:929–931.

52. Smith KR, et al. Methylphenidate use in geriatric depression: a systematic review. *Int J Geriatr Psychiatry* 2021; **36**:1304–1312.

53. Grade C, et al. Methylphenidate in early poststroke recovery: a double-blind, placebo-controlled study. *Arch Phys Med Rehabil* 1998; **79**:1047–1050.

54. Lazarus LW, et al. Efficacy and side effects of methylphenidate for poststroke depression. *J Clin Psychiatry* 1992; **53**:447–449.

55. Lingam VR, et al. Methylphenidate in treating poststroke depression. *J Clin Psychiatry* 1988; **49**:151–153.

56. Delbari A, et al. Effect of methylphenidate and/or levodopa combined with physiotherapy on mood and cognition after stroke: a randomized, double-blind, placebo-controlled trial. *Eur Neurol* 2011; **66**:7–13.

57. Sugden SG, et al. Modafinil monotherapy in poststroke depression. *Psychosomatics* 2004; **45**:80–81.

58. Rosenberg PB, et al. Methylphenidate in depressed medically ill patients. *J Clin Psychiatry* 1991; **52**:263–267.

59. Woods SW, et al. Psychostimulant treatment of depressive disorders secondary to medical illness. *J Clin Psychiatry* 1986; **47**:12–15.

60. Kaufmann MW, et al. The use of d-amphetamine in medically ill depressed patients. *J Clin Psychiatry* 1982; **43**:463–464.

61. Wagner GJ, et al. Dexamphetamine as a treatment for depression and low energy in AIDS patients: a pilot study. *J Psychosom Res* 1997; **42**:407–411.

62. Wagner GJ, et al. Effects of dextroamphetamine on depression and fatigue in men with HIV: a double-blind, placebo-controlled trial. *J Clin Psychiatry* 2000; **61**:436–440.

63. Cheng YS, et al. Therapeutic benefits of pharmacologic and nonpharmacologic treatments for depressive symptoms after traumatic brain injury: a systematic review and network meta-analysis. *J Psychiatry Neurosci* 2021; **46**:e196–e207.

Post-stroke depression

Depression is a well-established risk factor for stroke.[1,2] In addition, depression is seen in at least 30–40% of survivors of stroke[3,4] and post-stroke depression is known to slow functional rehabilitation.[5] Antidepressants may reduce depressive symptom severity[6] and thereby facilitate faster rehabilitation.[7] They may also improve global cognitive functioning,[8,9] enhance motor recovery[10] and even reduce mortality.[11] Despite these benefits, post-stroke depression often goes untreated.[12]

Prophylaxis of post-stroke depression

The high incidence of depression after stroke makes prophylaxis worthy of consideration. Pooled data suggest a prophylactic effect for antidepressants.[13,14] Nortriptyline, fluoxetine, escitalopram, duloxetine, mirtazapine and sertraline appear to prevent post-stroke depression.[13,14]

A large cohort study suggested that mirtazapine and venlafaxine may be associated with an increased risk of a new stroke compared with SSRIs or TCAs.[15]

Mianserin seems ineffective in the treatment of post-stroke depression.[16] Amitriptyline[17] and duloxetine are effective in treating central post-stroke pain.

Routine use of antidepressants for the prevention of post-stroke depression is, however, not recommended.[18] A Cochrane review[19] suggests that there may be a benefit but regards the supporting evidence as poor. RCTs published since the Cochrane review suggest that the risks of prescribing fluoxetine (bone fractures, falls, seizures) may outweigh uncertain reduction in incident depression.[20–22] Prophylactic use may be justified in individual cases.

Treatment of post-stroke depression

Treatment is complicated by medical comorbidity and by the potential for interaction with other co-prescribed drugs. Antidepressants that enhance serotonin release can be expected to reduce platelet adhesion and increase the risk of bleeding, especially when co-prescribed with aspirin or anticoagulants (see section on SSRIs and bleeding in this chapter). There is also potential for pharmacokinetic interaction between antidepressants and anticoagulants.

Overall, contraindication to antidepressant treatment is more likely with tricyclics than with SSRIs.[23] Fluoxetine,[24,25] citalopram/escitalopram[8,26–28] and nortriptyline[29,30] are probably the most studied[31] and seem to be effective and safe in respect to pharmacokinetic interaction. RCTs also support the use of other antidepressants, including sertraline,[27] mirtazapine[32] and agomelatine.[33] Reboxetine (which, like nortriptyline, does not affect platelet activity) may also be effective and well tolerated,[34] although its effects overall are doubtful.[35] Vortioxetine may be of particular benefit because of its additional benefits for cognition, independent of any effects on depressive symptoms. It also does not appear to adversely affect cardiovascular parameters or interact with warfarin or aspirin, but data to support its use specifically in post-stroke depression are limited to a single pilot study.[36]

Despite their anti-platelet effects, SSRIs seem not to increase risk of stroke[37,38] (at least post-stroke), although some doubt remains.[39,40] Depression itself increases the risk of stroke, so initiation of an antidepressant post-stroke may appear to be associated

---

Box 3.3 Post-stroke depression – recommended drugs

- SSRIs*
- Mirtazapine
- Nortriptyline*

---

*Caution is clearly required if the index stroke was known to be haemorrhagic because SSRIs increase the risk of de novo haemorrhagic stroke (although absolute risk is low), especially when combined with warfarin or other anti-platelet drugs.[41,42] If the patient is taking warfarin, suggest citalopram or escitalopram (probably lowest interaction potential[43]) and use the lowest effective dose.[40] Little is known of the pharmacokinetic interaction potential with direct-acting oral anticoagulants (DOACs). Citalopram or escitalopram may again be preferred, as neither drug affects the enzymes associated with DOAC metabolism.[44] The pharmacodynamic interaction always remains – SSRIs increase the risk of major bleeding when combined with anticoagulants.[45]

with a heightened risk of stroke recurrence for this reason. Stroke can be embolic or haemorrhagic – SSRIs may protect against the former[46,47] and provoke the latter,[48,49] although the evidence base for this is rather weak[50] (see section on SSRIs and bleeding in this chapter). Other adverse effects may also be problematic; specifically falls, bone fractures and seizures.[19,24] Agomelatine is better tolerated than SSRIs or SNRIs in the post-stroke population and seems not to affect clotting parameters.[33]

Antidepressants are clearly effective in post-stroke depression[51] and treatment should not usually be withheld.[52] Inadequate treatment of depression increases the risk of stroke.[11,53] Two network meta-analyses suggested that paroxetine might be the drug of choice when considering both efficacy and tolerability post-stroke, although small sample sizes and a lack of high-quality studies in this area limit the strength of this recommendation.[54,55] Each analysis included only one paroxetine trial, whereas a meta-analysis of four trials of paroxetine found no benefit.[56] A 2020 large network meta-analysis of 51 trials ranked mirtazapine first for response rate, followed by venlafaxine and escitalopram, although the studies were limited to Chinese participants and so may lack generalisability.[57] Box 3.3 shows recommended drugs for use in post-stroke depression.

Where SSRIs are given in any patient treated with anticoagulants or aspirin, consideration should be given to the prescription of a proton-pump inhibitor for gastric protection. Nortriptyline, which does not appear to increase risk of bleeding, is an alternative.

References

1. Murphy RP, et al. Depressive symptoms and risk of acute stroke: INTERSTROKE case-control study. *Neurology* 2023; 100:e1787–e1798.
2. Ashraf F, et al. Association between depression and stroke risk in adults: a systematic review and meta-analysis. *Front Neurol* 2024; 15:1331300.
3. Gainotti G, et al. Relation between depression after stroke, antidepressant therapy, and functional recovery. *J Neurol Neurosurg Psychiatry* 2001; 71:258–261.
4. Hayee MA, et al. Depression after stroke-analysis of 297 stroke patients. *Bangladesh Med Res Counc Bull* 2001; 27:96–102.
5. Paolucci S, et al. Post-stroke depression, antidepressant treatment and rehabilitation results: a case-control study. *Cerebrovasc Dis* 2001; 12:264–271.
6. Xu XM, et al. Efficacy and feasibility of antidepressant treatment in patients with post-stroke depression. *Medicine (Baltimore)* 2016; 95:e5349.
7. Gainotti G, et al. Determinants and consequences of post-stroke depression. *Curr Opin Neurol* 2002; 15:85–89.
8. Jorge RE, et al. Escitalopram and enhancement of cognitive recovery following stroke. *Arch Gen Psychiatry* 2010; 67:187–196.
9. Gu SC, et al. Early selective serotonin reuptake inhibitors for recovery after stroke: a meta-analysis and trial sequential analysis. *J Stroke Cerebrovasc Dis* 2018; 27:1178–1189.

10. Thilarajah S, et al. Factors associated with post-stroke physical activity: a systematic review and meta-analysis. *Arch Phys Med Rehabil* 2018; **27**:1178–1189.
11. Krivoy A, et al. Low adherence to antidepressants is associated with increased mortality following stroke: a large nationally representative cohort study. *Eur Neuropsychopharmacol* 2017; **27**:970–976.
12. El Husseini N, et al. Depression and antidepressant use after stroke and transient ischemic attack. *Stroke* 2012; **43**:1609–1616.
13. Farooq S, et al. Pharmacological interventions for prevention of depression in high risk conditions: systematic review and meta-analysis. *J Affect Disord* 2020; **269**:58–69.
14. Woranush W, et al. Preventive approaches for post-stroke depression: where do we stand? A systematic review. *Neuropsychiatr Dis Treat* 2021; **17**:3359–3377.
15. Coupland C, et al. Antidepressant use and risk of adverse outcomes in older people: population based cohort study. *BMJ* 2011; **343**:d4551.
16. Palomaki H, et al. Prevention of poststroke depression: 1 year randomised placebo controlled double blind trial of mianserin with 6 month follow up after therapy. *J Neurol Neurosurg Psychiatry* 1999; **66**:490–494.
17. Lampl C, et al. Amitriptyline in the prophylaxis of central poststroke pain. Preliminary results of 39 patients in a placebo-controlled, long-term study. *Stroke* 2002; **33**:3030–3032.
18. Masuccio FG, et al. Post-stroke depression in older adults: an overview. *Drugs Aging* 2024; **41**:303–318.
19. Legg LA, et al. Selective serotonin reuptake inhibitors (SSRIs) for stroke recovery. *Cochrane Database Syst Rev* 2021; **11**:CD009286.
20. Tay J, et al. Does fluoxetine reduce apathetic and depressive symptoms after stroke? An analysis of the efficacy of fluoxetine – a randomized controlled trial in stroke trial data set. *Int J Stroke* 2023; **18**:285–295.
21. AFFINITY Trial Collaboration. Safety and efficacy of fluoxetine on functional outcome after acute stroke (AFFINITY): a randomised, double-blind, placebo-controlled trial. *Lancet Neurol* 2020; **19**:651–660.
22. Almeida OP, et al. Depression outcomes among patients treated with fluoxetine for stroke recovery: the AFFINITY randomized clinical trial. *JAMA Neurol* 2021; **78**:1072–1079.
23. Cole MG, et al. Feasibility and effectiveness of treatments for post-stroke depression in elderly inpatients: systematic review. *J Geriatr Psychiatry Neurol* 2001; **14**:37–41.
24. Mead G, et al. Individual patient data meta-analysis of the effects of fluoxetine on functional outcomes after acute stroke. *Int J Stroke* 2024; **19**:798–808.
25. Wu J, et al. The efficacy and safety of fluoxetine versus placebo for stroke recovery: a meta-analysis of randomized controlled trials. *Int J Clin Pharm* 2023; **45**:839–846.
26. Cui M, et al. Efficacy and safety of citalopram for the treatment of poststroke depression: a meta-analysis. *J Stroke Cerebrovasc Dis* 2018; **27**:2905–2918.
27. Yan N, et al. The safety and efficacy of escitalopram and sertraline in post-stroke depression: a randomized controlled trial. *BMC Psychiatry* 2024; **24**:365.
28. Ece Çetin F, et al. Efficacy of citalopram on stroke recurrence: a randomized clinical trial. *J Clin Neurosci* 2022; **101**:168–174.
29. Robinson RG, et al. Nortriptyline versus fluoxetine in the treatment of depression and in short-term recovery after stroke: a placebo-controlled, double-blind study. *Am J Psychiatry* 2000; **157**:351–359.
30. Zhang Wh, et al. Nortriptyline protects mitochondria and reduces cerebral ischemia/hypoxia injury. *Stroke* 2008; **39**:455–462.
31. Starkstein SE, et al. Antidepressant therapy in post-stroke depression. *Expert Opin Pharmacother* 2008; **9**:1291–1298.
32. Niedermaier N, et al. Prevention and treatment of poststroke depression with mirtazapine in patients with acute stroke. *J Clin Psychiatry* 2004; **65**:1619–1623.
33. Chen Y, et al. Efficacy and safety of agomelatine versus SSRIs/SNRIs for post-stroke depression: a systematic review and meta-analysis of randomized controlled trials. *Int Clin Psychopharmacol* 2024; **39**:163–173.
34. Rampello L, et al. An evaluation of efficacy and safety of reboxetine in elderly patients affected by 'retarded' post-stroke depression: a random, placebo-controlled study. *Arch Gerontol Geriatr* 2005; **40**:275–285.
35. Eyding D, et al. Reboxetine for acute treatment of major depression: systematic review and meta-analysis of published and unpublished placebo and selective serotonin reuptake inhibitor controlled trials. *BMJ* 2010; **341**:c4737.
36. Gamberini G, et al. Safety and efficacy of vortioxetine on depressive symptoms and cognition in post-stroke patients: a pilot study. *J Affect Disord* 2021; **286**:108–109.
37. Broman J, et al. Association of post-stroke-initiated antidepressants with long-term outcomes in young adults with ischaemic stroke. *Ann Med* 2022; **54**:1757–1766.
38. Douglas I, et al. The use of antidepressants and the risk of haemorrhagic stroke: a nested case control study. *Br J Clin Pharmacol* 2011; **71**:116–120.
39. Trajkova S, et al. Use of antidepressants and risk of incident stroke: a systematic review and meta-analysis. *Neuroepidemiology* 2019; **53**:142–151.
40. Kim JH, et al. Major adverse cardiovascular events in antidepressant users within patients with ischemic heart diseases: a nationwide cohort study. *J Clin Psychopharmacol* 2020; **40**:475–481.
41. Jeong HE, et al. Risk of major adverse cardiovascular events associated with concomitant use of antidepressants and non-steroidal anti-inflammatory drugs: a retrospective cohort study. *CNS Drugs* 2020; **34**:1063–1074.
42. Quinn GR, et al. Effect of selective serotonin reuptake inhibitors on bleeding risk in patients with atrial fibrillation taking warfarin. *Am J Cardiol* 2014; **114**:583–586.
43. Sayal KS, et al. Psychotropic interactions with warfarin. *Acta Psychiatr Scand* 2000; **102**:250–255.
44. Fitzgerald JL, et al. Drug interactions of direct-acting oral anticoagulants. *Drug Saf* 2016; **39**:841–845.
45. Bakker S, et al. Selective serotonin reuptake inhibitor use and risk of major bleeding during treatment with vitamin K antagonists: results of a cohort study. *Thromb Haemost* 2023; **123**:245–254.

46. He Y, et al. Effect of fluoxetine on three-year recurrence in acute ischemic stroke: a randomized controlled clinical study. *Clin Neurol Neurosurg* 2018; **168**:1–6.

47. Douros A, et al. Degree of serotonin reuptake inhibition of antidepressants and ischemic risk: a cohort study. *Neurology* 2019; **93**:e1010–e1020.

48. Trifiro G, et al. Risk of ischemic stroke associated with antidepressant drug use in elderly persons. *J Clin Psychopharmacol* 2010; **30**:252–258.

49. Wu CS, et al. Association of cerebrovascular events with antidepressant use: a case-crossover study. *Am J Psychiatry* 2011; **168**:511–521.

50. Mortensen JK, et al. Safety of selective serotonin reuptake inhibitor treatment in recovering stroke patients. *Expert Opin Drug Saf* 2015; **14**:911–919.

51. Mead GE, et al. Selective serotonin reuptake inhibitors for stroke recovery. *JAMA* 2013; **310**:1066–1067.

52. Allida SM, et al. Pharmacological, non-invasive brain stimulation and psychological interventions, and their combination, for treating depression after stroke. *Cochrane Database Syst Rev* 2023; 7:CD003437.

53. Bangalore S, et al. Cardiovascular hazards of insufficient treatment of depression among patients with known cardiovascular disease: a propensity score adjusted analysis. *Eur Heart J Qual Care Clin Outcomes* 2018; **4**:258–266.

54. Sun Y, et al. Comparative efficacy and acceptability of antidepressant treatment in poststroke depression: a multiple-treatments meta-analysis. *BMJ Open* 2017; 7:e016499.

55. Deng L, et al. Interventions for management of post-stroke depression: a Bayesian network meta-analysis of 23 randomized controlled trials. *Sci Rep* 2017; 7:16466.

56. Li L, et al. Effectiveness of paroxetine for poststroke depression: a meta-analysis. *J Stroke Cerebrovasc Dis* 2020; **29**:104664.

57. Li X, et al. Comparative efficacy of nine antidepressants in treating Chinese patients with post-stroke depression: a network meta-analysis. *J Affect Disord* 2020; **266**:540–548.

Antidepressant prophylaxis

After first episode

A single episode of depression should be treated for at least 6–9 months after full remission.[1] If antidepressant therapy is stopped immediately on recovery, 50% of patients experience a return of depressive symptoms within 3–6 months.[1] A landmark study of fluoxetine maintenance[2] demonstrated that stopping successful treatment at 12 weeks produced the highest relapse rate, followed by withdrawal at 26 weeks, and then withdrawal at 50 weeks (at which point placebo and active treatment did not differ in respect to relapse risk). Another trial suggested that withdrawal should only be attempted when patients had been free of significant symptoms for 16–20 weeks.[3] Even non-continuous use of antidepressants during the first 6 months of treatment predicts higher rates of relapse.[4]

Recurrent depression

Major depressive disorder is unremitting in 15% of cases and recurrent in 35%. About 50% of those with a first-onset episode recover and have no further episodes when followed for over 20 years.[5] Many factors are known to increase the risk of recurrence, including a family history of depression, recurrent dysthymia, concurrent non-affective psychiatric illness, female gender, long episode duration, degree of treatment resistance,[6] chronic medical illness and social factors (e.g. lack of confiding relationships and psychosocial stressors). Some prescription drugs may precipitate depression.[6,7] Antidepressants are generally effective in the post-acute maintenance phase – the 6 months after remission.[8] Longer-term outcomes have also been examined.

Figure 3.4 outlines the risk of recurrence for patients who have multiple episodes of depression. Those recruited to the study had already experienced at least three episodes of depression, with 3 years or less between episodes.[9,10]

A meta-analysis of antidepressant continuation studies[11] concluded that continuing treatment with antidepressants reduces the odds of depressive relapse by around two-thirds

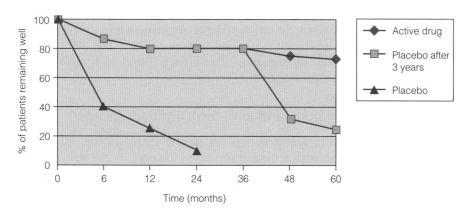

Figure 3.4 The risk of recurrence in patients who have several episodes of depression. Patients had experienced at least three episodes of depression with 3 years or fewer between episodes.

CHAPTER 3

(approximately equal to a halving of the absolute risk). A later meta-analysis of 54 studies suggested that odds of relapse were reduced by 65%.[12] The risk of relapse is greatest in the first few months after discontinuation and this holds true irrespective of the duration of prior treatment.[13] Benefits persist at 36 months and beyond and seem to be similar across heterogeneous patient groups (first episode, multiple episode and chronic).

An RCT of maintenance treatment in elderly patients, many of whom were first episode, found continuation treatment with antidepressants beneficial over 2 years, with a similar effect size to that seen in younger adults.[14] One small RCT (n = 22) demonstrated benefit from prophylactic antidepressants in adolescents.[15]

Many patients who might benefit from maintenance treatment with antidepressants do not receive them.[16] Assuring optimal management of long-term depression vastly reduces mortality associated with the condition.[17]

An alternative view is that the prophylactic effects of antidepressants have been overestimated because of confounding in maintenance trials. Effective drug treatment may be abruptly withdrawn, and it is the manner of this withdrawal (not necessarily the withdrawal itself) which increases the risk of relapse.[18,19] Most of the apparent relapse after stopping antidepressants occurs in the first 6 months.[20] Abrupt discontinuation increases the risk of relapse and exacerbates withdrawal symptoms (see below). It may be that at least part of the advantage reported for continuation treatment is derived from suboptimal treatment in patients switched to placebo. Some studies employ longer periods (a month or more) of withdrawal from active treatment[21] but even this may not be long enough to allow complete abolition of the negative effects of withdrawal.[22] There is also a minority school of thought which posits that antidepressants may ultimately worsen the conditions they treat.[23] Some tenuous support for this theory comes from the observation that response to antidepressants reduces in line with the number of antidepressants previously prescribed.[24]

Other disadvantages of long-term antidepressants include an increased risk of GI and cerebral haemorrhage (see section on SSRIs and bleeding in this chapter) and an additional risk of interaction with co-prescribed drugs likely to increase risk of bleeding or hyponatraemia.

These observations, alongside awareness that maintenance trials have been conducted largely in those in remission, strongly suggest that antidepressant treatment should be continued only where there is clear evidence of substantial efficacy. This may seem like an obvious point, but clinical experience suggests that long-term, ineffective or partially effective antidepressant treatment is commonplace. The aim of treatment should be the achieving and maintenance of remission. Residual symptoms portend poor outcome and higher risk of relapse.[25]

Discontinuation of medium- and long-term antidepressants

Stopping antidepressants in remitted patients clearly increases the risk of relapse compared with continuing with antidepressants.[26] However, as already noted, many studies may be confounded by abrupt discontinuation of active treatment, which worsens risk of relapse[27] and increases risk of withdrawal symptoms (which may mimic relapse).[28]

Two studies have tried to address these confounding influences. In the ANTLER trial, patients who were well after at least 2 years of treatment were randomised to continue treatment or to have antidepressants slowly stopped.[29] After 1 year, relapse occurred in 56% of stoppers and 39% of continuers. There was clear evidence of withdrawal symptoms despite the slow withdrawal (probably because alternate day dosing was used). In the REDUCE study,[30] patients receiving antidepressants for 1 year (first episode) or 2 years (multi-episode) were slowly withdrawn from treatment. Around 43% of patients were able to discontinue treatment without relapse by 6 months. The main finding from these studies, taken together, is that successful withdrawal from long-term antidepressants is possible, but that continued treatment is probably necessary (and somewhat effective) for a substantial proportion of people.

Dose for prophylaxis

Adults should receive the same dose as used for acute treatment.[31] There is some evidence to support the use of lower doses in elderly patients. Dosulepin 75mg/day offers effective prophylaxis[32] but is now rarely used and its relevance is dubious. There is no evidence to support the use of lower than standard doses of SSRIs.[33]

Relapse rates after ECT are similar to those after stopping antidepressants.[34] Antidepressant prophylaxis will be required, ideally with a different drug from the one that failed in the first instance, although good data in this area are lacking.

Lithium also has some efficacy in the prophylaxis of unipolar depression but efficacy relative to standard antidepressants is unknown.[35] Lithium treatment may have the best outcomes of any treatment for unipolar depression.[36] In the UK, NICE has recommended that lithium should not be used as the sole prophylactic drug in unipolar depression.[37] There is some support for the use of a combination of lithium and nortriptyline.[38] Maintenance treatment with lithium protects against suicide.[31]

References

1. Cleare A, et al. Evidence-based guidelines for treating depressive disorders with antidepressants: a revision of the 2008 British Association for Psychopharmacology guidelines. *J Psychopharmacol* 2015; **29**:459–525.
2. Reimherr FW, et al. Optimal length of continuation therapy in depression: a prospective assessment during long-term fluoxetine treatment. *Am J Psychiatry* 1998; **155**:1247–1253.
3. Prien RF, et al. Continuation drug therapy for major depressive episodes: how long should it be maintained? *Am J Psychiatry* 1986; **143**:18–23.
4. Kim KH, et al. The effects of continuous antidepressant treatment during the first 6 months on relapse or recurrence of depression. *J Affect Disord* 2011; **132**:121–129.
5. Eaton WW, et al. Population-based study of first onset and chronicity in major depressive disorder. *Arch Gen Psychiatry* 2008; **65**:513–520.
6. National Institute for Health and Care Excellence. Depression in adults with a chronic physical health problem: recognition and management. Clinical guideline [CG91]. 2009 (reviewed May 2024, last checked November 2024); https://www.nice.org.uk/guidance/CG91.
7. Patten SB, et al. Drug-induced depression. *Psychother Psychosom* 1997; **66**:63–73.
8. Kishi T, et al. Antidepressants for the treatment of adults with major depressive disorder in the maintenance phase: a systematic review and network meta-analysis. *Mol Psychiatry* 2023; **28**:402–409.
9. Frank E, et al. Three-year outcomes for maintenance therapies in recurrent depression. *Arch Gen Psychiatry* 1990; **47**:1093–1099.
10. Kupfer DJ, et al. Five-year outcome for maintenance therapies in recurrent depression. *Arch Gen Psychiatry* 1992; **49**:769–773.
11. Geddes JR, et al. Relapse prevention with antidepressant drug treatment in depressive disorders: a systematic review. *Lancet* 2003; **361**:653–661.
12. Glue P, et al. Meta-analysis of relapse prevention antidepressant trials in depressive disorders. *Aust N Z J Psychiatry* 2010; **44**:697–705.
13. Keller MB, et al. The Prevention of Recurrent Episodes of Depression with Venlafaxine for Two Years (PREVENT) study: outcomes from the 2-year and combined maintenance phases. *J Clin Psychiatry* 2007; **68**:1246–1256.
14. Reynolds CF, III, et al. Maintenance treatment of major depression in old age. *N Engl J Med* 2006; **354**:1130–1138.
15. Cheung A, et al. Maintenance study for adolescent depression. *J Child Adolesc Psychopharmacol* 2008; **18**:389–394.
16. Holma IA, et al. Maintenance pharmacotherapy for recurrent major depressive disorder: 5-year follow-up study. *Br J Psychiatry* 2008; **193**:163–164.

17. Gallo JJ, et al. Long term effect of depression care management on mortality in older adults: follow-up of cluster randomized clinical trial in primary care. *BMJ* 2013; **346**:f2570.

18. Cohen D, et al. Withdrawal effects confounding in clinical trials: another sign of a needed paradigm shift in psychopharmacology research. *Ther Adv Psychopharmacol* 2020; **10**:2045125320964097.

19. Hengartner MP. Editorial: Antidepressant prescriptions in children and adolescents. *Front Psychiatry* 2020; **11**:600283.

20. Zhou D, et al. Effects of antidepressant medicines on preventing relapse of unipolar depression: a pooled analysis of parametric survival curves. *Psychol Med* 2022; **52**:48–56.

21. DeRubeis RJ, et al. Prevention of recurrence after recovery from a major depressive episode with antidepressant medication alone or in combination with cognitive behavioral therapy: phase 2 of a 2-phase randomized clinical trial. *JAMA Psychiatry* 2020; **77**:237–245.

22. Horowitz MA, et al. Tapering of SSRI treatment to mitigate withdrawal symptoms. *Lancet Psychiatry* 2019; **6**:538–546.

23. Fava GA. May antidepressant drugs worsen the conditions they are supposed to treat? The clinical foundations of the oppositional model of tolerance. *Ther Adv Psychopharmacol* 2020; **10**:2045125320970325.

24. Amsterdam JD, et al. Prior antidepressant treatment trials may predict a greater risk of depressive relapse during antidepressant maintenance therapy. *J Clin Psychopharmacol* 2019; **39**:344–350.

25. Kennedy N, et al. Residual symptoms at remission from depression: impact on long-term outcome. *J Affect Disord* 2004; **80**:135–144.

26. Kato M, et al. Discontinuation of antidepressants after remission with antidepressant medication in major depressive disorder: a systematic review and meta-analysis. *Mol Psychiatry* 2021; **26**:118–133.

27. Van Leeuwen E, et al. Approaches for discontinuation versus continuation of long-term antidepressant use for depressive and anxiety disorders in adults. *Cochrane Database Syst Rev* 2021; **4**:CD013495.

28. Horowitz MA, et al. Distinguishing relapse from antidepressant withdrawal: clinical practice and antidepressant discontinuation studies. *BJPsych Advances* 2022; **28**:297–311.

29. Lewis G, et al. Maintenance or discontinuation of antidepressants in primary care. *N Engl J Med* 2021; **385**:1257–1267.

30. Kendrick T, et al. Internet and telephone support for discontinuing long-term antidepressants: the REDUCE cluster randomized trial. *JAMA Netw Open* 2024; **7**:e2418383.

31. Anderson IM, et al. Evidence-based guidelines for treating depressive disorders with antidepressants: a revision of the 2000 British Association for Psychopharmacology guidelines. *J Psychopharmacol* 2008; **22**:343–396.

32. Group OADI. How long should the elderly take antidepressants? A double-blind placebo-controlled study of continuation/prophylaxis therapy with dothiepin. *Br J Psychiatry* 1993; **162**:175–182.

33. Franchini L, et al. Dose-response efficacy of paroxetine in preventing depressive recurrences: a randomized, double-blind study. *J Clin Psychiatry* 1998; **59**:229–232.

34. Nobler MS, et al. *Refractory Depression and Electroconvulsive Therapy*. Chichester: Wiley; 1994.

35. Cipriani A, et al. Lithium versus antidepressants in the long-term treatment of unipolar affective disorder. *Cochrane Database Syst Rev* 2006; (4):CD003492.

36. Young AH. Lithium for long-term treatment of unipolar depression. *Lancet Psychiatry* 2017; **4**:511–512.

37. National Institute for Health and Care Excellence. Depression in adults: treatment and management. NICE guideline [NG222]. 2022 (last reviewed September 2024, last checked November 2024); https://www.nice.org.uk/guidance/ng222.

38. Sackeim HA, et al. Continuation pharmacotherapy in the prevention of relapse following electroconvulsive therapy: a randomized controlled trial. *JAMA* 2001; **285**:1299–1307.

Drug interactions with antidepressants

Antidepressants are involved in a number of both pharmacokinetic and pharmacodynamic interactions.

Pharmacokinetic interactions

Pharmacokinetic interactions occur when one drug interferes with the absorption, distribution, metabolism or elimination of another drug. This may result in a subtherapeutic effect or toxicity. The largest group of pharmacokinetic interactions involves drugs that inhibit or induce hepatic CYP enzymes (Tables 3.11 and 3.12). Other enzyme systems include the flavin-containing monooxygenase (FMO) and the uridine diphosphate (UDP)-glucuronosyltransferases (UGT).[1] While both these latter enzyme systems are involved in the metabolism of psychotropic drugs, the potential for drugs to inhibit or induce these enzyme systems has been less well studied.

The clinical consequences of pharmacokinetic interactions in an individual patient can be difficult to predict. Some could be highly clinically significant; for example, when paroxetine (a potent CYP2D6 inhibitor) is taken with tamoxifen, metabolism to its active metabolite is reduced, possibly increasing the risk of breast cancer recurrence.[2] The following factors affect outcome of interactions: the degree of enzyme inhibition or induction, the pharmacokinetic properties of the affected drug and other co-administered drugs, the relationship between plasma level and pharmacodynamic effect for the affected drug, and patient-specific factors such as genetic differences in metabolic enzymes variability[3] in the role of primary and secondary metabolic pathways and the presence of comorbid physical illness.[4]

Table 3.11 Summary of antidepressant effects on CYP enzymes.[5-7]

Antidepressant		Substrate for	Inhibits
SSRIs			
	Citalopram	**CYP2C19**, CYP2D6, CYP3A4	CYP2D6 (weak)
	Escitalopram	**CYP2C19**, CYP2D6, CYP3A4	CYP2D6 (weak)
	Fluoxetine	**CYP2D6**, CYP3A4	**CYP2D6** (moderate to potent), CYP2C9 (moderate), CYP3A4 (weak)
	Fluvoxamine	CYP2D6; others possibly involved	**CYP1A2** (potent), **CYP2C19** (potent), CYP3A4 (weak), CYP2C9 (weak)
	Paroxetine	**CYP2D6**	**CYP2D6** (potent)
	Sertraline	**CYP3A4**, CYP2D6 (minor) and possibly other pathways	**CYP2D6** (weak)
SNRIs			
	Desvenlafaxine	CYP3A4	CYP2D6 (weak)
	Duloxetine	**CYP1A2**, **CYP2D6**	CYP2D6 (moderate)
	Levomilnacipran	**CYP3A4**, CYP2C8, CYP2C19, CYP2D6	
	Venlafaxine	**CYP2D6**, CYP3A4	CYP2D6 (weak)

(Continued)

Table 3.11 (*Continued*)

Antidepressant	Substrate for	Inhibits
TCAs		
Amitriptyline	**CYP1A2**, **CYP2D6**, CYP3A4, CYP2C19	
Clomipramine		
Desipramine	**CYP2D6**	
Dosulepin	CYP2D6 and possibly other pathways	
Doxepin	CYP2D6, CYP1A2 (minor), CYP3A4 (minor)	
Imipramine	**CYP1A2**, **CYP2D6**, CYP3A4, CYP2C19	
Lofepramine	**2D6** (metabolised to desipramine)[8]	Not known[9]
Nortriptyline	**CYP2D6**	
Trimipramine	**CYP2D6**	
Others		
Agomelatine	**CYP1A2**	
Brexanolone[10]	Metabolised via non-CYP pathways	CYP2C9
Bupropion	**CYP2B6**	**CYP2D6** (potent)
Dextromethorphan/bupropion[11]	**CYP2B6**, **CYP2D6**	**CYP2D6** (potent)
Esketamine	**CYP3A4**, **CYP2B6**	
Mianserin	CYP2D6	
Mirtazapine	CYP1A2, CYP2D6, CYP3A4	CYP2D6 (weak)
Phenelzine		CYP2C19, CYP3A4
Reboxetine	**CYP3A4**	
Tranylcypromine[12]		**CYP2A6**, CYP2C19
Trazodone	CYP3A4	
Vortioxetine	**CYP2D6**, CYP2A6, CYP2B6, CYP2C8, CYP2C9, CYP2C19, CYP3A4	
Vilazodone	**CYP3A4**	CYP2C8

CYP enzymes highlighted in **bold** indicate predominant metabolic enzyme pathway or potent inhibition of enzyme activity.

Pharmacodynamic interactions

Pharmacodynamic interactions arise when the effects of one drug are altered by another drug via mechanisms such as direct competition at receptor sites (e.g. dopamine agonists with dopamine antagonists), augmentation of the same neurotransmitter pathway (e.g. fluoxetine with tramadol or a triptan can lead to serotonin syndrome) or an effect on the physiological functioning of an organ/organ system in different ways (e.g. SSRIs impair clotting and non-steroidal anti-inflammatory drugs [NSAIDs] irritate the gastric

Table 3.12 Pharmacokinetic interactions: a brief summary of important interactions.[13,14]

CYP1A2	CYP2B6	CYP2C9	CYP2C19	CYP2D6	CYP3A4/5/7
Genetic polymorphism. Ultra-rapid metabolisers possible.	2–10% of total hepatic CYP content[15]	5–10% of people of European descent poor metabolisers	~20% of Asian and 3–5% people of European descent poor metabolisers	3–5% of people of European descent poor metabolisers	60% p450 content
Induced by:	*Induced by:*	*Induced by:*	*Induced by:*	*Induced by:*	*Induced by:*
carbamazepine charcoal cooking tobacco smoke omeprazole phenobarbital phenytoin	carbamazepine efavirenz (chronically)[16] lopinavir rifampicin ritonavir	phenytoin rifampicin	apalutamide artemisinin efavirenz enzalutamide rifampicin	carbamazepine phenytoin	carbamazepine phenytoin prednisolone rifampicin St John's wort
Inhibited by:	*Inhibited by:*	*Inhibited by:*	*Inhibited by:*	*Inhibited by:*	*Inhibited by:*
cimetidine ciprofloxacin erythromycin fluvoxamine	clopidogrel efavirenz (acutely)[16] ticlopidine voriconazole	cimetidine fluoxetine fluvoxamine moclobemide sertraline	armodafinil etravirine fluconazole fluoxetine fluvoxamine esomeprazole isoniazid moclobemide modafinil omeprazole voriconazole cimetidine	bupropion citalopram chlorpromazine desvenlafaxine duloxetine escitalopram fluoxetine fluphenazine haloperidol paroxetine sertraline tricyclics	erythromycin fluoxetine fluvoxamine grapefruit juice ketoconazole norfluoxetine paroxetine sertraline tricyclics
Metabolises:	*Metabolises:*	*Metabolises:*	*Metabolises:*	*Metabolises:*	*Metabolises:*
agomelatine benzodiazepines caffeine clozapine duloxetine haloperidol mirtazapine olanzapine ramelteon theophylline tizanidine tricyclics warfarin	bupropion methadone tramadol	agomelatine bupropion citalopram diazepam escitalopram omeprazole phenytoin tricyclics warfarin	citalopram diazepam moclobemide	aripiprazole atomoxetine brexpiprazole clozapine codeine dextromethorphan donepezil duloxetine haloperidol phenothiazines risperidone tamoxifen tricyclics tramadol trazodone venlafaxine vortioxetine	calcium blockers carbamazepine clozapine donepezil erythromycin galantamine levomilnacipran methadone mirtazapine reboxetine risperidone statins tricyclics valproate venlafaxine vilazodone vortioxetine z-hypnotics

CHAPTER 3

mucosa so, when these drugs are used together, the risk of GI bleeds is increased). Here, we provide a broad summary of these interactions. Up-to-date interaction tables are readily available online and most known interactions are described in an individual product's literature.

Tricyclic antidepressants[7,17–19]

- are H1 antagonists (sedative). This effect can be exacerbated by other sedative drugs or alcohol. Beware respiratory depression.
- are anticholinergic (dry mouth, blurred vision, constipation). This effect can be exacerbated by other anticholinergic drugs such as antihistamines or antipsychotics. Also associated with cognitive impairment and GI obstruction.
- are adrenergic α1 blockers (postural hypotension). This effect can be exacerbated by other drugs that block α1 receptors and by antihypertensive drugs in general. As a consequence, falls may be more common.
- are arrhythmogenic. Caution is required with other drugs that can alter cardiac conduction directly or indirectly (see section on antidepressant-induced arrhythmia in this chapter).
- lower the seizure threshold. Caution is required with other proconvulsive drugs (e.g. some antipsychotics) and particularly if the patient is being treated for epilepsy (see section on epilepsy in Chapter 10).
- possess varying degrees of serotonin reuptake inhibition (amitriptyline and clomipramine in particular). There is the potential for these drugs to interact with other serotonergic drugs (e.g. tramadol, SSRIs, MAOIs, triptans) to cause serotonin syndrome.

SSRIs/SNRIs[7,17,18,20,21]

- increase serotonergic neurotransmission. The main concern when co-prescribed with other serotonergic drugs is serotonin syndrome.
- inhibit platelet aggregation and increase the risk of bleeding, particularly of the upper GI tract. This effect is exacerbated by aspirin and NSAIDs (see section on SSRIs and bleeding in this chapter).
- may be more likely than other antidepressants to cause hyponatraemia (see section on antidepressant-induced hyponatraemia in this chapter). This may exacerbate electrolyte disturbances caused by other drugs such as diuretics.
- are associated with a decrease in bone mineral density. This adds to the negative effects prolactin elevating drugs have on bone mineral density and increases the risks of clinical harm should the patient have a fall.

MAOIs[12,22,23]

- prevent the metabolism of monoamine neurotransmitters (e.g. serotonin). Co-prescription with serotonergic drugs (in particular, serotonin reuptake inhibitors or releasing agents) risks potentially fatal serotonin syndrome. Examples include SSRI and related antidepressants but also certain over-the-counter medicines (e.g. chlorphenamine, dextromethorphan), opioids (e.g. tramadol, pethidine), antipsychotics (lumateperone and ziprasidone) and drugs of misuse such as MDMA (3,4-methylene dioxymethamphetamine).

■ prevent the destruction of other monoamine neurotransmitters (e.g. catecholamines). Co-prescription with sympathomimetic drugs that raise blood pressure (e.g. psycho-stimulants) can cause hypertensive crises. MAOIs also prevent the breakdown of dietary tyramine (high levels present in aged and fermented foods), which acts as a catecholamine-releasing agent leading to similar hypertensive reactions.

References

1. Carvalho Henriques B, et al. How can drug metabolism and transporter genetics inform psychotropic prescribing? *Front Genet* 2020; **11**:491895.

2. Bradbury M, et al. Time to update evidence-based guideline recommendations about concurrent tamoxifen and antidepressant use? A systematic review. *Clin Breast Cancer* 2022; **22**:e362–e373.

3. Kleine Schaars K, et al. Pharmacogenomics and the management of mood disorders: a review. *J Pers Med* 2023; **13**:1183.

4. Devane CL. Antidepressant-drug interactions are potentially but rarely clinically significant. *Neuropsychopharmacology* 2006; **31**:1594–1604.

5. Andrade C. Ketamine for depression, 5: potential pharmacokinetic and pharmacodynamic drug interactions. *J Clin Psychiatry* 2017; **78**:e858–e861.

6. Preskorn SH. Drug–drug interactions (DDIs) in psychiatric practice, part 9: interactions mediated by drug-metabolizing cytochrome P450 enzymes. *J Psychiatr Pract* 2020; **26**:126–134.

7. Preston C, ed. *Stockley's Drug Interactions*. Medicines Complete. 2024; https://www.pharmaceuticalpress.com/products/stockleys-drug-interactions.

8. Generics UK T/A Mylan. Summary of Product Characteristics. Lofepramine 70 mg film-coated tablets. Electronic Medicines Compendium, 2017; https://web.archive.org/web/20170803211505/http://www.medicines.org.uk/emc/medicine/33411#companyDetails.=.

9. Lancaster SG, et al. Lofepramine: a review of its pharmacodynamic and pharmacokinetic properties, and therapeutic efficacy in depressive illness. *Drugs* 1989; **37**:123–140.

10. Edinoff AN, et al. Brexanolone, a GABA(A) modulator, in the treatment of postpartum depression in adults: a comprehensive review. *Front Psychiatry* 2021; **12**:699740.

11. Keam SJ. Dextromethorphan/bupropion: first approval. *CNS Drugs* 2022; **36**:1229–1238.

12. Van den Eynde V, et al. The prescriber's guide to classic MAO inhibitors (phenelzine, tranylcypromine, isocarboxazid) for treatment-resistant depression. *CNS Spectr* 2023; **28**:427–440.

13. Mitchell PB. Drug interactions of clinical significance with selective serotonin reuptake inhibitors. *Drug Saf* 1997; **17**:390–406.

14. Kelly CM, et al. Selective serotonin reuptake inhibitors and breast cancer mortality in women receiving tamoxifen: a population based cohort study. *BMJ* 2010; **340**:c693.

15. Hedrich WD, et al. Insights into CYP2B6-mediated drug-drug interactions. *Acta Pharm Sin B* 2016; **6**:413–425.

16. Gufford BT, et al. Influence of CYP2B6 pharmacogenetics on stereoselective inhibition and induction of bupropion metabolism by efavirenz in healthy volunteers. *J Pharmacol Exp Ther* 2022; **382**:313–326.

17. Preskorn SH. Drug–drug interactions (DDIs) in psychiatric practice, part 8: relative receptor binding affinity as a way of understanding the differential pharmacology of currently available antidepressants. *J Psychiatr Pract* 2020; **26**:46–51.

18. National Institute for Health and Care Excellence. *British National Formulary*. 2024; https://bnf.nice.org.uk.

19. Gillman PK. Tricyclic antidepressant pharmacology and therapeutic drug interactions updated. *Br J Pharmacol* 2007; **151**:737–748.

20. Preskorn SH. Drug–drug interactions (DDIs) in psychiatric practice, part 6: pharmacodynamic considerations. *J Psychiatr Pract* 2019; **25**:290–297.

21. Mercurio M, et al. The use of antidepressants is linked to bone loss: a systematic review and metanalysis. *Orthop Rev (Pavia)* 2022; **14**:38564.

22. Gillman PK. Advances pertaining to the pharmacology and interactions of irreversible nonselective monoamine oxidase inhibitors. *J Clin Psychopharmacol* 2011; **31**:66–74.

23. Grady MM, et al. Practical guide for prescribing MAOIs: debunking myths and removing barriers. *CNS Spectr* 2012; **17**:2–10.

Cardiac effects of antidepressants – summary

The cardiac effects of antidepressants are summarised in Table 3.13.

Table 3.13 Cardiac effects of antidepressants.

Drug	Heart rate	Blood pressure	QTc	Arrhythmia	Conduction disturbance	Licensed restrictions post-MI	Comments
Agomelatine[1,2]	No changes reported	No changes reported	Single case of QTc prolongation	No arrhythmia reported	Unclear	No specific contra-indication	Cautiously recommended
Bupropion[1,3,4]	Slight increase	Slight increases in blood pressure but can sometimes be significant. Rarely postural hypotension.	QTc shortening, but prolongation has been reported in cases of overdose[5]	No effect. Rare reports in overdose.	None	Well tolerated for smoking cessation in post-MI patients	Be aware of interaction potential. Monitor blood pressure
Brexanolone[6–8]	One case of tachycardia reported in trials	Small reduction in blood pressure possible	No effect on QTc interval	No arrythmia reported	None	No specific contraindication	Minimal effect on cardiac parameters in trial data
Citalopram[1,9–12] (assume same for **escitalopram**)	Small decrease in heart rate	Slight drop in systolic blood pressure	Dose-related increase in QTc	Torsade de Pointes reported, mainly in overdose	None	Caution in patients with recent MI or uncompensated heart failure. But some evidence of safety in CVD.	Minor metabolite which increases QTc interval. No clear evidence of increased risk of arrhythmia at any licensed dose.
Dextromethorphan + bupropion[13]	As per bupropion	As per bupropion	As per bupropion. QTc prolongation in dextromethorphan overdose.[14]	As per bupropion	As per bupropion	No specific contraindication	As per bupropion
Duloxetine[1,15–17]	Slight increase	Important effect (see SPC). Caution in hypertension.	Isolated reports of QT prolongation	Isolated reports of toxicity	Isolated reports of toxicity	Caution in patients 'whose conditions could be compromised by an increased heart rate or by an increase in blood pressure'	Not recommended in cardiac disease

Drug	Heart rate	Blood pressure	QTc interval	Arrhythmia	Cardiac conduction	Caution	Comment
Fluoxetine[12,18-20]	Small decrease in mean heart rate	Minimal effect on blood pressure	No effect on QTc interval	None	None	Caution in patients with acute MI or heart failure	Evidence of safety post MI
Fluvoxamine[21,22]	Minimal effect on heart rate	Small drop in systolic blood pressure	No significant effect on QTc	None	None	Caution	Limited changes in ECG have been observed
Levomilnacipran[23-25]	Slight increase	Small increase	No effect on QTc interval*	Pre-existing tachyarrhythmias should be treated before initiating treatment	None	Caution in patients with cardiac disease	Monitor heart rate and blood pressure
Lofepramine[26,27]	Modest increase in heart rate	Less decrease in postural blood pressure than other TCAs	May prolong QTc interval at higher doses	May occur at higher doses, but rare	Unclear	Coronary insufficiency in patients with recent MI	Less cardiotoxic than other TCAs. Reasons unclear
MAOIs[26,28]	Decrease in heart rate	Postural hypotension. Risk of hypertensive crisis.	Unclear but may shorten QTc interval	May cause arrhythmia and decrease LVF	No clear effect on cardiac conduction	Use with caution in patients with CVD	Not recommended in CVD
Milnacipran[1,29]	Slight increase in heart rate (c.10bpm)	Small increases in systolic and diastolic BP	No effect on QTc	None	None	Caution	Avoid in hypertension and heart failure
Mirtazapine[1,30]	Minimal change in heart rate	Minimal effect on BP	No effect on QTc	None	None	Caution in patients with recent MI	Evidence of safety post MI. Good alternative to SSRIs.
Moclobemide[31-33]	Marginal decrease in heart rate	Minimal effect on blood pressure. Isolated cases of hypertensive episodes.	No effect on QTc interval in normal doses. Prolongation in overdose.	None	None	General caution in patients with a history of cardiac disorders	Possibly arrhythmogenic in overdose
Paroxetine[12,34,35]	Small decrease in mean heart rate	Minimal effect on BP	No effect on QTc interval	None	None	General caution in patients with cardiac disease	Probably safe post MI
Reboxetine[36-38]	Significant increase in heart rate	Marginal increase in both systolic and diastolic BP. Postural decrease at higher doses.	No effect on QTc	Rhythm abnormalities may occur	Atrial and ventricular ectopic beats, especially in the elderly	Caution in patients with cardiac disease	Probably best avoided in IHD

Table 3.13 (Continued)

Drug	Heart rate	Blood pressure	QTc	Arrhythmia	Conduction disturbance	Licensed restrictions post-MI	Comments
Sertraline[12,39–42]	Minimal effect on heart rate	Minimal effect on BP	No effect on QTc interval at standard doses. Small increase (<10ms) at 400mg/day.[43]	None	None	Drug of choice post MI but formal labelling acknowledges effect on QT and cautions against use in patients with additional risk factors for QTc prolongation	Safe post MI and in heart failure
Trazodone[26,44–46]	Decrease in heart rate more common, although increase can also occur	Can cause significant postural hypotension	Can prolong QTc interval	Several case reports of prolonged QT and arrhythmia	Unclear	Contraindicated in patients with acute MI	May be arrhythmogenic in patients with pre-existing cardiac disease
Tricyclics[26,47,48]	Increase in heart rate	Postural hypotension	Prolongation of QTc interval[†] and QRS interval	Ventricular arrhythmia common in overdose. Torsade de Pointes reported.	Slows cardiac conduction; blocks cardiac Na/K channels	Contraindicated in patients with recent MI	TCAs affect cardiac contractility. Some TCAs linked to IHD and sudden cardiac death. Avoid in IHD.
Venlafaxine[15,49–53] (assume same for **desvenlafaxine**)	Marginally increased	Some increase in postural blood pressure. At higher doses increase in BP.	Possible prolongation in overdose, but very rare	Rare reports of cardiac arrhythmia in overdose	Rare reports of conduction abnormalities	Has not been evaluated in post-MI patients. Caution advised.	Evidence for arrhythmogenic potential is slim, but avoid in IHD
Vilazodone[54–56]	Increased in overdose	Increased in overdose	No effect, even in overdose	No reports, even in overdose	No effect	No specific contraindications	Probably no effect on CV function in clinical doses
Vortioxetine[57–59]	No effect	No effect	No effect	No effect	No effect	No specific contraindications	Trial data suggest no effect on QTc or on coagulation parameters

* Small increase in QTc reported when using Bazett's correction formula but not with Fridericia's.

† Possibly the result of overestimation that can occur when using Bazett's correction formula at high resting heart rates.

CV, cardiovascular; CVD, cardiovascular disease; IHD, ischaemic heart disease; LVF, left ventricular function; MI, myocardial infarction; SPC, summary of product characteristics.

SSRIs are generally recommended in cardiac disease but beware anti-platelet activity and CYP-medicated interactions with co-administered cardiac drugs. Mirtazapine has been suggested as a suitable alternative[60] but it is also associated with bleeding disorders.[61]

SSRIs may protect against myocardial infarction (MI),[62,63] and untreated depression worsens prognosis in cardiovascular disease.[64] Post MI, SSRIs and mirtazapine have either a neutral or beneficial effect on mortality.[65] Treatment of depression with SSRIs should not therefore be withheld post MI. Protective effects of treatment of depression post MI appear to relate to antidepressant administration, possibly because of an anti-coagulant effect or because of indirect reduction in arrhythmia frequency.[42,66] CBT may be ineffective in this respect.[67,68] Note that the anti-platelet effect of SSRIs may have adverse consequences too (see section on SSRIs and bleeding in this chapter).

References

1. Behlke LM, et al. The cardiovascular effects of newer antidepressants in older adults and those with or at high risk for cardiovascular diseases. *CNS Drugs* 2020; **34**:1133–1147.
2. Kozian R, et al. [QTc prolongation during treatment with agomelatine]. *Psychiatr Prax* 2010; **37**:405–407.
3. Dwoskin LP, et al. Review of the pharmacology and clinical profile of bupropion, an antidepressant and tobacco use cessation agent. *CNS Drug Rev* 2006; **12**:178–207.
4. Castro VM, et al. QT interval and antidepressant use: a cross sectional study of electronic health records. *BMJ* 2013; **346**:f288.
5. Robinson S. Treatment of status epilepticus and prolonged QT after massive intentional bupropion overdose with lidocaine. *Am J Emerg Med* 2022; **55**:232.e3–232.e4.
6. Sage Therapeutics. Highlights of prescribing information. ZULRESSO® (brexanolone) injection, for intravenous use. 2019 (last accessed November 2024); https://www.accessdata.fda.gov/drugsatfda_docs/label/2019/211371lbl.pdf.
7. Faden J, et al. Intravenous brexanolone for postpartum depression: what it is, how well does it work, and will it be used? *Ther Adv Psychopharmacol* 2020; **10**:2045125320968658.
8. Center for Drug Evaluation and Research. Risk Evaluation and Mitigation Strategy (REMS) Document ZULRESSO (brexanolone) REMS Program. 2019 (last accessed February 2025); https://www.accessdata.fda.gov/drugsatfda_docs/nda/2019/211371Orig1s000REMS.pdf.
9. Catalano G, et al. QTc interval prolongation associated with citalopram overdose: a case report and literature review. *Clin Neuropharmacol* 2001; **24**:158–162.
10. Astrom-Lilja C, et al. Drug-induced torsades de pointes: a review of the Swedish pharmacovigilance database. *Pharmacoepidemiol Drug Saf* 2008; **17**:587–592.
11. Zivin K, et al. Evaluation of the FDA warning against prescribing citalopram at doses exceeding 40mg. *Am J Psychiatry* 2013; **170**:642–650.
12. Calvi A, et al. Antidepressant drugs effects on blood pressure. *Front Cardiovasc Med* 2021; **8**:704281.
13. Axsome Therapeutics. Highlights of Prescribing Information. AUVELITY (dextromethorphan hydrobromide and bupropion hydrochloride) extended-release tablets for oral use. 2022 (last accessed November 2024); https://www.accessdata.fda.gov/drugsatfda_docs/label/2022/215430s000lblCorrect3.pdf.
14. Kaplan B, et al. QTc prolongation due to dextromethorphan. *Int J Cardiol* 2011; **148**:363–364.
15. Colucci VJ, et al. Heart failure worsening and exacerbation after venlafaxine and duloxetine therapy. *Ann Pharmacother* 2008; **42**:882–887.
16. Stuhec M. Duloxetine-induced life-threatening long QT syndrome. *WienKlinWochenschr* 2013; **125**:165–166.
17. Orozco BS, et al. Duloxetine: an uncommon cause of fatal ventricular arrhythmia. *Clin Toxicol* 2014; **51**:672.
18. Fisch C. Effect of fluoxetine on the electrocardiogram. *J Clin Psychiatry* 1985; **46**:42–44.
19. Roose SP, et al. Cardiovascular effects of fluoxetine in depressed patients with heart disease. *Am J Psychiatry* 1998; **155**:660–665.
20. Strik JJ, et al. Efficacy and safety of fluoxetine in the treatment of patients with major depression after first myocardial infarction: findings from a double-blind, placebo-controlled trial. *Psychosom Med* 2000; **62**:783–789.
21. Strik JJ, et al. Cardiac side-effects of two selective serotonin reuptake inhibitors in middle-aged and elderly depressed patients. *Int Clin Psychopharmacol* 1998; **13**:263–267.
22. Stirnimann G, et al. Brugada syndrome ECG provoked by the selective serotonin reuptake inhibitor fluvoxamine. *Europace* 2010; **12**:282–283.
23. Mago R, et al. Safety and tolerability of levomilnacipran ER in major depressive disorder: results from an open-label, 48-week extension study. *Clin Drug Investig* 2013; **33**:761–771.
24. Allergan USA. Highlights of prescribing information. Fetzima (levomilnacipran) extended-release capsules for oral use. 2019 (last accessed November 2024); https://www.accessdata.fda.gov/drugsatfda_docs/label/2019/204168s006lbl.pdf.
25. Huang Q, et al. Efficacy and safety of multiple doses of levomilnacipran extended-release for the treatment of major depressive disorder. *Neuropsychiatr Dis Treat* 2016; **12**:2707–2714.
26. Warrington SJ, et al. The cardiovascular effects of antidepressants. *Psychol Med Monogr Suppl* 1989; **16**:i–40.
27. Stern H, et al. Cardiovascular effects of single doses of the antidepressants amitriptyline and lofepramine in healthy subjects. *Pharmacopsychiatry* 1985; **18**:272–277.

28. Waring WS, et al. Acute myocarditis after massive phenelzine overdose. *Eur J Clin Pharmacol* 2007; **63**:1007–1009.

29. Forest Pharmaceuticals. Highlights of prescribing information. Savella (milnacipran HCl) tablets. 2011 (last accessed November 2024); https://www.accessdata.fda.gov/drugsatfda_docs/label/2011/022256s011lbl.pdf.

30. Aurobindo Pharma-Milpharm. Summary of product characteristics. Mirtazapine 30mg tablets. 2024 (last accessed November 2024); https://www.medicines.org.uk/emc/product/535/smpc.

31. Moll E, et al. Safety and efficacy during long-term treatment with moclobemide. *Clin Neuropharmacol* 1994; **17** Suppl 1:S74–S87.

32. Hilton S, et al. Moclobemide safety: monitoring a newly developed product in the 1990s. *J Clin Psychopharmacol* 1995; **15**:76S–83S.

33. Downes MA, et al. QTc abnormalities in deliberate self-poisoning with moclobemide. *Intern Med J* 2005; **35**:388–391.

34. Kuhs H, et al. Cardiovascular effects of paroxetine. *Psychopharmacology* 1990; **102**:379–382.

35. Roose SP, et al. Comparison of paroxetine and nortriptyline in depressed patients with ischemic heart disease. *JAMA* 1998; **279**:287–291.

36. Mucci M. Reboxetine: a review of antidepressant tolerability. *J Psychopharmacol* 1997; **11**:S33–S37.

37. Holm KJ, et al. Reboxetine: a review of its use in depression. *CNS Drugs* 1999; **12**:65–83.

38. Fleishaker JC, et al. Lack of effect of reboxetine on cardiac repolarization. *Clin Pharmacol Ther* 2001; **70**:261–269.

39. Shapiro PA, et al. An open-label preliminary trial of sertraline for treatment of major depression after acute myocardial infarction (the SADHAT Trial). Sertraline Anti-Depressant Heart Attack Trial. *Am Heart J* 1999; **137**:1100–1106.

40. Glassman AH, et al. Sertraline treatment of major depression in patients with acute MI or unstable angina. *JAMA* 2002; **288**:701–709.

41. Jiang W, et al. Safety and efficacy of sertraline for depression in patients with CHF (SADHART-CHF): a randomized, double-blind, placebo-controlled trial of sertraline for major depression with congestive heart failure. *Am Heart J* 2008; **156**:437–444.

42. Leftheriotis D, et al. The role of the selective serotonin re-uptake inhibitor sertraline in nondepressive patients with chronic ischemic heart failure: a preliminary study. *Pacing Clin Electrophysiol* 2010; **33**:1217–1223.

43. Abbas R, et al. A thorough QT study to evaluate the effects of a supratherapeutic dose of sertraline on cardiac repolarization in healthy subjects. *Clin Pharmacol Drug Dev* 2020; **9**:307–320.

44. Service JA, et al. QT prolongation and delayed atrioventricular conduction caused by acute ingestion of trazodone. *Clin Toxicol (Phila)* 2008; **46**:71–73.

45. Dattilo PB, et al. Prolonged QT associated with an overdose of trazodone. *J Clin Psychiatry* 2007; **68**:1309–1310.

46. Winkler D, et al. Trazodone-induced cardiac arrhythmias: a report of two cases. *Hum Psychopharmacol* 2006; **21**:61–62.

47. Hippisley-Cox J, et al. Antidepressants as risk factor for ischaemic heart disease: case–control study in primary care. *BMJ* 2001; **323**:666–669.

48. Taylor D, et al. The cardiovascular safety of tricyclic antidepressants in overdose and in clinical use. *Ther Adv Psychopharmacol* 2024; **14**:20451253241243297.

49. Khawaja IS, et al. Cardiovascular effects of selective serotonin reuptake inhibitors and other novel antidepressants. *Heart Dis* 2003; **5**:153–160.

50. Upjohn UK Limited. Summary of product characteristics. Efexor XL 75 mg (venlafaxine hydrochloride) hard prolonged release capsules. 2024 (last accessed November 2024); https://www.medicines.org.uk/emc/product/5474/smpc#gref.

51. Letsas K, et al. QT interval prolongation associated with venlafaxine administration. *Int J Cardiol* 2006; **109**:116–117.

52. Taylor D, et al. Volte-face on venlafaxine: reasons and reflections. *J Psychopharmacol* 2006; **20**:597–601.

53. Cooper JM, et al. Desvenlafaxine overdose and the occurrence of serotonin toxicity, seizures and cardiovascular effects. *Clin Toxicol (Phila)* 2017; **55**:18–24.

54. Edwards J, et al. Vilazodone lacks proarrhythmogenic potential in healthy participants: a thorough ECG study. *Int J Clin Pharmacol Ther* 2013; **51**:456–465.

55. Heise CW, et al. A review of vilazodone exposures with focus on serotonin syndrome effects. *Clin Toxicol (Phila)* 2017; **55**:1004–1007.

56. Gaw CE, et al. Evaluation of dose and outcomes for pediatric vilazodone ingestions. *Clin Toxicol (Phila)* 2018; **56**:113–119.

57. Citrome L. Vortioxetine for major depressive disorder: a systematic review of the efficacy and safety profile for this newly approved antidepressant: what is the number needed to treat, number needed to harm and likelihood to be helped or harmed? *Int J Clin Pract* 2014; **68**:60–82.

58. Takeda Pharmaceuticals America. Highlights of prescribing information. BRINTELLIX (vortioxetine) tablets. 2024 (last accessed February 2025); https://us.trintellix.com.

59. Baldwin DS, et al. The safety and tolerability of vortioxetine: analysis of data from randomized placebo-controlled trials and open-label extension studies. *J Psychopharmacol* 2016; **30**:242–252.

60. Honig A, et al. Treatment of post-myocardial infarction depressive disorder: a randomized, placebo-controlled trial with mirtazapine. *Psychosom Med* 2007; **69**:606–613.

61. Na K-S, et al. Can we recommend mirtazapine and bupropion for patients at risk for bleeding? A systematic review and meta-analysis. *J Affect Disord* 2018; **225**:221–226.

62. Alqdwah-Fattouh R, et al. Differential effects of antidepressant subgroups on risk of acute myocardial infarction: a nested case–control study. *Br J Clin Pharmacol* 2020; **86**:2040–2050.

63. Sauer WH, et al. Selective serotonin reuptake inhibitors and myocardial infarction. *Circulation* 2001; **104**:1894–1898.

64. Davies SJ, et al. Treatment of anxiety and depressive disorders in patients with cardiovascular disease. *BMJ* 2004; **328**:939–943.

65. Taylor D, et al. Pharmacological interventions for people with depression and chronic physical health problems: systematic review and meta-analyses of safety and efficacy. *Br J Psychiatry* 2011; **198**:179–188.

66. Chen S, et al. Serotonin and catecholaminergic polymorphic ventricular tachycardia: a possible therapeutic role for SSRIs? *Cardiovasc J Afr* 2010; **21**:225–228.

67. Berkman LF, et al. Effects of treating depression and low perceived social support on clinical events after myocardial infarction: the Enhancing Recovery in Coronary Heart Disease Patients (ENRICHD) randomized trial. *JAMA* 2003; **289**:3106–3116.

68. Zambrano J, et al. Psychiatric and psychological interventions for depression in patients with heart disease: a scoping review. *J Am Heart Assoc* 2020; **9**:e018686.

Antidepressant-induced arrhythmia

Depression confers an increased risk of cardiovascular disease[1] and sudden cardiac death.[2] Possible factors include platelet activation, decreased heart rate variability, reduced physical activity, and an association with an increased risk of diabetes.[3]

Tricyclic antidepressants have established arrhythmogenic activity, which arises as a result of potent blockade of cardiac sodium channels and variable activity at potassium channels.[4] ECG changes produced include PR, QRS and QT prolongation and the Brugada syndrome.[5] These actions are very evident in overdose but their effects in clinical doses is unclear. Normal clinical use of nortriptyline has been associated in one study with an increased risk of cardiac arrest,[6] although a large cohort study did not confirm this finding.[7] Lofepramine, for reasons unknown, seems to lack the overdose arrhythmogenicity of other TCAs, despite its major metabolite, desipramine, being a potent potassium channel blocker.[8] Oddly, in one study,[9] clinical use of lofepramine was associated with an increased risk of myocardial infarction (MI), whereas other antidepressants were not. Network meta-analysis suggests that TCAs have a very low risk of causing ventricular arrythmia or sudden cardiac death outside overdose or high-dose usage.[10] In patients taking tricyclics, ECG monitoring is a more meaningful and useful measure of toxicity than plasma level monitoring.

There is limited evidence that venlafaxine is a sodium channel antagonist[11] and a weak antagonist at hERG (human ether-a-go-go-related gene) potassium channels. Arrhythmia is a rare occurrence, even after massive overdose,[12–15] and ECG changes after overdose are no more common than with SSRIs.[16] No ECG changes are seen in therapeutic dosing[17] or even at supratherapeutic doses (450mg/day)[18] and sudden cardiac death in clinical use is no more common than with fluoxetine or citalopram.[7,19] Desvenlafaxine does not appear to prolong QT, even in overdose.[20]

Moclobemide,[21] citalopram,[22,23] escitalopram,[24] bupropion (amfebutamone),[25] trazodone[26,27] and sertraline,[28] among others,[1] have been reported to prolong the QTc interval in overdose but the clinical consequences of this are uncertain. Sertraline prolongs QT by 5–10ms at 400mg a day,[29] but QT changes are not usually seen with most SSRIs at normal clinical doses.[30,31] Nonetheless, an association between SSRIs (as a group) and QT changes in normal dosing can be shown[32] but this seems largely to be driven by the effects of citalopram and escitalopram.[33] The effect on QTc is dose related[33] but modest.[32]

Most studies have failed to find any association between citalopram or escitalopram treatment and arrhythmia or cardiac mortality in routine clinical practice,[7,34,35] although some have reported very small increases in mortality.[36] Genetic variation in CYP2I9 metabolic capacity may explain individual differences in cardiac toxicity, as it determines the serum concentration of citalopram metabolites,[37] but whether it is the parent compounds or their metabolites that are responsible for cardiotoxicity is unclear.[38]

Vortioxetine seems to have no effect on QT.[39–41] Similarly, agomelatine has no effect, even at supratherapeutic doses.[42] Vilazodone has no effect on cardiac conduction.[43] Levomilnacipran[44] and milnacipran[45] probably have no effect on QT, at least at therapeutic doses.

CHAPTER 3

Use in at-risk patients

There is clear evidence for the safety of sertraline[46] and mirtazapine[47] (and to a lesser extent, citalopram,[47] fluoxetine[48] and bupropion[49]) in people at risk of arrhythmia due to recent MI. One trial found that SSRIs and trazodone decrease the risk of MI,[50] another suggested no effect in either direction for any antidepressant.[51] Citalopram seems to be safe to use in patients with coronary artery disease[52] (despite its link to a risk of torsades de pointes).[53] Escitalopram did not affect mortality in a trial in patients with heart failure,[54] and a later systematic review found no adverse effect on mortality for any SSRIs in heart failure.[55] Sertraline may help improve cardiovascular risk factors.[56]

Recent pharmacovigilance database studies report some association between antidepressants and cardiac arrythmias and cardiovascular death.[57,58] Meta-analysis suggests that overall, antidepressants (SSRIs, SNRIs and TCAs) are associated with an increased risk of atrial fibrillation but not ventricular arrythmias or sudden cardiac death.[59] Conflicting results are reported in elderly patients, with cohort studies reporting both increased risk of arrythmias[60] and no increased risk.[61]

Relative cardiotoxicity

Relative cardiotoxicity of antidepressants is difficult to establish. Surveillance monitoring data suggest that many marketed antidepressants are linked to arrhythmia (ranging from clinically insignificant to life threatening) and sudden cardiac death. For a substantial proportion of drugs, these figures are perhaps more likely to reflect coincidence and/or confounding rather than causation.

The Fatal Toxicity Index (FTI) may provide some means for comparison, at least for overdose toxicity. This is a measure of the number of overdose deaths per million (FP10) prescriptions issued. FTI figures suggest high toxicity for all tricyclic drugs (but not lofepramine), medium toxicity for venlafaxine and moclobemide, and low toxicity for SSRIs, mirtazapine and reboxetine.[62–66] However, FTI does not necessarily reflect only cardiotoxicity (antidepressants also cause serotonin syndrome, seizures and coma, for example) and is, in any case, open to other influences. This is best evidenced in the change in FTI over time. A good example here is nortriptyline, the FTI of which has been estimated at 0.6[16] and 39.2[12] and several values in between.[67] This change probably reflects changes in the type of patient prescribed nortriptyline but double counting (nortriptyline is a metabolite of amitriptyline) at post mortem also plays a part. Venlafaxine is relatively more often prescribed to patients with more severe depression and who are relatively more likely to attempt suicide.[68–70] This is apt to inflate venlafaxine's FTI and erroneously suggest greater inherent toxicity. Drugs with consistently low FTIs can probably be assumed to have very low risk of arrhythmias.

Citalopram and escitalopram have surprisingly low overdose toxicity, despite QT prolongation occurring in about a third of reported overdoses.[71] Standard doses of citalopram may be causally associated with an increased risk of cardiac arrest[6] but, as mentioned earlier, other data suggest no increased risk of arrhythmia or death with standard and higher licensed doses of citalopram and escitalopram.[34] Citalopram and escitalopram are probably the most cardiotoxic of the SSRIs but their toxicity is modest at worst, and possibly insignificant in respect to risk of adverse outcomes.

Summary

- Tricyclics (but not lofepramine) have an established link to ion channel blockade and cardiac arrhythmia, especially in overdose.
- Non-tricyclics generally have a very low risk of inducing arrhythmia.
- Sertraline is recommended post MI, but other SSRIs and mirtazapine are also likely to be safe.
- Bupropion, citalopram, escitalopram, moclobemide and venlafaxine should be used with caution or avoided in those at risk of serious arrhythmia (those with heart failure, left ventricular hypertrophy, previous arrhythmia or MI). An ECG should be performed at baseline and 1 week after every increase in dose if any of these drugs are used in at-risk patients.
- TCAs (with the exception of lofepramine) are best avoided completely in patients at risk of serious arrhythmia. If use of a TCA cannot be avoided, an ECG should be performed at baseline, 1 week after each increase in dose and periodically throughout treatment. Frequency will be determined by the stability of the cardiac disorder. Advice from a cardiology specialist should be sought.
- The arrhythmogenic potential of TCAs and other antidepressants is dose related. Consideration should be given to ECG monitoring of all patients prescribed doses towards the top of the licensed range and those who are prescribed other drugs that, through pharmacokinetic (e.g. fluoxetine) or pharmacodynamic (e.g. diuretics) mechanisms, may add to the risk posed by the drug.

CHAPTER 3

References

1. Taylor D. Antidepressant drugs and cardiovascular pathology: a clinical overview of effectiveness and safety. *Acta Psychiatr Scand* 2008; 118:434–442.
2. Whang W, et al. Depression and risk of sudden cardiac death and coronary heart disease in women: results from the Nurses' Health Study. *J Am Coll Cardiol* 2009; 53:950–958.
3. Nemeroff CB, et al. Heartache and heartbreak: the link between depression and cardiovascular disease. *Nat Rev Cardiol* 2012; 9:526–539.
4. Thanacoody HK, et al. Tricyclic antidepressant poisoning: cardiovascular toxicity. *Toxicol Rev* 2005; 24:205–214.
5. Sicouri S, et al. Sudden cardiac death secondary to antidepressant and antipsychotic drugs. *Expert Opin Drug Saf* 2008; 7:181–194.
6. Weeke P, et al. Antidepressant use and risk of out-of-hospital cardiac arrest: a nationwide case–time–control study. *Clin Pharmacol Ther* 2012; 92:72–79.
7. Leonard CE, et al. Antidepressants and the risk of sudden cardiac death and ventricular arrhythmia. *Pharmacoepidemiol Drug Saf* 2011; 20:903–913.
8. Hong HK, et al. Block of the human ether-a-go-go-related gene (hERG) K+ channel by the antidepressant desipramine. *Biochem Biophys Res Commun* 2010; 394:536–541.
9. Coupland C, et al. Antidepressant use and risk of cardiovascular outcomes in people aged 20 to 64: cohort study using primary care database. *BMJ* 2016; 352:i1350.
10. Prasitlumkum N, et al. Antidepressants and risk of sudden cardiac death: a network meta-analysis and systematic review. *Med Sci (Basel)* 2021; 9:26.
11. Khalifa M, et al. Mechanism of sodium channel block by venlafaxine in guinea pig ventricular myocytes. *J Pharmacol Exp Ther* 1999; 291:280–284.
12. Colbridge MG, et al. Venlafaxine in overdose: experience of the National Poisons Information Service (London centre). *J Toxicol Clin Toxicol* 1999; 37:383.
13. Blythe D, et al. Cardiovascular and neurological toxicity of venlafaxine. *Hum Exp Toxicol* 1999; 18:309–313.
14. Combes A, et al. Conduction disturbances associated with venlafaxine. *Ann Intern Med* 2001; 134:166–167.
15. Isbister GK. Electrocardiogram changes and arrhythmias in venlafaxine overdose. *Br J Clin Pharmacol* 2009; 67:572–576.
16. Whyte IM, et al. Relative toxicity of venlafaxine and selective serotonin reuptake inhibitors in overdose compared to tricyclic antidepressants. *QJM* 2003; 96:369–374.
17. Feighner JP. Cardiovascular safety in depressed patients: focus on venlafaxine. *J Clin Psychiatry* 1995; 56:574–579.
18. Abbas R, et al. Lack of an effect of supratherapeutic dose of venlafaxine on cardiac repolarization in healthy subjects. *Clin Pharmacol Drug Dev* 2022; 11:100–111.

19. Martinez C, et al. Use of venlafaxine compared with other antidepressants and the risk of sudden cardiac death or near death: a nested case–control study. *BMJ* 2010; 340:c249.

20. Cooper JM, et al. Desvenlafaxine overdose and the occurrence of serotonin toxicity, seizures and cardiovascular effects. *Clin Toxicol (Phila)* 2017; 55:18–24.

21. Downes MA, et al. QTc abnormalities in deliberate self-poisoning with moclobemide. *Intern Med J* 2005; 35:388–391.

22. Kelly CA, et al. Comparative toxicity of citalopram and the newer antidepressants after overdose. *J Toxicol Clin Toxicol* 2004; 42:67–71.

23. Grundemar L, et al. Symptoms and signs of severe citalopram overdose. *Lancet* 1997; 349:1602.

24. Mohammed R, et al. Prolonged QTc interval due to escitalopram overdose. *J Miss State Med Assoc* 2010; 51:350–353.

25. Isbister GK, et al. Bupropion overdose: QTc prolongation and its clinical significance. *Ann Pharmacother* 2003; 37:999–1002.

26. Service JA, et al. QT prolongation and delayed atrioventricular conduction caused by acute ingestion of trazodone. *Clin Toxicol (Phila)* 2008; 46:71–73.

27. Dattilo PB, et al. Prolonged QT associated with an overdose of trazodone. *J Clin Psychiatry* 2007; 68:1309–1310.

28. de Boer RA, et al. QT interval prolongation after sertraline overdose: a case report. *BMC Emerg Med* 2005; 5:5.

29. Abbas R, et al. A thorough QT study to evaluate the effects of a supratherapeutic dose of sertraline on cardiac repolarization in healthy subjects. *Clin Pharmacol Drug Dev* 2020; 9:307–320.

30. Maljuric NM, et al. Use of selective serotonin re-uptake inhibitors and the heart rate corrected QT interval in a real-life setting: the population-based Rotterdam Study. *Br J Clin Pharmacol* 2015; 80:698–705.

31. van Haelst IM, et al. QT interval prolongation in users of selective serotonin reuptake inhibitors in an elderly surgical population: a cross-sectional study. *J Clin Psychiatry* 2014; 75:15–21.

32. Beach SR, et al. Meta-analysis of selective serotonin reuptake inhibitor-associated QTc prolongation. *J Clin Psychiatry* 2014; 75:e441–449.

33. Castro VM, et al. QT interval and antidepressant use: a cross sectional study of electronic health records. *BMJ* 2013; 346:f288.

34. Zivin K, et al. Evaluation of the FDA warning against prescribing citalopram at doses exceeding 40 mg. *Am J Psychiatry* 2013; 170:642–650.

35. Ray WA, et al. High-dose citalopram and escitalopram and the risk of out-of-hospital death. *J Clin Psychiatry* 2017; 78:190–195.

36. Lin YT, et al. Selective serotonin reuptake inhibitor use and risk of arrhythmia: a nationwide, population-based cohort study. *Clin Ther* 2019; 41:1128–1138.e8.

37. Farhat H, et al. Citalopram and escitalopram: mechanisms of cardiotoxicity, toxicology predisposition and risks of use in geriatric and hemodialysis populations. *Glob Cardiol Sci Pract* 2024; 2024:e202434.

38. Faraj P, et al. Pro-arrhythmic effect of escitalopram and citalopram at serum concentrations commonly observed in older patients: a study based on a cohort of 19,742 patients. *EBioMedicine* 2023; 95:104779.

39. Dubovsky SL. Pharmacokinetic evaluation of vortioxetine for the treatment of major depressive disorder. *Expert Opin Drug Metab Toxicol* 2014; 10:759–766.

40. Alam MY, et al. Safety, tolerability, and efficacy of vortioxetine (Lu AA21004) in major depressive disorder: results of an open-label, flexible-dose, 52-week extension study. *Int Clin Psychopharmacol* 2014; 29:36–44.

41. Wang Y, et al. Effect of vortioxetine on cardiac repolarization in healthy adult male subjects: results of a thorough QT/QTc study. *Clin Pharmacol Drug Dev* 2013; 2:298–309.

42. Donazzolo Y, et al. Evaluation of the effects of therapeutic and supra-therapeutic doses of agomelatine on the QT/QTc interval: a phase I, randomised, double-blind, placebo-controlled and positive-controlled, cross-over thorough QT/QTc study conducted in healthy volunteers. *J Cardiovasc Pharmacol* 2014; 64:440–451.

43. Edwards J, et al. Vilazodone lacks proarrhythmogenic potential in healthy participants: a thorough ECG study. *Int J Clin Pharmacol Ther* 2013; 51:456–465.

44. Mago R, et al. Safety and tolerability of levomilnacipran ER in major depressive disorder: results from an open-label, 48-week extension study. *Clin Drug Investig* 2013; 33:761–771.

45. Periclou A, et al. Effects of milnacipran on cardiac repolarization in healthy participants. *J Clin Pharmacol* 2010; 50:422–433.

46. Glassman AH, et al. Sertraline treatment of major depression in patients with acute MI or unstable angina. *JAMA* 2002; 288:701–709.

47. van Melle JP, et al. Effects of antidepressant treatment following myocardial infarction. *Br J Psychiatry* 2007; 190:460–466.

48. Strik JJ, et al. Efficacy and safety of fluoxetine in the treatment of patients with major depression after first myocardial infarction: findings from a double-blind, placebo-controlled trial. *Psychosom Med* 2000; 62:783–789.

49. Rigotti NA, et al. Bupropion for smokers hospitalized with acute cardiovascular disease. *Am J Med* 2006; 119:1080–1087.

50. Alqdwah-Fattouh R, et al. Differential effects of antidepressant subgroups on risk of acute myocardial infarction: a nested case–control study. *Br J Clin Pharmacol* 2020; 86:2040–2050.

51. Wu CS, et al. Use of antidepressants and risk of hospitalization for acute myocardial infarction: a nationwide case-crossover study. *J Psychiatr Res* 2017; 94:7–14.

52. Lesperance F, et al. Effects of citalopram and interpersonal psychotherapy on depression in patients with coronary artery disease: the Canadian Cardiac Randomized Evaluation of Antidepressant and Psychotherapy Efficacy (CREATE) trial. *JAMA* 2007; 297:367–379.

53. Astrom-Lilja C, et al. Drug-induced torsades de pointes: a review of the Swedish pharmacovigilance database. *Pharmacoepidemiol Drug Saf* 2008; 17:587–592.

54. Angermann CE, et al. Effect of escitalopram on all-cause mortality and hospitalization in patients with heart failure and depression: the MOOD-HF randomized clinical trial. *JAMA* 2016; 315:2683–2693.

55. Hedrick R, et al. The impact of antidepressants on depressive symptom severity, quality of life, morbidity, and mortality in heart failure: a systematic review. *Drugs Context* 2020; 9:2020-5-4.

CHAPTER 3

56. Sherwood A, et al. Effects of exercise and sertraline on measures of coronary heart disease risk in patients with major depression: results from the SMILE-II randomized clinical trial. *Psychosom Med* 2016; **78**:602–609.

57. Wang Z, et al. Exploring the correlation between cardiovascular adverse events and antidepressant use: a retrospective pharmacovigilance analysis based on the FDA Adverse Event Reporting System database. *J Affect Disord* 2024; **367**:96–108.

58. Yokohara S, et al. Psychotherapeutic drug-induced life-threatening arrhythmias: a retrospective analysis using the Japanese adverse drug event report database. *J Arrhythm* 2023; **39**:928–936.

59. Cao Y, et al. Associations of antidepressants with atrial fibrillation and ventricular arrhythmias: a systematic review and meta-analysis. *Front Cardiovasc Med* 2022; **9**:840452.

60. Biffi A, et al. Antidepressants and the risk of arrhythmia in elderly affected by a previous cardiovascular disease: a real-life investigation from Italy. *Eur J Clin Pharmacol* 2018; **74**:119–129.

61. Aakjaer M, et al. Serious arrhythmia in initiators of citalopram, escitalopram, and other selective serotonin reuptake inhibitors: a population-based cohort study in older adults. *Clin Transl Sci* 2022; **15**:2105–2115.

62. Crome P. The toxicity of drugs used for suicide. *Acta Psychiatr Scand Suppl* 1993; **371**:33–37.

63. Cheeta S, et al. Antidepressant-related deaths and antidepressant prescriptions in England and Wales, 1998–2000. *Br J Psychiatry* 2004; **184**:41–47.

64. Buckley NA, et al. Fatal toxicity of serotoninergic and other antidepressant drugs: analysis of United Kingdom mortality data. *BMJ* 2002; **325**:1332–1333.

65. Buckley NA, et al. Greater toxicity in overdose of dothiepin than of other tricyclic antidepressants. *Lancet* 1994; **343**:159–162.

66. Morgan O, et al. Fatal toxicity of antidepressants in England and Wales, 1993–2002. *Health Stat Q* 2004; (23):18–24.

67. Taylor D, et al. The cardiovascular safety of tricyclic antidepressants in overdose and in clinical use. *Ther Adv Psychopharmacol* 2024; **14**:20451253241243297.

68. Egberts ACG, et al. Channeling of three newly introduced antidepressants to patients not responding satisfactorily to previous treatment. *J Clin Psychopharmacol* 1997; **17**:149–155.

69. Mines D, et al. Prevalence of risk factors for suicide in patients prescribed venlafaxine, fluoxetine, and citalopram. *Pharmacoepidemiol Drug Saf* 2005; **14**:367–372.

70. Chan AN, et al. A comparison of venlafaxine and SSRIs in deliberate self-poisoning. *J Med Toxicol* 2010; **6**:116–121.

71. Hasnain M, et al. Escitalopram and QTc prolongation. *J Psychiatry Neurosci* 2013; **38**:E11.

CHAPTER 3

Antidepressant-induced hyponatraemia

Most antidepressants have been associated with hyponatraemia. Onset is usually within 30 days of starting treatment.[1-3] The effect appears not to be dose related,[1,4] although some case reports suggest otherwise. The most likely mechanism of this adverse effect is the syndrome of inappropriate secretion of antidiuretic hormone (SIADH). Risk of hospitalisation with hyponatraemia is elevated from 1 in 1,600 in the general population to 1 in 300 for those on any antidepressant.[5] Hyponatraemia is a potentially serious adverse effect of antidepressants that demands careful monitoring,[6] particularly in those patients at greatest risk. Hyponatraemia of all severities is associated with increased mortality.[7]

Which antidepressants?

No antidepressant has been definitively shown not to be linked with hyponatraemia and almost all have a reported association.[8] It has been suggested that serotonergic drugs are relatively more likely than noradrenergic drugs to cause hyponatraemia,[9,10] although this is disputed.[11] A 2024 meta-analysis suggests that the risk may be highest with SNRIs, followed by SSRIs,[12] and lowest with mirtazapine and trazodone. There are notably few reports for MAOIs,[13,14] but all marketed antidepressants have some association with hyponatraemia, even more recently introduced drugs such as vortioxetine,[15] desvenlafaxine[16] and vilazodone.[17]

Older women who are frail and/or prescribed other medication known to reduce plasma sodium are at greatest risk.[15,18] CYP2D6 poor metabolisers may be at increased risk of antidepressant-induced hyponatraemia,[19] although evidence is somewhat inconsistent.[20]

Database studies

A 2018 French pharmacovigilance database study found an association of hyponatraemia with agomelatine, a drug not previously reported to cause hyponatraemia.[21] Another database study using US Food and Drug Administration (FDA) data found the strongest association between hyponatraemia and antidepressants to be for mirtazapine, in contrast to most other reports,[22] and a further French database study found the greatest risk to be with duloxetine.[23] A 2022 Japanese study[24] found that SSRIs and SNRIs caused, on average, a 1mmol/L fall in plasma sodium, an effect not seen with other antidepressants examined. The effect on sodium was directly linked to a drug's binding affinity for the SERT transporter. The mean effect of antidepressants on sodium in this study suggests that clinical hyponatraemia might be an extreme of the normal distribution of effects rather than an idiosyncratic effect only seen in certain people.

Extrapolating from incident report databases to estimate relative or absolute risk of hyponatraemia is fraught with difficulty. Problems include disproportionate reporting for antidepressants for which the adverse effect is considered to be rare, the inability to adjust for confounding by indication (drugs perceived to be of low risk are more likely to be prescribed to patients at already at high risk of hyponatraemia) and the impact of concomitant prescriptions. Table 3.14 provides a summary of the risk of hyponatraemia with antidepressants.

Table 3.14 Summary of risk of hyponatraemia with antidepressants[5,12,24–26]

Drug/drug group	Risk of ↓Na	Level of supporting evidence
SNRIs	High	Strong
SSRIs	High	Strong
Tricyclics	Moderate	Strong
MAOIs	Low	Weak
NaSSas (mirtazapine, mianserin)	Low	Strong
Trazodone	Low	Strong
Bupropion	Low	Moderate
Agomelatine	Low	Moderate

MAOIs, monoamine oxidase inhibitors; NaSSas, noradrenergic and specific serotonergic antidepressants.

Monitoring[1,27,28]

All patients taking antidepressants should be informed of and observed for signs of hyponatraemia (dizziness, nausea, lethargy, confusion, cramps, seizures). The risk is highest in the first 4 weeks of starting antidepressants, and diminishes over time until by 3–6 months the risk is the same as for patients who do not take antidepressants.[18] Consequently, in patients treated with antidepressants for several months or years, other causes should be assumed in the event of hyponatraemia. Serum sodium should be determined (at baseline and 2 and 4 weeks, and then 3-monthly[29]) for those at high risk of drug-induced hyponatraemia. This frequency of electrolyte monitoring may not identify all cases as serum sodium may drop precipitously.[30] Box 3.4 lists high-risk factors for drug-induced hyponatraemia.

Box 3.4 High-risk factors for drug-induced hyponatraemia

- Older age
- Female sex
- Major surgery
- History of hyponatraemia or a low baseline sodium concentration
- Co-therapy with other drugs known to be associated with hyponatraemia (e.g. diuretics, NSAIDs, antipsychotics, carbamazepine, cancer chemotherapy, calcium antagonists, angiotensin-converting enzyme inhibitors and laxatives)
- Reduced renal function (glomerular filtration rate <50mL/minute)
- Medical comorbidity (e.g. hypothyroidism, diabetes, chronic obstructive pulmonary disease (COPD), hypertension, head injury, congestive cardiac failure, cardiovascular accident, various cancers)
- Low body weight

Age is perhaps the most important risk factor, so for older people (especially women) monitoring is essential.[27]

Treatment[28]

The normal range for serum sodium is 136–145mmol/L. It may be possible to manage mild hyponatraemia (>130 mmol/L) with fluid restriction. Some suggest increasing sodium intake,[4] although this is likely to be impractical. If symptoms persist, the antidepressant should be discontinued.

- If serum sodium is >125mmol/L – monitor sodium daily until normal. Symptoms include headache, nausea, vomiting, muscle cramps, restlessness, lethargy, confusion and disorientation. Withdraw the offending antidepressant as soon as possible.
- If serum sodium is <125 mmol/L – refer urgently to specialist medical care. The antidepressant should be discontinued immediately. There is an increased risk of life-threatening symptoms such as seizures, coma and respiratory arrest. Over-rapid correction of hyponatraemia may be harmful.

Restarting treatment

- Hyponatraemia may recur on rechallenge with the same or a different SSRI, but may be less likely with an antidepressant from another class.[27,31]
- Consider withdrawing other drugs associated with hyponatraemia (risk increases exponentially when antidepressants are combined with diuretics, etc.).
- Prescribe a drug from a different class. Consider noradrenergic drugs such as nortriptyline and lofepramine, or mirtazapine, or an MAOI such as moclobemide. Agomelatine or bupropion[32] might also be considered. Begin with a low dose, increase slowly and monitor closely. If hyponatraemia recurs and continued antidepressant use is essential, consider water restriction and/or careful use of demeclocycline.
- Consider (es)ketamine or ECT if a standard antidepressant cannot be given.

Other prescribed drugs

Carbamazepine has a well-known association with SIADH[33] and antipsychotic use has been linked to hyponatraemia (see section on hyponatraemia in psychosis in Chapter 1). Other commonly prescribed drugs such as thiazide diuretics, opiates, NSAIDs, tramadol, cytotoxics, omeprazole and trimethoprim can also cause hyponatraemia.[2,33]

References

1. Egger C, et al. A review on hyponatremia associated with SSRIs, reboxetine and venlafaxine. *Int J Psychiatry Clin Pract* 2006; **10**:17–26.
2. Liamis G, et al. A review of drug-induced hyponatremia. *Am J Kidney Dis* 2008; **52**:144–153.
3. Takeda K, et al. Analysis of the frequency and onset time of hyponatremia/syndrome of inappropriate antidiuretic hormone induced by antidepressants or antipsychotics. *Ann Pharmacother* 2022; **56**:303–308.
4. Kruger S, et al. Duloxetine and hyponatremia: a report of 5 cases. *J Clin Psychopharmacol* 2007; **27**:101–104.
5. Gandhi S, et al. Second-generation antidepressants and hyponatremia risk: a population-based cohort study of older adults. *Am J Kidney Dis* 2017; **69**:87–96.
6. Mohan S, et al. Prevalence of hyponatremia and association with mortality: results from NHANES. *Am J Med* 2013; **126**:1127–1137.e1.
7. Selmer C, et al. Hyponatremia, all-cause mortality, and risk of cancer diagnoses in the primary care setting: a large population study. *Eur J Intern Med* 2016; **36**:36–43.
8. Thomas A, et al. Hyponatraemia and the syndrome of inappropriate antidiuretic hormone secretion associated with drug therapy in psychiatric patients. *CNS Drugs* 1995; **5**:357–369.
9. Movig KL, et al. Serotonergic antidepressants associated with an increased risk for hyponatraemia in the elderly. *Eur J Clin Pharmacol* 2002; **58**:143–148.

10. Movig KL, et al. Association between antidepressant drug use and hyponatraemia: a case-control study. *Br J Clin Pharmacol* 2002; **53**:363–369.

11. Kirby D, et al. Hyponatraemia and selective serotonin re-uptake inhibitors in elderly patients. *Int J Geriatr Psychiatry* 2001; **16**:484–493.

12. Gheysens T, et al. The risk of antidepressant-induced hyponatremia: a meta-analysis of antidepressant classes and compounds. *Eur Psychiatry* 2024; **67**:e20.

13. Mercier S, et al. [Severe hyponatremia induced by moclobemide]. *Therapie* 1997; **52**:82–83.

14. Peterson JC, et al. Inappropriate antidiuretic hormone secondary to a monamine oxidase inhibitor. *JAMA* 1978; **239**:1422–1423.

15. Seifert J, et al. Psychotropic drug-induced hyponatremia: results from a drug surveillance program-an update. *J Neural Transm (Vienna)* 2021; **128**:1249–1264.

16. Liew ED, et al. Syndrome of inappropriate antidiuretic hormone secretion associated with desvenlafaxine. *Int J Clin Pharm* 2014; **36**:253–255.

17. Das S, et al. Dose dependent hyponatremia caused by vilazodone: a case report. *Asian J Psychiatr* 2019; **43**:213.

18. Mannheimer B, et al. Time-dependent association between selective serotonin reuptake inhibitors and hospitalization due to hyponatremia. *J Psychopharmacol* 2021; **35**:928–933.

19. Kwadijk-de GS, et al. Variation in the CYP2D6 gene is associated with a lower serum sodium concentration in patients on antidepressants. *Br J Clin Pharmacol* 2009; **68**:221–225.

20. Stedman CA, et al. Cytochrome P450 2D6 genotype does not predict SSRI (fluoxetine or paroxetine) induced hyponatraemia. *Hum Psychopharmacol* 2002; **17**:187–190.

21. Rochoy M, et al. [Antidepressive agents and hyponatremia: a literature review and a case/non-case study in the French Pharmacovigilance database]. *Therapie* 2018; **73**:389–398.

22. Mazhar F, et al. Association of hyponatraemia and antidepressant drugs: a pharmacovigilance-pharmacodynamic assessment through an analysis of the US Food and Drug Administration Adverse Event Reporting System (FAERS) database. *CNS Drugs* 2019; **33**:581–592.

23. Revol R, et al. [Hyponatremia associated with SSRI/NRSI: descriptive and comparative epidemiological study of the incidence rates of the notified cases from the data of the French National Pharmacovigilance Database and the French National Health Insurance]. *Encephale* 2018; **44**:291–296.

24. Nagashima T, et al. Identifying antidepressants less likely to cause hyponatremia: triangulation of retrospective cohort, disproportionality, and pharmacodynamic studies. *Clin Pharmacol Ther* 2022; **111**:1258–1267.

25. Leth-Moller KB, et al. Antidepressants and the risk of hyponatremia: a Danish register-based population study. *BMJ Open* 2016; **6**:e011200.

26. Moscona-Nissan A Sr, et al. Mirtazapine risk of hyponatremia and syndrome of inappropriate antidiuretic hormone secretion in adult and elderly patients: a systematic review. *Cureus* 2021; **13**:e20823.

27. Dirks AC, et al. Recurrent hyponatremia after substitution of citalopram with duloxetine. *J Clin Psychopharmacol* 2007; **27**:313.

28. Pinkhasov A, et al. Management of SIADH-related hyponatremia due to psychotropic medications: an expert consensus from the Association of Medicine and Psychiatry. *J Psychosom Res* 2021; **151**:110654.

29. Arinzon ZH, et al. Delayed recurrent SIADH associated with SSRIs. *Ann Pharmacother* 2002; **36**:1175–1177.

30. Lane NE, et al. Hyponatremia-associated hospital visits are not reduced by early electrolyte testing in older adults starting antidepressants. *J Am Geriatr Soc* 2024; **72**:1770–1780.

31. Bavbek N, et al. Recurrent hyponatremia associated with citalopram and mirtazapine. *Am J Kidney Dis* 2006; **48**:e61–e62.

32. Varela Piñón M, et al. Selective serotonin reuptake inhibitor-induced hyponatremia: clinical implications and therapeutic alternatives. *Clin Neuropharmacol* 2017; **40**:177–179.

33. Shepshelovich D, et al. Medication-induced SIADH: distribution and characterization according to medication class. *Br J Clin Pharmacol* 2017; **83**:1801–1807.

CHAPTER 3

Antidepressants and hyperprolactinaemia

Prolactin release is controlled by endogenous dopamine but is also indirectly modulated by serotonin via stimulation of $5HT_{1C}$ and $5HT_2$ receptors.[1,2] Long-standing increased plasma prolactin (with or without symptoms) is very occasionally seen with antidepressant use.[3] Where antidepressant-induced hyperprolactinaemia does occur, rises in prolactin are usually small and short-lived,[4] so symptoms are very rare. There is no association between SSRI use and breast cancer.[5]

Routine monitoring of prolactin is not recommended but where symptoms suggest the possibility of hyperprolactinaemia then measurement of plasma prolactin is essential. Where symptomatic hyperprolactinaemia is confirmed, a switch to mirtazapine is recommended (see below), although there is also evidence that switching to an alternative SSRI can resolve symptoms.[6,7]

Some details of associations between antidepressants and increased prolactin are given in Table 3.15.

Table 3.15 Reported associations between antidepressants and increased prolactin.

Drug/group	Prospective studies	Case reports/series
Agomelatine	No mention of prolactin changes in clinical trials[8] Melatonin itself may inhibit prolactin production[9]	None
Bupropion	Single doses of up to 100mg seem not to affect prolactin[10] May decrease prolactin[11]	None
Monoamine oxidase inhibitors	Small mean changes observed with phenelzine[11] and tranylcypromine[12]	Very occasional reports of increased prolactin[11]
Mirtazapine	Strong evidence that mirtazapine has no effect on prolactin[13]	Occasional reports of galactorrhoea[14] and gynaecomastia[15]
SNRIs	Clear association observed between venlafaxine and duloxetine and prolactin elevation[16–18]	Galactorrhoea reported with venlafaxine[19,20] and duloxetine.[21,22] Duloxetine-linked hyperprolactinaemia has been treated with aripiprazole.[16]
SSRIs	Prospective studies generally show no change in prolactin.[23–25] Some evidence from prescription event monitoring that SSRIs are associated with higher risk of non-puerperal lactation.[26] In a French study, 1.6% of adverse event reports for SSRIs were of hyperprolactinaemia.[3]	Galactorrhoea reported with fluoxetine,[6,27] paroxetine,[28–30] sertraline[31] and fluvoxamine[30] Euprolactinaemic galactorrhoea and amenorrhoea[32] reported with escitalopram[33] and fluvoxamine[34] Hyperprolactinaemia reported with sertraline[7,35]
Tricyclics	Small mean changes seen in some studies[11,36,37] but no changes in others[11,38]	Symptomatic hyperprolactinaemia reported with imipramine,[33] dosulepin[39] and clomipramine[40,41] Galactorrhoea reported with nortriptyline[42] and when trazodone was added to citalopram[43] Raised prolactin may be linked to response to amitriptyline[36,44]
Vortioxetine	No mention of prolactin changes in clinical trials[45]	None One review suggests 'probable relation between vortioxetine and galactorrhoea'[46]

References

1. Emiliano AB, et al. From galactorrhea to osteopenia: rethinking serotonin–prolactin interactions. *Neuropsychopharmacology* 2004; 29:833–846.

2. Rittenhouse PA, et al. Neurons in the hypothalamic paraventricular nucleus mediate the serotonergic stimulation of prolactin secretion via 5-HT1c/2 receptors. *Endocrinology* 1993; 133:661–667.

3. Trenque T, et al. Serotonin reuptake inhibitors and hyperprolactinaemia: a case/non-case study in the French pharmacovigilance database. *Drug Saf* 2011; 34:1161–1166.

4. Voicu V, et al. Drug-induced hypo- and hyperprolactinemia: mechanisms, clinical and therapeutic consequences. *Expert Opin Drug Metab Toxicol* 2013; 9:955–968.

5. Niu D, et al. The relationship between antidepressants and breast cancer: evidence from Mendelian randomization. *Cancer Causes Control* 2024; 35:55–62.

6. Mondal S, et al. A new logical insight and putative mechanism behind fluoxetine-induced amenorrhea, hyperprolactinemia and galactorrhea in a case series. *Ther Adv Psychopharmacol* 2013; 3:322–334.

7. Strzelecki D, et al. Hyperprolactinemia and bleeding following use of sertraline but not use of citalopram and paroxetine: a case report. *Arch Psychiatry Psychother* 2012; 1:45–48.

8. Taylor D, et al. Antidepressant efficacy of agomelatine: meta-analysis of published and unpublished studies. *BMJ* 2014; 348:g1888.

9. Chu YS, et al. Stimulatory and entraining effect of melatonin on tuberoinfundibular dopaminergic neuron activity and inhibition on prolactin secretion. *J Pineal Res* 2000; 28:219–226.

10. Whiteman PD, et al. Bupropion fails to affect plasma prolactin and growth hormone in normal subjects. *Br J Clin Pharmacol* 1982; 13:745.

11. Meltzer HY, et al. Effect of antidepressants on neuroendocrine axis in humans. *Adv Biochem Psychopharmacol* 1982; 32:303–316.

12. Price LH, et al. Effects of tranylcypromine treatment on neuroendocrine, behavioral, and autonomic responses to tryptophan in depressed patients. *Life Sci* 1985; 37:809–818.

13. Schule C, et al. The influence of mirtazapine on anterior pituitary hormone secretion in healthy male subjects. *Psychopharmacology (Berl)* 2002; 163:95–101.

14. Schroeder K, et al. Mirtazapine-induced galactorrhea: a case report. *J Neuropsychiatry Clin Neurosci* 2013; 25:E13–E14.

15. Lynch A, et al. [Gynecomastia-galactorrhea during treatment with mirtazapine]. *Presse Med* 2004; 33:458.

16. Luo T, et al. Aripiprazole for the treatment of duloxetine-induced hyperprolactinemia: a case report. *J Affect Disord* 2019; 250:330–332.

17. Daffner-Bugia C, et al. The neuroendocrine effects of venlafaxine in healthy subjects. *Hum Psychopharmacol* 1996; 11:1–9.

18. McGrane IR, et al. Probable galactorrhea associated with sequential trials of escitalopram and duloxetine in an adolescent female. *J Child Adolesc Psychopharmacol* 2019; 29:788–789.

19. Sternbach H. Venlafaxine-induced galactorrhea. *J Clin Psychopharmacol* 2003; 23:109–110.

20. Demir EY, et al. Hyperprolactinemia connected with venlafaxine: a case report. *Anatol J Psychiatry* 2014; 15:S10–S14.

21. Ashton AK, et al. Hyperprolactinemia and galactorrhea induced by serotonin and norepinephrine reuptake inhibiting antidepressants. *Am J Psychiatry* 2007; 164:1121–1122.

22. Korkmaz S, et al. Galactorrhea during duloxetine treatment: a case report. *Turk Psikiyatri Derg* 2011; 22:200–201.

23. Schlosser R, et al. Effects of subchronic paroxetine administration on night-time endocrinological profiles in healthy male volunteers. *Psychoneuroendocrinology* 2000; 25:377–388.

24. Nadeem HS, et al. Comparison of the effects of citalopram and escitalopram on 5-Ht-mediated neuroendocrine responses. *Neuropsychopharmacology* 2004; 29:1699–1703.

25. Masoudi M, et al. Effect of sertraline on depression severity and prolactin levels in women with polycystic ovary syndrome: a placebo-controlled randomized trial. *Int Clin Psychopharmacol* 2021; 36:238–243.

26. Egberts AC, et al. Non-puerperal lactation associated with antidepressant drug use. *Br J Clin Pharmacol* 1997; 44:277–281.

27. Peterson MC. Reversible galactorrhea and prolactin elevation related to fluoxetine use. *Mayo Clin Proc* 2001; 76:215–216.

28. Morrison J, et al. Galactorrhea induced by paroxetine. *Can J Psychiatry* 2001; 46:88–89.

29. Evrensel A, et al. A case of galactorrhea during paroxetine treatment. *Int J Psychiatry Med* 2016; 51:302–305.

30. Bhattacharjee S, et al. Selective serotonin reuptake inhibitor-induced galactorrhea with hyperprolactinemia. *Indian J Psychiatry* 2021; 63:613–616.

31. Moussaoui J, et al. Sertraline-induced galactorrhoea: a case report. *Cureus* 2024; 16:e62357.

32. Selvaraj V, et al. Escitalopram-induced amenorrhea and false positive urine pregnancy test. *Korean J Fam Med* 2017; 38:40–42.

33. Mahasuar R, et al. Euprolactinemic galactorrhea associated with use of imipramine and escitalopram in a postmenopausal woman. *Gen Hosp Psychiatry* 2010; 32:341–343.

34. Vispute C, et al. Fluvoxamine-induced reversible euprolactinemic galactorrhea in a case of obsessive-compulsive disorder. *Ann Indian Psychiatry* 2017; 1:127–128.

35. Ekinci N, et al. Sertraline-related amenorrhea in an adolescent. *Clin Neuropharmacol* 2019; 42:99–100.

36. Fava GA, et al. Prolactin, cortisol, and antidepressant treatment. *Am J Psychiatry* 1988; 145:358–360.

37. Orlander H, et al. Imipramine induced elevation of prolactin levels in patients with HIV/AIDS improved their immune status. *West Indian Med J* 2009; 58:207–213.

38. Meltzer HY, et al. Lack of effect of tricyclic antidepressants on serum prolactin levels. *Psychopharmacology (Berl)* 1977; 51:185–187.

39. Gadd EM, et al. Antidepressants and galactorrhoea. *Int Clin Psychopharmacol* 1987; 2:361–363.

40. Anand VS. Clomipramine-induced galactorrhoea and amenorrhoea. *Br J Psychiatry* 1985; 147:87–88.

41. Fowlie S, et al. Hyperprolactinaemia and nonpuerperal lactation associated with clomipramine. *Scott Med J* 1987; 32:52.

42. Kukreti P, et al. Rising trend of use of antidepressants induced non- puerperal lactation: a case report. *J Clin Diagn Res* 2016; **10**:Vd01–Vd02.

43. Arslan FC, et al. Trazodone induced galactorrhea: a case report. *Gen Hosp Psychiatry* 2015; **37**:373.e1–2.

44. Centner S, et al. Amitriptyline-induced hyperprolactinemia in a pediatric patient. *Cureus* 2024; **16**:e59604.

45. Mahableshwarkar AR, et al. A randomized, double-blind, fixed-dose study comparing the efficacy and tolerability of vortioxetine 2.5 and 10 mg in acute treatment of adults with generalized anxiety disorder. *Hum Psychopharmacol* 2014; **29**:64–72.

46. Verma A, et al. Risks associated with vortioxetine in the established therapeutic indication. *Curr Neuropharmacol* 2020; **19**:711–717.

Antidepressants and diabetes mellitus

Depression and diabetes

Prevalence rates of depression are high in both type I (22%) and type II (19%) diabetes.[1] Comorbid depression in type II diabetes is associated with *poorer* glycaemic control, increased hospital admissions, increased diabetic complications and poorer compliance to diabetes treatments and dietary recommendations.[1] The presence of depression has a negative impact on metabolic control and poor metabolic control may worsen depression.[2] Considering all of this, the treatment of comorbid depression in patients with diabetes is of vital importance and drug choice should take into account likely effects on metabolic control (Table 3.16). In 2012, Cochrane[3] concluded that antidepressants are effective in diabetes and moderately improve glycaemic control.

In contrast, there is some evidence that the association between diabetes and depression is in part a reflection of the use of antidepressants. That is, antidepressants as a group may cause diabetes,[4,5] although the association may not be present after adjusting for comorbidity.[6] Evidence relating to individual drugs is described in Table 3.16.

Table 3.16 Effect of antidepressants on glucose homeostasis and weight.

Antidepressant class	Effect on glucose homeostasis
SSRIs[7–19]	■ Studies indicate that SSRIs have a favourable effect on diabetic parameters in patients with type II diabetes. Insulin requirements may be decreased. ■ Fluoxetine has been associated with improvement in HbA_{1c} levels, reduced insulin requirements, weight loss and enhanced insulin sensitivity. Its effect on insulin sensitivity is independent of its effect on weight loss. Sertraline may also reduce HbA_{1c}. ■ Escitalopram also seems to improve glycaemic control ■ Some evidence that long-term SSRIs may increase the risk of diabetes in general[20] and gestational diabetes in particular[21] but there is also evidence of no effect either way[22]
TCAs[13,14,23–25]	■ TCAs are associated with increased appetite, weight gain and hyperglycaemia ■ Nortriptyline improved depression but worsened glycaemic control in diabetic patients in one study. Overall improvement in depression had a beneficial effect on HbA_{1c}. Clomipramine reported to precipitate diabetes. ■ Long-term use of TCAs seems to increase risk of diabetes[4]
MAOIs[26,27]	■ Irreversible MAOIs have a tendency to cause extreme hypoglycaemic episodes and weight gain ■ No known effects with moclobemide
SNRIs[24,28,29]	■ SNRIs do not appear to disrupt glycaemic control and have minimal impact on weight ■ Studies of duloxetine in the treatment of diabetic neuropathy show that it has little influence on glycaemic control. No data in depression and diabetes. ■ Limited data on venlafaxine but may slightly increase risk of incident diabetes[20] ■ One report of hyperglycaemia with desvenlafaxine[30]
Mirtazapine[31,32]	■ Mirtazapine does not appear to impair glucose tolerance in non-diabetic depressed patients ■ Improvement in HbA_{1c} was seen with short-term use but HbA_{1c} worsened during a 1-year follow-up ■ Mirtazapine was associated with an increase in body mass index in patients with diabetes both in the short and long term

(Continued)

Table 3.16 *(Continued)*

Antidepressant class	Effect on glucose homeostasis
Agomelatine[19]	■ A few studies suggest agomelatine is effective with some improvement or no worsening of glycaemic parameters ■ Agomelatine also demonstrated a minimum effect on body weight
Bupropion	■ Improved weight and HbA_{1c} in one open study[33]
Vortioxetine	■ No clinically relevant changes in weight or blood in one subgroup analysis of clinical trial data.[34] Limited evidence of an improvement in HbA_{1c}.[19]
Reboxetine, trazodone	■ No data in patients with diabetes ■ One study revealed 20% increased risk of type 2 diabetes in people prescribed trazodone[20]

HbA_{1c}, glycated haemoglobin; MAOI, monoamine oxidase inhibitor; TCA, tricyclic antidepressant.

Recommendations

■ All patients with a diagnosis of depression should be screened for diabetes.
■ In those who are diabetic:
  ■ use SSRIs first line; data support sertraline, escitalopram and fluoxetine
  ■ SNRIs, bupropion, vortioxetine and agomelatine are also likely to be safe but there are fewer supporting data
  ■ avoid TCAs and MAOIs if possible, because of their effects on weight and glucose homeostasis
  ■ monitor blood glucose and HbA_{1c} carefully when antidepressant treatment is initiated, when the dose is changed and after discontinuation
  ■ metformin may be a preferred diabetes treatment because of its putative beneficial effects on mood in type II diabetes.[35,36]

References

1. Berk M, et al. Comorbidity between major depressive disorder and physical diseases: a comprehensive review of epidemiology, mechanisms and management. *World Psychiatry* 2023; **22**:366–387.
2. Lustman PJ, et al. Depression in diabetic patients: the relationship between mood and glycemic control. *J Diabetes Complications* 2005; **19**:113–122.
3. Baumeister H, et al. Psychological and pharmacological interventions for depression in patients with diabetes mellitus and depression. *Cochrane Database Syst Rev* 2012; **12**:CD008381.
4. Wang Y, et al. Antidepressants use and the risk of type 2 diabetes mellitus: a systematic review and meta-analysis. *J Affect Disord* 2021; **287**:41–53.
5. Movahed F, et al. Incident diabetes in adolescents using antidepressant: a systematic review and meta-analysis. *Eur Child Adolesc Psychiatry* 2024; doi: 10.1007/s00787-024-02502-x [Online ahead of print].
6. Kim H, et al. Depression, antidepressant use, and the risk of type 2 diabetes: a nationally representative cohort study. *Front Psychiatry* 2023; **14**:1275984.
7. Maheux P, et al. Fluoxetine improves insulin sensitivity in obese patients with non-insulin-dependent diabetes mellitus independently of weight loss. *Int J Obes Relat Metab Disord* 1997; **21**:97–102.
8. Gulseren L, et al. Comparison of fluoxetine and paroxetine in type II diabetes mellitus patients. *Arch Med Res* 2005; **36**:159–165.
9. Lustman PJ, et al. Sertraline for prevention of depression recurrence in diabetes mellitus: a randomized, double-blind, placebo-controlled trial. *Arch Gen Psychiatry* 2006; **63**:521–529.
10. Gray DS, et al. A randomized double-blind clinical trial of fluoxetine in obese diabetics. *Int J Obes Relat Metab Disord* 1992; **16** Suppl 4:S67–S72.
11. Knol MJ, et al. Influence of antidepressants on glycaemic control in patients with diabetes mellitus. *Pharmacoepidemiol Drug Saf* 2008; **17**:577–586.

12. Briscoe VJ, et al. Effects of a selective serotonin reuptake inhibitor, fluoxetine, on counterregulatory responses to hypoglycemia in healthy individuals. *Diabetes* 2008; **57**:2453–2460.

13. Andersohn F, et al. Long-term use of antidepressants for depressive disorders and the risk of diabetes mellitus. *Am J Psychiatry* 2009; **166**:591–598.

14. Kivimaki M, et al. Antidepressant medication use, weight gain, and risk of type 2 diabetes: a population-based study. *Diabetes Care* 2010; **33**:2611–2616.

15. Rubin RR, et al. Antidepressant medicine use and risk of developing diabetes during the diabetes prevention program and diabetes prevention program outcomes study. *Diabetes Care* 2010; **33**:2549–2551.

16. Echeverry D, et al. Effect of pharmacological treatment of depression on A1C and quality of life in low-income Hispanics and African Americans with diabetes: a randomized, double-blind, placebo-controlled trial. *Diabetes Care* 2009; **32**:2156–2160.

17. Dhavale HS, et al. Depression and diabetes: impact of antidepressant medications on glycaemic control. *J Assoc Physicians India* 2013; **61**:896-899.

18. Mojtabai R. Antidepressant use and glycemic control. *Psychopharmacology (Berl)* 2013; **227**:467–477.

19. Srisurapanont M, et al. Antidepressants for depressed patients with type 2 diabetes mellitus: a systematic review and network meta-analysis of short-term randomized controlled trials. *Neurosci Biobehav Rev* 2022; **139**:104731.

20. Nguyen TTH, et al. Role of serotonin transporter in antidepressant-induced diabetes mellitus: a pharmacoepidemiological-pharmacodynamic study in VigiBase(®). *Drug Saf* 2018; **41**:1087–1096.

21. Dandjinou M, et al. Antidepressant use during pregnancy and the risk of gestational diabetes mellitus: a nested case–control study. *BMJ Open* 2019; **9**:e025908.

22. Kuo HY, et al. Antidepressants and risk of type 2 diabetes mellitus: a population-based nested case-control study. *J Clin Psychopharmacol* 2020; **40**:359–365.

23. Lustman PJ, et al. Effects of nortriptyline on depression and glycemic control in diabetes: results of a double-blind, placebo-controlled trial. *Psychosom Med* 1997; **59**:241–250.

24. McIntyre RS, et al. The effect of antidepressants on glucose homeostasis and insulin sensitivity: synthesis and mechanisms. *Expert Opin Drug Saf* 2006; **5**:157–168.

25. Mumoli N, et al. Clomipramine-induced diabetes. *Ann Intern Med* 2008; **149**:595–596.

26. Goodnick PJ. Use of antidepressants in treatment of comorbid diabetes mellitus and depression as well as in diabetic neuropathy. *Ann Clin Psychiatry* 2001; **13**:31–41.

27. McIntyre RS, et al. Mood and psychotic disorders and type 2 diabetes: a metabolic triad. *Can J Diabetes* 2005; **29**:122–132.

28. Raskin J, et al. Duloxetine versus routine care in the long-term management of diabetic peripheral neuropathic pain. *J Palliat Med* 2006; **9**:29–40.

29. Crucitti A, et al. Duloxetine treatment and glycemic controls in patients with diagnoses other than diabetic peripheral neuropathic pain: a meta-analysis. *Curr Med Res Opin* 2010; **26**:2579–2588.

30. Mekonnen AD, et al. Desvenlafaxine-associated hyperglycemia: a case report and literature review. *Ment Health Clin* 2020; **10**:85–89.

31. Song HR, et al. Does mirtazapine interfere with naturalistic diabetes treatment? *J Clin Psychopharmacol* 2014; **34**:588–594.

32. Song HR, et al. Effects of mirtazapine on patients undergoing naturalistic diabetes treatment: a follow-up study extended from 6 to 12 months. *J Clin Psychopharmacol* 2015; **35**:730–731.

33. Roopan S, et al. Use of antidepressants in patients with depression and comorbid diabetes mellitus: a systematic review. *Acta Neuropsychiatr* 2017; **29**:127–139.

34. Baldwin DS, et al. Efficacy and safety of vortioxetine in treatment of patients with major depressive disorder and common co-morbid physical illness. *J Affect Disord* 2022; **311**:588–594.

35. Zhang Y, et al. Effect of metformin on the risk of depression: a systematic review and meta-regression of observational studies. *Asian J Psychiatry* 2024; **92**:103894.

36. Yang Y, et al. Metformin treatment improves depressive symptoms associated with type 2 diabetes: a 24-week longitudinal study. *J Affect Disord* 2024; **365**:80–86.

CHAPTER 3

CHAPTER 3

Antidepressants and sexual dysfunction

Sexual dysfunction is common in the general population, although reliable frequency data are lacking.[1] Reported prevalence rates vary depending on how sexual dysfunction is defined, assessed and the method of data collection.[1] Physical illness, psychiatric illness, substance misuse and prescribed drug treatment can all cause sexual dysfunction.[2] People with depression are more likely to have obesity,[3] diabetes[4] and cardiovascular disease[5] than the general population, making them more likely to suffer sexual dysfunction without any influence of depression or antidepressants themselves.

Before beginning antidepressants, baseline sexual functioning should be determined to set a baseline against which the effect of antidepressants can be measured. Treatment-emergent sexual dysfunction adversely affects quality of life and may contribute to reduced compliance.[6] Questionnaires or rating scales can be useful (for example, the Arizona Sexual Experience Scale).[7] If scales are not used then direct questioning should be employed, as it is much more effective than relying on spontaneous patient reporting.[8] Complaints of sexual dysfunction may indicate progression or inadequate treatment of underlying medical or psychiatric conditions but may also be the result of drug treatment.[6]

Effects of depression

Both depression and the drugs used to treat depression can cause disorders of desire, arousal and orgasm. The precise nature of the sexual dysfunction may indicate whether depression or treatment is the more likely cause. For example, 40–50% of people with depression report diminished libido and problems regarding sexual arousal in the month before diagnosis (and therefore treatment), but only 15–20% experience orgasm problems before taking an antidepressant.[9] The degree of loss of libido appears to correlate with depression severity.[10]

Although many patients experience treatment-emergent sexual dysfunction while taking antidepressants, in others the reduction in depressive symptoms can be accompanied by improvements in sexual desire and satisfaction.[6,11] Improvements are more common among those who respond to antidepressant treatment.[6] For example, a post-hoc analysis of data from the STAR*D (Sequenced Treatment Alternatives to Relieve Depression) study revealed that sexual dysfunction was problematic in 21% of patients whose depression remitted with citalopram treatment compared with 61% of those whose depression did not remit.[12]

Effects of antidepressant drugs

Antidepressants can cause sedation, hormonal changes, disturbance of cholinergic/adrenergic balance, peripheral alpha-adrenergic agonism, inhibition of nitric oxide and increased serotonin neurotransmission. Any or all of these actions may result in sexual dysfunction. Sexual dysfunction has been reported as an adverse effect of all antidepressants, although rates vary and some have reported rates similar to or below that of placebo (Table 3.17). Individual susceptibility also varies and may be at least partly genetically determined.[13]

Not all of the sexual effects of antidepressants are undesirable. Serotonergic antidepressants, including clomipramine, are effective in the treatment of premature ejaculation[6,14]

Table 3.17 Relative frequency of sexual dysfunction (SD) with antidepressants.[10,13,15–17]

Antidepressant	Impact on sexual response			Comments[13]
	Sexual desire*	Sexual arousal[†]	Orgasm[‡]	
Agomelatine	–	–	–	Rates of SD similar to placebo[6]
Bupropion	–	+/–	–	Low rates of SD compared with most antidepressants.[18] Good evidence that SD occurs at or below the rate of placebo. Less robust evidence for dextromethorphan-bupropion but rates of SD also appear to be low.[19]
Duloxetine	++	+	++	Rate of SD similar to some SSRIs and venlafaxine[18]
Levomilnacipran	?	++	++	Limited comparative studies with other antidepressants[20] so relative frequency of SD is uncertain. Erectile dysfunction and disorders of ejaculation shown in RCTs.[21]
Monoamine oxidase inhibitors	++	++	++	Limited evidence though reported incidence of SD ranges from 20–42%. Rates of SD with transdermal selegiline are comparable to placebo.
Mirtazapine	+	–	–	Causes less SD than SSRIs[22]
Moclobemide	–	–	–	Consistently shown to have a low risk of SD
Reboxetine	–	+	–	Probably causes less SD than SSRIs/SNRIs though anti-depressant efficacy has been questioned[23]
SSRIs	++	++	++	High rates of SD with all SSRIs (although reported incidence varies widely).[13] Rates of anorgasmia may be lower with fluvoxamine.[24]
Trazodone	–	+	+	Priapism reported in case studies. However, overall reports of SD seem to be low. Early case reports documented increased sexual desire.
Tricyclics	++	++	++	SD more common with clomipramine (particularly anorgasmia), amitriptyline and imipramine. Less common with secondary amine TCAs (desipramine, nortriptyline, lofepramine).
Venlafaxine	++	++	++	High rates of SD. Isolated case reports of increased libido, orgasm and spontaneous erections.
Vilazodone	+	+	+	Rates of SD possibly lower than citalopram and similar to placebo in RCTs. However, a clear advantage over other antidepressants remains uncertain.[20]
Vortioxetine	–	+	+	Rates of SD probably lower than duloxetine and paroxetine,[25] and reportedly similar to placebo at doses 10mg/day or less[23,26]

Key: ++, common; +, may occur; –, absent or rare; ?, unknown/insufficient information.
* Or sex drive.
[†] Ease of arousal and ability to achieve lubrication or erections.
[‡] Ease of reaching orgasm and orgasm satisfaction.

CHAPTER 3

and may also be beneficial in paraphilias.[27] The short-acting SSRI dapoxetine is an effective treatment for premature ejaculation and is licensed for this indication in many countries.[6,28] A systematic review of RCTs with trazodone showed benefit for reducing so-called psychogenic erectile dysfunction.[6]

Sexual adverse effects can be minimised by careful selection of the antidepressant drug. Data mainly come from observational studies as the assessment of sexual adverse effects in early clinical trials was generally inadequate, often relying on spontaneous reports rather than using validated questionnaires and lacking positive controls.[29] Where possible, information contained in this section has been obtained from studies where sexual adverse effects are purposefully and directly investigated. Management strategies for people who do develop sexual dysfunction on antidepressants are summarised in Table 3.18. No single approach can be considered ideal,[6] so individual assessment is recommended.

Post-SSRI sexual dysfunction

Sexual dysfunction with antidepressants is largely dose dependent[13] and is generally considered to be fully reversible.[13] However, there have been reports of long-lasting sexual dysfunction where the symptoms have continued despite discontinuation of SSRIs/SNRIs.[30] The term post-SSRI sexual dysfunction (PSSD) has been used to describe these symptoms. Reported PSSD symptoms include decreased libido, erectile dysfunction, delayed ejaculation, anorgasmia and vaginal dryness.[31,32] In men, decreased genital sensation and numbness, pleasureless orgasm and premature ejaculation are also commonly reported symptoms of PSSD.[31] The prevalence and pathophysiology of

Table 3.18 Management of sexual adverse effects.

Strategy	Details
1. Rule out other possible causes[33]	■ Depressive symptoms are associated with impaired sexual functioning. Compare sexual functioning on antidepressants with sexual functioning before antidepressants, not before the onset of depressive illness. ■ Consider other possible contributing causes (e.g. alcohol/substance misuse, diabetes, atherosclerosis, cardiac disease, and central and peripheral nervous system conditions). Other medications could be implicated, including both non-psychotropics (e.g. diuretics, beta-blockers) and other psychotropics.
2. Switch to a lower-risk antidepressant[23]	■ Lower-risk antidepressants include agomelatine, bupropion, mirtazapine, vilazodone, vortioxetine and moclobemide.[13] Of these, agomelatine, bupropion and vortioxetine[34] have the best evidence supporting a more favourable sexual adverse effect profile.[13]
Non-pharmacological treatment strategies	■ Waiting for spontaneous remission: widely used, although least effective method.[24] Remission may occur in a small number of people (5–10%) but can take up to 4–6 months.[13] Impractical for many patients, although it might be considered in milder cases.[30] ■ Dose reduction: can be considered in patients who have achieved full remission on an antidepressant[6] ■ Drug holidays: intermittently missing one or two doses prior to planned sexual activity may possibly help but risks discontinuation symptoms.[13,35,36] Not an effective strategy with fluoxetine, owing to its long half-life.[13] Lowering doses by a half for two consecutive days prior to sexual activity is another possible strategy.[24]

(Continued)

Table 3.18 *(Continued)*

Strategy	Details
Pharmacological treatments	■ Phosphodiesterase inhibitors: both sildenafil and tadalafil have been shown to improve sexual functioning in men with antidepressant-related erectile dysfunction.[23,37] Sildenafil is supported by the most evidence.[38] Limited evidence in women, although one RCT found benefits.[23] ■ Bupropion: may be useful in women at higher doses (300mg/day).[37] Lower doses may be ineffective.[23] A positive RCT in men[39] was later retracted. ■ Mirtazapine: evidence is mixed. Open studies suggest some benefit for antidepressant-induced sexual dysfunction, but negative results were reported in one RCT.[33] ■ Transdermal testosterone: RCTs provide evidence of efficacy in women with SSRI/SNRI-emergent loss of libido[40] and in men who continue to take serotonergic antidepressants with low or low-normal testosterone levels[41] ■ Others:[13] many other agents have been studied; many have little effectiveness. Buspirone was effective in one study for citalopram- or paroxetine-induced sexual dysfunction, but ineffective in another study with fluoxetine. Cyproheptadine has been used successfully in case reports of SSRI-induced sexual dysfunction in men and for anorgasmia in women. Loratadine was effective in a small open study for men with SSRI-induced erectile dysfunction. Amantadine was effective in earlier studies for SSRI-induced sexual dysfunction, but recent results have been negative. Yohimbine may be effective for medication-induced sexual dysfunction and improvements were reported by patients in two small studies (although results were nonsignificant). Bethanechol appears to help with TCA-induced sexual dysfunction when taken before sexual activity. Granisetron has been superficially evaluated. Flibanserin and bremelanotide are approved by the FDA for treatment of hypoactive sexual desire disorder in premenopausal women[42] but there are no data to support use for antidepressant-induced sexual dysfunction. Pine bark extract was found to be superior to placebo in one meta-analysis.[38] ■ Augmenting agents in treatment-resistant depression: some drugs used as an adjunct for treatment-resistant depression have been associated with improvement in sexual functioning in secondary analyses. Aripiprazole improved sexual functioning and desire, though only in women.[24] Adjunctive brexpiprazole is associated with modest improvements.[43] Pimavanserin, used as an add-on treatment to SSRIs/SNRIs, improved sexual functioning.[44]

FDA, Food and Drug Administration; TCA, tricyclic antidepressant.

PSSD remain uncertain.[32,45,46] One estimate put the risk at 1 in 216 patients treated.[47] Diagnosis relies on taking an accurate history of medications, symptom onset, symptom profile and eliminating other possible causes.[31] Healy and co-workers have proposed diagnostic criteria for PSSD.[48] Treatment strategies for PSSD remain anecdotal and no definitive treatments exist, although serotonin antagonists, dopaminergic agents and vortioxetine have been used.[31] Multidisciplinary management is essential, possibly including urology and endocrinology.[31]

References

1. McCabe MP, et al. Incidence and prevalence of sexual dysfunction in women and men: a consensus statement from the Fourth International Consultation on Sexual Medicine 2015. *J Sex Med* 2016; **13**:144–152.
2. Chokka PR, et al. Assessment and management of sexual dysfunction in the context of depression. *Ther Adv Psychopharmacol* 2018; **8**:13–23.
3. Pereira-Miranda E, et al. Overweight and obesity associated with higher depression prevalence in adults: a systematic review and meta-analysis. *J Am Coll Nutr* 2017; **36**:223–233.
4. Semenkovich K, et al. Depression in type 2 diabetes mellitus: prevalence, impact, and treatment. *Drugs* 2015; **75**:577–587.
5. Cohen BE, et al. State of the art review: depression, stress, anxiety, and cardiovascular disease. *Am J Hypertens* 2015; **28**:1295–1302.
6. Montejo AL, et al. The impact of severe mental disorders and psychotropic medications on sexual health and its implications for clinical management. *World Psychiatry* 2018; **17**:3–11.
7. McGahuey CA, et al. The Arizona Sexual Experience Scale (ASEX): reliability and validity. *J Sex Marital Ther* 2000; **26**:25–40.
8. Papakostas GI. Identifying patients who need a change in depression treatment and implementing that change. *J Clin Psychiatry* 2016; **77**:e1009.
9. Kennedy SH, et al. Sexual dysfunction before antidepressant therapy in major depression. *J Affect Disord* 1999; **56**:201–208.
10. Clayton AH, et al. Antidepressants and sexual dysfunction: mechanisms and clinical implications. *Postgrad Med* 2014; **126**:91–99.
11. Weber S, et al. Sexual function improves as depressive symptoms decrease during treatment with escitalopram: results of a naturalistic study of patients with major depressive disorder. *J Sex Med* 2023; **20**:161–169.
12. Ishak WW, et al. Sexual satisfaction and quality of life in major depressive disorder before and after treatment with citalopram in the STAR*D study. *J Clin Psychiatry* 2013; **74**:256–261.
13. Clayton AH, et al. Sexual dysfunction due to psychotropic medications. *Psychiatr Clin North Am* 2016; **39**:427–463.
14. Sathianathen NJ, et al. Selective serotonin re-uptake inhibitors for premature ejaculation in adult men. *Cochrane Database Syst Rev* 2021; **3**:CD012799.
15. Serretti A, et al. Treatment-emergent sexual dysfunction related to antidepressants: a meta-analysis. *J Clin Psychopharmacol* 2009; **29**:259–266.
16. Chiesa A, et al. Antidepressants and sexual dysfunction: epidemiology, mechanisms and management. *J Psychopathol* 2010; **16**:104–113.
17. Lew-Starowicz M, et al. *Impact of Psychotropic Medications on Sexual Functioning*. Cham: Springer; 2021:353–371.
18. Reichenpfader U, et al. Sexual dysfunction associated with second-generation antidepressants in patients with major depressive disorder: results from a systematic review with network meta-analysis. *Drug Saf* 2014; **37**:19–31.
19. Tabuteau H, et al. Effect of AXS-05 (dextromethorphan-bupropion) in major depressive disorder: a randomized double-blind controlled trial. *Am J Psychiatry* 2022; **179**:490–499.
20. Wagner G, et al. Efficacy and safety of levomilnacipran, vilazodone and vortioxetine compared with other second-generation antidepressants for major depressive disorder in adults: a systematic review and network meta-analysis. *J Affect Disord* 2018; **228**:1–12.
21. Gommoll CP, et al. A randomized, double-blind, placebo-controlled study of flexible doses of levomilnacipran ER (40–120 mg/day) in patients with major depressive disorder. *J Drug Assess* 2014; **3**:10–19.
22. Watanabe N, et al. Mirtazapine versus other antidepressive agents for depression. *Cochrane Database Syst Rev* 2011; (12):CD006528.
23. Cleare A, et al. Evidence-based guidelines for treating depressive disorders with antidepressants: a revision of the 2008 British Association for Psychopharmacology guidelines. *J Psychopharmacol* 2015; **29**:459–525.
24. Montejo AL, et al. Management strategies for antidepressant-related sexual dysfunction: a clinical approach. *J Clin Med* 2019; **8**:1640.
25. De Diego-Adeliño J, et al. Vortioxetine in major depressive disorder: from mechanisms of action to clinical studies: an updated review. *Expert Opin Drug Saf* 2022; **21**:673–690.
26. Jacobsen PL, et al. Treatment-emergent sexual dysfunction in randomized trials of vortioxetine for major depressive disorder or generalized anxiety disorder: a pooled analysis. *CNS Spectr* 2016; **21**:367–378.
27. Culos C, et al. Pharmacological interventions in paraphilic disorders: systematic review and insights. *J Clin Med* 2024; **13**:1524.
28. McMahon CG. Dapoxetine: a new option in the medical management of premature ejaculation. *Ther Adv Urol* 2012; **4**:233–251.
29. Khin NA, et al. Regulatory and scientific issues in studies to evaluate sexual dysfunction in antidepressant drug trials. *J Clin Psychiatry* 2015; **76**:1060–1063.
30. Rothmore J. Antidepressant-induced sexual dysfunction. *Med J Aust* 2020; **212**:329–334.
31. Gül M, et al. A clinical guide to rare male sexual disorders. *Nat Rev Urol* 2024; **21**:35–49.
32. Tarchi L, et al. Selective serotonin reuptake inhibitors, post-treatment sexual dysfunction and persistent genital arousal disorder: a systematic review. *Pharmacoepidemiol Drug Saf* 2023; **32**:1053–1067.
33. Francois D, et al. Antidepressant-induced sexual side effects: incidence, assessment, clinical implications, and management. *Psychiatr Ann* 2017; **47**:154–160.
34. Montejo AL, et al. Switching to vortioxetine in patients with poorly tolerated antidepressant-related sexual dysfunction in clinical practice: a 3-month prospective real-life study. *J Clin Med* 2024; **13**:546.
35. Alipour-Kivi A, et al. The effect of drug holidays on sexual dysfunction in men treated with selective serotonin reuptake inhibitors (SSRIs) other than fluoxetine: an 8-week open-label randomized clinical trial. *BMC Psychiatry* 2024; **24**:67.
36. Lalegani E, et al. Safety and efficacy of drug holidays for women with sexual dysfunction induced by selective serotonin reuptake inhibitors (SSRIs) other than fluoxetine: an open-label randomized clinical trial. *Brain Sci* 2023; **13**:1397.
37. Taylor MJ, et al. Strategies for managing sexual dysfunction induced by antidepressant medication. *Cochrane Database Syst Rev* 2013; **5**:CD003382.

38. Luft MJ, et al. Pharmacologic interventions for antidepressant-induced sexual dysfunction: a systematic review and network meta-analysis of trials using the Arizona sexual experience scale. *CNS Spectr* 2021; doi: 10.1017/S1092852921000377.

39. Safarinejad MR. The effects of the adjunctive bupropion on male sexual dysfunction induced by a selective serotonin reuptake inhibitor: a double-blind placebo-controlled and randomized study. *BJU Int* 2010; **106**:840–847.

40. Montejo AL, et al. Sexual side-effects of antidepressant and antipsychotic drugs. *Curr Opin Psychiatry* 2015; **28**:418–423.

41. Amiaz R, et al. Testosterone gel replacement improves sexual function in depressed men taking serotonergic antidepressants: a randomized, placebo-controlled clinical trial. *J Sex Marital Ther* 2011; **37**:243–254.

42. Barakeh D, et al. Pharmacotherapy of hypoactive sexual desire disorder in premenopausal women. *Ann Pharmacother* 2025; **59**:148–161.

43. Clayton AH, et al. Effect of brexpiprazole on prolactin and sexual functioning: an analysis of short- and long-term study data in major depressive disorder. *J Clin Psychopharmacol* 2020; **40**:560–567.

44. Freeman MP, et al. Improvement of sexual functioning during treatment of MDD with adjunctive pimavanserin: a secondary analysis. *Depress Anxiety* 2020; **37**:485–495.

45. Bala A, et al. Post-SSRI sexual dysfunction: a literature review. *Sex Med Rev* 2018; **6**:29–34.

46. Peleg LC, et al. Post-SSRI sexual dysfunction (PSSD): biological plausibility, symptoms, diagnosis, and presumed risk factors. *Sex Med Rev* 2022; **10**:91–98.

47. Ben-Sheetrit J, et al. Estimating the risk of irreversible post-SSRI sexual dysfunction (PSSD) due to serotonergic antidepressants. *Ann Gen Psychiatry* 2023; **22**:15.

48. Healy D, et al. Diagnostic criteria for enduring sexual dysfunction after treatment with antidepressants, finasteride and isotretinoin. *Int J Risk Saf Med* 2022; **33**:65–76.

CHAPTER 3

SSRIs and bleeding

Serotonin is released from platelets in response to vascular injury, promoting vasoconstriction and morphological changes in platelets that lead to aggregation.[1] SSRIs inhibit the serotonin transporter, which is responsible for the uptake of serotonin into platelets (Table 3.19). The resultant depletion of platelet serotonin leads to a reduced ability to form clots and a subsequent increase in the risk of bleeding. Broadly speaking, the relative risk of any bleeding event compared with no use of SSRI/SNRI is around 1.4, with the absolute risk being between around 0.5% and 6%[2] (depending on numerous factors).

SSRIs may also increase gastric acid secretion and therefore may be indirectly irritant to the gastric mucosa,[3] increasing the risk of peptic ulcer.[4] The risk of abnormal bleeding of any kind with SSRIs is highest during the first 30 days of treatment.[5,6] The effect on bleeding is probably related to the affinity of individual SSRIs for the serotonin transporter.[7,8]

Table 3.19 Antidepressants and degree of serotonin reuptake inhibition.[6,9]

Degree of serotonin reuptake inhibition	Antidepressant
Strong	Sertraline, paroxetine, fluoxetine, duloxetine, clomipramine
Intermediate	Citalopram, escitalopram, fluvoxamine, vilazodone, vortioxetine, venlafaxine Amitriptyline, imipramine
Weak or none	Agomelatine, dosulepin, doxepin, lofepramine, mirtazapine, moclobemide, nortriptyline, reboxetine, mianserin

Risk factors for bleeding with SSRIs

- Age, particularly those over 65 years
- Alcohol misuse
- Coronary artery disease
- Drug misuse
- Hypertension
- History of GI bleed
- History of stroke
- History of major bleeding
- Liver disease
- Labile international normalised ratio (INR)
- Medication predisposing to bleeding
- Peptic ulcer
- Renal disease
- Smoking

Caution should be exercised when prescribing serotonergic antidepressants for people with medical conditions such as gout, asthma, COPD, lupus, psoriasis, interferon-induced depression in patients with hepatitis C[10] and arthritis, when patients might also be taking corticosteroids, aspirin or NSAIDS.

Gastrointestinal bleeding

The use of serotonergic antidepressants is an independent risk factor for all bleeding events. SSRIs increase the rate of upper GI bleeding (UGIB), with hazard ratio (HR) of 1.97, and lower GI bleeding (LGIB; HR 2.96) after adjusting for all relevant risk factors.[11] In absolute terms, it is likely that SSRIs are responsible for an additional 3 episodes of bleeding in every 1,000 patient years of treatment,[7,12,13] but this figure masks large variations in risk. For example, 1 in 85 patients with a history of GI bleeding will have a further bleed attributable to treatment with a SSRI.[14]

Gastroprotective drugs (proton-pump inhibitors, PPIs) decrease the risk of GI bleeds associated with SSRIs (either alone or in combination with NSAIDs), although not quite to control levels.[15] A 2020 study found that SSRIs increased the risk of GI bleeding in people taking direct-acting anticoagulants for atrial fibrillation and that this risk was increased further in those not prescribed PPIs.[16] Another found no increased risk of bleeding for SSRIs prescribed alongside any anticoagulants.[17]

People who take SSRIs are at significantly increased risk of being admitted to hospital with a UGIB compared with age- and sex-matched controls.[7,15,18,19] This association holds when age, gender and the effects of other drugs such as aspirin and NSAIDs are controlled for.[2] In addition to this, a meta-analysis of 22 studies concluded that current users of SSRIs are 55% more at risk of UGIB compared with those who do not take SSRIs. This risk was significantly and further increased by concurrent use of antiplatelet drugs or NSAIDs.[5]

Co-prescription of low-dose aspirin may double the risk of GI bleeding associated with SSRIs alone,[20] as does co-prescription of NSAIDs.[21] Combined use of SSRIs and NSAIDs greatly increases the use of anti-acid drugs.[22] The elderly and those with a history of GI bleeding are at greatest risk of GI bleeds.[14,15,19]

Early studies found that in patients who take warfarin, SSRIs increase the risk of a non-GI bleed two- to three-fold (similar to the effect size of NSAIDs) but did not seem to increase the risk of a GI bleed.[23,24] A later study[11] showed an increased risk of UGIB and LGIB in concomitant users of warfarin and serotonergic antidepressant (Table 3.20). This effect does not seem to be associated with any change in INR, making it difficult to identify those at highest risk.[24] In keeping with these findings, SSRI use in patients taking anticoagulants being treated for acute coronary syndromes may decrease the risk of minor cardiac events at the expense of an increased risk of a bleed.[25] SSRIs may decrease mortality overall in this group.[26] Thus, the increased risk of UGIBs associated with SSRIs may be balanced by a decreased risk of embolic events. One database study failed to find a reduction in the risk of a first MI in patients treated with SSRIs,[27] while another[28] found a reduction in the risk of being admitted to hospital with a first MI in smokers on SSRIs. The effect size in the second study was large: approximately 1 in 10 hospitalisations were avoided in patients treated with SSRIs.[28] This is similar to the effect size of other antiplatelet therapies such as aspirin.[29] A 2021 meta-analysis suggested that SSRIs halved the risk of MI in people with coronary artery disease.[26]

Table 3.20 Approximate absolute risk of GI bleeding with concomitant use of SSRIs.

Drug	Absolute risk of UGIB (%)*	Absolute risk of LGIB (%)*
Aspirin + SSRI	6	3
Warfarin + SSRI	4	3
NSAID + SSRI*	3	1
SSRI alone	2	1

LGIB, lower gastrointestinal bleeding; UGIB, upper gastrointestinal bleeding.
* Percentage figures rounded to nearest integer.
** A 2023 meta-analysis suggested that the risk of a GI bleed was over 40% for people on SSRI + NSAIDs.[30] This seems to be the result of erroneous interpretation of case–control study data.

Many studies do not state changes in absolute risk of intestinal bleeding and some of those that do fail to provide denominator details (i.e. duration of treatment). Ideally, risk should be defined as the number of additional cases per 1,000 patient years. Table 3.20 shows approximate absolute risks (without a denominator) derived from a single study[11] and a personal communication.[31]

Risk decreases to the same level as controls in past users of SSRIs, indicating that bleeding is likely to be associated with treatment itself rather than some inherent characteristic of the patients being treated.[7] It also means that the effect of SSRIs disappears after their withdrawal.

The excess risk of bleeding is not confined to UGIBs (Table 3.20). The risk of LGIBs may also be increased[32] and an increased risk of uterine bleeding (see later) has also been reported.[12]

Intracranial/intracerebral haemorrhage

There is a clear association between the use of SSRIs and intracranial/intracerebral haemorrhage (ICH) and risk is further increased by concomitant use of NSAIDs and anticoagulants. Elevated risk of ICH has been observed across all classes of antidepressants with serotonergic activity. In a cohort study of 1,363,990 users of antidepressants,[6] the overall rate of ICH was 3.8 per 10,000 patient years. Current use of SSRI increased the risk of ICH (relative risk 1.17) compared with TCA with an absolute adjusted rate difference of 6.7 per 100,000 persons per year. Among the SSRI group, the risk of ICH was 25% greater in those who used strong inhibitors of serotonin reuptake system in comparison with users of weak inhibitors (Table 3.20). This correlates to an absolute adjusted rate difference of 9.5 events per 100,000 persons per year. Overall risk was highest during the first 30 days of use. A 2018 meta-analysis of 12 studies confirmed an increased risk of ICH for SSRIs (OR 0.8–2.42), with an indication that stronger reuptake inhibitors had a greater effect.[33] Since then, one study reported no increased risk of ICH with SSRIs, either alone or alongside anticoagulants,[34] whereas another[35] found that SSRIs increased risk of recurrence of ICH by 31%. A 2022 meta-analysis including nearly 2 million patients found an increased risk of ICH only when SSRIs were prescribed with anticoagulants.[36]

Table 3.21 Absolute risk of intracranial haemorrhage with SSRI with or without anticoagulant or NSAIDs.

Study	Risk with SSRI alone	Risk with SSRI + NSAID	Risk with antidepressant + anticoagulant
Shin et al. 2015[37]	1 in 632* (0.16%)	1 in 175* (0.57%)	–
Renoux et al. 2017[6]	1 in 450** (0.22%)	–	1 in 260** (0.38%)
Smoller et al. 2009[38]	1 in 240*** (0.42%)	–	–

* Within 30 days of taking antidepressant.
** Incident users (no time limit).
*** Annual risk (older patients).

One database study[37] also identified an increased risk of ICH in those who have been taking SSRIs alone or in combination with NSAIDs. This and other studies providing data on absolute risk are summarised in Table 3.21, which gives estimates of absolute risk of ICH derived from three studies.

Gynaecological and obstetric haemorrhage

A multicentre cross-sectional study[39] found an association between the use of antidepressants and menstruation disorders (unusual or excess bleeding, irregular menstruation, menorrhagia, etc.). This study found that the prevalence of menstruation disorder in the study group who were taking SSRIs, venlafaxine or mirtazapine, either alone or in combination, was 24.6% compared with 12.2% in people not taking antidepressants.

Abnormal vaginal bleeding

Cases of abnormal vaginal bleeding associated with SSRIs have been reported in a young woman,[40] a postmenopausal woman[41] and a preadolescent girl aged 11.[42]

Postpartum haemorrhage

While one study[43] could not find an increased risk of postpartum haemorrhage (PPH) with the use of SSRI or non-SSRI antidepressants, a large cohort study[44] found an association between PPH and all classes of antidepressants, with a number needed to harm of 80 for current users of SSRIs and 97 for those on other antidepressants. One hospital-based cohort study[45] found an absolute risk of PPH of 18% and an absolute risk of postpartum anaemia of 12.8% after a non-surgical vaginal delivery in women who were current users of SSRIs. The absolute risk of both PPH and postpartum anaemia for those without any exposure to antidepressants was 8.7%. The blood loss during delivery was also higher for those who had SSRI exposure. The length of hospital stay was also significantly increased for those who had been taking an SSRI. A recent population study[46] identified that the use of serotonergic medications was associated with 1.5 times increased risk of PPH. This study highlighted that women who have been taking other psychoactive medications such as antipsychotics and mood stabilisers were three times more at risk of PPH compared with mothers who did not take any medications, suggesting that the occurrence of PPH might not be entirely due to serotonergic activity.

In 2021, the UK Medicines and Healthcare products Regulatory Agency issued a warning regarding the use of SSRIs and postpartum blood loss.[47] However, a 2024 meta-analysis of 20 studies concluded that SSRI use was a 'minor risk factor for postpartum haemorrhage'.[48]

Surgical and postoperative bleeding

Use of SSRIs in the preoperative period has been associated with a 20% increase in inpatient mortality (absolute risk 1 in 1,000), although patient factors rather than drug factors could not be excluded as the cause.[49] One study[50] found that patients prescribed SSRIs who underwent orthopaedic surgery had an almost four-fold risk of requiring a blood transfusion. This equated to 1 additional patient requiring transfusion for every 10 patients taking an SSRI and undergoing surgery and was double the risk of patients who were taking NSAIDs alone. It should be noted in this context that treatment with SSRIs has been associated with a 2.4-fold increase in the risk of hip fracture[51] and a two-fold increase of fracture in old age[51] (mirtazapine[52] and TCAs[50] also increase risk of hip fracture). One study recognised preoperative treatment with SSRIs, other antidepressants or antipsychotics as independent risk factors for blood transfusion in elective fast-track hip and knee arthroplasty.[54] Table 3.22 shows the risk of perioperative blood loss and blood transfusion in patients taking SSRIs compared with those not taking SSRIs.

The combination of advanced age, SSRI treatment, orthopaedic surgery and NSAIDs clearly presents a very high risk. However, there does not seem to be an increased risk of bleeding in patients who undergo coronary artery bypass surgery.[55]

During a 10-year review of women who underwent cosmetic breast surgery procedures, the use of SSRIs increased the risk of postoperative bleeding by a factor of 4.14 compared with those who did not take SSRIs. The authors emphasised the importance of balancing the risks and benefits of stopping antidepressants prior to elective surgeries, particularly in psychologically vulnerable patients.[56]

Table 3.22 Risk of perioperative blood loss and blood transfusion in SSRI users compared with non-SSRI users.[57]

Surgical procedure	Need for reoperation due to bleeding event in users of SADs vs non-users, OR (95% CI)	Need for blood product or red blood cell transfusion in users of SADs vs non-users, OR (95% CI)	Increased risk of mortality in users of SADs vs non-users, OR (95% CI)
CABG	1.07 (0.66–1.74)	1.06 (0.90–1.24)	1.53 (1.15–2.04)
Breast cancer-directed surgery	2.7 (1.6–4.56)	–	–
Orthopaedic surgery	–	1.61 (0.97–2.68)*	0.83 (0.69–1.00)
Major surgery	–	1.19 (1.15–1.23)	1.19 (1.03–1.37)

CABG, coronary artery bypass graft; CI, confidence interval; OR, odds ratio; SADs, serotonergic antidepressants.
* In one study,[58] absolute risk of blood transfusion was 5.7% for people on SSRIs and 5.1% for those not on SSRIs.

A review of 13 studies found an increased odds ratio (a range of 1.21 to 4.14) of perioperative bleeding with SSRIs.[59] One study noted an increased risk of bleeding in women undergoing breast surgery[60] and the authors suggest withholding SSRIs for 2 weeks prior to such planned surgery. Venlafaxine may have similar effects[59] but duloxetine may not affect bleeding risk.[61]

Alternatives to SSRIs/SNRIs

Non-SSRI antidepressants such as mirtazapine and bupropion have been suggested as safer alternatives to SSRIs and SNRIs.[62] Preliminary studies suggest mirtazapine, bupropion and nortriptyline have minimal effects on measurable clotting mechanisms.[63] However, there is little evidence that these drugs are safer and one meta-analysis found an increased risk of UGIB with mirtazapine (vs no treatment) and no difference in bleeding risk between mirtazapine or bupropion and SSRIs.[64]

Overall

Serotonergic antidepressants increase the risk of various types of bleeding, especially when prescribed alongside oral anticoagulants of any kind.[36,65,66] Evidence is strongest for SSRIs and it is likely that risk of bleeding is related to affinity for the serotonin transporter. SSRIs increase the risk of GI bleeding, haemorrhagic stroke, perioperative bleeding, postpartum haemorrhage and uterine bleeding. Their effect is exacerbated by co-prescription with aspirin, anticoagulants and NSAIDs. In most cases, the use of SSRIs increases the risk of an event by a clinically meaningful extent, but especially when co-prescribed with other drugs that affect clotting.

Summary

- SSRIs increase the risk of GI, uterine, cerebral and perioperative bleeding.
- Risk is increased still further in those also receiving aspirin, NSAIDs or oral anticoagulants.
- Try to avoid SSRIs/SNRIs in patients receiving NSAIDs, aspirin or oral anticoagulants or in those with a history of cerebral or GI bleeds.
- Safer alternatives have not been definitively identified but noradrenergic antidepressants (nortriptyline, bupropion) are preferred.
- If SSRI/SNRI use cannot be avoided, monitor closely and prescribe gastroprotective PPIs.
- Limited evidence suggests that bleeding risks may be lower with less potent serotonin reuptake inhibitors (Table 3.19).

References

1. Skop BP, et al. Potential vascular and bleeding complications of treatment with selective serotonin reuptake inhibitors. *Psychosomatics* 1996; 37:12–16.
2. Laporte S, et al. Bleeding risk under selective serotonin reuptake inhibitor (SSRI) antidepressants: a meta-analysis of observational studies. *Pharmacol Res* 2017; 118:19–32.
3. Andrade C, et al. Serotonin reuptake inhibitor antidepressants and abnormal bleeding: a review for clinicians and a reconsideration of mechanisms. *J Clin Psychiatry* 2010; 71:1565–1575.
4. Dall M, et al. There is an association between selective serotonin reuptake inhibitor use and uncomplicated peptic ulcers: a population-based case–control study. *Aliment Pharmacol Ther* 2010; 32:1383–1391.

5. Jiang HY, et al. Use of selective serotonin reuptake inhibitors and risk of upper gastrointestinal bleeding: a systematic review and meta-analysis. *Clin Gastroenterol Hepatol* 2015; **13**:42–50.

6. Renoux C, et al. Association of selective serotonin reuptake inhibitors with the risk for spontaneous intracranial hemorrhage. *JAMA Neurol* 2017; **74**:173–180.

7. Dalton SO, et al. Use of selective serotonin reuptake inhibitors and risk of upper gastrointestinal tract bleeding: a population-based cohort study. *Arch Intern Med* 2003; **163**:59–64.

8. Verdel BM, et al. Use of serotonergic drugs and the risk of bleeding. *Clin Pharmacol Ther* 2011; **89**:89–96.

9. Tatsumi M, et al. Pharmacological profile of antidepressants and related compounds at human monoamine transporters. *Eur J Pharmacol* 1997; **340**:249–258.

10. Weinrieb RM, et al. A critical review of selective serotonin reuptake inhibitor-associated bleeding: balancing the risk of treating hepatitis C-infected patients. *J Clin Psychiatry* 2003; **64**:1502–1510.

11. Cheng YL, et al. Use of SSRI, but not SNRI, increased upper and lower gastrointestinal bleeding: a nationwide population-based cohort study in Taiwan. *Medicine (Baltimore)* 2015; **94**:e2022.

12. Meijer WE, et al. Association of risk of abnormal bleeding with degree of serotonin reuptake inhibition by antidepressants. *Arch Intern Med* 2004; **164**:2367–2370.

13. Yuet WC, et al. Selective serotonin reuptake inhibitor use and risk of gastrointestinal and intracranial bleeding. *J Am Osteopath Assoc* 2019; **119**:102–111.

14. van Walraven C, et al. Inhibition of serotonin reuptake by antidepressants and upper gastrointestinal bleeding in elderly patients: retrospective cohort study. *BMJ* 2001; **323**:655–658.

15. de Abajo FJ, et al. Risk of upper gastrointestinal tract bleeding associated with selective serotonin reuptake inhibitors and venlafaxine therapy: interaction with nonsteroidal anti-inflammatory drugs and effect of acid-suppressing agents. *Arch Gen Psychiatry* 2008; **65**:795–803.

16. Lee MT, et al. Concomitant use of NSAIDs or SSRIs with NOACs requires monitoring for bleeding. *Yonsei Med J* 2020; **61**:741–749.

17. Quinn GR, et al. Selective serotonin reuptake inhibitors and bleeding risk in anticoagulated patients with atrial fibrillation: an analysis from the ROCKET AF trial. *J Am Heart Assoc* 2018; **7**:e008755.

18. de Abajo FJ, et al. Association between selective serotonin reuptake inhibitors and upper gastrointestinal bleeding: population based case–control study. *BMJ* 1999; **319**:1106–1109.

19. Lewis JD, et al. Moderate and high affinity serotonin reuptake inhibitors increase the risk of upper gastrointestinal toxicity. *Pharmacoepidemiol Drug Saf* 2008; **17**:328–335.

20. Axelsson MAB, et al. Bleeding in patients on concurrent treatment with a selective serotonin reuptake inhibitor (SSRI) and low-dose acetylsalicylic acid (ASA) compared with SSRI or low-dose ASA alone-a systematic review and meta-analysis. *Br J Clin Pharmacol* 2024; **90**:916–932.

21. Alam SM, et al. Selective serotonin reuptake inhibitors increase risk of upper gastrointestinal bleeding when used with NSAIDs: a systemic review and meta-analysis. *Sci Rep* 2022; **12**:14452.

22. de Jong JC, et al. Combined use of SSRIs and NSAIDs increases the risk of gastrointestinal adverse effects. *Br J Clin Pharmacol* 2003; **55**:591–595.

23. Schalekamp T, et al. Increased bleeding risk with concurrent use of selective serotonin reuptake inhibitors and coumarins. *Arch Intern Med* 2008; **168**:180–185.

24. Wallerstedt SM, et al. Risk of clinically relevant bleeding in warfarin-treated patients: influence of SSRI treatment. *Pharmacoepidemiol Drug Saf* 2009; **18**:412–416.

25. Ziegelstein RC, et al. Selective serotonin reuptake inhibitor use by patients with acute coronary syndromes. *Am J Med* 2007; **120**:525–530.

26. Fernandes N, et al. The impact of SSRIs on mortality and cardiovascular events in patients with coronary artery disease and depression: systematic review and meta-analysis. *Clin Res Cardiol* 2021; **110**:183–193.

27. Meier CR, et al. Use of selective serotonin reuptake inhibitors and risk of developing first-time acute myocardial infarction. *Br J Clin Pharmacol* 2001; **52**:179–184.

28. Sauer WH, et al. Selective serotonin reuptake inhibitors and myocardial infarction. *Circulation* 2001; **104**:1894–1898.

29. Antiplatelet Trialists' Collaboration. Collaborative overview of randomised trials of antiplatelet therapy I: prevention of death, myocardial infarction, and stroke by prolonged antiplatelet therapy in various categories of patients. *BMJ* 1994; **308**:81–106.

30. Haghbin H, et al. Risk of gastrointestinal bleeding with concurrent use of NSAID and SSRI: a systematic review and network meta-analysis. *Dig Dis Sci* 2023; **68**:1975–1982.

31. Cheng YL, personal communication, 2017.

32. Wessinger S, et al. Increased use of selective serotonin reuptake inhibitors in patients admitted with gastrointestinal haemorrhage: a multicentre retrospective analysis. *Aliment Pharmacol Ther* 2006; **23**:937–944.

33. Douros A, et al. Risk of intracranial hemorrhage associated with the use of antidepressants inhibiting serotonin reuptake: a systematic review. *CNS Drugs* 2018; **32**:321–334.

33. Liu L, et al. Selective serotonin reuptake inhibitors and intracerebral hemorrhage risk and outcome. *Stroke* 2020; **51**:1135–1141.

35. Kubiszewski P, et al. Association of selective serotonin reuptake inhibitor use after intracerebral hemorrhage with hemorrhage recurrence and depression severity. *JAMA Neurol* 2020; **78**:1–8.

36. Nochaiwong S, et al. Use of serotonin reuptake inhibitor antidepressants and the risk of bleeding complications in patients on anticoagulant or antiplatelet agents: a systematic review and meta-analysis. *Ann Med* 2022; **54**:80–97.

37. Shin JY, et al. Risk of intracranial haemorrhage in antidepressant users with concurrent use of non-steroidal anti-inflammatory drugs: nationwide propensity score matched study. *BMJ* 2015; **351**:h3517.

38. Smoller JW, et al. Antidepressant use and risk of incident cardiovascular morbidity and mortality among postmenopausal women in the Women's Health Initiative study. *Arch Intern Med* 2009; **169**:2128–2139.

39. Uguz F, et al. Antidepressants and menstruation disorders in women: a cross-sectional study in three centers. *Gen Hosp Psychiatry* 2012; **34**:529–533.

40. Andersohn F, et al. Citalopram-induced bleeding due to severe thrombocytopenia. *Psychosomatics* 2009; **50**:297–298.

41. Durmaz O, et al. Vaginal bleeding associated with antidepressants. *Int J Gynaecol Obstet* 2015; **130**:284.

42. Turkoglu S, et al. Vaginal bleeding and hemorrhagic prepatellar bursitis in a preadolescent girl, possibly related to fluoxetine. *J Child Adolesc Psychopharmacol* 2015; **25**:186–187.

43. Salkeld E, et al. The risk of postpartum hemorrhage with selective serotonin reuptake inhibitors and other antidepressants. *J Clin Psychopharmacol* 2008; **28**:230–234.

43. Palmsten K, et al. Use of antidepressants near delivery and risk of postpartum hemorrhage: cohort study of low income women in the United States. *BMJ* 2013; **347**:f4877.

45. Lindqvist PG, et al. Selective serotonin reuptake inhibitor use during pregnancy increases the risk of postpartum hemorrhage and anemia: a hospital-based cohort study. *J Thromb Haemost* 2014; **12**:1986–1992.

46. Heller HM, et al. Increased postpartum haemorrhage, the possible relation with serotonergic and other psychopharmacological drugs: a matched cohort study. *BMC Pregnancy Childbirth* 2017; **17**:166.

47. Medicines and Healthcare products Regulatory Agency. Drug Safety Update. SSRI/SNRI antidepressant medicines: small increased risk of postpartum haemorrhage when used in the month before delivery. 2021 (last accessed February 2025); https://www.gov.uk/drug-safety-update/ssri-slash-snri-antidepressant-medicines-small-increased-risk-of-postpartum-haemorrhage-when-used-in-the-month-before-delivery?utm_source=e-shot&utm_medium=email&utm_campaign=DSU_January2021split1.

48. Bobo WV, et al. The association of antidepressants in late pregnancy with postpartum hemorrhage: systematic review of controlled observational studies. *J Child Adolesc Psychopharmacol* 2024; **34**:428–466.

49. Auerbach AD, et al. Perioperative use of selective serotonin reuptake inhibitors and risks for adverse outcomes of surgery. *JAMA Intern Med* 2013; **173**:1075–1081.

50. Movig KL, et al. Relationship of serotonergic antidepressants and need for blood transfusion in orthopedic surgical patients. *Arch Intern Med* 2003; **163**:2354–2358.

51. Liu B, et al. Use of selective serotonin-reuptake inhibitors of tricyclic antidepressants and risk of hip fractures in elderly people. *Lancet* 1998; **351**:1303–1307.

52. Richards JB, et al. Effect of selective serotonin reuptake inhibitors on the risk of fracture. *Arch Intern Med* 2007; **167**:188–194.

53. Leach MJ, et al. The risk of hip fracture due to mirtazapine exposure when switching antidepressants or using other antidepressants as add-on therapy. *Drugs Real World Outcomes* 2017; **4**:247–255.

54. Gylvin SH, et al. Psychopharmacologic treatment and blood transfusion in fast-track total hip and knee arthroplasty. *Transfusion* 2017; **57**:971–976.

55. Andreasen JJ, et al. Effect of selective serotonin reuptake inhibitors on requirement for allogeneic red blood cell transfusion following coronary artery bypass surgery. *Am J Cardiovasc Drugs* 2006; **6**:243–250.

56. Basile FV, et al. Use of selective serotonin reuptake inhibitors antidepressants and bleeding risk in breast cosmetic surgery. *Aesthetic Plast Surg* 2013; **37**:561–566.

57. Singh I, et al. Influence of pre-operative use of serotonergic antidepressants (SADs) on the risk of bleeding in patients undergoing different surgical interventions: a meta-analysis. *Pharmacoepidemiol Drug Saf* 2015; **24**:237–245.

58. Hoveidaei AH, et al. Preoperative SSRI use increases perioperative transfusion need in patients undergoing surgical procedures on the hip joint. *Eur J Orthop Surg Traumatol* 2024; **34**:3903–3908.

59. Mahdanian AA, et al. Serotonergic antidepressants and perioperative bleeding risk: a systematic review. *Expert Opin Drug Saf* 2014; **13**:695–704.

60. Jeong BO, et al. Use of serotonergic antidepressants and bleeding risk in patients undergoing surgery. *Psychosomatics* 2014; **55**:213–220.

61. Perahia DG, et al. The risk of bleeding with duloxetine treatment in patients who use nonsteroidal anti-inflammatory drugs (NSAIDs): analysis of placebo-controlled trials and post-marketing adverse event reports. *Drug Healthc Patient Saf* 2013; **5**:211–219.

62. Bixby AL, et al. Clinical management of bleeding risk with antidepressants. *Ann Pharmacother* 2019; **53**:186–194.

63. Halperin D, et al. Influence of antidepressants on hemostasis. *Dialogues Clin Neurosci* 2007; **9**:47–59.

64. Na K-S, et al. Can we recommend mirtazapine and bupropion for patients at risk for bleeding? A systematic review and meta-analysis. *J Affect Disord* 2018; **225**:221–226.

65. Machado CM, et al. Impact of selective serotonin-reuptake inhibitors in hemorrhagic risk in anticoagulated patients taking non-vitamin K antagonist anticoagulants: a systematic review and meta-analysis. *J Clin Psychopharmacol* 2023; **43**:267–272.

66. Rahman AA, et al. Concomitant use of selective serotonin reuptake inhibitors and oral anticoagulants and risk of major bleeding: a systematic review and meta-analysis. *Thromb Haemost* 2023; **123**:54–63.

CHAPTER 3

St John's wort

St John's wort (SJW), *Hypericum perforatum*, contains a combination of at least 10 different components, including hypericin, hyperforin and various flavonoids.[1] Preparations of SJW are often unstandardised and this has complicated the interpretation of clinical trials. Both the active ingredient(s) and mechanism(s) of action of SJW are unclear.[1] Constituents of SJW may inhibit monoamine oxidase (MAO), inhibit the reuptake of noradrenaline and serotonin, upregulate serotonin receptors and decrease serotonin receptor expression.[1]

Some preparations of SJW have been granted a traditional herbal registration certificate,[2] but this is based on traditional use rather than proven efficacy and tolerability. SJW is licensed in Germany for the treatment of depression.[2]

Evidence for St John's wort in the treatment of depression

A number of trials have examined the efficacy of SJW in the treatment of depression. They have been extensively reviewed[3-7] and most authors conclude that SJW is likely to be effective in the treatment of mild to moderate depression.[3,5,6,8] Cochrane concludes that SJW is more effective than placebo in the treatment of mild to moderate depression, and is as effective as, and better tolerated than, standard antidepressants.[4] Some formal guidelines recommended its use in mild to moderate depression.[9] The supporting evidence, however, is not without several limitations. For example, studies in German-speaking countries showed more favourable results than studies elsewhere.[4] Concerns have also been raised about the inadequate dosing of SSRIs in comparative studies.[10,11] In two reanalyses of data from a large negative RCT of SJW, both participant and clinician beliefs about treatment assignment were more strongly associated with clinical outcomes than the actual treatment received: those who guessed randomisation to active treatment fared better than those who guessed randomisation to placebo.[12,13] Efficacy in severe depression remains uncertain.[4-6] Oddly, there appear to be no published studies of SJW in depression since 2020,[14] perhaps reflecting the difficulties inherent in marketing for a profit an unpatentable natural product.

There is a little evidence for SJW in postmenopausal depression[15] or in pain syndromes.[16] Other important observations include:

- The active component of SJW for treating depression has not yet been determined. Trials used different preparations of SJW, most of which were standardised according to their total content of hypericins. However, evidence suggests that hypericins alone do not treat depression.[5]
- Many SJW preparations bought over the internet are sold as unregulated food supplements and are often of poor quality and/or are adulterated.[2] One analysis of 47 different SJW preparations found that 36% were adulterated with other *Hypericum* species and 19% were adulterated with food dyes.[2]
- Published studies are generally acute treatment studies. There are only preliminary data to support the effectiveness of SJW in the medium term. Longer-term and relapse-prevention data are lacking.[17]

On balance, SJW should probably not be prescribed. We lack sufficient understanding of what the active ingredient is or what constitutes a therapeutic dose and most preparations of SJW are unlicensed.[3]

Adverse effects

SJW appears to be well tolerated.[5,6] In a systematic review of existing studies, adverse effects were significantly less common than with older antidepressants, slightly less than SSRIs and similar to placebo.[6] The most common, if infrequent, adverse effects are nausea, rash, fatigue, restlessness and photosensitivity.[18] Although severe phototoxic reactions seem to be rare, patients should be informed that SJW can increase light sensitivity.[18] SJW may also share the propensity of SSRIs to increase the risk of bleeding; a case report describes prolonged epistaxis after nasal insertion of SJW.[19] Case reports have also described mania, hypomania and mixed states associated with SJW.[20] Manic symptoms associated with SJW have been documented in patients both with[20,21] and without previously recognised bipolar affective disorder.[20] The onset of manic symptoms ranged from 3 days to 2 months.[20] Caution is advised with high doses and those with a known history of bipolar affective disorder.[22] A single case report documented supraventricular tachycardia associated with SJW.[23]

Drug interactions

SJW is a potent inducer of intestinal and hepatic CYP3A4, CYP2C9, CYP2C19, CYP2E1 and intestinal p-glycoprotein.[18,24] Hyperforin is responsible for this effect.[25] The hyperforin content of SJW preparations varies 50-fold, which will result in a different propensity for drug interactions between brands. Preparations providing a daily dose of less than 1mg hyperforin are less likely to induce CYP enzymes.[25,26] CYP3A4 activity is induced over 1–2 weeks and returns to normal approximately 7 days after SJW is discontinued.[27]

SJW significantly reduces plasma concentrations of warfarin,[28] hormonal contraceptives,[29] digoxin and indinavir.[18] According to case reports, SJW has lowered plasma concentrations of clozapine, theophylline, ciclosporin, gliclazide, rivaroxaban and statins.[18,24,30–32] There is a theoretical risk that SJW may interact with some antiseizure medications. It has also been reported that SJW can increase the effects of clopidogrel (a pro-drug).[24] Serotonin syndrome has been reported when SJW was taken together with sertraline, paroxetine, nefazodone and various triptans.[33,34] SJW should not be taken with any drugs that have a predominantly serotonergic action. Box 3.5 details the key points that patients should know about SJW.

Box 3.5 Key points that patients should know about St John's wort

- Evidence suggests that SJW may be effective in the treatment of mild to moderate depression, but we do not know enough about how much should be taken or what the adverse effects are. There is less evidence of benefit in severe depression.
- SJW is not a licensed medicine.
- Available preparations are not standardised and differ in potency.[3]
- SJW can interact with other medicine[3] resulting in serious adverse effects. Some important drugs may be metabolised more rapidly and therefore become ineffective with serious consequences (e.g. increased viral load in human immunodeficiency virus, failure of oral contraceptives leading to unwanted pregnancy, reduced anticoagulant effect with warfarin leading to thrombosis).
- The symptoms of depression can sometimes be caused by other physical or mental illness. It is important that these possible causes are investigated.
- It is always best to consult the doctor if any herbal or natural remedy is being taken or the patient is thinking of taking one.

People may regard herbal remedies as 'natural' and therefore harmless.[35] Many are not aware of the potential of such remedies for causing adverse effects or interacting with other drugs. A large study from Germany (*n* = 588), where SJW is a licensed antidepressant, found that for every prescription written for SJW, one person purchased SJW without seeking the advice of a doctor.[36] Many of these people had severe or persistent depression but few told their doctor that they took SJW. A small US study (*n* = 22) found that people tend to take SJW because it is easy to obtain alternative medicines and also because they perceive herbal medicines as being purer and safer than prescription medicines. Few would discuss this medication with their conventional healthcare provider.[37] Clinicians need to be proactive in asking patients if they use such treatments and try to dispel the myth that natural is a synonym for safe.

References

1. Velingkar VS, et al. A current update on phytochemistry, pharmacology and herb–drug interactions of *Hypericum perforatum*. *Phytochem Rev* 2017; **16**:725–744.
2. Booker A, et al. St John's wort (*Hypericum perforatum*) products: an assessment of their authenticity and quality. *Phytomedicine* 2018; **40**:158–164.
3. National Institute for Health and Care Excellence. Depression in adults: treatment and management. NICE guideline [NG222]. 2022 (last updated May 2024, last checked May 2024); https://www.nice.org.uk/guidance/ng222.
4. Linde K, et al. St John's wort for major depression. *Cochrane Database Syst Rev* 2008; (4):CD000448.
5. Ng QX, et al. Clinical use of Hypericum perforatum (St John's wort) in depression: a meta-analysis. *J Affect Disord* 2017; **210**:211–221.
6. Apaydin EA, et al. A systematic review of St. John's wort for major depressive disorder. *Syst Rev* 2016; **5**:148.
7. Sarris J, et al. Plant-based medicines (phytoceuticals) in the treatment of psychiatric disorders: a meta-review of meta-analyses of randomized controlled trials. *Can J Psychiatry* 2021; **66**:849–862.
8. Volz H.P. Hypericum and depression. In: Riederer P, Laux G, Nagatsu T, Le W, Riederer C (eds) *NeuroPsychopharmacotherapy*. Cham: Springer; 2020:1–8.
9. Sarris J, et al. Clinician guidelines for the treatment of psychiatric disorders with nutraceuticals and phytoceuticals: the World Federation of Societies of Biological Psychiatry and Canadian Network for Mood and Anxiety Treatments Taskforce. *World J Biol Psychiatry* 2022; **23**:424–455.
10. Asher GN, et al. Comparative benefits and harms of complementary and alternative medicine therapies for initial treatment of major depressive disorder: systematic review and meta-analysis. *J Altern Complement Med* 2017; **23**:907–919.
11. Gartlehner G, et al. Pharmacological and non-pharmacological treatments for major depressive disorder: review of systematic reviews. *BMJ Open* 2017; **7**:e014912.
12. Chen JA, et al. Association between patient beliefs regarding assigned treatment and clinical response: reanalysis of data from the Hypericum Depression Trial Study Group. *J Clin Psychiatry* 2011; **72**:1669–1676.
13. Chen JA, et al. Association between physician beliefs regarding assigned treatment and clinical response: re-analysis of data from the Hypericum Depression Trial Study Group. *Asian J Psychiatr* 2015; **13**:23–29.
14. Zhao X, et al. The efficacy and safety of St. John's wort extract in depression therapy compared to SSRIs in adults: a meta-analysis of randomized clinical trials. *Adv Clin Exp Med* 2023; **32**:151–161.
15. Eatemadnia A, et al. The effect of Hypericum perforatum on postmenopausal symptoms and depression: a randomized controlled trial. *Complement Ther Med* 2019; **45**:109–113.
16. Galeotti N. *Hypericum perforatum* (St John's wort) beyond depression: a therapeutic perspective for pain conditions. *J Ethnopharmacol* 2017; **200**:136–146.
17. Cleare A, et al. Evidence-based guidelines for treating depressive disorders with antidepressants: a revision of the 2008 British Association for Psychopharmacology guidelines. *J Psychopharmacol* 2015; **29**:459–525.
18. Russo E, et al. *Hypericum perforatum*: pharmacokinetic, mechanism of action, tolerability, and clinical drug–drug interactions. *Phytother Res* 2014; **28**:643–655.
19. Crampsey DP, et al. Nasal insertion of St John's wort: an unusual cause of epistaxis. *J Laryngol Otol* 2007; **121**:279–280.
20. Bostock E, et al. Mania associated with herbal medicines, other than cannabis: a systematic review and quality assessment of case reports. *Front Psychiatry* 2018; **9**:280.
21. Rodrigues Cordeiro C, et al. Triggers for acute mood episodes in bipolar disorder: a systematic review. *J Psychiatr Res* 2023; **161**:237–260.
22. Sarris J. Herbal medicines in the treatment of psychiatric disorders: 10-year updated review. *Phytother Res* 2018; **32**:1147–1162.
23. Fisher KA, et al. St. John's wort-induced supraventricular tachycardia. *Cureus* 2021; **13**:e14356.
24. Soleymani S, et al. Clinical risks of St John's wort (*Hypericum perforatum*) co-administration. *Expert Opin Drug Metab Toxicol* 2017; **13**:1047–1062.
25. Chrubasik-Hausmann S, et al. Understanding drug interactions with St John's wort (*Hypericum perforatum* L.): impact of hyperforin content. *J Pharm Pharmacol* 2018; **71**:129–138.

26. Nicolussi S, et al. Clinical relevance of St. John's wort drug interactions revisited. *Br J Pharmacol* 2020; **177**:1212–1226.
27. Imai H, et al. The recovery time-course of CYP3A after induction by St John's wort administration. *Br J Clin Pharmacol* 2008; **65**:701–707.
28. Choi S, et al. A systematic review of the pharmacokinetic and pharmacodynamic interactions of herbal medicine with warfarin. *PLoS One* 2017; **12**:e0182794.
29. Berry-Bibee EN, et al. Co-administration of St. John's wort and hormonal contraceptives: a systematic review. *Contraception* 2016; **94**:668–677.
30. Xu H, et al. Effects of St John's wort and CYP2C9 genotype on the pharmacokinetics and pharmacodynamics of gliclazide. *Br J Pharmacol* 2008; **153**:1579–1586.
31. Andren L, et al. Interaction between a commercially available St. John's wort product (Movina) and atorvastatin in patients with hypercholesterolemia. *Eur J Clin Pharmacol* 2007; **63**:913–916.
32. Scholz I, et al. Effects of *Hypericum perforatum* (St John's wort) on the pharmacokinetics and pharmacodynamics of rivaroxaban in humans. *Br J Clin Pharmacol* 2021; **87**:1466–1474.
33. Committee of Safety in Medicine and Medicines Control Agency. Reminder: St John's wort (*Hypericum perforatum*) interactions. *Curr Probl Pharmacovigilance* 2000; **26**:6–7.
34. Lantz MS, et al. St. John's wort and antidepressant drug interactions in the elderly. *J Geriatr Psychiatry Neurol* 1999; **12**:7–10.
35. Barnes J, et al. Different standards for reporting ADRs to herbal remedies and conventional OTC medicines: face-to-face interviews with 515 users of herbal remedies. *Br J Clin Pharmacol* 1998; **45**:496–500.
36. Linden M, et al. Self medication with St. John's wort in depressive disorders: an observational study in community pharmacies. *J Affect Disord* 2008; **107**:205–210.
37. Wagner PJ, et al. Taking the edge off: why patients choose St. John's wort. *J Fam Pract* 1999; **48**:615–619.

CHAPTER 3

Antidepressants: relative adverse effects – a rough guide

Table 3.23 gives a very approximate, unreferenced view of the absolute and relative risk of a small range of adverse effects associated with standard antidepressants. Further details can be found in specific sections in this chapter.

Table 3.23 Common adverse effects of antidepressants.

Drug	Sedation	Postural hypotension	Cardiac conduction disturbance	Anticholinergic effects	Nausea/ vomiting	Sexual dysfunction
Tricyclics						
Amitriptyline	+++	+++	+++	+++	+	+++
Clomipramine	++	+++	+++	++	++	+++
Dosulepin	+++	+++	+++	++	+	+
Doxepin	+++	++	+++	+++	+	+
Imipramine	++	+++	+++	+++	+	+
Lofepramine	+	+	+	++	+	+
Nortriptyline	+	++	++	+	+	+
Protriptyline	–	+	++	++	++	+
Trimipramine	+++	+++	++	++	+	+
Other antidepressants						
Agomelatine	+	–	–	–	–	–
Bupropion	–	–	+	–	+	–
Dextromethorphan/ bupropion	+	–	+	–	++	–
Duloxetine (SNRI)	–	–*	–	–	++	+++
Levomilnacipran (SNRI)	–	–*	–	–	++	++
Mianserin	++	–	–	–	–	–
Mirtazapine	+++	+	–	+	+	–
Reboxetine	+	–*	–	+	+	+
Trazodone	+++	+	+	+	+	+
Venlafaxine/ desvenlafaxine	–	–*	+	–	+++	+++
SSRIs						
Citalopram	–	–	+	–	++	+++
Escitalopram	–	–	+	–	++	+++

(Continued)

Table 3.23 (*Continued*)

Drug	Sedation	Postural hypotension	Cardiac conduction disturbance	Anticholinergic effects	Nausea/ vomiting	Sexual dysfunction
Fluoxetine	–	–	–	–	++	+++
Fluvoxamine	+	–	–	–	+++	+++
Paroxetine	+	–	–	+	++	+++
Sertraline	–	–	–	–	++	+++
Vilazodone	–	–	–	–	+	++
Vortioxetine	–	+	–	–	+	+
Monoamine oxidase inhibitors						
Isocarboxazid	+	++	+	++	+	+
Phenelzine	+	+	+	+	+	+
Tranylcypromine	–	+	+	+	+	+
Reversible inhibitor of monoamine oxidase A						
Moclobemide	–	–	–	–	+	+

Key: Incidence/severity: +++, high; ++, moderate; +, low; –, very low/none.
* Hypertension reported.

CHAPTER 3

Anxiety spectrum disorders

Anxiety disorders can occur in isolation, be comorbid with other psychiatric disorders (particularly depression), be a consequence of physical illness such as thyrotoxicosis or be drug-induced (e.g. by caffeine). Comorbidity with other psychiatric disorders is very common.

These disorders tend to be chronic and treatment is often only partially successful. People with anxiety disorders may be especially prone to adverse effects.[1] High initial doses of SSRIs in particular may be poorly tolerated, for example.

Benzodiazepines

Benzodiazepines provide rapid symptomatic relief from acute anxiety states.[2] Nearly all guidelines and consensus statements recommend that this group of drugs should be used only to treat anxiety that is severe, disabling or subjecting the individual to extreme distress. Because of their potential to cause physical dependence and withdrawal symptoms, these drugs should be used at the lowest effective dose for the shortest period of time (maximum 4 weeks), while longer-term treatment strategies are put in place. For the majority of patients these recommendations are sensible and should be followed. A very small number of patients with severely disabling anxiety may benefit from long-term treatment with a benzodiazepine and these patients should not normally be denied treatment. Benzodiazepines are, however, known to be over-prescribed in the long term for treatment of both anxiety[3] and depression,[4] perhaps especially in the USA, where attitudes to benzodiazepines differ markedly from other developed countries.[5]

In the UK, NICE recommends that benzodiazepines should not be used to treat panic disorder.[6] In other countries, alprazolam is widely used for this indication. Benzodiazepines should be used with some care in post-traumatic stress disorder (PTSD).[7]

SSRIs/SNRIs

When used to treat **generalised anxiety disorder (GAD)**, SSRIs should initially be prescribed at half the normal starting dose and titrated to the normal antidepressant dosage range as tolerated (initial worsening of anxiety may be seen when treatment is started).[8] The same advice applies to the use of venlafaxine and duloxetine. Modest benefit is usually seen within 6 weeks and continues to increase over time.[9] The optimal duration of treatment has not been determined but should probably be at least 1 year.[10,11] Effective treatment of GAD may prevent the development of major depression.[10]

An early network meta-analysis suggested that fluoxetine is the most effective SSRI in GAD and sertraline the best tolerated.[12] More recent analyses suggest that bupropion[13] or agomelatine[14] is the most effective drug in GAD. Neither analysis found clear effects over placebo for lorazepam or vortioxetine.

When used to treat **panic disorder,** the same starting dose and dosage titration should be used as for GAD. Doses of clomipramine,[15] citalopram[16] and sertraline[17] towards the bottom of the antidepressant range give the best balance between efficacy and adverse effects, whereas higher doses of paroxetine ($\geq$40mg) may be required.[18] Higher doses of all drugs may be effective when standard doses have failed. Efficacy of SSRIs (but not SNRIs) increases across the licensed dose range in anxiety disorders.[19] Onset of action may be as long as 6 weeks. Women may respond better to SSRIs than men.[20] Augmentation with clonazepam leads to a more rapid response but not a greater magnitude of response overall.[18] The optimal duration of treatment is unknown but should be at least 8 months.[21] A large naturalistic study showed convincing evidence of benefit for at least 3 years.[22] Less than half are likely to remain well after medication is withdrawn.[23]

Lower starting doses are also required in **PTSD**, although high doses (e.g. fluoxetine 60mg) are usually required for full effect. Response is usually seen within 8 weeks, but can take up to 12 weeks.[23] Treatment should be continued for at least 6 months and probably longer.[11,24,25]

Although the doses of SSRIs licensed for the treatment of **obsessive compulsive disorder (OCD)** are higher than those licensed for the treatment of depression (e.g. fluoxetine 60mg, paroxetine 40–60mg), lower (standard antidepressant) doses may be effective, particularly for maintenance treatment.[26] Initial response is usually slower to emerge than in depression (it can take 10–12 weeks). Dose should be increased to gain maximal benefit. Treatment should continue for at least 1 year.[11] The relapse rate in those who continue treatment for 2 years is half that of those who stop treatment after initial response (25–40% vs 80%).[27] In most people with OCD, the condition is persistent and symptom severity fluctuates over time.[28] Second-line treatment is usually the addition of either risperidone or aripiprazole. Very high doses of SSRIs have also been tried (e.g. 650mg/day sertraline), apparently without any major safety problems.[29]

Body dysmorphic disorder should be treated initially with CBT. If symptoms are moderate to severe, adding an SSRI may improve outcome.[30] Buspirone may usefully augment the SSRI,[30] although no RCT has been conducted.

Standard antidepressant starting doses are well tolerated in **social phobia**,[31,32] and dosage titration may benefit some patients but is not always required. Some benefit is usually seen within 8 weeks and treatment should be continued for at least 1 year and probably longer.[32] In the UK, NICE recommends CBT as first-line treatment for social anxiety.[33]

All patients treated with SSRIs should be monitored for the development of akathisia, increased anxiety and the emergence of suicidal ideation; the risk is greatest in those younger than 30 years, those with comorbid depression and those already known to be at higher risk of suicide.[30,34]

SSRIs should not be stopped abruptly, as patients with anxiety spectrum disorders are particularly sensitive to discontinuation symptoms (see section on stopping antidepressants in this chapter). The dose should be reduced as slowly as tolerated over several months.

Pregabalin

Pregabalin is licensed for the treatment of GAD. Several large RCTs have demonstrated its efficacy and tolerability and comparable speed of onset of action to a benzodiazepine.[2,35] The dose of pregabalin in GAD is initially 150mg, increased gradually to a maximum of 600mg in two to three divided doses. It is widely misused (often alongside opioids)[36] and there is a significant risk of diversion.[37] Pregabalin seems to worsen the overdose toxicity of opiates.[38] Pregabalin should not be stopped abruptly as it may precipitate a severe withdrawal syndrome that includes seizures.[39]

Psychological approaches

There is good evidence to support the efficacy of psychological interventions in anxiety spectrum disorders.[11,40] Examples include exposure therapy in OCD and social phobia. Initial drug therapy may be required to help the patient become more receptive to psychological input, although evidence to support this assumption is slim. Some studies suggest that optimal outcome is achieved by combining psychological and drug therapies,[6,41] but negative studies also exist.[42,43]

A discussion of the evidence base for psychological interventions is outside the scope of this text. It is recognised that for many patients psychological therapies are the appropriate first-line treatment, and this is supported by NICE.[6]

Summary of NICE guidelines for the treatment of GAD, panic disorder and OCD

- A 'stepped care' approach is recommended to help in choosing the most effective intervention for GAD,[6] panic disorder[6] and OCD.[30]
- A comprehensive assessment is recommended, which considers the degree of distress and functional impairment, the effect of any comorbid mental illness, substance misuse or medical condition, and past response to treatment.
- Treat the primary disorder first.
- Psychological therapy is more effective than pharmacological therapy and should be used as first-line therapy where possible. Details of the types of therapy recommended and their duration can be found in the NICE guidelines.
- Pharmacological therapy is also effective. Most evidence supports the use of the SSRIs (sertraline as first line).
- Provide information on the probable benefits and disadvantages of each mode of treatment.
- Consider combination therapy for complex anxiety disorders that are refractory to treatment.

Panic disorder

- Benzodiazepines should not be used except in a crisis.
- An SSRI should be used as first-line therapy. If SSRIs are contraindicated or there is no response, imipramine or clomipramine can be used.
- Self-help (based on CBT principles) should be encouraged, as should formal CBT.

GAD

- Benzodiazepines should not be used except for crises.
- An SSRI should be used as first-line treatment.
- SNRIs and pregabalin are second and third choices, respectively.
- High-intensity psychological intervention and self-help (based on CBT principles) should be encouraged.
- Antipsychotics should not be offered (presumably this includes quetiapine).

OCD (where there is moderate or severe functional impairment)

- Use an SSRI or intensive CBT.
- Combine the SSRI and CBT if the response to a single strategy is suboptimal.
- Use clomipramine if SSRIs fail.
- If response is still suboptimal, add an antipsychotic or combine clomipramine and citalopram.

Boxes 3.6–3.10 give details of specific drugs used in anxiety spectrum disorders.

Box 3.6 Generalised anxiety disorder

Drug	Comment
Crisis management	
Benzodiazepines	Normally for short-term use only, maximum 2–4 weeks, although some are of the opinion that risks are overstated[44]
First-line treatment (in order of preference)[30]	
SSRIs (up to maximum licensed dose)	May initially exacerbate symptoms. A lower starting dose is recommended. Fluoxetine and sertraline are preferred options.[12] Vortioxetine may not be effective.[45]
SNRIs[14] (up to maximum licensed dose)	May initially exacerbate symptoms. A lower starting dose is recommended.
Pregabalin 150–600mg/day in divided doses	Response may be seen in the first week of treatment.[46] Increasingly misused. Significant withdrawal syndrome. Overdose risk with opiates.
Second-line treatment (less well tolerated or weaker evidence base; no order of preference)	
Agomelatine[47] 10–50mg/day	Agomelatine has been shown to prevent relapse over a 6-month period[48,49]
Betablockers	
Propranolol 40–120mg/day in divided doses	Initiate at 40mg and titrate dose up to effect if needed. Useful for somatic symptoms, particularly tachycardia.[50] Otherwise has limited efficacy. Highly toxic in overdose.[51]
Buspirone 15–60mg/day in divided doses	Has a delayed onset of action; takes up to 6 weeks to show equal efficacy to benzodiazepines[52]
Hydroxyzine 50–100mg/day in divided doses	Unclear that hydroxyzine is effective due to a direct anxiolytic effect or to a broader sedative effect[53]
Quetiapine (MR, 50–300mg)	Recommended as monotherapy. Probably not effective as adjunctive therapy to SSRI/SNRI in treatment resistance.[54]
Tricyclic antidepressants	
Clomipramine 50–250mg/day[55–57]	Initiate at 10mg/day and increase the dose gradually
Imipramine 75–200mg/day in divided doses[58]	Initiate at 25mg/day every 4 days and when at 100mg can increase in 50mg increments[10]

(Continued)

Drug	Comment
Monoamine oxidase inhibitors	
Phenelzine 45–90mg/day in divided doses[59]	For mixed anxiety and depressive states. Patients need to avoid food high in tyramine.
Mirtazapine 15–30mg at night[60,61]	
Experimental	
Cannabidiol	Large effect size[62]
Chamomile 220–1500mg/day	Two RCTs, one positive, one negative using standardised doses of chamomile and placebo[63]
Gingko biloba 240–480mg/day	One positive RCT using standardised doses of Gingko biloba and placebo[64]
Ketamine	Seemingly rapidly effective[65]
Lavender oil preparation 80–160mg/day	Substantial supporting evidence[66]
Riluzole 50–100mg/day doses[67]	Liver function monitoring required

Box 3.7 Panic disorder

Drug	Comment
Crisis management	
Benzodiazepines	Rapid effect although panic symptoms return quickly if the drug is withdrawn.[68] NICE does not recommend.[6] Cochrane lukewarm.[69] Probably the most effective treatment.[70] Alprazolam is not superior to other benzodiazepines[71] and its effects may have been overestimated.[72]
First-line treatment (in order of preference)[6,73]	
SSRIs (up to maximum licensed dose)	Therapeutic effect can be delayed (this applies to all antidepressants)[74] and patients can experience an initial exacerbation of panic symptoms.[6] Use supported by Cochrane[75] and a 2022 meta-analysis.[76]
Venlafaxine MR 75–225mg[73]	Initiate at 37.5mg for 7 days

(Continued)

Drug	Comment
Second-line treatment (less well tolerated or weak evidence base; no order of preference)	
Mirtazapine 15–60mg/day[77]	A meta-analysis suggests that mirtazapine does not help with panic symptoms but with the anxiety associated with this disorder.[73] Rather limited data overall.[78]
Moclobemide 300–600mg/day[79]	One fixed dose study of 450mg/day and one flexible dose study suggest efficacy.[79,80] Brofaromine (a similar drug) is also effective.[70]
Monoamine oxidase inhibitors	
Phenelzine 10–60mg/day[74]	No long-term studies; reserve for treatment-resistant cases due to poor tolerability[74]
Tricyclic antidepressants	
Clomipramine 25–250mg/day[74]	Start with a low dose and increase dose according to response and tolerability. Good evidence of effectiveness.[70]
Imipramine 25–300mg/day[74]	
Lofepramine 70–210mg/day in divided doses[81]	
Experimental	
Gabapentin 600–3600mg/day	One RCT showed no difference between gabapentin and placebo. However, significant improvement was demonstrated in the more severely ill.[82]
Inositol 12g/day[83]	One positive RCT in 21 patients. Equivalent to fluvoxamine in one study.[84] Well tolerated.
Levetiracetam 250mg twice daily[78]	Usually well tolerated
Pindolol 7.5mg/day	Efficacy suggested in a small 21 patient RCT where 2.5mg tds was used to augment fluoxetine in treatment-resistant panic disorder[85]
Valproate 500–2250mg/day	Two very small positive open studies[86,87]
Hydrocortisone	Only acute treatment shown to prevent development of post-traumatic stress disorder[88]

CHAPTER 3

Box 3.8 Post-traumatic stress disorder

Drug	Comments
First-line treatment (in order of preference) (Psychological approaches should be used before drug treatments)[89,90]	
SSRIs (up to maximum licensed doses)	Paroxetine, sertraline or fluoxetine are the preferred SSRIs.[91,92] Recommended by NICE.[89] Good support but small effective size.[93,94]
Venlafaxine modified release 37.5–300mg[95]	Recommended by NICE[89] Supported by meta-analyses[93,96]
Second-line treatment (less well tolerated or weak evidence base; no order of preference)	
Antipsychotics	May be effective for the intrusion symptoms (flashbacks and nightmares) but not the avoidance and hyperarousal symptoms of post-traumatic stress disorder. Studies done as monotherapy or as adjunctive treatment.[97]
Olanzapine 5–20mg	May be the most effective treatment[96]
Risperidone 0.5–6mg	Specifically mentioned by NICE[89]
Quetiapine 50–800mg[98]	More robust support than for risperidone[93,96]
Mirtazapine 15–45mg/day[99]	Recommended by NICE[89] Second most effective drug in a network meta-analysis[100]
Monoamine oxidase inhibitors	
Phenelzine 15–75mg/day[101]	Recommended by NICE[89] Most effective drug in a network meta-analysis[100]
Prazosin 2–15mg at night[102]	For nightmares and sleep disturbances. Initiate at 1mg at night and titrate dose gradually to reduce the risk of hypotension. Supported by a systematic review[103] and meta-analysis.[93]
Tricyclic antidepressants	Start at a low dose and increase dose according to tolerability
Amitriptyline 50–300mg/day[104]	Recommended by NICE[89] For all TCAs start at a low dose and increase dose according to tolerability
Imipramine 50–300mg/day	Best supporting evidence is for desipramine but this drug is not widely available[100]
Ketamine IV[105,106]	Rapid reduction in symptom severity suggested. Developing evidence showing acute and chronic efficacy.[107–109]
Experimental	
Duloxetine 60–120mg	Two small open studies suggest efficacy. Start at 30mg for 1 week[110,111]
Lamotrigine up to 500mg/day	Small double-blind study in 15 patients[112]
MDMA-assisted therapy	Developing database[113]
Phenytoin plasma concentration 10–20ng/ml[114]	Open-label study in 12 patients
Valproate up to 2.5g[115]	Probably not effective[100]

MAOI, monoamine oxidase inhibitor; MDMA, 3,4-methylenedioxymethamphetamine.

Box 3.9 Obsessive–compulsive disorder

Drug	Comments
First-line treatment (in order of preference)	
Any SSRI[41] (up to maximum licensed dose)	If the first SSRI is not tolerated or has a poor response an alternative SSRI may be tried[30]
Clomipramine (up to 250mg)	Owing to poorer tolerability, recommended trying at least one SSRI first[30]
Second-line treatment (unlicensed or weaker evidence base; in no order of preference)	
Add antipsychotic to SSRI (low to moderate doses)[116,117]	Most evidence supports the use of aripiprazole or risperidone.[116] Some evidence for haloperidol.[117]
Citalopram 40mg with clomipramine 150mg	Based on small randomised open-label study.[118] Recommended by NICE.[30] ECG monitoring required.
Acetylcysteine[119] (up to 2400mg/day added to SSRI or clomipramine)	GI adverse effects may be problematic. Two of five controlled studies negative. Pooled effect shows benefit.[120]
Lamotrigine 100mg+ added to SSRI[121]	Dose must be titrated gradually as indicated in the summary of product characteristics. May worsen OCD in some.[122]
Topiramate up to 400mg added to SSRI[123,124]	Not well tolerated; suggested benefits for compulsion but not obsessions.[123] Two trials found it ineffective[125,126]
Experimental	
High-dose SSRIs	Dose titrated gradually according to tolerability. ECG monitoring recommended. Higher doses have been safely used[29] (e.g. sertraline 650mg, fluoxetine 120mg/day)
Escitalopram 25–50mg[127]	
Sertraline 250–400mg[128]	
Memantine	Good evidence for 20mg/day added to SSRIs.[129] Most effective add-on treatment in a 2023 meta-analysis.[130]
NSAIDs (e.g. celecoxib 400mg/day)	Some supporting evidence[126]
Amantadine 200mg/day	One positive RCT[131]
SNRIs	
Venlafaxine up to 375mg[132]	
Duloxetine 60mg[133]	
Mirtazapine 30–60mg[134]	Small trial in 30 patients
5HT$_3$ antagonists	
Granisetron 1mg with fluvoxamine 200mg[135]	Some evidence for each drug but ondansetron may be the more effective[130,137,138]
Ondansetron 4mg with fluoxetine 20mg[136]	

CHAPTER 3

(Continued)

Drug	Comments
Pregabalin 75–225mg/day added to sertraline	One small positive RCT[139]
Riluzole 50mg bd added to existing drug treatment[140]	Variable results in early trials[126]
Anti-androgen – triptorelin 3.75mg IM every 4 weeks added to existing drug treatment[141]	Open-label study done in six men
Psilocybin	Emerging evidence for effect[142,143]
IV treatment	Quicker onset of action suggested compared with oral treatments
Clomipramine IV[144]	IV may be more effective than oral clomipramine
Ketamine IV[145,146]	Developing evidence base[126]
Once-weekly morphine 15–45mg added to existing drug treatment[147]	Small study involving 23 treatment-resistant patients. Positive effects were transient.

Box 3.10 Social phobia (social anxiety disorder)

Drug	Comments
First line drug treatment[148] (in order of preference)	
SSRIs (up to maximum licensed dose)	If no response to the first SSRI, try an alternative SSRI. Supporting meta-analyses for fluvoxamine[149] and citalopram.[150] Emerging data for vilazodone.[151]
Venlafaxine modified release 75–225mg/day	Supporting meta-analysis[152]
Second line drug treatment (less well tolerated or weaker evidence base, no order of preference)	
Olanzapine 5–20mg[153]	Few studies with antipsychotics. Most evidence with olanzapine.
Atenolol 25–100mg/day	Reduces autonomic symptoms in performance situations.[153] Probably not effective in social phobia.[154]
Benzodiazepines: Clonazepam 0.3–6mg/day[153]	Helpful on prn basis. Most evidence for treatment with clonazepam and bromazepam. Switching an SSRI to venlafaxine no more effective than adding clonazepam to SSRI.[155]
Sertraline plus clonazepam up to 3mg/day[155]	
Gabapentin 900–3600mg/day[153]	

(Continued)

Drug	Comments
Levetiracetam 300–3000mg/day in divided doses[156]	
Moclobemide 600mg/day in divided doses	Initiate at 300mg/day in divided doses. Has a UK licence for social phobia. Recommended by NICE.[148]
Phenelzine 15–90mg/day[157]	Avoidance of tyramine-rich food important. Recommended by NICE.[148]
Pregabalin 150–600mg/day[153]	600mg/day superior to placebo[153]
Experimental	
Ketamine 0.5mg/kg IV	One good RCT,[158] one post hoc analysis[159]
Topiramate 25–400mg/day[160]	Small open-label study of 23 patients suggests efficacy but poorly tolerated
Valproate 500–2500mg/day[161]	Small open-label study of 17 patients suggests efficacy

References

1. Nash JR, et al. Pharmacotherapy of anxiety. *Handb Exp Pharmacol* 2005; (169):469–501.
2. Munkholm K, et al. Minor tranquillizers for short-term treatment of newly onset symptoms of anxiety and distress: a systematic review with network meta-analysis of randomized trials. *Eur Arch Psychiatry Clin Neurosci* 2024; **274**:475–486.
3. Benitez CI, et al. Use of benzodiazepines and selective serotonin reuptake inhibitors in middle-aged and older adults with anxiety disorders: a longitudinal and prospective study. *Am J Geriatr Psychiatry* 2008; **16**:5–13.
4. Demyttenaere K, et al. Clinical factors influencing the prescription of antidepressants and benzodiazepines: results from the European study of the epidemiology of mental disorders (ESEMeD). *J Affect Disord* 2008; **110**:84–93.
5. Hirschtritt ME, et al. Balancing the risks and benefits of benzodiazepines. *JAMA* 2021; **325**:347–348.
6. National Institute for Health and Care Excellence. Generalised anxiety disorder and panic disorder in adults: management. Clinical guideline [CG113]. 2011 (last updated June 2020, reviewed May 2024, last checked November 2024); https://www.nice.org.uk/guidance/cg113.
7. Davidson JR. Use of benzodiazepines in social anxiety disorder, generalized anxiety disorder, and posttraumatic stress disorder. *J Clin Psychiatry* 2004; **65** Suppl 5:29–33.
8. Scott A, et al. Antidepressant drugs in the treatment of anxiety disorders. *Adv Psychiatr Treat* 2001; **7**:275–282.
9. Ballenger JC. Remission rates in patients with anxiety disorders treated with paroxetine. *J Clin Psychiatry* 2004; **65**:1696–1707.
10. Davidson JR, et al. A psychopharmacological treatment algorithm for generalised anxiety disorder (GAD). *J Psychopharmacol* 2010; **24**:3–26.
11. Baldwin DS, et al. Evidence-based pharmacological treatment of anxiety disorders, post-traumatic stress disorder and obsessive-compulsive disorder: a revision of the 2005 guidelines from the British Association for Psychopharmacology. *J Psychopharmacol* 2014; **28**:403–439.
12. Baldwin D, et al. Efficacy of drug treatments for generalised anxiety disorder: systematic review and meta-analysis. *BMJ* 2011; **342**:d1199.
13. Slee A, et al. Pharmacological treatments for generalised anxiety disorder: a systematic review and network meta-analysis. *Lancet* 2019; **393**:768–777.
14. Kong W, et al. Comparative remission rates and tolerability of drugs for generalised anxiety disorder: a systematic review and network meta-analysis of double-blind randomized controlled trials. *Front Pharmacol* 2020; **11**:580858.
15. Caillard V, et al. Comparative effects of low and high doses of clomipramine and placebo in panic disorder: a double-blind controlled study. French University Antidepressant Group. *Acta Psychiatr Scand* 1999; **99**:51–58.
16. Wade AG, et al. The effect of citalopram in panic disorder. *Br J Psychiatry* 1997; **170**:549–553.
17. Londborg PD, et al. Sertraline in the treatment of panic disorder: a multi-site, double-blind, placebo-controlled, fixed-dose investigation. *Br J Psychiatry* 1998; **173**:54–60.
18. Pollack MH, et al. Combined paroxetine and clonazepam treatment strategies compared to paroxetine monotherapy for panic disorder. *J Psychopharmacol* 2003; **17**:276–282.

19. Jakubovski E, et al. Systematic review and meta-analysis: dose-response curve of SSRIs and SNRIs in anxiety disorders. *Depress Anxiety* 2019; **36**:198–212.

20. Clayton AH, et al. Sex differences in clinical presentation and response in panic disorder: pooled data from sertraline treatment studies. *Arch Womens Ment Health* 2006; **9**:151–157.

21. Rickels K, et al. Panic disorder: long-term pharmacotherapy and discontinuation. *J Clin Psychopharmacol* 1998; **18**:12S–18S.

22. Choy Y, et al. Three-year medication prophylaxis in panic disorder: to continue or discontinue? A naturalistic study. *Compr Psychiatry* 2007; **48**:419–425.

23. Michelson D, et al. Continuing treatment of panic disorder after acute response: randomised, placebo-controlled trial with fluoxetine. The Fluoxetine Panic Disorder Study Group. *Br J Psychiatry* 1999; **174**:213–218.

24. Davidson J, et al. Efficacy of sertraline in preventing relapse of posttraumatic stress disorder: results of a 28-week double-blind, placebo-controlled study. *Am J Psychiatry* 2001; **158**:1974–1981.

25. Williams T, et al. Pharmacotherapy for post traumatic stress disorder (PTSD). *Cochrane Database Syst Rev* 2022; **3**(3):CD002795.

26. Martenyi F, et al. Fluoxetine v. placebo in prevention of relapse in post-traumatic stress disorder. *Br J Psychiatry* 2002; **181**:315–320.

27. The Expert Consensus Panel for obsessive–compulsive disorder: treatment of obsessive–compulsive disorder. *J Clin Psychiatry* 1997; **58** Suppl 4:2–72.

28. Catapano F, et al. Obsessive–compulsive disorder: a 3-year prospective follow-up study of patients treated with serotonin reuptake inhibitors OCD follow-up study. *J Psychiatr Res* 2006; **40**:502–510.

29. Levy DM, et al. Off-label higher doses of serotonin reuptake inhibitors in the treatment of obsessive–compulsive disorder: safety and tolerability. *Compr Psychiatry* 2024; **133**:152486.

30. National Institute for Health and Care Excellence. Surveillance decision. Evidence: Obsessive-compulsive disorder and body dysmorphic disorder: treatment. Clinical Guidance [CG31]. 2005 (last updated February 2019); https://www.nice.org.uk/guidance/cg31/resources/2019-surveillance-of-obsessivecompulsive-disorder-and-body-dysmorphic-disorder-treatment-nice-guideline-cg31-6713804845/chapter/Surveillance-decision?tab=evidence.

31. Blomhoff S, et al. Randomised controlled general practice trial of sertraline, exposure therapy and combined treatment in generalised social phobia. *Br J Psychiatry* 2001; **179**:23–30.

32. Hood SD, et al. Psychopharmacological treatments: an overview. In: WR Crozier and LE Alden, eds. *International Handbook of Social Anxiety: Concepts, research and interventions relating to the self and shyness.* Oxford: Wiley; 2001:471–504.

33. Mayo-Wilson E, et al. Psychological and pharmacological interventions for social anxiety disorder in adults: a systematic review and network meta-analysis. *Lancet Psychiatry* 2014; **1**:368–376.

34. National Institute for Health and Care Excellence. Depression in adults: treatment and management. NICE guideline [NG222]. 2022 (last reviewed September 2024, last checked November 2024); https://www.nice.org.uk/guidance/ng222.

35. Pollack MH. Refractory generalized anxiety disorder. *J Clin Psychiatry* 2009; **70** Suppl 2:32–38.

36. Lancia M, et al. Pregabalin abuse in combination with other drugs: monitoring among methadone patients. *Front Psychiatry* 2019; **10**:1022.

37. Hägg S, et al. Current evidence on abuse and misuse of gabapentinoids. *Drug Saf* 2020; **43**:1235–1254.

38. Kalk NJ, et al. Fatalities associated with gabapentinoids in England (2004–2020). *Br J Clin Pharmacol* 2022; **88**:3911–3917.

39. Naveed S, et al. Pregabalin-associated discontinuation symptoms: a case report. *Cureus* 2018; **10**:e3425.

40. Roberts NP, et al. Early psychological interventions to treat acute traumatic stress symptoms. *Cochrane Database Syst Rev* 2010; (3):CD007944.

41. Skapinakis P, et al. Pharmacological and psychotherapeutic interventions for management of obsessive-compulsive disorder in adults: a systematic review and network meta-analysis. *Lancet Psychiatry* 2016; **3**:730–739.

42. van Apeldoorn FJ, et al. Is a combined therapy more effective than either CBT or SSRI alone? Results of a multicenter trial on panic disorder with or without agoraphobia. *Acta Psychiatr Scand* 2008; **117**:260–270.

43. Marcus SM, et al. A comparison of medication side effect reports by panic disorder patients with and without concomitant cognitive behavior therapy. *Am J Psychiatry* 2007; **164**:273–275.

44. Offidani E, et al. Efficacy and tolerability of benzodiazepines versus antidepressants in anxiety disorders: a systematic review and meta-analysis. *Psychother Psychosom* 2013; **82**:355–362.

45. Meza N, et al. Vortioxetine for generalised anxiety disorder in adults. *Medwave* 2021; **21**:e8172.

46. Generoso MB, et al. Pregabalin for generalized anxiety disorder: an updated systematic review and meta-analysis. *Int Clin Psychopharmacol* 2017; **32**:49–55.

47. Wang SM, et al. Agomelatine for the treatment of generalized anxiety disorder: a meta-analysis. *Clin Psychopharmacol Neurosci* 2020; **18**:423–433.

48. Stein DJ, et al. Agomelatine prevents relapse in generalized anxiety disorder: a 6-month randomized, double-blind, placebo-controlled discontinuation study. *J Clin Psychiatry* 2012; **73**:1002–1008.

49. Hood SD, et al. Systematic review and network meta-analysis of agomelatine for the treatment of generalized anxiety disorder in adult patients. *Int Clin Psychopharmacol* 2024; doi:10.1097/YIC.0000000000000551.

50. Hayes PE, et al. Beta-blockers in anxiety disorders. *J Affect Disord* 1987; **13**:119–130.

51. UK Health Security Agency. *National Poisons Information Service Report 2022 to 2023.* London: UKHSA; 2022 (last accessed February 2025); https://www.npis.org/Download/NPIS%20report%202022-23.pdf.

52. Chessick CA, et al. Azapirones for generalized anxiety disorder. *Cochrane Database Syst Rev* 2006; **3**:CD006115.

53. Guaiana G, et al. Hydroxyzine for generalised anxiety disorder. *Cochrane Database Syst Rev* 2010; (12):CD006815.

54. Khan A, et al. Extended-release quetiapine fumarate (quetiapine XR) as adjunctive therapy in patients with generalized anxiety disorder and a history of inadequate treatment response: a randomized, double-blind study. *Ann Clin Psychiatry* 2014; **26**:3–18.

55. Wingerson D, et al. Clomipramine treatment for generalized anxiety disorder. *J Clin Psychopharmacol* 1992; **12**:214–215.

56. den Boer JA, et al. Effect of serotonin uptake inhibitors in anxiety disorders; a double-blind comparison of clomipramine and fluvoxamine. *Int Clin Psychopharmacol* 1987; **2**:21–32.

57. Kahn RS, et al. Effect of a serotonin precursor and uptake inhibitor in anxiety disorders; a double-blind comparison of 5-hydroxytryptophan, clomipramine and placebo. *Int Clin Psychopharmacol* 1987; **2**:33–45.

58. Rickels K, et al. Antidepressants for the treatment of generalized anxiety disorder. A placebo-controlled comparison of imipramine, trazodone, and diazepam. *Arch Gen Psychiatry* 1993; **50**:884–895.

59. Robinson DS, et al. The monoamine oxidase inhibitor, phenelzine, in the treatment of depressive-anxiety states: a controlled clinical trial. *Arch Gen Psychiatry* 1973; **29**:407–413.

60. Gambi F, et al. Mirtazapine treatment of generalized anxiety disorder: a fixed dose, open label study. *J Psychopharmacol* 2005; **19**:483–487.

61. Sitsen JMA, et al. Mirtazapine, a novel antidepressant, in the treatment of anxiety symptoms. *Drug Investigation* 1994; **8**:339–344.

62. Han K, et al. Therapeutic potential of cannabidiol (CBD) in anxiety disorders: a systematic review and meta-analysis. *Psychiatry Res* 2024; **339**:116049.

63. Amsterdam JD, et al. A randomized, double-blind, placebo-controlled trial of oral Matricaria recutita (chamomile) extract therapy for generalized anxiety disorder. *J Clin Psychopharmacol* 2009; **29**:378–382.

64. Woelk H, et al. Ginkgo biloba special extract EGb 761 in generalized anxiety disorder and adjustment disorder with anxious mood: a randomized, double-blind, placebo-controlled trial. *J Psychiatr Res* 2007; **41**:472–480.

65. Hull TD, et al. At-home, sublingual ketamine telehealth is a safe and effective treatment for moderate to severe anxiety and depression: findings from a large, prospective, open-label effectiveness trial. *J Affect Disord* 2022; **314**:59–67.

66. Bartova L, et al. Beneficial effects of Silexan on co-occurring depressive symptoms in patients with subthreshold anxiety and anxiety disorders: randomized, placebo-controlled trials revisited. *Eur Arch Psychiatry Clin Neurosci* 2023; **273**:51–63.

67. Mathew SJ, et al. Open-label trial of riluzole in generalized anxiety disorder. *Am J Psychiatry* 2005; **162**:2379–2381.

68. Otto MW, et al. Discontinuation of benzodiazepine treatment: efficacy of cognitive-behavioral therapy for patients with panic disorder. *Am J Psychiatry* 1993; **150**:1485–1490.

69. Breilmann J, et al. Benzodiazepines versus placebo for panic disorder in adults. *Cochrane Database Syst Rev* 2019; (3):CD010677.

70. Guaiana G, et al. Pharmacological treatments in panic disorder in adults: a network meta-analysis. *Cochrane Database Syst Rev* 2023; (11):CD012729.

71. Moylan S, et al. The efficacy and safety of alprazolam versus other benzodiazepines in the treatment of panic disorder. *J Clin Psychopharmacol* 2011; **31**:647–652.

72. Ahn-Horst RY, et al. Unpublished trials of alprazolam XR and their influence on its apparent efficacy for panic disorder. *Psychol Med* 2024; **54**:1026–1033.

73. Andrisano C, et al. Newer antidepressants and panic disorder: a meta-analysis. *Int Clin Psychopharmacol* 2013; **28**:33–45.

74. Batelaan NM, et al. Evidence-based pharmacotherapy of panic disorder: an update. *Int J Neuropsychopharmacol* 2012; **15**:403–415.

75. Bighelli I, et al. Antidepressants versus placebo for panic disorder in adults. *Cochrane Database Syst Rev* 2018; (4):CD010676.

76. Chawla N, et al. Drug treatment for panic disorder with or without agoraphobia: systematic review and network meta-analysis of randomised controlled trials. *BMJ* 2022; **376**:e066084.

77. Boshuisen ML, et al. The effect of mirtazapine in panic disorder: an open label pilot study with a single-blind placebo run-in period. *Int Clin Psychopharmacol* 2001; **16**:363–368.

78. Zulfarina MS, et al. Pharmacological therapy in panic disorder: current guidelines and novel drugs discovery for treatment-resistant patient. *Clin Psychopharmacol Neurosci* 2019; **17**:145–154.

79. Tiller JW, et al. Moclobemide for anxiety disorders: a focus on moclobemide for panic disorder. *Int Clin Psychopharmacol* 1997; **12** Suppl 6:S27–S30.

80. Kruger MB, et al. The efficacy and safety of moclobemide compared to clomipramine in the treatment of panic disorder. *Eur Arch Psychiatry Clin Neurosci* 1999; **249** Suppl 1:S19–S24.

81. Fahy TJ, et al. The Galway Study of Panic Disorder. I: Clomipramine and lofepramine in DSM III-R panic disorder: a placebo controlled trial. *J Affect Disord* 1992; **25**:63–75.

82. Pande AC, et al. Placebo-controlled study of gabapentin treatment of panic disorder. *J Clin Psychopharmacol* 2000; **20**:467–471.

83. Benjamin J, et al. Double-blind, placebo-controlled, crossover trial of inositol treatment for panic disorder. *Am J Psychiatry* 1995; **152**:1084–1086.

84. Palatnik A, et al. Double-blind, controlled, crossover trial of inositol versus fluvoxamine for the treatment of panic disorder. *J Clin Psychopharmacol* 2001; **21**:335–339.

85. Hirschmann S, et al. Pindolol augmentation in patients with treatment-resistant panic disorder: a double-blind, placebo-controlled trial. *J Clin Psychopharmacol* 2000; **20**:556–559.

86. Woodman CL, et al. Panic disorder: treatment with valproate. *J Clin Psychiatry* 1994; **55**:134–136.

87. Primeau F, et al. Valproic acid and panic disorder. *Can J Psychiatry* 1990; **35**:248–250.

88. Astill Wright L, et al. Pharmacological prevention and early treatment of post-traumatic stress disorder and acute stress disorder: a systematic review and meta-analysis. *Transl Psychiatry* 2019; **9**:334.

89. National Institute for Health and Care Excellence. Post-traumatic stress disorder. NICE guideline [NG116]. 2018 (reviewed August 2024, last accessed November 2024); https://www.nice.org.uk/guidance/NG116.

90. Moore BA, et al. Management of post-traumatic stress disorder in veterans and military service members: a review of pharmacologic and psychotherapeutic interventions since 2016. *Curr Psychiatry Rep* 2021; **23**:9.

CHAPTER 3

91. Hoskins M, et al. Pharmacotherapy for post-traumatic stress disorder: systematic review and meta-analysis. *Br J Psychiatry* 2015; **206**:93–100.

92. Lee DJ, et al. Psychotherapy versus pharmacotherapy for posttraumatic stress disorder: systematic review and meta-analyses to determine first-line treatments. *Depress Anxiety* 2016; **33**:792–806.

93. Hoskins MD, et al. Pharmacological therapy for post-traumatic stress disorder: a systematic review and meta-analysis of monotherapy, augmentation and head-to-head approaches. *Eur J Psychotraumatol* 2021; **12**:1802920.

94. Williams T, et al. Pharmacotherapy for post traumatic stress disorder (PTSD). *Cochrane Database Syst Rev* 2022; (3):CD002795.

95. Davidson J, et al. Treatment of posttraumatic stress disorder with venlafaxine extended release: a 6-month randomized controlled trial. *Arch Gen Psychiatry* 2006; **63**:1158–1165.

96. Zhang ZX, et al. Clinical outcomes of recommended active pharmacotherapy agents from NICE guideline for post-traumatic stress disorder: network meta-analysis. *Prog Neuropsychopharmacol Biol Psychiatry* 2023; **125**:110754.

97. Han C, et al. The potential role of atypical antipsychotics for the treatment of posttraumatic stress disorder. *J Psychiatr Res* 2014; **56**:72–81.

98. Villarreal G, et al. Efficacy of quetiapine monotherapy in posttraumatic stress disorder: a randomized, placebo-controlled trial. *Am J Psychiatry* 2016; **173**:1205–1212.

99. Davidson JR, et al. Mirtazapine vs. placebo in posttraumatic stress disorder: a pilot trial. *Biol Psychiatry* 2003; **53**:188–191.

100. Cipriani A, et al. Comparative efficacy and acceptability of pharmacological treatments for post-traumatic stress disorder in adults: a network meta-analysis. *Psychol Med* 2018; **48**:1975–1984.

101. Kosten TR, et al. Pharmacotherapy for posttraumatic stress disorder using phenelzine or imipramine. *J Nerv Ment Dis* 1991; **179**:366–370.

102. George KC, et al. Meta-analysis of the efficacy and safety of prazosin versus placebo for the treatment of nightmares and sleep disturbances in adults with posttraumatic stress disorder. *J Trauma Dissociation* 2016; **17**:494–510.

103. Coventry PA, et al. Psychological and pharmacological interventions for posttraumatic stress disorder and comorbid mental health problems following complex traumatic events: systematic review and component network meta-analysis. *PLoS Med* 2020; **17**:e1003262.

104. Davidson J, et al. Treatment of posttraumatic stress disorder with amitriptyline and placebo. *Arch Gen Psychiatry* 1990; **47**:259–266.

105. Albott CS, et al. Efficacy, safety, and durability of repeated ketamine infusions for comorbid posttraumatic stress disorder and treatment-resistant depression. *J Clin Psychiatry* 2018; **79**:17m11634.

106. Feder A, et al. Efficacy of intravenous ketamine for treatment of chronic posttraumatic stress disorder: a randomized clinical trial. *JAMA Psychiatry* 2014; **71**:681–688.

107. Feder A, et al. A randomized controlled trial of repeated ketamine administration for chronic posttraumatic stress disorder. *Am J Psychiatry* 2021; **178**:193–202.

108. Sicignano DJ, et al. The impact of ketamine for treatment of post-traumatic stress disorder: a systematic review with meta-analyses. *Ann Pharmacother* 2024; **58**:669–677.

109. Rohde J, et al. Combined effects of nasal ketamine and trauma-focused psychotherapy in treatment-resistant post-traumatic stress disorder: a pilot case series. *Behav Sci (Basel)* 2024; **14**:717.

110. Walderhaug E, et al. Effects of duloxetine in treatment-refractory men with posttraumatic stress disorder. *Pharmacopsychiatry* 2010; **43**:45–49.

111. Villarreal G, et al. Duloxetine in military posttraumatic stress disorder. *Psychopharmacol Bull* 2010; **43**:26–34.

112. Hertzberg MA, et al. A preliminary study of lamotrigine for the treatment of posttraumatic stress disorder. *Biol Psychiatry* 1999; **45**:1226–1229.

113. Mitchell JM, et al. MDMA-assisted therapy for moderate to severe PTSD: a randomized, placebo-controlled phase 3 trial. *Nat Med* 2023; **29**:2473–2480.

114. Bremner DJ, et al. Treatment of posttraumatic stress disorder with phenytoin: an open-label pilot study. *J Clin Psychiatry* 2004; **65**:1559–1564.

115. Adamou M, et al. Valproate in the treatment of PTSD: systematic review and meta analysis. *Curr Med Res Opin* 2007; **23**:1285–1291.

116. Veale D, et al. Atypical antipsychotic augmentation in SSRI treatment refractory obsessive–compulsive disorder: a systematic review and meta-analysis. *BMC Psychiatry* 2014; **14**:317.

117. Dold M, et al. Antipsychotic augmentation of serotonin reuptake inhibitors in treatment-resistant obsessive-compulsive disorder: an update meta-analysis of double-blind, randomized, placebo-controlled trials. *Int J Neuropsychopharmacol* 2015; **18**:pyv047.

118. Pallanti S, et al. Citalopram for treatment-resistant obsessive–compulsive disorder. *Eur Psychiatry* 1999; **14**:101–106.

119. Costa DLC, et al. Randomized, double-blind, placebo-controlled trial of n-acetylcysteine augmentation for treatment-resistant obsessive–compulsive disorder. *J Clin Psychiatry* 2017; **78**:e766–e773.

120. Couto JP, et al. Oral N-acetylcysteine in the treatment of obsessive–compulsive disorder: a systematic review of the clinical evidence. *Prog Neuropsychopharmacol Biol Psychiatry* 2018; **86**:245–254.

121. Bruno A, et al. Lamotrigine augmentation of serotonin reuptake inhibitors in treatment-resistant obsessive-compulsive disorder: a double-blind, placebo-controlled study. *J Psychopharmacol* 2012; **26**:1456–1462.

122. Sharma V, et al. Lamotrigine-induced obsessive–compulsive disorder in patients with bipolar disorder. *CNS Spectr* 2019; **24**:390–394.

123. Berlin HA, et al. Double-blind, placebo-controlled trial of topiramate augmentation in treatment-resistant obsessive–compulsive disorder. *J Clin Psychiatry* 2011; **72**:716–721.

124. Mowla A, et al. Topiramate augmentation in resistant OCD: a double-blind placebo-controlled clinical trial. *CNS Spectr* 2010; **15**:613–617.

125. Afshar H, et al. Topiramate augmentation in refractory obsessive-compulsive disorder: a randomized, double-blind, placebo-controlled trial. *J Res Med Sci* 2014; **19**:976–981.

126. Grassi G, et al. Investigational and experimental drugs to treat obsessive–compulsive disorder. *J Exp Pharmacol* 2020; **12**:695–706.

127. Rabinowitz I, et al. High-dose escitalopram for the treatment of obsessive–compulsive disorder. *Int Clin Psychopharmacol* 2008; **23**:49–53.

128. Ninan PT, et al. High-dose sertraline strategy for nonresponders to acute treatment for obsessive-compulsive disorder: a multicenter double-blind trial. *J Clin Psychiatry* 2006; **67**:15–22.

129. Modarresi A, et al. A systematic review and meta-analysis: memantine augmentation in moderate to severe obsessive-compulsive disorder. *Psychiatry Res* 2019; **282**:112602.

130. Maiti R, et al. Pharmacological augmentation of serotonin reuptake inhibitors in patients with obsessive–compulsive disorder: a network meta-analysis. *Acta Psychiatr Scand* 2023; **148**:19–31.

131. Naderi S, et al. Amantadine as adjuvant therapy in the treatment of moderate to severe obsessive-compulsive disorder: a double-blind randomized trial with placebo control. *Psychiatry Clin Neurosci* 2019; **73**:169–174.

132. Dell'Osso B, et al. Serotonin-norepinephrine reuptake inhibitors in the treatment of obsessive-compulsive disorder: a critical review. *J Clin Psychiatry* 2006; **67**:600–610.

133. Mowla A, et al. Duloxetine augmentation in resistant obsessive–compulsive disorder: a double-blind controlled clinical trial. *J Clin Psychopharmacol* 2016; **36**:720–723.

134. Koran LM, et al. Mirtazapine for obsessive–compulsive disorder: an open trial followed by double-blind discontinuation. *J Clin Psychiatry* 2005; **66**:515–520.

135. Askari N, et al. Granisetron adjunct to fluvoxamine for moderate to severe obsessive–compulsive disorder: a randomized, double-blind, placebo-controlled trial. *CNS Drugs* 2012; **26**:883–892.

136. Soltani F, et al. A double-blind, placebo-controlled pilot study of ondansetron for patients with obsessive–compulsive disorder. *Hum Psychopharmacol* 2010; **25**:509–513.

137. Sharafkhah M, et al. Comparing the efficacy of ondansetron and granisetron augmentation in treatment-resistant obsessive–compulsive disorder: a randomized double-blind placebo-controlled study. *Int Clin Psychopharmacol* 2019; **34**:222–233.

138. Suhas S, et al. Treatment strategies for serotonin reuptake inhibitor-resistant obsessive–compulsive disorder: a network meta-analysis of randomised controlled trials. *World J Biol Psychiatry* 2023; **24**:162–177.

139. Mowla A, et al. Pregabalin augmentation for resistant obsessive–compulsive disorder: a double-blind placebo-controlled clinical trial. *CNS Spectr* 2020; **25**:552–556.

140. Coric V, et al. Riluzole augmentation in treatment-resistant obsessive–compulsive disorder: an open-label trial. *Biol Psychiatry* 2005; **58**:424–428.

141. Eriksson T. Anti-androgenic treatment of obsessive–compulsive disorder: an open-label clinical trial of the long-acting gonadotropin-releasing hormone analogue triptorelin. *Int Clin Psychopharmacol* 2007; **22**:57–61.

142. Owe-Larsson M, et al. Psilocybin in pharmacotherapy of obsessive–compulsive disorder. *Pharmacol Rep* 2024; **76**:911–925.

143. Moreno FA, et al. Safety, tolerability, and efficacy of psilocybin in 9 patients with obsessive–compulsive disorder. *J Clin Psychiatry* 2006; **67**:1735–1740.

144. Fallon BA, et al. Intravenous clomipramine for obsessive–compulsive disorder refractory to oral clomipramine: a placebo-controlled study. *Arch Gen Psychiatry* 1998; **55**:918–924.

145. Rodriguez CI, et al. Randomized controlled crossover trial of ketamine in obsessive–compulsive disorder: proof-of-concept. *Neuropsychopharmacology* 2013; **38**:2475–2483.

146. Bloch MH, et al. Effects of ketamine in treatment-refractory obsessive-compulsive disorder. *Biol Psychiatry* 2012; **72**:964–970.

147. Koran LM, et al. Double-blind treatment with oral morphine in treatment-resistant obsessive-compulsive disorder. *J Clin Psychiatry* 2005; **66**:353–359.

148. National Institute for Health and Care Excellence. Social anxiety disorder: recognition, assessment and treatment. Clinical guideline [CG159]. 2013 (reviewed May 2024, last accessed November 2024); https://www.nice.org.uk/guidance/cg159.

149. Liu X, et al. Efficacy and tolerability of fluvoxamine in adults with social anxiety disorder: a meta-analysis. *Medicine (Baltimore)* 2018; **97**:e11547.

150. Baldwin DS, et al. Efficacy of escitalopram in the treatment of social anxiety disorder: a meta-analysis versus placebo. *Eur Neuropsychopharmacol* 2016; **26**:1062–1069.

151. Careri JM, et al. A 12-week double-blind, placebo-controlled, flexible-dose trial of vilazodone in generalized social anxiety disorder. *Prim Care Companion CNS Disord* 2015; **17**:10.4088/PCC.4015m01831.

152. Mitsui N, et al. Antidepressants for social anxiety disorder: a systematic review and meta-analysis. *Neuropsychopharmacol Rep* 2022; **42**:398–409.

153. Blanco C, et al. The evidence-based pharmacotherapy of social anxiety disorder. *Int J Neuropsychopharmacol* 2013; **16**:235–249.

154. Archer C, et al. Beta-blockers for the treatment of anxiety disorders: a systematic review and meta-analysis. *J Affect Disord* 2025; **368**:90–99.

155. Pollack MH, et al. A double-blind randomized controlled trial of augmentation and switch strategies for refractory social anxiety disorder. *Am J Psychiatry* 2014; **171**:44–53.

156. Simon NM, et al. An open-label study of levetiracetam for the treatment of social anxiety disorder. *J Clin Psychiatry* 2004; **65**:1219–1222.

157. Blanco C, et al. A placebo-controlled trial of phenelzine, cognitive behavioral group therapy, and their combination for social anxiety disorder. *Arch Gen Psychiatry* 2010; **67**:286–295.

158. Taylor JH, et al. Ketamine for social anxiety disorder: a randomized, placebo-controlled crossover trial. *Neuropsychopharmacology* 2018; **43**:325–333.

159. Truppman Lattie D, et al. Anxiolytic effects of acute and maintenance ketamine, as assessed by the Fear Questionnaire subscales and the Spielberger State Anxiety Rating Scale. *J Psychopharmacol* 2021; **35**:137–141.

160. Van Ameringen M, et al. An open trial of topiramate in the treatment of generalized social phobia. *J Clin Psychiatry* 2004; **65**:1674–1678.

161. Kinrys G, et al. Valproic acid for the treatment of social anxiety disorder. *Int Clin Psychopharmacol* 2003; **18**:169–172.

CHAPTER 3

Benzodiazepines in the treatment of psychiatric disorders

Benzodiazepines have a valid place in the treatment of some forms of epilepsy and severe muscle spasm, and as premedication agents in some surgical procedures. However, the vast majority of prescriptions are written for their hypnotic and anxiolytic effects. They are also used for rapid tranquillisation and, usually as adjuncts, in the treatment of depression and schizophrenia. Benzodiazepines are commonly both prescribed and misused. A European study found that almost 10% of adults had taken a benzodiazepine over the previous year[1] and a 2019 US study reported past-year usage of 12.6% among adults.[2] Generally speaking, the use of benzodiazepines in psychiatric disorders has gradually become less supportable over the past few decades.[3]

Benzodiazepines are sometimes divided into two groups depending on their half-life: hypnotics (short half-life) or anxiolytics (long half-life), although there are many exceptions (for example, nitrazepam and alprazolam, respectively).

Anxiolytic effect

Benzodiazepines reduce pathological anxiety, agitation and tension. Although useful in the short-term management of generalised anxiety disorder,[4] either alone or to augment SSRIs, benzodiazepines are associated with tolerance and withdrawal. Despite awareness of this, many patients continue to take these drugs for years[5] with unknown benefits and many likely harms. Most authorities agree that, where a benzodiazepine is prescribed, this should not routinely be for longer than 4 weeks.[6]

In the UK, NICE recommends that benzodiazepines should not be used in patients with generalised anxiety disorder except as a short-term measure during crisis.[7] Evidence is mixed in other anxiety disorders, and potential benefits should be viewed in the context of the known problems associated with benzodiazepine use. A small number of trials report the efficacy of benzodiazepines in social anxiety disorder.[8] Benzodiazepines are useful in the short-term treatment of panic disorders,[9,10] but little is known about their efficacy and safety with long-term use.[10,11] Benzodiazepines are, with some exceptions, relatively ineffective in the treatment of PTSD[12,13] or phobias.[14]

Hypnotic effect

Benzodiazepines are effective hypnotics but they inhibit rapid eye movement (REM) sleep and REM rebound is seen when they are discontinued.[14] There is a debate over the clinical significance of this property.[15]

Benzodiazepines are effective in the short term.[16] RCTs support the effectiveness of Z hypnotics over a period of at least 6 months,[17] but it is unclear if this holds true for benzodiazepine hypnotics. Intermittent use probably extends the period over which benzodiazepines are effective as hypnotics.

Physical causes (pain, dyspnoea, etc.) or substance misuse (most commonly high caffeine consumption) should always be excluded before a hypnotic drug is prescribed. Where possible, behavioural therapies (e.g. CBT for insomnia or sleep restriction) should be offered before prescribing hypnotics.[17] A high proportion of hospitalised patients are prescribed hypnotics.[18,19] These drugs should not be routinely continued at discharge.

Use in depression

Benzodiazepines are not a treatment for major depressive illness. The only meta-analysis conducted found no advantage for benzodiazepines over placebo in depression.[20] However, there is some evidence that benzodiazepines may be helpful in preventing relapse of psychotic depression.[21] Combining benzodiazepines with antidepressants during the early phase of antidepressant treatment (1–4 weeks) may improve depression to a greater extent than antidepressants alone.[22] This improvement is not maintened with longer-term treatment.[22] In the UK, the National Service Framework for Mental Health[23] at one time emphasised this point by including a requirement that GPs audit the ratio of benzodiazepines to antidepressants prescribed in their practice. NICE suggests that a benzodiazepine may be helpful for up to 2 weeks early in treatment, particularly in combination with an SSRI (to help with sleep and the management of SSRI-induced agitation).[7] Use beyond this timeframe is discouraged. Limiting initial supply quantities to short periods (1–7 days) may reduce the risk of patients becoming long-term users of benzodiazepines.[24]

Use in psychosis

Benzodiazepines are commonly used for rapid tranquillisation, either alone or in combination with an antipsychotic.[25] However, a Cochrane review concluded that there is no convincing evidence that combining an antipsychotic and a benzodiazepine offers any advantage over the use of antipsychotics or benzodiazepines alone.[26]

A further Cochrane review in schizophrenia concluded that there are no proven benefits, outside short-term sedation.[27] In contrast, another systematic review using different outcome measures found superiority over placebo for global, psychiatric and behavioural outcomes, but inferiority to antipsychotics on longer-term global outcomes.[28] A significant minority of patients with established psychotic illness fail to respond adequately to antipsychotics alone, and this can result in benzodiazepines being prescribed on a chronic basis.[29] There is, however, no evidence to support benzodiazepine augmentation of antipsychotics in schizophrenia and use should be reserved for the short-term sedation of acutely agitated patients.[30] Evidence supporting the use of benzodiazepines in tardive dyskinesia is weak[31] but these drugs remain a treatment option in this condition.

Adverse effects

Headaches, confusion, ataxia, dysarthria, blurred vision, GI disturbances, jaundice and paradoxical excitement are all possible adverse effects. Benzodiazepines impair cognition, and long-term use has been associated with a range of cognitive deficits (e.g. memory, attention and processing speed), which may persist after withdrawal.[32,33] The use of benzodiazepines has been associated with at least a 50% increase in the risk of hip fracture in the elderly.[34] This is probably because benzodiazepines increase the risk of falls. Benzodiazepines often cause anterograde amnesia and can adversely affect driving performance.[35,36] Benzodiazepines can also cause disinhibition (see section on benzodiazepines and disinhibition in this chapter). Benzodiazepines have been linked to aggressive behaviour, although the association is modest and possibly related to dose and personality factors.[37]

Epidemiological research has linked benzodiazepine prescribing to serious medical conditions including dementia, infections and cancer.[38–41] However, a causal relationship has not been established and evidence is conflicting.[39,41] All studies in this area are confounded by the failure to include illicit use of benzodiazepines.

Respiratory depression is rare with oral therapy but is possible when parenteral routes are used.[25] Buccal and intranasal administration may also cause respiratory depression.[42,43] The use of the specific benzodiazepine antagonist flumazenil is effective in reversing respiratory[25] depression but is not without risk (e.g. convulsions and arrhythmia, particularly in mixed overdoses with TCAs) so selective use is recommended.[44] Flumazenil has a much shorter half-life than many benzodiazepines, making close observation of the patient essential for several hours after administration.

Intravenous injections of benzodiazepine can be painful and can lead to thrombophlebitis because of the low water solubility of benzodiazepines, so it is necessary to use solvents in the preparation of injectable forms. Diazepam is available in emulsion form (Diazemuls® in the UK) to overcome these problems.

Drug interactions

Benzodiazepines do not induce microsomal enzymes and so do not frequently precipitate pharmacokinetic interactions with any other drugs. Most benzodiazepines are metabolised by CYP3A4, which is inhibited by erythromycin, several SSRIs and ketoconazole. It is theoretically possible that co-administration of these drugs will result in higher serum levels of benzodiazepines. Pharmacodynamic interactions (usually increased sedation) can occur. Benzodiazepines are associated with an important interaction with methadone (see Chapter 5) and should be used with caution in patients prescribed clozapine (increased risk of cardiopulmonary depression) and not at all with intramuscular olanzapine.

References

1. Demyttenaere K, et al. Clinical factors influencing the prescription of antidepressants and benzodiazepines: results from the European study of the epidemiology of mental disorders (ESEMeD). *J Affect Disord* 2008; 110:84–93.
2. Maust DT, et al. Benzodiazepine use and misuse among adults in the United States. *Psychiatr Serv* 2019; 70:97–106.
3. Hirschtritt ME, et al. Balancing the risks and benefits of benzodiazepines. *JAMA* 2021; 325:347–348.
4. Slee A, et al. Pharmacological treatments for generalised anxiety disorder: a systematic review and network meta-analysis. *Lancet* 2019; 393:768–777.
5. Kurko TA, et al. Long-term use of benzodiazepines: definitions, prevalence and usage patterns – a systematic review of register-based studies. *Eur Psychiatry* 2015; 30:1037–1047.
6. Brandt J, et al. Prescribing and deprescribing guidance for benzodiazepine and benzodiazepine receptor agonist use in adults with depression, anxiety, and insomnia: an international scoping review. *EClinicalMedicine* 2024; 70:102507.
7. National Institute for Health and Care Excellence. Generalised anxiety disorder and panic disorder in adults: management. Clinical guideline [CG113]. 2011 (last updated 2020, last reviewed May 2024); https://www.nice.org.uk/guidance/cg113.
8. Williams T, et al. Pharmacotherapy for social anxiety disorder (SAnD). *Cochrane Database Syst Rev* 2017; 10:CD001206.
9. Guaiana G, et al. Pharmacological treatments in panic disorder in adults: a network meta-analysis. *Cochrane Database Syst Rev* 2023; 11:CD012729.
10. Breilmann J, et al. Benzodiazepines versus placebo for panic disorder in adults. *Cochrane Database Syst Rev* 2019; 3:CD010677.
11. Bighelli I, et al. Antidepressants and benzodiazepines for panic disorder in adults. *Cochrane Database Syst Rev* 2016; 9:CD011567.
12. Campos B, et al. To BDZ or not to BDZ? That is the question! Is there reliable scientific evidence for or against using benzodiazepines in the aftermath of potentially traumatic events for the prevention of PTSD? A systematic review and meta-analysis. *J Psychopharmacol* 2022; 36:449–459.
13. Guina J, et al. Benzodiazepines for PTSD: a systematic review and meta-analysis. *J Psychiatr Pract* 2015; 21:281–303.
14. Guina J, et al. Benzodiazepines I: upping the care on downers: the evidence of risks, benefits and alternatives. *J Clin Med* 2018; 7:17.

15. Roehrs T, et al. Drug-related sleep stage changes: functional significance and clinical relevance. *Sleep Med Clin* 2010; 5:559–570.
16. Yue JL, et al. Efficacy and tolerability of pharmacological treatments for insomnia in adults: a systematic review and network meta-analysis. *Sleep Med Rev* 2023; 68:101746.
17. Wilson S, et al. British Association for Psychopharmacology consensus statement on evidence-based treatment of insomnia, parasomnias and circadian rhythm disorders: an update. *J Psychopharmacol* 2019; 33:923–947.
18. Hallahan BP, et al. Benzodiazepine and hypnotic prescribing in an acute adult psychiatric in-patient unit. *Psychiatr Bull* 2009; 33:12–14.
19. Mahomed R, et al. Prescribing hypnotics in a mental health trust: what consultants say and what they do. *Pharmaceutical J* 2002; 268:657–659.
20. Benasi G, et al. Benzodiazepines as a monotherapy in depressive disorders: a systematic review. *Psychother Psychosom* 2018; 87:65–74.
21. Shiwaku H, et al. Benzodiazepines reduce relapse and recurrence rates in patients with psychotic depression. *J Clin Med* 2020; 9:1938.
22. Ogawa Y, et al. Antidepressants plus benzodiazepines for adults with major depression. *Cochrane Database Syst Rev* 2019; 6:CD001026.
23. Department of Health and Social Care. *A National Service Framework for Mental Health: Modern standards and service models.* London: DHSC; 1999 (last accessed February 2025); https://www.gov.uk/government/publications/quality-standards-for-mental-health-services.
24. Bushnell GA, et al. Simultaneous antidepressant and benzodiazepine new use and subsequent long-term benzodiazepine use in adults with depression, United States, 2001–2014. *JAMA Psychiatry* 2017; 74:747–755.
25. Patel MX, et al. Joint BAP NAPICU evidence-based consensus guidelines for the clinical management of acute disturbance: de-escalation and rapid tranquillisation. *J Psychopharmacol* 2018; 32:601–640.
26. Zaman H, et al. Benzodiazepines for psychosis-induced aggression or agitation. *Cochrane Database Syst Rev* 2017; 12:CD003079.
27. Dold M, et al. Benzodiazepines for schizophrenia. *Cochrane Database Syst Rev* 2012; 11:CD006391.
28. Sim F, et al. Re-examining the role of benzodiazepines in the treatment of schizophrenia: a systematic review. *J Psychopharmacol* 2015; 29:212–223.
29. Paton C, et al. Benzodiazepines in schizophrenia. Is there a trend towards long-term prescribing? *Psychiatr Bull* 2000; 24:113–115.
30. Dold M, et al. Benzodiazepine augmentation of antipsychotic drugs in schizophrenia: a meta-analysis and Cochrane review of randomized controlled trials. *Eur Neuropsychopharmacol* 2013; 23:1023–1033.
31. Bergman H, et al. Benzodiazepines for antipsychotic-induced tardive dyskinesia. *Cochrane Database Syst Rev* 2018; 1:CD000205.
32. Huff C, et al. Enduring neurological sequelae of benzodiazepine use: an Internet survey. *Ther Adv Psychopharmacol* 2023; 13:20451253221145561.
33. Crowe SF, et al. The residual medium and long-term cognitive effects of benzodiazepine use: an updated meta-analysis. *Arch Clin Neuropsychol* 2017; 33:901–911.
34. Poly TN, et al. Association between benzodiazepines use and risk of hip fracture in the elderly people: a meta-analysis of observational studies. *Joint Bone Spine* 2020; 87:241–249.
35. Barbone F, et al. Association of road-traffic accidents with benzodiazepine use. *Lancet* 1998; 352:1331–1336.
36. Rudisill TM, et al. Medication use and the risk of motor vehicle collisions among licensed drivers: a systematic review. *Accid Anal Prev* 2016; 96:255–270.
37. Albrecht B, et al. Benzodiazepine use and aggressive behaviour: a systematic review. *Aust N Z J Psychiatry* 2014; 48:1096–1114.
38. Kim DH, et al. Use of hypnotics and risk of cancer: a meta-analysis of observational studies. *Korean J Fam Med* 2018; 39:211–218.
39. Brandt J, et al. Benzodiazepines and Z-drugs: an updated review of major adverse outcomes reported on in epidemiologic research. *Drugs R D* 2017; 17:493–507.
40. Peng TR, et al. Hypnotics and risk of cancer: a meta-analysis of observational studies. *Medicina (Kaunas)* 2020; 56:513.
41. Wu CC, et al. Benzodiazepine use and the risk of dementia in the elderly population: an umbrella review of meta-analyses. *J Pers Med* 2023; 13:1485.
42. Mula M. The safety and tolerability of intranasal midazolam in epilepsy. *Expert Rev Neurother* 2014; 14:735–740.
43. Midazolam oral transmucosal route: an alternative to rectal diazepam for some children. *Prescrire Int* 2013; 22:173–177.
44. Penninga EI, et al. Adverse events associated with flumazenil treatment for the management of suspected benzodiazepine intoxication: a systematic review with meta-analyses of randomised trials. *Basic Clin Pharmacol Toxicol* 2016; 118:37–44.

CHAPTER 3

Benzodiazepines, z-drugs and gabapentinoids: dependence, withdrawal effects and discontinuation

In most developed countries, the use of benzodiazepines or z-drugs is restricted to a maximum 2–4 weeks.[1-3] However, long-term use remains common in the UK, with 300,000 adults taking either a benzodiazepine or z-drug for more than 12 months.[4] Most guidelines, including NICE in the UK, recommend that people on long-term benzodiazepines or z-drugs should be advised to stop because of tolerance to these drugs (which can develop after 2–4 weeks) because physical dependence (distinct from addiction) is likely to develop, and because of numerous adverse effects (Box 3.11).[5]

Gabapentinoids (GABA analogues) can also cause addiction, physical dependence and withdrawal over the same period.[6-8] In total, 1.5 million people in England are prescribed gabapentinoids,[9] and the number of prescriptions for these medications rose seven-fold between 2010 and 2020.[10]

Further details on withdrawal effects and safe deprescribing of these drug classes are outlined in the companion to this text, the *Maudsley Deprescribing Guidelines: Antidepressants, Benzodiazepines, Gabapentinoids and Z-drugs*.[11]

Physical dependence on these classes of drugs does not require misuse, abuse or addiction but simply repeated exposure.[12] The vast majority of people who experience withdrawal effects are taking drugs as prescribed by their physician (so-called 'iatrogenic dependence'). This is distinct from addiction, which involves craving and compulsion, and can be associated with misuse and abuse, occurring only in 2% of patients.[12]

Box 3.11 Adverse effects of benzodiazepines

Emotional[13]	Reactions which can be mistaken for a psychiatric disorder[14]
■ Depression/dysphoria	■ Agitation
■ Numbness/emotional anaesthesia	■ Emotional lability
■ Anxiety/phobias/panic	■ Restlessness
■ Anger/irritability/mood lability	■ Inter-dose withdrawal
■ Excitement/euphoria	

Physical[13]	Cognitive*[15-17]
■ Motor incoordination/ataxia	■ Deficits in memory
■ Dizziness	■ Deficits in attention
■ Slurred speech	■ Increased reaction time
■ Sensory alterations (tinnitus/strange tastes/ paraesthesia/numbness/burning)	■ Motor incoordination
	■ Drowsiness
■ Rash	■ Nightmares/intrusive thoughts
■ Autonomic dysfunction (tachycardia/bradycardia/ diaphoresis/hypotension/hypertension)	■ Impaired judgement
	■ Perceptual illusions/hallucinations

Increased morbidity[16,17]	Behavioural[13]
■ Increased risk of motor vehicle accidents	■ Insomnia
■ Higher risk of falls (elderly)	■ Avoidance/agoraphobia
■ Delirium (elderly)	■ Appetite/weight (anorexia, weight gain)
■ ? Dementia	■ Impulsivity/disinhibition
■ ? Cancer	■ Suicidality
■ ? Infections	■ Aggression

*Some of these impairments can persist after discontinuation.

Long-term use of benzodiazepines is associated with a number of problems (Box 3.10). Patients may be unaware of problems and may only appreciate the issue after stopping the drug.[18] Long-term z-drug use is associated with similar risks.[19] Gabapentinoids have been linked to increased risk of suicide, unintentional overdose, road traffic accidents, and head and body injuries,[20] suggesting that limitation of their long-term use may be prudent.

Withdrawal symptoms

Stopping these medications is often difficult (Box 3.12). One study found that 90% of patients experience withdrawal symptoms on stopping benzodiazepines, with 32% of people on long half-life benzodiazepines and 42% of people on short half-life benzodiazepines unable to cease their medication because of withdrawal symptoms.[21] Short-acting drugs such as lorazepam are associated with more severe problems on withdrawal than longer-acting drugs such as diazepam.[22,23] As these drugs are somewhat ineffective for anxiety and insomnia in the long term, symptoms that arise on stopping are perhaps just as likely to be withdrawal symptoms as opposed to relapse (though symptoms can be similar).[24] Mental state often improves after withdrawal symptoms abate.[25] Some of the worst consequences of benzodiazepine withdrawal are akathisia and new-onset suicidality, which are poorly recognised and often misdiagnosed.[11]

Withdrawal symptoms can last days or weeks but, for some people, they can last longer than a year, especially in the case of long-term use,[22,25] as highlighted by an FDA black box warning.[26] This is called a 'protracted withdrawal syndrome'.[27] The long-lasting effects on the nervous system, months or years after stopping benzodiazepines, have been termed 'benzodiazepine-induced neural dysfunction'.[28]

Box 3.12 Withdrawal effects from benzodiazepines[29,30]

Physical	Psychological
■ Stiffness	■ Anxiety/insomnia
■ Fatigue and weakness	■ Terror/panic attacks
■ GI disturbance	■ Nightmares
■ Paraesthesia	■ Depersonalisation/derealisation
■ Flu-like symptoms	■ Delusions and hallucinations
■ Visual disturbances	■ Depression
■ Sensory hypersensitivity	■ Psychosis*
■ Convulsions*	■ Mood instability
■ Cognitive impairment	■ Paranoia
■ Impaired memory	■ Obsessive-compulsive symptoms
■ Tremor	■ Suicidal ideation
■ Dizziness	■ Mania
■ Muscle spasms/cramps	
■ Chest pain	
■ Hypertension	
■ Tachycardia	
■ Photophobia	
■ Confusion, delirium*	
■ Akathisia	

* Usually only from very rapid withdrawal.

Stopping benzodiazepines

If the patient is in agreement, benzodiazepines should be withdrawn. Tapering can be difficult and should not be imposed on a patient against their will. A cluster randomised trial supports the effectiveness of a face-to-face educational intervention.[31] Continuing support can be required to prepare a patient for withdrawal and to support them through the process (e.g. psychological therapies or self-help groups).[32]

Dosage reduction (tapering)

Gradual reduction of benzodiazepine dose reduces the intensity of withdrawal symptoms by giving time for neural adaptations to the drug to resolve.[24] Meta-analysis has confirmed that gradual dose reduction ('tapering') improves drug cessation rates compared with routine clinical care.[33] Most studies find that a gradual withdrawal over at least 10 weeks is most successful in achieving cessation,[34] although many patients will require considerably longer (sometimes several years). Sudden benzodiazepine withdrawal has potentially fatal consequences, so tapering is always advisable.

Direct taper or switching to diazepam?

Patients who take short- or intermediate-acting benzodiazepines can be tapered off these drugs directly but more than once-a-day dosing might be required.

An alternative approach is to switch to an equivalent dose of diazepam, which has a long half-life and therefore might provoke less severe withdrawal.[22,29] Some patients report withdrawal symptoms from abrupt switches to diazepam and so a stepwise switch is probably prudent. Cochrane is lukewarm about switching to diazepam.[34] Approximate 'diazepam equivalent'[35] doses are shown in Table 3.24. Owing to individual differences some patients may require more or less diazepam to control withdrawal symptoms.

The list in Table 3.24 is an approximate guide only and adjustments should be made to manage withdrawal symptoms for the individual.[11] Extra precautions apply in

Table 3.24 Approximate 'diazepam equivalent' doses.[35]

Drug	Dose
Chlordiazepoxide	25mg
Clonazepam	0.5mg
Diazepam	10mg
Lorazepam	1mg
Lormetazepam	1–2mg
Nitrazepam	10mg
Oxazepam	20mg
Temazepam	20mg

CHAPTER 3

patients with hepatic dysfunction, as diazepam and other longer-acting drugs may accumulate to toxic levels.

Pattern of tapering

The relationship between dose of benzodiazepines and their effect on their principal target, the GABA-A receptor, is hyperbolic, as dictated by the law of mass action, with the following implications:

- Reducing dose by fixed amounts (e.g. 12.5mg in Figure 3.5a) will give rise to increasingly large reductions in GABA-A occupancy.
- This is consistent with clinical observation that withdrawal symptoms are nonlinearly related to dose reduction (e.g. a 1mg reduction of diazepam is tolerable from 20mg but intolerable from 5mg).[36]
- Reducing the diazepam dose by 5mg from 50mg will cause a reduction of 2.3 percentage points of GABA-A occupancy, but a 5mg reduction from 5mg will cause a reduction of 18.3 percentage points.

In order to reduce the dose of benzodiazepines by equal amounts of effect at their major target, hyperbolically reducing doses are required (Figure 3.5b):

- This means that the size of dose reductions should be smaller and smaller as the total dose gets smaller.
- In practice, these reductions can be most easily calculated based on a proportion of the most recent dose (an exponential pattern): for example, reductions of 10% of the *most recent* dose every month (so that reductions become smaller and smaller as total dose reduces).

Final doses before complete cessation may need to be very small (e.g. less than 1mg of diazepam equivalent).

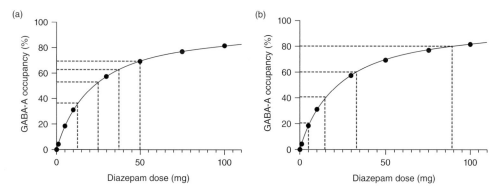

Figure 3.5 (a) Linear reductions of dose cause increasingly large reductions in effect on GABA-A receptor occupancy. (b) Reducing effect on GABA-A receptors by even amounts requires hyperbolically reducing doses of diazepam. Note how small the final doses will be required to be to prevent too large a final 'step down'. Source: Adapted from Brouillet et al. (1991).[37]

Practical application of these principles

Before tapering

- All patients should be informed of the risk of withdrawal symptoms on stopping any benzodiazepine, z-drug or gabapentinoid.
- The patient should be warned not to stop benzodiazepines abruptly, because this can cause seizures and can be fatal, and may be the method most likely to give rise to severe and long-lasting withdrawal symptoms.
- Although stopping benzodiazepines can cause unpleasant symptoms, if tapering is gradual and careful the process can be tolerable. Reassurance may be required for those that have rapidly tapered in the past.
- Most long-term users take months or years to taper. However, rate of reduction should be determined by what is tolerable for the patient, not externally imposed timetables.
- Preparation for benzodiazepine tapering may be required (e.g. lightening work or family duties or bolstering of non-pharmacological coping skills).[32,38]
- Gradual dose reduction is the most evidenced approach to cessation, with weaker evidence for adjunctive psychological interventions (relaxation, CBT).[33]
- Familiarity with the wide variety of withdrawal symptoms may help to mitigate unnecessary anxiety when symptoms arise.

The process of tapering

- Reductions in dosing for patients may be broadly risk stratified:
  - for low-risk patients (<6 months' use, long half-life benzodiazepine, no experience of significant withdrawal in the past), a test reduction could be made of 10–20%
  - for high-risk patients (>6 months use, short half-life benzodiazepine, past history of withdrawal symptoms), a test reduction of 5–10% could be recommended.
- Reductions should be made according to a proportion (e.g. 10%) of the last dose. This means that the reductions recommended will become smaller and smaller as the total dose is lowered. Most long-term users will be able to proceed between a rate of about 5–10% of their most recent dose per month (or perhaps more quickly).
- After reduction withdrawal symptoms should be monitored for 2–4 weeks, or until symptoms have resolved. Monitoring may take the form of simple measures of symptoms each day (e.g. out of 10) or using standardised benzodiazepine withdrawal scales.
- Further reduction should be titrated to the tolerability of this experience.

Troubleshooting

- If significant withdrawal symptoms emerge at any point, either hold the current dose to allow symptoms to resolve or, if that is intolerable, increase to the last dose at which the symptoms were tolerable and remain there until symptoms resolve. After stabilisation, tapering will need to be more gradual, with reductions being made in smaller amounts.
- The experience of distressing withdrawal symptoms does not necessarily indicate that a patient cannot stop benzodiazepines but that they will need to taper more slowly,

with smaller reductions than they have been undertaking (some need to taper at less than 5% of the most recent dose per month).

■ At very small doses, liquid formulations or specially compounded formulations may be required to allow small reductions.[11] Off-label options such as crushing and suspending tablets are sometimes used.[11]

■ Final doses before completely stopping the drug for some people will need to be very small to avoid a larger reduction in effect on the brain (e.g. as low as 0.1mg of diazepam).[11]

Further details of this process are provided in the *Maudsley Deprescribing Guidelines*.[11]

Reduction schedules

A guide to diazepam dose reductions:

■ Reduce by 5–10mg/day every 2–4 weeks, down to a daily dose of 50mg.

■ Reduce by 2–5mg/day every 2–4 weeks, down to a daily dose of 20mg.

■ Reduce by 1–2mg/day every 2–4 weeks, down to a daily dose of 10mg.

■ Reduce by 0.5–1mg/day every 2–4 weeks, down to a daily dose of 5mg.

■ Reduce by 0.25–0.5mg/day every 2–4 weeks, down to a daily dose of 2.5mg.

■ Reduce by 0.1–0.25mg/day every 2–4 weeks until stopped.

Tapering other drug classes

The same principles apply to tapering z-drugs or gabapentinoids. Gabapentinoids can cause severe withdrawal effects, although there is wide inter-individual variation. Tolerance and withdrawal are reported, even after brief or intermittent use for z-drugs as well.[39,40] Tapering according to a similar exponential scheme may be required for cessation. Again, specific reduction schedules for all licensed benzodiazepines, gabapentinoids and z-drugs are provided in the *Maudsley Deprescribing Guidelines*.[11]

References

1. National Institute for Health and Care Excellence. *British National Formulary*. 2024; https://bnf.nice.org.uk.

2. National Institute for Health and Care Excellence. Guidance on the use of zaleplon, zolpidem and zopiclone for the short-term management of insomnia. Technical Appraisal [TA77]. 2004 (reviewed August 2010, last checked July 2024); https://www.nice.org.uk/guidance/ta77.

3. National Institute for Health and Care Excellence. Generalised anxiety disorder and panic disorder in adults: management. Clinical guideline [CG113]. 2011 (last updated June 2020, last checked July 2024); https://www.nice.org.uk/guidance/cg113.

4. Davies J, et al. Long-term benzodiazepine and Z-drugs use in the UK: a survey of general practice. *Br J Gen Pract* 2017; **67**:e609–e613.

5. National Institute for Health and Care Excellence. Benzodiazepine and z-drug withdrawal. 2024 (last accessed July 2024); https://cks.nice.org.uk/topics/benzodiazepine-z-drug-withdrawal.

6. Schifano F, et al. An insight into z-drug abuse and dependence: an examination of reports to the European Medicines Agency Database of Suspected Adverse Drug Reactions. *Int J Neuropsychopharmacol* 2019; **22**:270–277.

7. Evoy KE, et al. Abuse and misuse of pregabalin and gabapentin. *Drugs* 2017; **77**:403–426.

8. Public Health England. Advice for prescribers on the risk of the misuse of pregabalin and gabapentin. 2014 (last accessed July 2024); https://assets.publishing.service.gov.uk/government/uploads/system/uploads/attachment_data/file/385791/PHE-NHS_England_pregabalin_and_gabapentin_advice_Dec_2014.pdf.

9. Marsden J, et al. Medicines associated with dependence or withdrawal: a mixed-methods public health review and national database study in England. *Lancet Psychiatry* 2019; **6**:935–950.

10. Public Health England. *Research and Analysis. Prescribed Medicines Review: Report*. 2020 (last accessed July 2024); https://www.gov.uk/government/publications/prescribed-medicines-review-report.

11. Horowitz M, et al. *The Maudsley Deprescribing Guidelines: Antidepressants, Benzodiazepines, Gabapentinoids and Z-drugs.* Oxford: Wiley-Blackwell; 2024.
12. Horowitz MA, et al. Addiction and physical dependence are not the same thing. *Lancet Psychiatry* 2023; 10:e23.
13. Guina J, et al. Benzodiazepines I: upping the care on downers: the evidence of risks, benefits and alternatives. *J Clin Med* 2018; 7:17.
14. Gutierrez MA, et al. Paradoxical reactions to benzodiazepines. *Am J Nurs* 2001; 101:34–40.
15. Crowe SF, et al. The residual medium and long-term cognitive effects of benzodiazepine use: an updated meta-analysis. *Arch Clin Neuropsychol* 2017; 33:901–911.
16. Brandt J, et al. Benzodiazepines and z-drugs: an updated review of major adverse outcomes reported on in epidemiologic research. *Drugs R D* 2017; 17:493–507.
17. Donnelly K, et al. Benzodiazepines, z-drugs and the risk of hip fracture: a systematic review and meta-analysis. *PLoS One* 2017; 12:e0174730.
18. Golombok S, et al. Cognitive impairment in long-term benzodiazepine users. *Psychol Med* 1988; 18:365–374.
19. Finkle WD, et al. Risk of fractures requiring hospitalization after an initial prescription for zolpidem, alprazolam, lorazepam, or diazepam in older adults. *J Am Geriatr Soc* 2011; 59:1883–1890.
20. Molero Y, et al. Associations between gabapentinoids and suicidal behaviour, unintentional overdoses, injuries, road traffic incidents, and violent crime: population based cohort study in Sweden. *BMJ* 2019; 365:l2147.
21. Schweizer E, et al. Long-term therapeutic use of benzodiazepines. II. Effects of gradual taper. *Arch Gen Psychiatry* 1990; 47:908–915.
22. Schweizer E, et al. Benzodiazepine dependence and withdrawal: a review of the syndrome and its clinical management. *Acta Psychiatr Scand* 1998; 98 Suppl 393:95–101.
23. Uhlenhuth EH, et al. International study of expert judgment on therapeutic use of benzodiazepines and other psychotherapeutic medications: IV. Therapeutic dose dependence and abuse liability of benzodiazepines in the long-term treatment of anxiety disorders. *J Clin Psychopharmacol* 1999; 19:23S–29S.
24. Ashton H. The diagnosis and management of benzodiazepine dependence. *Curr Opin Psychiatry* 2005; 18:249–255.
25. Ashton H. Benzodiazepine withdrawal: outcome in 50 patients. *Br J Addict* 1987; 82:665–671.
26. US Food and Drug Administration. FDA requiring boxed warning updated to improve safe use of benzodiazepine drug class: includes potential for abuse, addiction, and other serious risks 2020 (last accessed July 2024); https://www.fda.gov/drugs/drug-safety-and-availability/fda-requiring-boxed-warning-updated-improve-safe-use-benzodiazepine-drug-class#:~:text=FDA.
27. Ashton H. Protracted withdrawal from benzodiazepines: the post-withdrawal syndrome. *Psychiatr Ann* 1995; 1:174–179.
28. Ritvo AD, et al. Long-term consequences of benzodiazepine-induced neurological dysfunction: a survey. *PLoS One* 2023; 18:e0285584.
29. Soyka M. Treatment of benzodiazepine dependence. *N Engl J Med* 2017; 376:1147–1157.
30. Petursson H. The benzodiazepine withdrawal syndrome. *Addiction* 1994; 89:1455–1459.
31. Tannenbaum C, et al. Reduction of inappropriate benzodiazepine prescriptions among older adults through direct patient education: the EMPOWER cluster randomized trial. *JAMA Intern Med* 2014; 174:890–898.
32. Guy. A, et al. *Guidance for Psychological Therapists: Enabling Conversations with Clients Taking or Withdrawing from Prescribed Psychiatric Drugs.* London: APPG for Prescribed Drug Dependence; 2019.
33. Parr JM, et al. Effectiveness of current treatment approaches for benzodiazepine discontinuation: a meta-analysis. *Addiction* 2009; 104:13–24.
34. Denis C, et al. Pharmacological interventions for benzodiazepine mono-dependence management in outpatient settings. *Cochrane Database Syst Rev* 2006; (3):CD005194.
35. Ashton H. *Benzodiazepines: How They Work and How to Withdraw.* 2002 (last accessed February 2025); http://www.benzo.org.uk/manual/bzcha01.htm.
36. Ashton H. Benzodiazepine dependence. Adverse syndromes and psychiatric drugs. In: *Adverse Syndromes and Psychiatric Drugs: A Clinical Guide.* Oxford: Oxford University Press; 2004:239–260.
37. Brouillet E, et al. In vivo bidirectional modulatory effect of benzodiazepine receptor ligands on GABAergic transmission evaluated by positron emission tomography in non-human primates. *Brain Res* 1991; 557:167–176.
38. Inner Compass Initiative Inc. The Withdrawal Project. 2024; https://withdrawal.theinnercompass.org.
39. Pollmann AS, et al. Deprescribing benzodiazepines and Z-drugs in community-dwelling adults: a scoping review. *BMC Pharmacol Toxicol* 2015; 16:19.
40. Kales A, et al. Rebound insomnia after only brief and intermittent use of rapidly eliminated benzodiazepines. *Clin Pharmacol Ther* 1991; 49:468–476.

Benzodiazepines and disinhibition

Unexpected increases in aggressive or impulsive behaviour secondary to drug treatment are usually called disinhibitory or paradoxical reactions. These reactions may include acute excitement, hyperactivity, increased anxiety, vivid dreams, sexual disinhibition, aggression, hostility and rage. Examples of causative agents include amfetamines, methylphenidate, benzodiazepines and alcohol. Paradoxical reactions are an important consideration with benzodiazepines because these drugs are used to sedate and tranquillise – a paradoxical reaction is thus the polar opposite of the desired effect. These reactions are also a major problem in general medicine, where drugs such as midazolam are widely used for conscious sedation. In intensive care medicine, benzodiazepine-related disinhibition can be difficult to distinguish from hyperactive delirium.[1]

How common are disinhibitory reactions with benzodiazepines?

The incidence of disinhibitory reactions varies widely depending on the population studied (see 'Who is at risk?' below). For example, a meta-analysis of benzodiazepine RCTs that included many hundreds of patients with a wide range of diagnoses reported an incidence of less than 1% (the same as placebo).[2] Similarly, an analysis of behavioural disinhibition frequency in a psychiatric unit found no difference between those treated with benzodiazepines and those not.[3] However, a Norwegian study that reported on 415 cases of 'driving under the influence', in which flunitrazepam was the sole substance implicated, found that 6% of adverse effects could be described as disinhibitory reactions.[4] An RCT that recruited patients with panic disorder reported an incidence of disinhibition of 13%.[5] Authors of case series (often describing use in high-risk patients) reported rates of 10–20%,[2] and an RCT that included patients with borderline personality disorder reported a rate of 58%.[6] Most recently, a study of the use of parenteral midazolam for bronchoscopy found that almost 20% of patients exhibited moderate or severe disinhibition.[7]

Disinhibition is rather problematic to define, so incident rates are correspondingly difficult to determine. Aggression may be considered to be a disinhibition reaction but not defined as disinhibition per se. Aggression is robustly linked to benzodiazepine use both in the long term and after exposure to a single dose.[8,9]

Other GABA agonists, particularly zolpidem, have also been linked to disinhibition associated with somnambulism, automatism, amnesia and mania.[10–13]

Who is at risk?

Those at risk include people who have learning disabilities, neurological disorders or CNS degenerative diseases,[14] those who are young (children or adolescents) or elderly,[14–17] have a history of aggression or poor impulse control,[6,18] or are at increased risk of experiencing a disinhibitory reaction. The risk is further increased if the benzodiazepine is a high-potency drug (i.e. is active in doses below 1–2mg), has a short half-life, is given in a high dose or is administered intravenously.[14,19–21] Some people may be genetically predisposed to disinhibition reactions.[22]

Combinations of risk factors are clearly important. Low-risk long-acting benzodiazepines may cause disinhibition in high-risk populations such as children;[17] higher-risk, short-acting drugs given intravenously are extremely likely to cause disinhibition in personality disorder.

What is the mechanism?

Various theories of the mechanism have been proposed.[19,23–25] First, the anxiolytic and amnesic properties of benzodiazepines may lead to a loss of the restraint that governs normal social behaviour. Second, the sedative and amnesic properties of benzodiazepines may lead to a reduced ability to concentrate on the external social cues that guide appropriate behaviour. Last, benzodiazepine-mediated increases in GABA neurotransmission may lead to a reduction in the restraining influence of the cortex, resulting in untrammelled excitement, anxiety and hostility.

Flumazenil is usually used to reverse benzodiazepine sedation and respiratory depression, but it is also effective in treating disinhibition reactions.[26]

Subjective reports

People who take benzodiazepines rate themselves as being more tolerant and friendly, but respond more to provocation than patients treated with placebo.[27] People with impulse control problems who take benzodiazepines may self-report feelings of power and overwhelming self-esteem.[18] Psychology rating scales demonstrate increased suggestibility, failure to recognise anger in others and reduced ability to recognise social cues. The patient is usually completely unaware that their behaviour is bizarre or that it is the result of drug-induced disinhibition.

Clinical implications

Benzodiazepines are frequently used in rapid tranquillisation and the short-term management of disturbed behaviour. For the vast majority of treatment episodes, benzodiazepines produce sedation and reductions in anxiety and aggression. It is important to be aware, nonetheless, of their propensity to cause paradoxical disinhibitory reactions.

Suspected paradoxical reactions should be clearly documented in the clinical notes. In extreme cases, flumazenil can be used to reverse the reaction although its use is not without its own dangers (agitation, arrythmia, convulsions).[28] If the benzodiazepine was prescribed to control acute behavioural disturbance, future episodes should be managed with antipsychotic drugs[29] or other non-benzodiazepine sedatives.

Paradoxical disinhibitory/aggressive outbursts in the context of benzodiazepine use:

- Rare in the general population but more frequent in people with impulse control problems or central nervous system damage and in the very young or very old.
- Most often associated with high oral doses of high-potency drugs or with any dose of any drug administered parenterally.
- Usually occur in response to (often very mild) provocation, the exact nature of which is not always obvious to others.
- Recognised by others but often not by the sufferers, who often believe that they are friendly and tolerant.

References

1. Schieveld JNM, et al. On benzodiazepines, paradoxical agitation, hyperactive delirium, and chloride homeostasis. *Crit Care Med* 2018; **46**:1558–1559.

2. Dietch JT, et al. Aggressive dyscontrol in patients treated with benzodiazepines. *J Clin Psychiatry* 1988; **49**:184–188.

3. Rothschild AJ, et al. Comparison of the frequency of behavioral disinhibition on alprazolam, clonazepam, or no benzodiazepine in hospitalized psychiatric patients. *J Clin Psychopharmacol* 2000; **20**:7–11.

4. Bramness JG, et al. Flunitrazepam: psychomotor impairment, agitation and paradoxical reactions. *Forensic Sci Int* 2006; **159**:83–91.

5. O'Sullivan GH, et al. Safety and side-effects of alprazolam: controlled study in agoraphobia with panic disorder. *Br J Psychiatry* 1994; **165**:79–86.

6. Gardner DL, et al. Alprazolam-induced dyscontrol in borderline personality disorder. *Am J Psychiatry* 1985; **142**:98–100.

7. Matsumoto T, et al. Prevalence and characteristics of disinhibition during bronchoscopy with midazolam. *Respir Investig* 2022; **60**:345–354.

8. Albrecht B, et al. Motivational drive and alprazolam misuse: a recipe for aggression? *Psychiatry Res* 2016; **240**:381–389.

9. Albrecht B, et al. Benzodiazepine use and aggressive behaviour: a systematic review. *Aust N Z J Psychiatry* 2014; **48**:1096–1114.

10. Sabe M, et al. Zolpidem stimulant effect: induced mania case report and systematic review of cases. *Prog Neuropsychopharmacol Biol Psychiatry* 2019; **94**:109643.

11. Poceta JS. Zolpidem ingestion, automatisms, and sleep driving: a clinical and legal case series. *J Clin Sleep Med* 2011; **7**:632–638.

12. Pressman MR. Sleep driving: sleepwalking variant or misuse of z-drugs? *Sleep Med Rev* 2011; **15**:285–292.

13. Daley C, et al. 'I did what?' Zolpidem and the courts. *J Am Acad Psychiatry Law* 2011; **39**:535–542.

14. Bond AJ. Drug-induced behavioural disinhibition incidence, mechanisms and therapeutic implications. *CNS Drugs* 1998; **9**:41–57.

15. Hakimi Y, et al. Paradoxical adverse drug reactions: descriptive analysis of French reports. *Euro J Clin Pharmacol* 2020; **76**:1169–1174.

16. Hawkridge SM, et al. A risk–benefit assessment of pharmacotherapy for anxiety disorders in children and adolescents. *Drug Saf* 1998; **19**:283–297.

17. Kandemir H, et al. Behavioral disinhibition, suicidal ideation, and self-mutilation related to clonazepam. *J Child Adolesc Psychopharmacol* 2008; **18**:409.

18. Daderman AM, et al. Flunitrazepam (Rohypnol) abuse in combination with alcohol causes premeditated, grievous violence in male juvenile offenders. *J Am Acad Psychiatry Law* 1999; **27**:83–99.

19. van der Bijl P, et al. Disinhibitory reactions to benzodiazepines: a review. *J Oral Maxillofac Surg* 1991; **49**:519–523.

20. McKenzie WS, et al. Paradoxical reaction following administration of a benzodiazepine. *J Oral Maxillofac Surg* 2010; **68**:3034–3036.

21. Wilson KE, et al. Complications associated with intravenous midazolam sedation in anxious dental patients. *Prim Dent Care* 2011; **18**:161–166.

22. Short TG, et al. Paradoxical reactions to benzodiazepines: a genetically determined phenomenon? *Anaesth Intensive Care* 1987; **15**:330–331.

23. Weisman AM, et al. Effects of clorazepate, diazepam, and oxazepam on a laboratory measurement of aggression in men. *Int Clin Psychopharmacol* 1998; **13**:183–188.

24. Blair RJ, et al. Selective impairment in the recognition of anger induced by diazepam. *Psychopharmacology* 1999; **147**:335–338.

25. Wallace PS, et al. Reduction of appeasement-related affect as a concomitant of diazepam-induced aggression: evidence for a link between aggression and the expression of self-conscious emotions. *Aggress Behav* 2009; **35**:203–212.

26. Tae CH, et al. Paradoxical reaction to midazolam in patients undergoing endoscopy under sedation: incidence, risk factors and the effect of flumazenil. *Dig Liver Dis* 2014; **46**:710–715.

27. Bond AJ, et al. Behavioural aggression in panic disorder after 8 weeks' treatment with alprazolam. *J Affect Disord* 1995; **35**:117–123.

28. Penninga EI, et al. Adverse events associated with flumazenil treatment for the management of suspected benzodiazepine intoxication: a systematic review with meta-analyses of randomised trials. *Basic Clin Pharmacol Toxicol* 2016; **118**:37–44.

29. Paton C. Benzodiazepines and disinhibition: a review. *Psychiatr Bull* 2002; **26**:460–462.

CHAPTER 3

Premenstrual syndrome

Premenstrual syndrome (PMS) is a collection of mood and physical symptoms occurring during the luteal phase of the menstrual cycle. There are several definitions for PMS, which are differentiated by the severity of symptoms required. Premenstrual dysphoric disorder (PMDD), recently added to ICD-11,[1] exists at the more severe end of the diagnostic spectrum (see Craig et al. 2019[2] for review).

Pharmacological management of PMDD

The pharmacological management of PMDD can be divided into hormonal and non-hormonal treatments (Figure 3.6).

Non-hormonal

Guidelines published by the Royal College of Obstetricians and Gynaecologists in the UK[3] recommend SSRIs as first-line treatment. This is supported by a meta-analysis, which found similar efficacy between different SSRIs.[4] Intermittent, luteal phase dosing of SSRIs has been reported to be as effective as continuous prescribing.[5] During intermittent dosing, SSRIs appear to directly promote the conversion of progesterone to allopregnanolone (i.e. an allosteric modulator of the GABA-A receptor).[6]

Hormonal

The combined oral contraceptive pill (COCP) is another first-line treatment. It can be prescribed cyclically or back to back (typically for 3 months) to avoid symptoms associated with hormone withdrawal.[7] A 2021 meta-analysis reported that COCPs improved overall premenstrual symptomatology but not premenstrual depressive symptoms.[8] There is no evidence of one COCP being more efficacious than any other.

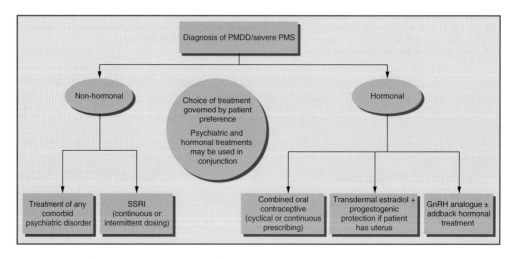

Figure 3.6 The pharmacological management of premenstrual dysphoric disorder.

If COCPs are ineffective, not tolerated, or contraindicated, a second-line approach is to prescribe continuous percutaneous bioidentical estradiol (i.e. implants or transdermal preparations).[9] In patients with a uterus, combination with a progestogen is required to reduce the risk of endometrial hyperplasia.

Gonadotrophin-releasing hormone agonists lead to (reversible) medical menopause. This can be used as a diagnostic test for PMDD and/or to determine the likely benefits of a hysterectomy and oophorectomy. Owing to the adverse effects typically associated with acute menopause, an 'addback' regime of estradiol alone or combined with a progestogen is required (i.e. dependent on whether the woman has a uterus).

References

1. World Health Organization. *International Classification of Diseases*, 11th revision. Geneva: WHO; 2024 (last accessed September 2024); https://icd.who.int/en.
2. Craig M, et al. Diagnosis and management of premenstrual syndrome. *Practitioner* 2019; **263**:15–19.
3. Green L, et al. Management of premenstrual syndrome. Green-top Guideline No. 48. *BJOG* 2017; **124**:e73–e105.
4. Marjoribanks J, et al. Selective serotonin reuptake inhibitors for premenstrual syndrome. *Cochrane Database Syst Rev* 2013; **2013**(6):CD001396.
5. Reilly TJ, et al. Intermittent selective serotonin reuptake inhibitors for premenstrual syndromes: a systematic review and meta-analysis of randomised trials. *J Psychopharmacol* 2023; **37**:261–267.
6. Hantsoo L, et al. Allopregnanolone in premenstrual dysphoric disorder (PMDD): evidence for dysregulated sensitivity to GABA-A receptor modulating neuroactive steroids across the menstrual cycle. *Neurobiol Stress* 2020; **12**:100213.
7. Noachtar IA, et al. Mental health symptoms in oral contraceptive users during short-term hormone withdrawal. *JAMA Netw Open* 2023; **6**:e2335957.
8. de Wit AE, et al. Efficacy of combined oral contraceptives for depressive symptoms and overall symptomatology in premenstrual syndrome: pairwise and network meta-analysis of randomized trials. *Am J Obstet Gynecol* 2021; **225**:624–633.
9. Naheed B, et al. Non-contraceptive oestrogen-containing preparations for controlling symptoms of premenstrual syndrome. *Cochrane Database Syst Rev* 2017; **3**:CD010503.

Chapter 4

Addictions and substance misuse

Introduction

Mental and behavioural problems caused by psychoactive substance use are common. The World Health Organization (WHO) in the ICD-11[1] identifies acute intoxication, harmful use, dependence syndrome, withdrawal state (with or without delirium), substance-induced psychotic disorder, substance-induced amnesic disorder, other mental and behavioural disorders and unspecified mental and behavioural disorders as substance-related disorders. A wide range of psychoactive substances may be problematic including alcohol, opioids, benzodiazepines, gamma-hydroxybutyrate/gamma-butyrolactone (GHB/GBL), stimulants, new psychoactive substances (NPS) (including cathinones, synthetic cannabinoids and phenylethylamines), khat, nitrates, hallucinogens, anabolic steroids, nitazenes and tobacco.

Substance misuse is frequently seen in people with severe mental illness (so-called dual diagnosis) and personality disorder. In many adult psychiatry settings, dual diagnosis is the norm rather than the exception. In many parts of the world substance misuse services may be provided separately from general psychiatric services. The model of care in most addiction services means that patients who are not motivated to engage will not be assertively treated and followed up. Dual diagnosis teams are not universally available, resulting in suboptimal treatment of substance misuse for many patients with mental illness.[2]

According to the ICD-11, dependence syndrome is 'a cluster of physiological, behavioural, and cognitive phenomena in which the use of a substance or a class of substances takes on a much higher priority for a given individual than other behaviours that once had greater value'. A definite diagnosis of dependence should only be made if at least three of the following have been present together in the last year:

- compulsion to take substance
- difficulties controlling substance-taking behaviour
- physiological withdrawal state

The Maudsley® Prescribing Guidelines in Psychiatry, Fifteenth Edition. David M. Taylor, Thomas R. E. Barnes and Allan H. Young.
© 2025 David M. Taylor. Published 2025 by John Wiley & Sons Ltd.

- evidence of tolerance
- neglect of alternative interests
- persistent use despite harm.

Substance use disorders should generally be treated with a combination of psychosocial and pharmacological interventions. This chapter concentrates on pharmacological interventions for alcohol, opioids and nicotine use. Treatments for people misusing benzodiazepines, GHB/GBL and stimulants are discussed briefly. Note that various National Institute for Health and Care Excellence (NICE) guidelines and technology appraisals and Department of Health substance misuse guidelines (the 'Orange Book')[3] provide a comprehensive overview of treatment options. UK national guidance on the treatment of alcohol-related problems is awaiting publication at the time of writing.[4]

References

1. World Health Organization. *International Statistical Classification of Diseases and Related Health Problems*. 2018 (last accessed September 2024); https://www.who.int/news-room/spotlight/international-classification-of-diseases.
2. Public Health England. Better care for people with co-occurring mental health and alcohol/drug use conditions. A guide for commissioners and service providers. 2017; https://www.gov.uk/government/uploads/system/uploads/attachment_data/file/625809/Co-occurring_mental_health_and_alcohol_drug_use_conditions.pdf.
3. Gov.UK Department of Health and Social Care. Drug misuse and dependence: UK guidelines on clinical management. 2017; https://www.gov.uk/government/publications/drug-misuse-and-dependence-uk-guidelines-on-clinical-management.
4. Gov.UK Department of Health and Social Care. Closed consultation. UK clinical guidelines for alcohol treatment: consultation document. 2023; https://www.gov.uk/government/consultations/uk-clinical-guidelines-for-alcohol-treatment/uk-clinical-guidelines-for-alcohol-treatment-consultation-document.

Alcohol dependence

In the UK 1 unit of alcohol is 10mL of ethanol or 1L of 1% alcohol. For example, 250mL of wine that is 10% alcohol contains 2.5 units. In the USA, one drink is defined as 14g (17.7mL) of ethanol (1.77 UK units). Other countries use somewhat different definitions based on volume or mass of alcohol.

The UK Department of Health has given the following advice and recommendations to minimise the health risks from alcohol consumption:[1]

- No more than 14 units should be consumed per week on a regular basis. This applies to both men and women.
- Harm is minimised when these units are spread across 3 or more days.
- Heavy, single-occasion drinking is associated with risk of harm, injury and accidents.
- The consumption of any volume of alcohol is still associated with a number of illnesses such as cancers of the throat, mouth and breast.
- There are no completely safe levels of drinking during pregnancy and precautionary avoidance of alcohol is recommended to reduce risk of harm to the baby.

Assessment and brief structured intervention

The UK NICE guideline on the diagnosis, assessment and management of harmful drinking and alcohol dependence recommends that staff working in services that might encounter problem drinkers should be competent in identifying and assessing harmful drinking and alcohol dependence.[2] The NICE public health guideline on reducing harmful drinking[3] recommends a session of brief structured advice based on FRAMES principles (feedback, responsibility, advice, menu, empathy, self-efficacy) as a useful intervention for everyone at increased risk of alcohol-related problems.

Where consumption above recommended levels has been identified, a more detailed clinical assessment is required. Depending on the context, this could include the following:

- History of alcohol use, including daily consumption and recent patterns of drinking.
- History of previous episodes of alcohol withdrawal.
- Time of most recent drink.
- Collateral history from a family member or carer.
- Other drug (illicit and prescribed) use.
- Severity of dependence and of withdrawal symptoms.
- Coexisting medical and psychiatric problems.
- Physical examination including cognitive function.
- Breathalyser: absolute breath alcohol level and whether rising or falling (take at least 20 minutes after last drink to avoid falsely high readings from the mouth, and 1 hour later).
- Laboratory investigations: full blood count (FBC), urea and electrolytes (U&E), liver function tests (LFTs), international normalised ratio (INR), prothrombin time (PT) and urinary drug screen.

CHAPTER 4

The following structured assessment tools are recommended:[2]

- The **Alcohol Use Disorders Identification Test (AUDIT)**[4] questionnaire is a 10-item questionnaire which is useful as a screening tool in those identified as being at increasing risk. Questions 1–3 address the quantity of alcohol consumed, 4–6 the signs and symptoms of dependence and 7–10 the behaviours and symptoms associated with harmful alcohol use. Each question is scored 0–4, giving a maximum total score of 40. A score of 8 or more is suggestive of hazardous or harmful alcohol use. Hazardous drinking = consumption of alcohol likely to cause harm. Harmful drinking = consumption already causing mental or physical health problems.
- The **Severity of Alcohol Dependence Questionnaire (SADQ)**[5] is a more detailed 20-item questionnaire with the score on each item ranging from 0 to 3, giving a maximum total score of 60.

Severity of alcohol dependence	
Mild	= SADQ score of 15 or less
Moderate	= SADQ score 15–30
Severe	= SADQ score >30

Alcohol withdrawal

In alcohol-dependent drinkers, the central nervous system (CNS) has adjusted to the constant presence of alcohol in the body (neuroadaptation). When the blood alcohol concentration (BAC) is suddenly lowered, the brain remains in a hyper-excited state, resulting in the withdrawal syndrome (Tables 4.1 and 4.2). There is no evidence to support prophylactic use of additional anticonvulsant medication to prevent seizures in high-risk individuals.

Table 4.1 Mild alcohol withdrawal.

Mild alcohol withdrawal manifestations	Usual timing of onset after last drink	Other information
Agitation/anxiety/irritability Tremor of hands, tongue, eyelids Sweating Nausea/vomiting/diarrhoea Fever Tachycardia Systolic hypertension General malaise	Onset at 3–12 hours Peak at 24–48 hours Duration up to 14 days	Symptoms are non-specific Absence does not exclude withdrawal May commence before blood alcohol levels reach zero

Management
- May be self-limiting but mitigated with adequate benzodiazepine cover and supportive treatment.
- Monitor vital signs. Use a withdrawal assessment scale.
- See Table 4.2 for the various benzodiazepine regimens recommended.

Table 4.2 Severe alcohol withdrawal.

Severe alcohol withdrawal complications	Usual timing of onset after last drink	Other information
Generalised seizures	12–18 hours	May commence before blood alcohol levels reach zero

Management
- The occurrence of a first seizure during medically assisted withdrawal requires investigation to rule out organic disease or idiopathic epilepsy.
- A meta-analysis of trials assessing the efficacy of drugs preventing alcohol withdrawal seizures demonstrated that benzodiazepines, particularly long-acting preparations such as diazepam, significantly reduced seizures *de novo*.[6,7]
- Long-acting benzodiazepine is recommended as prophylaxis in those with a previous history of seizures.[8]
- Some anticonvulsants are as effective as benzodiazepines, with some units recommending carbamazepine loading in patients with untreated epilepsy, or where seizures have occurred despite adequate benzodiazepine loading.[6]
- Phenytoin does not prevent alcohol withdrawal-related seizures when used on its own or in combination with benzodiazepines.[9] There is no need to continue anticonvulsants long term when used to prevent seizures in alcohol withdrawal.[9]

Delirium tremens	3–4 days (72–96 hours)	Develops in 3–5% of those admitted to hospital for alcohol withdrawal
Clouding of consciousness/confusion		
Vivid hallucinations, particularly in visual and tactile modalities		
Marked tremor		A medical emergency Mortality 10–20% if untreated
Other clinical features also include: autonomic hyperactivity (tachycardia, hypertension, sweating and fever), paranoid delusions, agitation and insomnia		
Prodromal symptoms include: night-time insomnia, restlessness, fear and confusion		
Risk factors: severe alcohol dependence, self-detoxification without medical input, multiple previous admissions for alcohol withdrawal, concurrent medical illness, previous history of delirium tremens and alcohol withdrawal seizures, low potassium, low magnesium, thiamine deficiency, inadequately treated withdrawal		
Recognition is important because treatment is different from delirium arising from other causes; delirium tremens needs **larger doses of benzodiazepines and more caution with antipsychotics**		

Management
- Delirium tremens is a medical emergency and requires prompt transfer to a general hospital,[9] preferably to a high-dependency setting.[10,11]

Pharmacologically assisted withdrawal (alcohol detoxification)

Alcohol withdrawal is associated with significant morbidity and mortality when improperly managed.

Pharmacologically assisted withdrawal is likely to be needed when:

- there has been regular consumption of >15 units/day
- AUDIT score >20
- there is a history of significant withdrawal symptoms.

Symptom scales can be helpful in determining the amount of pharmacological support required to manage withdrawal symptoms. The Clinical Institute Withdrawal Assessment of Alcohol Scale Revised (CIWA-Ar)[12] (Figure 4.1) and Short Alcohol Withdrawal Scale (SAWS)[13] (Table 4.3) are both 10-item scales that can be completed in around 5 minutes. The CIWA-Ar is an objective scale and the SAWS is a self-complete tool. A CIWA-Ar score >10 or a SAWS score >12 should prompt assisted withdrawal.

Community detoxification is usually possible when:

- There is a supervising carer, ideally 24 hours a day throughout the duration of the detoxification process.
- The treatment plan has been agreed with the patient, their carer and their GP.
- A contingency plan has been agreed with the patient, their carer and their GP.
- The patient is able to pick up medication daily and be reviewed by professionals regularly throughout the process.
- Out-patient/community-based programmes including psychosocial support are available.

Community detoxification should be stopped if the patient resumes drinking or fails to engage with the agreed treatment plan.

In-patient detoxification is likely to be required if:

- Regular consumption is >30 units/day.
- SADQ >30 (severe dependence).
- There is a history of seizures or delirium tremens.
- The patient is a minor or an older adult.
- There is current benzodiazepine use in combination with alcohol.
- Substances other than alcohol are also being misused.
- There is comorbid mental or physical illness, learning disability or cognitive impairment.
- The patient is pregnant.
- The patient is homeless or has no social support.
- There is a history of failed community detoxification.

In certain situations, there may be a clinical justification for undertaking a community detoxification in these patients, however the reasons must be clear and the decision made by an experienced clinician.

Patient:_____ Date: _____
Time: _____ (24 hours clock, midnight = 00:00)

Pulse or heart rate, taken for 1 minute:_____
Blood pressure:_____

NAUSEA AND VOMITING – Ask 'Do you feel sick to your stomach? Have you vomited?' Observation.
0 – no nausea and no vomiting
1 – mild nausea with no vomiting
2
3
4 – intermittent nausea with dry heaves
5
6
7 – constant nausea, frequent dry heaves and vomiting

TACTILE DISTURBANCES – Ask 'Have you any itching, pins and needles sensations, any burning, any numbness, or do you feel bugs crawling on or under your skin?' Observation.
0 – none
1 – very mild itching, pins and needles, burning or numbness
2 – mild itching, pins and needles, burning or numbness
3 – moderate itching, pins and needles, burning or numbness
4 – moderately severe hallucinations
5 – severe hallucinations
6 – extremely severe hallucinations
7 – continuous hallucinations

TREMOR – Arms extended and fingers spread apart. Observation.
0 – no tremor
1 – not visible, but can be felt fingertip to fingertip
2
3
4 – moderate, with patient's arms extended
5
6
7 – severe, even with arms not extended

AUDITORY DISTURBANCES – Ask 'Are you more aware of sounds around you? Are they harsh? Do they frighten you? Are you hearing anything that is disturbing to you? Are you hearing things you know are not there?' Observation.
0 – not present
1 – very mild harshness or ability to frighten
2 – mild harshness or ability to frighten
3 – moderate harshness or ability to frighten
4 – moderately severe hallucinations
5 – severe hallucinations
6 – extremely severe hallucinations
7 – continuous hallucinations

PAROXYSMAL SWEATS – Observation.
0 – no sweat visible
1 – barely perceptible sweating, palms moist
2
3
4 – beads of sweat obvious on forehead
5
6
7 – drenching sweats

VISUAL DISTURBANCES – Ask 'Does the light appear to be too bright? Is its colour different? Does it hurt your eyes? Are you seeing anything that is disturbing to you? Are you seeing things you know are not there?' Observation.
0 – not present
1 – very mild sensitivity
2 – mild sensitivity
3 – moderate sensitivity
4 – moderately severe hallucinations
5 – severe hallucinations
6 – extremely severe hallucinations
7 – continuous hallucinations

ANXIETY – Ask 'Do you feel nervous?' Observation.
0 – no anxiety, at ease
1 – mild anxious
2
3
4 – moderately anxious, or guarded, so anxiety is inferred
5
6
7 – equivalent to acute panic states as seen in severe delirium or acute schizophrenic reactions

HEADACHE, FULLNESS IN HEAD – Ask 'Does your head feel different? Does it feel like there is a band around your head?' Do not rate for dizziness or light-headedness. Otherwise, rate severity.
0 – not present
1 – very mild
2 – mild
3 – moderate
4 – moderately severe
5 – severe
6 – very severe
7 – extremely severe

AGITATION – Observation.
0 – normal activity
1 – somewhat more than normal activity
2
3
4 – moderately fidgety and restless
5
6
7 – paces back and forth during most of the interview, or constantly thrashes about

ORIENTATION AND CLOUDING OF SENSORIUM – Ask 'What day is this? Where are you? Who am I?'
0 – oriented and can do serial additions
1 – cannot do serial additions or is uncertain about date
2 – disoriented for date by no more than 2 calendar days
3 – disoriented for date by more than 2 calendar days
4 – disoriented for place or person

Scores
≤10 – mild withdrawal (do not need additional medication)
≤15 – moderate withdrawal
>15 – severe withdrawal

Total **CIWA-Ar** score _____
Rater's initials _____
Maximum possible score 67

Figure 4.1 Clinical Institute Withdrawal Assessment of Alcohol Scale, Revised (CIWA-Ar).[12] The CIWA-Ar is not copyrighted and may be reproduced freely.

Table 4.3 Short Alcohol Withdrawal Scale (SAWS).[13]

	None (0)	Mild (1)	Moderate (2)	Severe (3)
Anxious				
Sleep disturbance				
Problems with memory				
Nausea				
Restless				
Tremor (shakes)				
Feeling confused				
Sweating				
Miserable				
Heart pounding				

Table 4.4 summarises common interventions used in alcohol withdrawal.

Table 4.4 Alcohol withdrawal treatment interventions – a summary.

Severity	Supportive/ medical care	Pharmacotherapy for neuroadaptation reversal	Thiamine supplementation	Setting
Mild CIWA-Ar ≤10	Moderate- to high-level supportive care, little if any medical care required	Little to none required Simple remedies only (see below)	Oral likely to be sufficient if patient is well nourished	Home
Moderate CIWA-Ar ≤15	Moderate- to high-level supportive care, little medical care required	Little to none required Symptomatic treatment only	Intramuscular thiamine should be offered if the patient is malnourished followed by oral supplementation	Home or community team
Severe CIWA-Ar >15	High-level supportive care plus medical monitoring	Symptomatic and substitution treatment (chlordiazepoxide) probably required	Intramuscular thiamine should be offered followed by oral supplementation	Community team or hospital
CIWA-Ar >10 + comorbid alcohol-related medical problems	High-level supportive care plus specialist medical care	Symptomatic and substitution treatments usually required	Intramuscular thiamine followed by oral supplementation	Hospital

Benzodiazepines are the treatment of choice for alcohol withdrawal. They exhibit cross-tolerance with alcohol and have anticonvulsant properties. Their use is supported by NICE guidelines,[2,14] a Cochrane systematic review[7] and British Association for Psychopharmacology guidelines.[9] **Parenteral thiamine (vitamin B1)** and other vitamin replacement is an important adjunctive treatment for the prophylaxis and/or treatment of Wernicke–Korsakoff syndrome and other vitamin-related neuropsychiatric conditions.

In the UK, **chlordiazepoxide** is the benzodiazepine used for most patients in most centres as it is considered to have a relatively low dependence-forming potential. Some centres use diazepam. A short-acting benzodiazepine such as **oxazepam** or **lorazepam** may be used in individuals with impaired liver function or those who potentially may metabolise medication more slowly, such as older people.

There are three types of assisted withdrawal regimens: **fixed-dose reduction** (the most common in non-specialist settings), **variable-dose reduction** (usually results in less benzodiazepine being administered but best reserved for settings where staff have specialist skills in managing alcohol withdrawal) and finally **front-loading** (infrequently used, and reserved for severe alcohol withdrawal).[2,9] Assisted withdrawal regimens should never be started if the blood alcohol concentration is very high or is still rising. Monitor patients for oversedation/respiratory depression.

Fixed-dose reduction regimen

Fixed-dose regimens can be used in community or non-specialist in-patient/residential settings for uncomplicated patients. Patients should be started on a dose of benzodiazepine selected after an assessment of the severity of alcohol dependence (clinical history, number of units per drinking day and score on the SADQ). With respect to chlordiazepoxide, a general rule of thumb is that the starting dose can be estimated from current alcohol consumption. For example, if 20 units/day are being consumed, the starting dose should be 20mg four times a day. The dose is then tapered to zero over 5–10 days. Alcohol withdrawal symptoms should be monitored using a validated instrument such as the CIWA-Ar[12] or SAWS.[13]

Mild alcohol dependence usually requires very small doses of chlordiazepoxide or else may be managed without medication.

For **moderate alcohol dependence**, a typical regimen might be 10–20mg chlordiazepoxide four times a day, reducing gradually over 5–7 days (Table 4.5). This duration of treatment is usually adequate and longer treatment is rarely helpful or necessary. It is advisable to monitor withdrawal and BAC daily before providing the day's medication. This may mean that community pharmacologically assisted alcohol withdrawals should start on a Monday and last for 5 days.

Table 4.5 Moderate alcohol dependence: example of a fixed-dose chlordiazepoxide treatment regimen.

Day	Dose	Total daily dose (mg)
1	20mg four times a day	80
2	15mg four times a day	60
3	10mg four times a day	40
4	5mg four times a day	20
5	5mg twice a day	10

CHAPTER 4

Severe alcohol dependence usually requires in-patient treatment for assisted withdrawal because of the significant risk of life-threatening complications. However, there are rare occasions where a pragmatic community approach is required. In such situations, the decision to undertake a community-assisted withdrawal must be made by an experienced clinician. Intensive daily monitoring is advised for the first 2–3 days. This may require special arrangements over a weekend.

Prescribing should not start if the patient is intoxicated. In such circumstances, they should be reviewed at the earliest opportunity when not intoxicated. The dose of benzodiazepine may need to be reduced over a 7–10-day period in this group (occasionally longer if dependence is very severe or there is a history of complications during previous detoxifications) (Table 4.6).

Table 4.6 Severe alcohol dependence: example of a fixed-dose chlordiazepoxide regimen.

Day	Dose	Total daily dose (mg)
1 (first 24 hours)	40mg four times a day + 40mg when necessary	200
2	40mg four times a day	160
3	30mg four times a day	120
4	25mg four times a day	100
5	20mg four times a day	80
6	15mg four times a day	60
7	10mg four times a day	40
8	10mg four times a day	30
9	5mg four times a day	20
10	10mg at night	10

Symptom-triggered regimen

This should be reserved for managing assisted withdrawal in specialist alcohol in-patient or residential settings. Regular monitoring is required (e.g. pulse, blood pressure, temperature and level of consciousness). Medication is only given when withdrawal symptoms are observed as determined using CIWA-Ar, SAWS or an alternative validated measure. Symptom-triggered therapy is generally used in patients without a history of complications. A typical symptom-triggered regimen would be chlordiazepoxide 20–30mg hourly as needed. The total dose given each day would be expected to decrease from day 2 onwards. It is common for symptom-triggered treatment to last only 24–48 hours before switching to an individualised fixed-dose reducing schedule. Occasionally (e.g. in delirium tremens) the flexible regimen may need to be prolonged beyond the first 24 hours.

Example of a symptom-triggered chlordiazepoxide regimen[2]

- Days 1–5: 20–30mg chlordiazepoxide as needed, up to hourly, based on symptoms

Carbamazepine is an alternative to a benzodiazepine for managing withdrawal in situations where benzodiazepines are not a safe first-line option.[15,16] Examples include:

- A history of adverse reaction or allergy to benzodiazepine drugs.
- A preference for carbamazepine because of a history of harmful or dependent use of benzodiazepines.

Wernicke's encephalopathy

Wernicke's encephalopathy is an acute neuropsychiatric condition caused by thiamine deficiency. In alcohol dependence, thiamine deficiency is secondary to both reduced dietary intake and reduced absorption.

Risk factors for Wernicke's encephalopathy in alcohol dependence are:[16]

- acute withdrawal
- malnourishment
- decompensated liver disease
- emergency department attendance
- hospitalisation for comorbidity
- homelessness
- memory disturbance
- peripheral neuropathy
- previous history of Wernicke's encephalopathy.

The 'classic' triad of ophthalmoplegia, ataxia and confusion is rarely present in Wernicke's encephalopathy, and the syndrome is much more common than is recognised. A presumptive diagnosis of Wernicke's encephalopathy should therefore be made in any patient undergoing detoxification who experiences any of the following signs:

- ataxia
- hypothermia
- hypotension
- confusion
- ophthalmoplegia/nystagmus
- memory disturbance
- unconsciousness/coma.

Any history of malnutrition, recent weight loss, vomiting or diarrhoea or peripheral neuropathy should also be taken into consideration.[17]

Prophylactic thiamine

Low-risk drinkers without neuropsychiatric complications and with an adequate diet should be offered oral thiamine. The dose should be 300mg daily during assisted alcohol withdrawal and periods of continued alcohol intake.[9] As thiamine is required to utilise glucose, a glucose load in a thiamine-deficient patient can precipitate Wernicke's encephalopathy.

CHAPTER 4

Parenteral thiamine

Historically it has been advised that patients undergoing in-patient detoxification should be given parenteral thiamine as prophylaxis against Wernike's encephalopathy.[2,9,18,19] In many countries, there are no licensed forms of parenteral thiamine available.

In the UK, NICE[20] recommends offering prophylactic parenteral thiamine followed by oral thiamine to those defined as 'harmful or dependent drinkers' if they are also known to:

- be malnourished or at risk of malnourishment *or*
- have decompensated liver disease

and in addition:

- they attend an emergency department *or*
- are admitted to hospital with an acute injury or illness.

People at high risk of Wernicke's encephalopathy can have a range of conditions, including:

- significant weight loss
- poor diet
- low body mass index (BMI) (<18)
- other signs of malnutrition.

Consider offering prophylactic parenteral thiamine to people at high risk following the dosing below.

Community setting doses
■ Give intramuscular thiamine 200–300mg once daily for at least 3 days

Hospital setting doses
■ Give intramuscular or intravenous thiamine 200–300mg once daily for 3–5 days with daily review and monitoring for emergent signs of Wernicke's encephalopathy

If Wernicke's encephalopathy is suspected the patient should be transferred to a medical unit where intravenous thiamine can be administered. If untreated, Wernicke's encephalopathy progresses to Korsakoff's syndrome (permanent memory impairment, confabulation, confusion and personality changes).

Treatment of somatic symptoms

Somatic complaints are common during assisted withdrawal. Table 4.7 lists some remedies.

Table 4.7 Treatment of somatic symptoms.

Symptom	Recommended treatment
Dehydration	Ensure adequate fluid intake in order to maintain hydration and electrolyte balance; dehydration can precipitate life-threatening cardiac arrhythmia
Pain	Paracetamol (acetaminophen)
Nausea and vomiting	Metoclopramide 10mg or prochlorperazine 5mg 4–6 hourly
Diarrhoea	Diphenoxylate and atropine (Lomotil) or loperamide
Skin itching	Occurs commonly and not only in individuals with alcoholic liver disease: use oral antihistamines

Relapse prevention

There is no place for the continued use of benzodiazepines beyond treatment of the acute alcohol withdrawal syndrome. **Acamprosate** and supervised **disulfiram** are licensed in some countries for the treatment of alcohol dependence and may be offered in combination with psychosocial treatment.[2] Treatment should be initiated by a specialist service. After 12 weeks, transfer of the prescribing to primary care may be appropriate, although specialist care may continue. **Naltrexone** is also recommended as an adjunct in the treatment of moderate and severe alcohol dependence.[2] As it does not have marketing authorisation for the treatment of alcohol dependence in some countries, informed consent should be sought and documented prior to commencing treatment. A large number of new and repurposed agents are undergoing evaluation for the treatment of alcohol use disorder (AUD).[21,22]

Acamprosate

Acamprosate is a synthetic taurine analogue that acts as a functional glutamatergic N-methyl-D-aspartate (NMDA) antagonist and also increases gamma-aminobutyric acid (GABA) function. The number needed to treat (NNT) for the maintenance of abstinence has been calculated as 9–11.[9] Acamprosate should be initiated as soon as possible after abstinence has been achieved although the British Association for Psychopharmacology consensus guidelines[11] recommend that acamprosate should be started during detoxification because of its potential neuroprotective effect. In the UK, NICE[2] recommends that acamprosate should be continued for up to 6 months, with regular (monthly) supervision (Box 4.1). The summary of product characteristics (SPC) recommends that it is given for 1 year.

Box 4.1 Acamprosate: NICE Clinical guideline 115 (2011)[2,23]

Acamprosate should be offered for relapse prevention in moderately to severely dependent drinkers, in combination with psychosocial treatment. It should be prescribed for up to 6 months, or longer for those who perceive benefit and wish to continue taking it. The dose is 1998mg daily (666mg three times per day) for individuals over 60kg. For those under 60kg, the dose is 1332mg daily. Treatment should be stopped in those who continue to drink for 4–6 weeks after starting the drug.

Acamprosate is relatively well tolerated. Adverse effects include diarrhoea, abdominal pain, nausea, vomiting and pruritis.[2] It is contraindicated in severe renal or hepatic impairment, thus baseline liver and kidney function tests should be performed before commencing treatment. Acamprosate should be avoided in individuals who are pregnant or breastfeeding.

Naltrexone

Opioid blockade prevents increased dopaminergic activity after the consumption of alcohol, thus reducing its rewarding effects. Naltrexone, a non-selective opioid receptor antagonist, significantly reduces relapse to heavy drinking.[2,24] Although early trials used a dose of 50mg/day, later US studies have used 100mg/day. In the UK the usual dose is 50mg/day with a trial dose of 25mg for 2 days to evaluate for adverse effects (Box 4.2).

Box 4.2 Naltrexone: NICE Clinical guideline 115 (2011)[2,24]

Naltrexone (50mg/day) should be offered for relapse prevention in moderately to severely dependent drinkers in combination with psychosocial treatment. It should be prescribed for up to 6 months, or longer for those who perceive benefit and wish to continue taking it. Treatment should be stopped in those who continue to drink for 4–6 weeks after starting the drug or in those who feel unwell while taking it.

Naltrexone is well tolerated but adverse effects include nausea (especially in the early stages of treatment), headache, abdominal pain, reduced appetite and tiredness. A comprehensive medical assessment should be carried out prior to commencing naltrexone, together with baseline renal and liver function tests. Naltrexone can be started when patients are still drinking or during medically assisted withdrawal. There is no clear evidence as to the optimal duration of treatment but 6 months appears to be an appropriate period with follow-up, including monitoring liver function.[9]

Patients on naltrexone should not be given opioid agonist drugs for analgesia, non-opioid analgesics should be used instead. In the event that opioid analgesia is necessary, it can be instituted 48–72 hours after cessation of naltrexone. Hepatotoxicity has been described with high doses of naltrexone, so use should probably be avoided in acute liver failure.[25]

Long-acting injectable naltrexone has been developed to improve compliance.[26] Adverse effects are similar to those seen with the oral preparation.[27] In the UK, NICE concluded that the initial evidence was encouraging but not enough to support routine use.

Nalmefene

Nalmefene is also an opioid antagonist, recommended by NICE as an option for reducing alcohol consumption in people with alcohol dependence.[2,24] It has been shown in one meta-analysis to be superior to naltrexone in reducing heavy drinking.[28]

However, use of nalmefene remains controversial, with another meta-analysis suggesting that nalmefene had only limited efficacy in reducing alcohol consumption and that its value in treating alcohol addiction and relapse prevention is not fully established.[29] Nalmefene's efficacy is better than placebo[30] but its place in therapy has yet to be established.

Disulfiram (Antabuse)

Disulfiram is a second-line treatment for those with moderate or severe alcohol dependence who have successfully completed withdrawal and want to maintain abstinence.[31] It acts by inhibiting the enzyme aldehyde dehydrogenase, thus preventing complete metabolism of alcohol in the liver. This results in an accumulation of the toxic intermediate product, acetaldehyde, which causes the alcohol–disulfiram reaction, acting as a deterrent for further alcohol use (Table 4.8). Supervised medication optimises compliance and contributes to effectiveness.

The intensity of the intolerance reaction is dose-dependent, with regard to both the amount of alcohol consumed and the dose of disulfiram. However, it is thought that much of the therapeutic effect is mediated by the mental anticipation of the aversive reaction, rather than the pharmacological action itself. Sudden death can occur but is more prevalent at disulfiram doses above 1000mg.[31] With this in mind, the value of prescribing higher doses of disulfiram must be carefully considered.

The first dose is usually 800mg, reducing to 100–200mg daily for maintenance. In comorbid alcohol and cocaine dependence doses of 500mg daily have been given. Halitosis is a common adverse effect. If there is a sudden onset of jaundice (signalling the rare complication of hepatotoxicity), the patient should stop the drug and seek urgent medical attention.

The evidence for disulfiram is weaker than for acamprosate and naltrexone[2] although its effect size may be greater.[32] In the UK, NICE recommends its use 'as a second-line option for moderate to severe alcohol dependence for patients who are not suitable for acamprosate or naltrexone or have a specified preference for disulfiram and who aim to stay abstinent from alcohol' (Box 4.3).[2]

CHAPTER 4

Table 4.8 The alcohol–disulfiram reaction.

Mild alcohol–disulfiram reaction	Severe alcohol–disulfiram reaction	Contraindications
Facial flushing	Acute heart failure	Ingestion of alcohol within the previous
Sweating	Myocardial infarction	24 hours
Nausea	Arrhythmias	Cardiac failure
Hyperventilation	Bradycardia	Coronary artery disease
Dyspnea	Respiratory depression	Hypertension
Tachycardia	Severe hypotension	Cerebrovascular disease
Hypotenision		Pregnancy
		Breastfeeding
		Liver disease
		Peripheral neuropathy
		Severe mental illness

> **Box 4.3** Disulfiram: NICE Clinical guideline 115 (2011)[2]
>
> Disulfiram should be considered in combination with a psychological intervention for patients who wish to achieve abstinence, but for whom acamprosate or naltrexone are not suitable. Treatment should be started at least 24 hours after the last drink and should be overseen by a family member or carer. Monitoring is recommended every 2 weeks for the first 2 months, then monthly for the following 4 months. Medical monitoring should be continued at 6-monthly intervals after the first 6 months. Patients must not consume any alcohol while taking disulfiram.

Baclofen

Baclofen is a GABA-B agonist that does not have a licence for use in alcohol dependence but is nevertheless used by some clinicians as second-line treatment for those who have not responded to either naltrexone or acamprosate, or where there are contraindications for first-line treatment. A 2023 Cochrane review suggested that baclofen may help people with AUD in maintaining abstinence, particularly in people who are already detoxified.[33] A 2022 meta-analysis[32] also suggested baclofen is effective but is associated with higher rates of adverse effects including depression, vertigo, somnolence, numbness and muscle rigidity.

Antiseizure medications

There is currently insufficient evidence to support the use of antiseizure medications in the treatment of alcohol dependence, although they may reduce the number of drinks per drinking day compared with placebo.[34] The majority of the research has been carried out on topiramate. Topiramate acts as a GABA/glutamate modulator that has demonstrated safety and efficacy in reducing heavy drinking in patients without AUD.[35] It may as effective as naltrexone in AUD.[36]

There have been fewer studies on gabapentin,[37] valproate and levetiracetam.[30] Although these drugs have been used elsewhere in the world, they are not routinely used in the UK owing to lack of evidence and concerns regarding safety profiles for both gabapentin and valproate.

Pregnancy and alcohol use

Evidence indicates that alcohol consumption during pregnancy may cause harm to the fetus. The Department of Health advises that women should not drink any alcohol at all during pregnancy.[1] Drinking even 1–2 units/day during pregnancy can increase the risk of having a preterm, low birthweight or small for gestational age baby.

For alcohol-dependent pregnant women who have withdrawal symptoms, pharmacological cover for detoxification should be offered, ideally in an in-patient setting in collaboration with an antenatal team. The timing of detoxification in relation to the trimester of pregnancy should be risk-assessed against continued alcohol consumption and risks to the fetus.[9] Chlordiazepoxide has been suggested as being unlikely to pose a substantial risk, however dose-dependent malformations have been observed.[11] The UK Teratology Information Service (UKTIS)[38] provides national advice for healthcare professionals and likes to follow up on pregnancies that require alcohol detoxification. Specialist advice should always be sought. (See also Chapter 7.) No relapse prevention medication has been evaluated in pregnancy.[9]

Children and adolescents

The number of young people who are dependent and needing pharmacotherapy is small, but for those who are dependent there should be a lower threshold for admission to hospital. Doses of chlordiazepoxide for medically assisted withdrawal may need to be adjusted, but the general principles of withdrawal management are the same as for adults. All young people should have a full health screen carried out routinely to allow identification of physical and mental health problems. Relapse prevention medications are not licensed in the under 18 population due to lack of evidence. The evidence base for acamprosate, naltrexone and disulfiram in 16–19-year-olds is evolving,[9] but naltrexone is best supported in this age group.[39–41]

Older adults

For older adults, there should be a lower threshold for hospital admission for medically assisted alcohol withdrawal.[2] Benzodiazepines remain the treatment of choice but they may need to be prescribed in lower doses and in some situations shorter acting drugs may be preferred.[9] All older adults with AUD should have full routine health screens to identify physical and mental health problems. The evidence base for pharmacotherapy of AUD in older people is limited.[42]

Concurrent alcohol and substance use disorders

Where alcohol and drug use disorders are comorbid, treat both conditions actively.[2]

Coexisting alcohol and benzodiazepine dependence

This is best managed with one benzodiazepine, either chlordiazepoxide or diazepam. The starting dose should take into account the requirements for medically assisted alcohol withdrawal and the typical daily equivalent dose of the relevant benzodiazepine(s).[2,43] In-patient treatment should be carried out over a 2–3-week period, possibly longer.[2]

Coexisting alcohol dependence and cocaine use

In comorbid cocaine/alcohol dependence, naltrexone 150mg/day resulted in reduced cocaine and alcohol use in men but not in women.[44] Topiramate seems ineffective.[45]

Coexisting alcohol and opioid dependence

Both conditions should be treated and attention paid to the increased mortality of individuals withdrawing from both drugs.

CHAPTER 4

Coexisting alcohol and nicotine dependence

Encourage individuals to stop smoking. Refer for smoking cessation in primary care and other settings. In in-patient settings offer nicotine patches/inhalator during assisted alcohol withdrawal. Always promote vaping as a safer alternative to tobacco smoking.

Comorbid mental health disorders in AUD

People with AUD often present with other mental health disorders, particularly anxiety and depression. Public Health England has described it as 'the norm rather than the exception' and encourages a collaborative, effective and flexible approach between front-line services, stating that it is 'everyone's job' and that there is 'no wrong door'.[46]

Substance use disorders, including AUD, should never be a reason to exclude a patient from crisis or specialist psychiatric services after completion of detoxification.

Depression in AUD

Depressive and anxiety symptoms occur commonly during alcohol withdrawal, but usually diminish by the 3rd or 4th week of abstinence. Meta-analyses suggest that anti-depressants with mixed pharmacology (the tricyclics imipramine or trimipramine) perform better than selective serotonin reuptake inhibitors (SSRIs; fluoxetine or sertraline) in reducing depressive symptoms in individuals with AUD, but the antidepressant effect is modest.[2,9,47,48] Trazodone may also be effective.[49] A greater antidepressant effect was seen if the diagnosis of depression was made after at least 1 week of abstinence, thus excluding those with affective symptoms caused by alcohol withdrawal. There is stronger evidence for depression categorised as independent rather than substance-induced.[36] As treatment effects are masked by comparatively large placebo effects, which conceal improvements that would otherwise be attributed to medication, there is a need for larger randomised, placebo-controlled trials. Despite the evidence for tricyclics, they are rarely used in clinical practice because of their potential for cardiotoxicity and toxicity in overdose.[50] SSRIs may not be effective in depression in AUD and may worsen drinking behaviour.[51]

Relapse prevention medication should be considered in combination with anti-depressants. Pettinati et al.[52] showed that the combination of sertraline (200mg/day) with naltrexone (100mg/day) had superior outcomes – improved drinking outcomes and better mood – compared with placebo and compared with each drug alone. In contrast, citalopram showed no benefit when added to naltrexone.[53]

Secondary analyses of acamprosate and naltrexone trials suggest that:

- Acamprosate has an indirect modest beneficial effect on depression via increasing abstinence.
- In depressed alcohol-dependent patients, the combination of naltrexone and an antidepressant may be better than either drug alone,[9] but findings are not consistent.[53]

Ketamine is an emerging treatment for AUD[54] and may be helpful in comorbid depression.

Bipolar affective disorder in AUD

Bipolar patients tend to use alcohol to reduce symptoms of anxiety and depression, and comorbid AUD is common. Where there is comorbidity, it is important to treat the different phases of bipolar disorder as recommended elsewhere. It may be worth adding sodium valproate to lithium as the combination is associated with better drinking outcomes than lithium alone. However, the combination did not confer any extra benefit than lithium alone in improving mood (see British Association for Psychopharmacology consensus 2012).[9] In those who continue to drink, electrolyte imbalance may precipitate lithium toxicity. Lithium is probably best avoided completely in binge drinkers. Adding quetiapine to lithium or valproate has no effect.[55]

Naltrexone should be offered early to help bipolar patients reduce their alcohol consumption.[9] If naltrexone is not effective, then acamprosate should be offered. In the event that both naltrexone and acamprosate fail to promote abstinence, then disulfiram should be considered, and the risks made known to the patient.

Anxiety in AUD

Anxiety is commonly observed in alcohol-dependent individuals during intoxication, withdrawal and in the early days of abstinence. Alcohol is typically used to self-medicate anxiety disorders, particularly social anxiety. In alcohol-dependent individuals who experience anxiety it is often difficult to determine the extent to which the anxiety is a symptom of the AUD or whether it is an independent disorder. Medically assisted withdrawal and supported abstinence for up to 8 weeks are required before a full assessment can be made. If a medically assisted withdrawal is not possible then treatment of the anxiety disorder should still be attempted, following guidelines for the particular anxiety disorder.

The use of benzodiazepines is controversial[11] because of the increased risk of benzodiazepine misuse and dependence. Benzodiazepines should only be considered following assessment in a specialist addiction service. Long-term use is generally not recommended.[51]

One meta-analysis suggested that buspirone is effective in reducing symptoms of anxiety but not alcohol consumption.[9,56] Studies have also shown that paroxetine (up to 60mg/day) was superior to placebo in reducing social anxiety in AUD patients although alcohol consumption was not affected.[9,56]

Either naltrexone or disulfiram, alone or combined, improves drinking outcomes compared with placebo in patients with post-traumatic stress disorder (PTSD) and alcohol dependence.[57,58] Both acamprosate and baclofen have shown benefit in reducing anxiety in post hoc analyses of alcohol-dependence trials. It is therefore important to ensure that these patients are enabled to become abstinent and are prescribed relapse prevention medication. Anxiety should then be treated according to the appropriate NICE guidelines.

Schizophrenia in AUD

Patients with schizophrenia who also have AUD should be assessed and alcohol-specific relapse prevention treatment considered, usually either naltrexone or acamprosate. Disulfiram is contraindicated in psychosis.[59] Antipsychotic medication should be optimised[11] and clozapine may be considered. However, there is insufficient evidence to recommend the use of any one antipsychotic medication over another in AUD. Antipsychotics do not improve AUD itself.[51]

References

1. Gov.UK Department of Health and Social Care. UK Chief Medical Officers' low risk drinking guidelines. 2016 (last accessed August 2024); https://www.gov.uk/government/publications/alcohol-consumption-advice-on-low-risk-drinking.

2. National Institute for Health and Care Excellence. Alcohol-use disorders: diagnosis, assessment and management of harmful drinking (high-risk drinking) and alcohol dependence. Clinical guideline [CG115]. 2011 (last checked July 2019, last accessed August 2024); https://www.nice.org.uk/guidance/cg115.

3. National Institute for Health and Care Excellence. Alcohol-use disorders: prevention. Public health guideline [PH24]. 2010 (last checked July 2019, last accessed August 2024; updated 2010). https://www.nice.org.uk/guidance/ph24.

4. Babor T, et al. *AUDIT: The Alcohol Use Disorders Identification Test Guidelines for Use in Primary Care*, 2nd edn. 2001; https://iris.who.int/handle/10665/67205.

5. Stockwell T, et al. The severity of alcohol dependence questionnaire: its use, reliability and validity. *Br J Addict* 1983; **78**:145–155.

6. Minozzi S, et al. Anticonvulsants for alcohol withdrawal. *Cochrane Database Syst Rev* 2010; 3:CD005064.

7. Amato L, et al. Efficacy and safety of pharmacological interventions for the treatment of the alcohol withdrawal syndrome. *Cochrane Database Syst Rev* 2011; 6:CD008537.

8. Brathen G, et al. EFNS guideline on the diagnosis and management of alcohol-related seizures: report of an EFNS task force. *Eur J Neurol* 2005; **12**:575–581.

9. Lingford-Hughes AR, et al. Evidence-based guidelines for the pharmacological management of substance abuse, harmful use, addiction and comorbidity: recommendations from BAP. *J Psychopharmacol* 2012; **26**:899–952.

10. NSW Government. Clinical guidance for withdrawal from alcohol and other drugs. 2023 (last accessed August 2024); https://www.health.nsw.gov.au/aod/professionals/Pages/clinical-guidance.aspx.

11. Schuckit MA. Recognition and management of withdrawal delirium (delirium tremens). *N Engl J Med* 2014; **371**:2109–2113.

12. Sullivan JT, et al. Assessment of alcohol withdrawal: the revised clinical institute withdrawal assessment for alcohol scale (CIWA-Ar). *Br J Addict* 1989; **84**:1353–1357.

13. Gossop M, et al. A Short Alcohol Withdrawal Scale (SAWS): development and psychometric properties. *Addict Biol* 2002; **7**:37–43.

14. National Institute for Health and Care Excellence. Alcohol-use disorders: diagnosis and management of physical complications. Clinical guideline [CG100]. 2010 (last updated April 2017, last accessed August 2024); https://www.nice.org.uk/guidance/cg100.

15. Bahji A, et al. Comparative efficacy and safety of pharmacotherapies for alcohol withdrawal: a systematic review and network meta-analysis. *Addiction* 2022; **117**:2591–2601.

16. Fluyau D, et al. Beyond benzodiazepines: a meta-analysis and narrative synthesis of the efficacy and safety of alternative options for alcohol withdrawal syndrome management. *Eur J Clin Pharmacol* 2023; **79**:1147–1157.

17. Thomson AD, et al. Time to act on the inadequate management of Wernicke's encephalopathy in the UK. *Alcohol Alcohol* 2013; **48**:4–8.

18. Thomson AD, et al. The Royal College of Physicians report on alcohol: guidelines for managing Wernicke's encephalopathy in the accident and emergency department. *Alcohol Alcohol* 2002; **37**:513–521.

19. Day E, et al. Thiamine for prevention and treatment of Wernicke-Korsakoff syndrome in people who abuse alcohol. *Cochrane Database Syst Rev* 2013; 7:CD004033.

20. National Institute for Health and Care Excellence. CKS: Alcohol – problem drinking: supporting evidence. 2023 (last accessed September 2024); https://cks.nice.org.uk/topics/alcohol-problem-drinking/supporting-evidence.

21. Burnette EM, et al. Novel agents for the pharmacological treatment of alcohol use disorder. *Drugs* 2022; **82**:251–274.

22. Köhne S, et al. Emerging drugs in phase II and III clinical development for the treatment of alcohol use disorder. *Expert Opin Emerg Drugs* 2024; **29**:219–232.

23. Rösner S, et al. Acamprosate for alcohol dependence. *Cochrane Database Syst Rev* 2010; 9:CD004332.

24. Rösner S, et al. Opioid antagonists for alcohol dependence. *Cochrane Database Syst Rev* 2010; 12:CD001867.

25. AOP Orphan Ltd. Summary of product characteristics. Adepend (naltrexone hydrochloride) 50mg filmcoated tablets. 2020 (last accessed August 2024); https://www.medicines.org.uk/emc/product/3559/smpc.

26. Leighty AE, et al. Treatment outcomes of long-acting injectable naltrexone versus oral naltrexone in alcohol use disorder in veterans. *Ment Health Clin* 2019; **9**:392–396.

27. Krupitsky E, et al. Injectable extended-release naltrexone (XR-NTX) for opioid dependence: long-term safety and effectiveness. *Addiction* 2013; **108**:1628–1637.

28. Soyka M, et al. Comparing nalmefene and naltrexone in alcohol dependence: are there any differences? Results from an indirect meta-analysis. *Pharmacopsychiatry* 2016; **49**:66–75.

29. Palpacuer C, et al. Risks and benefits of nalmefene in the treatment of adult alcohol dependence: a systematic literature review and meta-analysis of published and unpublished double-blind randomized controlled trials. *PLoS Med* 2015; **12**:e1001924.

30. Kotake K, et al. Efficacy and safety of alcohol reduction pharmacotherapy according to treatment duration in patients with alcohol dependence or alcohol use disorder: a systematic review and network meta-analysis. *Addiction* 2024; **119**:815–832.

31. Mutschler J, et al. Current findings and mechanisms of action of disulfiram in the treatment of alcohol dependence. *Pharmacopsychiatry* 2016; **49**:137–141.

32. Bahji A, et al. Pharmacotherapies for adults with alcohol use disorders: a systematic review and network meta-analysis. *J Addict Med* 2022; **16**:630–638.

33. Agabio R, et al. Baclofen for alcohol use disorder. *Cochrane Database Syst Rev* 2023; **1**:CD012557.

34. Pani PP, et al. Anticonvulsants for alcohol dependence. *Cochrane Database Syst Rev* 2014; **2014**:CD008544.

35. Votaw VR, et al. An intensive longitudinal examination of topiramate treatment for alcohol use disorder: a secondary analysis of data from a randomized controlled trial. *Addiction* 2023; **118**:1040–1052.

36. Morley KC, et al. Topiramate versus naltrexone for alcohol use disorder: a genotype-stratified double-blind randomized controlled trial. *Am J Psychiatry* 2024; **181**:403–411.

37. Kranzler HR, et al. A meta-analysis of the efficacy of gabapentin for treating alcohol use disorder. *Addiction* 2019; **114**:1547–1555.

38. UK Teratology Information Service (UKTIS). 2024; www.UKTIS.org.

39. O'Malley SS, et al. Reduction of alcohol drinking in young adults by naltrexone: a double-blind, placebo-controlled, randomized clinical trial of efficacy and safety. *J Clin Psychiatry* 2015; **76**:e207–e213.

40. Miranda R, et al. Effects of naltrexone on adolescent alcohol cue reactivity and sensitivity: an initial randomized trial. *Addict Biol* 2014; **19**:941–954.

41. Roos CR, et al. Reward drinking and naltrexone treatment response among young adult heavy drinkers. *Addiction* 2021; **116**:2360–2371.

42. Joshi P, et al. Evaluation and management of alcohol use disorder among older adults. *Curr Geriatr Rep* 2021; **10**:82–90.

43. Gudin JA, et al. Risks, management, and monitoring of combination opioid, benzodiazepines, and/or alcohol use. *Postgrad Med* 2013; **125**:115–130.

44. Pettinati HM, et al. Gender differences with high-dose naltrexone in patients with co-occurring cocaine and alcohol dependence. *J Subst Abuse Treat* 2008; **34**:378–390.

45. Kampman KM, et al. A double-blind, placebo-controlled trial of topiramate for the treatment of comorbid cocaine and alcohol dependence. *Drug Alcohol Depend* 2013; **133**:94–99.

46. Public Health England. Better care for people with co-occurring mental health and alcohol/drug use conditions. A guide for commissioners and service providers. 2017; https://www.gov.uk/government/uploads/system/uploads/attachment_data/file/625809/Co-occurring_mental_health_and_alcohol_drug_use_conditions.pdf.

47. Agabio R, et al. Antidepressants for the treatment of people with co-occurring depression and alcohol dependence. *Cochrane Database Syst Rev* 2018; **4**:CD008581.

48. Stokes PRA, et al. Pharmacological treatment of mood disorders and comorbid addictions: a systematic review and meta-analysis: Traitement Pharmacologique des Troubles de L'humeur et des Dépendances Comorbides: une Revue Systématique et une Méta-Analyse. *Can J Psychiatry* 2020; **65**:749–769.

49. Di Nicola M, et al. Update on pharmacological treatment for comorbid major depressive and alcohol use disorders: the role of extended-release trazodone. *Curr Neuropharmacol* 2023; **21**:2195–2205.

50. Taylor D, et al. The cardiovascular safety of tricyclic antidepressants in overdose and in clinical use. *Ther Adv Psychopharmacol* 2024; **14**:20451253241243297.

51. Wood E, et al. Canadian guideline for the clinical management of high-risk drinking and alcohol use disorder. *CMAJ* 2023; **195**:E1364–E1379.

52. Pettinati HM, et al. A double-blind, placebo-controlled trial combining sertraline and naltrexone for treating co-occurring depression and alcohol dependence. *Am J Psychiatry* 2010; **167**:668–675.

53. Adamson SJ, et al. A randomized trial of combined citalopram and naltrexone for nonabstinent outpatients with co-occurring alcohol dependence and major depression. *J Clin Psychopharmacol* 2015; **35**:143–149.

54. Kelson M, et al. Ketamine treatment for alcohol use disorder: a systematic review. *Cureus* 2023; **15**:e38498.

55. Stedman M, et al. A double-blind, placebo-controlled study with quetiapine as adjunct therapy with lithium or divalproex in bipolar I patients with coexisting alcohol dependence. *Alcohol Clin Exp Res* 2010; **34**:1822–1831.

56. Ipser JC, et al. Pharmacotherapy for anxiety and comorbid alcohol use disorders. *Cochrane Database Syst Rev* 2015; **1**:CD007505.

57. Verplaetse TL, et al. Pharmacotherapy for co-occurring alcohol use disorder and post-traumatic stress disorder: targeting the opioidergic, noradrenergic, serotonergic, and GABAergic/glutamatergic systems. *Alcohol Res* 2018; **39**:193–205.

58. Morice CK, et al. Comorbid alcohol use and post-traumatic stress disorders: pharmacotherapy with aldehyde dehydrogenase 2 inhibitors versus current agents. *Prog Neuropsychopharmacol Biol Psychiatry* 2022; **115**:110506.

59. Brown & Burk UK Ltd. Summary of product characteristics. Disulfiram 200mg tablets. 2023 (last accessed August 2024); https://www.medicines.org.uk/emc/product/11168.

CHAPTER 4

Opioid dependence

Prescribing for opioid dependence

The treatment of opioid dependence is a rapidly changing and dynamic field. A decade or so ago, maintenance treatment with methadone was the dominant approach. The introduction of buprenorphine in different formulations, the positive experience of unsupervised consumption of opioids during the pandemic and the emergence of high-potency opioids in the illicit supply chain have contributed to a sea-change in practice.[1,2]

The pharmacological interventions used for opioid-dependent people in the UK and most developed countries include:

- Harm minimisation measures, e.g. take-home naloxone.
- Maintenance treatment with opioid substitution treatment (OST) such as methadone or buprenorphine (Box 4.4).
- Naltrexone for relapse prevention (although patient acceptability of this is low).

Box 4.4 Considerations when initiating opioid substitution treatment (OST)

- The aim of treatment is to minimise or abolish withdrawal symptoms without endangering the patient.
- All opioids are respiratory depressants.
- Prescribed opioids such as methadone and buprenorphine have low lethal doses in drug-naïve individuals.
- Even in patients prescribed them long term, tolerance can be lost over a matter of days.
- OST can be fatal, whereas opioid withdrawal is not life-threatening.
- The undoubted risk of opioid toxicity should be weighed against the risk of self-discharge from hospital against medical advice because of intolerable opiate withdrawal. Self-discharge carries risks, with an eightfold increased probability of drug-related death in the 2 days following self-discharge.[3] Opioid-dependent patients may also delay seeking care for their physical health problems because of the fear of withdrawal.[4]
- Non-specialist doctors should seek guidance either from established local protocols regarding initiation of opioid substitution (opioid agonist) treatment or from specialist drug services before prescribing opioid substitution treatment.
- The key patient safety questions to ask before you prescribe OST are:
  - *Is OST warranted (i.e. am I confident this patient is currently dependent on opioids)?*
  - *Am I confident that the patient will tolerate the dose of OST I am about to give them?*
  - It is important to document the reasoning for prescribing or not prescribing.

Treatment of opioid overdose

Opioid overdose is a preventable cause of death in the opioid-using population. This includes overdose of illicit opioids such as heroin and more potent opioids such as fentanyl and nitazenes, and overdose of prescribed opioids such as methadone or buprenorphine.

Opioid overdose is characterised clinically by the presence of:

- unconsciousness
- a low respiratory rate (<12)

- pin-point pupils
- cyanosis
- cold, clammy skin.

Naloxone is an opioid receptor antagonist that can reverse opioid overdose. It is available in pre-loaded syringes to give IM or IV or as a nasal spray.[4] For patients who have taken buprenorphine, fentanyl or nitazenes,[5,6] repeated naloxone boluses may be necessary to reverse toxicity because of their high affinity for opiate receptors.

Naloxone injection

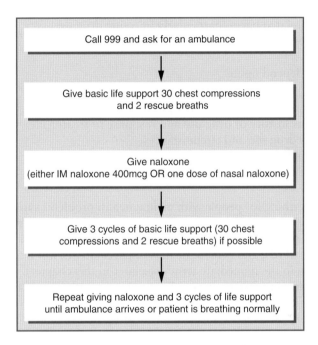

Figure 4.2 Flowchart for naloxone administration. Adapted from WHO (2014).[7]

Naloxone 400mcg IM/IV should be prescribed 'as required' for any in-patient with suspected harmful opioid use or dependence and should be kept in the resuscitation bag on the ward. *Anyone* can give naloxone to prevent an overdose death. Patients discharged from in-patient wards should be warned about loss of tolerance and they and their family members should be provided with naloxone training and take-home naloxone.[8] A summary of what to do in case of opioid overdose is shown in Figure 4.2 and training in take-home naloxone covers these actions.

Intranasal naloxone

Concentrated intranasal naloxone in doses of 2mg per kit is an alternative to intramuscular naloxone[4] with greater ease of use and acceptability to lay people.[9] The 2mg dose gives an equivalent time to onset of action to 400mcg IM but produces a longer lasting peak.[9,10]

CHAPTER 4

Opioid substitution treatment (OST)

The mainstay of pharmacological management of opioid dependence is OST. OST can be prescribed for detoxification, that is, at a dose to control withdrawal symptoms followed by progressive reduction and discontinuation. Alternatively, OST can be prescribed as 'maintenance', which refers to a longer period of months to years on a stable dose of OST.

The goals of OST are:

- To reduce or prevent withdrawal symptoms.
- To reduce or eliminate non-prescribed drug use.
- To stabilise drug intake and lifestyle.
- To reduce drug-related harm (particularly injecting drug use).
- To engage and provide an opportunity to work with the patient.

Treatment will depend upon:

- What pharmacotherapies and/or other interventions are available.
- Patient's previous history of drug use and response to treatment.
- Patient's current drug use and circumstances.
- Physical comorbidity.
- Location/service where treatment is initiated.

Most OST prescribing for people with mental health problems should be initiated by specialist addiction services alongside appropriate psychiatric care from mental health services.[8,11] Some people with opioid dependence will be admitted to psychiatric or general in-patient wards, and general or liaison psychiatrists will need to take over or initiate prescribing in the immediate term[8] (see later in this chapter).

Clinicians should take care to ensure that patients are physiologically dependent on opioids before initiating OST. There should be clear clinical evidence of opioid withdrawal and, if possible, a positive urine drug screen and documented *recent* on-going opioid substitution treatment (e.g. information from drug service or dispensing pharmacy, recently dated and named methadone bottles).

Assessment should involve the following:

- Which opioids the person is taking, and in what amounts.
- What other drugs are used, including alcohol and other depressants (e.g. gabapentinoids, benzodiazepines).
- Frequency, quantity and route of administration of all substances used.
- Time of last use.
- Physical comorbidity that may affect prescribing decisions such as chronic obstructive pulmonary disease (COPD) and cardiac conditions.
- Prescribed medication, which can interact with OST – such as respiratory depressants and those that prolong QT interval.
- Previous experience of treatment.
- Previous overdoses and whether these were intentional or accidental.
- Whether or not they have take-home naloxone.

- Whether or not there are objective signs of opioid withdrawal using a validated scale such as OOWS or COWS (see below).
- Examination of injection sites if they inject.
- Collateral information from addiction services and/or pharmacy in respect to usual dose of OST and most recently dispensed dose.

Timecourse of withdrawal symptoms

Withdrawal is dependent on duration of use, degree of dependence and type of opioid used (Table 4.9). Buprenorphine-related withdrawal symptoms tend to be milder than those from full agonist opioids, even when high-dose buprenorphine is abruptly discontinued.[12,13] Tapering over 4 weeks before complete discontinuation is associated with considerably less withdrawal than more rapid tapers.[14] Early indications are that buprenorphine long-acting injection is not associated with clinically significant withdrawal symptoms.[15]

Specific opioid withdrawal scales are freely available, such as the Clinical Opiate Withdrawal Scale (COWS)[16] or Objective Opiate Withdrawal Scale (OOWS)[17] which can be used to help assess withdrawal (Table 4.10).

Prescribing OST safely

- Use licensed medications for treatment of heroin dependence (i.e. methadone and buprenorphine).
- Ensure that the patient is dependent on opioids.
- Give a safe initial dose (see later in this chapter) and titrate cautiously.
- Use daily supervised consumption in those patients with a higher risk of overdose during dose initiation.

Induction and stabilisation of OST maintenance medication

Methadone and buprenorphine are the OST medications recommended by NICE in the UK for maintenance substitute prescribing and are effective in treating withdrawal symptoms and decreasing use of illicit opioids.[18] Methadone and buprenorphine are Controlled Drugs with high dependency potential. Methadone in particular has a low lethal dose. For these reasons, there are special documentation requirements, including specifying the patient's name, date of birth and address on prescriptions and writing the daily dose amount and total amount prescribed in both numbers and words. Instructions such as the requirement for consumption to be supervised should also be specified, for example 'daily supervised consumption'.[8]

Table 4.9 Timing of withdrawal symptoms of different opioids.

Drug	Onset	Peak	End
Heroin	4–6 hours	32–72 hours	5 days
Methadone	12–24 hours	4–6 days	Up to 40 days[19]
Buprenorphine (sublingual)	24–48 hours	3–5 days	8–10 days[13,20]

CHAPTER 4

Table 4.10 Clinical Opiate Withdrawal Scale (COWS).

Resting pulse rate: _____beats/min
Measured after patient is sitting or lying for 1 minute:
0 – pulse rate 80 or below
1 – pulse rate 81–100
2 – pulse rate 101–120
4 – pulse rate greater than 120

GI upset
Over last 30 minutes:
0 – no GI symptoms
1 – stomach cramps
2 – nausea or loose stool
3 – vomiting or diarrhoea
5 – multiple episodes of diarrhoea or vomiting

Sweating
Over past 30 minutes not accounted for by room temperature or patient activity:
0 – no report of chills or flushing
1 – subjective report of chills or flushing
2 – flushed or observable moistness on face
3 – beads of sweat on brow or face
4 – sweat streaming off face

Tremor
Observation of outstretched hands:
0 – no tremor
1 – tremor can be felt, but not observed
2 – slight tremor observable
4 – gross tremor or muscle twitching

Restlessness
Observation during assessment:
0 – able to sit still
1 – reports difficulty sitting still, but is able to do so
3 – frequent shifting or extraneous movements of legs/arms
5 – unable to sit still for more than a few seconds

Yawning
Observation during assessment:
0 – no yawning
1 – yawning once or twice during assessment
2 – yawning three or more times during assessment
4 – yawning several times/minute

Pupil size
0 – pupils pinned or normal size for room light
1 – pupils possibly larger than normal for room light
2 – pupils moderately dilated
5 – pupils so dilated that only the rim of the iris is visible

Anxiety or irritability
0 – none
1 – patient reports increasing irritability or anxiousness
2 – patient obviously irritable or anxious
4 – patient so irritable or anxious that participation in the assessment is difficult

Bone or joint aches
If patient was having pain previously, only the additional component attributed to opiates withdrawal is scored:
0 – not present
1 – mild diffuse discomfort
2 – patient reports severe diffuse aching of joints/muscles
4 – patient is rubbing joints or muscles and is unable to sit still because of discomfort

Gooseflesh skin:
0 – skin is smooth
3 – piloerection of skin can be felt or hairs standing up on arms
5 – prominent piloerection

Runny nose or tearing
Not accounted for by cold symptoms or allergies:
0 – not present
1 – nasal stuffiness or unusually moist eyes
2 – nose running or tearing
4 – nose constantly running or tears streaming down cheeks

Scores
5–12: mild withdrawal
13–24: moderate withdrawal
25–36: moderately severe withdrawal
More than 36: severe withdrawal

Total score: _____
(The total score is the sum of all 11 items)

The pharmacology of methadone and buprenorphine differs. Methadone is a full agonist at mu opioid receptors while buprenorphine is a partial agonist. This difference in pharmacology dictates the advantages and disadvantages of each drug (Table 4.11). The therapeutic dose (i.e. the dose at which treatment is associated with cessation of heroin use) for methadone is usually 60–100mg per day. The therapeutic dose for buprenorphine is between 12 and 24mg per day.

Table 4.11 Choosing between buprenorphine and methadone.

	Methadone	Sublingual buprenorphine
Safety	Associated with a reduced risk of mortality relative to being out of treatment[21] but with increased mortality during induction[22] Possible increased methadone-related mortality in those over 45[21] Increased risk of drug-related deaths in those with cardiovascular or respiratory comorbidity[21] Increased methadone-related death when directly supervised consumption (DSC) is replaced with take-home dosing[23]	No increased risk during induction[22] No increased mortality with age[21] Lower drug-related mortality than methadone in cardiovascular or respiratory comorbidity[21] No increase in buprenorphine-related deaths above expected trends when DSC replaced with take-home dosing[23]
Withdrawal syndrome	Appears to be more marked and prolonged	Has a milder withdrawal syndrome[19]
Titration	Associated with increased mortality during the titration phase[22] hence the need for gradual titration over a few weeks to reach therapeutic range (usually 60–100mg a day)	Able to reach therapeutic dose (12–16mg a day) within 2–3 days Risk of precipitated withdrawal if patients are not already in withdrawal when buprenorphine is initiated although this is infrequent (<1%)[24] and can be mitigated (see below)
Differences in retention	Greater retention in treatment than buprenorphine[25]	Associated with greater drop-out from treatment than methadone (applies to both high-dose and low-dose buprenorphine)
Differences in adverse effects	Risk of QT prolongation[26]	Less sedating than methadone (can be seen as undesirable by patients)[8]
Drug interactions	Methadone is largely metabolised by CYP3A4 and thus is affected by drugs that inhibit (e.g. cannabis[27,28]) or induce CYP3A4.[29]	As for methadone
Pregnancy	Widely used in pregnancy	Buprenorphine is associated with less severe neonatal withdrawal symptoms[30] and lower incidence of congenital abnormalities.[30] However, buprenorphine should not be initiated in pregnancy even if switching from methadone because of the risk of inducing withdrawal in the fetus.
Diversion	Patients at greater risk of diversion of medication (e.g. past history of this; treatment in a prison setting)[31] may be better served with methadone treatment (although buprenorphine long-acting injection has a low risk of buprenorphine diversion).	Sublingual buprenorphine tablets can be more easily diverted with the risk of tablets being injected.[32]

In rare cases, patients may be allergic to methadone or buprenorphine or to some of the constituents within the formulations.

Methadone

Initiation in all settings

- Do not prescribe/dispense to a patient who is clinically intoxicated with opioids or other drugs (including alcohol).
- Only prescribe as a 1mg/mL solution.
- Do not prescribe tablets as these can be crushed and injected.
- Describe supervision accurately, for example 'directly supervised consumption' or 'take away three times per week'.

Importance of context to methadone titration schedules

Methadone is associated with an increased risk of death during titration, because:

- It is a full agonist.
- Assessing dose equivalence with street heroin is difficult.
- There is wide inter-individual pharmacokinetic variation.
- Repeated dosing is associated with substantial accumulation with steady state only reached after about five doses of methadone.[33,34]

Thus for safety reasons, methadone titration schedules are usually conservative. However, ensuring safe methadone titration is context-dependent, in that the consequences of uncontrolled opioid withdrawal and consequent disengagement need to be considered.

Methadone in general hospital settings

Fear of inadequate treatment of opioid withdrawal during general hospital admissions has led to people with opioid dependence not seeking help for their physical health problems or seeking help only when desperate.[10] There is an elevated (fourfold) risk of drug-related death associated with hospital discharge and even more so for discharge against medical advice (almost eightfold increase).[3] The general hospital is also a setting where more doses can be administered within 24 hours (e.g. 4–6 hourly), where respiration and oxygen saturations can be monitored with a greater frequency than in other contexts and more sophisticated respiratory support and sustained naloxone reversal can be provided.

All these factors may allow a more aggressive methadone protocol (Table 4.12), with the caveat that a slower protocol may be necessary for those with head injuries, acute respiratory compromise, hepatic or renal failure, or co-prescription of other sedating drugs (e.g. medicated detoxification from alcohol using benzodiazepines).

Methadone in psychiatric hospital settings

Psychiatric hospital settings are different from general hospital settings in that familiarity with opioids and naloxone is lower, intensive physical health monitoring is less feasible and other sedating medications (antipsychotics, benzodiazepines) are routinely

Table 4.12 Methadone titration where extent of prior use is unknown or unconfirmed.

Setting	Procedure
General hospital	Initial dose of 10–20mg with further doses of 5–10mg every 6 hours if withdrawal persists (according to COWS or OOWS), up to 40mg in 24 hours. In the second 24 hours, the total dose used in the first 24 hours should be given as a split dose. Increase by 10mg every 2 days, monitoring withdrawal, sedation and respiratory depression. Maximum increase from day 1 dose over 1 week is 30mg. Consider split dosing.
Psychiatric hospital	Initial dose of 10–20mg on day 1. Increase by 10mg every 2 days, monitoring withdrawal, sedation and respiratory depression. Maximum increase from day 1 dose over 1 week is 30mg. Consider split dosing.
Community drug service	Initially, 10–30mg on day 1. Increase by 10mg every couple of days, monitoring withdrawal, sedation and respiratory depression. Maximum increase from day 1 dose over 1 week is 30mg.

given alongside methadone. This does *not* mean that methadone should be withheld – the risk of drug-related death following psychiatric hospital discharge is too great. All efforts should be directed at (re-)establishing methadone treatment and avoiding loss of tolerance to opioids. Generally, methadone titration in the psychiatric setting is more cautious (Table 4.12).

> **Important:** All patients starting a methadone treatment programme must be informed of the risks of toxicity and overdose, and the necessity for safe storage of any take-home medication.[8] Safe storage is vital, particularly if there are children in the household, as tragic deaths have occurred when children have ingested methadone. Prescribers should consider risks to children in all assessments and treatment plans of drug-using patients.

Cautions with methadone

Intoxication

Methadone should not be given to any patient showing signs of intoxication due to alcohol or other CNS depressant drugs (e.g. benzodiazepines)[35,36] as the risk of fatal overdose is greatly enhanced when concurrent methadone is taken.[37,38] Concurrent alcohol and both prescribed and illicit drug consumption must be borne in mind when considering subsequent prescribing of methadone. This is because of the increased risk of overdose associated with simultaneous use of several respiratory depressants.[39]

Severe hepatic/renal dysfunction

Metabolism and elimination of methadone may be affected in advanced liver disease.[40] The dose or dosing interval should be adjusted accordingly against clinical presentation. Because of extended plasma half-life, the interval between assessments during initial dosing may need to be extended. Around 20% of methadone is eliminated via the renal route. Renal disease does not affect methadone elimination as in such conditions it is excreted exclusively via the biliary route. However, patients with advanced renal disease are more sensitive to sedation caused by methadone. Thus, for those with glomerular filtration rate (GFR) <15mL/min or creatinine >700 mmol/L, a reduction of 50% in methadone dose should be considered.[41]

Methadone overdose

In the event of methadone overdose, **naloxone** should be administered as described in the section on opioid overdose earlier in this chapter.

Methadone and risk of torsades de pointes/QT interval prolongation

Methadone, either alone or combined with other QT-prolonging agents, may increase the likelihood of QT interval prolongation, which is associated with torsades de pointes and can be fatal.[26,42–44]

Recommended ECG monitoring

There is insufficient evidence to support the effectiveness of QT screening in preventing cardiac death in people prescribed methadone.[45] However, in the UK, the Medicines and Healthcare products Regulatory Agency (MHRA) recommends that patients with the following risk factors for QT interval prolongation receive regular electrocardiogram (ECG) monitoring while receiving methadone:

- heart disease
- liver disease
- dose of >100mg per day
- electrolyte abnormalities
- concomitant CYP3A4 inhibitor treatment
- concomitant medication that prolongs QT (e.g. certain antipsychotics and antidepressants, erythromycin).

Other factors that may also increase risk of QT prolongation are:

- cocaine use[46]
- synthetic cannabinoid receptor agonist (SCRA) use[47]
- eating disorder or malnutrition[48]
- human immunodeficiency virus (HIV) positive status.[48]

Individuals with the risk factors listed above should have a baseline ECG and subsequent ECG monitoring. This is especially the case in in-patient settings where ECGs are easily obtained. However, where patients refuse to attend for an ECG, the risk of stopping methadone should be weighed against the risk of continuing without QT data. There is no evidence base guiding frequency following initiation. Annual checks in the absence of cardiac symptomatology would be a reasonable minimum frequency. It is also important to check the actions of any medications being prescribed with methadone for CYP3A4 inhibitory activity, to inform the risk–benefit analysis when commencing methadone. Actions following a finding of prolonged QT interval are summarised in Table 4.13.

Buprenorphine

Buprenorphine is a synthetic partial opioid agonist with low intrinsic activity and high affinity at mu opioid receptors. This means that it produces less euphoria even at receptor-saturating doses and simultaneously blocks the action of other opioids. It is an effective treatment for heroin and prescribed opioid addiction although no more effective

Table 4.13 Recommended ECG monitoring for people taking methadone.

	Borderline prolonged QTc	Action	Prolonged QTc	Action	Very prolonged QTc	Action
Females	≥470ms	Repeat ECG Electrolytes Try to modify QT risk factors, e.g. cocaine use, SCRA use, methadone dose, psychotropic medications Regular ECG until normal	≥500ms	Repeat ECG Electrolytes Try to modify QT risk factors Seek cardiology and addictions advice Reduce methadone dose If long QTc despite reduction, switch to buprenorphine Regular ECGs until normal	≥550ms	Urgent cardiology and addictions advice Repeat ECG Electrolytes Try to modify QT risk factors Reduce methadone and re-evaluate within the week; switch to buprenorphine in in-patient setting
Males	≥440ms					

SCRA, synthetic cannabinoid receptor agonist.

than methadone.[49] It is associated with lower likelihood of retention in treatment than methadone[25] and clinical experience with buprenorphine suggests it can be difficult to initiate using conventional methods because of the need for sufficient withdrawal symptoms to start, but not so much withdrawal that it prevents attendance at the treatment centre. This has been addressed by novel micro- and macro-induction methods (see later). It has also been found to be effective in reducing prescription opioid use and improving treatment adherence in prescription opioid-dependent patients.

Sublingual buprenorphine

Buprenorphine is absorbed via the sublingual route, and this has long been the most used route of administration.[50,51] Each tablet takes approximately 5–10 minutes to disintegrate, dissolve and be absorbed. It is effective in treating opioid dependence because of the following:

- It alleviates/prevents opioid withdrawal and craving.
- It reduces the effects of additional opioid use because of its high receptor affinity – what patients refer to as a 'blocking' effect.[52,53]
- It is long-acting, allowing daily (or less frequent) dosing. The duration of action is related to the buprenorphine dose administered: low doses (e.g. 2mg) exert effects for up to 12 hours; higher doses (e.g. 16–32mg) exert effects for as long as 48–72 hours, allowing thrice weekly dosing.[54]

Different brands of oral buprenorphine and bioavailability

Espranor is a brand of buprenorphine that is increasingly used in UK community addictions services. Espranor is placed on the tongue, not under it. The pharmacokinetics of

Table 4.14 Conversion from buprenorphine to Espranor.

Buprenorphine sublingual	Espranor orodispersible
8mg	6mg
10mg	8mg
12mg	10mg
14/16mg	12mg
18mg	14mg
20/22mg	16mg
>26mg	18mg

buprenorphine show quite wide inter-individual variation and this variability is accommodated by titrating people against their personal therapeutic response. Table 4.14 shows the conversion from buprenorphine or other brands of buprenorphine to Espranor, based on clinical experience.

Given the uncertainty regarding dose equivalence, it is prudent not to switch between brands without good cause.

Conventional buprenorphine induction

The same principles apply as for methadone initiation. Proof of recent use is more difficult for buprenorphine because it is not included in standard multiple urine drug testing kits. It is commonly identified using a separate urine drug screen kit, which is not usually available outside addiction services. Therefore, collateral information from the addiction service or the dispensing pharmacy is essential if continuing buprenorphine in a non-specialist setting.

Of particular interest with buprenorphine is the phenomenon of *precipitated withdrawal*. Precipitated withdrawal occurs because buprenorphine is a partial agonist with a high receptor affinity. If it enters the brain when a full agonist (e.g. methadone or heroin) is still present it competes for binding at the opioid receptors and replaces the full agonist. Some receptors previously fully stimulated become partly stimulated. The patient experiences this change as opioid withdrawal. However, if the patient is *already in withdrawal*, they will experience the addition of a partial agonist as relief of that withdrawal. Patient education is an important factor in reducing the problems during induction.

To summarise, buprenorphine is a partial agonist with higher affinity for opioid receptors than pure agonists. If given to someone with high occupancy of opioid receptors by full agonists, the net effect will be a reduction in agonist activity and withdrawal symptoms may result. If receptor occupancy by pure agonists is so low that withdrawal symptoms are already evident, then giving buprenorphine will have the effect of increasing overall opioid receptor stimulation and withdrawal symptoms will abate. When a full agonist is given to someone maintained on buprenorphine, the net effect is usually nothing: buprenorphine cannot be dislodged by lower affinity agonists. This is the 'blocking effect' of buprenorphine. Adding a full agonist to buprenorphine does not (and indeed could not) precipitate withdrawal. This may seem obvious, but the belief that agonists can provoke withdrawal is apparently widely held.

The initial dose recommendations are as follows:[8]

- Patient in withdrawal and no risk factors: 8mg buprenorphine.
- Patient not experiencing withdrawal and no risk factors: 4mg buprenorphine.
- Patient has concomitant risk factors (e.g. medical condition, polydrug use, low or uncertain severity of dependence, psychiatric medications): 2–4mg buprenorphine.

No more than 8mg buprenorphine should be given on the first day in a non-specialist setting. In some cases, 8mg may be sufficient, but this may need to be increased to 12–16mg the following day if there is no evidence of intoxication. The doses can be given in divided doses so that they can be reviewed promptly in the event of any intoxication, although in practice this is difficult in the absence of on-site dispensing. For maintenance, the 'Orange Book'[8] recommends a dose between 12 and 24mg a day.

If patients are on other respiratory depressants such as benzodiazepines, the patient should be monitored for intoxication and respiratory depression.

Low-dose induction for buprenorphine initiation

In North America, the fentanyl epidemic has led to the development of innovations to facilitate initiation of buprenorphine. These include a low-dose induction technique that involves a slower titration of buprenorphine in a patient who is still actively using full opioid agonists and is not in withdrawal.[55] The protocols are similar to those discussed later in the section on methadone to buprenorphine transfer.

Prolonged-release buprenorphine injection

A prolonged-release subcutaneous buprenorphine injection (trade name Buvidal in the UK and EU, Sublocade and others in the USA and Australia) is licensed in the UK in weekly and monthly injectable form (Table 4.15). In Australia, the proportion of patients prescribed buprenorphine in depot form has grown from around 4% in 2019 to around 50% in 2022[51] and expansion of the use of buprenorphine long-acting injections is part of the 10-year drug strategy in England.[50]

Table 4.15 Conventional sublingual buprenorphine daily treatment doses and recommended corresponding doses of weekly and monthly Buvidal.

Dose of daily sublingual buprenorphine	Dose of weekly Buvidal	Dose of monthly Buvidal
2–6mg	8mg	
8–10mg	16mg	64mg
12–16mg	24mg	96mg
18–24mg	32mg	128mg

CHAPTER 4

Buprenorphine depot injection offers the same benefits as sublingual buprenorphine. It has a sustained release, and some patients find it reduces the noticeable peaks and troughs experienced on sublingual buprenorphine. Contraindications to prolonged-release buprenorphine injection are:

- Hypersensitivity or allergy to active substance or excipients.
- Severe hepatic impairment.
- Alcohol dependence and delirium tremens.

Adverse effects relate in the main to the delivery of the medication, with injection site reactions (pain, a lump) being the most common.

Long-acting buprenorphine may be more effective than sublingual buprenorphine. While early randomised controlled trials (RCTs) tested non-inferiority to sublingual buprenorphine, a recent trial testing superiority of Sublocade found superior retention, higher odds of early remission from opioid use disorder, reduced or absent craving and better clinician- and patient-reported outcomes for depot buprenorphine.[56] Sustained abstinence rates following buprenorphine depot medication were around 70% at 18 months. The longer the period on buprenorphine depot, the greater the proportion of patients who sustained abstinence.[57]

Transferring from methadone to buprenorphine

This should usually be done under the supervision of a specialist prescriber. Patients transferring from methadone are at risk of experiencing precipitated withdrawal symptoms that may continue at some level for 1–2 weeks. Available evidence, albeit of low quality, suggests that conventional methods, which involve stopping methadone either at the stable dose or following a fixed or flexible taper of methadone, are successful in the majority of cases.[58] Failure is associated with a methadone dose of >60mg per day.

Recently, different techniques have been tried to facilitate transfer without the need for precipitating withdrawal. These include:

- Bridging techniques, using opioids such as oxycodone or non-opioids such as ketamine.[59]
- Low-dose induction of buprenorphine, where buprenorphine is slowly titrated to a therapeutic dose while methadone remains at 100% of starting dose, with methadone tapered subsequently.[60]

Conventional transfer: transferring from methadone dose <40 mg to buprenorphine

Methadone should be ceased abruptly, and the first dose of buprenorphine given at least 24 hours after the last methadone dose. The following conversion rates at the start of treatment are recommended but higher buprenorphine doses may be subsequently needed depending on clinical presentation (Table 4.16).

Table 4.16 Transferring from methadone to oral buprenorphine.

Last methadone dose	Day 1: initial buprenorphine dose	Day 2: buprenorphine dose
20–40mg	4mg	6–8mg
10–20mg	4mg	4–8mg
1–10mg	2mg	2–4mg

Transferring from methadone 40–60mg to buprenorphine

Either immediately stop methadone and transfer directly to buprenorphine, or taper to 30mg methadone following a fixed or patient-led plan (evidence does not favour one over the other[58]). The first buprenorphine dose is usually delayed until the patient displays clear signs of withdrawal, generally 48–96 hours after the last dose of methadone.

An initial dose of 2–4mg should be given. The patient should then be reviewed 2–3 hours later. If withdrawal has been precipitated or worsened, further symptomatic medication can be prescribed. If there has been no precipitation or worsening of withdrawal, an additional 2–4mg of buprenorphine can be given on the same day. The patient should be reviewed the following day at which point the dose should be increased to between 8 and 12mg.

Alternatively, a technique of continuing to increase the buprenorphine on day 1 until withdrawal symptoms subside has also been reported as successful in a case report, but this relies on high levels of trust in the therapeutic relationship.[61]

Transferring from methadone doses >60mg to buprenorphine

Such transfers should not be attempted in an out-patient setting except in exceptional circumstances by an experienced practitioner. Usually, patients would be partially detoxified from methadone and transferred to buprenorphine when the methadone was at or below 30mg daily. However, if transfer from higher dose methadone to buprenorphine is required, a referral to a dedicated addictions in-patient unit should be considered where possible.

Transfer from low-dose methadone to buprenorphine

Case series of low-dose induction using varying protocols has been reported (Table 4.17). Most are in-patient based, although there is some evidence that it can also be done in the community with remote monitoring.[62] Protocols using transdermal buprenorphine patches initially or alongside sublingual buprenorphine have also been published.[63] The schedules for reducing methadone following establishment of therapeutic doses of buprenorphine also vary widely, some suggesting a dead stop from 100% original dose and some a rapid reduction (e.g. reduce to 50%, then stop). Few studies report withdrawal phenomena in detail or how these relate to the pharmacokinetics of the two opioids.

CHAPTER 4

Table 4.17 Example protocols for transition from low-dose methadone to buprenorphine.

Study	Daily dose (mg)									
	Day 1	2	3	4	5	6	7	8	9	10
Terasaki et al. 2019[64]	0.5	0.5 twice daily	1 twice daily	4 twice daily	8	8+4	12		Titrate	
Tay Wee Teck et al. 2021[62]	0.4	0.4	0.8	1.2	1.6	1.6	2	4	6	8–12
Weimer et al. 2021[65]	≈0.5 once daily (buccal 0.225 twice daily)	≈0.5 twice daily (buccal 0.225 twice daily)	≈1 twice daily (buccal 0.45 twice daily)	2 twice daily	4 twice daily	4 three times a day	4–8 twice daily			
Bhatraju et al. 2022[66]	0.5 once daily	0.5 twice daily	1 twice daily	2 twice daily	4 twice daily	8	8+4	8 twice daily		
Anderson et al. 2023[67]	0.5 once daily	0.5 twice daily	1 twice daily	2 twice daily	3 twice daily	4 twice daily	6 twice daily	8 twice daily	12/8	12/8

Transferring from prescription opioids to buprenorphine

Evidence is accruing in the treatment of prescribed opioid dependence with buprenorphine. Buprenorphine improves adherence to drug treatment and reduces prescription opioid misuse.[68] In the UK, the 'Orange Book' recommends that small divided doses are given to establish the dose required for stabilisation.[59]

Less than daily dosing with buprenorphine

Buprenorphine is licensed in most countries as a medication to be taken daily. International evidence and experience indicate that many clients can be comfortably maintained on one dose every 2–3 days.[54,69] This has been considered pertinent for patients in buprenorphine treatment who are considered unsuitable for take-away medication because of the risk of diversion but it may well be replaced by long-acting formulations.

The following conversion rate is recommended:

- 2-day buprenorphine dose = 2 x daily dose of buprenorphine (to a max. 32mg)
- 3-day buprenorphine dose = 3 x daily dose of buprenorphine (to a max. 32mg)

In the event of patients being unable to stabilise comfortably on buprenorphine (often those transferring from methadone), the option of transferring to methadone should be available. Methadone can be commenced 24 hours after the last buprenorphine dose. Doses should be titrated cautiously according to clinical response, being mindful of the residual 'blockade' effect of buprenorphine, which may last for several days, meaning that methadone toxicity can occur in a delayed manner.

Cautions with buprenorphine

Intoxication
Buprenorphine should normally not be given to any patient showing signs of intoxication, especially due to alcohol or other depressant drugs (e.g. benzodiazepines, sedating antipsychotics, pregabalin). Buprenorphine in combination with other sedative drugs can result in respiratory depression, sedation and coma. Nonetheless, buprenorphine is usually preferred to methadone in these clinical situations.

Liver function
There is some evidence suggesting that high-dose buprenorphine can cause changes in liver function in individuals with a history of liver disease and can rarely cause hepatitis.[70,71] Such patients should have LFTs measured before commencing with follow-up investigations conducted 6–12 weeks after commencing buprenorphine. More frequent testing should be considered in patients of particular concern (e.g. with severe liver disease). Elevated liver enzymes in the absence of clinically significant liver disease, however, does not necessarily contraindicate treatment with buprenorphine and if the patient refuses or it is practically difficult to obtain LFTs, the risk of withholding treatment should be weighed against the risk of prescribing without LFTs.

Overdose with buprenorphine
Buprenorphine (as a single drug in overdose) is generally regarded as safer than methadone and heroin because in experimental studies it causes no respiratory depression at up to 8mg[72] and is less likely to be associated with overdose death. However, in combination with other respiratory depressant drugs the effects may be harder to manage.[73] Higher than standard doses of naloxone may be needed to reverse buprenorphine overdose, with the optimal dose being between 2 and 4mg and a possible diminishing effect beyond 5mg.[6,74] As a consequence, ventilator support is often required in cases where buprenorphine is contributing to respiratory depression (e.g. in polydrug overdose).

Buprenorphine with naloxone (Suboxone)

Suboxone is a buprenorphine/naloxone combination preparation that may reduce the risk of diversion and injection. The different sublingual and parenteral absorption profiles of buprenorphine and naloxone are the key factor. If used sublingually, the naloxone component will have a negligible effect, but buprenorphine will be absorbed and act as usual. However, if Suboxone is injected, the naloxone will have a substantial antagonist effect and will attenuate the effects of the buprenorphine and is also likely to precipitate withdrawal in opioid-dependent individuals using full opioid agonists.

Alternative oral opioid preparations

Oral methadone and buprenorphine continue to be the mainstay of treatment.[8] Other oral options such as slow-release oral morphine (SROM) preparations and dihydrocodeine are not licensed in the UK for the treatment of opiate dependence. These alternatives can be considered in exceptional cases where clients are unable to tolerate methadone or buprenorphine. Note the short half-life, supervision requirements and diversion potential.[8]

SROM preparations have been shown elsewhere in Europe to be useful as maintenance therapy in those who fail to tolerate methadone, again only for prescribing by specialised clinicians.[8] A review of studies on SROM suggested that there was insufficient evidence to assess the effectiveness of this treatment.[75]

Injectable diamorphine

There is compelling evidence supporting the use of injectable diamorphine maintenance for the treatment of patients who fail to benefit from first-line OST.[76] Contemporary injectable prescribing differs from the earlier practice of prescribing unsupervised injectable opioids in that the patient must:

- Attend in person for their prescribed injectable opioid maintenance treatment – daily or more frequently, according to the treatment plan.
- Inject their dose under the direct supervision of a competent member of staff.
- Be given no take-away injectable medication.

In the UK the prescribing doctor must have a licence from the Home Office to prescribe diamorphine for opioid dependence. Oral OST is prescribed for those days when supervised injectable treatment is not available. This treatment differs from 'injecting rooms' – safe places with sterile equipment for people who use intravenous drugs but who are usually not in treatment – in that it is part of a holistic package of care with adjunctive psychosocial interventions. Although its cost-effectiveness has been demonstrated,[77] its implementation has been limited by various factors including high set-up costs.

At present, people should only be considered for injectable opioid prescribing in combination with psychosocial interventions, as part of a wider package of care. It is an option in cases where the individual has not responded adequately to oral opioid substitution treatment, where it can be supported by the necessary provisions for supervised consumption.[8,78] Patients are seen for supervised injecting in a specialist facility twice a day. Doctors caring for patients who are admitted to the acute hospital on diamorphine prescription will need to consult their local policies – ordinarily a documented conversation with the prescribing community addiction psychiatrist is sufficient to continue the prescription.

Where withdrawal symptoms occur on stopping OST or other opioids, Table 4.18 gives some advice on the treatment of specific symptoms.

Table 4.18 Treatment of withdrawal symptoms in people taking opioids. Adapted from Department of Health and Social Care (2017).[8]

Symptom	Treatment
Diarrhoea	Loperamide 4mg then 2mg after each loose stool; maximum 16mg daily for up to 5 days
Nausea, vomiting	Metoclopramide 10mg tds for a maximum of 5 days or prochlorperazine 5mg tds or 12.5mg IM bd
Abdominal cramps	Mebeverine 135mg tds
Agitation, anxiety and insomnia	Diazepam up to 5–10mg tds when required or zopiclone 7.5mg nocte for patients with a history of benzodiazepine dependence
Muscular pains and headaches	Paracetamol, aspirin or non-steroidal anti-inflammatories Topical rubefacients can be helpful in relieving muscle aches from methadone withdrawal.

Prescribing psychotropic medications in patients with opiate dependence

General psychiatrists often see and treat patients with addictions and psychiatric comorbidity. Prescribing guidelines regarding the treatment of comorbid psychiatric conditions pharmacologically can be found in the British Association of Psychopharmacology guidelines for substance misuse.[79]

Some general guidance is as follows:

- Prescribers should be cautious about prescribing sedating medications because of the increased risk of respiratory depression. For example, pregabalin greatly increases the risk of overdose death.[37,80] Pregabalin and olanzapine also appear to have an abuse liability in the opioid-dependent population.[81,82]
- Patients with opiate dependence suffer disproportionately from depression – about half of those entering treatment will meet the criteria for depression. They may require 20–50% higher doses of methadone than non-depressed patients to stabilise[83] but stabilisation may afford remission in a majority of cases.[84] There is limited clinical trial evidence of low to moderate quality regarding antidepressant use in opioid dependence which suggests that it is of limited benefit for either mood or drug use.[79,84] Positive studies have largely been those using medication with varied pharmacology such as tricyclic antidepressants (TCAs).[84] However, TCAs are not recommended in people with comorbid substance misuse because of their cardiotoxicity,[79] although lofepramine can probably be used if available.[85] The recommended approach to treatment of depression based on the evidence includes stabilising the patient on OST first, then if depression persists trying an SSRI because of their relative safety, but considering mixed pharmacology antidepressants as a second-line should the patient fail to respond.[84] Sertraline is probably the drug of choice in OST-treated patients as it has limited interaction potential.

CHAPTER 4

Opioid detoxification and reduction regimens

Opioid maintenance can be continued for a few weeks to almost indefinitely, depending on clinical need. Some patients are keen to detoxify after short periods of stability and other patients may decide to detoxify after longer periods on maintenance prescriptions. All detoxification programmes should be part of a care programme. Given the risk of serious fatal overdose after detoxification, services providing such treatment should educate the patient about these risks and supply them with naloxone and overdose training for emergency use.

In the UK, NICE guidelines state 'dose reduction can take place over anything from a few days to several months, with a higher initial stabilisation dose taking longer to taper' and indicate that 'up to 3 months is typical for methadone reduction, while buprenorphine reductions are typically carried out over 14 days to a few weeks'.[86] In practice, a detoxification in the community may extend over a longer period if this facilitates the client's comfort during the process, compliance with the care plan, continued abstinence from illicit use during detoxification and subsequent abstinence following detoxification.

Detoxification in an in-patient setting may take place over a shorter time than in the community (e.g. 14–21 days for methadone and 7–14 days for buprenorphine) 'as the supportive environment helps a service user to tolerate emerging withdrawal symptoms'.[87] As in the community, stabilisation on a dose of a substitute opioid is first achieved, followed by gradual dose reduction, with additive medications judiciously prescribed for withdrawal symptoms as needed.

Detoxification carries a recognised risk of relapse and fatal overdose. Therefore, if a patient is being detoxified there needs to be adequate aftercare in place, such as a rehabilitation programme and community support. For patients having emergency psychiatric or medical admissions, detoxification is not usually indicated unless with the support of specialist services and where aftercare arrangements are in place.

Opioid withdrawal in a community setting

Methadone withdrawal

Following a period of stabilisation with methadone or a longer period of maintenance, the patient and prescriber may agree a reduction programme as part of a care plan to reduce the daily methadone dose. The usual reduction would be by 5–10mg weekly or every 2 weeks, although there can be variation in the reduction and speed of reduction. In the community setting, patient preference is the most important variable in terms of dose reduction and rate of reduction. The detoxification programme should be reviewed regularly and remain flexible to adjustments and changes, such as relapse to illicit drug use or patient anxieties about speed of reduction. Factors such as an increase in heroin or other drug use or worsening of the patient's physical, psychological or social well-being may warrant a temporary increase or stabilisation of the dose or a slowing down of the reduction rate. Towards the end of the detoxification, the dose reduction may be slower: 1–2mg per week. A longer length of stability on maintenance treatment and prolonged reduction schedules (up to a year) substantially improve the chances of achieving abstinence.[88]

Buprenorphine withdrawal

The same principles as for methadone apply when planning a buprenorphine detoxification regimen. Dose reduction should be gradual to minimise withdrawal discomfort (Table 4.19).

Table 4.19 A suggested reduction regimen for buprenorphine.

Daily buprenorphine dose	Reduction rate
Above 16mg	4mg every 1–2 weeks
8–16mg	2–4mg every 1–2 weeks
2–8mg	2mg per week or fortnight
Below 2mg	0.4–0.8mg per week

Opioid withdrawal in a specialist addiction in-patient setting

Methadone

Patients should have a starting dose assessment of methadone over 48 hours by a specialist in-patient team. The dose may then be reduced following a linear regimen over up to 4 weeks.[86]

Buprenorphine

Buprenorphine can be used effectively for short-term in-patient detoxifications following the same principles as for methadone.

Naltrexone in relapse prevention

Trial evidence for the effectiveness of either oral or sustained-release naltrexone as a treatment for relapse prevention in opioid misusers has been inconclusive.[89,90] Naltrexone was found by NICE to be a cost-effective treatment strategy in aiding abstinence from opioid misuse for those who prefer an abstinence programme, are fully informed of the potential adverse effects and benefits of treatment, are highly motivated to remain on treatment, and have a partner supporting concordance.[91] Subsequently, Australian data indicated a threefold risk of mortality relative to methadone treatment following naltrexone cessation.[92] Almost all of the excess mortality was associated with overdose deaths after stopping naltrexone.

Close monitoring is particularly important when naltrexone is initiated because of the higher risk of fatal overdose at this and other times. Discontinuation of naltrexone is also associated with an increase in inadvertent overdose from illicit opioids. Postmortem data from Australia found that only 15.8% of those prescribed oral naltrexone had any naltrexone detected.[93] Thus, supervision of naltrexone administration and careful choice of who is prescribed it (those who are abstinence-focused and motivated) are very important. Although there have been concerns about people taking naltrexone experiencing adverse effects of unease (dysphoria), depression and insomnia, potentially leading to relapse to illicit opioid use or failure to continue on treatment, real-world evidence is mixed, with two studies finding no effect of naltrexone on mood and sleep[94,95] and one finding higher insomnia and distress in those patients who discontinued naltrexone.[96]

Initiating naltrexone

Naltrexone has the propensity to cause a severe withdrawal reaction in patients who are either currently taking opioid drugs or who were previously taking opioid drugs and in whom there has not been a sufficient wash-out period before administering naltrexone.

The minimum recommended interval between stopping the opioid and starting naltrexone depends on the opioid used, duration of use and the amount taken as a last dose. Opioid agonists with long half-lives such as methadone will require a wash-out period of up to 10 days, whereas shorter acting opioids such as heroin, morphine or fentanyl may only require up to 7 days. Experience with buprenorphine indicates that a wash-out period of up to 7 days is sufficient if the final buprenorphine dose is >2mg and duration of use >2 weeks. In some cases naltrexone may be started within 2–3 days of a patient stopping (e.g. if final buprenorphine dose <2mg and duration of use <2 weeks).

A test dose of naloxone (0.2–0.8mg) (which has a much shorter half-life than naltrexone) may be given to the patient as an IM dose before starting naltrexone treatment. Any withdrawal symptoms precipitated will be of shorter duration than if precipitated by naltrexone.

Patients *must* be advised of the risk of withdrawal before giving the dose (Box 4.5). It is worth thoroughly questioning the patient as to whether they have taken any opioid-containing preparation unknowingly (e.g. over-the-counter analgesic).

Box 4.5 Important points regarding prescribing naltrexone

- Ensure the recipient is fully informed of the increased risk of fatal opioid overdose.
- Following detoxification and any period of abstinence, an individual's tolerance to opioids will decrease markedly. At such a time, using opioids puts the individual at greatly increased risk of overdose.
- Discontinuation of naltrexone may also be associated with an increase in inadvertent overdose from illicit opioids, emphasising the need for close monitoring and support of the client at this time.

Dose of naltrexone

An initial dose of 25mg naltrexone should be administered after a suitable opioid-free interval (and naloxone challenge if appropriate). The patient should be monitored for 4 hours after the first dose for symptoms of opioid withdrawal. Symptomatic medication for withdrawal should be available for use, if necessary, on the first day of naltrexone dosing (withdrawal symptoms may last up to 4–8 hours). Once the patient has tolerated this low naltrexone dose, subsequent doses can be increased to 50mg daily as a maintenance dose.

Naltrexone is contraindicated in patients with hepatic dysfunction and liver function tests should be monitored during treatment.

Pain control in patients on OST

Analgesia for methadone-prescribed patients

Non-opioid analgesics should be used in preference (e.g. paracetamol, non-steroidal anti-inflammatory drugs [NSAIDs]) initially where appropriate. If opioid analgesia (e.g. codeine, dihydrocodeine, morphine) is indicated due to the type and severity of the pain then this should be titrated accordingly for pain relief in line with usual analgesic protocols. If an opioid analgesic is appropriate, a non-methadone opioid may be co-prescribed, i.e. it is not necessary to 'rationalise' the patient's entire opioid requirements to one drug.[97]

Analgesia for buprenorphine-prescribed patients

Patients taking buprenorphine will have a reduced effect of opioids including those prescribed for analgesia. While there are case reports detailing resolution of acute pain, or easier management of it, following buprenorphine discontinuation, head-to-head comparisons of stopping buprenorphine versus continuing buprenorphine show no superiority of one strategy over the other and there is no expert consensus. The British Peri-operative Pain and Addiction Interdisciplinary Network (PAIN) guidelines state that buprenorphine should be continued during periods of acute pain, for example perioperatively.[98] If a patient on buprenorphine requires treatment for acute pain, non-opioid analgesia and regional anaesthetic techniques should be used and an additional opioid added if needed.[98] The Australian guidelines include an option to use a more potent opioid (e.g. fentanyl) with the rationale that it may displace buprenorphine.[99] The PAIN guidelines state that there is insufficient evidence to choose one full agonist over another.

If standard pain approaches do not cause a resolution of the pain, consider reducing the dose of buprenorphine. The Australian guidelines state that second-line adjuvant non-opioid analgesia can also be considered such as ketamine as a potential third step.[99]

If buprenorphine is stopped during the period when acute pain relief is required, use of low-dose induction to re-establish buprenorphine treatment has been described as acceptable and tolerable.[100,101] From an implementation perspective, it is a practical option in the acute hospital as it does not rely on careful monitoring of withdrawal severity and awareness of medications prescribed on the 'prn' side, both of which can be missed on a busy ward.

The primary objectives during the period of acute pain are to manage the pain and avoid the consequences of withdrawal (e.g. discharge against medical advice), so it is important to maintain sufficient background medication to achieve both. Liaison with both the in-patient pain team and the local addictions services, as well as collaborative discussion with the patient, is important.

In palliative care, the principles of providing analgesia in substance misusers are no different from those for other adult patients needing palliative care, although increased liaison with substance misuse services is essential. Those who are opioid-dependent may receive maintenance therapy from a substance misuse service. For the purposes of palliative care, this should be regarded as a separate prescription from that for analgesia when attending a pain clinic. During admission all medication would usually be received from the in-patient unit, but there should be a clear plan for separate follow-ups for substance misuse and symptom palliation.[97] Pregabalin may be used for pain relief but there have been concerns regarding both the abuse potential of the drug[81] and the potential for co-prescription of pregabalin and opioids to increase the potential for fatal overdose.[102]

References

1. Scott G, et al. Patients' perceptions of self-administered dosing to opioid agonist treatment and other changes during the COVID-19 pandemic: a qualitative study. *BMJ Open* 2023; **13**:e069857.
2. Adams KK, et al. Initiating buprenorphine to treat opioid use disorder without prerequisite withdrawal: a systematic review. *Addict Sci Clin Pract* 2021; **16**:36.
3. Lewer D, et al. Fatal opioid overdoses during and shortly after hospital admissions in England: a case-crossover study. *PLoS Med* 2021; **18**:e1003759.
4. Strang J, et al. Naloxone without the needle – systematic review of candidate routes for non-injectable naloxone for opioid overdose reversal. *Drug Alcohol Depend* 2016; **163**:16–23.
5. Amaducci A, et al. Naloxone use in novel potent opioid and fentanyl overdoses in emergency department patients. *JAMA Netw Open* 2023; **6**:e2331264.
6. Van Dorp E, et al. Naloxone reversal of buprenorphine-induced respiratory depression. *Anesthesiology* 2006; **105**:51–57.
7. World Health Organization. Community management of opioid overdose. 2014; http://www.who.int/substance_abuse/publications/management_opioid_overdose/en.
8. Department of Health and Social Care. Drug misuse and dependence: UK guidelines on clinical management. 2017; https://www.gov.uk/government/publications/drug-misuse-and-dependence-uk-guidelines-on-clinical-management.
9. McDonald R, et al. Take-home naloxone kits: attitudes and likelihood-of-use outcomes from a European survey of potential overdose witnesses. *Eur Addict Res* 2022; **28**:220–225.
10. Harris M. Normalised pain and severe health care delay among people who inject drugs in London: adapting cultural safety principles to promote care. *Soc Sci Med* 2020; **260**:113183.
11. National Institute for Health and Care Excellence. Coexisting severe mental illness and substance misuse: community health and social care services. NICE Guideline [NG58]. 2016 (last accessed August 2024); https://www.nice.org.uk/guidance/ng58.
12. Tompkins DA, et al. A double blind, within subject comparison of spontaneous opioid withdrawal from buprenorphine versus morphine. *J Pharmacol Exp Ther* 2014; **348**:217–226.
13. San L, et al. Assessment and management of opioid withdrawal symptoms in buprenorphine-dependent subjects. *Br J Addict* 1992; **87**:55–62.
14. Dunn KE, et al. Characterizing opioid withdrawal during double-blind buprenorphine detoxification. *Drug Alcohol Depend* 2015; **151**:47–55.
15. Melichar J, et al. Abstract: Dramatically improved detoxification outcomes using long-acting injectable buprenorphine (LAIB) in the UK's first shared-care GP-led LAIB service. *J Psychopharm* 2023; **37** Suppl.
16. Tompkins DA, et al. Concurrent validation of the Clinical Opiate Withdrawal Scale (COWS) and single-item indices against the Clinical Institute Narcotic Assessment (CINA) opioid withdrawal instrument. *Drug Alcohol Depend* 2009; **105**:154–159.
17. Handelsman L, et al. Two new rating scales for opiate withdrawal. *Am J Drug Alcohol Abuse* 1987; **13**:293–308.
18. National Institute for Health and Care Excellence. Methadone and buprenorphine for the management of opioid dependence. Technology appraisal [TA114]. 2007 (reviewed February 2016, last accessed August 2024); https://www.nice.org.uk/guidance/ta114.
19. Farrell M. Opiate withdrawal. *Addiction* 1994; **89**:1471–1475.
20. Fudala PJ, et al. Use of buprenorphine in the treatment of opioid addiction. II. Physiologic and behavioral effects of daily and alternate-day administration and abrupt withdrawal. *Clin Pharmacol Ther* 1990; **47**:525–534.
21. Larney S, et al. Does opioid agonist treatment reduce overdose mortality risk in people who are older or have physical comorbidities? Cohort study using linked administrative health data in New South Wales, Australia, 2002–17. *Addiction* 2023; **118**:1527–1539.
22. Sordo L, et al. Mortality risk during and after opioid substitution treatment: systematic review and meta-analysis of cohort studies. *BMJ* 2017; **357**:j1550.
23. Aldabergenov D, et al. Methadone and buprenorphine-related deaths among people prescribed and not prescribed opioid agonist therapy during the COVID-19 pandemic in England. *Int J Drug Policy* 2022; **110**:103877.
24. D'Onofrio G, et al. Incidence of precipitated withdrawal during a multisite emergency department-initiated buprenorphine clinical trial in the era of fentanyl. *JAMA Netw Open* 2023; **6**:e236108.
25. Klimas J, et al. Retention in opioid agonist treatment: a rapid review and meta-analysis comparing observational studies and randomized controlled trials. *Syst Rev* 2021; **10**:216.
26. Treece JM, et al. Comprehensive review on methadone-induced QT prolongation and torsades. *J Pharmacol Pharmacother* 2018; **9**:66–75.
27. Vierke C, et al. Buprenorphine–cannabis interaction in patients undergoing opioid maintenance therapy. *Eur Arch Psychiatry Clin Neurosci* 2021; **271**:847–856.
28. Madden K, et al. Clinically significant drug-drug interaction between methadone and cannabidiol. *Pediatrics* 2020; **145**:e20193256.
29. McCance-Katz EF, et al. Drug interactions of clinical importance among the opioids, methadone and buprenorphine, and other frequently prescribed medications: a review. *Am J Addict* 2010; **19**:4–16.
30. Jones HE, et al. Neonatal abstinence syndrome after methadone or buprenorphine exposure. *N Engl J Med* 2010; **363**:2320–2331.
31. Winstock AR, et al. Diversion and injection of methadone and buprenorphine among clients in public opioid treatment clinics in New South Wales, Australia. *Subst Use Misuse* 2010; **45**:240–252.
32. Winstock AR, et al. What is diversion of supervised buprenorphine and how common is it? *J Addict Dis* 2009; **28**:269–278.
33. Leslie ST, et al. Methadone: evidence of accumulation. *BMJ* 1977; **1**:1284.
34. Verebely K, et al. Methadone in man: pharmacokinetic and excretion studies in acute and chronic treatment. *Clin Pharmacol Ther* 1975; **18**:180–190.

35. White JM, et al. Mechanisms of fatal opioid overdose. *Addiction* 1999; **94**:961–972.

36. Farrell M, et al. Suicide and overdose among opiate addicts. *Addiction* 1996; **91**:321–323.

37. Abrahamsson T, et al. Benzodiazepine, z-drug and pregabalin prescriptions and mortality among patients in opioid maintenance treatment – a nation-wide register-based open cohort study. *Drug Alcohol Depend* 2017; **174**:58–64.

38. Pierce M, et al. Impact of treatment for opioid dependence on fatal drug-related poisoning: a national cohort study in England. *Addiction* 2016; **111**:298–308.

39. Macleod J, et al. Prescription of benzodiazepines, z-drugs, and gabapentinoids and mortality risk in people receiving opioid agonist treatment: observational study based on the UK Clinical Practice Research Datalink and Office for National Statistics death records. *PLoS Med* 2019; **16**:e1002965.

40. Ključević Ž, et al. Liver damage indices as a tool for modifying methadone maintenance treatment: a cross-sectional study. *Croat Med J* 2018; **59**:298–306.

41. Odoma VA, et al. Opioid prescription in patients with chronic kidney disease: a systematic review of comparing safety and efficacy of opioid use in chronic kidney disease patients. *Cureus* 2023; **15**:e45485.

42. Krantz MJ, et al. Torsade de pointes associated with very-high-dose methadone. *Ann Intern Med* 2002; **137**:501–504.

43. Kornick CA, et al. QTc interval prolongation associated with intravenous methadone. *Pain* 2003; **105**:499–506.

44. Martell BA, et al. The impact of methadone induction on cardiac conduction in opiate users. *Ann Intern Med* 2003; **139**:154–155.

45. Pani PP, et al. QTc interval screening for cardiac risk in methadone treatment of opioid dependence. *Cochrane Database Syst Rev* 2013; **6**:CD008939.

46. Mayet S, et al. Methadone maintenance, QTc and torsade de pointes: who needs an electrocardiogram and what is the prevalence of QTc prolongation? *Drug Alcohol Rev* 2011; **30**:388–396.

47. Hancox JC, et al. Synthetic cannabinoids and potential cardiac arrhythmia risk: an important message for drug users. *Ther Adv Drug Saf* 2020; **11**:2042098620913416.

48. Isbister GK, et al. Drug induced QT prolongation: the measurement and assessment of the QT interval in clinical practice. *Br J Clin Pharmacol* 2013; **76**:48–57.

49. Mattick RP, et al. Buprenorphine maintenance versus placebo or methadone maintenance for opioid dependence. *Cochrane Database Syst Rev* 2014; **2**:CD002207.

50. Gov.UK. From harm to hope: a 10-year drugs plan to cut crime and save lives. First Annual Report 2022-23. 2023 (last assessed August 2024); https://assets.publishing.service.gov.uk/media/65dc7655529bfa0011e95508/E02949325_15.109_HO_Harm_to_Hope_AR_2022-23_Web+Accessible_v02.pdf.

51. Lintzeris N, et al. The uptake of long-acting depot buprenorphine for treating opioid dependence in Australia, 2019-2022: longitudinal sales data analysis. *Med J Aust* 2024; **220**:339–340.

52. Walsh SL, et al. Acute administration of buprenorphine in humans: partial agonist and blockade effects. *J Pharmacol Exp Ther* 1995; **274**:361–372.

53. Bickel WK, et al. Buprenorphine: dose-related blockade of opioid challenge effects in opioid dependent humans. *J Pharmacol Exp Ther* 1988; **247**:47–53.

54. Marsch LA, et al. Buprenorphine treatment for opioid dependence: the relative efficacy of daily, twice and thrice weekly dosing. *Drug Alcohol Depend* 2005; **77**:195–204.

55. Edinoff AN, et al. Low-dose initiation of buprenorphine: a narrative review. *Curr Pain Headache Rep* 2023; **27**:175–181.

56. Marsden J, et al. Extended-release pharmacotherapy for opioid use disorder (EXPO): protocol for an open-label randomised controlled trial of the effectiveness and cost-effectiveness of injectable buprenorphine versus sublingual tablet buprenorphine and oral liquid methadone. *Trials* 2022; **23**:697.

57. Boyett B, et al. Continued posttrial benefits of buprenorphine extended release: RECOVER study findings. *J Addict Med* 2023; **17**:182–189.

58. Lintzeris N, et al. Strategies for transfer from methadone to buprenorphine for treatment of opioid use disorders and associated outcomes: a systematic review. *J Addict Med* 2022; **16**:143–151.

59. Omoigui S, et al. Use of ketamine in ameliorating opioid withdrawal symptoms during an induction phase of buprenorphine. *Open Pain J* 2011; **4**:1–3.

60. Hämmig R, et al. Use of microdoses for induction of buprenorphine treatment with overlapping full opioid agonist use: the Bernese method. *Subst Abuse Rehabil* 2016; **7**:99–105.

61. Oakley B, et al. Managing opioid withdrawal precipitated by buprenorphine with buprenorphine. *Drug Alcohol Rev* 2021; **40**:567–571.

62. Tay Wee Teck J, et al. Using microdosing to induct patients into a long-acting injectable buprenorphine depot medication in low threshold community settings: a case study. *Front Pharmacol* 2021; **12**:631784.

63. Tang VM, et al. Case series: limited opioid withdrawal with use of transdermal buprenorphine to bridge to sublingual buprenorphine in hospitalized patients. *Am J Addict* 2020; **29**:73–76.

64. Terasaki D, et al. Transitioning hospitalized patients with opioid use disorder from methadone to buprenorphine without a period of opioid abstinence using a microdosing protocol. *Pharmacotherapy* 2019; **39**:1023–1029.

65. Weimer MB, et al. Hospital-based buprenorphine micro-dose initiation. *J Addict Med* 2021; **15**:255–257.

66. Bhatraju EP, et al. Low dose buprenorphine induction with full agonist overlap in hospitalized patients with opioid use disorder: a retrospective cohort study. *J Addict Med* 2022; **16**:461–465.

67. Anderson C, et al. Transitioning from high-dose methadone to buprenorphine using a microdosing approach: unique considerations at ASAM level 3 facilities. *J Addict Med* 2023; **17**:241–244.

68. Nielsen S, et al. Opioid agonist treatment for pharmaceutical opioid dependent people. *Cochrane Database Syst Rev* 2016; **5**:CD011117.

CHAPTER 4

69. Amass L, et al. Alternate-day buprenorphine dosing is preferred to daily dosing by opioid-dependent humans. *Psychopharmacology* 1998; **136**:217–225.

70. Kothadia JP, et al. Acute hepatitis after oral buprenorphine use in a heroin addict: 1838. *Am J Gastroenterol* 2016; **111**:S881.

71. Berson A, et al. Hepatitis after intravenous buprenorphine misuse in heroin addicts. *J Hepatol* 2001; **34**:346–350.

72. Comer SD, et al. Abuse liability of prescription opioids compared to heroin in morphine-maintained heroin abusers. *Neuropsychopharmacology* 2008; **33**:1179–1191.

73. Hickman M, et al. The impact of buprenorphine and methadone on mortality: a primary care cohort study in the United Kingdom. *Addiction* 2018; **113**:1461–1476.

74. Sarton E, et al. Naloxone reversal of opioid-induced respiratory depression with special emphasis on the partial agonist/antagonist buprenorphine. *Adv Exp Med Biol* 2008; **605**:486–491.

75. Ferri M, et al. Slow-release oral morphine as maintenance therapy for opioid dependence. *Cochrane Database Syst Rev* 2013; **6**:CD009879.

76. Strang J, et al. Heroin on trial: systematic review and meta-analysis of randomised trials of diamorphine-prescribing as treatment for refractory heroin addictiondagger. *Br J Psychiatry* 2015; **207**:5–14.

77. Byford S, et al. Cost-effectiveness of injectable opioid treatment v. oral methadone for chronic heroin addiction. *Br J Psychiatry* 2013; **203**:341–349.

78. Strang J, et al. Supervised injectable heroin or injectable methadone versus optimised oral methadone as treatment for chronic heroin addicts in England after persistent failure in orthodox treatment (RIOTT): a randomised trial. *Lancet* 2010; **375**:1885–1895.

79. Lingford-Hughes AR, et al. BAP updated guidelines: evidence-based guidelines for the pharmacological management of substance abuse, harmful use, addiction and comorbidity: recommendations from BAP. *J Psychopharmacol* 2012; **26**:899–952.

80. Kalk NJ, et al. Fatalities associated with gabapentinoids in England (2004–2020). *Br J Clin Pharmacol* 2022; **88**:3911–3917.

81. Bonnet U, et al. How addictive are gabapentin and pregabalin? A systematic review. *Eur Neuropsychopharmacol* 2017; **27**:1185–1215.

82. James PD, et al. Non-medical use of olanzapine by people on methadone treatment. *BJPsych Bull* 2016; **40**:314–317.

83. Tenore PL. Psychotherapeutic benefits of opioid agonist therapy. *J Addict Dis* 2008; **27**:49–65.

84. Nunes EV, et al. Treatment of co-occurring depression and substance dependence: using meta-analysis to guide clinical recommendations. *Psychiatr Ann* 2008; **38**:nihpa128505.

85. Taylor D, et al. The cardiovascular safety of tricyclic antidepressants in overdose and in clinical use. *Ther Adv Psychopharmacol* 2024; **14**:20451253241243297.

86. National Institute for Heath and Care Excellence. Drug misuse in over 16s: opioid detoxification. Clinical guideline [CG52]. 2007 (checked January 2019, last accessed August 2024; updated 2007); https://www.nice.org.uk/guidance/cg52.

87. National Institute for Health and Care Excellence. Drug misuse in over 16s: psychosocial interventions. Clinical guideline [CG51]. 2007 (last checked July 2016, last accessed August 2024; updated 2007); https://www.nice.org.uk/guidance/cg51.

88. Nosyk B, et al. Defining dosing pattern characteristics of successful tapers following methadone maintenance treatment: results from a population-based retrospective cohort study. *Addiction* 2012; **107**:1621–1629.

89. Minozzi S, et al. Oral naltrexone maintenance treatment for opioid dependence. *Cochrane Database Syst Rev* 2011; **4**:CD001333.

90. Lobmaier P, et al. Sustained-release naltrexone for opioid dependence. *Cochrane Database Syst Rev* 2008; **2**:CD006140.

91. National Institute for Health and Care Excellence. Naltrexone for the management of opioid dependence. Technology apprasial [TA115]. 2007 (last reviewed November 2010, last checked August 2024); https://www.nice.org.uk/guidance/ta115.

92. Degenhardt L, et al. Excess mortality among opioid-using patients treated with oral naltrexone in Australia. *Drug Alcohol Rev* 2015; **34**:90–96.

93. Darke S, et al. Circumstances of death of opioid users being treated with naltrexone. *Addiction* 2019; **114**:2000–2007.

94. Latif ZE, et al. Anxiety, depression, and insomnia among adults with opioid dependence treated with extended-release naltrexone vs buprenorphine-naloxone: a randomized clinical trial and follow-up study. *JAMA Psychiatry* 2019; **76**:127–134.

95. Dean AJ, et al. Does naltrexone treatment lead to depression? Findings from a randomized controlled trial in subjects with opioid dependence. *J Psychiatry Neurosci* 2006; **31**:38–45.

96. Carroll KM, et al. Accounting for the uncounted: physical and affective distress in individuals dropping out of oral naltrexone treatment for opioid use disorder. *Drug Alcohol Depend* 2018; **192**:264–270.

97. British Pain Society, et al. Pain and substance misuse: improving the patient experience. A consensus statement prepared by The British Pain Society in collaboration with The Royal College of Psychiatrists, The Royal College of General Practitioners and The Advisory Council on the Misuse of Drugs. 2007 (updated 2007); https://www.britishpainsociety.org/static/uploads/resources/misuse_0307_v13_FINAL.pdf.

98. Goel A, et al. Perioperative Pain and Addiction Interdisciplinary Network (PAIN): protocol of a practice advisory for the perioperative management of buprenorphine using a modified Delphi process. *BMJ Open* 2019; **9**:e027374.

99. Goverment of Western Australia. Clinical guidelines for use of depot buprenorphine (Buvidal® and Sublocade®) in the treatment of opioid dependence. 2024; https://www.mhc.wa.gov.au/media/4919/mhc24-32319-cpop-clinical-guidelines-for-the-use-of-depot-buprenorphine-in-the-treatment-of-opioid-dependence-march-2024.pdf.

100. Shelton T, et al. Case report. Successful induction of buprenorphine in medically complex patients concurrently on opioids: a case series at a tertiary care center. *Front Pharmacol* 2024; **15**:1335345.

101. DeWeese JP, et al. Rapid buprenorphine microdosing for opioid use disorder in a hospitalized patient receiving very high doses of full agonist opioids for acute pain management: titration, implementation barriers, and strategies to overcomes. *Subst Abus* 2021; **42**:506–511.

102. Lyndon A, et al. Risk to heroin users of polydrug use of pregabalin or gabapentin. *Addiction* 2017; **112**:1580–1589.

Nicotine and smoking cessation

Tobacco smoking is the leading preventable cause of illness and premature death worldwide. Smoking cessation interventions are clinically and cost effective for people with and without a mental illness.

In the UK, NICE recommends that every person who smokes, including those receiving community and in-patient mental healthcare, should be offered support to stop smoking. For those people who feel unable or who are unwilling to give up, they should be provided with treatment to temporarily abstain from smoking.[1]

NICE recommends that bupropion, nicotine replacement therapy (NRT), varenicline and nicotine-containing vaping devices should be accessible to adults who smoke.[1] It advises that when combined with behavioural support, varenicline, a combination of short-acting (e.g. mouth spray, lozenges) and long-acting (e.g. skin patches) NRT, or nicotine-containing vaping devices are more likely to help people successfully stop smoking, whereas behavioural support combined with either bupropion or single NRT is less likely to help people stop smoking.

A component network mental analysis to assess the comparative benefits and harms of vaping and different licensed smoking cessation pharmacotherapies found the most effective interventions were nicotine vaping devices (odds ratio [OR] 2.37), varenicline (OR 2.33), cytisine (OR 2.21) and combination NRT (OR 1.93).[2]

The effectiveness of smoking cessation treatments appears not to be reduced in patients with a variety of mental health problems.[3]

Smoking induces CYP1A2, and so stopping smoking may result in increased plasma levels of CYP1A2 substrates. See 'Smoking and psychotropic drugs' in Chapter 11.

Nicotine replacement therapy (NRT)

In the UK, NRT is licensed for smokers over the age of 12 years to help those who want to stop smoking, to reduce before stopping or during a temporary period of enforced abstinence when a person is unable to smoke. NRT is also indicated for pregnant and breastfeeding women attempting to stop smoking. Clinical guidelines in other countries recommend NRT as first-line treatment for people seeking pharmacological help to stop smoking. In recent years, vaping has become the most often used alternative to tobacco smoking in many countries.

The aim of NRT in those stopping smoking is to assist the transition from cigarette smoking to complete abstinence. It may also be used for those who wish to stop vaping. This is achieved by temporarily replacing some of the nicotine obtained from tobacco cigarettes with NRT products and minimising nicotine withdrawal symptoms and the motivation to smoke. People who have stopped smoking can safely use NRT if they wish to continue using nicotine recreationally or to prevent relapse back to smoking.

There are eight licensed NRT products in the UK: transdermal patches, lozenges, gum, sublingual tablets, inhalator, nasal spray, mouth spray and oral strips. All these products are General Sales List medicines and can be bought over the counter in the UK. NRT is formulated for systemic absorption through either the skin in the case of patches or the oral or nasal mucosa in the case of all the other products. This means that absorption of nicotine from NRT is much slower than nicotine from inhaling tobacco smoke and the risk of becoming addicted to NRT is lower.[4]

CHAPTER 4

Clinical effectiveness

A Cochrane review of NRT suggests combination NRT (i.e. two formulations such as a patch and an oral/nasal product) is associated with higher long-term abstinence rates than using a single NRT product (risk ratio [RR] 1.27).[5] Higher dose nicotine patches (25mg patches worn for 16 hours, or 21mg patches worn for 24 hours) are more likely to help people stop smoking compared with using lower dose patches (15mg patches worn for 16 hours, or 14mg patches worn for 24 hours).[5]

Studies with smokers from the general population suggest that each cigarette provides a smoker with approximately 1–2.9mg of nicotine, depending on the frequency and intensity of smoking.[6] Findings from studies in people with schizophrenia who smoke suggest they take more frequent puffs over a shorter period of time and, as a result, extract more nicotine from cigarettes compared with those without a mental health condition.[7] It is therefore plausible that these smokers may require higher doses of nicotine replacement. However, in general population studies, there is no clear evidence of superiority for higher dose NRT patches (42/44mg) over 21/22mg (24-hour) patches.[5]

The nicotine from oral products has to be absorbed through the cheeks, gums and back of the lips. The correct technique is to chew the gum/suck the lozenge until the taste becomes strong and then rest it between the cheek and gum. When the taste starts to fade, it is advised to repeat this process for about 20–30 minutes. Many gum users press the gum down against the (buccal) gum to increase the surface area of contact and hence the rate of nicotine absorption. Lozenges also allow sublingual absorption of nicotine but their physical size usually precludes this method unless the lozenge is broken into smaller pieces. Sublingual tablets are much smaller in size.

Drinking coffee and carbonated drinks may block the absorption of nicotine from oral nicotine products.[8]

Preparations and dose

Table 4.20 details preparations and doses of different types of NRT.

Adverse effects

Adverse effects from using NRT are related to the type of product and include skin irritation from patches and irritation to the inside of the mouth and coughs from oral products. Nausea may occur if the patient is still smoking. Some sleep disturbance can be expected in the early days of treatment, though this is also a symptom of nicotine withdrawal. NRT has no known pharmacokinetic interactions with psychotropic medication. Overdosing on nicotine is very rare (and usually intentional). Initial signs include nausea, vomiting, headache and diarrhoea. It has been estimated that the lower limit for causing a fatal outcome is 0.5–1g of ingested nicotine.[9]

Varenicline

Varenicline is a selective nicotinic acetylcholine receptor partial agonist. It mimics the action of nicotine and causes a sustained release of dopamine in the mesolimbic pathway. It also blocks dopamine release resulting from subsequent nicotine intake.

Table 4.20 Nicotine preparations and doses.

	Smoking <20 cigarettes/day	Smoking >20 cigarettes/day or people who smoke within 30 minutes of waking up
Topical patch 24-hour formulation (21mg, 14mg, 7mg) 16-hour formulation (25mg, 15mg, 10mg)	If smoking >20 cigarettes/day use 21mg (24-hour) or 25mg (16-hour) patch. There is no difference in efficacy between 16-hour and 24-hour formulations. The 16-hour patch should be removed at bedtime.	
Nasal spray (0.5mg/spray)	One spray in each nostril when craving; no more than twice per hour; maximum 64 sprays/day	
Oral spray (1mg/spray)	1–2 sprays when craving; no more than 2 sprays per episode; no more than 4 sprays/h; maximum 64 sprays/day	
Lozenge (1mg, 2mg, 4mg)	One 1mg lozenge hourly to prevent craving	One 2mg or 4mg lozenge hourly to prevent craving; usually no more than 15 lozenges/day
Gum (2mg, 4mg, 6mg)	One piece of 2mg hourly to prevent craving	One piece of 4mg or 6mg hourly to prevent craving; no more than 15 pieces 4mg/day
Inhalator (15mg)	No more than 6 cartridges of 15mg/day	
Sublingual tablet	1–2 tablets hourly to prevent craving	2 tablets hourly to prevent craving; no more than 40 tablets/day
Mouth strips (2.5mg)	One strip hourly to prevent craving	One strip hourly to prevent craving; no more than 15 strips/day

This means if it is taken as prescribed, any attempt to smoke a cigarette will be less pharmacologically rewarding and feel less satisfying to a smoker. Varenicline is indicated for smokers over the age of 18 who are motivated to stop smoking. It should be avoided in pregnancy and breastfeeding. In 2021, Pfizer recalled varenicline because it exceeded acceptable intake limits of a nitrosamine impurity (N-nitroso-varenicline). Generic versions of varenicline are available in some countries (e.g. USA).

Clinical effectiveness

A 2023 Cochrane review[10] found high-certainty evidence that varenicline is more effective than placebo (RR 2.32), bupropion (RR 1.36) and single-product NRT (RR 1.25), and is similarly effective to combination NRT.[11,12] Varenicline is more effective than placebo among patients with cardiovascular disease, COPD, severe mental illness, depression and HIV.[10] In smokers with serious mental illness, varenicline improved the odds of stopping smoking by 4–5 times compared with placebo.[13,14] There is inconclusive evidence for its effectiveness compared with placebo among people with asthma, substance use disorder and alcohol dependence.[10]

Preparations and dose

People who smoke should set a target stopping date between 1 and 2 weeks after starting varenicline treatment. Those who are not willing or able to set a target date within 1–2 weeks can start treatment and then choose their own stopping date within 5 weeks. Dosage regimens can be found in the treatment algorithm for those people making an attempt to stop smoking at the end of this section (Table 4.21).

Adverse effects

Very common adverse effects include nausea, strange dreams, sleep disturbance and headache, all occurring in more than 1 in 10 people. Varenicline has no known pharmacokinetic interaction with psychotropic medication.

Varenicline does not significantly increase the risk of neuropsychiatric adverse events (including anxiety, depression, aggression, psychosis and suicidal behaviour) when compared with placebo or nicotine patches in patients with or without a history of psychiatric disorders.[10,15]

Cytisine

Cytisine has a similar mechanism of action as varenicline and although it has been available as a smoking cessation aid in Eastern Europe since the 1960s, it has only latterly received marketing approval in the UK and other countries. It is indicated for smokers over the age of 18 who are motivated to stop smoking. It is contraindicated during pregnancy and breastfeeding.

Clinical effectiveness

A Cochrane review[10] found moderate-certainty evidence that cytisine is more effective than placebo (RR 1.30) or NRT (RR 1.43). Pooled results from two studies that compared cytisine with varenicline found no significant difference between the two drugs. The review did not identify studies among people with mental illness.

Preparations and dose

A course of treatment lasts 25 days, which is shorter than the recommended length of treatment for NRT, varenicline and bupropion with a multiple dosing regimen. A stopping date no later than the fifth day of treatment should be aimed for. Dosage regimens can be found in the treatment algorithm for those people making an attempt to stop smoking at the end of this section (Table 4.21).

Adverse effects

Very common adverse effects include increased appetite, weight gain, dizziness, irritability, mood changes, anxiety, drowsiness, fatigue, abnormal dreams, tachycardia, hypertension, dry mouth and nausea, although the latter may be less common than in patients taking varenicline and more common than in those using NRT. The SPC states that cytisine should not be used with antituberculous drugs.

Bupropion

Bupropion is an antidepressant with dopaminergic and adrenergic actions and is additionally an antagonist at the nicotinic acetylcholine receptor. It is indicated for smokers over the age of 18 who are motivated to stop smoking.

Clinical effectiveness

A Cochrane review[16] found high-certainty evidence that bupropion is more effective than placebo (RR 1.60). Bupropion was of similar efficacy to single-product NRT and less effective for quitting compared with varenicline and combination NRT. In smokers with serious mental illness, bupropion improved the odds of stopping by 3–4 times compared with placebo.[13,14]

Preparations and dose

People who smoke should set a target stopping date in the first 2 weeks of starting bupropion treatment. Dosage regimens can be found in the treatment algorithm for those people making an attempt to stop smoking at the end of this section (Table 4.21).

Adverse effects

Bupropion is contraindicated in those with seizure disorders, eating disorders and alcohol dependence. Clinicians should be cautious of the potential for manic switch in patients with bipolar affective disorder (very low risk but it can occur[17]). Common adverse effects include dizziness, taste changes, gastrointestinal disturbance and insomnia, which can be reduced by avoiding a dose close to bedtime. Unlike NRT and varenicline, bupropion is known to interact with psychotropic medicines. It is metabolised by the cytochrome CYP2B6. Caution is advised when bupropion is co-administered with medicines known to induce (e.g. carbamazepine, phenytoin) or inhibit (e.g. valproate) its metabolism as this may affect the efficacy of bupropion or increase the risk of adverse effects. Bupropion and its main metabolite (hydroxybupropion) are inhibitors of the CYP2D6 enzyme. It has been shown to increase the levels of medicines metabolised by CY2D6 (e.g. imipramine, risperidone, haloperidol) and so caution is required particularly with narrow therapeutic index drugs (lower starting doses are recommended).

Electronic nicotine vaping devices and vaping

Also referred to as vapes (formerly known as electronic cigarettes or e-cigarettes), electronic nicotine vaping devices produce an inhalable aerosol (vapour) which is formed by heating an e-liquid using a battery-powered heating coil. Vaping devices are activated by a switch or by suction as the user draws on the device's mouthpiece. They do not contain tobacco, are not combusted and do not produce smoke or sidestream vapour. Regulation of vaping devices varies across different countries and states, ranging from total bans to the absence of regulation. In the UK and European Union there are controls on quality standards (e.g. ingredients, packaging and advertising) and manufacturers have to notify the competent authority in each country (the MHRA in the UK) of the ingredients in nicotine vaping devices before they are placed on the market. Notified nicotine-containing vaping devices can only be sold to people over the age of 18 in the UK. Vaping devices

CHAPTER 4

that do not contain nicotine are regulated by Trading Standards in the UK. The Office for Health Improvement and Disparities, NHS England and the Care Quality Commission (CQC) support the use of vaping devices in mental health in-patient settings.[18-20]

Clinical effectiveness

Since 2013, electronic devices have been the most popular quitting aid in England. A Cochrane review of the effect of e-cigarettes for smoking cessation found high-certainty evidence that nicotine-containing vaping devices were more effective than NRT (RR 1.59) and moderate-certainty evidence that they were more effective than vaping devices without nicotine (RR 1.46).[2] There is a small evidence base that they are also effective for helping people with a mental health condition reduce smoking.[21]

Preparations and dose

The e-liquid is made up of nicotine, flavourings, propylene glycol (PG) and vegetable glycerine (VG). Single-use devices, prefilled cartridges or pods, and bottles of e-liquids are labelled with how many milligrams (mg) of nicotine there are per millilitre (mL), or as the percentage weight per volume (%w/v). In the UK, and several other countries, nicotine content ranges from zero (0%) to a maximum of 20mg/mL (or 2%). Nicotine is incorporated as freebase or nicotine salts; the latter has a lower pH than freebase nicotine, enabling a smoother throat-hit. Additionally, nicotine salts allow vaporisation at a lower temperature and enable higher nicotine levels to be inhaled,[21] which may help with switching from smoking to vaping. Access to a variety of flavours can encourage the uptake of vaping as an aid to stopping smoking and vaping non-tobacco flavours is associated with increased smoking cessation in adults.[22] The label on the vaping product packaging includes the ratio of VG to PG (VG/PG). PG is the carrier for the flavourings and nicotine and is also responsible for the throat-hit. VG has a natural sweetness and is responsible for the majority of aerosol (vapour). A 50/50 ratio is the most common. For smokers who miss the throat-hit or harsh feeling at the back of the throat from tobacco smoking, an e-liquid with a high PG ratio may be preferable (e.g. PG 70/VG 30). If big vapour clouds are preferred, then a high VG ratio needs to be used (e.g. PG 30/VG 70), though this is best suited to particular vaping devices (modular).

Adverse effects

Mouth and throat irritation, cough, headache and nausea are the most commonly reported symptoms of vaping and these subside over time. The Royal College of Physicians,[23] Office for Health Improvement and Disparities[22] and Committee on Toxicity of Chemicals in Food, Consumer Products and the Environment[24] advise that regulated vaping devices are a much less harmful alternative to tobacco smoking for dependent smokers and bystanders. Concurrent smoking and vaping (dual use) may not reduce the risk of adverse health effects, and people who vape should be encouraged to stop smoking completely, whereas people who have never smoked should be encouraged not to smoke or vape.[22,24]

Treatment algorithms

Tables 4.21 and 4.22 outline treatment algorithms for people making an attempt to stop smoking and those wanting to abstain or reduce their smoking level.

Table 4.21 Treatment algorithm for people making an attempt to stop smoking.

First-line pharmacological treatment is **combination NRT** or **varenicline** or **a nicotine-containing vaping device**[1] weekly by a trained tobacco-dependence treatment advisor for the duration of the attempt at stopping and for at least 4 weeks after discharge from hospital.

Combination NRT	Varenicline
For people who smoke more than 20 cigarettes/day or who smoke within 30 minutes of waking up:	
Start 21mg (24-hour) or 25mg (16-hour) patch and an oral/nasal NRT product of the person's choice	Set target stopping date between 1 and 2 weeks of starting varenicline treatment.
Continue patch use for up to 12 weeks, aiming to reduce patch dosage every 4 weeks	Start 0.5mg PO varenicline once daily on days 1–3.
Continue oral/nasal product use while experiencing craving.	Increase to 0.5mg PO varenicline twice daily on days 4–7.
For people who smoke less than 20 cigarettes/day and do not smoke within 30 minutes of waking up:	Increase to 1mg PO varenicline twice daily on days 8–84.
Start 14mg (24-hour) or 15mg (16-hour) patch and/or an oral/nasal NRT product of the person's choice	Consider 1mg varenicline PO twice daily for an additional 12 weeks for maintenance of abstinence in people who have successfully stopped smoking at the end of the initial 12 week course of varenicline.
Continue patch use for up to 12 weeks, aiming to reduce patch dosage every 4 weeks	
Continue oral/nasal product use while experiencing craving.	

People who want to use a nicotine vaping device to quit should generally set a stopping date and use the device to stop in one go by replacing all their tobacco cigarettes with it as soon as possible. Alternatively, they can gradually reduce the amount of tobacco they smoke over several weeks and increase the use of the vape until they have completely switched. Similar to the use of NRT, advise the service user to start with a higher strength of nicotine. There is no contraindication to using NRT and a nicotine vaping device simultaneously (if people find this beneficial).

Cytisine

Set target stopping date within 5 days of starting cytisine treatment

Days of treatment	Recommended dosing	Maximum daily dose
Days 1–3	**1.5mg** (1 tablet) every 2 hours	9mg (6 tablets)
Days 4–12	**1.5mg** (1 tablet) every 2.5 hours	7.5mg (5 tablets)
Days 13–16	**1.5mg** (1 tablet) every 3 hours	6mg (4 tablets)
Days 17–20	**1.5mg** (1 tablet) every 5 hours	4.5mg (3 tablets)
Days 21–25	**1.5–3mg (1–2 tablets)** a day	3mg (2 tablets)

Bupropion

Bupropion could be considered second line or where people who smoke express a preference for bupropion therapy.

Set target stopping date between 1 and 2 weeks of bupropion treatment.

Start 150mg PO bupropion daily on days 1–6.

Increase to 150mg PO bupropion twice daily on days 7–49 (with an interval of at least 8 hours between doses, and avoiding bedtime dosing to reduce risk of insomnia).

Maintain dose at 150mg PO bupropion on days 50–63 (otherwise discontinue if person has not stopped).

Table 4.22 Treatment algorithm for people not making an attempt to stop, i.e. those people temporarily abstaining or aiming to reduce their cigarette consumption.

Those who are unwilling or feel unable to quit should be encouraged to minimise harm and substitute nicotine from tobacco cigarettes with either **combination NRT** or a **vaping device**

Combination NRT	Vaping devices
For people who smoke more than 20 cigarettes/day or who smoke within 30 minutes of waking up:	
Start 21mg (24-hour) or 25mg (16-hour) patch and an oral/nasal NRT product of the person's choice	The dose of nicotine a vaper extracts from a vaping device varies depending on the device, the volume of e-liquid, other ingredients in the liquid and the frequency, size and depth of inhalation.
Continue to offer NRT products even if met with initial refusal	
Smokers should have fingertip control over NRT products at times of craving.	The more dependent a smoker is, the higher the strength of nicotine is recommended.
For people who smoke less than 20 cigarettes/day and do not smoke within 30 minutes of waking up:	A rough guide is that smokers of 20 tobacco cigarettes/day may require up to 20mg of nicotine/day.
Start 14mg (24-hour) or 15mg (16-hour) patch and/or an oral/nasal NRT product of the person's choice	Smokers should have fingertip control over their vaping device at times of craving.
Continue to offer NRT products even if met with initial refusal	Similar to NRT, people who smoke should be encouraged to regularly use a vaping device between smoking episodes to promote smoke-free intervals.
Smokers should have fingertip control over NRT products at times of craving.	

There are currently no medicinally licensed nicotine vaping devices and therefore it is not possible to prescribe them in most countries. Practitioners should consult local smoke-free policies to establish which type of vaping device is permitted in individual mental health in-patient settings and how to access them.

References

1. National Institute for Health and Care Excellence. Tobacco: preventing uptake, promoting quitting and treating dependence. NICE guideline [NG209]. 2021 (last updated 2023, last accessed March 2024); https://www.nice.org.uk/guidance/ng209.
2. Lindson N, et al. Pharmacological and electronic cigarette interventions for smoking cessation in adults: component network meta-analyses. *Cochrane Database Syst Rev* 2023; 9:CD015226.
3. Tidey JW, et al. Smoking cessation and reduction in people with chronic mental illness. *BMJ* 2015; 351:h4065.
4. Hajek P, et al. Dependence potential of nicotine replacement treatments: effects of product type, patient characteristics, and cost to user. *Prev Med* 2007; 44:230–234.
5. Theodoulou A, et al. Different doses, durations and modes of delivery of nicotine replacement therapy for smoking cessation. *Cochrane Database Syst Rev* 2023; 6:CD013308.
6. Henningfield JE, et al. Pharmacotherapy for nicotine dependence. *CA Cancer J Clin* 2005; 55:281–299; quiz 322–323, 325.
7. Williams JM, et al. Increased nicotine and cotinine levels in smokers with schizophrenia and schizoaffective disorder is not a metabolic effect. *Schizophr Res* 2005; 79:323–335.
8. Henningfield JE, et al. Drinking coffee and carbonated beverages blocks absorption of nicotine from nicotine polacrilex gum. *JAMA* 1990; 264:1560–1564.
9. Mayer B. How much nicotine kills a human? Tracing back the generally accepted lethal dose to dubious self-experiments in the nineteenth century. *Arch Toxicol* 2014; 88:5–7.
10. Livingstone-Banks J, et al. Nicotine receptor partial agonists for smoking cessation. *Cochrane Database Syst Rev* 2023; 5:CD006103.
11. Cahill K, et al. Nicotine receptor partial agonists for smoking cessation. *Cochrane Database Syst Rev* 2016:CD006103.
12. Howes S, et al. Antidepressants for smoking cessation. *Cochrane Database Syst Rev* 2020; 4:CD000031.
13. Roberts E, et al. Efficacy and tolerability of pharmacotherapy for smoking cessation in adults with serious mental illness: a systematic review and network meta-analysis. *Addiction* 2016; 111:599–612.
14. Siskind DJ, et al. Pharmacological interventions for smoking cessation among people with schizophrenia spectrum disorders: a systematic review, meta-analysis, and network meta-analysis. *Lancet Psychiatry* 2020; 7:762–774.

15. Anthenelli RM, et al. Neuropsychiatric safety and efficacy of varenicline, bupropion, and nicotine patch in smokers with and without psychiatric disorders (EAGLES): a double-blind, randomised, placebo-controlled clinical trial. *Lancet* 2016; 387:2507–2520.

16. Hajizadeh A, et al. Antidepressants for smoking cessation. *Cochrane Database Syst Rev* 2023; 5:CD000031.

17. Giasson-Gariepy K, et al. A case of hypomania during nicotine cessation treatment with bupropion. *Addict Sci Clin Pract* 2013; 8:22.

18. Care Quality Commission. Brief guide: the use of 'blanket restrictions' in mental health wards. 2020; https://www.cqc.org.uk/sites/default/files/20191125_900767_briefguide-blanket-restrictions_mental_health_wards_v3.pdf.

19. Health and Social Care. Using electronic cigarettes in NHS mental health organisations. 2020; https://www.gov.uk/government/publications/e-cigarettes-use-by-patients-in-nhs-mental-health-organisations/using-electronic-cigarettes-in-nhs-mental-health-organisations.

20. NHS England. Long term plan. 2019; https://www.longtermplan.nhs.uk/wp-content/uploads/2019/08/nhs-long-term-plan-version-1.2.pdf.

21. McNeill A, et al. Vaping in England: an evidence update including mental health and pregnancy, March 2020: a report commissioned by Public Health England. London: Public Health England. 2020; https://assets.publishing.service.gov.uk/government/uploads/system/uploads/attachment_data/file/869401/Vaping_in_England_evidence_update_March_2020.pdf.

22. Gov.UK. Research and analysis. Nicotine vaping in England: 2022 evidence update main findings. 2022; https://www.gov.uk/government/publications/nicotine-vaping-in-england-2022-evidence-update/nicotine-vaping-in-england-2022-evidence-update-main-findings.

23. Royal College of Physicians. Nicotine without smoke: tobacco harm reduction. A report by the Tobacco Advisory Group of the Royal College of Physicians. 2016; https://www.rcplondon.ac.uk/projects/outputs/nicotine-without-smoke-tobacco-harm-reduction-0.

24. Committee on Toxicity of Chemicals in Food Consumer Products and the Environment (COT). Statement on the potential toxicological risks from electronic nicotine (and non-nicotine) delivery systems (E(N)NDS – e-cigarettes). 2020; https://cot.food.gov.uk/sites/default/files/2020-09/COT%20E%28N%29NDS%20statement%202020-04.pdf.

Stimulant use disorder (SUD)

Stimulants, as a group, encompass a wide range of synthetics (amfetamine, methamphetamine, methylphenidate, mephedrone) and naturally derived substances (cocaine and crack, ephedrine, khat) broadly described as sympathomimetic. Ingestion creates characteristic euphoric effects thought to be mediated by release of the monoamines norepinephrine, serotonin and dopamine.[1] Cocaine and amfetamine use are the most common with a global prevalence rate of 0.4% and 0.7%, respectively. It is estimated that dependence will develop in 16% of people using cocaine and 11% of those who use amfetamines.[2]

Acute intoxication and chronic use of these substances can present with cardiovascular symptoms, movement disorders and a range of psychiatric symptoms including agitation, enhanced anxiety, paranoia, panic attacks and psychosis. Associations with violent behaviour, high-risk sexual activity and the injecting of stimulants further underline the implications of stimulant use at the public health level.[2–4]

Tolerance and dependence can be expected to develop following regular, long-term use. For patients dependent on stimulants, a withdrawal syndrome of approximately 1 week's duration marked by craving, fatigue, agitation, insomnia and increased appetite can follow on from abstinence.[5,6]

Recreationally, patterns of SUD vary from use of a single stimulant, several different stimulants and simultaneous or sequential use of drugs from different classes. Combinations of different drugs may be explored by patients as a means of shaping the overall psychoactive experience.[3] Stimulant use among people with opiate use disorder is common and linked to poor engagement with opiate agonist therapy and the increased risk of overdose that follows.[7,8]

Overview of treatment

After decades of research there are, at the time of writing, no pharmacological agents approved in the treatment of SUD.[9–12] It is worth mentioning explicitly that there is also limited evidence to support the prescribing of stimulants themselves (so-called agonist replacement therapy) for patients with SUD.[10,13] There is a need for rigorous, high-quality clinical trials that can overcome the historical methodological challenges.[11]

Stimulant use for many will be self-limiting without treatment beyond the provision of harm minimisation advice and psychoeducation. For those who use stimulants in combination with alcohol, heroin or GBL, effective treatment of the co-occurring dependency may enable reductions in stimulant use. Successful care of patients dependent on stimulants should involve a comprehensive treatment approach that includes psychosocial interventions that reflect the complexity of factors behind SUD. While a range of therapeutic modalities are recommended, there is particularly good evidence for contingency management.[2,11]

For many the route to abstinence is through mutual aid and peer support such as Cocaine Anonymous, Crystal Meth Anonymous or Rational Recovery. Further information on the treatment of cocaine dependence can be found in UK clinical guidelines.[14] The limited effective interventions available for SUD have prompted the exploring of other treatment modalities.

There is a small developing evidence base for the potential of interventions based on neuromodulation such as transcranial magnetic stimulation (tMS) in SUD. This is an area of research in its early stages, without consensus on an appropriate cortical target or optimal frequency of TMS.[15]

An important area of consideration is the management of patients with SUD and suspected or verified attention deficit hyperactivity disorder (ADHD). As might be expected, ADHD is more common in patients with substance use disorder.[16] There is limited guidance to support clinicians in making a definitive diagnosis of ADHD in this group of patients or to navigate the risk–benefit balance of commencing treatment with stimulants compared with second-line non-stimulant-based alternatives.[17,18]

Cocaine

Cocaine is a naturally derived compound found in the coca plant. Aside from application as a topical anaesthetic, it is primarily used recreationally. Once extracted, cocaine's properties are enhanced when processed into cocaine hydrochloride, a powdered form that is commonly insufflated (snorted). Removal of the hydrochloride creates a water-insoluble base form (freebase) known as 'crack' that can be smoked. Both forms of cocaine can be injected although as a freebase it must first be dissolved in an acid. An epidemiological study from 2023 suggests an increase in rates of crack injection in both England and Wales.[19]

Detoxification

Symptoms of withdrawal include depressed mood, agitation and insomnia. These are usually self-limiting. It should be noted that given cocaine's short half-life and the binge nature of cocaine use, many patients essentially detoxify themselves regularly, with no pharmacological therapy. Symptomatic relief such as the short-term use of hypnotics may be helpful in some, but these agents may become agents of dependence themselves for some patients.[14]

Substitution treatment

There is little evidence for substitution therapy for the treatment of cocaine misuse and it should not usually be prescribed.[1,9,11]

Amfetamines

Amfetamine-type substances were first synthesised in the early 20th century initially having a wide range of applications. Currently, their clinical use is restricted to the treatment of ADHD and narcolepsy.[20] Amfetamine as a salt, usually amfetamine sulphate, the cathinone mephedrone and the more potent, long-acting methamphetamine are most commonly associated with significant misuse.

Within a recreational context, amfetamine sulphate is known as 'speed' and mephedrone as 'drone' or 'meow meow'; names for methamphetamine include 'meth', 'crystal' or 'tina'. These substances can be ingested as tablets or 'pills', insufflated as powders and, less commonly, injected or 'slammed'. Methamphetamine, when in its crystalline form 'ice', can also be inhaled.

CHAPTER 4

Detoxification and dependence

A withdrawal syndrome is common in those who are dependent. Treatment should focus on symptomatic relief, although many symptoms of amfetamine withdrawal (low mood, listlessness, agitation, irritability, fatigue, etc.) are short-lived and may not be amenable to pharmacological treatment. Insomnia can be treated with short courses of hypnotics, again noting the risk of dependence on these agents.[1,9,11] A 2022 systemic review and meta-analysis observed that mirtazapine may reduce the amount of meth-amphetamine consumed by patients with methamphetamine use disorder.[21]

Polysubstance abuse

In those who are dependent on opioids and cocaine, the provision of effective substitution therapy for treatment of the opioid dependence with either methadone or buprenorphine can lead to a reduction in cocaine use.[14]

Psychosis associated with stimulant drugs

Psychotic symptoms in association with methamphetamine are related to frequency of use and severity of methamphetamine dependence.[22] In many, perhaps most, cases psychotic symptoms can resolve with the resolution of intoxication – i.e. over the course of a day or so. The majority of patients attending an emergency setting with acute psychotic symptoms in the context of very recent methamphetamine use can be managed with simple sedation (e.g. diazepam 5–10mg as needed 4–6 hourly for agitation) and therapeutic rest.[23] Some patients, however, may need more intensive treatment in line with the treatment of acute psychosis in Chapter 2.

It should be noted that psychotic symptoms in the context of stimulant use are progressive with continued use – they tend to start earlier in each binge and to last longer. A median of 25% of patients report on-going symptoms 1 month after meth-amphetamine consumption.[24] Psychosis in the context of intoxication is associated with persecutory delusions and tactile hallucinations, while more persistent methamphetamine-associated psychosis is characterised by delusions of persecution and auditory hallucinations and is largely indistinguishable from a primary psychotic disorder.[24] In the emergency department it can be difficult to make a clear diagnosis. Between 16% and 38% of patients initially diagnosed with methamphetamine psychosis are later diagnosed as having schizophrenia.[24]

In the acute setting, another important differential diagnosis in methamphetamine users presenting with agitated psychosis is GBL withdrawal delirium (where stimulant/GBL polysubstance use is prevalent). There is symptomatic overlap between stimulant intoxication – autonomic hyperactivity, agitation, hallucinations – and GBL withdrawal delirium. The latter requires higher doses of benzodiazepines and more prolonged treatment (see 'GHB and GBL dependence' later in this chapter).

As already stated, in the emergency setting, simple sedation with benzodiazepines for agitation is often sufficient initially. If antipsychotics are indicated, the fourfold increased odds of developing extrapyramidal side effects (EPSEs) in patients who use methamphetamine should be borne in mind.[25] Agents with a low propensity to cause EPSEs should be used and there is evidence for efficacy of olanzapine. Aripiprazole may be preferred for rapid tranquillisation as olanzapine and benzodiazepines cannot be co-administered. Haloperidol should not be used because of the risk of dystonia. Early review regarding continuation is important as for most patients their symptoms resolve within 2 or 3 weeks, and there is no evidence to support the benefit of prophylactic prescription of antipsychotics in methamphetamine-related psychosis.[26]

Stimulant-associated depression

Anhedonia can be profound in early abstinence from stimulants. For many, low mood will resolve in line with duration of abstinence and supportive psychosocial interventions.[19] For those in whom it endures psychological treatments are effective but may be difficult for addiction patients to access because of institutional barriers.[2]

Antidepressants have primarily been evaluated as treatment for the substance dependence itself, with depression as a secondary outcome. There is some evidence for TCAs in reducing depressive symptoms.[27] However, TCAs are not recommended in those with on-going comorbid substance misuse because of their cardiotoxicity.[28] There is no evidence to support the use of SSRIs and indeed these are associated with significant interactions with stimulants[19] and increased disengagement.[2]

References

1. Murnane KS, et al. Selective serotonin 2A receptor antagonism attenuates the effects of amphetamine on arousal and dopamine overflow in non-human primates. *J Sleep Res* 2013; **22**:581–588.

2. Farrell M, et al. Responding to global stimulant use: challenges and opportunities. *Lancet* 2019; **394**:1652–1667.

3. United Nations Office on Drugs and Crime. Treatment of stimulant use disorders: current practices and promising perspectives. United Nations Office on Drugs and Crime Vienna, Austria. 2019 (last checked May 2024); https://www.unodc.org/documents/drug-prevention-and-treatment/Treatment_of_PSUD_for_website_24.05.19.pdf.

4. Moradi S, et al. The association between methamphetamine use and number of sexual partners in men who have sex with men: a systematic review and meta-analysis. *Subst Abuse Treat Prevention Policy* 2022; **17**:27.

5. Substance Abuse and Mental Health Services Administration (SAMHSA). Treatment of stimulant use disorders. SAMSHA publication PEP 20-06-01-001. 2020; https://store.samhsa.gov/sites/default/files/pep20-06-01-001.pdf.

6. McGregor C, et al. The nature, time course and severity of methamphetamine withdrawal. *Addiction* 2005; **100**:1320–1329.

7. Mintz CM, et al. Analysis of stimulant prescriptions and drug-related poisoning risk among persons receiving buprenorphine treatment for opioid use disorder. *JAMA Netw Open* 2022; **5**:e2211634.

8. Cicero TJ, et al. Polysubstance use: a broader understanding of substance use during the opioid crisis. *Am J Public Health* 2020; **110**:244–250.

9. Siefried KJ, et al. Pharmacological treatment of methamphetamine/amphetamine dependence: a systematic review. *CNS Drugs* 2020; **34**:337–365.

10. Bahji A, et al. Navigating evidence, challenges, and caution in the treatment of stimulant use disorders. *Brain Sci* 2023; **13**:1416.

11. Ronsley C, et al. Treatment of stimulant use disorder: a systematic review of reviews. *PLoS One* 2020; **15**:e0234809.

12. Liu MT. Pharmacotherapy treatment of stimulant use disorder. *Ment Health Clin* 2021; **11**:347–357.

13. Stoops WW, et al. Agonist replacement for stimulant dependence: a review of clinical research. *Curr Pharm Des* 2013; **19**:7026–7035.

14. Department of Health and Social Care. Drug misuse and dependence: UK guidelines on clinical management. 2017; https://www.gov.uk/government/publications/drug-misuse-and-dependence-uk-guidelines-on-clinical-management.

15. Edinoff AN, et al. Transcranial stimulation for the treatment of stimulant use disorder. *Neurol Int* 2023; **15**:325–338.

16. Rohner H, et al. Prevalence of attention deficit hyperactivity disorder (ADHD) among substance use disorder (SUD) populations: meta-analysis. *Int J Environ Res Public Health* 2023; **20**:1275.

17. Ward B, et al. Managing adult attention-deficit/hyperactivity disorder with comorbid substance use disorder. *Can J Addict* 2023; **13**:6–12.

18. Levin FR. Diagnosing attention-deficit/hyperactivity disorder in patients with substance use disorders. *J Clin Psychiatry* 2007; **68** Suppl 11:9–14.

19. Edmundson C, et al. Recent increases in crack injection and associated risk factors among people who inject psychoactive drugs in England and Wales. *Int J Drug Policy* 2023:104262.

20. Heal DJ, et al. Amphetamine, past and present – a pharmacological and clinical perspective. *J Psychopharmacol* 2013; **27**:479–496.

21. Naji L, et al. Mirtazapine for the treatment of amphetamine and methamphetamine use disorder: a systematic review and meta-analysis. *Drug Alcohol Depend* 2022; **232**:109295.

22. Arunogiri S, et al. A systematic review of risk factors for methamphetamine-associated psychosis. *Aust NZ J Psychiatry* 2018; **52**:514–529.

CHAPTER 4

23. Isoardi KZ, et al. Methamphetamine presentations to an emergency department: management and complications. *Emerg Med Australas* 2019; **31**:593–599.

24. Voce A, et al. A systematic review of the symptom profile and course of methamphetamine-associated psychosis(substance use and misuse). *Subst Use Misuse* 2019; **54**:549–559.

25. Temmingh HS, et al. Methamphetamine use and antipsychotic-related extrapyramidal side-effects in patients with psychotic disorders. *J Dual Diagn* 2020; **16**:208–217.

26. Shoptaw SJ, et al. Treatment for amphetamine psychosis. *Cochrane Database Syst Rev* 2009; **1**:CD003026.

27. Pani PP, et al. Antidepressants for cocaine dependence and problematic cocaine use. *Cochrane Database Syst Rev* 2011; **12**:CD002950.

28. Lingford-Hughes AR, et al. BAP updated guidelines: evidence-based guidelines for the pharmacological management of substance abuse, harmful use, addiction and comorbidity: recommendations from BAP. *J Psychopharmacol* 2012; **26**:899–952.

GHB and GBL dependence

GHB and GBL misuse is uncommon but medically important because, in dependent users, withdrawal can proceed rapidly to life-threatening agitated delirium. Complications include seizures, bradycardia, cardiac arrest and renal failure. Professionals in acute and psychiatric hospitals need to be able to recognise and manage acute withdrawal.

Gamma-hydroxybutyrate (GHB) and gamma-butyrolactone (GBL, a pro-drug of GHB) are colloquially often referred to as 'G'. They reduce anxiety and produce disinhibition and sedation, primarily through actions at the GABA-B receptor. These drugs are used recreationally for socialising and occasionally to aid sleep. Among men who have sex with men (MSM) they can be used, often alongside stimulants such as mephedrone and crystal methamphetamine, to facilitate sex in the context of potential high-risk sexual behaviour ('chemsex'). Both GHB and GBL have a narrow therapeutic index and overdose is not uncommon. Dependence is rare, but in dependent users withdrawal has a rapid onset and can produce severe delirium with paranoid delusions and life-threatening complications.[1]

The withdrawal syndrome[1,2]

Dependent users take doses 'round the clock' (consuming doses day and night, typically every 1–3 hours). The onset of withdrawal symptoms occurs a few hours following the last dose. This withdrawal syndrome is similar to alcohol withdrawal and may include symptoms such as tachycardia, insomnia, anxiety, sweating and fine tremors.[1] Untreated, it can progress to agitated delirium, often with psychotic features (including paranoid delusions and hallucinations) later followed by severe tremors, muscle rigidity and seizures.[1] Muscle rigidity may be so severe as to produce fever, rhabdomyolysis and acute renal failure. The requirement for medication to manage symptoms eases over 4–6 days, although there are case reports of more prolonged withdrawal.

Withdrawal management

The evidence base for detoxification is limited. The core principle of managing withdrawal is to treat early and so prevent the development of delirium and other complications. Once established, delirium can be difficult to control.[3] Early treatment with benzodiazepines is required, and baclofen (a GABA-B agonist) and phenobarbital have also been used effectively as adjunctive medications.[1,4] Antipsychotic drugs are used in some countries.[5] Baclofen is freely available online and may be obtained by users for unsupervised withdrawal,[6] something which, given the dangers involved in withdrawal, should be unequivocally discouraged.

There is as yet no validated screening tool to determine when patients should receive pharmacological treatment for withdrawal symptoms. However, two case reports suggest that the CIWA-Ar scale can be used in the assessment of patients withdrawing from GHB.[7,8]

GHB itself has also been successfully used to aid withdrawal[9] with reducing doses given every 3 hours over up to 2 weeks. Pharmaceutical GHB may be more effective than benzodiazepines in managing withdrawal.[10]

CHAPTER 4

For up-to-date guidance on the management of GHB/GBL withdrawal, it is recommended in the UK that information be sought from the National Poisons Information Service (NPIS),[11] specifically the NPIS 24-hour telephone service and the poisons information database TOXBASE.[12]

The two scenarios with which clinicians should be conversant are unplanned acute withdrawal (Box 4.6) and planned elective withdrawal (Box 4.7).

Box 4.6 Management of unplanned acute withdrawal	
Setting	▪ Acute unplanned withdrawal is a medical emergency and should be managed in the acute hospital inpatient setting ▪ Severe withdrawal may require admission to ICU
Initial pharmacotherapy	▪ Initiate diazepam 20mg PO as soon as withdrawal symptoms are observed ▪ Diazepam can be repeated at 30 minutes to 4-hourly intervals until symptoms are controlled ▪ Most cases of GBL withdrawal require 60–80mg diazepam in the first 24 hours ▪ Higher daily dosages of up to 300mg PO diazepam may be necessary ▪ If on assessment the patient is drowsy, withhold diazepam dose, monitor respiratory signs and review once sedation attenuates ▪ One-to-one nursing care may assist in managing severe cases ▪ If there are concerns about the level of drowsiness from treatment with benzodiazepines then early discussion with anaesthetics/ICU team is advised to consider need for airway support ▪ From day 2 a tapering regimen of diazepam is started based on the total diazepam administered in the first 24 hours
Ajunctive pharmacotherapy	▪ Initiate baclofen 10mg PO tds in combination with benzodiazepine withdrawal regimen where benzodiazepines prove inadequate ▪ This can be titrated to 20mg PO tds in cases of continued anxiety and agitation ▪ In cases of severe withdrawal consider addition of phenobarbital in doses of 150–450mg/day oral or IV* (ICU only)[13] ▪ In cases where severe withdrawal remains uncontrolled, IV anaesthetics such as propofol* may be required (ICU only) ▪ Thiopental* coma has also been used in severe resistant withdrawal[10]

*The respiratory depressant effects of phenobarbital, thiopental and propofol cannot be reversed; facilities for mechanical ventilation should be available.
GBL, gamma-butyrolactone; ICU, intensive care unit; PO, by mouth; tds, three times a day.

Box 4.7 Management of planned elective withdrawal	
Setting	▪ All patients undergoing planned withdrawal should be medically supervised ▪ Ambulatory community detoxification should be attempted only where there is no history of delirium or psychosis. A responsible third party should be at home who is able to monitor and support the withdrawal process. There should be the option of transferring the patient to an in-patient unit if symptoms are not well controlled

Pre-withdrawal	■ Discuss treatment plan with the patient and person who will be supporting them
	■ Encourage patient to keep a week-long diary of GBL use including dose frequency and quantity
	■ Encourage patient to cease 'on-top' drug use such as mephedrone and crystal methamphetamine before elective withdrawal
	■ Start baclofen 10mg PO tds 3–7 days before target withdrawal date
	■ Encourage patients to reduce GBL dose as much as tolerable either by reducing each dose by 0.1mL every 1–2 days or increasing the time period between doses
Withdrawal	■ On day 1 of planned ambulatory withdrawal, ask patient to attend having used no GBL for a minimum of 2 hours, and advise them to dispose of their remaining supplies of GBL
	■ Advise patients they will need to stay at the clinic for up to 4 hours on day 1, that they cannot drive motor vehicles during withdrawal, and should not drink alcohol or take other sedatives during withdrawal
	■ Increase baclofen to 20mg PO tds
	■ Initiate benzodiazepine treatment once signs and symptoms of withdrawal develop – tachycardia, sweaty palms, fine tremor and anxiety. Start diazepam 20mg, review after 2 hours and monitor for anxiety/sedation/respiratory depression. Repeat up to 20mg PO diazepam if indicated
	■ Once 6 hours have passed since last GBL usage the patient may be given up to a further 40mg diazepam, and then seen daily on the following 2 days
	■ At each daily visit, review diazepam dosage and titrate to symptoms. Diazepam is seldom needed beyond 7 days. Typical initial daily doses of diazepam are around 40–60mg/day
Post-withdrawal	■ Continue baclofen 20mg PO tds following benzodiazepine withdrawal, reducing over 4–6 weeks. One of the few trials in this area successfully used 45–60mg a day for 3 months for relapse prevention[11]
	■ After withdrawal, persisting anxiety and insomnia are common, and there is a high risk of relapse. Before initiating elective withdrawal management, a plan should be in place to monitor and support patients for a minimum of 4 weeks to minimise risk of relapse

GBL, gamma-butyrolactone; PO, by mouth; tds, three times a day.

References

1. Kamal RM, et al. Pharmacological treatment in gamma-hydroxybutyrate (GHB) and gamma-butyrolactone (GBL) dependence: detoxification and relapse prevention. *CNS Drugs* 2017; **31**:51–64.
2. Bell J, et al. Gamma-butyrolactone (GBL) dependence and withdrawal. *Addiction* 2011; **106**:442–447.
3. Abdulrahim D, et al. *Textbook of Clinical Management of Club Drugs and Novel Psychoactive Substances: NEPTUNE Clinical Guidance.* Cambridge: Cambridge University Press; 2022.
4. LeTourneau JL, et al. Baclofen and gamma-hydroxybutyrate withdrawal. *Neurocrit Care* 2008; **8**:430–433.
5. Siefried KJ, et al. Inpatient GHB withdrawal management in an inner-city hospital in Sydney, Australia: a retrospective medical record review. *Psychopharmacology (Berl)* 2023; **240**:127–135.
6. Floyd CN, et al. Baclofen in gamma-hydroxybutyrate withdrawal: patterns of use and online availability. *Eur J Clin Pharmacol* 2018; **74**:349–356.
7. Liao PC, et al. Clinical management of gamma-hydroxybutyrate (GHB) withdrawal delirium with CIWA-Ar protocol. *J Formos Med Assoc* 2018; **117**:1124–1127.
8. Habibian S, et al. Successful management of gamma-hydroxybutyrate (GHB) withdrawal using baclofen as a standalone therapy: a case report. *J Addict Med* 2019; **13**:415–417.
9. Dijkstra BA, et al. Detoxification with titration and tapering in gamma-hydroxybutyrate (GHB) dependent patients: the Dutch GHB monitor project. *Drug Alcohol Depend* 2017; **170**:164–173.
10. Beurmanjer H, et al. Tapering with pharmaceutical GHB or benzodiazepines for detoxification in GHB-dependent patients: a matched-subject observational study of treatment-as-usual in Belgium and the Netherlands. *CNS Drugs* 2020; **34**:651–659.
11. National Poisons Information Service. 2024; https://www.npis.org.
12. TOXBASE®. 2024; https://www.toxbase.org.
13. Freeman G, et al. Phenobarbital to manage severe gamma-hydroxybutyrate withdrawal: a case series. *Drug Alcohol Rev* 2023; **42**:27–32.

CHAPTER 4

Benzodiazepine misuse

Benzodiazepine prescribing reached its peak during the 1960s and 1970s. Prescriptions that were originally started for disorders such as anxiety, depression and insomnia were often continued long term and led to the development of dependence. Benzodiazepines are still widely used in the USA: 5.2% of adults were prescribed a benzodiazepine in 2008,[1] just over 4% in 2018 and just less than 4% in 2021.[2]

There are a growing number of novel or 'designer' illicit benzodiazepines (e.g. diclazepam, etizolam, flualprazolam, flunitrazolam and norfludiazepam). There is limited information available about the health consequences and social harms of these substances, but they are likely to be similar to or worse than the established benzodiazepines.[3] As well as being prescribed, benzodiazepines can be acquired via the illicit market, diversion of prescriptions and internet purchasing (thought to be a rising trend).[4,5]

Benzodiazepine dependence can be thought of as either iatrogenic (low daily doses prescribed over many years) or non-iatrogenic (high doses, illicitly obtained, often consumed intermittently).

Withdrawal management

The UK NICE guideline on safe prescribing and withdrawal management of medicines associated with dependence recommends a shared decision-making approach with the individual.[6] Detailed information regarding benefits of discontinuation, the withdrawal process and possible symptoms should be discussed over the course of regular scheduled reviews. Withdrawal from benzodiazepines usually involves conversion to an equivalent dose of diazepam because its long duration of action may mitigate withdrawal symptoms.

Dose reduction recommendations include:

- Gradual reduction rather than abrupt discontinuation.[6]
- 'Slow, step-wise rate of reduction proportionate to the existing dose, so that decrements become smaller as the dose is lowered' (unless there is clinical risk and rapid withdrawal is needed).[6]
- Individualise according to the drug, dose, duration of treatment, history of dependence, withdrawal symptoms and re-emergence of underlying conditions (such as anxiety or insomnia).
- Withdrawal over a period of less than 6 months is appropriate for some patients.[7]
- Some guidelines suggest a reduction of about one-eighth of the daily dose every 2 weeks.[8]
- If reduction is unsuccessful aim to review regularly, stop further escalation in dose and consider reduction again later.

Additional interventions are given in Table 4.23.

Table 4.23 Psychosocial and pharmacological interventions in benzodiazepine withdrawal.

Psychosocial	Pharmacological
Contingency management and patient education have had some success at reducing benzodiazepine use	A 2018 Cochrane review could find no pharmaceutical add-on that could help facilitate the withdrawal process[12]
A Cochrane review found evidence that supported the use of cognitive behavioural therapy (CBT) alongside dose reduction[9]	Withdrawal symptoms should **not** be treated with another dependence-forming medicine or sodium valproate or buspirone[6]
Evidence suggests targeted interventions with non-pharmacological supportive therapies are more likely to result in successful deprescription[10]	
Multifaceted prescribing interventions (usually including psychological interventions/support) are recommended for older patients[11]	

Polysubstance use

Illicit benzodiazepines are often used in addition to a primary substance of abuse. People with non-iatrogenic benzodiazepine dependence often consume doses greater than 100mg diazepam equivalent a day. There is no evidence that substitute prescribing of benzodiazepines ultimately reduces benzodiazepine misuse. Benzodiazepine dependence as part of polysubstance dependence should also be treated by a gradual withdrawal of the medication. Benzodiazepines prescribed at greater than 30mg diazepam equivalent per day may cause harm[8] and so this should be avoided if at all possible.

Pregnancy and benzodiazepine misuse

Benzodiazepines are not major human teratogens but should ideally be gradually discontinued before a planned pregnancy. If a woman is prescribed benzodiazepines and found to be pregnant, the prescription should be gradually withdrawn over as short a time as possible, being mindful of the risk of withdrawal seizures and the potential consequences for the pregnant woman and fetus. A risk–benefit analysis should be undertaken and specialist advice sought (see pregnancy section in Chapter 7). As for all patients, it may be appropriate for a woman dependent on benzodiazepines to be stabilised on diazepam before any dose reduction.[8]

Summary

- Benzodiazepines should be withdrawn using a hyperbolic tapering schedule (Table 4.24).
- Discontinuation can sometimes be completed within 6 months.
- Switching to an equivalent dose of diazepam before withdrawal is commonplace but not always effective.

CHAPTER 4

■ Benzodiazepine misuse is frequently seen in multisubstance misuse where opioids may be the primary drug of dependence.

■ Consider cognitive behavioural therapy (CBT) when withdrawing from benzodiazepines.

Table 4.24 Typical diazepam withdrawal schedule for iatrogenic dependence.

Week	Dose
Baseline	30mg/day
Week 2	25mg/day
Week 4	20mg/day
Week 6	18mg/day
Week 8	16mg/day
Week 10	14mg/day
Week 12	12mg/day
Week 14	10mg/day
Then reduce by 2mg/day every 2 weeks if tolerated.	

More detailed information on benzodiazepine withdrawal is given in *The Maudsley Deprescribing Guidelines.*[13]

References

1. Olfson M, et al. Benzodiazepine use in the United States. *JAMA Psychiatry* 2015; **72**:136–142.
2. Milani SA, et al. Trends in the use of benzodiazepines, Z-hypnotics, and serotonergic drugs among US women and men before and during the COVID-19 pandemic. *JAMA Netw Open* 2021; **4**:e2131012.
3. Advisory Council on the Misuse of Drugs (ACMD). A review of the evidence of use and harms of novel benzodiazepines. London: Home Office. 2020; https://assets.publishing.service.gov.uk/government/uploads/system/uploads/attachment_data/file/881969/ACMD_report_-_a_review_of_the_evidence_of_use_and_harms_of_novel_benzodiazepines.pdf.
4. Manchester KR, et al. The emergence of new psychoactive substance (NPS) benzodiazepines: a review. *Drug Test Anal* 2018; **10**:392–393.
5. Sarker A, et al. Evidence of the emergence of illicit benzodiazepines from online drug forums. *Eur J Public Health* 2022; **32**:939–941.
6. National Institute for Health and Care Excellence. Medicines associated with dependence or withdrawal symptoms: safe prescribing and withdrawal management for adults. NICE guideline [NG215]. 2022 (last checked April 2024); https://www.nice.org.uk/guidance/ng215.
7. Lader M, et al. Withdrawing benzodiazepines in primary care. *CNS Drugs* 2009; **23**:19–34.
8. Department of Health. Drug misuse and dependence: UK guidelines on clinical management. London: Department of Health. 2017; https://assets.publishing.service.gov.uk/government/uploads/system/uploads/attachment_data/file/673978/clinical_guidelines_2017.pdf.
9. Darker CD, et al. Psychosocial interventions for benzodiazepine harmful use, abuse or dependence. *Cochrane Database Syst Rev* 2015; **5**:CD009652.
10. Soni A, et al. Feasibility and effectiveness of deprescribing benzodiazepines and Z-drugs: systematic review and meta-analysis. *Addiction* 2023; **118**:7–16.
11. Gould RL, et al. Interventions for reducing benzodiazepine use in older people: meta-analysis of randomised controlled trials. *Br J Psychiatry* 2014; **204**:98–107.
12. Baandrup L, et al. Pharmacological interventions for benzodiazepine discontinuation in chronic benzodiazepine users. *Cochrane Database Syst Rev* 2018; **3**:CD011481.
13. Horowitz M, et al. *The Maudsley Deprescribing Guidelines: Antidepressants, Benzodiazepines, Gabapentinoids and Z-drugs.* Oxford: Wiley-Blackwell; 2024.

CHAPTER 4

Drug-induced excited state

A drug-induced excited state is an under-recognised and potentially life-threatening syndrome of agitation, aggression and dysregulated physiological responses.[1] Illicit drugs are the most common cause, notably cocaine and New Psychoactive Substances including synthetic cannabinoids and stimulants such as mephedrone. There are also other causes of a drug-induced excited state.[2]

This section draws attention to the approach required for people whose behaviour presents a danger to themselves or others because of the acute effect of illicit substances, and who are at significant risk of physiological harm. The terms 'acute behavioural disturbance' or 'excited delirium' are not used because they are not recognised diagnoses and because they are highly controversial terms that are suspected of being misused in respect to deaths in police custody.[3-5]

Early intervention and de-escalation are crucial to effective and safe treatment. It cannot be overemphasised that physical restraint should be avoided whenever possible because of the substantial risk to life presented by restraint in these patients. Where restraint cannot be avoided, it should be used carefully and safely: avoiding restraint in the prone position and employing it for the briefest possible time (i.e. for seconds, not minutes).

Pathophysiology

Various components of the drug-induced excited state and its treatment (including restraint) lead to disorientation and a 'fight or flight' response. The physical exertion employed to 'escape' results in hyperthermia and catecholamine release.[6] Hyperthermia in turn leads to rhabdomyolysis (with raised creatine kinase)[7] as well as worsening delirium.[8] Excess sympathetic catecholamines prolong the cardiac QT interval and may adversely affect myocardial function.[9] Excess muscle activity, raised catecholamines, hyperthermia and dehydration contribute to a metabolic acidosis and the production of carbon dioxide. This manifests with tachypnoea and may herald pending cardiovascular collapse. It cannot be overemphasised that restraint grossly exacerbates risks in this cascade of events, especially if restraint is prolonged.

Identification

A drug-induced excited state is not a distinct diagnosis, but a term used to encapsulate a range of situations in which a person experiences distress, displays agitation or aggression and is at risk of physiological dysregulation. Perhaps the most common symptoms are violent behaviour, increased pain tolerance and constant activity.[10] Rapid breathing, a lack of fatigue, hyperpyrexia and tactile hyperthermia are also frequently observed.[11] A cascade of events may develop and may be provoked or worsened by restraint, leading to increased fear, then protracted physical struggle, hypoxia due to restraint, catecholamine release, lactic acidosis, and so on.

Management

Verbally de-escalate and try to ensure environmental safety for the individual and others. It bears repeating that restraint may exacerbate hyperthermia and catecholamine release, worsening outcomes.[12] Sedation is important to calm aggression and to reduce heat generation and catecholamine release. There is evidence to support intramuscular use of benzodiazepines (including lorazepam and midazolam[13]), antipsychotics (including haloperidol, droperidol, olanzapine and chlorpromazine[13,14]) and their combination.[15] Caution is required with antipsychotics because of the risk of acute dystonia and neuroleptic malignant syndrome.

Record pulse, blood pressure and temperature where and when safe to do so. Basic urinary drug screens have limited validity for New Psychoactive Substances but many clinical laboratories can identify potentially causative compounds (albeit with a time lag). An ECG is desirable but unlikely to be possible until individuals have been sedated. Full assessment and treatment require urgent ambulance transfer to an emergency department.[16] Psychiatric nursing personnel might be required to contain and support the individual. In the emergency department, intramuscular ketamine is the preferred sedative, with a predictable dose–response effect at 2–4mg/kg.[17] Antipyretics are ineffective cooling agents. Cooled intravenous fluids, water sprays and ice to the whole body may be required.

Outcomes

Mortality rates are not known, with the only source of data available being uncontrolled observations.[18] Risk of death is related to the duration of hyperthermia and peak temperature reached – body temperatures over 42°C usually have very poor outcomes. A body mass index of more than 25kg/m^2 is also associated with worse outcome. In non-fatal instances, most cases of drug-induced excited state are brief and fully resolve within 48 hours. Longer-term cardiac, renal and hepatic damage can occasionally occur.

References

1. Stevenson R, et al. Acute behavioural disturbance: a physical emergency psychiatrists need to understand. *BJPsych Advances* 2021; 27:333–342.
2. Kennedy DB, et al. Delayed in-custody death involving excited delirium. *J Correct Health Care* 2018; 24:43–51.
3. Tracy DK. Acute behavioural disturbance: what's in a name? *BJPsych Open* 2024; 10:e38.
4. Polling C, et al. Use of 'acute behavioural disturbance' in mental health records: differences over time and by ethnicity. *BJPsych Open* 2023; 9:e133.
5. Humphries C, et al. Consensus on acute behavioural disturbance in the UK: a multidisciplinary modified Delphi study to determine what it is and how it should be managed. *Emerg Med J* 2023; 41:4–12.
6. Bunai Y, et al. Fatal hyperthermia associated with excited delirium during an arrest. *Leg Med (Tokyo)* 2008; 10:306–309.
7. Borek HA, et al. Hyperthermia and multiorgan failure after abuse of 'bath salts' containing 3,4-methylenedioxypyrovalerone. *Ann Emerg Med* 2012; 60:103–105.
8. Otahbachi M, et al. Excited delirium, restraints, and unexpected death: a review of pathogenesis. *Am J Forensic Med Pathol* 2010; 31:107–112.
9. Wittstein IS, et al. Neurohumoral features of myocardial stunning due to sudden emotional stress. *N Engl J Med* 2005; 352:539–548.
10. Hall CA, et al. Frequency of signs of excited delirium syndrome in subjects undergoing police use of force: descriptive evaluation of a prospective, consecutive cohort. *J Forensic Leg Med* 2013; 20:102–107.
11. Baldwin S, et al. Distinguishing features of excited delirium syndrome in non-fatal use of force encounters. *J Forensic Leg Med* 2016; 41:21–27.
12. Stratton SJ, et al. Factors associated with sudden death of individuals requiring restraint for excited delirium. *Am J Emerg Med* 2001; 19:187–191.
13. Isbister GK, et al. Randomized controlled trial of intramuscular droperidol versus midazolam for violence and acute behavioral disturbance: the DORM study. *Ann Emerg Med* 2010; 56:392–401 e391.
14. Page CB, et al. A prospective study of the safety and effectiveness of droperidol in children for prehospital acute behavioral disturbance. *Prehosp Emerg Care* 2019; 23:519–526.
15. O'Connor N, et al. Pharmacological management of acute severe behavioural disturbance: a survey of current protocols. *Australas Psychiatry* 2017; 25:395–398.
16. Wetli CV, et al. Cocaine-associated agitated delirium and the neuroleptic malignant syndrome. *Am J Emerg Med* 1996; 14:425–428.
17. Li M, et al. Evaluation of ketamine for excited delirium syndrome in the adult emergency department. *J Emerg Med* 2020; 58:100–105.
18. Baldwin S, et al. Excited delirium syndrome (ExDS): situational factors and risks to officer safety in non-fatal use of force encounters. *Int J Law Psychiatry* 2018; 60:26–34.

Interactions between illicit drugs and prescribed psychotropic drugs

Interactions between drugs of misuse and prescribed psychotropics are common, not least because of the high rates of psychotropic prescribing in such patients.[1] Information on adverse interactions is derived largely from case reports and theoretical assumptions and rarely from systematic investigation. A summary of major interactions can be found in Table 4.25.

In all patients who misuse illicit drugs:

- Infection with hepatitis B and C is more common. The associated liver damage may lead to a reduced ability to metabolise other drugs and increased sensitivity to adverse effects.
- Infection with HIV is relatively common.[2,3] Antiretroviral drugs are involved in pharmacokinetic interactions with a number of prescribed and non-prescribed drugs.[4] For example, ritonavir can decrease the metabolism of ecstasy and precipitate toxicity, and a number of antiretrovirals can increase or decrease methadone metabolism.[5]
- Prescribed drugs may be used in the same way as illicit drugs (i.e. erratically and not as intended). Large quantities of prescribed drugs should not be given to out-patients.
- Additive or synergistic effects of respiratory depressants may play a contributory role in deaths from overdose with methadone or other opioid agonists.[6] Caution is needed in prescribing sedative medicines such as benzodiazepines and gabapentinoids.

CHAPTER 4

Table 4.25 Interactions between illicit drugs and psychotropics.

	Cannabis	Heroin/methadone[6]	Cocaine, amfetamines, ecstasy, MDA, 6-APD	Alcohol	Ketamine[7]
General considerations	■ Usually smoked in cigarettes (induces CYP1A2) ■ Can be sedative ■ Dose-related tachycardia ■ THC/CBD inhibit CYP3A4, CYP2C19 and CYP2D6[8,9]	■ Can produce sedation/ respiratory depression ■ QTc prolongation with methadone (see section on methadone earlier in this chapter)	■ Stimulants (cocaine can be sedative in higher doses) ■ Arrhythmia possible ■ Cerebral/cardiac ischaemia with cocaine – may be fatal ■ MDMA inhibits CYP2D6/CYP3A4 ■ Hyperthermia/dehydration with ecstasy[10]	■ Sedative ■ Liver damage possible ■ Induces various enzymes	■ Sedative readily causes unconciousness ■ Onset of effects may be rapid if snorted or injected
Older antipsychotics	■ Antipsychotics reduce the psychotropic effects of almost all drugs of abuse by blocking dopamine receptors (dopamine is the neurotransmitter responsible for 'reward') (e.g. haloperidol and MDMA[11]) ■ Patients prescribed antipsychotics may increase their consumption of illicit substances to compensate ■ Patients who have taken ecstasy may be more prone to EPSEs ■ Cardiotoxic or very sedative antipsychotics are best avoided, at least initially. Sulpiride is a reasonably safe first choice ■ Methamphetamines increase risk of EPSEs with haloperidol[12]				
Second-generation antipsychotics	■ Risk of additive sedation ■ Cannabis smoking in tobacco can reduce plasma levels of olanzapine and clozapine via induction of CYP1A2[13] ■ Clozapine might reduce cannabis and alcohol consumption[14] ■ Outcome of THC/CBD inhibition of CYP1A2 unknown	■ Risk of additive sedation ■ Case report of methadone withdrawal being precipitated by risperidone[15] ■ Isolated report of quetiapine increasing methadone levels, especially in those with slowed CYP2D6 hepatic metabolism[16]	■ Antipsychotics may reduce craving and cocaine-induced euphoria[17–21] ■ Olanzapine may worsen cocaine dependency[22] ■ Clozapine may increase cocaine levels but diminish subjective response[23]	■ Increased risk of hypotension with olanzapine (and possibly other beta-blockers)	■ Increased sedation ■ Possible interaction between risperidone and ketamine[24]

Antidepressants	■ Tachycardia has been reported (monitor pulse and take care with TCAs[25]) ■ Complex, unpredictable effects of CYP induction (tobacco) and CYP inhibition (THC/CBD)	■ Avoid very sedative antidepressants ■ Some SSRIs can increase methadone plasma levels[26] (citalopram is SSRI of choice but note the small risk of additive QTc prolongation) ■ Case report of serotonin syndrome occurring when sertraline prescribed with methadone for a palliative care patient[27]	■ Avoid TCAs (arrhythmia risk) ■ MAOIs contraindicated (hypertension) ■ Combining moclobemide and MDMA can be fatal[28] ■ SSRIs may increase plasma concentrations of MDMA[29] but reduce subjective effects[30] ■ Risk of SSRIs increasing cocaine levels, especially fluoxetine[31] ■ Concomitant use of SSRIs or aripiprazole and lamotrigine with cocaine or other stimulants (especially MDA and 6-APD) could precipitate a serotonin syndrome[32,33] ■ SSRIs may enhance subjective reaction to cocaine[34]	■ Avoid very sedative antidepressants ■ Avoid antidepressants that are toxic in overdose ■ Impaired psychomotor skills (not SSRIs)	■ Inhibitors of CYP3A4 (e.g. fluoxetine/paroxetine) will lengthen ketamine half-life ■ Beware hypertension with SNRIs and reboxetine
Anticholinergics		■ Misuse is likely. Try to avoid if at all possible (by using a second-generation drug if an antipsychotic is required) ■ Can cause hallucinations, elation and cognitive impairment			
Lithium		■ Very toxic if taken erratically ■ Always consider the effects of dehydration (particularly problematic with alcohol or ecstasy)			
Carbamazepine/ valproate	■ Carbamazepine may decrease THC concentrations via induction of CYP3A4[35]	■ Carbamazepine decreases methadone levels[36] (danger if carbamazepine stopped suddenly) ■ Valproate seems less likely to interact		■ Monitor LFTs	■ Carbamazepine decreases ketamine plasma concentrations via CYP3A4 induction
Benzodiazepines	■ Monitor level of sedation	■ Oversedation (and respiratory depression possible) ■ Concomitant use can lead to accidental overdose ■ Possible pharmacokinetic interaction (increased methadone levels)	■ Oversedation (if high doses of cocaine have been taken) ■ Widely used after cocaine intoxication ■ Future misuse possible	■ Oversedation (and respiratory depression) possible ■ Widely used in alcohol detoxification	■ Oversedation and respiratory depression
Gabapentinoids	■ Monitor level of sedation	■ Large increase in risk of death in overdose[37,38]	■ Does not reduce cocaine use[39]	■ Oversedation and respiratory depression possible	■ No interaction reported[24]

6-APD, 6-(2-aminopropyl)benzofuran; CBD, cannabidiol; EPSEs, extrapyramidal side effects; MAOIs, monoamine oxidase inhibitors, MDA, 3,4-methylenedioxyamphetamine; MDMA, 3,4-methylene dioxymethamphetamine; TCAs, tricyclic antidepressants; THC, tetrahydrocannabinol.

References

1. Zapelini do Nascimento D, et al. Potential psychotropic drug interactions among drug-dependent people. *J Psychoactive Drugs* 2021; **53**:168–176.

2. Vocci FJ, et al. Medication development for addictive disorders: the state of the science. *Am J Psychiatry* 2005; **162**:1432–1440.

3. Tsuang J, et al. Pharmacological treatment of patients with schizophrenia and substance abuse disorders. *Addict Disord Treat* 2005; **4**:127–137.

4. Bracchi M, et al. Increasing use of 'party drugs' in people living with HIV on antiretrovirals: a concern for patient safety. *Aids* 2015; **29**:1585–1592.

5. Gruber VA, et al. Methadone, buprenorphine, and street drug interactions with antiretroviral medications. *Curr HIV/AIDS Rep* 2010; **7**:152–160.

6. Department of Health and Social Care. Drug misuse and dependence: UK guidelines on clinical management. 2017; https://www.gov.uk/government/publications/drug-misuse-and-dependence-uk-guidelines-on-clinical-management.

7. Pfizer Ltd. Summary of product characteristics. Ketalar (ketamine hydrochloride) 10mg/ml injection. 2024 (last accessed July 2024); https://www.medicines.org.uk/emc/medicine/12939.

8. Arellano AL, et al. Neuropsychiatric and general interactions of natural and synthetic cannabinoids with drugs of abuse and medicines. *CNS Neurol Disord Drug Targets* 2017; **16**:554–566.

9. Abbott KL, et al. Adverse pharmacokinetic interactions between illicit substances and clinical drugs. *Drug Metab Rev* 2020; **52**:44–65.

10. Gowing LR, et al. The health effects of ecstasy: a literature review. *Drug Alcohol Rev* 2002; **21**:53–63.

11. Liechti ME, et al. Acute psychological and physiological effects of MDMA ('Ecstasy') after haloperidol pretreatment in healthy humans. *Eur Neuropsychopharmacol* 2000; **10**:289–295.

12. Matthew BJ, et al. Drug-induced parkinsonism following chronic methamphetamine use by a patient on haloperidol decanoate. *Int J Psychiatry Med* 2015; **50**:405–411.

13. Zullino DF, et al. Tobacco and cannabis smoking cessation can lead to intoxication with clozapine or olanzapine. *Int Clin Psychopharmacol* 2002; **17**:141–143.

14. Green AI, et al. Alcohol and cannabis use in schizophrenia: effects of clozapine vs. risperidone. *Schizophr Res* 2003; **60**:81–85.

15. Wines JD, Jr., et al. Opioid withdrawal during risperidone treatment. *J Clin Psychopharmacol* 1999; **19**:265–267.

16. Uehlinger C, et al. Increased (R)-methadone plasma concentrations by quetiapine in cytochrome P450s and ABCB1 genotyped patients. *J Clin Psychopharmacol* 2007; **27**:273–278.

17. Poling J, et al. Risperidone for substance dependent psychotic patients. *Addict Disord Treat* 2005; **4**:1–3.

18. Albanese MJ, et al. Risperidone in cocaine-dependent patients with comorbid psychiatric disorders. *J Psychiatr Pract* 2006; **12**:306–311.

19. Sattar SP, et al. Potential benefits of quetiapine in the treatment of substance dependence disorders. *J Psychiatry Neurosci* 2004; **29**:452–457.

20. Grabowski J, et al. Risperidone for the treatment of cocaine dependence: randomized, double-blind trial. *J Clin Psychopharmacol* 2000; **20**:305–310.

21. Kishi T, et al. Antipsychotics for cocaine or psychostimulant dependence: systematic review and meta-analysis of randomized, placebo-controlled trials. *J Clin Psychiatry* 2013; **74**:e1169–e1180.

22. Kampman KM, et al. A pilot trial of olanzapine for the treatment of cocaine dependence. *Drug Alcohol Depend* 2003; **70**:265–273.

23. Farren CK, et al. Significant interaction between clozapine and cocaine in cocaine addicts. *Drug Alcohol Depend* 2000; **59**:153–163.

24. Veraart JKE, et al. Pharmacodynamic interactions between ketamine and psychiatric medications used in the treatment of depression: a systematic review. *Int J Neuropsychopharmacol* 2021; **24**:808–831.

25. Benowitz NL, et al. Effects of delta-9-tetrahydrocannabinol on drug distribution and metabolism. Antipyrine, pentobarbital, and ethanol. *Clin Pharmacol Ther* 1977; **22**:259–268.

26. Hemeryck A, et al. Selective serotonin reuptake inhibitors and cytochrome P-450 mediated drug-drug interactions: an update. *Curr Drug Metab* 2002; **3**:13–37.

27. Bush E, et al. A case of serotonin syndrome and mutism associated with methadone. *J Palliat Med* 2006; **9**:1257–1259.

28. Vuori E, et al. Death following ingestion of MDMA (ecstasy) and moclobemide. *Addiction* 2003; **98**:365–368.

29. Rietjens SJ, et al. Pharmacokinetics and pharmacodynamics of 3,4-methylenedioxymethamphetamine (MDMA): interindividual differences due to polymorphisms and drug-drug interactions. *Crit Rev Toxicol* 2012; **42**:854–876.

30. Papaseit E, et al. MDMA interactions with pharmaceuticals and drugs of abuse. *Expert Opin Drug Metab Toxicol* 2020; **16**:357–369.

31. Fletcher PJ, et al. Fluoxetine, but not sertraline or citalopram, potentiates the locomotor stimulant effect of cocaine: possible pharmacokinetic effects. *Psychopharmacology (Berl)* 2004; **174**:406–413.

32. Silins E, et al. Qualitative review of serotonin syndrome, ecstasy (MDMA) and the use of other serotonergic substances: hierarchy of risk. *Aust NZ J Psychiatry* 2007; **41**:649–655.

33. Kotwal A, et al. Serotonin syndrome in the setting of lamotrigine, aripiprazole, and cocaine use. *Case Rep Med* 2015; **2015**:769531.

34. Soto PL, et al. Citalopram enhances cocaine's subjective effects in rats. *Behav Pharmacol* 2009; **20**:759–762.

35. GW Pharma Ltd. Summary of product characteristics. Sativex (delta-9-tetrahydrocannabinol, cannabidiol) oromucosal spray. 2022 (last accessed July 2024); https://www.medicines.org.uk/emc/product/602.

36. Miller BL, et al. Neuropsychiatric effects of cocaine: SPECT measurements. In: Paredes A, Gorelick DA, eds. *Cocaine: Physiological and Physiopathological Effects*, 1st edn. New York: Haworth Press; 1993:47–58.

37. Kalk NJ, et al. Fatalities associated with gabapentinoids in England (2004–2020). *Br J Clin Pharmacol* 2022; **88**:3911–3917.

38. Bonnet U, et al. Gabapentinoid-related deaths: an alarming global trend or just a special challenge within the long tail of the giant opioid epidemic? *Lancet Reg Health Am* 2022; **11**:100309.

39. Quintero Garzola GC. Reviewing treatments for cocaine consume problems: the gabapentinoid alternative. *Open Access J Clin Trials* 2021; **13**:45–60.

CHAPTER 4

Drugs of misuse – a summary

Urine testing for illicit drugs is routine on many psychiatric wards and in out-patient settings and doctors' offices. It is important to be aware of the duration of ability to detect drugs in urine and of other commonly used substances and of drugs that can give a false positive result. Some false positives are unpredictable (i.e. not related to chemical similarity), for example amisulpride can give a false positive for buprenorphine.[1] False positive results are most likely with point-of-care immunoassay kits. If a positive result has implications for a patient's liberty, and the patient denies use of substances, a second sample should be sent to the laboratory for definitive testing by liquid chromatography and mass spectrometry (LC-MS).

Table 4.26 gives a basic summary of the features of drugs of misuse.

Table 4.26 Summary of drugs of misuse.

Drug	Physical signs/ symptoms of intoxication	Most common mental state changes[2]	Withdrawal symptoms	Duration of withdrawal	Duration of detection in the urine[3,4]	Other substances that give a positive urine test result[5-7]
Amfetamine-type stimulants[8]	Tachycardia, increased BP; anorexia, tremor, restlessness	Visual/tactile/olfactory/ auditory hallucinations, paranoia, elation	Fatigue, hunger, depression, irritability, craving, social withdrawal	Peaks 7–34 hours, lasts maximum of 5 days	Depends on half-life, mostly 48–72 hours	Cough and decongestant preparations, bupropion, chloroquine, chlorpromazine, labetalol, promethazine, ranitidine, selegiline, large quantities of tyramine, tranylcypromine, trazodone and many others Desvenlafaxine may give a positive result for PCP[9]
Benzodiazepines	Sedation, disinhibition	Relaxation, visual hallucinations, disorientation, sleep disturbance	Anxiety, insomnia, delirium, seizures, visual/tactile/ olfactory/auditory hallucinations, psychosis	Usually short-lived but may last weeks to months	Up to 28 days depending on half-life of drug taken	Nefopam, sertraline, zopiclone, efavirenz
Cannabis[10-16]	Tachycardia, lack of co-ordination, red eyes, postural hypotension	Elation, psychosis, perceptual distortions, disturbance of memory/judgement, twofold increase in risk of developing schizophrenia	Restlessness, irritability, insomnia, anxiety	Uncertain, probably less than 1 month (longer in heavy users)	Single use: 3 days Chronic heavy use: up to 30 days	Passive 'smoking' of cannabis Efavirenz, ibuprofen, naproxen
Cocaine	Tachycardia/tachypnoea, increased BP/headache, respiratory depression, chest pain	Euphoria, paranoid psychosis, panic attacks, anxiety, insomnia, excitement	Fatigue, hunger, depression, irritability, craving, social withdrawal	12–18 hours	Up to 96 hours	Food/tea containing coco leaves, codeine, ephedrine/ pseudoephedrine

GHB/GBL	Drowsiness, coma, disinhibition	Sociability, confidence	Tremor, tachycardia, paranoia, delirium, psychosis, visual/tactile/olfactory/auditory hallucinations	3–4 days	8–10 hours[17]	Not known. Usually (and reliably) measured by LC-MS[18]
Heroin (diamorphine)	Pinpoint pupils, clammy skin, respiratory depression	Drowsiness, euphoria, hallucinations	Dilated pupils, nausea, diarrhoea, generalised pains, gooseflesh, runny nose/eyes	Peaks after 36–72 hours	Up to 72 hours	Diphenoxylate, naltrexone, naloxone, opiate analgesics, food/tea containing poppy seed, amisulpride, diphenhydramine, 4-quinolones, tramadol
Ketamine[19–22]	Increased HR, increased BP, palpitations, dizziness, abdominal discomfort, lower urinary tract symptoms, ataxia	Impaired consciousness, dissociation, hallucinations, ego diffusion	Fatigue, poor appetite, drowsiness, craving, anxiety, dysphoria, restlessness, palpitations, tremor, sweating	48 hours	Ketamine: up to 2 days. Norketamine: up to 14 days	Quetiapine
LSD[23]	Variable. Dilated pupils, moderate increase in HR and BP, flushing, sweating, hypersalivation, increased tendon reflexes	Euphoria, introspection, illusions, pseudo-hallucinations, altered sense of time, altered thought processes, altered perception of body, vivid recollections of significant memories	None	N/A	Up to 4 days	Ambroxol, amitriptyline, brompheniramine, bupropion, buspirone, cephadrine, chlorpromazine, desipramine, diltiazem, doxepin, ergonovine, fentanyl, fluoxetine, haloperidol, imipramine, labetalol, lysergol, methylphenidate, metoclopramide, prochlorperazine, risperidone, sertraline, thioridazine, trazodone, verapamil

(Continued)

Table 4.26 (Continued)

Drug	Physical signs/ symptoms of intoxication	Most common mental state changes[2]	Withdrawal symptoms	Duration of withdrawal	Duration of detection in the urine[3,4]	Other substances that give a positive urine test result[5-7]
Methadone	Pinpoint pupils, respiratory depression, pulmonary oedema	As for heroin	As for heroin but milder and longer lasting	Peaks after 4–6 days, can last 6 weeks	Up to 7 days with chronic use	Quetiapine
Other opioids such as nitazenes, fentanyls and oxycodone[24,25]	As for heroin, higher potency than heroin, faster onset of action, overdose common, seen as adulterants to street heroin	As for heroin	As for heroin	As for heroin, faster peak	Fentanyl: up to 72 hours Oxycodone: 2–4 days Nitazenes: variable	Fentanyls – ascorbic acid
Synthetic cannabinoid receptor agonists (SCRAs)	Tachycardia, hypertension, red eyes, agitation	Anxiety, agitation, aggression, psychotic symptoms, clouded consciousness	Anxiety, sleep disturbance, headache	Uncertain	Difficult to detect using conventional screening methods because of chemical heterogeneity	Too chemically diverse for urine screens, e.g. AB-fubinaca, ADB-fubinaca, AB-chminaca 3-methyl-butanoic acid, ADB-chminaca and 5-flouro-PB-22 are all classed as SCRAs Best detected and measured by LC-MS[26]*
Xylazine[27]	Bradycardia, hypotension, sedation, respiratory depression Rarely taken alone – usually an adulterant of opioids	Sedation, muscle relaxation	Hypertension, anxiety, irritability	Unclear	Unclear; probably a few hours Urine testing not common	Unclear LC-MS testing available[28]*

*For more detail on cross-reacting substances in urine testing, see Moeller et al. (2017).[29]

GBL/GHB, gamma-hydroxybutyrate/gamma-butyrolactone; HR, heart rate; LC-MS, liquid chromatography and mass spectrometry; LSD, lysergic acid diethylamide; N/A, not applicable; PCP, phencyclidine.

References

1. Couchman L, et al. Amisulpride and sulpiride interfere in the CEDIA DAU buprenorphine test. *Ann Clin Psychiatry* 2008; 45 Suppl 1.

2. Merative US L.P. Micromedex. 2024; https://www.micromedexsolutions.com/home/dispatch/.

3. Substance Abuse and Mental Health Services Administration (US). *Substance Abuse: Clinical Issues in Intensive Outpatient Treatment.* Treatment Improvement Protocol (TIP) Series, No. 47. 2006.

4. Vandevenne M, et al. Detection time of drugs of abuse in urine. *Acta Clin Belg* 2000; 55:323–333.

5. Brahm NC, et al. Commonly prescribed medications and potential false-positive urine drug screens. *Am J Health Syst Pharm* 2010; 67:1344–1350.

6. Saitman A, et al. False-positive interferences of common urine drug screen immunoassays: a review. *J Anal Toxicol* 2014; 38:387–396.

7. Liu CH, et al. False positive ketamine urine immunoassay screen result induced by quetiapine: a case report. *J Formos Med Assoc* 2017; 116:720–722.

8. Shoptaw SJ, et al. Treatment for amphetamine psychosis. *Cochrane Database Syst Rev* 2009; 1:CD003026.

9. Farley TM, et al. False-positive phencyclidine (PCP) on urine drug screen attributed to desvenlafaxine (Pristiq) use. *BMJ Case Rep* 2017; 2017:bcr-2017-222106.

10. Johns A. Psychiatric effects of cannabis. *Br J Psychiatry* 2001; 178:116–122.

11. Hall W, et al. Long-term cannabis use and mental health. *Br J Psychiatry* 1997; 171:107–108.

12. Murray RM, et al. Traditional marijuana, high-potency cannabis and synthetic cannabinoids: increasing risk for psychosis. *World Psychiatry* 2016; 15:195–204.

13. Marconi A, et al. Meta-analysis of the association between the level of cannabis use and risk of psychosis. *Schizophr Bull* 2016; 42:1262–1269.

14. Arseneault L, et al. Causal association between cannabis and psychosis: examination of the evidence. *Br J Psychiatry* 2004; 184:110–117.

15. Budney AJ, et al. Review of the validity and significance of cannabis withdrawal syndrome. *Am J Psychiatry* 2004; 161:1967–1977.

16. Bonnet U, et al. The cannabis withdrawal syndrome: current insights. *Subst Abuse Rehabil* 2017; 8:9–37.

17. Schröck A, et al. Pharmacokinetics of GHB and detection window in serum and urine after single uptake of a low dose of GBL – an experiment with two volunteers. *Drug Test Anal* 2014; 6:363–366.

18. Busardò FP, et al. Ultra-high performance liquid chromatography tandem mass spectrometry (UHPLC-MS/MS) for determination of GHB, precursors and metabolites in different specimens: application to clinical and forensic cases. *J Pharm Biomed Anal* 2017; 137:123–131.

19. Bowden-Jones O, et al. on behalf of the NEPTUNE Expert Group. *Guidance on the Clinical Management of Acute and Chronic Harms of Club Drugs and Novel Psychoactive Substances.* London: Novel Psychoactive Treatment UK Network (NEPTUNE); 2015.

20. Chen WY, et al. Gender differences in subjective discontinuation symptoms associated with ketamine use. *Subst Abuse Treat Prev Policy* 2014; 9:39.

21. Critchlow DG. A case of ketamine dependence with discontinuation symptoms. *Addiction* 2006; 101:1212–1213.

22. Adamowicz P, et al. Urinary excretion rates of ketamine and norketamine following therapeutic ketamine administration: method and detection window considerations. *J Anal Toxicol* 2005; 29:376–382.

23. Passie T, et al. The pharmacology of lysergic acid diethylamide: a review. *CNS Neurosci Ther* 2008; 14:295–314.

24. Gov.UK Advisory Council on Misuse of Drugs. Research and analysis: ACMD advice on 2-benzyl benzimidazole and piperidine benzimidazolone opioids (accessible version). 2024; https://www.gov.uk/government/publications/acmd-advice-on-2-benzyl-benzimidazole-and-piperidine-benzimidazolone-opioids/acmd-advice-on-2-benzyl-benzimidazole-and-piperidine-benzimidazolone-opioids-accessible-version.

25. Advisory Council on the Misuse of Drugs. ACMD report – misuse of fentanyl and fentanyl analogues. 2020; https://assets.publishing.service.gov.uk/media/5e0f5952e5274a0f9bccd774/ACMD_Report_-_Misuse_of_fentanyl_and_fentanyl_analogues.pdf.

26. Tebo C, et al. Suspected synthetic cannabinoid receptor agonist intoxication: does analysis of samples reflect the presence of suspected agents? *Am J Emerg Med* 2019; 37:1846–1849.

27. Malaca S, et al. Pharmacology and toxicology of xylazine: quid novum? *Eur Rev Med Pharmacol Sci* 2023; 27:7337–7345.

28. Truver MT, et al. A quantitative LC-MS/MS analysis of xylazine, p-fluorofentanyl, fentanyl and fentanyl-related compounds in postmortem blood. *J Chromatogr B Analyt Technol Biomed Life Sci* 2024; 1237:124059.

29. Moeller KE, et al. Clinical interpretation of urine drug tests: what clinicians need to know about urine drug screens. *Mayo Clin Proc* 2017; 92:774–796.

Substance misuse in pregnancy

Substance misuse in pregnancy has a wide range of adverse obstetric and fetal outcomes (Table 4.27). The overall quality of evidence is poor and based on small-scale observational studies. In the UK, the two main sources of information are the UK Teratology Information Service[1] and NICE guidance for pregnancy and complex social factors.[2] Outside the UK, WHO guidelines are available.[3]

Table 4.27 Risks and management of various drugs in pregnancy.

Substance	Associated risks	Management
Alcohol	Alcohol is a teratogen, even 1–2 units can increase the risk of having a preterm, low birthweight or small for gestational age baby.[4] In utero exposure can cause fetal alcohol spectrum disorders (FASDs) which include neurodevelopmental impairment, facial dysmorphology, congenital abnormalities and poor growth. These are dependent on dose, pattern timing, duration of exposure, fetal and maternal genetics, maternal nutrition, concurrent substance use and epigenetic response.[5] Neonates can experience withdrawal symptoms, including hyperactivity, crying, irritability, poor sucking, tremors, seizures, poor sleeping pattern hyperphagia and diaphoresis.[6]	Pregnant patients should be encouraged to cease alcohol consumption. **Medically assisted withdrawal** ■ Those who experience withdrawal symptoms should have benzodiazepine-assisted withdrawal.[3] ■ The timing of detoxification in relation to the trimester of pregnancy should be risk-assessed against continued alcohol consumption and risks to the fetus.[7] ■ Benzodiazepines are not known to be major teratogens and the duration of their use in medically assisted alcohol withdrawal is short. Diazepam and chlordiazepoxide are the benzodiazepines of choice.[8] ■ Specialist advice should usually be sought. **Relapse prevention medications** ■ No relapse prevention medications are advised in pregnancy, owing to the lack of safety data. However, given the teratogenicity of alcohol, there is debate over whether the benefit might outweigh the risk in certain circumstances.[9] ■ Acamprosate – fetal malformation and increased stillbirth are observed in animal studies with greater doses than in human therapy. One retrospective cohort study did not find an increased rate of congenital malformation, preterm delivery, low birthweight or neonatal complications. A small sample (n = 32) of unpublished data has observed congenital malformations, miscarriage and neurodevelopmental impacts; the results are confounded by maternal alcohol use and therefore cannot be reliably interpreted.[1] ■ Naltrexone – in animal studies it was not found to be teratogenic, however increased early fetal loss was observed at higher than recommended therapeutic doses. Clinical data relate to naltrexone use in opioid use disorder (OUD), and therefore are difficult to apply to alcohol use disorder. One study identified increased rates of pregnancy and labour complications for those with a naltrexone implant, compared with women without OUD, although this may be related to their OUD.[9] ■ Disulfiram – very limited data. There are concerns over the autonomic instability caused by the disulfiram-alcohol reaction.[1] Animal studies have not demonstrated the safety of disulfiram in pregnancy.[9] **Breastfeeding** ■ Alcohol is excreted in breast milk in similar concentrations to those in maternal blood. Alcohol is at its highest concentration in breast milk 30–60 minutes after ingestion and declines at the same rate as in maternal blood. Therefore, pregnant patients are advised to wait before breastfeeding. One study demonstrated that alcohol decreased lactation.[10] The safest option is to not drink alcohol, but if an individual chooses to drink, then they should drink no more than the recommended weekly intake and spread the drinks across the week.[11]

(Continued)

Table 4.27 (Continued)

Substance	Associated risks	Management
Tobacco	Miscarriage, low birthweight, prematurity and stillbirth[7]	Patients should be encouraged to cease smoking completely. **Pharmacological treatment** ■ Nicotine replacement therapy (NRT) probably does not have adverse effects on the fetus or infant.[12] NRT should be offered at the earliest opportunity and provided if desired throughout the pregnancy.[13] ■ Vaping may be preferred but its effect on the fetus has not been established, with few studies available. There is some evidence that vaping has no impact on birthweight.[14] ■ NRT should be offered alongside behavioural support.[13] ■ Bupropion and varenicline are not recommended.[13] Bupropion, when used to treat depression, may be continued after a risk–benefit analysis. Available human pregnancy exposure data have not indicated an increased risk of miscarriage, major congenital malformations, intrauterine death, impaired fetal growth or preterm delivery for bupropion or varenicline. One single case–control study of bupropion has suggested possible associations with cardiac malformations, but this has not been replicated.[1]
Opioids	Heroin dependence: sixfold increase in maternal obstetric complications and increased risk of neonatal complications including low birthweight, neonatal abstinence syndrome (NAS) and sudden infant death syndrome.[15] Dependence on other opioids: low birthweight, toxaemia, third trimester bleeding, malpresentation, puerperal morbidity, fetal distress, meconium aspiration, NAS, postnatal growth deficiency, microcephaly, neurobiological problems, increased neonatal mortality, increased sudden infant death syndrome (74-fold increase).[15]	Treatment should take place within a multidisciplinary team (including obstetric team, anaesthetists, neonatologists and addiction specialists) delivering a holistic package of care. **Opioid substitution treatment (OST)** ■ It is advised that methadone/buprenorphine (OST) be commenced or continued in pregnancy. It carries a significantly lower risk than continued illicit use despite the known risks of these medications.[3] ■ Buprenorphine is associated with a lower risk of NAS than methadone.[16] ■ Buprenorphine and methadone increase the risk of preterm delivery, small for gestational age and low birthweight. Buprenorphine carries a relatively lower risk of these.[16] ■ Buprenorphine has been associated with a lower risk of congenital malformations than methadone.[17] ■ Buprenorphine and methadone have the same rates of severe maternal complications and caesarean sections.[16] ■ Methadone-exposed babies have a higher rate of mortality in the first 2 years when compared with buprenorphine and naltrexone exposed babies.[18] ■ A Cochrane review found no difference in treatment retention between methadone and buprenorphine during pregnancy.[15] However, a larger systematic review and meta-analysis not focused on pregnancy found greater treatment retention for methadone.[19] ■ Pregnant patients are not advised to switch from methadone to buprenorphine because of the risk of withdrawal.[3]

- In the past, guidelines recommended that patients who take buprenorphine-naloxone (e.g. Suboxone) be switched to buprenorphine owing to there being inadequate safety data for the former.[20] However, a 2020 systematic review and meta-analysis identified no difference in outcomes for pregnant patients receiving buprenorphine-naloxone and that neonates were less likely to require treatment for NAS.[21] A 2023 systematic review confirmed that Suboxone was no less safe than buprenorphine alone (or methadone).[22]

- Metabolism of methadone is increased in the third trimester so it may be necessary to split the dose to twice daily or increase the dose.[4]

- Pregnancy increases the metabolism of buprenorphine. Increased frequency of dosing is required to maintain plasma levels, reducing the risk of withdrawals and increasing adherence to treatment.[23]

- Buvidal (long-acting buprenorphine injection) – there are very limited safety data available, and any benefits of use should be balanced with possible risks.[24]

Detoxification

- Detoxification is associated with a higher rate of relapse and mortality.[3] It should be driven by informed patient choice. If desired, detoxification is safest in the second trimester, as in the first it is associated with spontaneous abortion and in the third with preterm delivery, fetal distress and stillbirth.[4]

- Detoxification medications should be employed in small, frequent decrements, e.g. 2–3mg of methadone every 3–5 days.[4]

- Cycling between abstinence, relapse and intoxication results in fluctuating opioid concentrations, which increases the risk of maternal, obstetric, fetal and neonatal complications.[25]

Naltrexone

- There are limited human data that suggest similar findings with regard to safety as for methadone and buprenorphine.[18]

Other considerations

- It is useful to anticipate potential problems in pain management for pregnant patients prescribed opioids who are likely to require opioid pain relief. Such patients should be managed in specialist antenatal clinics due to the increased associated risks.

- Antenatal assessment by anaesthetists is recommended to anticipate any anaesthetic risks, analgesic requirements and problems with venous access.

Breastfeeding

- Patients prescribed methadone or buprenorphine should be encouraged to breastfeed even if they continue to use illicit opioids.[1] The level of buprenorphine and methadone in breast milk is low.[18]

- Breastfeeding brings general health benefits to mother and infant, low concentrations of methadone and buprenorphine are transferred to infant, and it reduces admission length and need for intervention in NAS.

- Patients should be advised to discontinue breastfeeding gradually as abrupt cessation can cause a delayed NAS.[26]

(Continued)

Table 4.27 (Continued)

Substance	Associated risks	Management
Cannabis	Associations with stillbirth, fetal growth restriction, impaired fetal neurodevelopment, preterm delivery, neonatal intensive care unit admissions and small for gestational age infants, neonatal withdrawal-like syndrome, increased aggressive behaviour and attention deficits.[27]	Abstinence should be encouraged. CBT, motivational enhancement therapy and abstinence-based incentives can be used. There are no pharmacological treatments currently available.[27] **Breastfeeding** ■ There are limited data. Avoid or reduce use during breastfeeding.[27]
Benzodiazepines	No conclusive evidence of congenital defects. Associations have been found with increased risk of spontaneous abortion and preterm labour.[28] Prolonged use of benzodiazepines in the near-term period, especially high doses, is associated with a neonatal withdrawal syndrome and 'floppy baby syndrome'.[1]	Ideally, benzodiazepines should be discontinued before pregnancy. Abrupt withdrawal of benzodiazepines is not advised because of the possibility of destabilisation, and the risk that it could lead to alcohol being substituted, which could pose a considerable risk to the fetus.[1] The consensus is that those dependent on illicit benzodiazepines should be stabilised on long-acting benzodiazepines (e.g. diazepam) at the lowest dose possible to prevent withdrawal symptoms. The dose should be gradually reduced, as long as it does not result in illicit use.[4] **Breastfeeding** ■ People taking high doses of benzodiazepines should not breastfeed.[4]
Stimulants	Increased risk of miscarriage, placental abruption, preterm birth, decreased birthweight, disturbed neurobehaviour at birth, poorer medical/behavioural/cognitive and motor problems.[29]	There are no effective pharmacological interventions and detoxification is the primary aim. **Breastfeeding** ■ Breastfeeding is not advised.[3]

References

1. UK Health Security Agency. UK Teratology Information Service. 2024; https://uktis.org.
2. National Institute for Health and Care Excellence. Pregnancy and complex social factors: a model for service provision for pregnant women with complex social factors. Clinical guideline [CG110]. 2010 (last checked March 2024); https://www.nice.org.uk/guidance/CG110.
3. World Health Organization. *Guidelines for the Identification and Management of Substance Use and Substance Use Disorders in Pregnancy.* Geneva: World Health Organization; 2014.
4. Department of Health. Drug misuse and dependence: UK guidelines on clinical management. London: Department of Health. 2017; https://assets.publishing.service.gov.uk/government/uploads/system/uploads/attachment_data/file/673978/clinical_guidelines_2017.pdf.
5. Popova S, et al. Fetal alcohol spectrum disorders. *Nat Rev Dis Primers* 2023; 9:11.
6. Hudak ML, et al. Neonatal drug withdrawal. *Pediatrics* 2012; 129:e540–e560.
7. Lingford-Hughes AR, et al. Evidence-based guidelines for the pharmacological management of substance abuse, harmful use, addiction and comorbidity: recommendations from BAP. *J Psychopharmacol* 2012; 26:899–952.
8. McAllister-Williams RH, et al. British Association for Psychopharmacology consensus guidance on the use of psychotropic medication preconception, in pregnancy and postpartum 2017. *J Psychopharmacol* 2017; 31:519–552.
9. Kelty E, et al. Pharmacotherapies for the treatment of alcohol use disorders during pregnancy: time to reconsider? *Drugs* 2021; 81:739–748.
10. Haastrup MB, et al. Alcohol and breastfeeding. *Basic Clin Pharmacol Toxicol* 2014; 114:168–173.
11. Royal College of Obstetricians and Gynaeocologists. Alcohol and pregnancy. 2018 (last accessed March 2024); https://www.rcog.org.uk/for-the-public/browse-our-patient-information/alcohol-and-pregnancy.
12. Taylor L, et al. Fetal safety of nicotine replacement therapy in pregnancy: systematic review and meta-analysis. *Addiction* 2021; 116:239–277.
13. National Institute for Health and Care Excellence. Tobacco: preventing uptake, promoting quitting and treating dependence. NICE guideline [NG209]. 2021 (last updated 2023, last accessed March 2024); https://www.nice.org.uk/guidance/ng209.
14. Calder R, et al. Vaping in pregnancy: a systematic review. *Nicotine Tob Res* 2021; 23:1451–1458.
15. Minozzi S, et al. Maintenance agonist treatments for opiate-dependent pregnant women. *Cochrane Database Syst Rev* 2020; 11:CD006318.
16. HalesMeds.com. Hale's medications and mothers' milk. 2024; https://www.halesmeds.com.
17. Suarez EA, et al. First trimester use of buprenorphine or methadone and the risk of congenital malformations. *JAMA Intern Med* 2024; 184:242–251.
18. Suarez EA, et al. Buprenorphine versus methadone for opioid use disorder in pregnancy. *N Engl J Med* 2022; 387:2033–2044.
19. Degenhardt L, et al. Buprenorphine versus methadone for the treatment of opioid dependence: a systematic review and meta-analysis of randomised and observational studies. *Lancet Psychiatry* 2023; 10:386–402.
20. Edge R, et al. *Buprenorphine for Opioid Use Disorders during Pregnancy: a Review of Comparative Clinical Effectiveness, Safety, Cost-Effectiveness, and Guidelines.* CADTH Rapid Response Reports. Ottawa: Canadian Agency for Drugs and Technologies in Health; 2019.
21. Link HM, et al. Buprenorphine-naloxone use in pregnancy: a systematic review and metaanalysis. *Am J Obstet Gynecol MFM* 2020; 2:100179.
22. Ordean A, et al. Safety and efficacy of buprenorphine-naloxone in pregnancy: a systematic review of the literature. *Pathophysiology* 2023; 30:27–36.
23. Caritis SN, et al. An evidence-based recommendation to increase the dosing frequency of buprenorphine during pregnancy. *Am J Obstet Gynecol* 2017; 217:459.e451–459.e456.
24. Camurus Ltd. Buvidal in pregnancy and breastfeeding. Personal communication, 2024.
25. Rausgaard NLK, et al. Management and monitoring of opioid use in pregnancy. *Acta Obstet Gynecol Scand* 2020; 99:7–15.
26. Holmes AP, et al. Breastfeeding considerations for mothers of infants with neonatal abstinence syndrome. *Pharmacotherapy* 2017; 37:861–869.
27. Hayer S, et al. Cannabis and pregnancy: a review. *Obstet Gynecol Surv* 2023; 78:411–428.
28. Shyken JM, et al. Benzodiazepines in pregnancy. *Clin Obstet Gynecol* 2019; 62:156–167.
29. Wouldes TA, et al. Stimulants: how big is the problem and what are the effects of prenatal exposure? *Semin Fetal Neonatal Med* 2019; 24:155–160.

Gambling disorder

At the time of writing, no medicines are licensed for the treatment of problem gambling. However, international guidelines and draft NICE guidance recommend naltrexone off-label to reduce gambling severity in people with gambling problems.[1,2] A 2017 meta-analysis demonstrated that when people receiving psychological therapy for problem gambling were given naltrexone there was a greater reduction in gambling than with those given placebo.[3] Naltrexone is the only drug with likely effectiveness in problem gambling. Other drugs that have been evaluated include nalmefene, serotonin reuptake inhibitors, glutamatergic agents (e.g. N-acetylcysteine, acamprosate, memantine), mood stabilisers (e.g. topiramate, carbamazepine, lithium) and modafinil, olanzapine, haloperidol, tolcapone and bupropion.[4]

Naltrexone should only be initiated in specialist gambling clinics following a discussion of efficacy and adverse effects. Patients should be told about the interaction with concomitant opioids. Following baseline biochemistry analysis to exclude severe renal or hepatic impairment, naltrexone should be initiated at a dose of 25mg, increasing to 50mg with a review of efficacy at 4–6 weeks. Prescriptions could then be transferred to primary care with continuation for as long as the person continues to report benefit, alongside 6-monthly monitoring of renal and liver function.

Clinicians should be aware of the known risks of developing or worsening of impulse control disorders with dopaminergic agents and aripiprazole (and probably other dopamine partial agonists),[5–7] particularly in individuals at increased risk for problem gambling.[8]

References

1. National Institute for Health and Care Excellence. Harmful gambling: identification, assessment and management. In development [GID-NG10210]. https://www.nice.org.uk/guidance/indevelopment/gid-ng10210.
2. Thomas SA, et al. Australian guideline for treatment of problem gambling: an abridged outline. *Med J Aust* 2011; **195**:664–665.
3. Mouaffak F, et al. Naltrexone in the treatment of broadly defined behavioral addictions: a review and meta-analysis of randomized controlled trials. *Eur Addict Res* 2017; **23**:204–210.
4. Mestre-Bach G, et al. Pharmacological management of gambling disorder: an update of the literature. *Expert Rev Neurother* 2024; **24**:391–407.
5. Akbari M, et al. Aripiprazole and its adverse effects in the form of impulsive-compulsive behaviors: a systematic review of case reports. *Psychopharmacology (Berl)* 2024; **241**:209–223.
6. Wolfschlag M, et al. Drug-induced gambling disorder: epidemiology, neurobiology, and management. *Pharmaceut Med* 2023; **37**:37–52.
7. Williams BD, et al. Aripiprazole and other third-generation antipsychotics as a risk factor for impulse control disorders: a systematic review and meta-analysis. *J Clin Psychopharmacol* 2024; **44**:39–48.
8. Medicines and Healthcare products Regulatory Agency. Aripiprazole (Abilify): reminder on known risk of gambling disorder. 2023; https://www.gov.uk/government/news/aripiprazole-abilify-reminder-on-known-risk-of-gambling-disorder.

Chapter 5

Prescribing in children and adolescents

Principles of prescribing practice in childhood and adolescence

Diagnosis can be difficult in children and comorbidity is very common. Treatment should generally target key symptoms rather than specific conditions. While a working diagnosis is beneficial to frame expectations and help communication with patients and parents, it should be kept in mind that it could take some time for the illness to evolve.[1]

Differences in pharmacokinetics and pharmacodynamics compared with adults can explain the more pronounced or unforeseen adverse reactions to medication in the young, as well as the differences in dose–effect relationships compared with those in adults.[2]

- **Start low, go slow and monitor**
  Depending on the age, dose starts lower than in adults or may be calculated in mg/kg per day terms.[1,2] Titration of dose should proceed slowly, aiming for the minimum dose that adequately controls symptoms and has minimum adverse reactions. Regular reviewing of efficacy and tolerability should guide if treatment is necessary and requires continuation.
- **Polypharmacy in the severely ill**
  Monotherapy is ideal. However, childhood-onset illness can be severe and may require treatment with psychosocial approaches in combination with more than one medication.[1] Co-prescribing of medication for different disorders or symptoms is common. This complicates the interpretation of efficacy of each medicine[1] and requires care with drug interactions and dose adjustments.
- **Adequate treatment duration**
  Children are generally relatively more ill than their adult counterparts and will often require longer periods of treatment before responding. An adequate trial of treatment for those who are admitted for in-patient care may well be 8 weeks or more for depression or schizophrenia.

The Maudsley® Prescribing Guidelines in Psychiatry, Fifteenth Edition. David M. Taylor, Thomas R. E. Barnes and Allan H. Young.
© 2025 David M. Taylor. Published 2025 by John Wiley & Sons Ltd.

- **Change one drug at a time**
  Ideally changes should be made to one drug at a time and, if possible, remove a drug when adding a new one.

- **Monitor outcome in more than one setting**
  For symptomatic treatments (such as stimulants for attention deficit hyperactivity or ADHD), bear in mind that the expression of problems may be different in different settings (e.g. home and school). For example, a dose titrated against parent reports may be too high for the daytime at school.

- **Educate the child and parents on the treatment**
  For some, the need for medication will be life-long. The first experiences with medications are crucial to long-term outcomes and adherence. Education regarding the target symptoms of the medication, likely adverse reactions and medication adherence should be addressed. Provide information on the monitoring required and how to identify adverse reactions. Patients and their guardians should be encouraged to ask for changes to their treatment regimen where they consider them ineffective or poorly tolerated.

- **Review long-term treatment**
  As children develop and grow through adolescence, dose changes may be required and adverse reactions may emerge or wane.

- **Transition from paediatric to adult services**
  It is essential that continuity of care is not lost when moving from paediatric to adult services as this can be distressing and increase the risk of relapse. Planning and co-ordination should start at an early stage to achieve a smooth transition.[3]

- **Technical aspects of paediatric prescribing**
  Most psychotropic drugs used in adults are not licensed for use in children or adolescents.[4] The Medicines Act 1968 and European legislation make provision for doctors to use medicines in an off-label or out-of-licence capacity or to use unlicensed medicines. Where possible a licensed preparation should be prescribed (Table 5.1), however it is recognised that the informed use of unlicensed medicines, or of licensed medicines in an 'off-label' way, is often necessary in paediatric practice. Individual prescribers are always responsible for ensuring that there is adequate information to support the quality, efficacy, safety and intended use of a drug before prescribing it.[5]

  When writing a prescription in most countries, inclusion of age is a legal requirement in the case of prescription-only medicines for children under 12 years of age, but it is preferable to state the age for all prescriptions for children.

Table 5.1 Psychotropic medications approved by the UK Medicines and Healthcare products Regulatory Agency (MHRA), European Medicines Agency and the US Food and Drug Administration for children and adolescents (January 2024).[6-9]

Condition	UK MHRA approval only; age (years)	European Medicine Agency;* age (years)	US Food and Drug Administration; age (years)
ADHD			
Amfetamine–dexamfetamine mixed salts	–	–	3+
Amfetamine–dexamfetamine mixed salts extended release	–	–	6+
Atomoxetine	6+	6+	6+
Clonidine extended release	–	–	6–17
Dexamfetamine	6–17	6–17	3–16
Dexamfetamine sustained release	–	–	6–16
Dexmethylphenidate	–	–	6+
Guanfacine extended release	6–17	6–17	6–17
Lisdexamfetamine	6+	6+	6–17
Methamfetamine	–	–	6–17
Methylphenidate	6+	6–18	6+
Viloxazine	–	–	6+
Anxiety disorders			
Duloxetine	–	–	GAD 7+
Escitalopram	–	–	GAD 7+
Autism spectrum disorder (irritability)			
Aripiprazole	–	–	6–17
Risperidone	–	–	5–17
Bipolar disorder (depressive episodes)			
Lurasidone	–	–	10+
Olanzapine–fluoxetine combination	–	–	10+
Bipolar disorder (manic or mixed episodes)			
Aripiprazole	Manic episodes 13+	Manic episodes 13+	Manic or mixed episodes 10+
Asenapine	–	–	10+
Lithium	–	–	7+
Lithium extended release	–	–	12+
Olanzapine	–	–	13+
Quetiapine extended release	–	–	10+

(Continued)

CHAPTER 5

Table 5.1 *(Continued)*

Condition	UK MHRA approval only; age (years)	European Medicine Agency;* age (years)	US Food and Drug Administration; age (years)
Risperidone	–	–	10+
Ziprasidone	–	10+	–
Conduct disorder			
Risperidone	5–18	5–18	–
Depressive disorder			
Amitriptyline	–	–	12+
Escitalopram	–	–	12+
Fluoxetine	8+	8+	8+
Enuresis			
Amitriptyline	6–17	6–17	–
Imipramine	6–17	5–18	6–17
Insomnia (in autism spectrum disorder or Smith Magenis syndrome)			
Melatonin extended release	6–17	2–18	–
Insomnia (in ADHD)			
Melatonin immediate release	6–17	–	–
Insomnia (short term)			
Promethazine	5+	–	–
Obsessive compulsive disorder			
Clomipramine	–	–	10+
Fluoxetine	–	–	7+
Fluvoxamine	8+	8+	8+
Sertraline	6+	6+	6+
Schizophrenia			
Aripiprazole	15+	15+	13+
Brexpiprazole	–	–	13+
Lurasidone	13+	–	13+
Olanzapine	–	–	13+
Paliperidone	15+	15+	12+
Quetiapine	–	–	13+
Risperidone	–	–	13+
Sulpiride	14+	6+	–
Tourette's disorder			
Aripiprazole	–	–	6–18

*Approvals may differ in individual countries.
GAD, generalised anxiety disorder.

References

1. Gerlach M, et al. *Psychiatric Drugs in Children and Adolescents. Basic Pharmacology and Practical Applications.* Vienna: Springer-Verlag; 2014.

2. Turner M, et al. *Prescribing Medicines for Children: From drug development to practical administration.* London: Pharmaceutical Press. Royal Pharmaceutical Society; 2019.

3. Paediatric Formulary Committee. *BNF for Children (online).* London: BMJ, Pharmaceutical Press, and RCPCH Publications; http://www.medicinescomplete.com.

4. Smogur M, et al. Psychotropic drug prescription in children and adolescents: approved medications in European countries and the United States. *J Child Adolesc Psychopharmacol* 2022; **32**:80–88.

5. Sharma AN, et al. BAP position statement: off-label prescribing of psychotropic medication to children and adolescents. *J Psychopharmacol* 2016; **30**:416–421.

6. Cortese S, et al. Psychopharmacology in children and adolescents: unmet needs and opportunities. *Lancet Psychiatry* 2023; **11**:143–154.

7. EMC. *Summaries of Product Characteristics.* 2024; https://www.medicines.org.uk/emc/.

8. IBM Watson Health. *IBM Micromedex Solutions.* 2024; https://www.ibm.com/watson-health/about/micromedex.

9. Gelbe Liste Pharmindex. *Gelbe Liste Online. News, Infos und Datenbanken für Ärzte, Apotheker und Fachpersonal aus Medizin und Pharmazie.* 2024; https://www.gelbe-liste.de/.

CHAPTER 5

Depression in children and adolescents

Diagnostic issues

Approximately 15% of young people experience depression by age 18 years and these young people often have significant functional impairment and risk of harm.[1] Compared with depressed adults, young people with depression tend to experience more irritability, loss of energy, insomnia and weight change, and less anhedonia and concentration problems.[2] These symptoms can overlap with and appear similar to other disorders or can be minimised and incorrectly attributed to typical teenage development, making diagnosis challenging. Assessments should therefore be undertaken by clinicians who understand developmental variations and can accurately identify depression in young people.[3]

Clinical guidance

For mild depression in children and adolescents, the UK National Institute for Health and Care Excellence (NICE) guidelines[4] and American Academy of Child and Adolescent Psychiatry (AACAP) practice parameter[3] recommend that supportive care or psychological intervention should be considered as first-line treatment, and that antidepressant medication should not be prescribed.

For moderate to severe depression in young people, these same guidelines recommend offering psychological therapy, either alone or in combination with antidepressant medication. In addition, the AACAP practice parameter recommends that antidepressant medication alone could be considered, particularly if the presentation is severe and the patient is unable to engage in talking therapy, if psychological interventions are not available or if this is the patient's and family's preference.

These guidelines were informed by research evidence for the effectiveness of selective serotonin reuptake inhibitors (SSRIs) in treating depression in young people. For example, a seminal large UK National Institute of Mental Health (NIMH) funded randomised controlled trial (RCT) – the Treatment of Adolescents With Depression Study (TADS)[5] – found a fluoxetine response rate of 61% over the acute (12-week) phase, which was significantly higher than the placebo response rate of 35%, giving a number needed to treat (NNT) of 4.[5] Subsequent systematic reviews and meta-analyses, which include this trial and others, have provided further evidence demonstrating that SSRIs are effective at improving symptoms and functioning, and are largely acceptable treatments for depression in young people. However, several individual studies and systematic reviews studies report less certain effects[6–10] and a 2021 Cochrane review described antidepressant effects as 'small and unimportant'.[11]

The current evidence base is unclear about whether SSRI medications alone, psychological therapy alone or combined treatment is most effective for treating depression in children and adolescents. TADS found that fluoxetine alone or in combination with cognitive behavioural therapy (CBT) might accelerate treatment response, and that adding CBT might decrease adverse effects including suicidality, so enhancing the safety of fluoxetine.[5,12] However, other studies have not replicated this finding,[13,14] including the Adolescent Depression Antidepressants and Psychotherapy Trial (ADAPT), which found no benefit in combining fluoxetine with CBT over fluoxetine alone.[15] A network meta-analysis comparing several treatments for depression in children and adolescents also found that combined fluoxetine and CBT was no more effective than fluoxetine alone but found that this combination was more effective than CBT alone.[16]

Prescribing for depression in children and adolescents

Before prescribing

- Undertake a comprehensive assessment: Establish a clinical diagnosis of depression. Exclude differential diagnoses, including psychiatric disorders (such as bipolar affective disorder), medical disorders (such as endocrine disorders) and medication-related effects (such as steroid adverse effects). Identify any comorbid psychiatric or medical conditions. Consider contraindications to SSRIs and potential interactions. Assess risk of harm to self and others. Formulate considering factors that could predispose, precipitate and perpetuate depression, such as family history of psychiatric disorders (including depression and bipolar affective disorder) and environmental stressors (including victimisation and other adverse experiences). If any co-occurring problems are identified, these should be addressed and prioritised based on a comprehensive formulation.
- Measure baseline severity: Measures of depression symptoms include the clinician-administered Children's Depression Rating Scale-Revised (CDRS-R)[17,18] and the child- and parent-reported Mood and Feelings Questionnaire (MFQ)[19] or Revised Children's Anxiety and Depression Scale (RCADS).[20] Measures of functional impairment include the Children's Global Assessment Scale (CGAS).[21]
- Obtain informed consent: Discuss the nature, course and treatment of depression, potential adverse effects of medication, delay in onset of treatment effects, plan for monitoring and maintenance of medication and potential discontinuation effects.
- Develop a safety plan: In all but exceptional circumstances, a parent or carer should be responsible for the secure storage of medication for a child or adolescent. Advise the young person and their parent/carer of professionals or services they should contact if they experience significant adverse effects, risk of harm or worsening symptoms.

What to prescribe

- **Fluoxetine** is the recommended first-line medication for depression in children and adolescents.[3,4] It has the strongest current evidence for efficacy,[6,9,11,16,22,23] showing moderate effects in reducing depression symptoms versus placebo (standardised mean difference = 0.51).[16] In the UK, NICE states that fluoxetine is the only antidepressant for which clinical trial evidence shows that benefits outweigh risks.[4] Fluoxetine should be started at a dose of 10mg daily which can be increased after 1 week to the minimum therapeutic dose of 20mg daily. Higher doses (up to 40–60mg daily) may be considered, particularly in older children of higher body weight or when, in severe illness, an early clinical response is considered a priority.[4,5,15,24] The long half-life of fluoxetine may be beneficial for adolescents because it confers a reduced risk of discontinuation effects or relapse if doses are delayed or missed.[25] Fluoxetine is approved for treatment of depression in patients aged 8 years and over by the US Food and

Drug Administration (FDA), and by the European Medicines Agency and the UK Medicines and Healthcare products Regulatory Agency (MHRA) if the young person has moderate to severe depression and has not responded to psychological therapy.[26]

- **Sertraline** and **escitalopram** have also been found to be more effective than placebo for treating depression in young people[6,22] and should be considered as alternatives if fluoxetine is not tolerated. Sertraline and escitalopram should also be started at low doses (25–50mg daily and 5–10mg daily, respectively) and titrated to therapeutic doses (50–200mg daily and 10–20mg daily, respectively). The half-lives of sertraline, escitalopram and some other antidepressants may be shorter in young people than adults, so twice daily dosing could be considered to prevent discontinuation symptoms.[27] Escitalopram is approved by the FDA for treatment of depression in patients aged 12 years and over.
- **Duloxetine** and **venlafaxine** may be effective but are relatively poorly tolerated.[28]
- **Agomelatine** was more effective than placebo in children aged 7–11 years and showed similar efficacy to fluoxetine. A dose of 10mg seems to be effective. Agomelatine is extremely well tolerated but not licensed for children or adolescents. Liver function test (LFT) changes occurred in 1% of participants.[29] **Vortioxetine** was no more effective than placebo in a large study of 12–17-year-old children.[30]
- For children and adolescents who have significant depressive symptoms resulting in distress or impairment despite an adequate trial of an SSRI alone, consider combination SSRI and psychological therapy. There is some limited evidence that combination treatment may be more beneficial than SSRI alone for some young people.[6,31–33]
- For children and adolescents who have significant depressive symptoms resulting in distress or impairment despite adequate trials of an SSRI (fluoxetine) *and* psychological therapy, consider a switch to a different SSRI (sertraline, escitalopram).[4,31] This guidance is largely based on the Treatment of Resistant Depression in Adolescents (TORDIA) trial,[24] the only RCT that has examined the comparative efficacy of different treatment strategies for SSRI-resistant depression in young people.[24] This trial found that many participants improved when switched to another SSRI or venlafaxine (response rate 47% and 48%, respectively) and improved even more when this medication switch was combined with starting concurrent CBT (response rate 55% vs 41% without CBT) after 12 weeks of treatment. A switch to an SSRI was just as efficacious as a switch to venlafaxine but had less frequent and severe side effects, so an SSRI switch is preferred.
- If limited response despite adequate trials of these medications and psychological therapy, consider augmenting SSRI treatment with another medication such as a second-generation antipsychotic or lithium. (Also consider augmentation if there has been partial response to an SSRI.[31]) Alternatively, consider switching to an antidepressant from a different class, for example mirtazapine[34] – especially if poor sleep is a problem. There are no RCTs testing the effectiveness of these strategies in children or adolescents, and so this guidance is largely based on evidence from studies of adults with treatment-resistant depression, in addition to very limited follow-up of TORDIA participants receiving open-label treatment.[31,35]
- Finally, if still no response to these medications and the young person's depression is very severe, ketamine, repetitive transcranial magnetic stimulation (rTMS) or electroconvulsive therapy can be considered. These interventions have an evidence base and

are approved for use in adults with treatment-resistant depression, but there is no substantial evidence in children and adolescents.[31] With regard to ketamine, or its enantiomer esketamine, emerging evidence suggests that it may be effective and adequately tolerated in adolescents with treatment-resistant depression based on a small number of studies, including two small RCTs.[36–38] Considering rTMS, initial evidence suggested that it may be effective, again based on a small number of studies and a small RCT, but a larger RCT found no evidence of effectiveness.[39] Electroconvulsive therapy (ECT) has limited evidence of effectiveness in young people, although one randomised trial in adolescents showed good effect against both depression and suicide.[40] Therefore, these treatments' unknown potential effects on the developing brain need to be considered carefully and weighed up against the risks of not attempting these treatments.[41] Further research is greatly needed to inform clinical decisions.[42]

- NICE warns against prescribing paroxetine, venlafaxine, tricyclic antidepressants or St John's wort for depression in young people, because of potential adverse effects and interactions.[4]

Table 5.2 summarises medication treatment for depression in children and adolescents.

Table 5.2 Summary of pharmacotherapy for depression in children and adolescents.[3,4,6,31]

	Medication	Starting dose	Therapeutic dose range
First line	Fluoxetine	10mg/day	20–60mg/day
Second line	Sertraline	25–50mg/day	50–200mg/day
	Escitalopram	5–10mg/day	10–20mg/day
	Citalopram*	10mg/day	20–40mg/day
Subsequently	Consider augmentation of antidepressant with second-generation antipsychotic or lithium.†		
	Consider switching to an antidepressant from a different class, such as mirtazapine.		

*Caution advised in cardiac or hepatic disease.
†No randomised controlled trials available in young people (but there is evidence from adult trials).

After prescribing

Acute phase

- Monitor for adverse effects regularly, for example weekly for the first 4 weeks. Children and adolescents generally tolerate SSRIs well. Potential adverse effects include those experienced by adults, described in Chapter 3. Additionally, young people taking SSRIs have a small increased risk of suicidality and switch to mania, as well as activation effects (see 'Specific issues' later in this chapter). Therefore, risk of harm, mood and behaviour should be monitored closely and addressed.[3,4,6,31]
- After 4 weeks of SSRI treatment at a therapeutic dose, assess response including depression severity using the measures completed at baseline. Most therapeutic effects appear by 4 weeks.[43]
- If partial or non-response, consider the possibility of poor treatment adherence, inaccurate diagnosis, comorbidity or modifiable maintaining factors.

CHAPTER 5

- If none of these factors explains the continued depressive symptoms and the young person does not have adverse effects, consider increasing the dose. Reassess every 4 weeks.[3,31] This recommendation is largely based on evidence from adult depression trials, which have demonstrated small but significant improvements in depression symptoms with higher doses of SSRIs,[44] as there has been only limited research on this topic in children and adolescents.[45]
- If adverse effects develop, consider reducing the dose to the highest tolerated dose.
- If partial or non-response after 8 weeks of the maximum recommended (or highest tolerated) therapeutic dose of an SSRI, consider the medication changes outlined earlier.[31]

Maintenance phase

Continue medication for 6–12 months after remission to reduce the risk of relapse. Consider a longer maintenance phase if depressive episodes were recurrent or chronic.[3,4,6,31] Again, this recommendation is largely based on evidence from adult depression trials, in addition to very limited research in children and adolescents.[46,47]

Discontinuation phase

Discontinuation may be considered after the maintenance phase. This is best undertaken during a period of low stress. Taper medications slowly and hyperbolically (see Chapter 3) to minimise the risk of discontinuation symptoms.[3,4,6,31]

Specific issues

- Age
  The evidence base for these recommendations is stronger for adolescents than for children, so caution should be higher when considering prescribing for children. There has been no research investigating antidepressant medication use in pre-school children, and medications are not recommended for this age group.[4,22]
- Suicidality
  Antidepressant medication has been linked to an increased risk of suicidality in young people, which led to warnings issued by the US FDA, the European Medicines Agency and the UK MHRA in 2003–2005. Subsequent meta-analyses have also found evidence of this association with reported suicidality,[11,22,48] particularly for venlafaxine,[16,23] as well as a link with aggression.[49] A meta-analysis of reported suicidal thoughts or attempts in depression trials found a pooled absolute rate in antidepressant-treated young people of 3% and in those receiving placebo of 2%, giving a number needed to harm (NNH) of 112 (note these rates are low, probably because those with high risk of suicidality were often excluded from trials).[50] Concern has also been expressed about emergent suicidality with escitalopram.[51] To date, there has been no link between antidepressant use and *completed* suicides, but extreme care should be exercised.
  Untreated depression is a significant risk factor for suicidality. After the FDA warning on antidepressant use in children and adolescents, antidepressant use declined, untreated depression increased and suicide rates increased.[52,53] Given the risks of untreated depression, including completed suicide and impaired functioning, and that many more patients benefit from SSRIs than those who experience these serious adverse events, it is thought that the benefits of antidepressants, particularly fluoxetine, are

likely to outweigh these risks in moderate to severe depression. Nonetheless, it bears repeating that the risk of suicide should be very carefully monitored.[3,4,6,31]

■ **Activation and manic switch**

Activation adverse effects of antidepressant medication – including increased activity, restlessness and agitation – occur more commonly in children than in adolescents or adults. These effects, including mild symptoms, may occur in about 10% of children with depression taking SSRIs.[54,55] They are usually a transient response to starting medication or increasing dose and should be differentiated from manic switch. Conversion to mania is rarer but is observed more often in young people taking antidepressants than in adults.[56,57] However, there is no clear evidence that this switch is caused by antidepressants.

References

1. Avenevoli S, et al. Major depression in the national comorbidity survey-adolescent supplement: prevalence, correlates, and treatment. *J Am Acad Child Adolesc Psychiatry* 2015; **54**:37–44.e32.
2. Rice F, et al. Adolescent and adult differences in major depression symptom profiles. *J Affect Disord* 2019; **243**:175–181.
3. Birmaher B, et al. Practice parameter for the assessment and treatment of children and adolescents with depressive disorders. *J Am Acad Child Adolesc Psychiatry* 2007; **46**:1503–1526.
4. National Institute for Health and Care Excellence (NICE). Depression in children and young people: identification and management. NICE Guideline [NG134]. 2019 (last checked December 2023). www.nice.org.uk/guidance/ng134.
5. March J, et al. Fluoxetine, cognitive-behavioral therapy, and their combination for adolescents with depression: Treatment for Adolescents with Depression Study (TADS) randomized controlled trial. *JAMA* 2004; **292**:807–820.
6. Goodyer IM, et al. Practitioner Review: Therapeutics of unipolar major depressions in adolescents. *J Child Psychol Psychiatry* 2019; **60**:232–243.
7. Locher C, et al. Efficacy and safety of selective serotonin reuptake inhibitors, serotonin-norepinephrine reuptake inhibitors, and placebo for common psychiatric disorders among children and adolescents: a systematic review and meta-analysis. *JAMA Psychiatry* 2017; **74**:1011–1020.
8. Teng T, et al. Effect of antidepressants on functioning and quality of life outcomes in children and adolescents with major depressive disorder: a systematic review and meta-analysis. *Transl Psychiatry* 2022; **12**:183.
9. Vitiello B, et al. Pharmacological treatment of children and adolescents with depression. *Expert Opin Pharmacother* 2016; **17**:2273–2279.
10. Walkup JT. Antidepressant efficacy for depression in children and adolescents: industry- and NIMH-funded studies. *Am J Psychiatry* 2017; **174**:430–437.
11. Hetrick SE, et al. New generation antidepressants for depression in children and adolescents: a network meta-analysis. *Cochrane Database Syst Rev* 2021; **5**:CD013674.
12. Treatment for Adolescents With Depression Study (TADS) Team. The Treatment for Adolescents With Depression Study (TADS): long-term effectiveness and safety outcomes. *Arch Gen Psychiatry* 2007; **64**:1132–1143.
13. Cox GR, et al. Psychological therapies versus antidepressant medication, alone and in combination for depression in children and adolescents. *Cochrane Database Syst Rev* 2014; **11**:CD008324.
14. Dubicka B, et al. Combined treatment with cognitive-behavioural therapy in adolescent depression: meta-analysis. *Br J Psychiatry* 2010; **197**:433–440.
15. Goodyer I, et al. Selective serotonin reuptake inhibitors (SSRIs) and routine specialist care with and without cognitive behaviour therapy in adolescents with major depression: randomised controlled trial. *BMJ* 2007; **335**:142.
16. Zhou X, et al. Comparative efficacy and acceptability of antidepressants, psychotherapies, and their combination for acute treatment of children and adolescents with depressive disorder: a systematic review and network meta-analysis. *Lancet Psychiatry* 2020; **7**:581–601.
17. Poznanski EO, et al. *Children's Depression Rating Scale, Revised (CDRS-R)*. Los Angeles: Western Psychological Services; 1996.
18. Mayes TL, et al. Psychometric properties of the Children's Depression Rating Scale-Revised in adolescents. *J Child Adolesc Psychopharmacol* 2010; **20**:513–516.
19. Angold A, et al. Development of a short questionnaire for use in epidemiological studies of depression in children and adolescents. *Int J Methods Psychiatr Res* 1995; **5**:237–249.
20. Chorpita BF, et al. Assessment of symptoms of DSM-IV anxiety and depression in children: a revised child anxiety and depression scale. *Behav Res Ther* 2000; **38**:835–855.
21. Shaffer D, et al. A children's global assessment scale (CGAS). *Arch Gen Psychiatry* 1983; **40**:1228–1231.
22. Hetrick SE, et al. Newer generation antidepressants for depressive disorders in children and adolescents. *Cochrane Database Syst Rev* 2012; **11**:CD004851.
23. Cipriani A, et al. Comparative efficacy and tolerability of antidepressants for major depressive disorder in children and adolescents: a network meta-analysis. *Lancet* 2016; **388**:881–890.
24. Brent D, et al. Switching to another SSRI or to venlafaxine with or without cognitive behavioral therapy for adolescents with SSRI-resistant depression: the TORDIA Randomized Controlled Trial. *JAMA* 2008; **299**:901–913.
25. Wilens TE, et al. Fluoxetine pharmacokinetics in pediatric patients. *J Clin Psychopharmacol* 2002; **22**:568–575.

CHAPTER 5

26. Aurobindo Pharma – Milpharm Ltd. Summary of product characteristics. Fluoxetine 20mg capsules. 2020 (last checked December 2023); https://www.medicines.org.uk/emc/product/11909/smpc#gref.

27. Findling RL, et al. The relevance of pharmacokinetic studies in designing efficacy trials in juvenile major depression. *J Child Adolesc Psychopharmacol* 2006; **16**:131–145.

28. Rao Y, et al. Efficacy and tolerability of antidepressant drugs in treatment of depression in children and adolescents: a network meta-analysis. *Zhejiang Da Xue Xue Bao Yi Xue Ban* 2022; **51**:480–490.

29. Arango C, et al. Safety and efficacy of agomelatine in children and adolescents with major depressive disorder receiving psychosocial counselling: a double-blind, randomised, controlled, phase 3 trial in nine countries. *Lancet Psychiatry* 2022; **9**:113–124.

30. Findling RL, et al. Vortioxetine for major depressive disorder in adolescents: 12-week randomized, placebo-controlled, fluoxetine-referenced, fixed-dose study. *J Am Acad Child Adolesc Psychiatry* 2022; **61**:1106–1118.e1102.

31. Dwyer JB, et al. Annual research review: defining and treating pediatric treatment-resistant depression. *J Child Psychol Psychiatry* 2020; **61**:312–332.

32. Asarnow JR, et al. Treatment of selective serotonin reuptake inhibitor-resistant depression in adolescents: predictors and moderators of treatment response. *J Am Acad Child Adolesc Psychiatry* 2009; **48**:330–339.

33. Curry J, et al. Predictors and moderators of acute outcome in the Treatment for Adolescents with Depression Study (TADS). *J Am Acad Child Adolesc Psychiatry* 2006; **45**:1427–1439.

34. Haapasalo-Pesu KM, et al. Mirtazapine in the treatment of adolescents with major depression: an open-label, multicenter pilot study. *J Child Adolesc Psychopharmacol* 2004; **14**:175–184.

35. Emslie GJ, et al. Treatment of Resistant Depression in Adolescents (TORDIA): week 24 outcomes. *Am J Psychiatry* 2010; **167**:782–791.

36. Dwyer JB, et al. Efficacy of intravenous ketamine in adolescent treatment-resistant depression: a randomized midazolam-controlled trial. *Am J Psychiatry* 2021; **178**:352–362.

37. Di Vincenzo JD, et al. The effectiveness, safety and tolerability of ketamine for depression in adolescents and older adults: a systematic review. *J Psychiatr Res* 2021; **137**:232–241.

38. Zhou Y, et al. Effect of repeated intravenous esketamine on adolescents with major depressive disorder and suicidal ideation: a randomized active-placebo-controlled trial. *J Am Acad Child Adolesc Psychiatry* 2024; **63**:507–518.

39. Sigrist C, et al. Transcranial magnetic stimulation in the treatment of adolescent depression: a systematic review and meta-analysis of aggregated and individual-patient data from uncontrolled studies. *Eur Child Adolesc Psychiatry* 2022; **31**:1501–1525.

40. Cai H, et al. Suicidal ideation and electroconvulsive therapy: outcomes in adolescents with major depressive disorder. *J ECT* 2023; **39**:166–172.

41. Zimmermann KS, et al. Esketamine as a treatment for paediatric depression: questions of safety and efficacy. *Lancet Psychiatry* 2020; **7**:827–829.

42. Ayvaci ER, et al. Special populations: treatment-resistant depression in children and adolescents. *Psychiatr Clin North Am* 2023; **46**:359–370.

43. Varigonda AL, et al. Systematic review and meta-analysis: early treatment responses of selective serotonin reuptake inhibitors in pediatric major depressive disorder. *J Am Acad Child Adolesc Psychiatry* 2015; **54**:557–564.

44. Jakubovski E, et al. Systematic review and meta-analysis: dose-response relationship of selective serotonin reuptake inhibitors in major depressive disorder. *Am J Psychiatry* 2016; **173**:174–183.

45. Heiligenstein JH, et al. Fluoxetine 40-60 mg versus fluoxetine 20 mg in the treatment of children and adolescents with a less-than-complete response to nine-week treatment with fluoxetine 10-20 mg: a pilot study. *J Child Adolesc Psychopharmacol* 2006; **16**:207–217.

46. Emslie GJ, et al. Fluoxetine treatment for prevention of relapse of depression in children and adolescents: a double-blind, placebo-controlled study. *J Am Acad Child Adolesc Psychiatry* 2004; **43**:1397–1405.

47. Emslie GJ, et al. Fluoxetine versus placebo in preventing relapse of major depression in children and adolescents. *Am J Psychiatry* 2008; **165**:459–467.

48. Li K, et al. Risk of suicidal behaviors and antidepressant exposure among children and adolescents: a meta-analysis of observational studies. *Front Psychiatry* 2022; **13**:880496.

49. Sharma T, et al. Suicidality and aggression during antidepressant treatment: systematic review and meta-analyses based on clinical study reports. *BMJ* 2016; **352**:i65.

50. Bridge JA, et al. Clinical response and risk for reported suicidal ideation and suicide attempts in pediatric antidepressant treatment: a meta-analysis of randomized controlled trials. *JAMA* 2007; **297**:1683–1696.

51. Plöderl M, et al. Re: "A multicenter double-blind, placebo-controlled trial of escitalopram in children and adolescents with generalized anxiety disorder" by Strawn et al. – Concerning harm-benefit ratio in a recent trial about escitalopram for generalized anxiety disorder. *J Child Adolesc Psychopharmacol* 2023; **33**:295–296.

52. Gibbons RD, et al. Early evidence on the effects of regulators' suicidality warnings on SSRI prescriptions and suicide in children and adolescents. *Am J Psychiatry* 2007; **164**:1356–1363.

53. Libby AM, et al. Decline in treatment of pediatric depression after FDA advisory on risk of suicidality with SSRIs. *Am J Psychiatry* 2007; **164**:884–891.

54. Offidani E, et al. Excessive mood elevation and behavioral activation with antidepressant treatment of juvenile depressive and anxiety disorders: a systematic review. *Psychother Psychosom* 2013; **82**:132–141.

55. Safer DJ, et al. Treatment-emergent adverse events from selective serotonin reuptake inhibitors by age group: children versus adolescents. *J Child Adolesc Psychopharmacol* 2006; **16**:159–169.

56. Baldessarini RJ, et al. Antidepressant-associated mood-switching and transition from unipolar major depression to bipolar disorder: a review. *J Affect Disord* 2013; **148**:129–135.

57. Virtanen S, et al. Antidepressant use and risk of manic episodes in children and adolescents with unipolar depression. *JAMA Psychiatry* 2024; **81**:25–33.

Bipolar disorder in children and adolescents

Clinical guidance

Before prescribing

- Establish clinical diagnosis informed by structured instrument assessment if possible. Symptom checklists should be avoided, especially in primary care. Try to monitor symptom patterns prospectively with mood or sleep diaries. If in doubt, seek specialist advice early on.
- Explain the diagnosis to the patient and family and invest time and effort in psychoeducation. This is likely to improve adherence and help children and adolescents and their families appreciate early warning signs of a relapse. Furthermore, there is evidence that such approaches reduce relapse rates, at least in adults.[1]
- Measure baseline symptoms of mania (e.g. Young Mania Rating Scale[2] [YMRS] and the parent YMRS[3]), depression (e.g. Children's Depression Rating Scale[4] [CDRS]) and impairment (e.g. Clinical Global Impression – BD version[5]). Use these to set clear and realistic treatment goals.
- Measure baseline height, weight, waist and hip circumference, pulse, blood pressure and electrocardiogram (ECG) and obtain baseline bloods as appropriate (fasting blood glucose, HbA_{1c}, fasting lipid profile, full blood count [FBC], urea and electrolytes [U&E], creatine kinase, LFTs, prolactin and thyroid function).

What to prescribe

- Tables 5.3, 5.4, 5.5 and 5.6 summarise medication use in bipolar mania and depression and acute mania.
- For the treatment of mania and hypomania in children and adolescents, UK NICE guidelines suggest following the same recommendations as for adults – second-generation antipsychotics (SGAs) may be used as first-line treatment, and mood stabilisers (MS) can be added after a failure of two trials of SGAs.[6] The difference in comparison with adult guidelines is that NICE recommends that SGAs should not be routinely offered for more than 12 weeks. This information should be shared with the child or adolescent and their family.
- SGAs seem to show greater short-term efficacy (effect size [ES] = 0.65 compared with placebo) than MS (ES = 0.20 compared with placebo) in youth, according to a 2010 meta-analysis.[7]
- SGAs produce significantly greater weight gain (particularly olanzapine) and somnolence in children and adolescents compared with adults,[7] although weight gain assessment is made complicated by normal growth at this time of life.
- Valproate should be **completely avoided** in all adolescents.
- Adherence to lithium cannot be assumed and blood level testing may be difficult in adolescents.
- Overall, we recommend the use of SGAs as first line for the acute treatment of mania in children and adolescents (Tables 5.3 and 5.5).
- It is helpful to document family history of response and non-response to pharmacological treatment as there is evidence to suggest that pharmacological response, at least for lithium, runs in families.[8]

CHAPTER 5

After prescribing

- Assess and measure symptoms on a regular basis to establish effectiveness.
- Monitor weight, height and waist to hip circumference at each visit and repeat all fasting bloods at 3 months (then every 6 months). Offer advice on healthy lifestyle and exercise.
- The duration of most medication trials is 3–5 weeks – this is the period over which most improvement is anticipated to occur. This should guide decisions about how long to try a single drug in a patient. A complete absence of response at 2 weeks should prompt consideration of a switch to another SGA (or a dose increase where labelling allows).
- If there is no response, check adherence, measure blood levels where possible and consider increasing the dose. Consider concurrent use of an SGA and MS.
- Judicious extrapolation of the evidence from adults[9] is required because of the very limited evidence base in youths with bipolar disorder. This includes treatment duration and prophylaxis.[6,7,10] Maintenance treatment should follow adult guidelines. Consider the use of lithium early in the course of treatment, either by switching to lithium monotherapy prophylaxis or as an adjunct to a successful acute medication. Lithium has therapeutic advantages over other options in adults but should only be used where adherence is assured.

Specific issues

- Bipolar depression is a common clinical challenge and its treatment has been studied much less in youths than in adults (Tables 5.4 and 5.6). Antidepressants should be used rarely and with care for the minimum duration possible and only in the presence of an antimanic agent.[6] There is limited evidence for the benefit of antidepressants in bipolar depression in adults.[11] Because of the dearth of trials in youth, we are compelled to extrapolate from adult studies,[6] which suggest use of the olanzapine/fluoxetine combination as the most effective treatment, along with lurasidone, which is supported by evidence from several trials in children aged 10–17 years.[12–14] The metabolic effects of olanzapine arguably make it a second-line choice after lurasidone.
- The exact relationship between ADHD and bipolar depression is still debated. Some evidence suggests that stimulants in children with ADHD and manic symptoms may be well tolerated[15] and that they may be safe and effective to use after mood stabilisation.[15] Caution and experience with prescribing these drugs are required.
- The DSM-5 category of disruptive mood dysregulation disorder (DMDD) includes severely irritable children (who were commonly misdiagnosed as having bipolar depression in the USA). There is no established treatment for DMDD. Lithium is ineffective[16] but SSRIs and psychological treatment options, such as parenting interventions, may be considered.[17]

Other treatments

- Adjunct treatments including psychoeducation, CBT and especially family-focused interventions can enhance treatment and reduce depression relapse rates in bipolar disorder.[18]

- There is emerging evidence that a combination of omega-3 fatty acids with inositol is effective in mania and hypomania in children aged 5–12 years.[19] Confirmatory trials are needed.
- Cariprazine may be effective in young people but evidence is limited.[20]
- The use of high-frequency rTMS in adolescents with treatment-resistant unipolar depression is only supported by open-label studies[21] and no RCT has been done in youth with either unipolar or bipolar depression. Therefore, its use is still considered experimental. One randomised sham-controlled study found rTMS ineffective in treating acute mania in youth (as an add-on to standard pharmacotherapy).[22]
- One small trial supported the adjunctive use of melatonin (6mg/day) in adults with mania.[23] Evidence is not yet sufficient to recommend its use in children.

Table 5.3 Pharmacological treatments of mania in children and adolescents.

Medication	Comment
Lithium	Lithium is cleared relatively quickly in children so twice daily dosing will be required, especially when using liquid or non-modified-release preparations.[24] One double-blind placebo-controlled randomised trial[25] showed *significant* reductions in substance use and clinical ratings after 6 weeks in adolescents with bipolar disorder and comorbid substance misuse. In a double-blind placebo-controlled discontinuation trial (N = 40) over 2 weeks, *no significant difference* in relapse rates were found between lithium and placebo.[26]
	A later double-blind placebo-controlled study (N = 81), over 8 weeks, demonstrated a *significantly larger* change in YMRS score in lithium-treated youths. There was a significant increase in thyrotropin with lithium, but no difference in weight gain.[27]
	Lithium and divalproex did not differ in an 18-month maintenance trial in youths (N = 60) who initially stabilised on combination pharmacotherapy of lithium and divalproex.[28] However, given the compelling evidence for lithium maintenance and prophylaxis in adults, we recommend that clinicians consider its use in adolescents in preference to valproate. Valproate should be avoided in adolescents in any case.
	A meta-analysis[29] found lithium to be 'clearly inferior' to risperidone in mania. Lithium may also be inferior to quetiapine in the treatment of mania in children and adolescents.[30]
	One small 6-month study found higher relapse rates in those who discontinued lithium compared with those who continued.[31] Another naturalistic 8-month study showed lithium to be effective and well tolerated.[32]
Valproate	In an RCT (N = 150)[33] divalproex ER (titrated to clinical response or 80–125mg/L) did not lead to significant differences in mean YMRS compared with placebo at 4 weeks. (Also see risperidone and quetiapine sections below.) **Valproate should be avoided in all peri- and post-pubertal children and adolescents.**
Oxcarbazepine	A double-blind placebo-controlled study (N = 116) did not show significant differences between placebo and oxcarbazepine (mean dose 1515mg/day) in reducing mania rating at 7 weeks.[34]

(Continued)

CHAPTER 5

Table 5.3 (Continued)

Medication	Comment
Olanzapine	A double-blind placebo-controlled study (N = 161)[35] showed olanzapine (5–20mg/day) to be significantly more effective than placebo over a period of 3 weeks. There was greater weight gain in the treatment group (weight gain was 3.7kg for olanzapine vs 0.3kg for placebo) and associated significantly increased fasting glucose, total cholesterol, AST, ALT and uric acid. The addition of topiramate reduces weight gain by more than a half.[36]
Risperidone	A double-blind placebo-controlled study (N = 169) showed risperidone (at doses 0.5–2.5 or 3–6mg) to be more effective than placebo in YMRS mean score reduction in a 3-week follow-up.[37] The lower dose led to the same benefits at a lower risk of adverse effects. Sleepiness and fatigue were common. Mean weight increase in treatment groups was 0.7kg vs 1.7kg for the low-dose arm and 1.4kg for the high-dose arm.
	In the Treatment of Early Age Mania (TEAM) study, higher response rates (and metabolic side effects) occurred with risperidone (mean dose 2.57mg) than with lithium (mean level 1.09mmol/L) and divalproex sodium (mean level 113.6mg/L).[38] A randomised follow-up of this study showed again the superiority of risperidone as an alternative treatment for non-responders to lithium and divalproex sodium, and as an add-on treatment to partial responders to the two drugs.[39] These results need to be interpreted with caution as the definition of mania was broader than that used in some countries. The same caveat applies when considering another double-blind placebo-controlled trial showing significantly better results for risperidone (mean dose 0.5mg) than for valproic acid (mean level 81mg/L) in 3–7-year-old children supposedly diagnosed with mania.[40]
Quetiapine	A double-blind placebo-controlled study (N = 277)[41] showed quetiapine (at doses of 400 or 600mg/day) to be significantly better than placebo in reducing mean YMRS scores at 3 weeks. The most common side effects included somnolence and sedation. Weight gain was 1.7kg in the quetiapine group and 0.4kg for placebo.
	Quetiapine is effective as an adjunct to valproate compared with valproate alone (N = 30, 6 weeks)[42] and was as effective as valproate in a double-blind trial (N = 50, 4 weeks).[43]
Aripiprazole	A double-blind placebo-controlled study[44,45] showed aripiprazole (at doses 10 or 30mg/day) to be significantly better than placebo at both 4 weeks (N = 296)[44] and 30 weeks (N = 210).[45] There was a higher incidence of extrapyramidal side effects in the treatment groups (especially the higher dose). Weight gain was significantly more common in the treatment groups compared with placebo (3.0kg for placebo; 6.5kg for the low-dose arm and 6.6kg for the high-dose arm) at week 30.
Ziprasidone	A double-blind placebo-controlled trial (N = 237)[46] showed ziprasidone (at flexible doses 40–160mg) to be more effective than placebo in reducing mean YMRS scores at 4 weeks. Sedation and somnolence were the most common side effects, while it demonstrated a neutral metabolic profile and no QTc prolongation. A second RCT of 171 participants showed broadly similar outcomes.[47]
Asenapine	A 3-week double-blind placebo-controlled study (N = 350) demonstrated statistical superiority of asenapine over placebo for each of the doses used (2.5, 5 or 10mg BD), with significant difference as early as day 4. However, many side effects were reported, including weight gain of more than 7% of baseline in 8–12% of the asenapine group vs 1.1% in the placebo group, metabolic changes (increase in insulin, lipids, glucose), as well as somnolence, sedation, oral hypoaesthesia and paraesthesia.[48]

ALT, alanine transaminase; AST, aspartate aminotransferase; ER, extended release; MS, mood stabilisers; YMRS, Young Mania Rating Scale.

Table 5.4 Pharmacological treatments of bipolar depression in children and adolescents.

Medication	Comment
Olanzapine/ fluoxetine combination	A large study (N = 255) of the olanzapine/fluoxetine combination (either 6/25 or 12/50mg daily) for 8 weeks[49] showed an advantage for the combination. Most frequent side effects were weight gain (4.4kg for olanzapine/fluoxetine and 0.5kg for placebo), somnolence and hyperlipidaemia. The olanzapine/fluoxetine combination is recommended by UK NICE guidelines,[6] along with quetiapine, as first-line treatment for bipolar depression in children and adolescents, as in adults. Although the olanzapine/fluoxetine combination is not currently available as a single preparation in the UK or European Union, its effects can be achieved by combining olanzapine and fluoxetine (e.g. 5/20 or 10/40mg).
Lurasidone	Lurasidone has been shown to be effective in bipolar depression in adults[50–52] and it does not seem to cause weight gain and other metabolic disturbances. It is also safe and effective in treating schizophrenia in adolescents.[53] Lurasidone was effective in bipolar depression in children (10–17 years) both acutely[12] and in a 2-year follow-up study.[14] Dose ranged from 18.5mg (20mg) to 74mg (80mg). Lurasidone may be the preferred antipsychotic in children on account of its good tolerability.[54] In fact, a 2022 network meta-analysis[14] considered lurasidone to be the optimal treatment for bipolar depression in youths.
Quetiapine	A small study in 32 adolescents,[55] followed by a larger RCT (N = 193),[56] failed to show effectiveness. The second study had a very high placebo response, which is not usually seen in adult quetiapine studies[57] and which may reflect issues in diagnosing mood disorders in multisite studies.[58] A 2022 meta-analysis suggested quetiapine was ineffective in bipolar depression in young people.[14]
Lamotrigine	Lamotrigine has only modest, if any, effects in adult bipolar depression[59] and it has not been studied in RCTs for the treatment of acute bipolar depression in children and adolescents and is, therefore, not recommended as a first-line drug. Moreover, a placebo-controlled randomised withdrawal study of adjunctive lamotrigine for bipolar disorder in youth, lasting over 36 weeks, failed to show any benefit in preventing time to occurrence of a bipolar event.[60]

CHAPTER 5

Table 5.5 Recommended first-line treatments for acute mania.*

Aripiprazole	10mg daily
Risperidone	0.5–2.5mg daily
Olanzapine	5–20mg daily
Quetiapine	Up to 400mg daily
Asenapine	2.5–10mg twice daily

*Continue acutely effective dosing regimen as prophylaxis and consider need for lithium if not already prescribed.

Table 5.6 Recommended first-line treatments for bipolar depression.*

Lurasidone	18.5mg (20mg) to 74mg (80mg) daily
Olanzapine/fluoxetine	6/25mg to 12/50mg daily

*Continue acutely effective dosing regimen as prophylaxis and consider need for lithium if not already prescribed.

References

1. Colom F, et al. A randomized trial on the efficacy of group psychoeducation in the prophylaxis of recurrences in bipolar patients whose disease is in remission. *Arch Gen Psychiatry* 2003; **60**:402–407.

2. Young RC, et al. A rating scale for mania: reliability, validity and sensitivity. *Br J Psychiatry* 1978; **133**:429–435.

3. Gracious BL, et al. Discriminative validity of a parent version of the Young Mania Rating Scale. *J Am Acad Child Adolesc Psychiatry* 2002; **41**:1350–1359.

4. Poznanski EO, et al. Preliminary studies of the reliability and validity of the children's depression rating scale. *J Am Acad Child Psychiatry* 1984; **23**:191–197.

5. Spearing MK, et al. Modification of the Clinical Global Impressions (CGI) Scale for use in bipolar illness (BP): the CGI-BP. *Psychiatry Res* 1997; **73**:159–171.

6. National Institute for Health and Care Excellence. Bipolar disorder: assessment and management. Clinical Guidance [CG185]. 2014 (last updated December 2023); https://www.nice.org.uk/guidance/cg185.

7. Correll CU, et al. Antipsychotic and mood stabilizer efficacy and tolerability in pediatric and adult patients with bipolar I mania: a comparative analysis of acute, randomized, placebo-controlled trials. *Bipolar Disord* 2010; **12**:116–141.

8. Duffy A, et al. A prospective study of the offspring of bipolar parents responsive and nonresponsive to lithium treatment. *J Clin Psychiatry* 2002; **63**:1171–1178.

9. Geddes JR, et al. Treatment of bipolar disorder. *Lancet* 2013; **381**:1672–1682.

10. Diaz-Caneja CM, et al. Practitioner review: long-term pharmacological treatment of pediatric bipolar disorder. *J Child Psychol Psychiatry* 2014; **55**:959–980.

11. Pacchiarotti I, et al. The International Society for Bipolar Disorders (ISBD) task force report on antidepressant use in bipolar disorders. *Am J Psychiatry* 2013; **170**:1249–1262.

12. DelBello MP, et al. Efficacy and safety of lurasidone in children and adolescents with bipolar I depression: a double-blind, placebo-controlled study. *J Am Acad Child Adolesc Psychiatry* 2017; **56**:1015–1025.

13. Singh MK, et al. Lurasidone in children and adolescents with bipolar depression presenting with mixed (subsyndromal hypomanic) features: post hoc analysis of a randomized placebo-controlled trial. *J Child Adolesc Psychopharmacol* 2020; **30**:590–598.

14. DelBello MP, et al. Tolerability, safety, and effectiveness of two years treatment with lurasidone in children and adolescents with bipolar depression. *J Am Acad Child Adolesc Psychiatry* 2021; **31**:494–503.

15. Goldsmith M, et al. Antidepressants and psychostimulants in pediatric populations: is there an association with mania? *Paediatr Drugs* 2011; **13**:225–243.

16. Dickstein DP, et al. Randomized double-blind placebo-controlled trial of lithium in youths with severe mood dysregulation. *J Child Adolesc Psychopharmacol* 2009; **19**:61–73.

17. Vidal-Ribas P, et al. The status of irritability in psychiatry: a conceptual and quantitative review. *J Am Acad Child Adolesc Psychiatry* 2016; **55**:556–570.

18. Miklowitz DJ. Evidence-based family interventions for adolescents and young adults with bipolar disorder. *J Clin Psychiatry* 2016; 77 Suppl E1:e5.

19. Wozniak J, et al. A randomized, double-blind, controlled clinical trial of omega-3 fatty acids and inositol as monotherapies and in combination for the treatment of pediatric bipolar spectrum disorder in children age 5-12. *Psychopharmacol Bull* 2022; **52**:31–51.

20. Riccobene T, et al. Pharmacokinetics, safety, and tolerability of cariprazine in pediatric patients with bipolar I disorder or schizophrenia. *J Child Adolesc Psychopharmacol* 2022; **32**:434–443.

21. Wall CA, et al. Magnetic resonance imaging-guided, open-label, high-frequency repetitive transcranial magnetic stimulation for adolescents with major depressive disorder. *J Child Adolesc Psychopharmacol* 2016; **26**:582–589.

22. Pathak V, et al. Efficacy of adjunctive high frequency repetitive transcranial magnetic stimulation of right prefrontal cortex in adolescent mania: a randomized sham-controlled study. *Clin Psychopharmacol Neurosci* 2015; **13**:245–249.

23. Moghaddam HS, et al. Efficacy of melatonin as an adjunct in the treatment of acute mania: a double-blind and placebo-controlled trial. *Int Clin Psychopharmacol* 2020; **35**:81–88.

24. Grant B, et al. Using lithium in children and adolescents with bipolar disorder: efficacy, tolerability, and practical considerations. *Paediatr Drugs* 2018; **20**:303–314.

25. Geller B, et al. Double-blind and placebo-controlled study of lithium for adolescent bipolar disorders with secondary substance dependency. *J Am Acad Child Adolesc Psychiatry* 1998; **37**:171–178.

26. Kafantaris V, et al. Lithium treatment of acute mania in adolescents: a placebo-controlled discontinuation study. *J Am Acad Child Adolesc Psychiatry* 2004; **43**:984–993.

27. Findling RL, et al. Lithium in the acute treatment of bipolar I disorder: a double-blind, placebo-controlled study. *Pediatrics* 2015; **136**:885–894.

28. Findling RL, et al. Double-blind 18-month trial of lithium versus divalproex maintenance treatment in pediatric bipolar disorder. *J Am Acad Child Adolesc Psychiatry* 2005; **44**:409–417.

29. Duffy A, et al. Efficacy and tolerability of lithium for the treatment of acute mania in children with bipolar disorder: a systematic review: a report from the ISBD-IGSLi joint task force on lithium treatment. *Bipolar Disord* 2018; **20**:583–593.

30. Patino LR, et al. A randomized, double-blind, controlled trial of lithium versus quetiapine for the treatment of acute mania in youth with early course bipolar disorder. *J Child Adolesc Psychopharmacol* 2021; **31**:485–493.

31. Findling RL, et al. Lithium for the maintenance treatment of bipolar I disorder: a double-blind, placebo-controlled discontinuation study. *J Am Acad Child Adolesc Psychiatry* 2019; **58**:287–296.e284.

32. Masi G, et al. Lithium treatment in bipolar adolescents: a follow-up naturalistic study. *Neuropsychiatr Dis Treat* 2018; **14**:2749–2753.

33. Wagner KD, et al. A double-blind, randomized, placebo-controlled trial of divalproex extended-release in the treatment of bipolar disorder in children and adolescents. *J Am Acad Child Adolesc Psychiatry* 2009; **48**:519–532.

34. Wagner KD, et al. A double-blind, randomized, placebo-controlled trial of oxcarbazepine in the treatment of bipolar disorder in children and adolescents. *Am J Psychiatry* 2006; **163**:1179–1186.

35. Tohen M, et al. Olanzapine versus placebo in the treatment of adolescents with bipolar mania. *Am J Psychiatry* 2007; **164**:1547–1556.

36. DelBello MP, et al. A double-blind placebo-controlled pilot study of topiramate in manic adolescents treated with olanzapine. *J Child Adolesc Psychopharmacol* 2023; **33**:126–133.

37. Haas M, et al. Risperidone for the treatment of acute mania in children and adolescents with bipolar disorder: a randomized, double-blind, placebo-controlled study. *Bipolar Disord* 2009; **11**:687–700.

38. Geller B, et al. A randomized controlled trial of risperidone, lithium, or divalproex sodium for initial treatment of bipolar I disorder, manic or mixed phase, in children and adolescents. *Arch Gen Psychiatry* 2012; **69**:515–528.

39. Walkup JT, et al. Treatment of early-age mania: outcomes for partial and nonresponders to initial treatment. *J Am Acad Child Adolesc Psychiatry* 2015; **54**:1008–1019.

40. Kowatch RA, et al. Placebo-controlled trial of valproic acid versus risperidone in children 3-7 years of age with bipolar I disorder. *J Child Adolesc Psychopharmacol* 2015; **25**:306–313.

41. Pathak S, et al. Efficacy and safety of quetiapine in children and adolescents with mania associated with bipolar I disorder: a 3-week, double-blind, placebo-controlled trial. *J Clin Psychiatry* 2013; **74**:e100–e109.

42. Delbello MP, et al. A double-blind, randomized, placebo-controlled study of quetiapine as adjunctive treatment for adolescent mania. *J Am Acad Child Adolesc Psychiatry* 2002; **41**:1216–1223.

43. Delbello MP, et al. A double-blind randomized pilot study comparing quetiapine and divalproex for adolescent mania. *J Am Acad Child Adolesc Psychiatry* 2006; **45**:305–313.

44. Findling RL, et al. Acute treatment of pediatric bipolar I disorder, manic or mixed episode, with aripiprazole: a randomized, double-blind, placebo-controlled study. *J Clin Psychiatry* 2009; **70**:1441–1451.

45. Findling RL, et al. Aripiprazole for the treatment of pediatric bipolar I disorder: a 30-week, randomized, placebo-controlled study. *Bipolar Disord* 2013; **15**:138–149.

46. Findling RL, et al. Ziprasidone in adolescents with schizophrenia: results from a placebo-controlled efficacy and long-term open-extension study. *J Child Adolesc Psychopharmacol* 2013; **23**:531–544.

47. Findling RL, et al. Efficacy, safety, and tolerability of flexibly dosed ziprasidone in children and adolescents with mania in bipolar I disorder: a randomized placebo-controlled replication study. *J Child Adolesc Psychopharmacol* 2022; **32**:143–152.

48. Findling RL, et al. Asenapine for the acute treatment of pediatric manic or mixed episode of bipolar I disorder. *J Am Acad Child Adolesc Psychiatry* 2015; **54**:1032–1041.

49. Detke HC, et al. Olanzapine/fluoxetine combination in children and adolescents with bipolar I depression: a randomized, double-blind, placebo-controlled trial. *J Am Acad Child Adolesc Psychiatry* 2015; **54**:217–224.

50. Loebel A, et al. Lurasidone monotherapy in the treatment of bipolar I depression: a randomized, double-blind, placebo-controlled study. *Am J Psychiatry* 2014; **171**:160–168.

51. Suppes T, et al. Lurasidone adjunctive with lithium or valproate for bipolar depression: a placebo-controlled trial utilizing prospective and retrospective enrolment cohorts. *J Psychiatr Res* 2016; **78**:86–93.

52. Suppes T, et al. Lurasidone for the treatment of major depressive disorder with mixed features: a randomized, double-blind, placebo-controlled study. *Am J Psychiatry* 2016; **173**:400–407.

53. Goldman R, et al. Efficacy and safety of lurasidone in adolescents with schizophrenia: a 6-week, randomized placebo-controlled study. *J Child Adolesc Psychopharmacol* 2017; **27**:516–525.

54. Solmi M, et al. Safety of 80 antidepressants, antipsychotics, anti-attention-deficit/hyperactivity medications and mood stabilizers in children and adolescents with psychiatric disorders: a large scale systematic meta-review of 78 adverse effects. *World Psychiatry* 2020; **19**:214–232.

55. Delbello MP, et al. A double-blind, placebo-controlled pilot study of quetiapine for depressed adolescents with bipolar disorder. *Bipolar Disord* 2009; **11**:483–493.

56. Findling RL, et al. Efficacy and safety of extended-release quetiapine fumarate in youth with bipolar depression: an 8 week, double-blind, placebo-controlled trial. *J Child Adolesc Psychopharmacol* 2014; **24**:325–335.

57. Suttajit S, et al. Quetiapine for acute bipolar depression: a systematic review and meta-analysis. *Drug Des Devel Ther* 2014; **8**:827–838.

58. Bridge JA, et al. Clinical response and risk for reported suicidal ideation and suicide attempts in pediatric antidepressant treatment: a meta-analysis of randomized controlled trials. *JAMA* 2007; **297**:1683–1696.

59. Calabrese JR, et al. Lamotrigine in the acute treatment of bipolar depression: results of five double-blind, placebo-controlled clinical trials. *Bipolar Disord* 2008; **10**:323–333.

60. Findling RL, et al. Adjunctive maintenance lamotrigine for pediatric bipolar I disorder: a placebo-controlled, randomized withdrawal study. *J Am Acad Child Adolesc Psychiatry* 2015; **54**:1020–1031.e1023.

CHAPTER 5

Psychosis in children and adolescents

Schizophrenia is rare in children, but the incidence increases rapidly in adolescence. A detailed developmental and physical assessment is always needed before the diagnosis is made.[1,2] Early-onset schizophrenia spectrum (EOSS) disorder is often chronic and in the majority of cases requires long-term treatment with antipsychotic medication.[3] However, there is very limited RCT evidence for maintenance treatment with antipsychotics beyond 8 weeks,[4] although there are supportive open-label studies.[5]

There have been several RCTs of first-generation antipsychotics, many of them using very high doses and all of them showing high rates of extrapyramidal side effects (EPSEs) and significant sedation.[5] Treatment-emergent dyskinesias can also be problematic[6] even when smaller doses are used.[7] First-generation antipsychotics should be avoided in children and adolescents.

There have also been a number of RCTs of SGAs in EOSS disorder. Olanzapine,[8–10] risperidone,[8,9,11,12] aripiprazole,[13,14] quetiapine,[14,15] paliperidone[16] and lurasidone[17] have all been shown to be effective in the treatment of psychosis in younger people. There is meta-analytical evidence suggesting broadly comparable efficacy of individual SGAs, with the exception of ziprasidone and asenapine which are relatively less effective.[18,19] Importantly, neither aripiprazole nor lurasidone seems to have an effect on QT in adolescents.[20,21] At the time of writing there is no RCT evidence supporting any additional benefit for long-acting antipsychotic injections in younger people, although advantages observed in adults might be assumed to be relevant in younger people. Indeed, a 2023 review of 119 reported adolescent cases suggested good outcomes.[22]

Children and adolescents are at greater risk than adults for adverse effects such as extrapyramidal symptoms, raised prolactin, sedation (even with aripiprazole[14]), weight gain and metabolic effects.[23] Metformin has RCT evidence for the reduction of antipsychotic-related overweight/obesity in children and adolescents with EOSS disorder, while healthy lifestyle education alone does not.[24]

There is evidence that clozapine is effective in treatment-resistant psychosis in adolescents, although this population may be somewhat more prone to neutropenia and seizures than adults.[25–29] Based on data obtained from the treatment of younger adults, olanzapine should probably be tried before moving to clozapine[30] because there is a palpable chance that it will be effective, although clozapine is clearly more effective than olanzapine in adolescents.[26,27]

Overall, algorithms for treating psychosis in children and adolescents are the same as those for adult patients. In the UK, NICE[31] recommends oral antipsychotics in conjunction with family interventions, individual CBT and art therapy. Starting doses should be at the lower end of, or below, the adult range. Antipsychotics should not be offered with the aim of decreasing the risk of developing psychosis;[31–33] they are indicated only in the treatment of psychosis.

When prescribing antipsychotics in children and adolescents always measure baseline parameters and monitor as outlined in the guidance in the chapter on schizophrenia (see Chapter 1). For children and adolescents also include waist and hip circumference, assessment of any movement disorders and assessment of nutritional status, diet and level of physical activity.[31]

References

1. Pina-Camacho L, et al. Autism spectrum disorder and schizophrenia: boundaries and uncertainties. *BJPsych Advances* 2016; **22**:316–324.
2. Hayes D, et al. Dilemmas in the treatment of early-onset first-episode psychosis. *Ther Adv Psychopharmacol* 2018; **8**:231–239.
3. Kumra S, et al. Efficacy and tolerability of second-generation antipsychotics in children and adolescents with schizophrenia. *Schizophr Bull* 2008; **34**:60–71.
4. Singappuli P, et al. Antipsychotic long-term treatment in children and young people: a systematic review and meta-analysis of efficacy and tolerability across mental health and neurodevelopmental conditions. *CNS Spectr* 2022; **27**:570–587.
5. Lee ES, et al. Psychopharmacologic treatment of schizophrenia in adolescents and children. *Child Adolesc Psychiatr Clin N Am* 2020; **29**:183–210.
6. Connor DF, et al. Neuroleptic-related dyskinesias in children and adolescents. *J Clin Psychiatry* 2001; **62**:967–974.
7. Campbell M, et al. Neuroleptic-related dyskinesias in autistic children: a prospective, longitudinal study. *J Am Acad Child Adolesc Psychiatry* 1997; **36**:835–843.
8. Sikich L, et al. A pilot study of risperidone, olanzapine, and haloperidol in psychotic youth: a double-blind, randomized, 8-week trial. *Neuropsychopharmacology* 2004; **29**:133–145.
9. Sikich L, et al. Double-blind comparison of first- and second-generation antipsychotics in early-onset schizophrenia and schizo-affective disorder: findings from the treatment of early-onset schizophrenia spectrum disorders (TEOSS) study. *Am J Psychiatry* 2008; **165**:1420–1431.
10. Kryzhanovskaya L, et al. Olanzapine versus placebo in adolescents with schizophrenia: a 6-week, randomized, double-blind, placebo-controlled trial. *J Am Acad Child Adolesc Psychiatry* 2009; **48**:60–70.
11. Haas M, et al. A 6-week, randomized, double-blind, placebo-controlled study of the efficacy and safety of risperidone in adolescents with schizophrenia. *J Child Adolesc Psychopharmacol* 2009; **19**:611–621.
12. Haas M, et al. Efficacy, safety and tolerability of two dosing regimens in adolescent schizophrenia: double-blind study. *Br J Psychiatry* 2009; **194**:158–164.
13. Findling RL, et al. A multiple-center, randomized, double-blind, placebo-controlled study of oral aripiprazole for treatment of adolescents with schizophrenia. *Am J Psychiatry* 2008; **165**:1432–1441.
14. Pagsberg AK, et al. Quetiapine extended release versus aripiprazole in children and adolescents with first-episode psychosis: the multicentre, double-blind, randomised tolerability and efficacy of antipsychotics (TEA) trial. *Lancet Psychiatry* 2017; **4**:605–618.
15. Findling RL, et al. Efficacy and safety of quetiapine in adolescents with schizophrenia investigated in a 6-week, double-blind, placebo-controlled trial. *J Child Adolesc Psychopharmacol* 2012; **22**:327–342.
16. Singh J, et al. A randomized, double-blind study of paliperidone extended-release in treatment of acute schizophrenia in adolescents. *Biol Psychiatry* 2011; **70**:1179–1187.
17. Arango C, et al. Lurasidone compared to other atypical antipsychotic monotherapies for adolescent schizophrenia: a systematic literature review and network meta-analysis. *Eur Child Adolesc Psychiatry* 2019; **29**:1195–1205.
18. Pagsberg AK, et al. Acute antipsychotic treatment of children and adolescents with schizophrenia-spectrum disorders: a systematic review and network meta-analysis. *J Am Acad Child Adolesc Psychiatry* 2017; **56**:191–202.
19. Lopez-Morinigo JD, et al. Pharmacological treatment of early-onset schizophrenia: a critical review, evidence-based clinical guidance and unmet needs. *Pharmacopsychiatry* 2022; **55**:233–245.
20. Jensen KG, et al. Change and dispersion of QT interval during treatment with quetiapine extended release versus aripiprazole in children and adolescents with first-episode psychosis: results from the TEA trial. *Psychopharmacology (Berl)* 2018; **235**:681–693.
21. Goldman R, et al. Efficacy and safety of lurasidone in adolescents with schizophrenia: a 6-week, randomized placebo-controlled study. *J Child Adolesc Psychopharmacol* 2017; **27**:516–525.
22. Baeza I, et al. What role for long-acting injectable antipsychotics in managing schizophrenia spectrum disorders in children and adolescents? A systematic review. *Paediatr Drugs* 2023; **25**:135–149.
23. Sunshine A, et al. Practitioner review: psychosis in children and adolescents. *J Child Psychol Psychiatry* 2023; **64**:980–988.
24. Correll CU, et al. Metformin add-on vs. antipsychotic switch vs. continued antipsychotic treatment plus healthy lifestyle education in overweight or obese youth with severe mental illness: results from the IMPACT trial. *World Psychiatry* 2020; **19**:69–80.
25. Kumra S, et al. Childhood-onset schizophrenia. A double-blind clozapine-haloperidol comparison. *Arch Gen Psychiatry* 1996; **53**:1090–1097.
26. Shaw P, et al. Childhood-onset schizophrenia: a double-blind, randomized clozapine-olanzapine comparison. *Arch Gen Psychiatry* 2006; **63**:721–730.
27. Kumra S, et al. Clozapine and 'high-dose' olanzapine in refractory early-onset schizophrenia: a 12-week randomized and double-blind comparison. *Biol Psychiatry* 2008; **63**:524–529.
28. Schneider C, et al. Systematic review of the efficacy and tolerability of clozapine in the treatment of youth with early onset schizophrenia. *Eur Psychiatry* 2014; **29**:1–10.
29. Adnan M, et al. Clozapine for management of childhood and adolescent-onset schizophrenia: a systematic review and meta-analysis. *J Child Adolesc Psychopharmacol* 2022; **32**:2–11.
30. Agid O, et al. An algorithm-based approach to first-episode schizophrenia: response rates over 3 prospective antipsychotic trials with a retrospective data analysis. *J Clin Psychiatry* 2011; **72**:1439–1444.
31. National Institute for Health and Care Excellence. Psychosis and schizophrenia in children and young people: recognition and management. Clinical Guidance [CG155]. 2013 (last updated October 2016, last checked October 2023); https://www.nice.org.uk/guidance/cg155.
32. Catalan A, et al. Annual research review: prevention of psychosis in adolescents – systematic review and meta-analysis of advances in detection, prognosis and intervention. *J Child Psychol Psychiatry* 2021; **62**:657–673.
33. Láng U, et al. Systematic review and meta-analysis: psychosis risk in children and adolescents with an at-risk mental state. *J Am Acad Child Adolesc Psychiatry* 2022; **61**:615–625.

CHAPTER 5

Anxiety disorders in children and adolescents

Diagnostic issues

Fear and worry are common in children and they are part of normal development. At the same time, anxiety disorders often begin in childhood and adolescence[1] and they are the most common psychiatric disorders in this age group, with overall prevalence between 8% and 30% depending on the impairment cut-offs used.[2] Anxiety disorders may be even more common in children with neurodevelopmental disorders.[3]

In children, the more obvious clinical presentation with distress and avoidance may be masked by prominent behavioural symptoms (e.g. irritability and angry outbursts linked to avoidance). Therefore, the assessment and treatment of anxiety disorders in children need to be undertaken by clinicians who can discriminate normal, developmentally appropriate worries, fears and shyness from anxiety disorders that significantly impair a child's functioning, and who can appreciate developmental variations in the presentation of symptoms.

Clinical guidance

Anxiety symptoms in children and adolescents often improve with age, presumably in parallel to the development of the prefrontal cortex and, in particular, executive function. However, anxiety disorders are distressing and impairing conditions that need to be treated promptly. Chronic stress mediators may have significant impact on brain development[4] and functional impairment linked to anxiety symptoms may prevent young people from accessing normative experiences that are critical for social, emotional and cognitive development. Finally, early and effective treatment may prevent continuity of psychopathology into adulthood: for example, young people with anxiety disorders are three times more likely to have anxiety and depression in adult life compared with non-anxious youth.[5]

Guidelines for the treatment of anxiety disorders in children and adolescents have been made available in the UK and the USA. NICE guidelines focus on the treatment of social anxiety disorder in children and adolescents, suggesting the use of cognitive behavioural therapy and cautioning against the routine use of pharmacological treatment for social anxiety in this age group.[6] Guidelines from AACAP cover the treatment of all anxiety disorders except post-traumatic stress disorder (PTSD) and obsessive compulsive disorder (OCD) (which are classified separately according to DSM).[7] AACAP guidelines suggest multimodal treatment including psychoeducation, psychotherapy (e.g. a 12-session course of exposure-based CBT) and pharmacotherapy. Drug treatment is endorsed for moderate-to-severe anxiety symptoms, when impairment makes participation in psychotherapy difficult, or when psychotherapy leads to only partial response.

Prescribing for anxiety disorders in children and adolescents

Before prescribing

- **Exclude other diagnoses**: Anxiety symptoms can be mimicked by a range of psychiatric disorders including depression (inattention, sleep problems), bipolar disorder (irritability, sleep problems, restlessness), oppositional-defiant disorder (irritability, oppositional behaviour), psychotic disorders (social withdrawal, restlessness), ADHD (inattention, restlessness), autism spectrum disorder (social withdrawal, poor social skills, repetitive behaviours and routines) and learning disabilities. They may also be mimicked by a range of endocrine (hyperthyroidism, hypoglycaemia, phaeochromocytoma), neurological (migraine, seizures, delirium, brain tumours), cardiovascular (cardiac arrhythmias) and respiratory (asthma) conditions and lead intoxication. Anxiety-like symptoms can be observed in response to several drugs and substances including anti-asthma medications, sympathomimetics, steroids, SSRIs, antipsychotics (akathisia), diet pills, cold medicines, caffeine and energy drinks.

- **Beware contraindications to SSRIs and potential interactions.**
- **Measure baseline severity:** Use structured interviews including the Anxiety Disorders Interview Schedule (ADIS) and the Kiddie-Schedule for Affective Disorders and Schizophrenia (Kiddie-SADS); questionnaires including the Revised Children's Anxiety and Depression Scale (RCADS), Screen for Child Anxiety and Related Emotional Disorders (SCARED) or the Multidimensional Anxiety Scale for Children (MASC); and measures of functional impairment including the Children's Global Assessment Scale (CGAS).
- **Obtain consent:** Discuss treatment with the young person and the family (e.g. name of medication, starting/estimated ending dose, titration timeline, possible side effects and strategies to monitor/minimise them, strategies to monitor progress, interventions for treatment-resistant cases). Document consent in writing.

What to prescribe

- **SSRIs:** These are the medications of choice for the treatment of anxiety disorders in children and adolescents. SSRI treatment is at least as effective as non-drug treatments.[8] A 2019 meta-analysis identified seven short-term RCTs (<16 weeks; n treatment = 446, n control = 386) testing the efficacy of SSRIs (fluoxetine, fluvoxamine, paroxetine, sertraline) on changes in severity of anxiety in young people (Clinical Global Impression I [CGI-I] scale). The odds ratio (vs placebo) of overall treatment response was 4.6 (95%CI = 3.1–7.5) and, in anxiety symptoms specifically, 5.2 (95%CI = 2.8–8.8).[9] The Childhood Anxiety Multimodal Study (CAMS) showed that monotherapy with sertraline (55% response) is as effective as CBT for anxiety (60% response) and better than placebo (24% response), and that combined therapy with sertraline and CBT is most likely to be successful (81% response).[10] A 2017 network meta-analysis found that SSRIs significantly reduce clinician-reported and parent-reported (but not child-reported) anxiety symptoms and increased rates of remission.[11] Another network meta-analysis found that the likelihood of treatment response was higher for SSRI compared with the following other medications;[9] a standard meta-analysis showed that clinically significant treatment effects typically emerge by week 6 of treatment, and that SSRIs are associated with more rapid and greater improvement than these other medications.[12] The most recent meta-analysis (11 studies, 2122 participants [2023])[13] suggests broadly similar efficacy for SSRIs/serotonin–noradrenaline reuptake inhibitors (SNRIs). With regard to tolerability, SSRIs are the best tolerated class of medications, particularly escitalopram and fluoxetine.[14]

Sertraline, fluoxetine and fluvoxamine have been approved by the US FDA for treatment of paediatric OCD, and fluoxetine and escitalopram have been approved for treatment of paediatric depression. The FDA issued in 2004 a black box warning for concerns related to worsening of depression, agitation and suicidal ideation linked to SSRIs. These concerns were based on a review of studies of adolescents with depression rather than young people with anxiety.

- **SNRIs:** Venlafaxine was tested in two short-term RCTs (n treatment = 294, n control = 311), duloxetine was tested in one short-term RCT (n treatment = 135, n control = 137) and atomoxetine was tested in one short-term RCT. The overall odds ratio of treatment response for SNRIs was 2.4 (95%CI = 1.7–3.6) over placebo.[9] However, SNRIs did not show statistically significant effects on improvement in anxiety symptoms over placebo.[9] The network meta-analysis mentioned earlier found that SNRIs significantly reduce clinician-reported (but not parent-reported or child-reported) anxiety symptoms.[11] SSRIs are more effective and better tolerated[9] so SNRIs could be considered a third-line treatment for anxiety disorders when two trials with different SSRIs prove ineffective.
- **Others:** The 5HT$_{1A}$ agonist **buspirone** has been examined in one short-term RCT (n treatment = 334, n control = 225) and found not to be effective.[15] The alpha$_2$ agonist **guanfacine** was evaluated in one short-term RCT (n treatment = 62, n control = 21) and found to be associated with an increased odds ratio for treatment response (5.6 [95%CI = 1.4–26.8]) but not for improvement in anxiety symptoms.[16]
- Neither **benzodiazepine** nor **tricyclic antidepressant** use is supported by controlled trials in children.[9] Benzodiazepine may also lead to paradoxical disinhibition in some children. Nevertheless, use of longer-acting benzodiazepines is at times considered in clinical practice either to alleviate disabling anxiety during initial titration of SSRIs or for rapid tranquillisation.

Table 5.7 lists the doses for treating anxiety disorders in children and adolescents.

After prescribing

Acute phase
- Start at the lowest available dose.
- Monitor side effects. SSRIs are generally well tolerated during treatment for anxiety disorders in young people. Psychological side effects include worsening of anxiety symptoms, agitation and disinhibition. Physical side effects including gastrointestinal symptoms (e.g. nausea, vomiting, dyspepsia, abdominal pain, diarrhoea, constipation), headache, increased motor activity and insomnia may occur, often in mild and transient form.
- After 1 week of treatment with SSRIs (2 weeks for SNRIs) when the child is compliant with medications and does not manifest more than minimal side effects, titrate incrementally with weekly intervals to the minimal therapeutic dose.
- Monitor side effects and response (e.g. RCADS, SCARED, MASC, CGAS, CGI-I) frequently and systematically.
- Dosage for treatment with SSRIs is often similar to dosage in adults because of faster metabolism in children.
- Therapeutic effect should appear by 6–8 weeks of treatment. It is important to communicate this to families.
- If partial or non-response, consider accuracy of diagnosis, adequacy of medication trial and compliance of patient.

Table 5.7 Typical dosage of medications for treatment of anxiety disorders in children and adolescents.

Medication	Starting dose (mg)	Dose range (mg/day)
SSRI		
Sertraline	12.5–25	25–200
Fluoxetine	5–10	10–60
Fluvoxamine	12.5–25	50–200 (bd if >50)
Paroxetine	5–10	10–40
Citalopram*	5–10	10–40
SNRI		
Venlafaxine XR	37.5	37.5–225
Duloxetine	30	30–120
Alpha$_2$ agonist		
Guanfacine	1	1–6
5HT$_{1A}$ partial agonist		
Buspirone*	5 tds	15–60
Benzodiazepine (prn)		
Clonazepam*	0.25–0.5	–
Lorazepam*	0.5–1	–

Note: always check dose with latest formal guidance, e.g. *British National Formulary for Children* (in the UK).
*Treatments not supported by randomised controlled trial evidence.
bd, twice daily; prn, as required; tds, three times daily.

- To improve response, consider adding CBT, changing medication (e.g. switch SSRIs, other classes) or combining medications (e.g. for comorbidities, to treat side effects, to potentiate action). Augmentation strategies with buspirone, benzodiazepines, atypical antipsychotics and stimulant medications have been proposed but lack empirical support.[7]

Maintenance phase
- Continue maintenance treatment for at least 1 year of stable improvement.
- Monitor response and side effects regularly.

Discontinuation phase
- Because of lack of information on long-term safety and possible improvement in symptoms with age and learning, consider discontinuing treatment after a period of stable improvement. A trial of medication withdrawal should be started at a period of low stress/demands. Discontinuation should also be considered if the medication is no longer working or the side effects are too severe. Taper SSRIs slowly (e.g. 25% of previous dose weekly) to minimise the risk of discontinuation symptoms. Monitor closely for recurrence of symptoms/relapse and, if deterioration is noted, consider restarting medication.

Pre-school children

Treatment of anxiety disorders in pre-school children must routinely focus on psychotherapy. In rare cases when a very young child has extreme ongoing symptoms and impairment, clinicians should reconsider diagnosis and case formulation, and reassess the adequacy of the psychotherapy trial. There are no RCTs of pharmacological interventions for anxiety in pre-school children, but case reports suggest a potential benefit of fluoxetine and buspirone.[17] Any prescription in pre-school children is off-label.[18]

References

1. Kessler RC, et al. Lifetime prevalence and age-of-onset distributions of DSM-IV disorders in the National Comorbidity Survey Replication. *Arch Gen Psychiatry* 2005; **62**:593–602.
2. Merikangas KR, et al. Lifetime prevalence of mental disorders in U.S. adolescents: results from the National Comorbidity Survey Replication – Adolescent Supplement (NCS-A). *J Am Acad Child Adolesc Psychiatry* 2010; **49**:980–989.
3. Simonoff E, et al. Psychiatric disorders in children with autism spectrum disorders: prevalence, comorbidity, and associated factors in a population-derived sample. *J Am Acad Child Adolesc Psychiatry* 2008; **47**:921–929.
4. Danese A, et al. Adverse childhood experiences, allostasis, allostatic load, and age-related disease. *Physiol Behav* 2012; **106**:29–39.
5. Pine DS, et al. The risk for early-adulthood anxiety and depressive disorders in adolescents with anxiety and depressive disorders. *Arch Gen Psychiatry* 1998; **55**:56–64.
6. National Institute for Health and Clinical Excellence. Social anxiety disorder: recognition, assessment and treatment. Clinical Guidance [CG159]. 2013 (last updated 2017, last checked December 2023); https://www.nice.org.uk/guidance/cg159.
7. Connolly SD, et al. Practice parameter for the assessment and treatment of children and adolescents with anxiety disorders. *J Am Acad Child Adolesc Psychiatry* 2007; **46**:267–283.
8. Arnardóttir A, et al. Comparative effectiveness of cognitive behavioral treatment, serotonin, and serotonin noradrenaline reuptake inhibitors for anxiety in children and adolescents: a network meta-analysis. *Nord J Psychiatry* 2023; **77**:118–126.
9. Dobson ET, et al. Efficacy and tolerability of pharmacotherapy for pediatric anxiety disorders: a network meta-analysis. *J Clin Psychiatry* 2019; **80**:17r12064.
10. Walkup JT, et al. Cognitive behavioral therapy, sertraline, or a combination in childhood anxiety. *N Engl J Med* 2008; **359**:2753–2766.
11. Wang Z, et al. Comparative effectiveness and safety of cognitive behavioral therapy and pharmacotherapy for childhood anxiety disorders: a systematic review and meta-analysis. *JAMA Pediatrics* 2017; **171**:1049–1056.
12. Strawn JR, et al. The impact of antidepressant dose and class on treatment response in pediatric anxiety disorders: a meta-analysis. *J Am Acad Child Adolesc Psychiatry* 2018; **57**:235–244.e232.
13. Stefánsdóttir ÍH, et al. Efficacy and safety of serotonin reuptake inhibitors (SSRI) and serotonin noradrenaline reuptake inhibitors (SNRI) for children and adolescents with anxiety disorders: a systematic review and meta-analysis. *Nord J Psychiatry* 2023; **77**:137–146.
14. Solmi M, et al. Safety of 80 antidepressants, antipsychotics, anti-attention-deficit/hyperactivity medications and mood stabilizers in children and adolescents with psychiatric disorders: a large scale systematic meta-review of 78 adverse effects. *World Psychiatry* 2020; **19**:214–232.
15. Strawn JR, et al. Buspirone in children and adolescents with anxiety: a review and Bayesian analysis of abandoned randomized controlled trials. *J Child Adolesc Psychopharmacol* 2018; **28**:2–9.
16. Strawn JR, et al. Extended release guanfacine in pediatric anxiety disorders: a pilot, randomized, placebo-controlled trial. *J Child Adolesc Psychopharmacol* 2017; **27**:29–37.
17. Gleason MM, et al. Psychopharmacological treatment for very young children: contexts and guidelines. *J Am Acad Child Adolesc Psychiatry* 2007; **46**:1532–1572.
18. Mohatt J, et al. Treatment of separation, generalized, and social anxiety disorders in youths. *Am J Psychiatry* 2014; **171**:741–748.

Obsessive compulsive disorder (OCD) and body dysmorphic disorder (BDD) in children and adolescents

The treatment of OCD and BDD in children and young people largely follows the same principles as those for adults.[1] BDD is recognised by both DSM-5 and ICD-11 as one of the obsessive compulsive disorders. Cognitive behavioural therapy is effective for both conditions in this age group and is recommended in the UK by NICE as the first-choice treatment, although it may be combined with medication for optimal effect.[2]

While CBT is the mainstay of treatment for OCD and BDD, medication alone may be the only viable therapeutic option in some cases. Some children are reluctant to engage with CBT, some may find it difficult to access or they may have very poor insight. This last situation may arise in the autism spectrum disorder alongside comorbid OCD or BDD. Insight in BDD is characteristically poorer than in OCD, with up to 50% of cases having beliefs about their appearance which are of delusional intensity. This too can affect motivation to engage with psychological therapy. Where medication is being used as the only evidence-based treatment, it is essential that this remains under review so that motivation and ability to engage with CBT are regularly revisited.

Drug treatment in obsessive compulsive disorder (OCD)

Sertraline (from age 6 years) and fluvoxamine (from age 8 years) are the SSRIs licensed in the UK for the treatment of OCD in young people. Studies have established the efficacy of SSRIs in the child and adolescent population in several placebo-controlled trials.[3–5]

SSRIs have a medium to large effect size in the treatment of OCD in children and young people.[6] A meta-analysis of 12 RCTs of pharmacotherapy in young people under 19 years of age showed that medication is consistently more effective than placebo. Fluoxetine is the most efficacious SSRI for treatment of depression.[7] Many young people presenting with OCD have a diagnosis of comorbid depression, so fluoxetine could be considered as an alternative SSRI to sertraline or fluvoxamine in these cases. Paroxetine is not recommended for use in children and young people.

Clomipramine remains a useful drug for some individuals and is debatably more efficacious than the SSRIs in treating OCD in children and young people.[8] However, clomipramine's side effect profile (sedation, dry mouth, potential for cardiac side effects) tends to limit its use in this age group and, as a consequence, SSRIs remain the first-line choice in OCD.

SNRIs are not recommended for treatment of OCD in children and young people, with no clear evidence of efficacy and poorer tolerability than SSRIs.

Drug treatment in body dysmorphic disorder (BDD)

No treatment is licensed in the UK for either adults or children with BDD. However, evidence shows significant improvements with SSRIs, both in terms of BDD symptoms, suicidality and often comorbid depressive symptoms (80–90% of people with BDD also have a comorbid diagnosis of depression[9]). In the UK, NICE recommends fluoxetine as the SSRI of choice for treating BDD in children. Although BDD cases have delusional intensity beliefs about their appearance, antipsychotics are not effective and are

CHAPTER 5

not recommended. Research in adult patients shows that BDD patients with delusional intensity appearance beliefs are as likely to respond to SSRI monotherapy as are non-delusional patients.[9]

Prescribing SSRIs in children

In 2004, the UK MHRA cautioned against the use of SSRIs in children and young people owing to a possible increased risk of suicidal ideation.[10] Careful re-analysis of treatment data suggests that SSRIs are clearly more efficacious in OCD than they are in moderate depressive episodes in children and young people.[6] Investigators concluded that within the paediatric OCD group, the pooled risk for suicidal ideation and attempts was less than 1% across all studies. This of course is an important risk and should be explained and carefully monitored. Nonetheless, the naturalistic course of untreated OCD and BDD is that patients tend not to spontaneously remit, and they have tremendous associated morbidity. It is also known that untreated OCD and BDD are associated with a 10-fold increased risk of completed suicide compared with the general population in OCD.[9,11] The risk of suicide in BDD is higher, with roughly one in three patients with BDD attempting suicide.[12] These factors need to be carefully considered and discussed with the patient and their carers or family in making informed choices about treatment.

On occasion, medications other than sertraline and fluvoxamine may be used 'off-label' with the appropriate and suitable cautions. NICE guidance[13] for the treatment of OCD recommends the use of maximum tolerated dose strategies of two SSRIs before the use of clomipramine, owing to the latter drug's greater propensity for side effects and need for cardiac monitoring. The alternative to clomipramine is augmentation with a low-dose antipsychotic. Factors guiding the choice of other medications may include issues such as the presence of other disorders; response to a certain drug in other family members; and cost and availability. Compliance with medication can be an issue with some young people, which can guide the choice of preparation. For instance, young people with poor compliance may be better suited to treatment with fluoxetine considering its long half-life compared with other SSRIs. A 2020 meta-analysis showed fluoxetine and sertraline to be more effective in OCD treatment than fluvoxamine.[8] Some children can find tablets or capsules hard to swallow and the availability of licensed liquid formulations is limited in most countries.

NICE guidelines for the assessment and treatment of OCD and BDD

NICE published guidelines in 2005 on evidence-based treatment options for OCD and BDD for young people and adults.[13] NICE recommends a 'stepped care' model, with increasing intensity of treatment according to clinical severity and complexity.[13] Assessment of the severity and impact of OCD or BDD can be aided by the use of the Children's Yale-Brown Obsessive Compulsive Scale (CY-BOCS) or BDD-YBOCS questionnaires, respectively, or other quantitative measures, both at baseline and as a helpful monitoring tool.[14]

The summary treatment algorithm from the NICE guideline is shown in Figure 5.1.

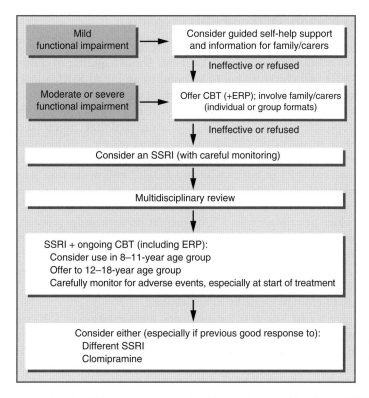

Figure 5.1 Treatment options for children and young people with obsessive compulsive disorder. CBT, cognitive behaviour therapy; ERP, exposure and response prevention. Adapted from NICE guidance.[13] Reprinted with permission.[15]

Initiation of treatment with medication

Clomipramine and SSRIs show a similar incremental effect on obsessions and compulsions from as early as 1–2 weeks after initiation and placebo-referenced improvements continue for at least 24 weeks. In some cases, a positive impact on mood may be seen before the initial changes in OCD symptoms.[16] In the UK, NICE therefore recommends two treatment trials of SSRIs for OCD and BDD of 3 months and increasing towards the maximum tolerated effective dosage. Carefully explaining these temporal effects to patients can be important in sustaining compliance. In addition, the earliest signs of improvement may be apparent to an informant before the patient. Use of an observer-rated quantitative measure such as the CY-BOCS or BDD-YBOCS may therefore be helpful to monitor progress in clinical settings.[17] Expert consensus typically suggests starting at the lowest dose known to be effective, titrating upwards and waiting for up to 12 weeks before evaluating effectiveness.[18] Careful dose titration is particularly recommended if there is insufficient clinical response. In clinical practice a balance must clearly be struck between tolerability and the rate of dosage increase. It is worth noting that the majority of young people with OCD will require a higher dose of SSRI, and as such it may well be clinically indicated to increase the dose more quickly after starting an SSRI.

CHAPTER 5

Treatment-refractory OCD and BDD in children

Evidence from randomised trials suggests that up to three-quarters of medicated patients have an adequate response to treatment. About a quarter of children and young people with OCD will therefore fail to respond to an initial SSRI, administered for at least 12 weeks at the maximum tolerated dose, in combination with an adequate trial of CBT and exposure and response prevention (ERP). These children should be reassessed and compliance clarified, and it should be ensured that clinical comorbidities are not being missed. In such cases, children and young people should usually have additional trials of at least one other SSRI. Research suggests that approximately 40% respond to a second SSRI in both OCD and BDD.[19] Following this, if the response is limited, consideration should be given to referral to a specialist centre.

In OCD, trials of clomipramine may be considered and/or augmentation with a low dose of risperidone or aripiprazole.[13,20] Augmentation with antipsychotics is not recommended in the treatment of BDD.

The combination of fluvoxamine and clomipramine has been used in refractory cases[21,22] but, given the dangers of serotonin syndrome, these regimens should be reserved for specialist centres. Improved efficacy seems to be linked to the altering of the metabolism of clomipramine by fluvoxamine.

There is evidence that low-dose antipsychotic augmentation of SSRI treatment as an off-label therapy can benefit patients whose response to treatment has been inadequate despite at least 3 months of two maximal tolerated separate SSRIs. There is a more robust evidence base in adult cohorts than in younger people. Only a third of treatment-resistant adult cases of OCD showed a meaningful response to this augmentation strategy. Small studies conducted on children and young people showed a clinical improvement for OCD, with a larger evidence base available for aripiprazole compared with risperidone.[23–25] A 6–8-week trial of low-dose antipsychotic augmentation is typically sufficient to assess efficacy. In practice, doses no larger than aripiprazole 2.5–5mg daily or risperidone 0.5mg daily should be used. It is important to discontinue the antipsychotic if no response is noted after this trial of SSRI augmentation. Antipsychotics alone are not efficacious treatments for obsessive compulsive disorders.

Often children and young people whose OCD or BDD has been difficult to treat have comorbidities such as autism spectrum disorder, ADHD or tic disorders. The response to medication can be differentially affected by these comorbidities. For instance, patients with tic disorders may benefit somewhat more from augmentation with second-generation antipsychotics.[26] Untreated ADHD can also commonly interfere with engagement with CBT due to poor focus. Very often efforts to address ADHD with appropriate treatments including medication can dramatically improve engagement with CBT. However, caution is required with regard to stimulant use, particularly for young people who are not 'fighting back' against compulsions. In this group, one can see an increase in compulsions as concentration improves.

Careful clinical review and reformulation are important in treatment-resistant OCD and BDD. Comorbidities and wider psychosocial factors need to be considered for their impact on the treatment response overall. The evidence base around systemic factors and their application in OCD is poor. Very often clinical experience shows that it can be vital to support families and carers during treatment.

Alternative experimental and adult treatments are given in Tables 5.8 and 5.9.

Duration of treatment and long-term follow-up

Untreated OCD runs a chronic course. A series of adult studies have shown that discontinuation of medication tends to result in a varying degree of symptomatic relapse.[27] Some authors have suggested that those with comorbidities are at the greatest risk of relapse.[28] Given that studies frequently exclude cases with additional comorbidities, it is likely that the relapse rates have been underestimated. In the UK, NICE guidelines recommend that if a young person has responded to medication, treatment for OCD or BDD should continue for at least 6 months after remission. This recommendation was based on clinical consensus rather than the product of carefully conducted research trials. Clinical experience would also suggest that when discontinuation of treatment is attempted it should be done slowly, cautiously and in a transparent manner with the patient and their family. Once again, the careful use of clinical outcome measures should be considered when stopping medication. There is a considerable evidence base and expert clinical consensus suggesting that discontinuing medication is associated with a deterioration in symptoms of either OCD or BDD. Increasingly adults and young people are being counselled to consider whether they wish to remain on SSRI medication longer term to mitigate the substantial risk of relapse of OCD or BDD symptoms. Thoughtful and honest discussion about the potential risks of stopping medication should be an active part of any care plan in OCD.

Individuals with developmental disabilities often struggle to generalise the lessons taken from successful CBT. They also have a higher propensity for adverse effects such as activation syndromes with SSRIs, therefore titration may need to be slower.[29] It is important that throughout childhood, adolescence and into adult life individuals with OCD or BDD should have rapid access to healthcare professionals, treatment opportunities and other support as needed. NICE recommends that if relapse occurs, people with OCD or BDD should be seen as soon as possible rather than placed on a routine waiting list because of the propensity for rapid deterioration of symptoms.

CHAPTER 5

Table 5.8 Alternative and experimental treatment of OCD in children and young people.

Treatment	Comment
Aripiprazole augmentation of SSRI	Evidence of clinical improvement in children and young people with OCD[23,24,26,30] No evidence base for use in BDD
Risperidone augmentation of SSRI	Fewer studies than aripiprazole augmentation in children and young people[25]
Fluvoxamine with low-dose clomipramine	Better tolerated than clomipramine monotherapy[31]
N-acetylcysteine (NAC)	Limited evidence suggests children and adolescents with OCD refractory to SSRIs or CBT may benefit from NAC augmentation.[32]
Memantine	Limited evidence suggests potential benefit.[33-35]
Lamotrigine	Case studies have reported response.[36]

BDD, body dysmorphic disorder; CBT, cognitive behavioural therapy; OCD, obsessive compulsive disorder.

Table 5.9 Treatments of OCD used in adults that may be effective in children.

Treatment	Comment
Topiramate augmentation of SSRI	Case studies suggest this may be beneficial and one RCT showed an effect for compulsions but not obsessions.[37,38] Other trials have not found it to be effective.[39] Not to be used in female adolescents.
High-dose SSRI (with ECG monitoring)	Higher than licensed maximum dose SSRI associated with clinical improvement and well tolerated in a retrospective case note survey, double-blind trial and open-label study[40-42]
SNRIs	Duloxetine shown to be as effective as sertraline in a small RCT, and an open-label trial suggested it could reduce symptoms of OCD[43,44]
Mirtazapine	Superior to placebo in an open trial[45]
Pregabalin	Augmentation of sertraline was more effective than augmentation with placebo.[46]
5HT$_3$ antagonists	Ondansetron is effective as add-on treatment.[47] Note risk of QT prolongation
Ketamine IV	Case report showed rapid resolution of symptoms[48]
Tolcapone (catechol-O-methyltransferase inhibitor)	One small trial showed benefit over placebo.[49]
Methylphenidate	Small study showed some benefit for OCD in combination with fluvoxamine[50]
Deep brain stimulation	Could be effective treatment for resistant OCD.[51]
Transcranial magnetic stimulation (TMS)	Meta-analysis showed that TMS can reduce the severity of OCD.[52]

References

1. Bandelow B, et al. World Federation of Societies of Biological Psychiatry (WFSBP) guidelines for treatment of anxiety, obsessive-compulsive and posttraumatic stress disorders – version 3. Part II: OCD and PTSD. *World J Biol Psychiatry* 2023; **24**:118–134.
2. Tao Y, et al. Comparing the efficacy of pharmacological and psychological treatment, alone and in combination, in children and adolescents with obsessive-compulsive disorder: a network meta-analysis. *J Psychiatr Res* 2022; **148**:95–102.
3. Pediatric OCD Treatment Study Team (POTS). Cognitive-behavior therapy, sertraline, and their combination for children and adolescents with obsessive-compulsive disorder: the Pediatric OCD Treatment Study (POTS) randomized controlled trial. *JAMA* 2004; **292**:1969–1976.
4. Geller DA, et al. Which SSRI? A meta-analysis of pharmacotherapy trials in pediatric obsessive-compulsive disorder. *Am J Psychiatry* 2003; **160**:1919–1928.
5. March JS, et al. Treatment benefit and the risk of suicidality in multicenter, randomized, controlled trials of sertraline in children and adolescents. *J Child Adolesc Psychopharmacol* 2006; **16**:91–102.
6. Garland J, et al. Update on the use of SSRIs and SNRIs with children and adolescents in clinical practice. *J Can Acad Child Adolesc Psychiatry* 2016; **25**:4–10.
7. National Institute for Clinical Excellence. Depression in children and young people: identification and management. NICE Guideline [NG134]. 2019 (last checked December 2023); https://www.nice.org.uk/guidance/ng134.
8. Boaden K, et al. Antidepressants in children and adolescents: meta-review of efficacy, tolerability and suicidality in acute treatment. *Front Psychiatry* 2020; **11**:717.
9. Phillips KA, et al. Treating body dysmorphic disorder with medication: evidence, misconceptions, and a suggested approach. *Body Image* 2008; **5**:13–27.
10. Weller IVD, et al. Report of the CSM expert working group on the safety of selective serotonin reuptake inhibitor antidepressants. 2005; https://www.neuroscience.ox.ac.uk/publications/474047.
11. Fernández de la Cruz L, et al. Suicide in obsessive-compulsive disorder: a population-based study of 36 788 Swedish patients. *Mol Psychiatry* 2017; **22**:1626–1632.
12. Pellegrini L, et al. Suicidality in patients with obsessive-compulsive and related disorders (OCRDs): a meta-analysis. *Compr Psychiatry* 2021; **108**:152246.

13. National Institute for Clinical Excellence. Obsessive-compulsive disorder and body dysmorphic disorder: treatment. Clinical Guideline [CG31]. 2005 (last checked December 2023); https://www.nice.org.uk/guidance/cg31.

14. Fernández de la Cruz L, et al. Suicide in obsessive-compulsive disorder: a population-based study of 36 788 Swedish patients. *Mol Psychiatry* 2017; 22:1626–1632.

15. Heyman I, et al. Obsessive-compulsive disorder. *BMJ* 2006; 333:424–429.

16. Scahill L, et al. Children's Yale-Brown Obsessive Compulsive Scale: reliability and validity. *J Am Acad Child Adolesc Psychiatry* 1997; 36:844–852.

17. Baldwin DS, et al. Evidence-based pharmacological treatment of anxiety disorders, post-traumatic stress disorder and obsessive-compulsive disorder: a revision of the 2005 guidelines from the British Association for Psychopharmacology. *J Psychopharmacol* 2014; 28:403–439.

18. Bloch MH, et al. Assessment and management of treatment-refractory obsessive-compulsive disorder in children. *J Am Acad Child Adolesc Psychiatry* 2015; 54:251–262.

19. Grados M, et al. Pharmacotherapy in children and adolescents with obsessive-compulsive disorder. *Child Adolesc Psychiatr Clin N Am* 1999; 8:617–634, x.

20. Bloch MH, et al. A systematic review: antipsychotic augmentation with treatment refractory obsessive-compulsive disorder. *Mol Psychiatry* 2006; 11:622–632.

21. Fung R, et al. Retrospective review of fluvoxamine-clomipramine combination therapy in obsessive-compulsive disorder in children and adolescents. *J Can Acad Child Adolesc Psychiatry* 2021; 30:150–155.

22. Hardy NE, et al. Clomipramine in combination with fluvoxamine: a potent medication combination for severe or refractory pediatric OCD. *J Can Acad Child Adolesc Psychiatry* 2021; 30:273–277.

23. Masi G, et al. Aripiprazole augmentation in 39 adolescents with medication-resistant obsessive-compulsive disorder. *J Clin Psychopharmacol* 2010; 30:688–693.

24. Ardic UA, et al. Successful treatment response with aripiprazole augmentation of SSRIs in refractory obsessive–compulsive disorder in childhood. *Child Psychiatry Hum Dev* 2017; 48:699–704.

25. Simeon J, et al. A retrospective chart review of risperidone use in treatment-resistant children and adolescents with psychiatric disorders. *Prog Neuropsychopharmacol Biol Psychiatry* 2002; 26:267–275.

26. Masi G, et al. Antipsychotic augmentation of selective serotonin reuptake inhibitors in resistant tic-related obsessive-compulsive disorder in children and adolescents: a naturalistic comparative study. *J Psychiatr Res* 2013; 47:1007–1012.

27. Fineberg NA, et al. Sustained response versus relapse: the pharmacotherapeutic goal for obsessive-compulsive disorder. *Int Clin Psychopharmacol* 2007; 22:313–322.

28. Fineberg NA, et al. Pharmacotherapy of obsessive-compulsive disorder: evidence-based treatment and beyond. *Austr N Z J Psychiatry* 2013; 47:121–141.

29. Kolevzon A, et al. Selective serotonin reuptake inhibitors in autism: a review of efficacy and tolerability. *J Clin Psychiatry* 2006; 67:407–414.

30. Ercan ES, et al. A promising preliminary study of aripiprazole for treatment-resistant childhood obsessive-compulsive disorder. *J Child Adolesc Psychopharmacol* 2015; 25:580–584.

31. Fung R, et al. Retrospective review of fluvoxamine-clomipramine combination therapy in obsessive-compulsive disorder in children and adolescents. *J Can Acad Child Adolesc Psychiatry* 2021; 30:150–155.

32. Parli GM, et al. N-acetylcysteine for obsessive-compulsive and related disorders in children and adolescents: a review. *Ann Pharmacother* 2023; 57:847–854.

33. Hosenbocus S, et al. Memantine: a review of possible uses in child and adolescent psychiatry. *J Can Acad Child Adolesc Psychiatry* 2013; 22:166–171.

34. Häge A, et al. Glutamatergic medication in the treatment of obsessive compulsive disorder (OCD) and autism spectrum disorder (ASD) – study protocol for a randomised controlled trial. *Trials* 2016; 17:141.

35. Niemeyer L, et al. Memantine as treatment for compulsivity in child and adolescent psychiatry: descriptive findings from an incompleted randomized, double-blind, placebo-controlled trial. *Contemp Clin Trials Commun* 2022; 29:100982.

36. Naguy A, et al. Lamotrigine augmentation in treatment-resistant pediatric obsessive-compulsive disorder with a 16 month follow-up. *J Child Adolesc Psychopharmacol* 2016; 26:769–772.

37. Berlin HA, et al. Double-blind, placebo-controlled trial of topiramate augmentation in treatment-resistant obsessive-compulsive disorder. *J Clin Psychiatry* 2011; 72:716–721.

38. Van Ameringen M, et al. Topiramate augmentation in treatment-resistant obsessive-compulsive disorder: a retrospective, open-label case series. *Depress Anxiety* 2006; 23:1–5.

39. Afshar H, et al. Topiramate augmentation in refractory obsessive-compulsive disorder: a randomized, double-blind, placebo-controlled trial. *J Res Med Sci* 2014; 19:976–981.

40. Pampaloni I, et al. High-dose selective serotonin reuptake inhibitors in OCD: a systematic retrospective case notes survey. *J Psychopharmacol* 2010; 24:1439–1445.

41. Ninan PT, et al. High-dose sertraline strategy for nonresponders to acute treatment for obsessive-compulsive disorder: a multicenter double-blind trial. *J Clin Psychiatry* 2006; 67:15–22.

42. Rabinowitz I, et al. High-dose escitalopram for the treatment of obsessive–compulsive disorder. *Int Clin Psychopharmacol* 2008; 23:49–53.

43. Mowla A, et al. Duloxetine augmentation in resistant obsessive-compulsive disorder: a double-blind controlled clinical trial. *J Clin Psychopharmacol* 2016; 36:720–723.

CHAPTER 5

44. Dougherty DD, et al. Open-label study of duloxetine for the treatment of obsessive-compulsive disorder. *Int J Neuropsychopharmacol* 2015; 18:pyu062.

45. Koran LM, et al. Mirtazapine for obsessive-compulsive disorder: an open trial followed by double-blind discontinuation. *J Clin Psychiatry* 2005; 66:515–520.

46. Mowla A, et al. Pregabalin augmentation for resistant obsessive-compulsive disorder: a double-blind placebo-controlled clinical trial. *CNS Spectr* 2020; 25:552–556.

47. Eissazade N, et al. Efficacy and safety of 5-hydroxytryptamine-3 (5-HT3) receptor antagonists in augmentation with selective serotonin reuptake inhibitors (SSRIs) in the treatment of moderate to severe obsessive-compulsive disorder: a systematic review and meta-analysis of randomized clinical trials. *Sci Rep* 2023; 13:20837.

48. Rodriguez CI, et al. Rapid resolution of obsessions after an infusion of intravenous ketamine in a patient with treatment-resistant obsessive-compulsive disorder. *J Clin Psychiatry* 2011; 72:567–569.

49. Grant JE, et al. Tolcapone in obsessive-compulsive disorder: a randomized double-blind placebo-controlled crossover trial. *Int Clin Psychopharmacol* 2021; 36:225–229.

50. Zheng H, et al. Combined fluvoxamine and extended-release methylphenidate improved treatment response compared to fluvoxamine alone in patients with treatment-refractory obsessive-compulsive disorder: a randomized double-blind, placebo-controlled study. *Eur Neuropsychopharmacol* 2019; 29:397–404.

51. Abdelnaim MA, et al. Deep brain stimulation for treatment resistant obsessive compulsive disorder; an observational study with ten patients under real-life conditions. *Front Psychiatry* 2023; 14:1242566.

52. Patel S, et al. Effectiveness of repetitive transcranial magnetic stimulation in depression, schizophrenia, and obsessive-compulsive disorder: an umbrella meta-analysis. *Prim Care Companion CNS Disord* 2023; 25:22r03423.

Post-traumatic stress disorder (PTSD) in children and adolescents

Diagnostic issues

Traumatic events and PTSD are common in young people. One in three children experiences traumatic events[1] and about 1 in 13 children develops PTSD before age 18.[1] The prevalence of PTSD in adolescents can be much higher in at-risk groups, for example those attending emergency departments, in forensic settings or among refugee/asylum seekers. Young people with PTSD are at high risk of self-harm (nearly 50%) and suicide attempt (20%) and are often functionally impaired, for example not being in education, employment or education (NEET) (more than 25%).[1] Of note, more than three out of four young people with PTSD have comorbid psychiatric diagnoses, most commonly depression, conduct disorder, alcohol dependence or generalised anxiety disorder.[1] Furthermore, PTSD is not the most common diagnosis in trauma-exposed young people – disorders that are most prevalent in the general population (e.g. depression, conduct disorder, alcohol dependence) are also more prevalent in trauma-exposed young people.[1]

A diagnosis of PTSD is based on the triad of intrusive re-experiencing, avoidance of stimuli associated with the trauma and hyper-arousal after trauma exposure. Because of the abnormal processing of traumatic memories, young people with PTSD may suffer persistent *re-experiencing* of the traumatic event(s) through nightmares or unwanted and distressing memories, which are often experienced as if they were happening in the 'here and now' and often do not appear as frank dissociative symptoms or flashbacks. In order to minimise *re-experiencing* symptoms, young people with PTSD often develop overt or covert *avoidance* strategies, keeping themselves busy or distracted or staying away from people or places that remind them of the traumatic event. As a result of the symptoms, young people with PTSD often feel under continued threat and, therefore, display *physiological hyper-arousal*, appearing alert and vigilant for danger, irritable and struggling to concentrate on daily tasks. Because of the varied clinical manifestations, the assessment and treatment of PTSD in children and adolescents should be undertaken by clinicians who have expertise in the clinical presentations seen in trauma-exposed children and can appreciate developmental variations in the manifestation of symptoms.

Clinical guidance

The UK NICE guidelines[2] advise that treatment of PTSD in young people should focus on psychotherapy, with 12 sessions of trauma-focused CBT (TF-CBT) for PTSD resulting from a single traumatic event or longer for chronic or recurrent events. If TF-CBT is not effective, or based on the young person's preference, treatment may also include eye movement desensitisation and reprocessing (EMDR).

Based on the current evidence in NICE guidelines,[2] the AACAP[3] and the International Society for Traumatic Stress Studies (ISTSS),[4] pharmacotherapy is not recommended for treatment of PTSD in young people. The evidence for efficacy of pharmacotherapy (SSRIs and SGAs) in adults is also somewhat limited at present.[5,6] However, because of the high rates of comorbidity,[1] pharmacotherapy may be needed to target co-occurring psychiatric disorders. In adult PTSD, the best supported treatments are fluoxetine, paroxetine and

CHAPTER 5

venlafaxine.[7] 3,4-Methylenedioxymethamphetamine (MDMA),[8] ketamine[9] and psychedelic drugs[10] also show promise. Prazosin appears to be effective in reducing PTSD-related nightmares in children aged 4–18 years.[11] None of these agents is currently used to any extent in children and adolescents.

References

1. Lewis SJ, et al. The epidemiology of trauma and post-traumatic stress disorder in a representative cohort of young people in England and Wales. *Lancet Psychiatry* 2019; 6:247–256.
2. National Institute for Clinical Excellence. Post-traumatic stress disorder. NICE Guideline [NG116]. 2018 (last checked December 2023); https://www.nice.org.uk/guidance/NG116.
3. Cohen JA, et al. Practice parameter for the assessment and treatment of children and adolescents with posttraumatic stress disorder. *J Am Acad Child Adolesc Psychiatry* 2010; 49:414–430.
4. International Society for Traumatic Stress Studies (ISTSS). Posttraumatic stress disorder prevention and treatment guidelines: methodology and recommendations. 2019; https://istss.org/getattachment/Treating-Trauma/New-ISTSS-Prevention-and-Treatment-Guidelines/ISTSS_PreventionTreatmentGuidelines_FNL-March-19-2019.pdf.aspx.
5. Cipriani A, et al. Comparative efficacy and acceptability of pharmacological treatments for post-traumatic stress disorder in adults: a network meta-analysis. *Psychol Med* 2018; 48:1975–1984.
6. Huang ZD, et al. Comparative efficacy and acceptability of pharmaceutical management for adults with post-traumatic stress disorder: a systematic review and meta-analysis. *Front Pharmacol* 2020; 11:559.
7. Ehret M. Treatment of posttraumatic stress disorder: focus on pharmacotherapy. *Ment Health Clin* 2019; 9:373–382.
8. Jerome L, et al. Long-term follow-up outcomes of MDMA-assisted psychotherapy for treatment of PTSD: a longitudinal pooled analysis of six phase 2 trials. *Psychopharmacology (Berl)* 2020; 237:2485–2497.
9. Fremont R, et al. Ketamine for treatment of posttraumatic stress disorder: state of the field. *Focus (Am Psychiatr Publ)* 2023; 21:257–265.
10. Krediet E, et al. Reviewing the potential of psychedelics for the treatment of PTSD. *Int J Neuropsychopharmacol* 2020; 23:385–400.
11. Hudson N, et al. Evaluation of low dose prazosin for PTSD-associated nightmares in children and adolescents. *Ment Health Clin* 2021; 11:45–49.

CHAPTER 5

Attention deficit hyperactivity disorder (ADHD) in children and adolescents

- A diagnosis of ADHD should be made only after a comprehensive assessment by a specialist with expertise in ADHD.[1] Appropriate psychological, psychosocial and behavioural interventions should be put in place. Drug treatments should be only a part of the overall treatment plan.

- The indication for drug treatment is the presence of impairment resulting from ADHD despite environmental modifications, parent training (if appropriate), advice on parenting strategies and liaison with school.

- **Methylphenidate** is the first-line treatment when medication is indicated. It is a central nervous system (CNS) stimulant with a large evidence base from trials. Most common adverse effects include insomnia, appetite suppression, raised blood pressure, raised pulse rate and growth deceleration. These adverse effects can usually be managed by treatment breaks or dose reduction, depending on the side effect. Long-term use in children is associated with lower height and weight.[2] In the UK and elsewhere, there are several modified-release preparations with different release profiles available, including generic options.

- **Dexamfetamine** is an alternative CNS stimulant. Effects and adverse reactions are broadly similar to methylphenidate, but there is somewhat less evidence for efficacy and safety than exists for methylphenidate. Dexamfetamine is probably more likely to be diverted and misused. Both methylphenidate and dexamfetamine are Controlled Drugs in most countries. This makes prescribing and dispensing more complex.

- **Lisdexamfetamine** is a pro-drug – dexamfetamine is complexed with the amino acid lysine and in this form is inactive. It is broken down in red blood cells so that dexamfetamine is gradually made available. It therefore has a similar practical role to extended-release preparations of methylphenidate and, like them, is unlikely to be abused for recreational or dependency-driven purposes. Several RCTs have established it as superior to placebo in children[3,4] and adolescents.[5] Effect size from preliminary research appears to be at least as great as that of osmotic-controlled release oral delivery system (OROS)-methylphenidate[4] and it seems to have a similar range of adverse effects.[6,7] Network meta-analyses found lisdexamfetamine to be more effective than methylphenidate[8,9] and long-term data suggest that it can be considered as an alternative to extended-release methylphenidate.[10] Lisdexamfetamine is also effective in pre-school children[11] although it is not licensed for this age group.

- **Atomoxetine** is a non-stimulant alternative.[12-15] It may be particularly useful for children who do not respond to stimulants, where stimulant diversion is a problem or when 'dopaminergic' adverse effects (such as tics, anxiety and stereotypies) become problematic on stimulants. Parents should be warned of the possibilities of suicidal thinking and emerging liver disease and advised of the possible features that they might notice. Atomexetine is less effective than stimulants.[9,13,16,17]

CHAPTER 5

- A licensed modified-release preparation of **guanfacine** is approved in the UK and elsewhere for use in children with ADHD. Guanfacine is an α2 agonist medication and can be considered as an alternative non-stimulant medication to atomoxetine.[18] It is broadly as effective as atomoxetine.[19] Although not licensed for adults in most countries, children started on guanfacine should probably continue as adults.
- Another non-stimulant medication with evidence of effectiveness in the treatment for ADHD is the α2 agonist **clonidine**.[20] Extended-release clonidine is widely used for ADHD in the USA but not licensed in most countries.
- There is some evidence supporting the efficacy of **tricyclic antidepressants**[21,22] but these are not recommended in clinical practice.
- **Bupropion**[9,23,24] seems to be efficacious and well tolerated. **Modafinil** also appears to have useful activity in children but not in adults with ADHD.[9,25,26] Evidence supporting the use of these drugs is somewhat limited compared with standard treatments.[9] **Viloxazine** is also effective[27] and approved in the USA.
- The use of **second-generation antipsychotics**[28,29] for ADHD is not recommended.[28,29] These may reduce hyperactivity in autism spectrum disorders[30] but should not be prescribed for this indication.
- Emerging ADHD pharmacotherapies[31] include the SNRIs **venlafaxine** and **duloxetine, agomelatine, dasotraline** (a serotonin, noradrenaline and dopamine reuptake inhibitor) and **tipepidine** (potassium channel inhibitor).
- Comorbid psychiatric illness is common in children with ADHD. Stimulants are often helpful overall but are unlikely to be appropriate for children who have a psychotic illness. Problems with substance misuse should be managed in their own right alongside ADHD treatment[32] and treatments need to be chosen carefully.
- Combinations of stimulants and atomoxetine have been used, but there are few trials and no clear evidence for improved efficacy.[33]
- Combinations of stimulants and guanfacine are approved in some countries. There is some evidence that the combination might have additive effects on symptoms control.[34]
- Once stimulant treatment has been established, it is appropriate for repeat prescriptions to be supplied through general practitioners[1] with reviews at least once a year by a healthcare professional with training and expertise in managing ADHD.

Box 5.1 summarises the NICE guidelines for treating children with ADHD and Table 5.10 summarises prescribing in ADHD.

Box 5.1 Summary of UK NICE guidance for ADHD in children[1]

- Drug treatment should only be initiated by a specialist and only after comprehensive assessment of mental and physical health and social influences. In children under 5 years, medication should be initiated after a second specialist opinion from an ADHD service with expertise in managing ADHD in younger children (ideally a tertiary service)
- An ADHD-focused group parent-training programme should be offered for parents or carers of children aged less than 5 years with ADHD. Environmental modifications need to be implemented in all cases. If ADHD symptoms are still causing a persistent significant impairment in at least one domain despite environmental modifications, medication can be offered following a baseline assessment
- Methylphenidate, lisdexamfetamine, dexamfetamine, atomoxetine and guanfacine are recommended within their licensed indications
- Methylphenidate (either short or long acting) is the first choice of medication
- Consider switching to lisdexamfetamine for children aged 5 years and over and young people who have had a 6-week trial of methylphenidate at an adequate dose and not derived enough benefit in terms of reduced ADHD symptoms and associated impairment
- Consider dexamfetamine for children aged 5 years and over and young people whose ADHD symptoms are responding to lisdexamfetamine but who cannot tolerate the longer effect profile
- Offer atomoxetine or guanfacine to children aged 5 years and over and young people if they cannot tolerate methylphenidate or lisdexamfetamine or their symptoms have not responded to separate 6-week trials of lisdexamfetamine and methylphenidate, having considered alternative preparations and adequate doses
- Monitoring should include measurement of height and weight (with entry on growth charts) and recording of blood pressure and heart rate. An electrocardiogram is not needed before starting stimulants* atomoxetine or guanfacine unless the person has any of the following:
- History of congenital heart disease or previous cardiac surgery
  - history of sudden death in a first-degree relative under 40 years suggesting a cardiac disease
  - shortness of breath on exertion compared with peers
  - fainting on exertion or in response to fright or noise
  - palpitations that are rapid, regular and start and stop suddenly
  - chest pain suggesting cardiac origin
  - signs of heart failure
  - a murmur heard on cardiac examination
  - blood pressure that is classified as hypertensive for adults
  - a coexisting condition that is being treated with a medicine that may pose an increased cardiac risk

A cardiology opinion should be sought if any of the above apply

*The cardiovascular toxicity of stimulants remains poorly quantified. Some analyses show no adverse effect[35] while population studies suggest increased risk of hypertension and other adverse outcomes.[36]

CHAPTER 5

Table 5.10 Prescribing in attention deficit hyperactivity disorder (ADHD).

Medication	Onset and duration of action	Dose	Notes	Recommended monitoring/general notes
Methylphenidate immediate release Branded products (Ritalin, Medikinet, Tranquilyn) and various generic preparations available[37–39]	Onset: 20–60 minutes Duration: 2–4 hours	Initially 5–10mg daily titrated up in weekly increments of 5–10mg, to a maximum of 2.1mg/kg/day in divided doses. Licensed maximum dose 60mg daily (or after specialist review up to 90mg daily)[1]	Methylphenidate usually first-line treatment in ADHD. Generally well tolerated[40]	For methylphenidate, dexamfetamine and lisdexamfetamine Monitor: ■ Blood pressure[41] ■ Pulse ■ Height ■ Weight Monitor for insomnia, mood and appetite change and the development of tics,[42] although some evidence suggests tics are not associated with psychostimulants[43] Discontinue if no benefits seen in 1 month Controlled Drugs
Methylphenidate modified release*			An afternoon dose of immediate-release methylphenidate may be necessary in some children to optimise treatment.	
Concerta XL[37,38,44–46] Bioequivalent versions: Affenid XL, Xaggitin XL, Matoride XL, Xenidate XL, Delmosart modified release	Onset: 0.5 –2 hours Duration: 12 hours	Initially 18mg in the morning, titrated up to a licensed maximum dose of 54mg daily (or after specialist review up to 108mg daily; NB unlicensed) 18mg = 15mg methylphenidate immediate release	Consists of an immediate-release component (22% of the dose) and a modified-release component (78% of the dose).	
Equasym XL[47,48]	Onset: 20–60 minutes Duration: 8 hours	Initially 10mg in the morning, titrated up to a licensed maximum dose of 60mg daily	Consists of an immediate-release component (30% of the dose) and a modified-release component (70% of the dose). Capsules can be opened and sprinkled.	
Medikinet XL Bioequivalent versions: Metyrol XL and Meflynate	Onset: 20–60 minutes Duration: up to 8 hours	Dose as for Equasym XL	Consists of an immediate-release component (50% of the dose) and a modified-release component (50% of the dose). Capsules can be opened and sprinkled.[49]	

Table 5.10 (*Continued*)

Medication	Onset and duration of action	Dose	Notes	Recommended monitoring/general notes
Ritalin XL[50]	Onset: 60 minutes Duration: 8–12 hours	Dose as for Equasym XL	Consists of an immediate-release component (50% of the dose) and a modified-release component (50% of the dose).	
Dexamfetamine immediate release[40,51]	Onset: 20–60 minutes Duration: 3–6 hours	Initially 2.5–10mg daily, titrated up in weekly increments of 2.5–5mg, to a maximum of 20mg daily in divided doses (occasionally up to 40mg daily is necessary)	Considered to be less well tolerated than methylphenidate.[40]	
Lisdexamfetamine (Elvanse)[3–5]	Onset: 20–60 minutes Duration: 13+ hours	Initially 20 or 30mg in the morning, titrated up to a licensed maximum dose of 70mg daily	Pro-drug, gradually hydrolysed to dexamfetamine Capsules can be opened and sprinkled.[52] Licensed in adults	
Atomoxetine[53,54]	Approximately 4–6 weeks (atomoxetine is a noradrenaline reuptake inhibitor)	When switching from a stimulant, continue stimulant for first 4 weeks of therapy. For children <70kg: Initially 0.5mg/kg/day for 7 days, then increase according to response. Recommended maintenance dose 1.2mg/kg/day (in single or divided doses) and up to 1.8mg/kg/day, to a maximum of 120mg daily if necessary[1] For children >70kg: Initially 40mg daily for 7 days, then increase according to response. Recommended maintenance dose 80mg daily	Less effective than stimulants (see text).[13,17] May be useful where stimulant diversion is a problem.[55] Licensed in adults	Monitor: ■ Blood pressure[56] ■ Pulse ■ Height ■ Weight Monitor for insomnia, mood and appetite change and the development of tics. Monitor young people and adults with ADHD for sexual dysfunction (that is, erectile and ejaculatory dysfunction) as potential adverse effects of atomoxetine. Not a Controlled Drug

CHAPTER 5

(*Continued*)

Table 5.10 (*Continued*)

Medication	Onset and duration of action	Dose	Notes	Recommended monitoring/general notes
Guanfacine modified release[9,57]	Approximately 1– 5 weeks[58] (guanfacine is a central alpha2A-adrenergic receptor agonist)	For child 6–12 years (body weight 25kg and above): Initially 1mg once daily; adjusted in steps of 1mg every week if necessary and if tolerated; maintenance 0.05–0.12mg/kg once daily (max. per dose 4mg)	Efficacy and tolerability data should be interpreted with caution.[9]	Similar monitoring to other medication for ADHD.
		For child 13–17 years (body weight 34–41.4kg): Initially 1mg once daily; adjusted in steps of 1mg every week if necessary and if tolerated; maintenance 0.05–0.12mg/kg once daily (max. per dose 4mg)		
		For child 13–17 years (body weight 41.5–49.4kg): Initially 1mg once daily; adjusted in steps of 1mg every week if necessary and if tolerated; maintenance 0.05–0.12mg/kg once daily (max. per dose 5mg)		
		For child 13–17 years (body weight 49.5–58.4kg): Initially 1mg once daily; adjusted in steps of 1mg every week if necessary and if tolerated; maintenance 0.05–0.12mg/kg once daily (max. per dose 6mg)		
		For child 13–17 years (body weight 58.5kg and above): Initially 1mg once daily; adjusted in steps of 1mg every week if necessary and if tolerated; maintenance 0.05–0.12mg/kg once daily (max. per dose 7mg)		

*For details of other preparations available outside the UK, see Cortese et al., 2017.[59]

References

1. National Institute for Health and Clinical Excellence. Attention deficit hyperactivity disorder: diagnosis and management. NICE Guideline [NG87]. 2018 (last updated September 2019, last accessed December 2023); https://www.nice.org.uk/guidance/NG87.
2. Carucci S, et al. Long term methylphenidate exposure and growth in children and adolescents with ADHD. A systematic review and meta-analysis. *Neurosci Biobehav Rev* 2021; **120**:509–525.
3. Biederman J, et al. Lisdexamfetamine dimesylate and mixed amphetamine salts extended-release in children with ADHD: a double-blind, placebo-controlled, crossover analog classroom study. *Biol Psychiatry* 2007; **62**:970–976.
4. Coghill D, et al. European, randomized, phase 3 study of lisdexamfetamine dimesylate in children and adolescents with attention-deficit/hyperactivity disorder. *Eur Neuropsychopharmacol* 2013; **23**:1208–1218.
5. Findling RL, et al. Efficacy and safety of lisdexamfetamine dimesylate in adolescents with attention-deficit/hyperactivity disorder. *J Am Acad Child Adolesc Psychiatry* 2011; **50**:395–405.
6. Heal DJ, et al. Amphetamine, past and present – a pharmacological and clinical perspective. *J Psychopharmacol* 2013; **27**:479–496.
7. Coghill DR, et al. Long-term safety and efficacy of lisdexamfetamine dimesylate in children and adolescents with ADHD: a phase IV, 2-year, open-label study in Europe. *CNS Drugs* 2017; **31**:625–638.
8. Joseph A, et al. Comparative efficacy and safety of attention-deficit/hyperactivity disorder pharmacotherapies, including guanfacine extended release: a mixed treatment comparison. *Eur Child Adolesc Psychiatry* 2017; **26**:875–897.
9. Cortese S, et al. Comparative efficacy and tolerability of medications for attention-deficit hyperactivity disorder in children, adolescents, and adults: a systematic review and network meta-analysis. *Lancet Psychiatry* 2018; **5**:727–738.
10. Findling RL, et al. Long-term effectiveness and safety of lisdexamfetamine dimesylate in school-aged children with attention-deficit/hyperactivity disorder. *CNS Spectr* 2008; **13**:614–620.
11. Childress AC, et al. Efficacy and safety of lisdexamfetamine in preschool children with attention-deficit/hyperactivity disorder. *J Am Acad Child Adolesc Psychiatry* 2022; **61**:1423–1434.
12. Michelson D, et al. Once-daily atomoxetine treatment for children and adolescents with attention deficit hyperactivity disorder: a randomized, placebo-controlled study. *Am J Psychiatry* 2002; **159**:1896–1901.
13. Kratochvil CJ, et al. Atomoxetine and methylphenidate treatment in children with ADHD: a prospective, randomized, open-label trial. *J Am Acad Child Adolesc Psychiatry* 2002; **41**:776–784.
14. Weiss M, et al. A randomized, placebo-controlled study of once-daily atomoxetine in the school setting in children with ADHD. *J Am Acad Child Adolesc Psychiatry* 2005; **44**:647–655.
15. Kratochvil CJ, et al. A double-blind, placebo-controlled study of atomoxetine in young children with ADHD. *Pediatrics* 2011; **127**:e862–e868.
16. Catala-Lopez F, et al. The pharmacological and non-pharmacological treatment of attention deficit hyperactivity disorder in children and adolescents: a systematic review with network meta-analyses of randomised trials. *PLoS One* 2017; **12**:e0180355.
17. Liu Q, et al. Comparative efficacy and safety of methylphenidate and atomoxetine for attention-deficit hyperactivity disorder in children and adolescents: meta-analysis based on head-to-head trials. *J Clin Exp Neuropsychol* 2017; **39**:854–865.
18. Yu S, et al. Guanfacine for the treatment of attention-deficit hyperactivity disorder: an updated systematic review and meta-analysis. *J Child Adolesc Psychopharmacol* 2023; **33**:40–50.
19. Radonjić NV, et al. Nonstimulant medications for attention-deficit/hyperactivity disorder (ADHD) in adults: systematic review and meta-analysis. *CNS Drugs* 2023; **37**:381–397.
20. Connor DF, et al. A meta-analysis of clonidine for symptoms of attention-deficit/hyperactivity disorder. *J Am Acad Child Adolesc Psychiatry* 1999; **38**:1551–1559.
21. Hazell P. Tricyclic antidepressants in children: is there a rationale for use? *CNS Drugs* 1996; **5**:233–239.
22. Otasowie J, et al. Tricyclic antidepressants for attention deficit hyperactivity disorder (ADHD) in children and adolescents. *Cochrane Database Syst Rev* 2014; **9**:CD006997.
23. Gorman DA, et al. Canadian guidelines on pharmacotherapy for disruptive and aggressive behaviour in children and adolescents with attention-deficit hyperactivity disorder, oppositional defiant disorder, or conduct disorder. *Can J Psychiatry* 2015; **60**:62–76.
24. Ng QX. A systematic review of the use of bupropion for attention-deficit/hyperactivity disorder in children and adolescents. *J Child Adolesc Psychopharmacol* 2017; **27**:112–116.
25. Biederman J, et al. A comparison of once-daily and divided doses of modafinil in children with attention-deficit/hyperactivity disorder: a randomized, double-blind, and placebo-controlled study. *J Clin Psychiatry* 2006; **67**:727–735.
26. Wang SM, et al. Modafinil for the treatment of attention-deficit/hyperactivity disorder: a meta-analysis. *J Psychiatr Res* 2017; **84**:292–300.
27. Nasser A, et al. A phase III, randomized, double-blind, placebo-controlled trial assessing the efficacy and safety of viloxazine extended-release capsules in adults with attention-deficit/hyperactivity disorder. *CNS Drugs* 2022; **36**:897–915.
28. Einarson TR, et al. *Novel Antipsychotics for Patients with Attention-Deficit Hyperactivity Disorder: a Systematic Review.* Technology Report No. 17. Ottawa: Canadian Coordinating Office for Health Technology Assessment (CCOHTA); 2001.
29. Pringsheim T, et al. The pharmacological management of oppositional behaviour, conduct problems, and aggression in children and adolescents with attention-deficit hyperactivity disorder, oppositional defiant disorder, and conduct disorder: a systematic review and meta-analysis. Part 2: antipsychotics and traditional mood stabilizers. *Can J Psychiatry* 2015; **60**:52–61.
30. Ji N, et al. An update on pharmacotherapy for autism spectrum disorder in children and adolescents. *Curr Opin Psychiatry* 2015; **28**:91–101.
31. Pozzi M, et al. Emerging drugs for the treatment of attention-deficit hyperactivity disorder (ADHD). *Expert Opin Emerg Drugs* 2020; **25**:395–407.
32. Humphreys KL, et al. Stimulant medication and substance use outcomes: a meta-analysis. *JAMA Psychiatry* 2013; **70**:740–749.

33. Treuer T, et al. A systematic review of combination therapy with stimulants and atomoxetine for attention-deficit/hyperactivity disorder, including patient characteristics, treatment strategies, effectiveness, and tolerability. *J Child Adolesc Psychopharmacol* 2013; 23:179–193.

34. McCracken JT, et al. Combined stimulant and guanfacine administration in attention-deficit/hyperactivity disorder: a controlled, comparative study. *J Am Acad Child Adolesc Psychiatry* 2016; 55:657–666.e651.

35. Zhang L, et al. Risk of cardiovascular diseases associated with medications used in attention-deficit/hyperactivity disorder: a systematic review and meta-analysis. *JAMA Network Open* 2022; 5:e2243597.

36. Zhang L, et al. Attention-deficit/hyperactivity disorder medications and long-term risk of cardiovascular diseases. *JAMA Psychiatry* 2024; 81:178–187.

37. Wolraich ML, et al. Pharmacokinetic considerations in the treatment of attention-deficit hyperactivity disorder with methylphenidate. *CNS Drugs* 2004; 18:243–250.

38. Joint Formulary Committee. *British National Formulary (online)*. London: BMJ and Pharmaceutical Press; http://www.medicinescomplete.com.

39. Janssen-Cilag Ltd. Summary of product characteristics. Concerta XL 18mg, 27mg, 36mg and 54mg prolonged-release tablets. 2023; https://www.medicines.org.uk/emc/product/6872/smpc.

40. Efron D, et al. Side effects of methylphenidate and dexamphetamine in children with attention deficit hyperactivity disorder: a double-blind, crossover trial. *Pediatrics* 1997; 100:662–666.

41. Hennissen L, et al. Cardiovascular effects of stimulant and non-stimulant medication for children and adolescents with ADHD: a systematic review and meta-analysis of trials of methylphenidate, amphetamines and atomoxetine. *CNS Drugs* 2017; 31:199–215.

42. Gadow KD, et al. Efficacy of methylphenidate for attention-deficit hyperactivity disorder in children with tic disorder. *Arch Gen Psychiatry* 1995; 52:444–455.

43. Cohen SC, et al. Meta-analysis: risk of tics associated with psychostimulant use in randomized, placebo-controlled trials. *J Am Acad Child Adolesc Psychiatry* 2015; 54:728–736.

44. Hoare P, et al. 12-month efficacy and safety of OROS MPH in children and adolescents with attention-deficit/hyperactivity disorder switched from MPH. *Eur Child Adolesc Psychiatry* 2005; 14:305–309.

45. Remschmidt H, et al. Symptom control in children and adolescents with attention-deficit/hyperactivity disorder on switching from immediate-release MPH to OROS MPH. Results of a 3-week open-label study. *Eur Child Adolesc Psychiatry* 2005; 14:297–304.

46. Wolraich ML, et al. Randomized, controlled trial of OROS methylphenidate once a day in children with attention-deficit/hyperactivity disorder. *Pediatrics* 2001; 108:883–892.

47. Findling RL, et al. Comparison of the clinical efficacy of twice-daily Ritalin and once-daily Equasym XL with placebo in children with attention deficit/hyperactivity disorder. *Eur Child Adolesc Psychiatry* 2006; 15:450–459.

48. Anderson VR, et al. Spotlight on methylphenidate controlled-delivery capsules (Equasym XL™) in the treatment of children and adolescents with attention-deficit hyperactivity disorder. *CNS Drugs* 2007; 21:173–175.

49. Flynn Pharma Ltd. Summary of product characteristics. Medikinet XL 5mg, 10mg, 20mg, 30mg, 40mg, 50mg and 60mg modified release capsules (methylphenidate hydrochloride). 2023; https://www.medicines.org.uk/emc/product/313/smpc.

50. Medicines and Healthcare products Regulatory Agency. Public assessment report. Ritalin XL 10mg, 20mg, 30mg, 40mg, 60mg modified-release hard capsules (last updated March 2014); https://mhraproductsproduction.blob.core.windows.net/docs/4781baf366b1fafd0ea20396 2ccb54faadcdcfcc.

51. Cyr M, et al. Current drug therapy recommendations for the treatment of attention deficit hyperactivity disorder. *Drugs* 1998; 56:215–223.

52. Takeda UK Ltd. Summary of product characteristics. Elvanse 20mg, 30mg, 40mg, 50mg, 60mg and 70mg capsules, hard (lisdexafetamine). 2023; https://www.medicines.org.uk/emc/product/14091/smpc.

53. Kelsey DK, et al. Once-daily atomoxetine treatment for children with attention-deficit/hyperactivity disorder, including an assessment of evening and morning behavior: a double-blind, placebo-controlled trial. *Pediatrics* 2004; 114:e1–e8.

54. Wernicke JF, et al. Cardiovascular effects of atomoxetine in children, adolescents, and adults. *Drug Saf* 2003; 26:729–740.

55. Heil SH, et al. Comparison of the subjective, physiological, and psychomotor effects of atomoxetine and methylphenidate in light drug users. *Drug Alcohol Depend* 2002; 67:149–156.

56. Reed VA, et al. The safety of atomoxetine for the treatment of children and adolescents with attention-deficit/hyperactivity disorder: a comprehensive review of over a decade of research. *CNS Drugs* 2016; 30:603–628.

57. Childress A, et al. Evaluation of the current data on guanfacine extended release for the treatment of ADHD in children and adolescents. *Expert Opin Pharmacother* 2020; 21:417–426.

58. Takeda UK Ltd. Guanfacine modified-release. Personal communication, 2020.

59. Cortese S, et al. New formulations of methylphenidate for the treatment of attention-deficit/hyperactivity disorder: pharmacokinetics, efficacy, and tolerability. *CNS Drugs* 2017; 31:149–160.

Autism spectrum disorder (ASD) in children and adolescents

Autism spectrum disorder is a complex condition characterised by core deficits in social communication development and behaviour (stereotypies and/or restricted and unusual patterns of interests) as well as sensory difficulties. ICD-11 now matches DSM-5 in removing the subtypes of autism (e.g. the term Asperger's syndrome has been discontinued). In addition, ICD-11 distinguishes between ASD with or without intellectual development. DSM-5 recommends recording whether or not there is accompanying intellectual impairment.

The heterogeneity of ASD poses assessment and treatment challenges. Co-occurring mental health conditions are highly prevalent in ASD[1] with 69–79% of individuals experiencing at least one in their lifetime.[2,3] These include attention deficit hyperactivity disorder (ADHD), disruptive behavioural disorders, anxiety and obsessive compulsive and mood disorders. Other associated problems include intellectual disability, epilepsy, sleep disturbance, self-harm, irritability and aggression towards others. Associated neurodevelopmental, medical and psychiatric disorders complicate the symptom profile and affect overall outcome. Evaluating and optimally treating co-occurring conditions and/or associated problem behaviours are, therefore, essential.

Currently there are no validated or licensed pharmacological treatments that alleviate core ASD symptoms.[4,5] Targeting problem behaviours and comorbid psychiatric conditions with pharmacological interventions is, however, common practice.

Pharmacotherapies are commonly used in individuals with ASD as adjuncts to psychological interventions. The evidence to date[4,6] shows reasonable efficacy of risperidone and aripiprazole for irritability and aggression; supports the use of methylphenidate, atomoxetine and guanfacine for ADHD and melatonin for sleep problems; but shows limited efficacy of SSRIs for anxiety, depression and repetitive behaviours. The evidence for antiepileptics remains inconsistent. There is a potential role for α2 agonists, cholinergic agonists, glutamatergic agents, gamma-aminobutyric acid (GABA) agonists and oxytocin but these require further investigation.[4,6]

Individuals with ASD are likely to experience more severe adverse effects than typically developing individuals.[4–6] Therefore, achieving an effective dose with minimum adverse effects can be a challenging task. Treatment should be initiated in small doses and increased about every five half-lives of the drug, and it may take 4–6 weeks of titration to determine the therapeutic dose for each individual case.[7] Excluding any medical conditions, the presence of pain or any other physical discomfort such as gastro-esophageal reflux must be a priority before managing problem behaviour with psychotropic drugs. A comprehensive physical examination should be part of standard practice.

The efficacy and adverse effects associated with pharmacotherapy in individuals with ASD should be systematically monitored in view of their impaired communication and the increased propensity for more adverse effects. Standardised behaviour rating scales and adverse effect checklists are essential tools in monitoring progress.[8]

Pharmacological treatment of core ASD symptoms

Evidence from clinical trials to date has not demonstrated clear efficacy of any psychotropic agent in routinely treating core symptoms of ASD.[4,6]

Restricted repetitive behaviours and interests (RRBIs)

RRBIs are distressing and disruptive to functioning and therefore an important treatment target to improve overall outcomes in ASD.[9] Behavioural therapies should be used as first line. When RRBIs are severe with significant impact on functioning and/or pose risks to others or self then pharmacotherapy can be considered.

A Cochrane review (last updated in 2013) found 'no evidence of effect of SSRIs on reducing RRBIs in children and emerging evidence of harm' although there are data that support their use in adults.[10] A 2022 meta-analysis of 16 studies demonstrated a small effect size for antidepressants in treating restricted and repetitive behaviours. Subgroup analyses indicated that clomipramine had a higher efficacy than SSRIs and adults had a better response than adolescents and children.[11] Risperidone is probably effective in reducing RRBIs in children who have high levels of irritability or aggression[12] (any specific efficacy for repetitive behaviours is doubtful). Reductions in stereotypical behaviours have also been reported[13–16] albeit in studies with methodological limitations.[6] A 2020 meta-analysis of studies on a wide range of currently available pharmacological agents showed evidence supporting only antipsychotic medication,[17] whereas another recent meta-analysis of nine studies found no evidence for any pharmacological agent in reducing RRBIs.[18] Overall, given the profile of adverse effects of dopamine-blocking agents, consensus guidance from the British Association for Psychopharmacology[6] rightly cautions against their routine use for the treatment of RRBIs. If they are used, they should be prescribed in small doses and as part of a carefully considered, time-limited and monitored overall treatment plan.

Social and communication impairment

Currently, no drug has been consistently shown to improve the core social and communication impairments in ASD.[7] **Risperidone** may have a secondary effect through improvement in irritability.[19] Analysis of data from two multicentre trials suggested that risperidone was effective for the treatment of social disability in children with ASD.[20] Glutamatergic drugs and oxytocin looked promising.[21] However, two meta-analyses and two recent double-blind placebo-controlled trials suggested that **oxytocin** has no significant effect on social communication.[22–25] Larger studies with better methodology are needed.[23,26] **Sulforaphane** has shown mixed results with both positive and negative trials.[27–29] **Insulin growth factor 1** (IGF-1)[30] awaits further work to prove its efficacy in modifying ASD core symptoms, as do **glutamatergic agents**.[31–33] **Acetylcysteine**[34] is probably not effective. Three small double-blind placebo-controlled trials using **folinic acid** for language impairment look encouraging.[35]

There is growing but inconsistent evidence for dietary interventions reducing ASD core symptoms.[36,37] The targeting of the gut microbiome, including probiotic treatment and faecal microbiota transplants, has drawn much interest.[38] However, there is little evidence to support the use of nutritional supplements or dietary therapies for children with ASD[36] or indeed any relationship between maternal food intake and child's diet and the development of ASD/symptoms severity.[37]

Pharmacological treatment of co-occurring disorders and problem behaviours in ASD

Inattention, overactivity and impulsiveness in ASD (symptoms of ADHD)

Individuals with ASD have high rates of inattention, overactivity and impulsiveness and in around a third of patients these symptoms merit the diagnosis of ADHD.[1,39]

The largest controlled trial to date has been with **methylphenidate**, conducted by the Research Units on Paediatric Psychopharmacology (RUPP) Autism Network.[40,41] In a previous retrospective and prospective study of children with ASD, Santosh and colleagues[42] reported positive benefits of treatment with methylphenidate. In general, methylphenidate produces highly variable responses in children with ASD and ADHD symptoms, ranging from marked improvement with few adverse effects to poor response with or without problematic adverse effects. A large double-blind placebo-controlled trial of methylphenidate in children with intellectual disability and ADHD showed that optimal dosing with methylphenidate was effective in some.[43] Adverse effects are more commonly reported than in children with ADHD alone.[44-46] However, where ADHD symptoms are severe and/or disabling, it is reasonable to proceed with a treatment trial of methylphenidate. It is advisable to warn parents of the lower likelihood of response and the potential adverse effects and to proceed with low initial doses (around 0.125mg/kg three times daily, depending on the preparation) increasing by small increments. Treatment should be stopped immediately if behaviour deteriorates or there are unacceptable adverse effects. A systematic review[6] confirms that, although effective, the efficacy of methylphenidate for treatment of ADHD in ASD is less than in ADHD alone and that more adverse effects (decreased appetite, sleeping difficulties, abdominal discomfort, social withdrawal, irritability and emotional outbursts) should be expected in ASD. A 2021 meta-analysis supports the efficacy of methylphenidate and atomoxetine.[47]

There are no published data on the efficacy of **amfetamines** in children with ASD even though they have been used to treat ADHD in these patients as well as in typically developed children. **Lisdexamfetamine** (a pro-drug containing d-amfetamine bound to amino acid lysine) has been found to have efficacy and tolerability in treating ADHD in children and young people[48] but with no specific data about those with ASD.

Atomoxetine is a noradrenergic reuptake inhibitor licensed to treat ADHD with similar efficacy to methylphenidate.[6] Preliminary evidence from small open-label trials and a handful of randomised double-blind trials[49,50] showed that it may be useful in children with ASD, with the most common adverse effects being nausea, fatigue and sleep difficulties. These studies were followed by a larger trial that confirmed that atomoxetine (alone and combined with parent training) significantly reduced ADHD symptoms.[51] In a 24-week extension of the same study, atomoxetine combined with parent training was superior in reducing ADHD symptoms to atomoxetine alone.[52]

There is evidence that **α2 agonists** (clonidine and guanfacine) can be used as alternative treatments. A multisite RCT of extended-release guanfacine compared with placebo in children with ASD (mean age 8.5 years) over a period of 8 weeks showed that it is safe and effective in managing hyperactivity in this group.[53] No serious adverse events except for drowsiness, fatigue and decreased appetite were reported.

There are reports from controlled studies supporting the use of **risperidone** or **aripiprazole** for ADHD symptoms. However, these were not primary outcomes of the studies and therefore need further investigation.

Irritability (aggression, self-injurious behaviour, severe disruptive behaviours)

Aggression towards others and self, frequently underlined by irritability, is a common problem in ASD. Although behavioural and environmental approaches should be first-line treatments, more severe and dangerous behaviours usually necessitate pharmaco-therapy.[54] The duration of recommended treatment is difficult to derive from published evidence but treatment appears to be beneficial for up to 6–12 months.[55] Efforts to reduce and possibly discontinue such treatment at the end of this period should be strongly considered.[54,55]

SGAs are the first-line pharmacological treatment for children and adolescents with ASD and associated irritability.[55–58] **Risperidone**[59,60] and **aripiprazole**[61] have been reliably shown to help with irritability and associated disruptive behaviours[5] in ASD and have been approved for this use by the US FDA. In a meta-analysis of data from 46 RCTs[62] comparing efficacy of risperidone, aripiprazole and other compounds with placebo, risperidone and aripiprazole were the most effective, with moderate to large effect sizes. Another meta-analysis of short-term (8 weeks) aripiprazole in the treatment of irritability in ASD children aged 6–17 years[63] found similar results when compared with placebo. The most recent Cochrane review[64] concluded that aripiprazole and risperidone probably reduce both irritability and self-injury with a large effect size. However, no effect was shown for aggression. The usual recommended dose of aripiprazole for maintenance is between 5 and 15mg daily.[55] The starting dose is 2mg/day. The dosing of risperidone is rather more complicated – FDA-recommended dosages for risperidone are outlined in Box 5.2.

Despite their promising efficacy, adverse effects such as weight gain and metabolic changes, increased appetite and somnolence (even with aripiprazole) can be problematic.[16,65–68] Research is underway to determine if therapeutic drug monitoring of risperidone and aripiprazole will help in optimising treatment while minimising weight gain.[69] One long-term placebo discontinuation study found that relapse rates did not differ between those who stayed on aripiprazole versus those randomised to switch to only placebo, suggesting that re-evaluation of aripiprazole use after a period of stabilisation in irritability symptoms is warranted.[70] There is only one study that makes a direct head-to-head comparison[71] showing similar tolerability and efficacy profiles for risperidone and aripiprazole. Risperidone usually causes hyperprolactinaemia which, although it may be asymptomatic, may have longer-term effects, therefore necessitating close monitoring. Aripiprazole has no effect on prolactin, which makes it a preferred option. Aripiprazole may on the other hand be ineffective for self-injurious behaviours.[6]

Lurasidone, in fixed doses of 20 or 60mg/day, has been shown to be ineffective in a randomised double-blind trial over 6 weeks.[72] The effectiveness of other SGAs such as **olanzapine**,[73] **quetiapine**, **ziprasidone** and **clozapine** has not been tested in adequately powered RCTs. While controlled studies support the use of mood stabilisers such as **lithium**[74,75] and **sodium valproate**[76] in the treatment of persistent aggression in children they are not as effective as SGAs for the treatment of irritability in ASD.[77] Limited data support the combination of **risperidone** and **topiramate** being better than risperidone alone.[78] Further RCTs are probably warranted of brain-derived neurotrophic factor stimulators such as loxapine and amitriptyline.[79]

Use of risperidone in children and adolescents

Box 5.2 US Food and Drug Administration guidance for risperidone dosing in children and adolescents[80]

- Risperidone is indicated for the treatment of irritability associated with autistic spectrum disorder (ASD) in children (aged 5 years and over) and adolescents in the UK/EU and USA
- The dosage of risperidone should be individualised according to the response of the patient

Doses of risperidone in paediatric patients with autism spectrum disorders (by total mg/day)

Weight categories	Days 1–3	Days 4–18	Increments if dose increases are needed	Dose range
<20kg*	0.25mg	0.5mg	+0.25mg at ≥2-week intervals	0.5–3mg†
≥20kg	0.5mg	1.0mg	+0.5mg at ≥2-week intervals	1.0–3mg‡

*Caution should be exercised for children <15kg – no dosing data available
†Therapeutic effect plateaus at 1mg/day
‡Those weighing >45kg may require higher doses – therapeutic effect plateaus at 3mg

General considerations

- Risperidone can be administered once daily or twice daily
- Patients experiencing somnolence may benefit from taking the whole daily dose at bedtime
- Once sufficient clinical response has been achieved and maintained, consideration may be given to gradually lowering the dose to achieve the optimal balance of efficacy and safety
- There is insufficient evidence from controlled trials to indicate how long treatment should continue

Adverse effects

- Weight gain, somnolence and hyperglycaemia require monitoring
- Long-term safety of risperidone in children and adolescents with ASD remains to be fully determined

---

Using **benzodiazepines** to manage irritability and aggression in ASD is not recommended. However, it may be necessary to manage acute aggression with a benzodiazepine. The possibility of behavioural disinhibition that may worsen aggression must be borne in mind.

The use of **minocycline, arbaclofen** or **amantadine** for irritability is not recommended unless better evidence from double-blind RCTs is available.[6]

Sleep disturbance

Children with ASD have significant sleep problems,[81] with sleep-onset insomnia, sleep-maintenance insomnia and irregularities of the sleep–wake cycle being the typical problems encountered. It is essential to understand the aetiology of the sleep problem before embarking on a course of treatment. Abnormalities in the melatonin system have received some attention.[82]

Melatonin has been shown in 17 studies to be beneficial in children with ASD.[83] A meta-analysis of five studies showed good efficacy with doses ranging from 1mg to 10mg and treatment lasting from 14 days to over 4 years.[84] Melatonin is usually very well tolerated.[84,85] One RCT showed that, while melatonin improved sleep onset, the child's behaviour during the day did not improve.[86] There is also evidence that melatonin combined with CBT is superior to melatonin only, CBT only and placebo in reducing symptoms of insomnia.[87]

Risperidone may benefit sleep difficulties in those with extreme irritability. In the anxious or depressed child, antidepressants may be beneficial. Insomnia due to hyperarousal may benefit from **clonidine** or **clonazepam**.[88]

Anxiety, OCD and depression

SSRIs have yet to show specific efficacy in ASD. Preliminary data from a randomised placebo-blind clinical trial showed beneficial effects of **fluoxetine** in reducing OCD symptoms in children with ASD, although confounding factors precluded firm conclusions.[89] In a systematic review,[6] although **risperidone** was reported by several studies to reduce OCD and anxiety symptoms in young people with ASD, the selection of participants with high levels of irritability did not allow firm conclusions to be drawn about specific effects of risperidone on OCD and anxiety. There is little or no evidence for treating anxiety or OCD symptoms with risperidone, clomipramine or an SSRI. There are some data on **buspirone** effectively targeting anxiety in ASD[90] and **propranolol** showing positive cognitive effects in ASD.[91] However, further evaluation is needed. Guidance on doses of fluoxetine can be found in Box 5.3.

Use of fluoxetine in children and adolescents

When using fluoxetine to treat repetitive behaviours in ASD patients, doses much lower than those used to treat depression are normally required. It is advisable to use a liquid preparation and begin at the lowest possible dose, monitoring for adverse effects. A suitable regimen is outlined in Box 5.3.

Box 5.3 Use of fluoxetine in children and adolescents

- **Liquid fluoxetine** (as hydrochloride): 20mg/5mL
- 2.5mg/day a day for 1 week; note that 2.5mg = 0.625mL, which is difficult to measure accurately
- Follow with a flexible titration schedule based on weight, tolerability and adverse effects up to a maximum dose of 0.8mg/kg/day (0.3mg/kg/day for week 2, 0.5mg/kg/day for week 3 and 0.8mg/kg/day subsequently)
- Reduction may be indicated if adverse effects are problematic

Adverse effects

- Monitor for treatment-emergent **suicidal** behaviour, self-harm and hostility, particularly at the beginning of treatment
- Hyponatraemia is also possible – see Chapter 3

References

1. Lai MC, et al. Prevalence of co-occurring mental health diagnoses in the autism population: a systematic review and meta-analysis. *Lancet Psychiatry* 2019; 6:819–829.

2. Lever AG, et al. Psychiatric co-occurring symptoms and disorders in young, middle-aged, and older adults with autism spectrum disorder. *J Autism Dev Disord* 2016; 46:1916–1930.

3. Buck TR, et al. Psychiatric comorbidity and medication use in adults with autism spectrum disorder. *J Autism Dev Disord* 2014; 44:3063–3071.

4. Goel R, et al. An update on pharmacotherapy of autism spectrum disorder in children and adolescents. *Int Rev Psychiatry* 2018; 30:78–95.

5. Accordino RE, et al. Psychopharmacological interventions in autism spectrum disorder. *Expert Opin Pharmacother* 2016; 17:937–952.

6. Howes OD, et al. Autism spectrum disorder: consensus guidelines on assessment, treatment and research from the British Association for Psychopharmacology. *J Psychopharmacol* 2018; 32:3–29.

7. Santosh P. Medication in autism spectrum disorder. *Cut Edge Psychiatry Pract* 2014; 1:143–155.

8. Greenhill LL. Assessment of safety in pediatric psychopharmacology. *J Am Acad Child Adolesc Psychiatry* 2003; 42:625–626.

9. Leekam SR, et al. Restricted and repetitive behaviors in autism spectrum disorders: a review of research in the last decade. *Psychol Bull* 2011; 137:562–593.

10. Williams K, et al. Selective serotonin reuptake inhibitors (SSRIs) for autism spectrum disorders (ASD). *Cochrane Database Syst Rev* 2013; 8:CD004677.

11. Liang SC, et al. Therapeutic effects of antidepressants for global improvement and subdomain symptoms of autism spectrum disorder: a systematic review and meta-analysis. *J Psychiatry Neurosci* 2022; 47:e299–e310.

12. McDougle CJ, et al. A double-blind, placebo-controlled study of risperidone addition in serotonin reuptake inhibitor-refractory obsessive-compulsive disorder. *Arch Gen Psychiatry* 2000; 57:794–801.

13. McDougle CJ, et al. Risperidone for the core symptom domains of autism: results from the study by the Autism Network of the Research Units on Pediatric Psychopharmacology. *Am J Psychiatry* 2005; 162:1142–1148.

14. McCracken JT, et al. Risperidone in children with autism and serious behavioral problems. *N Engl J Med* 2002; 347:314–321.

15. Arnold LE, et al. Parent-defined target symptoms respond to risperidone in RUPP autism study: customer approach to clinical trials. *J Am Acad Child Adolesc Psychiatry* 2003; 42:1443–1450.

16. Dinnissen M, et al. Clinical and pharmacokinetic evaluation of risperidone for the management of autism spectrum disorder. *Expert Opin Drug Metab Toxicol* 2015; 11:111–124.

17. Zhou MS, et al. Meta-analysis: pharmacologic treatment of restricted and repetitive behaviors in autism spectrum disorders. *J Am Acad Child Adolesc Psychiatry* 2020; 60:35–45.

18. Yu Y, et al. Pharmacotherapy of restricted/repetitive behavior in autism spectrum disorder: a systematic review and meta-analysis. *BMC Psychiatry* 2020; 20:121.

19. Canitano R, et al. Risperidone in the treatment of behavioral disorders associated with autism in children and adolescents. *Neuropsychiatr Dis Treat* 2008; 4:723–730.

20. Scahill L, et al. Brief report: social disability in autism spectrum disorder: results from Research Units on Pediatric Psychopharmacology (RUPP) Autism Network trials. *J Autism Dev Disord* 2013; 43:739–746.

21. Posey DJ, et al. Developing drugs for core social and communication impairment in autism. *Child Adolesc Psychiatr Clin N Am* 2008; 17:787–801.

22. Ooi YP, et al. Oxytocin and autism spectrum disorders: a systematic review and meta-analysis of randomized controlled trials. *Pharmacopsychiatry* 2017; 50:5–13.

23. Hu L, et al. Oxytocin treatment for core symptoms in children with autism spectrum disorder: a systematic review and meta-analysis. *Eur J Clin Pharmacol* 2023; 79:1357–1363.

24. Guastella AJ, et al. The effect of oxytocin nasal spray on social interaction in young children with autism: a randomized clinical trial. *Mol Psychiatry* 2023; 28:834–842.

25. Sikich L, et al. Intranasal oxytocin in children and adolescents with autism spectrum disorder. *N Engl J Med* 2021; 385:1462–1473.

26. Alvares GA, et al. Beyond the hype and hope: critical considerations for intranasal oxytocin research in autism spectrum disorder. *Autism Res* 2017; 10:25–41.

27. McGuinness G, et al. Sulforaphane treatment for autism spectrum disorder: a systematic review. *EXCLI J* 2020; 19:892–903.

28. Magner M, et al. Sulforaphane treatment in children with autism: a prospective randomized double-blind study. *Nutrients* 2023; 15:718.

29. Zimmerman AW, et al. Randomized controlled trial of sulforaphane and metabolite discovery in children with autism spectrum disorder. *Mol Autism* 2021; 12:38.

30. Riikonen R. Treatment of autistic spectrum disorder with insulin-like growth factors. *Eur J Paediatr Neurol* 2016; 20:816–823.

31. Fung LK, et al. Developing medications targeting glutamatergic dysfunction in autism: progress to date. *CNS Drugs* 2015; 29:453–463.

32. Aye SZ, et al. The effectiveness and adverse effects of D-cycloserine compared with placebo on social and communication skills in individuals with autism spectrum disorder. *Cochrane Database Syst Rev* 2021; 2:CD013457.

33. Brignell A, et al. Memantine for autism spectrum disorder. *Cochrane Database Syst Rev* 2022; 8:CD013845.

34. Dean OM, et al. A randomised, double blind, placebo-controlled trial of a fixed dose of N-acetyl cysteine in children with autistic disorder. *Aust N Z J Psychiatry* 2017; 51:241–249.

35. Thom RP, et al. Recent updates in psychopharmacology for the core and associated symptoms of autism spectrum disorder. *Curr Psychiatry Rep* 2021; 23:79.

36. Sathe N, et al. Nutritional and dietary interventions for autism spectrum disorder: a systematic review. *Pediatrics* 2017; 139:e20170346.

CHAPTER 5

37. Peretti S, et al. Diet: the keystone of autism spectrum disorder? *Nutr Neurosci* 2019; **22**:825–839.

38. Yang Y, et al. Targeting gut microbiome: a novel and potential therapy for autism. *Life Sci* 2018; **194**:111–119.

39. Lee YJ, et al. Advanced pharmacotherapy evidenced by pathogenesis of autism spectrum disorder. *Clin Psychopharmacol Neurosci* 2014; **12**:19–30.

40. Research Units on Pediatric Psychopharmacology (RUPP) Autism Network. Randomized, controlled, crossover trial of methylphenidate in pervasive developmental disorders with hyperactivity. *Arch Gen Psychiatry* 2005; **62**:1266–1274.

41. Posey DJ, et al. Positive effects of methylphenidate on inattention and hyperactivity in pervasive developmental disorders: an analysis of secondary measures. *Biol Psychiatry* 2007; **61**:538–544.

42. Santosh PJ, et al. Impact of comorbid autism spectrum disorders on stimulant response in children with attention deficit hyperactivity disorder: a retrospective and prospective effectiveness study. *Child Care Health Dev* 2006; **32**:575–583.

43. Simonoff E, et al. Randomized controlled double-blind trial of optimal dose methylphenidate in children and adolescents with severe attention deficit hyperactivity disorder and intellectual disability. *J Child Psychol Psychiatry* 2013; **54**:527–535.

44. Sung M, et al. What's in the pipeline? Drugs in development for autism spectrum disorder. *Neuropsychiatr Dis Treat* 2014; **10**:371–381.

45. Siegel M, et al. Psychotropic medication in children with autism spectrum disorders: a systematic review and synthesis for evidence-based practice. *J Autism Dev Disord* 2012; **42**:1592–1605.

46. Williamson ED, et al. Psychotropic medications in autism: practical considerations for parents. *J Autism Dev Disord* 2012; **42**:1249–1255.

47. Rodrigues R, et al. Practitioner review: pharmacological treatment of attention-deficit/hyperactivity disorder symptoms in children and youth with autism spectrum disorder: a systematic review and meta-analysis. *J Child Psychol Psychiatry* 2021; **62**:680–700.

48. Coghill D, et al. European, randomized, phase 3 study of lisdexamfetamine dimesylate in children and adolescents with attention-deficit/hyperactivity disorder. *Eur Neuropsychopharmacol* 2013; **23**:1208–1218.

49. Arnold LE, et al. Atomoxetine for hyperactivity in autism spectrum disorders: placebo-controlled crossover pilot trial. *J Am Acad Child Adolesc Psychiatry* 2006; **45**:1196–1205.

50. Harfterkamp M, et al. A randomized double-blind study of atomoxetine versus placebo for attention-deficit/hyperactivity disorder symptoms in children with autism spectrum disorder. *J Am Acad Child Adolesc Psychiatry* 2012; **51**:733–741.

51. Handen BL, et al. Atomoxetine, parent training, and their combination in children with autism spectrum disorder and attention-deficit/hyperactivity disorder. *J Am Acad Child Adolesc Psychiatry* 2015; **54**:905–915.

52. Smith T, et al. Atomoxetine and parent training for children with autism and attention-deficit/hyperactivity disorder: a 24-week extension study. *J Am Acad Child Adolesc Psychiatry* 2016; **55**:868–876.e862.

53. Scahill L, et al. Extended-release guanfacine for hyperactivity in children with autism spectrum disorder. *Am J Psychiatry* 2015; **172**:1197–1206.

54. National Institute for Health and Care Excellence. Autism spectrum disorder in under 19s: support and management. Clinical Guidance 170 [CG170]. 2013 (last updated June 2021, last checked February 2024); https://www.nice.org.uk/guidance/CG170.

55. Kaplan G, et al. Psychopharmacology of autism spectrum disorders. *Pediatr Clin North Am* 2012; **59**:175–187, xii.

56. McDougle CJ, et al. Atypical antipsychotics in children and adolescents with autistic and other pervasive developmental disorders. *J Clin Psychiatry* 2008; **69** Suppl 4:15–20.

57. Parikh MS, et al. Psychopharmacology of aggression in children and adolescents with autism: a critical review of efficacy and tolerability. *J Child Adolesc Psychopharmacol* 2008; **18**:157–178.

58. DeVane CL, et al. Pharmacotherapy of autism spectrum disorder: results from the randomized BAART clinical trial. *Pharmacotherapy* 2019; **39**:626–635.

59. Jesner OS, et al. Risperidone for autism spectrum disorder. *Cochrane Database Syst Rev* 2007; **2007**:CD005040.

60. Scahill L, et al. Risperidone approved for the treatment of serious behavioral problems in children with autism. *J Child Adolesc Psychiatr Nurs* 2007; **20**:188–190.

61. Curran MP. Aripiprazole: in the treatment of irritability associated with autistic disorder in pediatric patients. *PaediatrDrugs* 2011; **13**:197–204.

62. Fung LK, et al. Pharmacologic treatment of severe irritability and problem behaviors in autism: a systematic review and meta-analysis. *Pediatrics* 2016; **137** Suppl 2:S124–S135.

63. Douglas-Hall P, et al. Aripiprazole: a review of its use in the treatment of irritability associated with autistic disorder patients aged 6-17. *J Cent Nerv Syst Dis* 2011; **3**:1–11.

64. Iffland M, et al. Pharmacological intervention for irritability, aggression, and self-injury in autism spectrum disorder (ASD). *Cochrane Database Syst Rev* 2023; **10**:CD011769.

65. Caccia S. Safety and pharmacokinetics of atypical antipsychotics in children and adolescents. *Paediatr Drugs* 2013; **15**:217–233.

66. Sharma A, et al. Efficacy of risperidone in managing maladaptive behaviors for children with autistic spectrum disorder: a meta-analysis. *J Pediatr Health Care* 2012; **26**:291–299.

67. Kent JM, et al. Risperidone dosing in children and adolescents with autistic disorder: a double-blind, placebo-controlled study. *J Autism Dev Disord* 2013; **43**:1773–1783.

68. Maayan L, et al. Weight gain and metabolic risks associated with antipsychotic medications in children and adolescents. *J Child Adolesc Psychopharmacol* 2011; **21**:517–535.

69. Hermans RA, et al. The effect of therapeutic drug monitoring of risperidone and aripiprazole on weight gain in children and adolescents: the SPACe 2: STAR (trial) protocol of an international multicentre randomised controlled trial. *BMC Psychiatry* 2022; **22**:814.

70. Hirsch LE, et al. Aripiprazole for autism spectrum disorders (ASD). *Cochrane Database Syst Rev* 2016; **2016**:CD009043.

71. Ghanizadeh A, et al. A head-to-head comparison of aripiprazole and risperidone for safety and treating autistic disorders, a randomized double blind clinical trial. *Child Psychiatry Hum Dev* 2014; **45**:185–192.

72. Loebel A, et al. Lurasidone for the treatment of irritability associated with autistic disorder. *J Autism Dev Disord* 2016; **46**:1153–1163.

73. Hollander E, et al. A double-blind placebo-controlled pilot study of olanzapine in childhood/adolescent pervasive developmental disorder. *J Child Adolesc Psychopharmacol* 2006; **16**:541–548.

74. Campbell M, et al. Lithium in hospitalized aggressive children with conduct disorder: a double-blind and placebo-controlled study. *J Am Acad Child Adolesc Psychiatry* 1995; **34**:445–453.

75. Malone RP, et al. A double-blind placebo-controlled study of lithium in hospitalized aggressive children and adolescents with conduct disorder. *Arch Gen Psychiatry* 2000; **57**:649–654.

76. Donovan SJ, et al. Divalproex treatment for youth with explosive temper and mood lability: a double-blind, placebo-controlled crossover design. *Am J Psychiatry* 2000; **157**:818–820.

77. Stigler KA, et al. Pharmacotherapy of irritability in pervasive developmental disorders. *Child Adolesc Psychiatr Clin N Am* 2008; **17**:739–752.

78. Rezaei V, et al. Double-blind, placebo-controlled trial of risperidone plus topiramate in children with autistic disorder. *Prog Neuropsychopharmacol Biol Psychiatry* 2010; **34**:1269–1272.

79. Hellings JA, et al. Dopamine antagonists for treatment resistance in autism spectrum disorders: review and focus on BDNF stimulators loxapine and amitriptyline. *Expert Opin Pharmacother* 2017; **18**:581–588.

80. Janssen Pharmaceutical Companies. Highlights of prescribing information. Risperdal® (risperidone) tablets, for oral use, Risperdal® (risperidone) oral solution, Risperdal® M-TAB® (risperidone) orally disintegrating tablets. 2019; https://www.accessdata.fda.gov/drugsatfda_docs/label/2019/020272s082,020588s070,021444s056lbl.pdf.

81. Krakowiak P, et al. Sleep problems in children with autism spectrum disorders, developmental delays, and typical development: a population-based study. *J Sleep Res* 2008; **17**:197–206.

82. Sanchez-Barcelo EJ, et al. Clinical uses of melatonin in pediatrics. *Int J Pediatr* 2011; **2011**:892624.

83. Doyen C, et al. Melatonin in children with autistic spectrum disorders: recent and practical data. *Eur Child Adolesc Psychiatry* 2011; **20**:231–239.

84. Rossignol DA, et al. Melatonin in autism spectrum disorders: a systematic review and meta-analysis. *Dev Med Child Neurol* 2011; **53**:783–792.

85. Andersen IM, et al. Melatonin for insomnia in children with autism spectrum disorders. *J Child Neurol* 2008; **23**:482–485.

86. Gringras P, et al. Melatonin for sleep problems in children with neurodevelopmental disorders: randomised double masked placebo controlled trial. *BMJ* 2012; **345**:e6664.

87. Cortesi F, et al. Controlled-release melatonin, singly and combined with cognitive behavioural therapy, for persistent insomnia in children with autism spectrum disorders: a randomized placebo-controlled trial. *J Sleep Res* 2012; **21**:700–709.

88. Johnson KP, et al. Sleep in children with autism spectrum disorders. *Curr Treat Options Neurol* 2008; **10**:350–359.

89. Reddihough DS, et al. Effect of fluoxetine on obsessive-compulsive behaviors in children and adolescents with autism spectrum disorders: a randomized clinical trial. *JAMA* 2019; **322**:1561–1569.

90. Buitelaar JK, et al. Buspirone in the management of anxiety and irritability in children with pervasive developmental disorders: results of an open-label study. *J Clin Psychiatry* 1998; **59**:56–59.

91. Narayanan A, et al. Effect of propranolol on functional connectivity in autism spectrum disorder – a pilot study. *Brain Imaging Behav* 2010; **4**:189–197.

CHAPTER 5

Tics and Tourette's syndrome in children and adolescents

Transient tics occur in 5–20% of children. Tourette's syndrome (TS) occurs in about 0.7% of children and adolescents and is defined by persistent motor and vocal tics. As many as 65% of individuals with TS will have no tics or only very mild tics by adult life. Tics wax and wane over time and are variably exacerbated by external factors such as stress, inactivity and fatigue, depending on the individual. Tics are about two to three times more common in boys than girls.[1] Functional tic disorders (involuntary physical movements, often related to anxiety) have also been described in recent years.[2] These are typically seen in teenage girls.

Detection and treatment of comorbidity

Comorbid OCD, ADHD, ASD, depression, anxiety and behavioural problems are more prevalent than would be expected by chance, and often cause the major impairment in people with tic disorders.[3] These comorbid conditions are usually treated first before assessing the level of disability caused by the tics.

Education and behavioural treatments

Most people with tics do not require pharmacological treatment. Education is crucial for the individual with tics, their family and the people they interact with, especially at school (Figure 5.2). Treatment aimed primarily at reducing tics is warranted if the tics cause distress to the patient or are functionally disabling. Behavioural interventions have been found to be effective with similar effect sizes to antipsychotic medication.[4,5] Habit reversal, comprehensive behavioural intervention for tics and exposure and response prevention are the behavioural treatments of choice.[6]

Pharmacological treatments

Studies of pharmacological interventions in TS are difficult to interpret for several reasons:

- There is a large inter-individual variation in tic frequency and severity. Small, randomised studies may include patients who are very different at baseline.
- The severity of tics in a given individual varies markedly over time, making it difficult to separate drug effect from natural variation.
- The bulk of the literature consists of case reports, case series, open studies and underpowered, randomised studies. Publication bias is also likely to be an issue.
- A high proportion of patients have comorbid psychiatric illness. It can be difficult to disentangle any direct effect on tics from an effect on the comorbid illness. This makes it difficult to interpret studies that report improvements in global functioning rather than specific reductions in tics.
- Large numbers of individuals attending clinics with TS appear to use complementary or alternative therapies, with the majority reporting benefits and up to half finding

these more helpful compared with medication.[7] Robust research about the use of complementary or alternative therapies, their efficacy and potential adverse effects is lacking[8] and certainty of evidence for their use is very low.[9]

Adrenergic α2 agonists

Clonidine has been shown in open studies to reduce the severity and frequency of tics but in one study this effect did not seem to be convincingly larger than placebo.[10] Other studies have shown more substantial reductions in tics.[11-14] Therapeutic doses of clonidine are in the order of 3–5mcg/kg, and the dose should be built up gradually. A transdermal patch has also shown effectiveness.[15] The main adverse effects are sedation, postural hypotension and depression. Patients and their families should be informed not to stop clonidine suddenly because of the risk of rebound hypertension. Guanfacine also has some evidence of effectiveness in the treatment of tics.[16,17] The efficacy of clonidine (but not of guanfacine) was demonstrated in a 2023 systematic review and network meta-analysis of double-blind RCTs in TS which included children, adolescents and adults.[9] Adrenergic α2 agonists may also be used in children with ADHD whose tics deteriorate with stimulant medication.[18]

Antipsychotics

Adverse effects of antipsychotics may outweigh their beneficial effects in the treatment of tics so it is recommended that clonidine or guanfacine is generally tried first (Figure 5.2). Antipsychotics may, however, be more effective than adrenergic α2 agonists in alleviating tics.[9]

A number of first-generation antipsychotics have been used in TS. In a Cochrane review, **pimozide** demonstrated robust efficacy in a meta-analysis of six trials.[19] In these trials, pimozide was compared with haloperidol (one trial), placebo (one trial), haloperidol and placebo (two trials) and risperidone (two trials) and was found to be more effective than placebo, as effective as risperidone and slightly less effective than haloperidol in reducing tics. It was associated with less severe adverse effects than haloperidol but did not differ from risperidone in that respect. ECG monitoring is essential for pimozide and haloperidol. **Haloperidol** is often poorly tolerated. **Tiapride** may also be effective, but evidence may not be generalisable and it has limited availability.[9]

SGAs, in particular aripiprazole, have in recent years been used more commonly for the treatment of TS.[20] **Aripiprazole** is an effective and well-tolerated treatment of children with TS (and also tics[21]). A 10-week multicentre double-blind randomised placebo-controlled trial (N = 61) demonstrated the efficacy of aripiprazole in tic reduction in TS. Treatment was associated with significantly decreased serum prolactin concentration, increased mean body weight (by 1.6kg), body mass index and waist circumference.[22] Aripiprazole was also found to be effective in another randomised double-blind placebo-controlled trial (N = 133) comparing low-dose aripiprazole (5mg/day if <50kg; 10mg/day if ≥50kg), high-dose aripiprazole (10mg/day if <50kg; 20mg/day if ≥50kg) or placebo for 8 weeks.[23] At week 8, tics were reduced in both the high-dose group and the low-dose group, with 69% of patients in the low-dose group and 74% in the high-dose group being very much improved or much improved, compared with 38% in the placebo group. Surprisingly, a higher proportion of children in the low-dose group (18.2%) compared with the high-dose group (9.3%) and placebo group (9.1%) gained clinically significant weight (≥7%) which may have been related to a lower average baseline weight in this group.

Several case series also support the use of aripiprazole.[24–27] A study evaluating the metabolic side effects of aripiprazole (N = 25) and pimozide (N = 25) in TS over a 24-month period demonstrated that treatment was not associated with significant increase in body mass index. However, pimozide treatment was associated with increases in blood glucose that did not plateau from 12 to 24 months, aripiprazole treatment was associated with increased cholesterol and both medications were associated with increased triglycerides.[28] Two meta-analyses support the efficacy of aripiprazole.[29,30] One study[31] suggests twice-weekly administration may be better tolerated than daily dosing. A small RCT (N = 24) comparing aripiprazole with sodium valproate in children with TS demonstrated a statistically significant difference in tic reduction favouring aripiprazole.[32]

Risperidone has, in addition to the studies mentioned, also been shown to be more effective than placebo in a small (N = 34) randomised study.[33] Fatigue and increased appetite were problematic in the risperidone arm and a mean weight gain of 2.8kg over 8 weeks was reported. One small RCT found risperidone and clonidine to be equally effective.[34] A small double-blind crossover study suggested that **olanzapine**[35] may be more effective than pimozide. **Sulpiride** has been shown to be effective and relatively well tolerated,[36] as has **ziprasidone**.[37] Open studies support the efficacy of **quetiapine**[38] and **olanzapine**.[39,40] One very small crossover study (N = 7) found no effect for **clozapine**.[41] Antipsychotic medications may not differ from each other in terms of efficacy for tics, with low to very low certainty of evidence for this comparison.[9]

Overall, metabolic side effects and weight gain are common with second-generation antipsychotics, even aripiprazole, so benefit/risk ratios need careful discussion.[42]

Other drugs

A small, double-blind placebo-controlled crossover trial of **baclofen** was suggestive of beneficial effects in overall impairment rather than a specific effect on tics.[43] The numerical benefits shown in this study did not reach statistical significance. Similarly, a double-blind placebo-controlled trial of **nicotine** augmentation of haloperidol found beneficial effects in overall impairment rather than a specific effect on tics.[44] These benefits persisted for several weeks after nicotine (in the form of patches) was withdrawn. Nicotine patches were associated with a high prevalence of nausea and vomiting (71% and 40%, respectively). The authors suggest that use as required may be appropriate. **Flutamide**, an antiandrogen, has been the subject of a small RCT in adults with TS. Modest, short-lived effects were seen in motor but not phonic tics.[45] A small RCT showed significant advantages for **metoclopramide** over placebo[46] and for **topiramate** over placebo. A meta-analysis identified 14 RCTs (all from China) comparing topiramate with haloperidol or tiapride. It concluded that owing to the overall low quality of the study designs, there is not enough evidence to support the routine use of topiramate in clinical practice.[47] **Tetrabenazine** may be useful as an add-on treatment.[48] **Ecopipam**, a D1 receptor antagonist, was also found to be effective in the treatment of tics in a randomised placebo-controlled crossover study including children and adolescents with TS.[49] A second trial (n = 153)[50] confirmed the efficacy of ecopipam. The monoamine depleting agents **deutetrabenazine** and **valbenazine**, the selective serotonin 5-HT3 receptor antagonist **ondansetron** and **pergolide**, a D1-D2-D3 agonist, are probably not effective.[9,51]

Case reports or case series describing positive effects have been published for **clomiphene**,[52] **tramadol**,[53] **ketanserin**,[54] **cyproterone**,[55] **levetiracetam**,[56] **pregabalin**[57] and **cannabis**.[58] A Cochrane review of cannabinoids concluded that there was little if any current evidence for efficacy[59] and, despite a strong biological rationale for use, their overall efficacy and safety remain largely unknown.[60] Many other drugs have been reported to be effective in single case reports. Patients in these reports all had comorbid psychiatric illness, making it difficult to determine the effect of these drugs on TS alone.

Botulinum toxin has been used to treat bothersome or painful focal motor tics, particularly those affecting neck muscles.[42] However, a 2018 Cochrane review expressed uncertainty about its place in the treatment of tics owing to the low quality of available evidence.[61]

There may be a subgroup of children who develop tics and/or OCD in association with streptococcal or other infections or triggers. This group has been given (in the case of *Streptococcus*) the acronym PANDAS (paediatric autoimmune neuropsychiatric disorder associated with *Streptococcus*)[62] or, more broadly, PANS (paediatric acute-onset neuropsychiatric syndrome).[63] This is thought to be an autoimmune-mediated effect, and there have been trials of immune-modulatory therapy in these children as well as treatment with antibiotics for active infections and also as preventative treatment. More research in this area is warranted.

CHAPTER 5

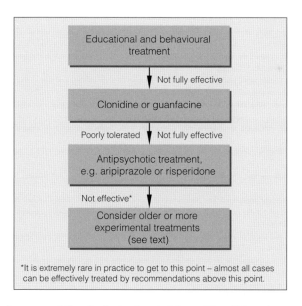

Figure 5.2 Summary of recommendations for the treatment of tics and Tourette's syndrome.

References

1. Murphy TK, et al. Practice parameter for the assessment and treatment of children and adolescents with tic disorders. *J Am Acad Child Adolesc Psychiatry* 2013; **52**:1341–1359.
2. Pringsheim T, et al. European Society for the Study of Tourette Syndrome 2022 criteria for clinical diagnosis of functional tic-like behaviours: international consensus from experts in tic disorders. *Eur J Neurol* 2023; **30**:902–910.
3. Szejko N, et al. European clinical guidelines for Tourette syndrome and other tic disorders – version 2.0. Part I: assessment. *Eur Child Adolesc Psychiatry* 2022; **31**:383–402.
4. McGuire JF, et al. A meta-analysis of behavior therapy for Tourette syndrome. *J Psychiatr Res* 2014; **50**:106–112.
5. Rizzo R, et al. A randomized controlled trial comparing behavioral, educational, and pharmacological treatments in youths with chronic tic disorder or Tourette syndrome. *Front Psychiatry* 2018; **9**:100.
6. Andrén P, et al. European clinical guidelines for Tourette syndrome and other tic disorders – version 2.0. Part II: psychological interventions. *Eur Child Adolesc Psychiatry* 2022; **31**:403–423.
7. Patel H, et al. Use of complementary and alternative medicine in children with Tourette syndrome. *J Child Neurol* 2020; **35**:512–516.
8. Kumar A, et al. A comprehensive review of Tourette syndrome and complementary alternative medicine. *Curr Dev Disord Rep* 2018; **5**:95–100.
9. Farhat LC, et al. Comparative efficacy, tolerability, and acceptability of pharmacological interventions for the treatment of children, adolescents, and young adults with Tourette's syndrome: a systematic review and network meta-analysis. *Lancet Child Adolesc Health* 2023; **7**:112–126.
10. Goetz CG, et al. Clonidine and Gilles de la Tourette's syndrome: double-blind study using objective rating methods. *Ann Neurol* 1987; **21**:307–310.
11. Leckman JF, et al. Clonidine treatment of Gilles de la Tourette's syndrome. *Arch Gen Psychiatry* 1991; **48**:324–328.
12. Tourette's Syndrome Study Group. Treatment of ADHD in children with tics: a randomized controlled trial. *Neurology* 2002; **58**:527–536.
13. Du YS, et al. Randomized double-blind multicentre placebo-controlled clinical trial of the clonidine adhesive patch for the treatment of tic disorders. *Aust N Z J Psychiatry* 2008; **42**:807–813.
14. Hedderick EF, et al. Double-blind, crossover study of clonidine and levetiracetam in Tourette syndrome. *Pediatr Neurol* 2009; **40**:420–425.
15. Song PP, et al. The efficacy and tolerability of the clonidine transdermal patch in the treatment for children with tic disorders: a prospective, open, single-group, self-controlled study. *Front Neurol* 2017; **8**:32.
16. Scahill L, et al. A placebo-controlled study of guanfacine in the treatment of children with tic disorders and attention deficit hyperactivity disorder. *Am J Psychiatry* 2001; **158**:1067–1074.
17. Cummings DD, et al. Neuropsychiatric effects of guanfacine in children with mild Tourette syndrome: a pilot study. *Clin Neuropharmacol* 2002; **25**:325–332.
18. Osland ST, et al. Pharmacological treatment for attention deficit hyperactivity disorder (ADHD) in children with comorbid tic disorders. *Cochrane Database Syst Rev* 2018; **6**:CD007990.
19. Pringsheim T, et al. Pimozide for tics in Tourette's syndrome. *Cochrane Database Syst Rev* 2009; **2009**:CD006996.
20. Roessner V, et al. European clinical guidelines for Tourette syndrome and other tic disorders – version 2.0. Part III: pharmacological treatment. *Eur Child Adolesc Psychiatry* 2022; **31**:425–441.
21. Yoo HK, et al. An open-label study of the efficacy and tolerability of aripiprazole for children and adolescents with tic disorders. *J Clin Psychiatry* 2007; **68**:1088–1093.
22. Yoo HK, et al. A multicenter, randomized, double-blind, placebo-controlled study of aripiprazole in children and adolescents with Tourette's disorder. *J Clin Psychiatry* 2013; **74**:e772–e780.
23. Sallee F, et al. Randomized, double-blind, placebo-controlled trial demonstrates the efficacy and safety of oral aripiprazole for the treatment of Tourette's disorder in children and adolescents. *J Child Adolesc Psychopharmacol* 2017; **27**:771–781.
24. Davies L, et al. A case series of patients with Tourette's syndrome in the United Kingdom treated with aripiprazole. *Hum Psychopharmacol* 2006; **21**:447–453.
25. Seo WS, et al. Aripiprazole treatment of children and adolescents with Tourette disorder or chronic tic disorder. *J Child Adolesc Psychopharmacol* 2008; **18**:197–205.
26. Murphy TK, et al. Open label aripiprazole in the treatment of youth with tic disorders. *J Child Adolesc Psychopharmacol* 2009; **19**:441–447.
27. Wenzel C, et al. Aripiprazole for the treatment of Tourette syndrome: a case series of 100 patients. *J Clin Psychopharmacol* 2012; **32**:548–550.
28. Rizzo R, et al. Metabolic effects of aripiprazole and pimozide in children with Tourette syndrome. *Pediatr Neurol* 2012; **47**:419–422.
29. Liu Y, et al. Effectiveness and tolerability of aripiprazole in children and adolescents with Tourette's disorder: a meta-analysis. *J Child Adolesc Psychopharmacol* 2016; **26**:436–441.
30. Wang S, et al. The efficacy and safety of aripiprazole for tic disorders in children and adolescents: a systematic review and meta-analysis. *Psychiatry Res* 2017; **254**:24–32.
31. Ghanizadeh A. Twice-weekly aripiprazole for treating children and adolescents with tic disorder, a randomized controlled clinical trial. *Ann Gen Psychiatry* 2016; **15**:21.
32. Tao D, et al. Randomized controlled clinical trial comparing the efficacy and tolerability of aripiprazole and sodium valproate in the treatment of Tourette syndrome. *Ann Gen Psychiatry* 2019; **18**:24.
33. Scahill L, et al. A placebo-controlled trial of risperidone in Tourette syndrome. *Neurology* 2003; **60**:1130–1135.

34. Gaffney GR, et al. Risperidone versus clonidine in the treatment of children and adolescents with Tourette's syndrome. *J Am Acad Child Adolesc Psychiatry* 2002; **41**:330–336.

35. Onofrj M, et al. Olanzapine in severe Gilles de la Tourette syndrome: a 52-week double-blind cross-over study vs. low-dose pimozide. *J Neurol* 2000; **247**:443–446.

36. Robertson MM, et al. Management of Gilles de la Tourette syndrome using sulpiride. *Clin Neuropharmacol* 1990; **13**:229–235.

37. Sallee FR, et al. Ziprasidone treatment of children and adolescents with Tourette's syndrome: a pilot study. *J Am Acad Child Adolesc Psychiatry* 2000; **39**:292–299.

38. Mukaddes NM, et al. Quetiapine treatment of children and adolescents with Tourette's disorder. *J Child Adolesc Psychopharmacol* 2003; **13**:295–299.

39. Budman CL, et al. An open-label study of the treatment efficacy of olanzapine for Tourette's disorder. *J Clin Psychiatry* 2001; **62**:290–294.

40. McCracken JT, et al. Effectiveness and tolerability of open label olanzapine in children and adolescents with Tourette syndrome. *J Child Adolesc Psychopharmacol* 2008; **18**:501–508.

41. Caine ED, et al. The trial use of clozapine for abnormal involuntary movement disorders. *Am J Psychiatry* 1979; **136**:317–320.

42. Roessner V, et al. Pharmacological treatment of tic disorders and Tourette syndrome. *Neuropharmacology* 2013; **68**:143–149.

43. Singer HS, et al. Baclofen treatment in Tourette syndrome: a double-blind, placebo-controlled, crossover trial. *Neurology* 2001; **56**:599–604.

44. Silver AA, et al. Transdermal nicotine and haloperidol in Tourette's disorder: a double-blind placebo-controlled study. *J Clin Psychiatry* 2001; **62**:707–714.

45. Peterson BS, et al. A double-blind, placebo-controlled, crossover trial of an antiandrogen in the treatment of Tourette's syndrome. *J Clin Psychopharmacol* 1998; **18**:324–331.

46. Nicolson R, et al. A randomized, double-blind, placebo-controlled trial of metoclopramide for the treatment of Tourette's disorder. *J Am Acad Child Adolesc Psychiatry* 2005; **44**:640–646.

47. Yang CS, et al. Topiramate for Tourette's syndrome in children: a meta-analysis. *Pediatr Neurol* 2013; **49**:344–350.

48. Porta M, et al. Tourette's syndrome and role of tetrabenazine: review and personal experience. *Clin Drug Invest* 2008; **28**:443–459.

49. Gilbert DL, et al. Ecopipam, a D1 receptor antagonist, for treatment of Tourette syndrome in children: a randomized, placebo-controlled crossover study. *Mov Disord* 2018; **33**:1272–1280.

50. Gilbert DL, et al. Ecopipam for Tourette syndrome: a randomized trial. *Pediatrics* 2023; **151**:e2022059574.

51. Chou CY, et al. Emerging therapies and recent advances for Tourette syndrome. *Heliyon* 2023; **9**:e12874.

52. Sandyk R. Clomiphene citrate in Tourette's syndrome. *Int J Neurosci* 1988; **43**:103–106.

53. Shapira NA, et al. Novel use of tramadol hydrochloride in the treatment of Tourette's syndrome. *J Clin Psychiatry* 1997; **58**:174–175.

54. Bonnier C, et al. Ketanserin treatment of Tourette's syndrome in children. *Am J Psychiatry* 1999; **156**:1122–1123.

55. Izmir M, et al. Cyproterone acetate treatment of Tourette's syndrome. *Can J Psychiatry* 1999; **44**:710–711.

56. Awaad Y, et al. Use of levetiracetam to treat tics in children and adolescents with Tourette syndrome. *Mov Disord* 2005; **20**:714–718.

57. Hienert M, et al. Pregabalin in Tourette's syndrome: a case series. *Am J Psychiatry* 2016; **173**:1242–1243.

58. Sandyk R, et al. Marijuana and Tourette's syndrome. *J Clin Psychopharmacol* 1988; **8**:444–445.

59. Curtis A, et al. Cannabinoids for Tourette's syndrome. *Cochrane Database Syst Rev* 2009; **2009**:CD006565.

60. Artukoglu BB, et al. The potential of cannabinoid-based treatments in Tourette syndrome. *CNS Drugs* 2019; **33**:417–430.

61. Pandey S, et al. Botulinum toxin for motor and phonic tics in Tourette's syndrome. *Cochrane Database Syst Rev* 2018; **1**:CD012285.

62. Martino D, et al. The PANDAS subgroup of tic disorders and childhood-onset obsessive-compulsive disorder. *J Psychosom Res* 2009; **67**:547–557.

63. Chang K, et al. Clinical evaluation of youth with pediatric acute-onset neuropsychiatric syndrome (PANS): recommendations from the 2013 PANS Consensus Conference. *J Child Adolesc Psychopharmacol* 2015; **25**:3–13.

CHAPTER 5

Melatonin in the treatment of insomnia in children and adolescents

Insomnia is a common symptom in childhood. Underlying causes may be behavioural (inappropriate sleep associations or bedtime resistance), physiological (delayed sleep phase syndrome) or related to underlying mood disorders (anxiety, depression and bipolar disorder). All forms of insomnia are more common in children with learning difficulties, autism, ADHD and sensory impairments (particularly visual). Although behavioural interventions should be the primary intervention and have a robust evidence base, exogenous melatonin is now the first-line medication prescribed for childhood insomnia (Figure 5.3).[1]

Melatonin is a hormone that is produced by the pineal gland in a circadian manner. The evening rise in melatonin, enabled by darkness, precedes the onset of natural sleep by about 2 hours.[2] Melatonin is involved in the induction of sleep and in synchronisation of the circadian system.

There is a wide variety of unlicensed fast-release, slow-release and liquid preparations of melatonin. Many products rely on food grade rather than pharmaceutical grade melatonin and some are expensive. In 2018 the European Medicines Agency and UK MHRA approved Slenyto, a paediatric-appropriate prolonged-release melatonin minitablet, for children with autism and insomnia. This approval was on the basis of a phase III multicentre randomised placebo-controlled study of children with autism. Results of the study included clinically significant improvement in caregivers' diary-reported sleep latency, total sleep time and longest sleep period.[3] Effects were maintained in the long term. The medication was well tolerated and no unexpected safety issues were reported. The study was the only 'class 1' rated study in the 2020 America Academy of Neurology practice guideline on the treatment for insomnia and disrupted sleep behaviour in children and adolescents with ASD.[4] Secondary outcomes showed improvements in children's social functioning and behaviour, and caregivers' well-being. A meta-analysis of melatonin in ASD came to similar, positive conclusions.[5]

Two RCTs[6,7] showed melatonin had comparable benefits when used to treat children with ADHD and insomnia. On this basis, the MHRA in the UK has approved various immediate-release (tablet, e.g. Adaflex) and liquid (e.g. Colonis, Ceyesto) melatonin preparations for the management of sleep-onset insomnia in children with ADHD.

There is less evidence (and clinical consensus) for the use of melatonin in typically developing children, although a 2023 meta-analysis provided a conditional recommendation 'for use of melatonin in children and adolescents 2–20 years, who despite optimisation of sleep hygiene practices, continue to present with difficulties in daily functioning, due to chronic insomnia attributed to an underlying disorder'.[8]

Efficacy

A meta-analysis that included adult and paediatric studies of melatonin in primary sleep disorders demonstrated that melatonin modestly decreases sleep-onset latency, increases total sleep time and improves overall sleep quality; effects that appear not to dissipate with continued melatonin use.[9] A more recent (2022) analysis confirmed benefits only for sleep latency and sleep duration.[10]

CHAPTER 5

Adverse effects

Many of the children who have received melatonin in RCTs and published case series had developmental problems and/or sensory deficits. The scope for detecting subtle adverse effects in this population is limited. Screening for adverse effects was not routine in all studies. In early published accounts, melatonin was reported to worsen seizures[11] and exacerbate asthma.[12,13] Other reported adverse effects included headache, depression, restlessness, confusion, nausea, tachycardia and pruritis.[14,15] However, in more recent and larger placebo-controlled studies involving children with learning difficulty, autism and epilepsy,[3,16-18] there were no excess adverse effects in the treatment group over placebo and, in particular, seizures were not worsened. A Cochrane review also found no worsening of seizure frequency in patients with epilepsy who were given melatonin.[19] Melatonin has no detectable impact on puberty.[20]

Dose

The cut-off point between physiological and pharmacological doses in children is less than 500mcg. Physiological doses (i.e. <500mcg) of melatonin may result in very high receptor occupancy. The doses used in RCTs and published case series vary hugely with between 500mcg and 5mg doses usually being used, although much lower and higher doses have been studied. In one large RCT, 18% of children seemed to respond to a 500mcg dose but others seemed to require much higher doses (12mg).[18] Increasing doses above 5mg is likely to provoke the direct sedative effects of melatonin rather than its sleep phase-shifting properties. This might be necessary and helpful for some children with severe and bilateral brain injury.

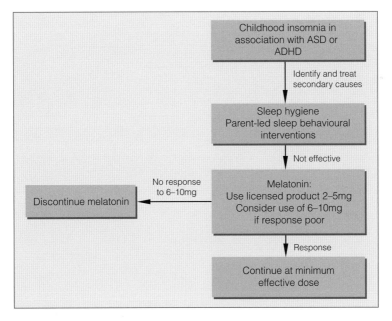

Figure 5.3 Summary of recommendations in the treatment of insomnia.

CHAPTER 5

References

1. Gringras P. When to use drugs to help sleep. *Arch Dis Child* 2008; **93**:976–981.
2. Macchi MM, et al. Human pineal physiology and functional significance of melatonin. *Front Neuroendocrinol* 2004; **25**:177–195.
3. Gringras P, et al. Efficacy and safety of pediatric prolonged-release melatonin for insomnia in children with autism spectrum disorder. *J Am Acad Child Adolesc Psychiatry* 2017; **56**:948–957.e944.
4. Williams Buckley A, et al. Practice guideline: treatment for insomnia and disrupted sleep behavior in children and adolescents with autism spectrum disorder: report of the Guideline Development, Dissemination, and Implementation Subcommittee of the American Academy of Neurology. *Neurology* 2020; **94**:392–404.
5. Xiong M, et al. Efficacy of melatonin for insomnia in children with autism spectrum disorder: a meta-analysis. *Neuropediatrics* 2023; **54**:167–173.
6. Van der Heijden KB, et al. Effect of melatonin on sleep, behavior, and cognition in ADHD and chronic sleep-onset insomnia. *J Am Acad Child Adolesc Psychiatry* 2007; **46**:233–241.
7. Weiss MD, et al. Sleep hygiene and melatonin treatment for children and adolescents with ADHD and initial insomnia. *J Am Acad Child Adolesc Psychiatry* 2006; **45**:512–519.
8. Edemann-Callesen H, et al. Use of melatonin for children and adolescents with chronic insomnia attributable to disorders beyond indication: a systematic review, meta-analysis and clinical recommendation. *EClinicalMedicine* 2023; **61**:102049.
9. Ferracioli-Oda E, et al. Meta-analysis: melatonin for the treatment of primary sleep disorders. *PLoS One* 2013; **8**:e63773.
10. Salanitro M, et al. Efficacy on sleep parameters and tolerability of melatonin in individuals with sleep or mental disorders: a systematic review and meta-analysis. *Neurosci Biobehav Rev* 2022; **139**:104723.
11. Sheldon SH. Pro-convulsant effects of oral melatonin in neurologically disabled children. *Lancet* 1998; **351**:1254.
12. Maestroni GJ. The immunoneuroendocrine role of melatonin. *J Pineal Res* 1993; **14**:1–10.
13. Sutherland ER, et al. Elevated serum melatonin is associated with the nocturnal worsening of asthma. *J Allergy Clin Immunol* 2003; **112**:513–517.
14. Chase JE, et al. Melatonin: therapeutic use in sleep disorders. *Ann Pharmacother* 1997; **31**:1218–1226.
15. Jan JE, et al. Melatonin treatment of sleep-wake cycle disorders in children and adolescents. *Dev Med Child Neurol* 1999; **41**:491–500.
16. Coppola G, et al. Melatonin in wake-sleep disorders in children, adolescents and young adults with mental retardation with or without epilepsy: a double-blind, cross-over, placebo-controlled trial. *Brain Dev* 2004; **26**:373–376.
17. Garstang J, et al. Randomized controlled trial of melatonin for children with autistic spectrum disorders and sleep problems. *Child Care Health Dev* 2006; **32**:585–589.
18. Gringras P, et al. Melatonin for sleep problems in children with neurodevelopmental disorders: randomised double masked placebo controlled trial. *BMJ* 2012; **345**:e6664.
19. Brigo F, et al. Melatonin as add-on treatment for epilepsy. *Cochrane Database Syst Rev* 2016; **2016**:CD006967.
20. Malow BA, et al. Sleep, growth, and puberty after 2 years of prolonged-release melatonin in children with autism spectrum disorder. *J Am Acad Child Adolesc Psychiatry* 2012; **60**:252–261.e3.

Rapid tranquillisation (RT) in children and adolescents

As in adults, a comprehensive assessment and effective treatment plan undertaken by staff skilled in the use of de-escalation techniques and appropriate placement of the patient are key to minimising the need for enforced parenteral medication. The differential diagnoses for agitated or challenging behaviour can be broad, but there is concern that RT may be disproportionately used in a neurodiverse population where other strategies may be more appropriate and the outcome more predictable.[1,2]

Healthcare professionals undertaking RT and/or restraint in children and adolescents should be trained and competent in undertaking these procedures in this population and should be clear about the legal context for any restrictive practices they employ. Be particularly cautious when considering high-potency antipsychotic medication (e.g. haloperidol) especially for those who are neuroleptic naïve, because of the increased risk of acute dystonic reactions in this age group.[3] Children are particularly prone to acute extrapyramidal effects of psychotropic and physical medication.[4] In the UK, NICE recommends using intramuscular lorazepam (and recommends no other drug).[5] Evidence suggests that lorazepam is effective (at a median dose of 1mg) and rarely causes respiratory depression resulting in oxygen desaturation.[1] Reviews support the use of a range of SGA drugs[6] with the most frequently used agent being olanzapine, which has evidence of its safety and efficacy.[7]

A wide dose range is given here for medication used in RT. This is partly a consequence of the wide range of body mass in individuals aged from under 10 to 18 years. Caution is required, especially for younger children, but in older adolescents consider the use of adult doses, especially in those who are not drug naïve and where doses at the lower end of the quoted dose range have proved ineffective.

A summary is given in Table 5.11.

Table 5.11 Recommended drugs for rapid tranquillisation if the oral route is refused or has proven ineffective.

Medication	Dose	Onset of action	Comment
Olanzapine IM[8,9]	2.5–10mg	15–30 minutes	Possibly increased risk of respiratory depression when administered with benzodiazepines, particularly if alcohol has been consumed. Separate administration by at least 1 hour.
Haloperidol IM[10]	0.025–0.075mg/kg/dose (max. 2.5mg) IM Adolescents >12 years can receive the adult dose (2.5–5mg)	20–30 minutes	Must have parenteral anticholinergics present in case of laryngeal spasm or other dystonia (young people more vulnerable to severe dystonia). Adult data suggest co-administration of promethazine may reduce EPS risk.[11] **ECG is essential**
Lorazepam* IM[12]	<12 years: 0.5–1mg; >12 years: 0.5-2mg	20–40 minutes	Slower onset of action than midazolam Only treatment recommended by NICE Flumazenil is the reversing agent for all benzodiazepines.

(Continued)

Table 5.11 (*Continued*)

Medication	Dose	Onset of action	Comment
Midazolam* IM, IV or buccal[12]	0.1–0.15mg/kg IM Buccal midazolam 300–500mcg/kg or 6–10 years = 7.5mg; >10 years = 10mg	10–20 min IM (1–3 min IV)	Quicker onset and shorter duration of action than lorazepam or diazepam IV administration should only be used (usually as a last resort) with extreme caution and where resuscitation facilities are available. Quicker onset and shorter duration of action than haloperidol When given as buccal liquid, onset of action is 15–30 minutes.[13] There are some published data of its use in mental health but only in adults;[14] buccal liquid is unlicensed for this use.
Diazepam* IV (not for IM administration)[15]	0.1mg/kg/dose by slow IV injection Max. 40mg total daily dose <12 years and 60mg >12 years	1–3 minutes	Long half-life that does not correlate with length of sedation Possibility of accumulation **Never give as IM injection.**
Ziprasidone IM[16,17]	10–20mg	15–30 minutes IM	Apparently effective QT prolongation is of concern in this patient group. **ECG is essential.**
Aripiprazole IM[18,19]	9.75mg	15–30 minutes	Evidence of effectiveness in adults but no clinical trial data for children and adolescents
Promethazine IM	<12 years: 5–25mg (max. 50mg/day) >12 years: 25–50mg (max. 100mg/day)	Up to 60 minutes	An effective sedative, although has a slow onset of action. Useful if the cause of behavioural disturbance is unknown and there is concern about the use of antipsychotic medication in a child or young person.

*Note that young people are particularly vulnerable to disinhibitory reactions with benzodiazepines. EPS, extrapyramidal symptoms.

Oral medication should always be offered (and repeated if necessary if the young person is willing to take it) before resorting to parenteral treatment. Oral alternatives such as buccal midazolam[14] and inhaled loxapine[20] have not been widely investigated in children in RT and have limited availability. Buccal midazolam is commonly used for seizures in children.

Monitoring after RT is the same as in adults (see Chapter 3).

References

1. Kendrick JG, et al. Pharmacologic management of agitation and aggression in a pediatric emergency department – a retrospective cohort study. *J Pediatric Pharmacol Therapeutics* 2018; **23**:455–459.
2. Wolpert KH, et al. Behavioral management of children with autism in the emergency department. *Pediatr Emerg Care* 2023; **39**:45–50.
3. National Institute for Health and Care Excellence. Psychosis and schizophrenia in children and young people: recognition and management. Clinical Guidance [CG155]. 2013 (last updated October 2016, last checked October 2023); https://www.nice.org.uk/guidance/cg155.
4. Chang MY, et al. Drug-induced extrapyramidal symptoms at the pediatric emergency department. *Pediatr Emerg Care* 2020; **36**:468–472.
5. National Institute for Health and Care Excellence. Violence and aggression: short-term management in mental health, health and community settings. NICE Guideline [NG10]. 2015 (last checked October 2023); https://www.nice.org.uk/guidance/ng10.
6. Rudolf F, et al. A retrospective review of antipsychotic medications administered to psychiatric patients in a tertiary care pediatric emergency department. *J Pediatric Pharmacol Therapeutics* 2019; **24**:234–237.
7. Cole JB, et al. The use, safety, and efficacy of olanzapine in a level I pediatric trauma center emergency department over a 10-year period. *Pediatr Emerg Care* 2020; **36**:70–76.
8. Breier A, et al. A double-blind, placebo-controlled dose-response comparison of intramuscular olanzapine and haloperidol in the treatment of acute agitation in schizophrenia. *Arch Gen Psychiatry* 2002; **59**:441–448.
9. Lindborg SR, et al. Effects of intramuscular olanzapine vs. haloperidol and placebo on QTc intervals in acutely agitated patients. *Psychiatry Res* 2003; **119**:113–123.
10. Powney MJ, et al. Haloperidol for psychosis-induced aggression or agitation (rapid tranquillisation). *Cochrane Database Syst Rev* 2012; **11**:CD009377.
11. TREC Collaborative Group. Rapid tranquillisation for agitated patients in emergency psychiatric rooms: a randomised trial of midazolam versus haloperidol plus promethazine. *BMJ* 2003; **327**:708–713.
12. Nobay F, et al. A prospective, double-blind, randomized trial of midazolam versus haloperidol versus lorazepam in the chemical restraint of violent and severely agitated patients. *Acad Emerg Med* 2004; **11**:744–749.
13. Schwagmeier R, et al. Midazolam pharmacokinetics following intravenous and buccal administration. *Br J Clin Pharmacol* 1998; **46**:203–206.
14. Taylor D, et al. Buccal midazolam for agitation on psychiatric intensive care wards. *Int J Psychiatry Clin Pract* 2008; **12**:309–311.
15. Nunn K, et al. Medication table. In: Nunn KP, Dey C, eds. *The Clinician's Guide to Psychotropic Prescribing in Children and Adolescents*, 1st edn. Sydney: Glad Publishing 2003:383–452.
16. Khan SS, et al. A naturalistic evaluation of intramuscular ziprasidone versus intramuscular olanzapine for the management of acute agitation and aggression in children and adolescents. *J Child Adolesc Psychopharmacol* 2006; **16**:671–677.
17. Staller JA. Intramuscular ziprasidone in youth: a retrospective chart review. *J Child Adolesc Psychopharmacol* 2004; **14**:590–592.
18. Sanford M, et al. Intramuscular aripiprazole: a review of its use in the management of agitation in schizophrenia and bipolar I disorder. *CNS Drugs* 2008; **22**:335–352.
19. National Institute for Health and Clinical Excellence. Aripiprazole for schizophrenia in people aged 15 to 17 years. Technology Appraisal [TA213]. 2011 (last checked October 2023); https://www.nice.org.uk/guidance/ta213.
20. Lesem MD, et al. Rapid acute treatment of agitation in individuals with schizophrenia: multicentre, randomised, placebo-controlled study of inhaled loxapine. *Br J Psychiatry* 2011; **198**:51–58.

CHAPTER 5

Doses of commonly used psychotropic drugs in children and adolescents

Commonly used psychotropic drugs are presented in Table 5.12.

Table 5.12 Starting doses of commonly used psychotropic drugs in children and adolescents.[1,2]

Drug	Starting dose*	Comment
Antipsychotics		
Aripiprazole	2mg	Adjust dose according to response and adverse effects.
Clozapine	6.25–12.5mg	Use plasma levels to determine maintenance dose.
Lurasidone	18.5mg (20mg) to 37mg (40mg)	Adjust dose according to response and adverse effects.
Olanzapine	2.5–5mg	Adjust dose according to response and adverse effects.
Quetiapine	25mg	Effective dose usually in the range 150–200mg daily.
Risperidone	0.25–2mg	Adjust dose according to response and adverse effects.
Antidepressants		
Citalopram	10mg daily	Effective dose 10–40mg (note QT effects)
Escitalopram	5mg/day	Effective dose 10–20mg (note QT effects)
Fluoxetine	5–10mg/day	Adjust dose according to response and adverse effects.
Sertraline	25mg daily	Effective dose usually in the range 50–100mg daily.
Other drugs		
Lithium	100–200mg/day lithium carbonate	Use plasma levels to determine maintenance dose.
Melatonin	1–2mg at night	Effective dose 2–10mg
Valproate	10–20mg/kg/day in divided doses	Use plasma levels to determine maintenance dose. Do not offer valproate to girls or young women of child-bearing potential unless there is a pregnancy prevention programme (PPP) in place.[1,3]

*Suggested approximate oral starting doses (see primary literature for doses in individual indications). Lower dose in suggested range is for children weighing less than 25kg.

References

1. Paediatric Formulary Committee. *BNF for Children (online)*. London: BMJ, Pharmaceutical Press, and RCPCH Publications; http://www.medicinescomplete.com.
2. Merative US LP. Micromedex. 2024; https://www.micromedexsolutions.com/home/dispatch/.
3. Gov.UK. Guidance: Valproate use by women and girls. 2018 (last updated January 2024); https://www.gov.uk/guidance/valproate-use-by-women-and-girls.

Chapter 6

Prescribing in older people

General principles in prescribing in older adults

General principles

The pharmacokinetics and pharmacodynamics of most drugs are altered to an important extent in older people. These changes in drug handling and action must be taken into account if treatment is to be effective and adverse effects minimised. Older people often have a number of concurrent illnesses and may require treatment with several drugs. This leads to a greater chance of problems arising because of drug interactions and a higher rate of drug-induced problems in general.[1] It is reasonable to assume that all drugs are more likely to cause adverse effects in older patients than in younger patients (Box 6.1).

Box 6.1 Reducing drug-related risk in older people

Adherence to the following principles will reduce drug-related morbidity and mortality:
- Use drugs only when absolutely necessary
- Avoid, if possible, drugs that block α1 adrenoceptors, have anticholinergic adverse effects, are very sedative, have a long half-life or are potent inhibitors of hepatic metabolising enzymes
- Start with a low dose and increase slowly but do not undertreat. Some drugs still require the full adult dose
- Try not to treat the adverse effects of one drug with another drug. Find a better-tolerated alternative
- Keep therapy simple; that is, once-daily administration whenever possible

---

How drugs affect the ageing body (altered pharmacodynamics)

As we age, control over reflex actions such as blood pressure and temperature regulation is reduced. Receptors may become more sensitive. This results in an increased incidence and severity of adverse effects. For example, drugs that decrease gut motility are more likely to cause constipation (e.g. anticholinergics and opioids) and drugs that affect blood pressure are more likely to cause falls (e.g. tricyclic antidepressants [TCAs]

The Maudsley® Prescribing Guidelines in Psychiatry, Fifteenth Edition. David M. Taylor, Thomas R. E. Barnes and Allan H. Young.
© 2025 David M. Taylor. Published 2025 by John Wiley & Sons Ltd.

and diuretics). Older people demonstrate an exaggerated response to central nervous system (CNS)-active drugs such as benzodiazepines and opioids. This is partly because of an age-related decline in CNS function and partly due to increased pharmacodynamic sensitivity to these drugs (due to increased blood–brain barrier permeability).[2,3] Therapeutic response to medication can also be delayed; for example, older adults may take longer to respond to antidepressants than younger adults.[4]

Older people may be more prone to developing serious adverse effects such as agranulocytosis[5] and neutropenia[6] with clozapine, stroke with antipsychotic drugs[7] and bleeding with selective serotonin reuptake inhibitors (SSRIs).[8]

How ageing affects drug therapy (altered pharmacokinetics)[9,10]

Absorption
Gut motility decreases with age, as does secretion of gastric acid. This leads to drugs being absorbed more slowly, resulting in a slower onset of action. In general, the same *amount* of drug is absorbed as in a younger adult, but the rate of absorption is slower.

Distribution
Older adults have more body fat, less body water and less albumin than younger adults. This leads to an increased volume of distribution and a longer duration of action for some fat-soluble drugs (e.g. diazepam), higher concentrations of some drugs at the site of action (e.g. digoxin) and a reduction in the amount of drug bound to albumin (increased amounts of active 'free drug'; e.g. warfarin, phenytoin).

Metabolism
The majority of drugs are hepatically metabolised. Liver size is reduced in the elderly, but in the absence of hepatic disease or significantly reduced hepatic blood flow, there is no significant reduction in metabolic capacity. The magnitude of pharmacokinetic interactions is unlikely to be altered but the pharmacodynamic consequences of these interactions may be amplified.

Excretion
Renal function declines with age: 35% of function is lost by the age of 65 years and 50% by the age of 80.

More function is lost if there are concurrent medical problems such as heart disease, diabetes or hypertension. Measurement of serum creatinine or urea can be misleading in the elderly because muscle mass is reduced, so less creatinine is produced. It is particularly important that estimated glomerular filtration rate (eGFR)[11] is used as a measure of renal function in this age group. It is best to assume that all elderly patients have at most two-thirds of normal renal function.

Most drugs are eventually (after metabolism) excreted by the kidney. A few do not undergo biotransformation first. Lithium and sulpiride are important examples. Drugs primarily excreted via the kidney will accumulate in the elderly, leading to toxicity and adverse effects. Dosage reduction is likely to be required (see Chapter 8).

Drug interactions

Some drugs have a narrow therapeutic index (a small increase in dose can cause toxicity and a small reduction in dose can cause a loss of therapeutic action). The most commonly prescribed ones are digoxin, warfarin, theophylline, phenytoin and lithium.

Changes in the way these drugs are handled in older people and the greater chance of interaction with other drugs mean that toxicity and therapeutic failure are more likely. These drugs can be used safely but extra care must be taken and blood concentrations should be measured where possible.

Some drugs inhibit or induce hepatic metabolising enzymes. Important examples include some SSRIs, erythromycin and carbamazepine. This may lead to the metabolism of another drug being altered. Many drug interactions occur through this mechanism. Details of individual interactions and their consequences can be found in the *British National Formulary (BNF)* online for individual drugs.[12] Most can be predicted by a sound knowledge of pharmacology.

Administering medicines in foodstuffs[13–16]

Sometimes patients refuse treatment with medicines, even when such treatment is thought to be in their best interests. In the UK, where the patient has a mental illness or has capacity, the Mental Health Act should be used, but if the patient lacks capacity this option may not be desirable. Medicines should never be administered covertly to older patients with dementia without a full discussion with the multidisciplinary team (MDT) and the patient's relatives. The outcome of this discussion should be clearly documented in the patient's clinical notes. Medicines should be administered covertly only if the clear and express purpose is to reduce suffering for the patient. (For further information, see 'Covert administration of medicines within food and drink' later in this chapter.)

For advice on dosing of psychotropics in older people, see 'A guide to medication doses of commonly used psychotropics in older adults' later in this chapter.

References

1. Royal College of Physicians. Medication for older people. Summary and recommendations of a report of a working party of The Royal College of Physicians. *J R Coll Physicians Lond* 1997; **31**:254–257.
2. Bowie MW, et al. Pharmacodynamics in older adults: a review. *Am J Geriatr Pharmacother* 2007; **5**:263–303.
3. Cleare A, et al. Evidence-based guidelines for treating depressive disorders with antidepressants: a revision of the 2008 British Association for Psychopharmacology guidelines. *J Psychopharmacol* 2015; **29**:459–525.
4. Baldwin R, et al. Management of depression in later life. *Adv Psychiatr Treat* 2004; **10**:131–139.
5. Munro J, et al. Active monitoring of 12,760 clozapine recipients in the UK and Ireland. Beyond pharmacovigilance. *Br J Psychiatry* 1999; **175**:576–580.
6. O'Connor DW, et al. The safety and tolerability of clozapine in aged patients: a retrospective clinical file review. *World J Biol Psychiatry* 2010; **11**:788–791.
7. Douglas IJ, et al. Exposure to antipsychotics and risk of stroke: self controlled case series study. *BMJ* 2008; **337**:a1227.
8. Paton C, et al. SSRIs and gastrointestinal bleeding. *BMJ* 2005; **331**:529–530.
9. Mayersohn M. Special pharmacokinetic considerations in the elderly. In: Evans W, Schentage J, Jusko J, eds. *Applied Pharmacokinetics: Principles of Therapeutic Drug Monitoring*. Vancouver, WA: Applied Therapeutics Inc; 1992.
10. Dening T, Thomas A, Stewart R, Taylor JP, eds. *Oxford Textbook of Old Age Psychiatry*. Oxford: Oxford University Press; 2020.
11. Morriss R, et al. Lithium and eGFR: a new routinely available tool for the prevention of chronic kidney disease. *Br J Psychiatry* 2008; **193**:93–95.
12. Joint Formulary Committee. *British National Formulary (online)*. London: BMJ and Pharmaceutical Press; http://www.medicinescomplete.com.
13. Royal College of Psychiatrists. College statement on covert administration of medicines. *Psychiatric Bull* 2004; **28**:385–386.
14. Haw C, et al. Administration of medicines in food and drink: a study of older inpatients with severe mental illness. *Int Psychogeriatr* 2010; **22**:409–416.
15. Haw C, et al. Covert administration of medication to older adults: a review of the literature and published studies. *J Psychiatr Ment Health Nurs* 2010; **17**:761–768.
16. Specialist Pharmacy Service. Covert administration of medicines in adults: pharmaceutical issues 2022 (last updated June 2023); https://www.sps.nhs.uk/articles/covert-administration-of-medicines-in-adults-pharmaceutical-issues/.

CHAPTER 6

Dementia

Dementia is a progressive syndrome affecting around 5% of those aged over 65 years, rising to 20% in the over 80s. The disorder is characterised by cognitive decline, impaired memory and thinking and a gradual loss of skills needed to carry out activities of daily living (ADL). Changes in mood, personality and social behaviour are frequent.[1]

The various types of dementia are classified according to the different disease processes affecting the brain. The most common cause of dementia is Alzheimer's disease (AD), accounting for around 60% of all cases. Vascular dementia (VaD) and dementia with Lewy bodies (DLB) are responsible for most other cases. AD and VaD may coexist and are often difficult to separate clinically. Dementia is also encountered in about 30–70% of patients with Parkinson's disease[1] (see Chapter 10).

Alzheimer's disease (AD)

Mechanism of action of cognitive enhancers used in AD

Acetylcholinesterase (AChE) inhibitors

The cholinergic hypothesis of AD is predicated on the observation that the cognitive deterioration associated with the disease results from progressive loss of cholinergic neurons and decreasing levels of acetylcholine (ACh) in the brain.[2] However, it is no longer widely believed that cholinergic depletion alone is responsible for the symptoms of AD.[3]

Three inhibitors of AChE are currently licensed in the UK and elsewhere for the treatment of mild to moderate dementia in AD: donepezil, rivastigmine and galantamine. These three drugs are also recommended in severe AD. In addition, rivastigmine is licensed in some countries for the treatment of mild to moderate dementia associated with Parkinson's disease.

Both AChE and butyrylcholinesterase (BuChE) have been found to play an important role in the degradation of ACh.[4] Cholinesterase inhibitors differ in pharmacological action: donepezil selectively inhibits AChE, rivastigmine affects both AChE and BuChE and galantamine selectively inhibits AChE and also has nicotinic receptor agonist properties.[5] To date, these differences have not been shown to result in important differences in efficacy or tolerability (see Table 6.1 for a comparison of AChE inhibitors).

Memantine

Memantine is licensed in the UK and elsewhere for the treatment of moderate to severe dementia in AD. It is believed to exert its therapeutic effect by acting as a low to moderate affinity, non-competitive N-methyl-D-aspartate (NMDA) receptor antagonist that binds preferentially to open NMDA receptor-operated calcium channels. This activity-dependent binding blocks NMDA-mediated ion flux and is thought to mitigate the effects of sustained and pathologically elevated levels of glutamate (and this excitotoxicity) that may lead to neuronal dysfunction (Table 6.1).[6]

Table 6.1 Characteristics of cognitive enhancers.[7–14]

Characteristic	Donepezil	Rivastigmine	Galantamine	Memantine
Primary mechanism	AChE-I (selective and reversible)	AChE-I (reversible, non-competitive inhibitor)	AChE-I (competitive and reversible)	Glutamate receptor antagonist
Other mechanism	None	BuChE-I	Nicotine receptor agonist	$5HT_3$ receptor antagonist
Starting dose	5mg daily	1.5mg bd (oral) (or 4.6mg/24 hours patch)	8mg XL daily (or 4mg bd solution) (immediate-release tablets largely discontinued)	5mg daily
Usual treatment dose	10mg daily	3–6mg bd (oral) (or 9.5mg/24 hours patch)	16–24mg XL daily (or 8–12mg bd solution)	20mg daily (or 10mg bd)
Recommended minimum interval between dose increases	4 weeks (increase by 5mg daily)	2 weeks for oral (increase by 1.5mg twice a day) 4 weeks for patch (increase to 9.5mg/24 hours) Consider increase to 13.3mg/24 hours after 6 months	4 weeks (increase by 8mg XL daily or by 4mg bd for solution)	1 week (increase by 5mg weekly)
Adverse effects[7–13] (*very common: ≥1/10 and common: ≥1/100)	Diarrhoea,* nausea,* headache,* common cold, anorexia, hallucinations, agitation, aggressive behaviour, abnormal dreams and nightmares, syncope, dizziness, insomnia, vomiting, rash, pruritis, muscle cramps, urinary incontinence, fatigue, pain, falls	Anorexia,* dizziness,* nausea,* vomiting,* diarrhoea,* decreased appetite, nightmares, agitation, confusion, anxiety, headache, somnolence, tremor, abdominal pain and dyspepsia, sweating, fatigue and asthenia, malaise, weight loss (frequency of adverse effects with the patch may differ)	Nausea,* vomiting,* decreased appetite, hallucination, depression, syncope, dizziness, tremor, headache, somnolence, lethargy, bradycardia, hypertension, abdominal pain and discomfort, diarrhoea, dyspepsia, muscle spasms, fatigue, asthenia, malaise, weight loss, fall, laceration	Drug hypersensitivity, somnolence, dizziness, balance disorders, hypertension, dyspnoea, constipation, elevated liver function test, headache
Half-life (hours)	~70	~1 (oral) 3.4 (patch)	7–8 (oral solution) 8–10 (XL capsules)	60–100
Metabolism	CYP3A4 CYP2D6 (minor)	Minimal involvement of CYP isoenzymes	CYP3A4 CYP2D6	Primarily non-hepatic
Drug–drug interactions	Yes (see Table 6.2)	Interactions unlikely	Yes (see Table 6.2)	Yes (see Table 6.2)
Effect of food on absorption	None	Delays rate and extent of absorption	Delays rate but not extent of absorption	None

AChE-I, acetylcholinesterase inhibitor; bd, twice a day; BuChE, butyrylcholinesterase.

CHAPTER 6

Efficacy of cognitive enhancers used in AD

Currently, no treatments exist that unequivocally reverse disease progression in dementia. Therapeutic interventions are therefore targeted at specific symptoms or at improving or slowing the decline in cognitive function. AChE inhibitors (AChE-Is) may provide some modest cognitive, functional and global benefits in mild to moderate AD.[15]

The three AChE-Is seem to have broadly similar clinical effects; estimates of the number needed to treat (NNT) (for an improvement of >4 points in the AD Assessment Scale – cognitive subscale [ADAS-cog]) range from 4 to 12.[16]

An analysis of memantine studies found estimated NNT ranged from 3 to 8[17] for improved cognitive function. A Cochrane review of memantine in dementia confirmed that there was a small clinical benefit of memantine in people with moderate to severe AD, which occurs irrespective of whether they are also taking a cholinesterase inhibitor, but no benefit in people with mild AD.[17]

A 2021 study[18] investigated the 'real world' effectiveness of cholinesterase inhibitors and memantine. The study found that, in general, the initial decline in Mini Mental State Examination (MMSE) and Montreal Cognitive Assessment (MoCA) scores occurred approximately 2 years before medication was eventually initiated. Medication stabilised cognitive performance for the ensuing 2–5 months. The effect was enhanced in more cognitively impaired cases and attenuated in those taking antipsychotics. Importantly, patients who were switched between agents at least once tended to continue to decline at their pre-medication rate (i.e. did not benefit from pharmacological interventions). Those who remained on the same agent tended to respond better and to stabilise in respect to cognitive changes for a period once the medication was prescribed. Of course, switching might be more common in non-responders, so the act of switching itself may not be detrimental to outcome. Overall, 68% of individuals experienced a period of cognitive stabilisation before continuing to decline at the pre-treatment rate. Other studies have found similar benefits alongside evidence that AChE-Is may reduce overall mortality.[19]

Switching between drugs used in dementia

The benefits of treatment with AChE-Is are rapidly lost when drug administration is interrupted[20] and may not be fully regained when drug treatment is reinitiated.[21] Poor tolerability with one agent does not rule out good tolerability with another.[22] The British Association for Psychopharmacology (BAP) guidelines for dementia confirm that previous comparative trials have failed to consistently demonstrate any significant differences in efficacy between the three AChE-Is, the main differences found being in frequency and type of adverse events. As a result, their recommendation remains valid that a significant proportion of patients (up to 50%) appear to both tolerate and benefit from switching between AChE-Is if they cannot tolerate one.[23]

Several cases of discontinuation syndrome upon stopping donepezil have been published[24,25] suggesting that a gradual withdrawal should be carried out where possible. However, a study comparing abrupt versus stepwise switching from donepezil to memantine found no clinically relevant differences in adverse effects despite patients in the abrupt group experiencing more frequent adverse effects than the stepwise discontinuation group (46% vs 32%, respectively).[26] (For switching to rivastigmine patch see 'Tolerability' later in this chapter.)

Following a systematic review of the literature,[27] a practical approach to switching between AChE-Is has been proposed. In the case of intolerance, switching to another agent should be done only after complete resolution of side effects following discontinuation of the initial agent. In the case of lack of efficacy, switching can be done overnight, with a quicker titration scheme thereafter. Switching to another AChE-I is not recommended in individuals who show loss of benefit several years after initiation of therapy.

Other effects

AChE-Is may also affect non-cognitive aspects of AD and other dementias. For more information about the management of these symptoms, see 'Management of behavioural and psychological symptoms of dementia (BPSD)' later in this chapter.

Dosing and formulations

For dosing information see Table 6.1 and up-to-date manufacturers' literature.

Rivastigmine transdermal patches (9.5mg/24 hours) have been shown to be as effective as the highest doses of capsules but with a superior tolerability profile in a 6-month double-blind placebo-controlled randomised controlled (RCT).[28] This has been confirmed in a Chinese study.[29] A nasal spray has also been developed.[30]

The US Food and Drug Administration (FDA) has approved a higher daily dose of **donepezil sustained release (23mg)** for moderate to severe AD. In the approval trial there was a small statistically significant improvement in cognition (a 2.2 improvement over the 10mg dose on the Severe Impairment Battery [SIB] scale) but no difference in global functioning (a 0.06 improvement on the Clinician's Interview-Based Impression of Change plus caregiver input [CIBIC-plus] scale). Furthermore, the higher dose was not superior on either of the prespecified secondary outcome measures and the rate of gastrointestinal adverse effects was over three times higher (21%) in the first month in the group receiving donepezil 23mg than in the 10mg group (5.9%).[31]

The **memantine extended release (ER) 28mg once-daily capsule** formulation was approved in the USA in 2010. Its efficacy was demonstrated in a large, multinational, phase III trial which showed that the addition of memantine ER to ongoing cholinesterase inhibitors improved key outcomes compared with cholinesterase inhibitor monotherapy, including measures of cognition and global status. The most common adverse events were headache, diarrhoea and dizziness.[32] While the FDA chose to approve memantine ER based on efficacy data from this study, the European Medicines Agency decided against approval. It questioned the clinical relevance of the drug given the small differences on the co-primary endpoints and the non-significant differences on the functional measure. In addition, since no comparison studies were performed between memantine immediate release (IR) and memantine ER, the risk–benefit ratio could not be fully evaluated.[33]

CHAPTER 6

These high doses of donepezil and memantine have not yet been approved in the UK and many other countries. In addition, most older people seen in practice with AD are likely to be frailer and have more comorbidities than patients in clinical trials and may therefore be less likely to tolerate the higher doses.

Combination treatment

Guidelines and the UK's National Institute for Health and Care Excellence (NICE)[1] recommend the use of a combination of AChE-I plus memantine rather than AChE-I alone in patients with moderate to severe AD. A network meta-analysis of 54 trials found that memantine plus donepezil showed superior outcomes for cognition, global assessment, daily activities and neuropsychiatric symptoms, but lower acceptability than monotherapy and placebo. A 2022 analysis observed broadly similar outcomes.[34] Combination therapy may be more cost-effective because memantine slows the progression of AD.[35] A Cochrane review has confirmed these recommendations for combined therapy.[36] Studies have also shown that there are no pharmacokinetic or pharmacodynamic interactions between AChE-Is and memantine.[37,38]

Drug tolerability

Drug tolerability may differ between AChE-Is, but, in the absence of sufficient direct comparisons, it is difficult to draw conclusions. Overall tolerability can be broadly evaluated by reference to the numbers withdrawing from clinical trials. Withdrawal rates in trials of donepezil[39,40] ranged from 4% to 16% (placebo 1–7%), 7% to 29% (placebo 7%) with rivastigmine[41,42] and 7% to 23% (placebo 7–9%) with galantamine.[43–45] These figures relate to withdrawals specifically associated with adverse effects. The number needed to harm (NNH) has been reported to be 12.[16] A study of the French pharmacovigilance database identified age and the use of antipsychotic drugs, antihypertensives and drugs targeting the alimentary tract and metabolism as factors associated with serious reactions to AChE-Is.[46] It has also been suggested that donepezil and rivastigmine are active centrally (CNS events, extrapyramidal symptoms, sleep disturbances and cardiorespiratory events), in contrast to galantamine, which is more active peripherally (muscle cramps and weakness, cardiorespiratory events and urinary incontinence).[47]

Tolerability seems to be affected by the speed of titration and, perhaps less clearly, by dose. Most adverse effects occurred in trials during titration, and slower titration schedules are recommended in clinical use. This may mean that these drugs are equally well tolerated in practice.

Rivastigmine patches offer convenience and a superior tolerability profile to rivastigmine capsules.[28,29] Data from three trials found that rivastigmine patches were better tolerated than the capsules with fewer gastrointestinal adverse effects and fewer discontinuations due to these adverse effects.[48] Data support recommendations for patients on high doses of rivastigmine capsules (>6mg/day) to switch directly to the 9.5mg/24 hours patch, while those on lower doses (≤6mg/day) should start on 4.6mg/hour patch for 4 weeks before increasing to the 9.5mg/hour patch. This latter switch is also recommended for patients switching from other oral cholinesterase inhibitors to the rivastigmine patch (with a 1-week washout period in patients sensitive to adverse effects or who have very low body weight or a history of bradycardia).[49] It is possible to consider increasing the dose to 13.3mg/24 hours after 6 months on 9.5mg/24 hours if tolerated and cognitive or functional decline occurs on the lower dose. A 48-week RCT found the higher-strength patch (13.3mg) significantly reduced deterioration in instrumental activities of daily living (IADL) compared with the 9.5mg/24 hours patch and was well tolerated.[50]

Patients and caregivers should be instructed on important administration details for the rivastigmine patch:[9]

- The transdermal patch should not be applied to skin that is red, irritated or cut.
- Reapplication to the exact same skin location within 14 days should be avoided to minimise the potential **risk of skin irritation.**
- The previous day's patch must be removed before applying a new one every day.
- Only one patch should be worn at a time.
- The patch should not be cut into pieces.

The following cautions exist for the use of AChE-Is: asthma, chronic obstructive pulmonary disease (COPD), sick sinus syndrome, supraventricular conduction abnormalities, susceptibility to peptic ulcers, history of seizures, bladder (or gastrointestinal) outflow obstruction, cardiac disease, congestive heart failure, unstable angina, electrolyte disturbances; and for rivastigmine patches: risk of fatal overdose with patch administration errors.[7]

Memantine appears to be well tolerated[51,52] and the only conditions associated with warnings include severe hepatic impairment and epilepsy/seizures.[53] (See *BNF* or equivalent for required dosage adjustments in renal impairment.) Isolated cases of international normalised ratio (INR) increases have been reported when memantine is co-administered with warfarin.

Adverse effects of drugs

Cholinesterase inhibitors

When adverse effects occur with AChE-Is they are largely predictable: excess cholinergic stimulation leads to nausea, vomiting, dizziness, insomnia and diarrhoea.[54] Such effects are most likely to occur at the start of therapy or when the dose is increased. They are dose related and tend to be transient. Urinary incontinence has also been reported.[55]

A network meta-analysis[56] compared efficacy and safety with these agents and found the following hierarchy in terms of tolerability:

- Withdrawals from studies due to adverse effects: donepezil > galantamine > rivastigmine patch > rivastigmine (meaning donepezil is best tolerated and so on).
- Nausea: rivastigmine patch > donepezil > galantamine > rivastigmine.
- Vomiting: donepezil > rivastigmine patch > galantamine > rivastigmine.
- Diarrhoea: galantamine > rivastigmine > rivastigmine patch > donepezil.
- Dizziness: rivastigmine patch > galantamine > donepezil > rivastigmine.

CHAPTER 6

An analysis of 16 years of individual case safety reports from VigiBase found that the most common adverse effects reported with AChE-Is were neuropsychiatric symptoms (31.4%), gastrointestinal disorders (15.9%) and general disorders and administration site conditions (11.9%). Cardiovascular adverse drug reactions (ADRs) accounted for 11.7% of ADRs.[57]

In view of their pharmacological action, AChE-Is can be expected to have vagotonic effects on the heart rate (i.e. bradycardia). The potential for this action may be of particular importance in patients with sick sinus syndrome or other supraventricular cardiac conduction disturbances, such as sinoatrial or atrioventricular block.[7-12]

Concerns over the potential cardiac adverse effects associated with AChE-Is were raised following findings from controlled trials of galantamine in mild cognitive impairment (MCI) in which increased mortality was associated with galantamine compared with placebo (1.5% vs 0.5%).[58] Although no specific cause of death was dominant, half the deaths reported were due to cardiovascular disorders. As a result, the FDA issued a warning restricting galantamine in patients with MCI. The relevance to AD remains unclear.[59]

The most prominent cardiovascular adverse effects of AChE-Is are bradycardia and syncope, which can result in serious outcomes such as falls, fractures and other trauma as well as necessitate pacemaker placement. If these adverse effects are experienced, patients should undergo a thorough history/evaluation, including a medication review, rhythm monitoring, consideration of neurological symptoms, lowering the doses of other medications that might contribute to bradycardia, stopping or reducing the AChE-I dose or even pacemaker placement. Many of these factors should be considered before the initiation of these medications and periodically thereafter to optimise patient care and mitigate possible adverse events[60,61] (Figure 6.1). There are also a few reports that they may occasionally be associated with QT prolongation and torsades de pointes.[62]

It seems that patients with DLB are more susceptible to the bradyarrhythmic adverse effects of these drugs owing to the autonomic insufficiency associated with the disease.[63]

The manufacturers of all three agents advise that the drugs should be used with caution in patients with cardiovascular disease or in those taking concurrent medicines that reduce heart rate (e.g. digoxin or β blockers). Although a pre-treatment mandatory electrocardiogram (ECG) has been suggested,[59] a review of published evidence showed that the incidence of cardiovascular side effects is low and that serious adverse effects are rare. In addition, the value of pre-treatment screening and routine ECGs is questionable and is not currently recommended by NICE. However, in patients with a history of cardiovascular disease or who are prescribed concomitant negative chronotropic drugs with AChE-Is, an ECG is advised.[60]

Memantine

Although little is known about the cardiovascular effects of memantine, there have been reports of bradycardia and reduced cardiovascular survival associated with its use.[64]

An analysis of pooled prospective data for memantine revealed that the most frequently reported adverse effects in placebo-controlled trials included agitation

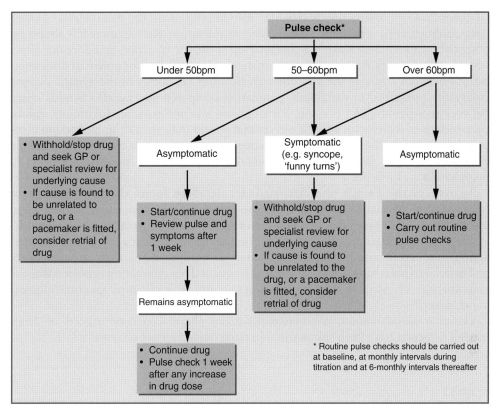

Figure 6.1 Suggested guidelines for managing cardiovascular risk prior to and during treatment with acetylcholinesterase inhibitors (AChE-Is) in Alzheimer's disease.[60,61] bpm, beats per minute. Reproduced with permission from Rowland et al. 2007, © 2007 by The Royal College of Psychiatrists.

(7.5% memantine vs 12% placebo), falls (6.8% vs 7.1%), dizziness (6.3% vs 5.7%), accidental injury (6.0% vs 7.2%), influenza-like symptoms (6.0% vs 5.8%), headache (5.2% vs 3.7%) and diarrhoea (5.0% vs 5.6%).[65] Given the higher or similar rates seen with placebo, few conclusions can be drawn.

The French pharmacovigilance database compared adverse effects reported with donepezil with memantine. The most frequent ADRs with donepezil alone and memantine alone were respectively bradycardia (10% vs 7%), weakness (5% vs 6%) and convulsions (4% vs 3%). Although it is well known that donepezil is often associated with bradycardia and memantine associated with seizures, this analysis suggested that memantine can also induce bradycardia and donepezil seizures, thus highlighting the care required when treating patients with dementia who have a history of bradycardia or epilepsy.[66]

Drug interactions

Potential for interaction may also differentiate currently available cholinesterase inhibitors. Donepezil[67] and galantamine[68] are metabolised by cytochromes 2D6 and 3A4 so drug levels may be altered by other drugs affecting the function of these enzymes.

Cholinesterase inhibitors themselves may also interfere with the metabolism of other drugs, although this is perhaps a theoretical consideration. Rivastigmine has almost no potential for interaction since it is metabolised at the site of action and does not affect hepatic cytochromes. A prospective pharmacodynamic analysis of potential drug interactions between rivastigmine and other medications (22 different therapeutic classes) commonly prescribed in the elderly population compared adverse effects odds ratios between rivastigmine and placebo. Rivastigmine was not associated with any significant pattern of increase in adverse effects that would indicate a drug interaction compared with placebo.[69] Rivastigmine thus appears to be least likely to cause problematic drug interactions, a factor that may be important in an elderly population subject to polypharmacy (Table 6.2).

Analysis of the French pharmacovigilance database found that the majority of reported drug interactions concerning AChE-Is were pharmacodynamic in nature and most frequently involved the combination of AChE-I and bradycardic drugs (β blockers, digoxin, amiodarone, calcium channel antagonists). Almost a third of these interactions resulted in cardiovascular ADRs such as bradycardia, atrioventricular block and arterial hypotension. The second most frequent drug interaction reported was the combination of AChE-I with anticholinergic drugs leading to pharmacological antagonism.[70]

The pharmacodynamics, pharmacokinetic and pharmacogenetic aspects of drugs used in dementia have been summarised in two comprehensive reviews.[71,72]

Table 6.2 Drug–drug interactions.[8–12,73,74]

Drug	Metabolism	Plasma levels increased by	Plasma levels decreased by	Pharmacodynamic interactions
Donepezil (Aricept®)	Substrate at 3A4 and 2D6	Ketoconazole Itraconazole Erythromycin Quinidine Fluoxetine Paroxetine	Rifampicin Phenytoin Carbamazepine Alcohol	Antagonistic with anticholinergic drugs and competitive neuromuscular blockers (e.g. tubocurarine). Potential for synergistic activity with cholinomimetics such as depolarising neuromuscular blocking agents (e.g. succinylcholine), cholinergic agonists and peripherally acting cholinesterase inhibitors (e.g. neostigmine). Beta blockers, amiodarone or calcium channel blockers may have additive effects on cardiac conduction. Caution with concomitant use of drugs known to induce QT prolongation and/or torsades de pointes. Movement disorders and neuroleptic malignant syndrome have occurred with concomitant use of antipsychotics and cholinesterase inhibitors. Concurrent use with seizure lowering agents may result in reduced seizure threshold.

CHAPTER 6

Table 6.2 (*Continued*)

Drug	Metabolism	Plasma levels increased by	Plasma levels decreased by	Pharmacodynamic interactions
Rivastigmine (Exelon®)	Non-hepatic metabolism	Metabolic interactions appear unlikely Smoking tobacco increases the clearance of rivastigmine		Antagonistic effects with anticholinergic and competitive neuromuscular blockers (e.g. tubocurarine). Potential for synergistic activity with cholinomimetics such as depolarising neuromuscular blocking agents (e.g. succinylcholine), cholinergic agonists (e.g. bethanecol) or peripherally acting cholinesterase inhibitors (e.g. neostigmine). Synergistic effects on cardiac conduction with β blockers, amiodarone and calcium channel blockers. Caution with concomitant use of drugs known to induce QT prolongation and/or torsades de pointes. Movement disorders and neuroleptic malignant syndrome have occurred with concomitant use of antipsychotics and cholinesterase inhibitors. Concurrent use with metoclopramide may result in increased risk of EPSEs.
Galantamine (Reminyl®)	Substrate at 3A4 and 2D6	Ketoconazole Erythromycin Ritonavir Quinidine Paroxetine Fluoxetine Fluvoxamine Amitriptyline	None known	Antagonistic effects with anticholinergic and competitive neuromuscular blockers (e.g. tubocurarine). Potential for synergistic activity with cholinomimetics such as depolarising neuromuscular blocking agents (e.g. succinylcholine), cholinergic agonists and peripherally acting cholinesterase inhibitors (e.g. neostigmine). Possible interaction with agents that significantly reduce heart rate such as digoxin, β blockers, certain calcium channel blockers and amiodarone. Caution with concomitant use of drugs known to induce QT prolongation and/or torsades de pointes (manufacturer recommends ECG in such cases). Movement disorders and neuroleptic malignant syndrome have occurred with concomitant use of antipsychotics and cholinesterase inhibitors.

(Continued)

Table 6.2 (*Continued*)

Drug	Metabolism	Plasma levels increased by	Plasma levels decreased by	Pharmacodynamic interactions
Memantine (Exiba®)	Primarily non-hepatic metabolism Renally eliminated	Cimetidine Ranitidine Procainamide Quinidine Quinine Nicotine Trimethoprim Isolated cases of INR increases reported with concomitant warfarin (close monitoring of prothrombin time or INR advisable) Drugs that alkalinise urine (pH ~8) may reduce renal elimination of memantine, e.g. carbonic anhydrase inhibitors, sodium bicarbonate	None known (Possibility of reduced serum level of hydrochlorothiazide when co-administered with memantine)	Effects of L-dopa, dopaminergic agonists, selegiline and anticholinergics may be enhanced. Effects of barbiturates and antipsychotics may be reduced. Avoid concomitant use with amantadine, ketamine and dextromethorphan – increased risk of CNS toxicity. One published case report on possible risk for phenytoin and memantine combination. Dosage adjustment may be necessary for antispasmodic agents, dantrolene or baclofen when administered with memantine. A single case report of myoclonus and confusion when co-administered with co-trimoxazole or trimethoprim

NB This list is not exhaustive. Take caution with other drugs that are also inhibitors or enhancers of CYP3A4 and CYP2D6 enzymes.
EPSEs, extrapyramidal side effects; INR, international normalised ratio.

When to stop treatment

A large multicentre study[75] of community-dwelling patients with moderate or severe AD investigated the long-term effects of donepezil over 12 months compared with stopping donepezil after 3 months, switching to memantine or combining donepezil with memantine. Continued treatment with donepezil was associated with continued cognitive benefits, and patients with an MMSE score as low as 3 also benefitted from treatment. This suggests that patients should continue treatment with AChE-Is for as long as possible and there should not be a cut-off MMSE score where treatment is stopped automatically. Moreover, secondary and post-hoc analyses of this study found that withdrawal of donepezil in patients with moderate to severe AD increased the risk of nursing home placement during 12 months of treatment but made no difference during the following 3 years of follow-up. This highlights the point that decisions to stop or continue treatment should be informed by potential risks of withdrawal, even if the perceived benefits of continued treatment are not clear.[76] A 2021 Cochrane review came to similar conclusions.[36]

The consensus opinion is that if the drug is well tolerated and the patient's physical health is stable, then it is probably best to continue the drug. The risks of discontinuation of dementia medication should be balanced against the adverse effects.[77]

In addition to this, a meta-analysis evaluating the efficacy of the three AChE-Is and memantine in relation to the severity of AD found that the efficacy of all drugs except memantine was independent of dementia severity in all domains. The effect of memantine on functional impairment was actually better in patients with more severe AD. This suggests that the severity of a patient's illness should not preclude treatment with these drugs.[78]

Guidance for discontinuation of dementia medication in clinical practice is summarised here.[79]

Reasons for stopping treatment
- When the patient/caregiver decides to stop (after being advised on the risks and benefits of stopping treatment).
- When the patient refuses to take the medication (but see 'Covert administration of medicines within food and drink' later in this chapter).
- When there are problems with patient compliance which cannot be reasonably resolved.
- When the patient's cognitive, functional or behavioural decline is worsened by treatment.
- When there are intolerable adverse effects.
- When comorbidities make treatment risky or futile (e.g. terminal illness).
- Where there is no clinically meaningful benefit to continuing therapy (clinical judgement should be used here rather than ceasing treatment when a patient reaches a certain score on a cognitive outcome or when they are institutionalised).
- When dementia has progressed to a severely impaired stage (Global Deterioration Scale stage 7: development of swallowing difficulties).

When a decision is made to stop therapy (for reasons other than lack of tolerability), tapering of the dose and monitoring the patient for evidence of significant decline during the next 1–3 months are advised. If such decline occurs, reinstatement of therapy should be considered.

NICE recommendations

NICE guidance on dementia[80] was last updated in June 2018 (Box 6.2).

Other treatments *(where the evidence remains less certain)*

A 2009 Cochrane review[81] concluded that **Ginkgo biloba** appears to be safe in use with no excess adverse effects compared with placebo, but the evidence that it has predictable and clinically significant benefit for people with dementia or cognitive impairment is inconsistent and unreliable. In contrast, a 2015 systematic review and meta-analysis[82]

Box 6.2 Summary of NICE guidance for the treatment of AD[80,83]

- The three AChE-Is donepezil, galantamine and rivastigmine are recommended for managing mild to moderate AD
- Memantine is recommended for managing moderate AD for people who are intolerant of or have a contraindication to AChE-Is or for managing severe AD
- For people with an established diagnosis of AD who are already taking an AChE-I:
  - consider memantine in addition to an AChE-I if they have moderate disease
  - offer memantine in addition to an AChE-I if they have severe disease
- For people who are not taking an AChE-I or memantine, prescribers should only start treatment with these on the advice of a clinician who has the necessary knowledge and skills. This could include:
  - secondary care medical specialists such as psychiatrists, geriatricians and neurologists
  - other healthcare professionals (such as GPs, nurse consultants and advanced nurse practitioners) if they have specialist expertise in diagnosing and treating AD
- Once a decision has been made to start an AChE-I or memantine, the first prescription may be made in primary care
- For people with an established diagnosis of AD who are already taking an AChE-I, primary care prescribers may start treatment with memantine without taking advice from a specialist clinician
- Ensure that local arrangements for prescribing, supply and treatment review follow the NICE guideline on medicines optimisation[84]
- Do not stop AChE-Is in people with AD because of disease severity alone
- Therapy with an AChE-I should be initiated with a drug with the lowest acquisition cost (taking into account required daily dose and the price per dose once shared care has started). An alternative may be considered on the basis of adverse effects profile, expectations about adherence, medical comorbidity, possibility of drug interactions and dosing profiles

Summary of NICE guidance for the treatment of non-AD dementia[80,83]

- Offer donepezil or rivastigmine to people with mild to moderate DLB
- Only consider galantamine for people with mild to moderate DLB if donepezil and rivastigmine are not tolerated
- Consider donepezil or rivastigmine for people with severe DLB
- Consider memantine for people with DLB if AChE-Is are not tolerated or are contraindicated
- Only consider AChE-Is or memantine for people with VaD if they have suspected comorbid AD, Parkinson's disease dementia or DLB
- Do not offer AChE-Is or memantine to people with frontotemporal dementia
- Do not offer AChE-Is or memantine to people with cognitive impairment caused by multiple sclerosis
- For guidance on pharmacological management of Parkinson's disease dementia, see Parkinson's disease dementia in the NICE guideline on Parkinson's disease

Medicines that may cause cognitive impairment[1]

- Be aware that some commonly prescribed medicines are associated with increased anticholinergic burden, and therefore cognitive impairment
- Consider minimising the use of medicines associated with increased anticholinergic burden, and if possible look for alternatives:
  - when assessing whether to refer a person with suspected dementia for diagnosis
  - during medication reviews with people living with dementia
- Be aware that there are validated tools for assessing anticholinergic burden but there is insufficient evidence to recommend one over the others (see 'Safer prescribing for physical conditions in dementia' later in this chapter).
- For guidance on carrying out medication reviews, see the medication review in the NICE guideline on medicines optimisation[84]

NB The Anticholinergic Effect on Cognition (AEC) scale can be accessed at www.medichec.com.

AChE-I, acetylcholinesterase inhibitors; AD, Alzheimer's disease; DLB, dementia with Lewy bodies; VaD, vascular dementia.

found that Ginkgo biloba 240mg/day was able to stabilise or slow decline in cognition, function, behaviour and global change at 22–26 weeks in patients with cognitive impairment and dementia, especially for patients with neuropsychiatric symptoms. A 2022 umbrella review confirmed the efficacy of Ginkgo.[85] Several reports have noted that Ginkgo may increase the risk of bleeding.[86]

The findings of a systematic review[87] suggest that supplementation of **B complex vitamins**, especially **folic acid**, may have a positive effect on delaying and preventing the risk of cognitive decline. **Ascorbic acid** and a high dose of **vitamin E**, when given separately, also showed positive effects on cognitive performance, but there is not sufficient evidence to support their use. The results of **vitamin D** supplementation trials are not conclusive in assessing the potential benefits that vitamin D might have on cognition.

A Cochrane review of **omega-3 fatty acids** for the treatment of dementia (632 people with mild to moderate AD) found that taking omega-3 polyunsaturated fatty acid supplements for 6 months had no effect on cognition (learning and understanding), everyday functioning, quality of life or mental health. The trials did not report side effects very well, but none of the studies described significant harmful effects on health.[88]

A systematic review and meta-analysis including four RCTs involving 259 participants suggested that the effects of **ginseng** on AD remain unproven.[89]

Natural **hirudin**, isolated from the salivary gland of the medicinal leech, is a direct thrombin inhibitor and has been used for many years in China. A small 20-week open-label RCT of 84 patients receiving donepezil or donepezil plus hirudin (3g/day) found that patients on the combination showed significant decrease in ADAS-cog scores and significant increase in ADL scores compared with donepezil alone. However, haemorrhage and hypersensitivity reactions were more common in the combination group than in the donepezil group (11.9% and 7.1% vs 2.4% and 2.4%, respectively).[77] The potential haemorrhagic effects of hirudin need further exploration before it can be considered for clinical use.

Huperzine A, an alkaloid isolated from the Chinese herb *Huperzia serrata*, is a potent, highly selective, reversible AChE-I used for treating AD since 1994 in China and available as a nutraceutical in the USA. Despite its promising effects on cognition and ADLs, there is insufficient evidence to support its use in dementia[90] or MCI[90,91] due to the high heterogeneity of reviews and low quality of primary studies. High-quality, large, multi-centre RCTs with long-term follow-up in different settings are warranted but no studies have been published since 2020. A Cochrane review of huperzine A in VaD found no convincing evidence for its value in VaD.[92]

There is increasing evidence to suggest possible efficacy of *Crocus sativus* (**saffron**) in the management of AD. A systematic review and meta-analysis of RCTs revealed that saffron significantly improves cognitive function measured by ADAS-cog and the Clinical Dementia Rating Scale – Sums of Boxes (CDR-SB) compared with placebo groups. In addition, there was no difference between saffron and conventional medicines (donepezil, memantine). No serious adverse events were reported in the included studies. Saffron may be beneficial in improving cognitive function in patients with MCI and AD, however no evidence was found to support its effects on other types of dementia. More high-quality randomised placebo-controlled trials are needed to further confirm the efficacy and safety of saffron for MCI and dementia.[93]

Cerebrolysin is a parenterally administered, porcine brain-derived peptide preparation that has pharmacodynamic properties similar to those of endogenous neurotrophic

CHAPTER 6

factors. A meta-analysis included six RCTs comparing cerebrolysin 30mg/day with placebo in mild to moderate AD. Cerebrolysin was more effective than placebo at 4 weeks regarding cognitive function and at 4 weeks and 6 months regarding global clinical change and 'global benefit'. Its safety was comparable with placebo. In addition, a large 28-week RCT comparing cerebrolysin, donepezil or combination therapy showed (i) higher improvements in global outcome for cerebrolysin and the combination therapy than for donepezil alone at study endpoint; (ii) a lack of significant group differences in cognitive, functional and behavioural domains at the endpoint; and (iii) best scores of cognitive improvement in the combination therapy group at all study visits.[94] This therapeutic option requires further investigation in large trials.

A Cochrane review assessing cerebrolysin in VaD found that intravenous courses improved cognition and general function in people living with VaD, with no suggestion of adverse effects. However, these data are not definitive. The analyses were limited by heterogeneity, and studies had high risk of bias. If there are benefits, the effects may be too small to be clinically meaningful. Cerebrolysin continues to be used and promoted as a treatment for VaD, but the supporting evidence base is weak. The most commonly reported non-serious adverse events were headache, aesthenia, dizziness, hypertension and hypotension.[95]

For information on **statins** see 'Safer prescribing for physical conditions in dementia' later in this chapter.

A longitudinal prospective study examined the relationship between **chocolate** consumption and cognitive decline in an elderly cognitively healthy population. A total of 531 participants aged ≥65 years with normal MMSE scores were followed for a median of 48 months. Dietary habits were evaluated at baseline and the MMSE was used to assess global cognitive function at baseline and at follow-up. After adjustment for confounders, chocolate intake was associated with a 41% lower risk of cognitive decline. This protective effect was observed only among subjects with an average daily consumption of caffeine lower than 75mg.[96]

Souvenaid is a medical food for the dietary management of early AD. A Cochrane review[97] concluded that it probably does not reduce the risk of progression to dementia, there is no convincing evidence that it affects other outcomes important to people with AD (in the prodromal stage or mild to moderate stages) and its effects in more severe AD remain unclear.

Idalopirdine is a $5HT_6$ receptor antagonist. The $5HT_6$ receptor is expressed in areas of the CNS involved with memory and there is evidence suggesting that blocking of these receptors induces acetylcholine release and could restore ACh levels in a deteriorated cholinergic system.[98] A systematic review and meta-analysis analysed four RCTs with 2803 patients with AD. Idalopirdine was not shown to be effective for AD patients and is associated with a risk of elevated liver enzymes and vomiting. Although idalopirdine might be more effective at high doses and in moderate AD subgroups, the effect size is small.[99]

A large number of RCTs of **anti-inflammatory drugs** in AD have failed to reach primary outcomes. Large-scale studies of non-steroidal anti-inflammatory drugs (NSAIDs) including indomethacin, naproxen and rofecoxib in AD have been unsuccessful. RCTs with a range of other anti-inflammatory drugs including prednisolone, hydroxychloroquine, simvastatin, atorvastatin, aspirin and rosiglitazone have also shown no clinically significant changes in primary cognitive outcomes in patients with AD.[23] A 2020 Cochrane review evaluated aspirin and other NSAIDs for the prevention of dementia and found no evidence to support the use of low-dose aspirin or other NSAIDs of any class (celecoxib, rofecoxib, naproxen) for the prevention of dementia. There was, however, evidence of harm including higher rates of death and major bleeding compared with placebo with aspirin, and in one of the studies more people developed dementia in the NSAID group. More stomach bleeding and other stomach problems, such as pain, nausea and gastritis, were also reported with NSAIDs.[100]

Two existing compounds, trazodone and dibenzoylmethane, were found to be markedly neuroprotective in mouse models of neurodegeneration, using clinically relevant doses over a prolonged period of time, without systemic toxicity. **Trazodone**, a serotonin antagonist and reuptake antidepressant with additional anxiolytic and hypnotic effects, was associated with delayed cognitive decline in a small retrospective study examining its long-term use. Trazodone non-users had a 2.6-fold faster decline in MMSE (primary outcome) assessment than trazodone users.[101] However, a study of UK population-based electronic health records found no association between trazodone use and a reduced risk of dementia compared with other antidepressants. These results suggest that the clinical use of trazodone is not associated with a reduced risk of dementia.[102] Similarly, three identical naturalistic cohort studies using UK clinical registers found no evidence of cognitive benefit from trazodone compared with other antidepressants in people with dementia.[104] Despite pre-clinical evidence, trazodone should not be prescribed for cognition in dementia.[103] There are no observational data suggesting trazodone reduces risk of dementia but some data that suggest important adverse outcomes in older people.[104] **Dibenzoylmethane** (DBM) is a minor constituent of liquorice that has been found to have antineoplastic effects, with efficacy against prostate and mammary tumours. In prion-diseased mice, both trazodone and DBM treatment restored memory deficits, abrogated the development of neurological signs, prevented neurodegeneration and significantly prolonged survival. In tauopathy-frontotemporal dementia mice, both drugs were neuroprotective, rescued memory deficits and reduced hippocampal atrophy. Further, trazodone reduced p-tau burden.[105]

KarXT (xanomeline plus trospium (Cobenfy)) is an investigational treatment that has shown early promise in the treatment of positive and negative symptoms of schizophrenia. Unlike all currently approved treatments for schizophrenia, KarXT does not directly bind to dopamine receptors; instead, the therapeutic effects of KarXT appear to be mediated through direct agonism of muscarinic acetylcholine receptors. To mitigate the cholinomimetic effects of xanomeline (e.g. vomiting), trospium is combined with xanomeline. Findings suggest that KarXT may have a separable and meaningful impact on cognition, particularly among patients with cognitive impairment.[106]

Quercetin is a flavonoid widely distributed among plants and found commonly in our daily diet (fruits and vegetables). It has beneficial properties against general mechanisms of AD aetiology; it protects neuronal cells by attenuating oxidative stress and neuroinflammation. Quercetin inhibits β-amyloid (Aβ) aggregation and tau phosphorylation and restores acetylcholine levels through the inhibition of hydrolysis of acetylcholine by AChE enzyme. Although showing neuroprotective efficacy in several in vitro and animal models, in vivo studies have reported that it is extensively metabolised upon absorption from the gut, affecting its bioavailability, and has low blood–brain barrier penetrability, thus limiting its efficacy in combating neurodegenerative disorders. Therefore, future clinical trials must improve its bioavailability, developing related molecules with greater gut and brain penetrability, which will likely improve clinical efficacy.[107]

CHAPTER 6

Novel treatments

Amyloid plaques are composed of β-amyloid (Aβ) in the extracellular space. Aβ is derived from the amyloid precursor protein (APP), a transmembrane protein. B secretase and γ secretase cleave the APP and generate pathological Aβ, and accumulation of Aβ results in neurotoxicity. Reducing the accumulation of Aβ has become a therapeutic purpose of AD. Antiamyloid therapy consists of three strategies: secretase inhibitors, Aβ aggregation inhibitors and Aβ immunotherapy.[108]

Aducanumab is an antibody that works by targeting Aβ and preferentially binds to the aggregated Aβ. Through this interaction, aducanumab could reduce the build-up of Aβ and therefore the number of amyloid plaques present in the brain, thus potentially slowing neurodegeneration and disease progression. Although in early 2019 the manufacturers (Biogen) announced that aducanumab failed futility analyses in two identically designed phase III AD trials and discontinued its development, later in the year they made the announcement that they were applying for US FDA marketing approval. They explained they had reanalysed data from the trials to include patients who had continued in the studies after the cut-off date for the futility analyses and stated that one trial showed significant findings and a subset from the second trial supports these positive findings.[109] One concern with aducanumab was the frequency of adverse effects, particularly amyloid-related imaging abnormalities (ARIAs). In June 2021, the FDA made the decision to grant conditional accelerated approval for aducanumab to treat AD patients. Aducanumab was not approved in Europe.

The phase III trial of **lecanemab** (Clarity-AD trial) was more encouraging. Lecanemab lowers brain Aβ plaque burden through binding to soluble Aβ protofibrils as well as (to a variable extent) other forms of Aβ. The study included 1795 participants with MCI or early AD plus evidence of amyloid on a positron emission tomography (PET) scan or by cerebrospinal fluid testing. They were randomly assigned to receive 10mg/kg body weight of lecanemab via intravenous infusion every 2 weeks or matched placebo. After 18 months, lecanemab reduced cognitive decline, as measured by CDR-SB, which quantifies symptom severity across a range of cognitive and functional domains, by 27% compared with placebo; an absolute difference of 0.45 points (change from baseline 1.21 for lecanemab vs 1.66 with placebo, p <0.001). All key secondary endpoints were also met. The incidence of ARIAs, which manifest as oedema or microhaemorrhages, was 21% of the lecanemab group. Most cases were asymptomatic and detected incidentally. However, reports of deaths in the open-label extension phase of the study (possibly linked to co-administration of the thrombolytic drug alteplase) have heightened concerns about lecanemab's safety in patients taking thrombolytic drugs.[110,111] Lecanemab has been approved by the FDA and was undergoing a full evaluation by the European Medicines Agency at the time of writing.[112]

Donanemab is another high-potency antiamyloid drug infused intravenously every 4 weeks. In 2022, results were announced for the phase III trial (TRAILBLAZER-ALZ 2 trial) which included 1736 participants with early symptomatic AD (MCI/mild dementia) with amyloid and low/medium or high tau pathology based on PET imaging. Compared with placebo, donanemab treatment over 18 months resulted in slowing of cognitive and functional decline by approximately 35% in the primary target population studied. In addition, 52% of treated participants converted to amyloid PET-negative status by 12 months. ARIA-E (with oedema) and ARIA-H (with microhaemorrhage/haemosiderosis) occurred in

24.0% and 31.4% of treated individuals, respectively.[113,114] Donanemab is, at the time of writing, undergoing a full evaluation by the FDA and NICE.

The development of three monoclonal antibodies, **gosuranemab, tilavonemab** and **zagotenemab**, was terminated due to negative results. A phase II study of **semorinemab**, an anti-tau monoclonal antibody, was negative. While semorinemab had a significant effect on cognition measured by the ADAS-Cog11, this effect did not extend to improved functional or global outcomes.[115] Further exploration is required. Clinical trials of anti-tau vaccines are underway.

In addition to the above, results of recent trials of **solanezumab, crenezumab** and **gantenerumab** were all negative.

Vascular dementia (VaD)

Vascular dementia comprises 10–50% of dementia cases and is the second most common type of dementia after AD. It is caused by ischaemic damage to the brain and is associated with cognitive impairment and behavioural disturbances. The management options are currently very limited and focus on controlling the underlying risk factors for cerebrovascular disease.[116]

Note that it is impossible to diagnose with certainty vascular or Alzheimer's dementia and much dementia has mixed causation. This might explain why certain AChE-Is do not always provide consistent results in probable VaD and the data indicating efficacy in cognitive outcomes were derived from older patients, who were therefore likely to have concomitant AD pathology.[117]

None of the currently available drugs is formally licensed in the UK for VaD. The management of VaD has been summarised.[118,119] Unlike the situation with stroke, there is no conclusive evidence that treatment of hyperlipidaemia with statins or treatment of blood clotting abnormalities with acetylsalicylic acid has an effect on VaD incidence or disease progression.[120] Similarly, a Cochrane review found that there were no studies supporting the role of statins in the treatment of VaD.[121] A Cochrane review of cholinesterase inhibitors for VaD and other vascular cognitive impairments found moderate- to high-certainty evidence that donepezil 5mg, donepezil 10mg and galantamine 16–24mg have a slight beneficial effect on cognition in people with vascular cognitive impairment, although the size of the change is unlikely to be clinically important. Donepezil 10mg and galantamine 16–24mg are probably associated with more adverse events than placebo. The evidence for rivastigmine was less certain. Data suggest that donepezil 10mg has the greatest effect on cognition, but at the cost of adverse effects. The effect is modest, but in the absence of any other treatments, these agents may be considered in people living with vascular cognitive impairments. Further research into rivastigmine is needed, including the use of transdermal patches.[122]

A meta-analysis of RCTs found that cholinesterase inhibitors and memantine produce small benefits in cognition of uncertain clinical significance and concluded that data were insufficient to support widespread use of these agents in VaD; the effect is lower than that seen in AD, although no direct comparison has been made.[116] A systematic review and Bayesian network meta-analysis comparing the efficacy and safety of cognitive enhancers for treating vascular cognitive impairment found significant efficacy for donepezil, galantamine and memantine on cognition. Memantine was found to provide significant efficacy in global status. They were all safe and well tolerated.[123]

CHAPTER 6

Dementia with Lewy bodies (DLB)

DLB may account for 15–25% of cases of dementia. Characteristic symptoms are dementia with fluctuation of cognitive ability, early and persistent visual hallucinations and spontaneous motor features of parkinsonism. Falls, syncope, transient disturbances of consciousness, neuroleptic sensitivity and hallucinations in other modalities are also common.[124]

There are significant complexities in managing an individual with DLB. Presentation varies between patients and can vary over time within an individual. Treatments can address one symptom but worsen another, which makes disease management difficult. Symptoms are often managed in isolation and by different specialists, which makes high-quality care difficult to accomplish. Clinical trials and meta-analyses now provide an evidence base for the treatment of cognitive, neuropsychiatric and motor symptoms in patients with DLB.[125] In summary, robust evidence exists for the efficacy of rivastigmine and donepezil in the treatment of cognitive symptoms in patients with DLB, but high-quality RCTs of galantamine are needed. Memantine could have some benefits, but further studies with larger numbers of patients are also needed to determine whether there is an improvement and, if so, which specific symptoms are improved. Whether memantine should be used as a monotherapy or whether it should be combined with cholinesterase inhibitors is also unclear.[125,126]

For a helpful guide on the management of specific symptoms in DLB see the management of DLB summary sheets.[127]

The 2018 update of the NICE guidelines[1] recommends the use of AChE-Is and memantine (if AChE-Is are not tolerated) in DLB and Parkinson's disease dementia (see Box 6.2).

Mild cognitive impairment (MCI)

Mild cognitive impairment is hypothesised to represent a pre-clinical stage of dementia but forms a heterogeneous group with variable prognosis. A Cochrane review assessing the safety and efficacy of AChE-Is in MCI found there was very little evidence that they affect progression to dementia or cognitive test scores. This weak evidence was countered by the increased risk of adverse effects, particularly gastrointestinal effects, meaning that AChE-Is could not be recommended in MCI.[128] A systematic review[129] found that there was no replicated evidence that any intervention was effective for MCI including AChE-Is and the NSAID rofecoxib. A further systematic review and meta-analysis found that although AChE-Is have a slight efficacy in the treatment of MCI, there are many safety issues, therefore they are difficult to recommend for MCI.[130] Experts from several different countries have reviewed the available evidence for the pharmacological and non-pharmacological treatment for MCI.[131,132]

Other dementias

A systemic review of RCTs for **frontotemporal dementias** showed that certain drugs may be effective in reducing behavioural symptoms (e.g. SSRIs, trazodone) but none of these had an effect on cognition.[133] Due to new techniques in neuroimaging, genetics and biomarker analysis, much has been discovered about the phenomena underlying frontotemporal lobar degeneration. This has allowed the design of new molecule-based therapies that are still in the early stages of research but may show promise.[134]

A Cochrane review assessed the efficacy and safety of AChE-Is for **rare dementias associated with neurological conditions**. The sample sizes of most trials were very small and efficacy on cognitive function was found to be unclear, although AChE-Is were associated with more gastrointestinal adverse effects than placebo.[135]

Summary of clinical practice guidance for use of anti-dementia drugs

AChE-Is and memantine are effective in AD of a broad range of severity. Other drugs including statins, anti-inflammatory drugs, vitamin E, nutritional supplements and Gingko cannot be recommended either for the treatment or prevention of AD. Neither AChE-Is nor memantine are effective in MCI. AChE-Is are not effective in frontotemporal dementia and may cause agitation. AChE-Is may be used for people with Lewy body dementia (both Parkinson's disease dementia and DLB), and memantine may be helpful. No drugs are clearly effective in VaD, though AChE-Is are beneficial in mixed dementia. Early evidence suggests multifactorial interventions may have the potential to prevent or delay the onset of dementia. Many novel pharmacological approaches involving strategies to reduce amyloid and/or tau deposition in those with or at high risk of AD are in progress. Although results of pivotal studies in early (prodromal/mild) AD are awaited, results to date in more established (mild to moderate) AD have been equivocal and no disease-modifying agents are either licensed or can be currently recommended for clinical use.

Table 6.3 summarises the clinical practice guidelines from BAP.[23]

Table 6.3 Summary of British Association for Psychopharmacology recommendations.

	First choice	Second choice
Alzheimer's disease	AChE-Is	Memantine
Vascular dementia	None (some benefit with donepezil 10mg – but risk of adverse effects)	None
Mixed dementia	AChE-Is	Memantine
Dementia with Lewy bodies	AChE-Is	Memantine
Mild cognitive impairment	None	None
Dementia with Parkinson's disease	AChE-Is	Memantine
Frontotemporal dementia	None	None

AChE-Is, acetylcholinesterase inhibitors.

References

1. National Institute for Health and Care Excellence. Dementia: assessment, management and support for people living with dementia and their carers. NICE Guideline [NG97]. 2018 (checked September 2023, last accessed December 2023); https://www.nice.org.uk/guidance/ng97.

2. Francis PT, et al. The cholinergic hypothesis of Alzheimer's disease: a review of progress. *J Neurol Neurosurg Psychiatry* 1999; **66**:137–147.

3. Craig LA, et al. Revisiting the cholinergic hypothesis in the development of Alzheimer's disease. *Neurosci Biobehav Rev* 2011; **35**:1397–1409.

4. Mesulam M, et al. Widely spread butyrylcholinesterase can hydrolyze acetylcholine in the normal and Alzheimer brain. *Neurobiol Dis* 2002; **9**:88–93.

5. Weinstock M. Selectivity of cholinesterase inhibition: clinical implications for the treatment of Alzheimer's disease. *CNS Drugs* 1999; **12**:307–323.

6. Matsunaga S, et al. Memantine monotherapy for Alzheimer's disease: a systematic review and meta-analysis. *PLoS One* 2015; **10**:e0123289.

7. Joint Formulary Committee. *British National Formulary (online)*. London: BMJ and Pharmaceutical Press; http://www.medicinescomplete.com.

8. Eisai Ltd. Summary of product characteristics. Aricept 5mg, 10mg tablets (donepezil). 2023; https://www.medicines.org.uk/emc/product/3776/smpc.

9. Novartis Pharmaceuticals UK Ltd. Summary of product characteristics. Exelon 4.6mg/24h, 9.5mg/24h, 13.3mg/24h transdermal patch. 2023; https://www.medicines.org.uk/emc/product/7764/smpc.

10. Sandoz Ltd. Summary of product characteristics. Rivastigmine Sandoz 1.5mg, 3mg, 4.5mg, 6mg hard capsules. 2021; https://www.medicines.org.uk/emc/product/8407/smpc.

11. Takeda UK Ltd. Summary of product characteristics. Reminyl XL 8mg, 16mg, 24mg prolonged release capsules. 2022; https://www.medicines.org.uk/emc/product/3934/smpc.

12. Takeda UK Ltd. Summary of product characteristics. Reminyl oral solution. 2022; https://www.medicines.org.uk/emc/medicine/10337.

13. Lundbeck Ltd. Summary of product characteristics. Ebixa 5mg/pump actuation oral solution, 20mg and 10 mg tablets and treatment initiation pack. 2021; https://www.medicines.org.uk/emc/product/8222/smpc.

14. NHS Prescription Services. *Electronic Drug Tariff*. 2020; http://www.drugtariff.nhsbsa.nhs.uk/#/00791628-DD/DD00791615/Home2020.

15. Buckley JS, et al. A risk-benefit assessment of dementia medications: systematic review of the evidence. *Drugs Aging* 2015; **32**:453–467.

16. Lanctot KL, et al. Efficacy and safety of cholinesterase inhibitors in Alzheimer's disease: a meta-analysis. *CMAJ* 2003; **169**:557–564.

17. McShane R, et al. Memantine for dementia. *Cochrane Database Syst Rev* 2019; **3**:CD003154.

18. Vaci N, et al. Real-world effectiveness, its predictors and onset of action of cholinesterase inhibitors and memantine in dementia: retrospective health record study. *Br J Psychiatry* 2021; **218**:261–267.

19. Zuin M, et al. Acetyl-cholinesterase-inhibitors slow cognitive decline and decrease overall mortality in older patients with dementia. *Sci Rep* 2022; **12**:12214.

20. Burns A, et al. Efficacy and safety of donepezil over 3 years: an open-label, multicentre study in patients with Alzheimer's disease. *Int J Geriatr Psychiatry* 2007; **22**:806–812.

21. Doody RS, et al. Open-label, multicenter, phase 3 extension study of the safety and efficacy of donepezil in patients with Alzheimer disease. *Arch Neurol* 2001; **58**:427–433.

22. Farlow MR, et al. Effective pharmacologic management of Alzheimer's disease. *Am J Med* 2007; **120**:388–397.

23. O'Brien JT, et al. Clinical practice with anti-dementia drugs: a revised (third) consensus statement from the British Association for Psychopharmacology. *J Psychopharmacol* 2017; **31**:147–168.

24. Singh S, et al. Discontinuation syndrome following donepezil cessation. *Int J Geriatr Psychiatry* 2003; **18**:282–284.

25. Bidzan L, et al. Withdrawal syndrome after donepezil cessation in a patient with dementia. *Neurol Sci* 2012; **33**:1459–1461.

26. Waldemar G, et al. Tolerability of switching from donepezil to memantine treatment in patients with moderate to severe Alzheimer's disease. *Int J Geriatr Psychiatry* 2008; **23**:979–981.

27. Massoud F, et al. Switching cholinesterase inhibitors in older adults with dementia. *Int Psychogeriatr* 2011; **23**:372–378.

28. Winblad B, et al. A six-month double-blind, randomized, placebo-controlled study of a transdermal patch in Alzheimer's disease – rivastigmine patch versus capsule. *Int J Geriatr Psychiatry* 2007; **22**:456–467.

29. Zhang ZX, et al. Rivastigmine patch in Chinese patients with probable Alzheimer's disease: a 24-week, randomized, double-blind parallel-group study comparing rivastigmine patch (9.5 mg/24 h) with capsule (6 mg twice daily). *CNS Neurosci Ther* 2016; **22**:488–496.

30. Morgan TM, et al. Absolute bioavailability and safety of a novel rivastigmine nasal spray in healthy elderly individuals. *Br J Clin Pharmacol* 2017; **83**:510–516.

31. Knopman DS. Donepezil 23 mg: an empty suit. *Neurol Clin Pract* 2012; **2**:352–355.

32. Plosker GL. Memantine extended release (28 mg once daily): a review of its use in Alzheimer's disease. *Drugs* 2015; **75**:887–897.

33. Deardorff WJ, et al. A fixed-dose combination of memantine extended-release and donepezil in the treatment of moderate-to-severe Alzheimer's disease. *Drug Des Devel Ther* 2016; **10**:3267–3279.

34. Veroniki AA, et al. Comparative safety and efficacy of cognitive enhancers for Alzheimer's dementia: a systematic review with individual patient data network meta-analysis. *BMJ Open* 2022; **12**:e053012.

35. Guo J, et al. Memantine, donepezil, or combination therapy – what is the best therapy for Alzheimer's disease? A network meta-analysis. *Brain Behav* 2020; **10**:e01831.

36. Parsons C, et al. Withdrawal or continuation of cholinesterase inhibitors or memantine or both, in people with dementia. *Cochrane Database Syst Rev* 2021; **2**:CD009081.

37. Periclou AP, et al. Lack of pharmacokinetic or pharmacodynamic interaction between memantine and donepezil. *Ann Pharmacother* 2004; **38**:1389–1394.

38. Grossberg GT, et al. Rationale for combination therapy with galantamine and memantine in Alzheimer's disease. *J Clin Pharmacol* 2006; **46**:17S–26S.

39. Rogers SL, et al. Donepezil improves cognition and global function in Alzheimer disease: a 15-week, double-blind, placebo-controlled study. Donepezil Study Group. *Arch Intern Med* 1998; **158**:1021–1031.

40. Rogers SL, et al. A 24-week, double-blind, placebo-controlled trial of donepezil in patients with Alzheimer's disease. Donepezil Study Group. *Neurology* 1998; **50**:136–145.

41. Corey-Bloom J, et al. A randomized trial evaluating the efficacy and safety of ENA 713 (rivastigmine tartrate), a new acetylcholinesterase inhibitor, in patients with mild to moderately severe Alzheimer's disease. *Int J Geriatr Psychopharmacol* 1998; **1**:55–64.

42. Rosler M, et al. Efficacy and safety of rivastigmine in patients with Alzheimer's disease: international randomised controlled trial. *BMJ* 1999; **318**:633–638.

43. Tariot PN, et al. A 5-month, randomized, placebo-controlled trial of galantamine in AD. The Galantamine USA-10 Study Group. *Neurology* 2000; **54**:2269–2276.

44. Raskind MA, et al. Galantamine in AD: a 6-month randomized, placebo-controlled trial with a 6-month extension. The Galantamine USA-1 Study Group. *Neurology* 2000; **54**:2261–2268.

45. Wilcock GK, et al. Efficacy and safety of galantamine in patients with mild to moderate Alzheimer's disease: multicentre randomised controlled trial. Galantamine International-1 Study Group. *BMJ* 2000; **321**:1445–1449.

46. Pariente A, et al. Factors associated with serious adverse reactions to cholinesterase inhibitors: a study of spontaneous reporting. *CNS Drugs* 2010; **24**:55–63.

47. Inglis F. The tolerability and safety of cholinesterase inhibitors in the treatment of dementia. *Int J Clin Pract Suppl* 2002; **127**:45–63.

48. Sadowsky CH, et al. Safety and tolerability of rivastigmine transdermal patch compared with rivastigmine capsules in patients switched from donepezil: data from three clinical trials. *Int J Clin Pract* 2010; **64**:188–193.

49. Sadowsky C, et al. Switching from oral cholinesterase inhibitors to the rivastigmine transdermal patch. *CNS Neurosci Ther* 2010; **16**:51–60.

50. Cummings J, et al. Randomized, double-blind, parallel-group, 48-week study for efficacy and safety of a higher-dose rivastigmine patch (15 vs. 10 cm^2) in Alzheimer's disease. *Dement Geriatr Cogn Disord* 2012; **33**:341–353.

51. Parsons CG, et al. Memantine is a clinically well tolerated N-methyl-D-aspartate (NMDA) receptor antagonist – a review of preclinical data. *Neuropharmacology* 1999; **38**:735–767.

52. Reisberg B, et al. Memantine in moderate-to-severe Alzheimer's disease. *N Engl J Med* 2003; **348**:1333–1341.

53. Jones RW. A review comparing the safety and tolerability of memantine with the acetylcholinesterase inhibitors. *Int J Geriatr Psychiatry* 2010; **25**:547–553.

54. Dunn NR, et al. Adverse effects associated with the use of donepezil in general practice in England. *J Psychopharmacol* 2000; **14**:406–408.

55. Hashimoto M, et al. Urinary incontinence: an unrecognised adverse effect with donepezil. *Lancet* 2000; **356**:568.

56. Kobayashi H, et al. The comparative efficacy and safety of cholinesterase inhibitors in patients with mild-to-moderate Alzheimer's disease: a Bayesian network meta-analysis. *Int J Geriatr Psychiatry* 2016; **31**:892–904.

57. Kroger E, et al. Adverse drug reactions reported with cholinesterase inhibitors: an analysis of 16 years of individual case safety reports from VigiBase. *Ann Pharmacother* 2015; **49**:1197–1206.

58. FDA Alert for Healthcare Professionals. Galantamine hydrobromide (marketed as Razadyne, formerly Reminyl). 2005; https://www.fda.gov/Drugs/DrugSafety/ucm109350.htm.

59. Malone DM, et al. Cholinesterase inhibitors and cardiovascular disease: a survey of old age psychiatrists' practice. *Age Ageing* 2007; **36**:331–333.

60. NHS Yorkshire and Humber Clinical Networks. The assessment of cardiac status before prescribing acetyl cholinesterase inhibitors for dementia. Version 1. 2016; http://www.yhscn.nhs.uk/media/PDFs/mhdn/Dementia/ECG%20Documents/ACHEIGuidance%20V1_Final.pdf.

61. Rowland JP, et al. Cardiovascular monitoring with acetylcholinesterase inhibitors: a clinical protocol. *Adv Psychiatric Treat* 2007; **13**:178–184.

62. Young S, et al. Cardiovascular complications of acetylcholinesterase inhibitors in patients with Alzheimer's disease: a narrative review. *Ann Geriatr Med Res* 2021; **25**:170–177.

63. Rosenbloom MH, et al. Donepezil-associated bradyarrhythmia in a patient with dementia with Lewy bodies (DLB). *Alzheimer Dis Assoc Disord* 2010; **24**:209–211.

64. Howes LG. Cardiovascular effects of drugs used to treat Alzheimer's disease. *Drug Saf* 2014; **37**:391–395.

65. Farlow MR, et al. Memantine for the treatment of Alzheimer's disease: tolerability and safety data from clinical trials. *Drug Saf* 2008; **31**:577–585.

66. Babai S, et al. Comparison of adverse drug reactions with donepezil versus memantine: analysis of the French pharmacovigilance database. *Therapie* 2010; **65**:255–259.

67. Dooley M, et al. Donepezil: a review of its use in Alzheimer's disease. *Drugs Aging* 2000; **16**:199–226.

68. Scott LJ, et al. Galantamine: a review of its use in Alzheimer's disease. *Drugs* 2000; **60**:1095–1122.

69. Grossberg GT, et al. Lack of adverse pharmacodynamic drug interactions with rivastigmine and twenty-two classes of medications. *Int J Geriatr Psychiatry* 2000; **15**:242–247.

70. Tavassoli N, et al. Drug interactions with cholinesterase inhibitors: an analysis of the French pharmacovigilance database and a comparison of two national drug formularies (Vidal, British National Formulary). *Drug Saf* 2007; **30**:1063–1071.

71. Noetzli M, et al. Pharmacodynamic, pharmacokinetic and pharmacogenetic aspects of drugs used in the treatment of Alzheimer's disease. *Clin Pharmacokinet* 2013; **52**:225–241.

72. Pasqualetti G, et al. Potential drug-drug interactions in Alzheimer patients with behavioral symptoms. *Clin Interv Aging* 2015; **10**:1457–1466.

CHAPTER 6

73. Medicines Complete. Stockley's drug interactions. 2023; https://www.medicinescomplete.com/.

74. Merative US LP. Micromedex. 2023; https://www.micromedexsolutions.com/home/dispatch/.

75. Howard R, et al. Donepezil and memantine for moderate-to-severe Alzheimer's disease. *N Engl J Med* 2012; **366**:893–903.

76. Howard R, et al. Nursing home placement in the Donepezil and Memantine in Moderate to Severe Alzheimer's Disease (DOMINO-AD) trial: secondary and post-hoc analyses. *Lancet Neurol* 2015; **14**:1171–1181.

77. Li DQ, et al. Donepezil combined with natural hirudin improves the clinical symptoms of patients with mild-to-moderate Alzheimer's disease: a 20-week open-label pilot study. *Int J Med Sci* 2012; **9**:248–255.

78. Di Santo SG, et al. A meta-analysis of the efficacy of donepezil, rivastigmine, galantamine, and memantine in relation to severity of Alzheimer's disease. *J Alzheimers Dis* 2013; **35**:349–361.

79. Parsons C. Withdrawal of antidementia drugs in older people: who, when and how? *Drugs Aging* 2016; **33**:545–556.

80. National Institute for Health and Care Excellence. Dementia: assessment, management and support for people living with dementia and their carers. NICE Guideline [NG97]. 2018 (checked September 2023, last accessed December 2023); https://www.nice.org.uk/guidance/ng97.

81. Birks J, et al. Ginkgo biloba for cognitive impairment and dementia. *Cochrane Database Syst Rev* 2009; **2**:CD003120.

82. Tan MS, et al. Efficacy and adverse effects of ginkgo biloba for cognitive impairment and dementia: a systematic review and meta-analysis. *J Alzheimers Dis* 2015; **43**:589–603.

83. National Institute for Health and Clinical Excellence. Donepezil, galantamine, rivastigmine and memantine for the treatment of Alzheimer's disease. Technology Appraisal [TA217]. 2011 (last updated June 2018, last accessed December 2023); https://www.nice.org.uk/guidance/ta217.

84. National Institute for Health and Clinical Excellence. Medicines optimisation: the safe and effective use of medicines to enable the best possible outcomes. NICE Guideline [NG5]. 2015 (checked March 2019, last accessed January 2024); https://www.nice.org.uk/guidance/ng52015.

85. Fan F, et al. The efficacy and safety of Alzheimer's disease therapies: an updated umbrella review. *J Alzheimers Dis* 2022; **85**:1195–1204.

86. Bent S, et al. Spontaneous bleeding associated with ginkgo biloba: a case report and systematic review of the literature: a case report and systematic review of the literature. *J Gen Intern Med* 2005; **20**:657–661.

87. Gil Martínez V, et al. Vitamin supplementation and dementia: a systematic review. *Nutrients* 2022; **14**:1033.

88. Burckhardt M, et al. Omega-3 fatty acids for the treatment of dementia. *Cochrane Database Syst Rev* 2016; **4**:CD009002.

89. Wang Y, et al. Ginseng for Alzheimer's disease: a systematic review and meta-analysis of randomized controlled trials. *Curr Top Med Chem* 2016; **16**:529–536.

90. Ghassab-Abdollahi N, et al. The effects of Huperzine A on dementia and mild cognitive impairment: an overview of systematic reviews. *Phytother Res* 2021; **35**:4971–4987.

91. Yue J, et al. Huperzine A for mild cognitive impairment. *Cochrane Database Syst Rev* 2012; **12**:CD008827.

92. Hao Z, et al. Huperzine A for vascular dementia. *Cochrane Database Syst Rev* 2009; **2**:CD007365.

93. Ayati Z, et al. Saffron for mild cognitive impairment and dementia: a systematic review and meta-analysis of randomised clinical trials. *BMC Complement Med Ther* 2020; **20**:333.

94. Gavrilova SI, et al. Cerebrolysin in the therapy of mild cognitive impairment and dementia due to Alzheimer's disease: 30 years of clinical use. *Med Res Rev* 2021; **41**:2775–2803.

95. Cui S, et al. Cerebrolysin for vascular dementia. *Cochrane Database Syst Rev* 2019; **11**:CD008900.

96. Moreira A, et al. Chocolate consumption is associated with a lower risk of cognitive decline. *J Alzheimers Dis* 2016; **53**:85–93.

97. Burckhardt M, et al. Souvenaid for Alzheimer's disease. *Cochrane Database Syst Rev* 2020; **12**:CD011679.

98. Galimberti D, et al. Idalopirdine as a treatment for Alzheimer's disease. *Expert Opin Investig Drugs* 2015; **24**:981–987.

99. Matsunaga S, et al. Efficacy and safety of idalopirdine for Alzheimer's disease: a systematic review and meta-analysis. *Int Psychogeriatr* 2019; **31**:1627–1633.

100. Jordan F, et al. Aspirin and other non-steroidal anti-inflammatory drugs for the prevention of dementia. *Cochrane Database Syst Rev* 2020; **4**:CD011459.

101. La AL, et al. Long-term trazodone use and cognition: a potential therapeutic role for slow-wave sleep enhancers. *J Alzheimers Dis* 2019; **67**:911–921.

102. Brauer R, et al. Trazodone use and risk of dementia: a population-based cohort study. *PLoS Med* 2019; **16**:e1002728.

103. Sommerlad A, et al. Effect of trazodone on cognitive decline in people with dementia: cohort study using UK routinely collected data. *Int J Geriatr Psychiatry* 2021; **37**:doi: 10.1002/gps.5625.

104. Coupland C, et al. Antidepressant use and risk of adverse outcomes in older people: population based cohort study. *BMJ* 2011; **343**:d4551.

105. Halliday M, et al. Repurposed drugs targeting eIF2alpha-P-mediated translational repression prevent neurodegeneration in mice. *Brain* 2017; **140**:1768–1783.

106. Sauder C, et al. Effectiveness of KarXT (xanomeline-trospium) for cognitive impairment in schizophrenia: post hoc analyses from a randomised, double-blind, placebo-controlled phase 2 study. *Transl Psychiatry* 2022; **12**:491.

107. Khan H, et al. Neuroprotective effects of quercetin in Alzheimer's disease. *Biomolecules* 2019; **10**:59.

108. Yu TW, et al. Novel therapeutic approaches for Alzheimer's disease: an updated review. *Int J Mol Sci* 2021; **22**:8208.

109. Schneider L. A resurrection of aducanumab for Alzheimer's disease. *Lancet Neurol* 2020; **19**:111–112.

110. The Lancet. Lecanemab for Alzheimer's disease: tempering hype and hope. *Lancet* 2022; **400**:1899.

111. Van Dyck CH, et al. Lecanemab in early Alzheimer's disease. *N Engl J Med* 2023; **388**:9–21.

112. Jönsson L, et al. The affordability of lecanemab, an amyloid-targeting therapy for Alzheimer's disease: an EADC-EC viewpoint. *Lancet Reg Health Eur* 2023; **29**:100657.

113. Sims JR, et al. Donanemab in early symptomatic Alzheimer disease: the TRAILBLAZER-ALZ 2 randomized clinical trial. *JAMA* 2023; **330**:512–527.

114. Ramanan VK, et al. Antiamyloid monoclonal antibody therapy for Alzheimer disease: emerging issues in neurology. *Neurology* 2023; **101**:842–852.

115. Monteiro C, et al. Randomized phase II study of the safety and efficacy of semorinemab in participants with mild-to-moderate Alzheimer disease: Lauriet. *Neurology* 2023; **101**:e1391–e1401.

116. Kavirajan H, et al. Efficacy and adverse effects of cholinesterase inhibitors and memantine in vascular dementia: a meta-analysis of randomised controlled trials. *Lancet Neurol* 2007; **6**:782–792.

117. Wang J, et al. Cholinergic deficiency involved in vascular dementia: possible mechanism and strategy of treatment. *Acta Pharmacol Sin* 2009; **30**:879–888.

118. Bocti C, et al. Management of dementia with a cerebrovascular component. *Alzheimers Dementia* 2007; **3**:398–403.

119. Demaerschalk BM, et al. Treatment of vascular dementia and vascular cognitive impairment. *Neurologist* 2007; **13**:37–41.

120. Baskys A, et al. Pharmacological prevention and treatment of vascular dementia: approaches and perspectives. *Exp Gerontol* 2012; **47**:887–891.

121. McGuinness B, et al. Statins for the prevention of dementia. *Cochrane Database Syst Rev* 2016; **1**:CD003160.

122. Battle CE, et al. Cholinesterase inhibitors for vascular dementia and other vascular cognitive impairments: a network meta-analysis. *Cochrane Database Syst Rev* 2021; **2**:CD013306.

123. Jin BR, et al. Comparative efficacy and safety of cognitive enhancers for treating vascular cognitive impairment: systematic review and Bayesian network meta-analysis. *Neural Regen Res* 2019; **14**:805–816.

124. Wild R, et al. Cholinesterase inhibitors for dementia with Lewy bodies. *Cochrane Database Syst Rev* 2003; **3**:CD003672.

125. Taylor JP, et al. New evidence on the management of Lewy body dementia. *Lancet Neurol* 2020; **19**:157–169.

126. McKeith IG, et al. Diagnosis and management of dementia with Lewy bodies: fourth consensus report of the DLB Consortium. *Neurology* 2017; **89**:88–100.

127. Newcastle University. Management of Lewy body dementia summary sheet. Diamond Lewy. 2019; https://research.ncl.ac.uk/media/sites/researchwebsites/diamond-lewy/One%20page%20symptom%20LBD%20management%20summaries.pdf.

128. Russ TC, et al. Cholinesterase inhibitors for mild cognitive impairment. *Cochrane Database Syst Rev* 2012; **9**:CD009132.

129. Cooper C, et al. Treatment for mild cognitive impairment: systematic review. *Br J Psychiatry* 2013; **203**:255–264.

130. Matsunaga S, et al. Efficacy and safety of cholinesterase inhibitors for mild cognitive impairment: a systematic review and meta-analysis. *J Alzheimers Dis* 2019; **71**:513–523.

131. Kasper S, et al. Management of mild cognitive impairment (MCI): the need for national and international guidelines. *World J Biol Psychiatry* 2020; **21**:579–594.

132. Petersen RC, et al. Practice guideline update summary: mild cognitive impairment. Report of the Guideline Development, Dissemination, and Implementation Subcommittee of the American Academy of Neurology. *Neurology* 2018; **90**:126–135.

133. Nardell M, et al. Pharmacological treatments for frontotemporal dementias: a systematic review of randomized controlled trials. *Am J Alzheimers Dis Other Demen* 2014; **29**:123–132.

134. Boeve BF, et al. Advances and controversies in frontotemporal dementia: diagnosis, biomarkers, and therapeutic considerations. *Lancet Neurol* 2022; **21**:258–272.

135. Li Y, et al. Cholinesterase inhibitors for rarer dementias associated with neurological conditions. *Cochrane Database Syst Rev* 2015; **3**:CD009444.

CHAPTER 6

Safer prescribing for physical conditions in dementia

People with dementia are susceptible to cognitive adverse effects of drugs. Drugs may affect cognition through their action on cholinergic, histaminergic, opioid or other neurotransmitter pathways. Some medications may also interact with cognitive-enhancing medication.

Anticholinergic drugs

Anticholinergic drugs reduce the efficacy of acetylcholinesterase inhibitors[1] and cause sedation, delirium and falls.[2] These effects are more severe in older patients with dementia.[3] A high anticholinergic burden is associated with cognitive decline[4] and increased hospitalisation and mortality.[4,5] The Anticholinergic Effect on Cognition (AEC)[6] scale can be used to calculate the anticholinergic burden of drugs in patients. Table 6.4 lists the AEC scores of drugs commonly prescribed for older adults in the UK.[6] Combining several drugs with anticholinergic activity increases the total anticholinergic burden for an individual.

It is good practice to keep the anticholinergic burden to a minimum in older people and those with dementia. Where possible, drugs with no anticholinergic action and an equivalent therapeutic effect should be used. If this is not possible, the prescription of a drug with low anticholinergic activity or high specificity to the site of action (and thus minimal central activity) should be encouraged. Anticholinergic drugs that do not cross the blood–brain barrier (BBB) have less profound effects on cognitive function.[7] The AEC takes all of these factors into account.

The following are recommendations for using AEC scores:[6]

- All individual drugs with an AEC score of 2 or 3 in older people presenting with symptoms of cognitive impairment, dementia or delirium should either be:
  - stopped, or
  - switched to an alternative drug with a lower AEC score (preferably 0).
- In patients who are not receiving any individual drug with an AEC score of 2 or 3 but who have a *total* AEC score of 3 or above, a patient–clinician review should take place.
- If withdrawal of the drug is deemed appropriate, this should be gradual (where possible) to avoid rebound (nausea, sweating, urinary frequency, diarrhoea).

Table 6.4 Anticholinergic Effect on Cognition (AEC) scale scores (Adapted from [6]). *

Adcal – 0	Clarithromycin – NK	**Gabapentin** – 0	**Naproxen** – 0	Sitagliptin – 0
Agomelatine – 0	Clemastine – 3	Galantamine – 0	Nifedipine – 0	Solifenacin – 1
Alendronic acid (alendronate) – 0	Clomipramine – 3	Gaviscon – 0	Nimodipine – 0	Sotalol – 0
Alfuzosin – 0	Clonazepam – NK	Gliclazide – 0	Nitrofurantoin – NK	Spironolactone – NK
Alimemazine (trimeprazine) – 3	Clonidine – NK	Granisetron – 0	Nortriptyline – 3	Sulphasalazine – 0
Allopurinol – NK	Clopidogrel – 0	**Haloperidol** – 0	**Olanzapine** – 2	Sulpiride – 0
Alprazolam – 0	Clozapine – 3	Heparin – 0	Omeprazole – 0	**Tamoxifen** – NK
Alverine – 0	Co-beneldopa – 0	Hydrochlorothiazide – 0	Ondansetron – 0	Tamsulosin – 0
Amantadine – 2	Co-careldopa – 0	Hydrocodone – NK	Orlistat – 0	Temazepam – 1
Amiloride – 0	Codeine – NK	Hydrocortisone – NK	Orphenadrine – 3	Tetracycline – 0
Aminophylline – 0	Colchicine – NK	Hydroxyzine – 1	Oxcarbazepine – NK	Theophylline – 0
Amiodarone – 1	Co-tenidone – 0	Hyoscine butylbromide (buscopan) – 1	Oxybutynin – 3	Thiamine – 0
Amisulpride – 0	Cyclizine – 1	Hyoscine hydrobromide – 3	Oxycodone – NK	Tiotropium bromide (inhalation) – 0
Amitriptyline – 3	Cyproheptadine – 3	Ibuprofen – 0	**Paliperidone** – 1	Tizanidine – NK
Amlodipine – 0	**Dabigatran** – NK	Iloperidone – 1	Pantoprazole – 0	Tolcapone – 0
Amoxicillin – 0	Darifenacin – 0	Imipramine – 3	Paracetamol – 0	Tolterodine – 2
Anastrozole – NK	Desipramine – 2	Indapamide – 0	Paroxetine – 2	Topiramate – NK
Apixaban – NK	Dexamethasone – NK	Insulin – 0	Penicillin – 0	Tramadol – 0
Apomorphine – 0	Dexamfetamine – 0	Ipratropium bromide – 0	Peppermint oil – 0	Tranylcypromine – 0
Aripiprazole – 1	Dextropropoxyphene – NK	Irbesartan – NK	Pergolide – 0	Trazodone – 0
Asenapine – 1	Diazepam – 1	Isocarboxazid – 1	Perindopril – 0	Trifluoperazine – 2
Aspirin – 0	Diclofenac – 0	Isosorbide dinitrate – 0	Perphenazine – 1	Trihexyphenidyl (benzhexol) – 3

(Continued)

Table 6.4 (*Continued*)

Atenolol – 0	Dicycloverine (dicyclomine) – 2	Isosorbide mononitrate – 0	Pethidine – 2	Trimethoprim – 0
Atomoxetine – 0	Digoxin – NK	Ketorolac – 0	Phenelzine – 1	Trimipramine – 3
Atorvastatin – 0	Dihydrocodeine – NK	Labetalol – 0	Phenytoin – NK	Trospium – 0
Atropine – 3	Diltiazem – 0	Lactulose – 0	Pimozide – 2	Valproate – 0
Atropine eye drops – 1	Dimenhydrinate – 2	Lamotrigine – 0	Pirenzepine – 1	Venlafaxine – 0
Azathioprine – 0	Diphenhydramine – 2	Lansoprazole – NK	Pravastatin – 0	Verapamil – NK
Baclofen – NK	Dipyridamole – 0	Lercanidipine – 0	Prazosin – 0	Vitamin B12 – 0
Beclometasone dipropionate (inhaler) – 0	Disopyramide – 2	Levetiracetam – NK	Prednisolone – 1	Vitamins – 0
Bendroflumethiazide – 0	Docusate sodium – 0	Levodopa – 0	Pregabalin – NK	Vortioxetine – 0
Benztropine – 3	Domperidone – 1	Levomepromazine (methotrimeprazine) – 2	Prochlorperazine – 2	Warfarin – 0
Betahistine – 0	Donepezil – 0	Levothyroxine (thyroxine) – 0	Procyclidine – 3	Ziprasidone – 0
Bezafibrate – 0	Dothiepin (dosulepin) – 3	Liraglutide – 0	Promazine – 2	Zolpidem – 0
Bisacodyl – 0	Doxazosin – 0	Lisinopril – 0	Promethazine – 3	Zopiclone – NK
Bisoprolol – NK	Doxepin – 3	Lithium – 1	Propantheline – 2	Zotepine – 2
Bromocriptine – 1	Doxycycline – 0	Lofepramine – 3	Propranolol – 0	Zuclopentixol (zuclopenthixol) – 1
Budesonide (inhaler) – 0	Dulaglutide – 0	Loperamide – 0	Quetiapine – 2	
Bumetanide – NK	Duloxetine – 0	Loratadine – 0	Quinidine – 1	
Buprenorphine – 0	Escitalopram – 1	Lorazepam – 0	Quinine – 1	
Bupropion – 0	Enalapril – 0	Losartan – 0	Rabeprazole – 0	
Buspirone – 1	Enoxaparin – 0	Lovastatin – 0	Ramipril – NK	
Cabergoline – 0	Entacapone – 0	Lurasidone – 0	Ranitidine – 0	

Calcium – 0	Erythromycin – NK	Macrogol – 0	Rasagiline – 0
Calcium and vitamin D – 0	Exanatide – 0	Magnesium – 0	Reboxetine – 0
Candesartan – 0	Ezetimibe – 0	Mebeverine – 0	Risedronate – 0
Captopril – NK	Felodipine – 0	Melatonin – 0	Risperidone – 0
Carbachol – 0	Fentanyl – 1	Meloxicam – 0	Rivaroxaban – NK
Carbamazepine – 1	Ferrous sulphate – 0	Memantine – 0	Rivastigmine – 0
Carbimazole – NK	Fesoterodine – 0	Mesalazine – 0	Ropinirole – 0
Carbocisteine – 0	Fexofenadine – 0	Metformin – NK	Rosiglitazone – 0
Cariprazine – 0	Finasteride – 0	Methocarbamol – NK	Rosuvastatin – NK
Carvedilol – NK	Flavoxate – NK	Methotrexate – NK	Salbutamol – 0
Cefalexin (cephalexin) – 0	Flecainide – 0	Metoclopramide – 0	Salmeterol (inhaler) – 0
Cetirizine – 0	Flucloxacillin – 0	Metoprolol – 0	Selegiline – 0
Chloral hydrate – NK	Fludrocortisone – NK	Mianserin – 2	Senna – 0
Chlordiazepoxide – 0	Fluoxetine – 1	Midazolam – 1	Sertindole – 1
Chlorphenamine – 2	Flupentixol (flupenthixol) – 1	Minocycline – 0	Sertraline – 1
Chlorpromazine – 3	Fluphenazine – 1	Mirabegron – 0	Sildenafil – 0
Chlortalidone – NK	Fluvoxamine – 0	Mirtazapine – 1	Simvastatin – 0
Cimetidine – 0	Folic acid – 0	Moclobemide – 0	
Cinnarizine – 1	Furosemide – 0	Morphine – 0	
Ciprofloxacin – 0			
Citalopram – 1			

*The AEC scale is available as a regularly updated web-based app. Please go to www.medichec.com. This site has been updated to include the identification of medications that are reported to cause dizziness and drowsiness since these adverse effects can add to cognitive impairment and confusion in older people and can increase the risk of falls. Medichec also identifies medications that are reported to cause QTc prolongation, hyponatraemia, bleeding risk and constipation.
1–3, scores 1 to 3; NK, not known.

Safety of physical health medication prescribed in dementia

Anticholinergic drugs used in urinary incontinence

Oxybutynin penetrates the CNS and is associated with cognitive decline. Although studies of **tolterodine** found no adverse CNS effects,[8] case reports have described memory loss, hallucinations and delirium.[9–11] **Darifenacin**, an M_3 selective receptor antagonist, has shown no effects on cognitive function tests compared with placebo,[12,13] although studies in dementia are lacking. **Solifenacin** may cause memory impairment[14] although it did not affect cognition in patients with a stroke.[15]

Trospium[16–18] and **fesoterodine**[19] do not seem to cause cognitive changes.[17,18,20,21] Tertiary amine drugs (i.e. oxybutynin, tolterodine, solifenacin, fesoterodine, darifenacin) are metabolised by cytochrome P450 (CYP) enzymes. Increasing age or co-administration of drugs that inhibit these enzymes (e.g. erythromycin, fluoxetine) can lead to higher serum levels and increased adverse effects. The metabolism of trospium is unknown, although metabolism via the CYP system does not occur, meaning that pharmacokinetic drug interactions are unlikely with this drug.[8]

Alpha blockers for urinary retention

Alpha blockers such as **tamsulosin**, **alfuzosin** and **prazosin** cause drowsiness, dizziness and depression.[22] There is no published literature reporting their effects on cognition, but α blockers are not thought to have any anticholinergic action.

Drugs used in gastrointestinal disorders

Loperamide

Although loperamide may have some anticholinergic activity, there are no data to suggest that it can worsen cognitive function in patients with dementia. It may add to the anticholinergic cognitive burden if used in conjunction with other anticholinergic drugs.

Laxatives

Laxatives do not have any negative impact on cognitive function. In fact, since constipation can lead to delirium and behavioural and psychological symptoms of dementia, treating it may improve these symptoms.

Antiemetics

Cyclizine is a first-generation histamine antagonist and can impair cognitive and psychomotor performance (see 'Antihistamines' later in this chapter).[23]

Metoclopramide has little anticholinergic action, but the D_2 receptor antagonism of both metoclopramide and prochlorperazine can produce movement disorders and so these drugs must be used with caution in people with dementia.

Domperidone is a dopamine D_2 receptor antagonist that does not usually cross the BBB. However, since BBB alterations can occur in dementia, CNS penetration of domperidone and resulting adverse effects can occur.[24] There is a small increased risk of serious cardiac adverse effects with domperidone, especially in older people. Domperidone is now contraindicated in those with underlying cardiac conditions or

severe hepatic impairment and in patients receiving other medications known to prolong QT interval or potent CYP3A4 inhibitors; treatment should not exceed 1 week.[25]

Serotonin 5HT$_3$ receptor antagonists, used for treating chemotherapy-induced nausea and vomiting, do not have adverse effects on cognition, and may have some
cognitive-enhancing action.[26] These drugs should be used cautiously in patients with
cardiac comorbidities or taking concomitant arrhythmogenic drugs or drugs known to
prolong QT interval. **Granisetron** can be administered once daily, which is preferable in
people with dementia or swallowing difficulties. Granisetron is metabolised exclusively via a single CYP family (CYP3A4), and thus has a lower propensity for drug
interactions.[27]

Antispasmodics

Hyoscine hydrobromide (scopolamine) is a centrally acting lipophilic anticholinergic
which penetrates the BBB. It impairs memory, speed of processing and attention. Older
patients suffer these symptoms at lower doses and are more vulnerable to confusion
and hallucinations.[28] People with Alzheimer's disease experience clinically significant
cognitive impairment at lower doses compared with healthy, aged-matched controls.[3]
The effect that hyoscine has on cognition is so significant that it is used in trials to produce memory deficits similar to those seen in dementia (the scopolamine challenge
test).[29] There is rarely a good reason to use this drug in people with dementia.

Hyoscine butylbromide (Buscopan) exerts topical spasmolytic action on smooth
muscle of the gastrointestinal tract. Hyoscine butylbromide is not thought to enter the
CNS, so central anticholinergic adverse effects are rare.[30]

Alverine, mebeverine and **peppermint oil** are relaxants of intestinal smooth muscle
with no effect on cognition.

Bronchodilators

Beta agonists

In patients with Parkinson's disease or essential tremor, tremor induced by β agonists
may result in misdiagnosis and over-treatment of Parkinson's disease.[31] Tremor is a
common adverse effect of cholinesterase inhibitors so caution should be exercised when
used with β agonists.

Anticholinergic bronchodilators

Inhaled anticholinergic drugs have few systemic side effects.[31] A placebo-controlled
comparison of ipratropium and theophylline treatment was unable to detect a negative
effect with either drug on the cognitive function of older patients. This suggests that
treatment with inhaled ipratropium is not associated with significant cognitive impairment in older people.[32]

Theophylline

As with cholinesterase inhibitors, nausea and vomiting are common adverse effects of
theophylline. Neurological effects such as headaches, anxiety, behavioural disturbances,
depression and seizures can occur in 50% of patients on theophylline. Although seizures are rare, they are much more likely in older people. Theophylline does not cause
significant cognitive impairment.[32]

CHAPTER 6

Hypersalivation

Oral anticholinergic agents used for hypersalivation (e.g. hyoscine hydrobromide) should be avoided in older people because of the risk of cognitive impairment, delirium and constipation (see 'Anticholinergic drugs' and 'Antispasmodics' earlier in this chapter). Pirenzepine is a relatively selective M_1 and M_4 muscarinic receptor antagonist which is not thought to cross the BBB and therefore has little CNS penetration.[33]

Atropine solution given sublingually or used as a mouthwash is sometimes used to manage hypersalivation. There are no data available on the extent of penetration through the BBB when atropine is administered by this route.

Myasthenia gravis

Unlike acetylcholinesterase inhibitors used in Alzheimer's disease (donepezil, rivastigmine, galantamine), those used in myasthenia gravis (**pyridostigmine, neostigmine**) act peripherally and do not cross the BBB.[34] Combining peripheral and central acetylcholinesterase inhibitors may add to the cholinomimetic adverse effect burden (e.g. nausea, vomiting, diarrhoea, abdominal cramps, increased salivation). Memantine may be an alternative to cholinesterase inhibitors in cases where the combined cholinomimetic effects of drugs used for myasthenia gravis and Alzheimer's disease are not tolerated.

Analgesics

NSAIDs and paracetamol

Paracetamol (acetaminophen) does not cause cognitive impairment other than in overdose, when it may cause delirium.[35] There is some evidence that the chronic use of aspirin can cause confusional states.[36] Case reports implicate NSAIDs in causing delirium and psychosis[37] although clinical trials have not demonstrated significant adverse effects on cognition with naproxen[38] or indomethacin.[39] NSAIDs are difficult to use in older people due to their cardiovascular risk and risk of gastrointestinal bleeding.[40] It is good practice to prescribe gastroprotection with these drugs or consider using topical NSAIDs (if clinically appropriate) to reduce the risk of gastrointestinal bleeding.

Opiates

Sedation is a potential problem with all opiates.[41] Delirium induced by opioids may be associated with agitation, hallucinations or delusions.[41] **Pethidine** is associated with a high risk of cognitive impairment as its metabolites have anticholinergic properties and accumulate rapidly if renal function is impaired.[42] **Codeine** may increase the risk of falls, and both tramadol and codeine have a high risk of drug–drug interactions as well as considerable variation in response and adverse effects.[43] **Fentanyl patches** should not be used to initiate opioid analgesia in frail older people[44] because of their long duration of action even after the patch is removed, making the treatment of adverse effects more difficult.[43] **Morphine** is an effective analgesic but is likely to cause cognitive problems and other adverse effects in older patients.[45] **Oxycodone** has a short half-life (at least in non-modified-release tablets), few drug–drug interactions and more predictable dose–response relationships than other opiates. It is therefore, theoretically, a good candidate for oral analgesia in dementia.[43] Caution, however, should be used owing to its addictive potential. **Buprenorphine** transdermal patches probably have less severe adverse effects than many other opiates.

Antihistamines

First-generation H_1 antihistamines include **chlorpheniramine, hydroxyzine, cyclizine** and **promethazine.** They are non-selective, have anticholinergic activity and readily penetrate the BBB. They can impair cognitive performance and can trigger seizures, dyskinesia, dystonia and hallucinations. The second-generation H_1 antihistamines (such as **loratadine, cetirizine** and **fexofenadine**) penetrate poorly into the CNS and should be the preferred choice because of their lack of sedative, cognitive and psychomotor impairment and anticholinergic adverse effects.

Statins

A Cochrane review assessed the clinical efficacy and tolerability of statins in the *treatment* of dementia[46] and showed that there was no significant benefit from statins in terms of cognitive function, but equally no evidence that statins were detrimental to cognition. Earlier case reports had highlighted subjective complaints of memory loss associated with the use of statins.[47] These tended to occur within 2 months of starting the drug and were most commonly associated with simvastatin. If cognitive problems occur on simvastatin, it may be worth first stopping the drug, and if the complaint resolves, try atorvastatin or pravastatin instead as these drugs are less likely to cross the BBB. However, in a large prospective cohort study of patients without dementia, baseline statin use was not associated with incident dementia or MCI, nor was statin use associated with decline in cognitive function over time and results did not differ by statin lipophilicity.[48] Another Cochrane review[49] assessed the efficacy of statins in the *prevention* of dementia and concluded that there was no evidence that statins given in late life to people at risk of vascular disease prevented cognitive decline or dementia. A meta-analysis of observational studies found that similar risks were observed for lipophilic and hydrophilic statins for both dementia and Alzheimer's disease, while high-potency statins showed a 20% reduction of dementia risk compared with a 16% risk reduction associated with low-potency statins, suggesting a greater efficacy of the former. While evidence has been mixed, it suggests that statins are unlikely to cause dementia or cognitive decline, but they may not prevent it either. Nevertheless, indications for statin treatment to prevent cardiovascular events remain.[50]

Antihypertensives

Mid-life hypertension has negative effects on cognition and increases the risk of a person developing dementia.[51] There is no evidence that antihypertensive treatment worsens cognition; it appears to have a positive effect on global cognition and long-term treatment of hypertension can reduce the risk of dementia.[52,53]

Anticoagulants

Several systematic reviews concluded that oral anticoagulation reduced significantly the incidence of cognitive impairment and dementia in patients with atrial fibrillation, probably due to the reduction of ischaemic cerebrovascular events. It appears that direct oral anticoagulant therapy is associated with a significant decrease in the risk of dementia when compared with vitamin K antagonist therapy, however further studies are needed to confirm these findings.[54]

Other cardiac drugs

Digoxin has been associated with acute confusional states at therapeutic drug concentrations.[55] It has also been reported to cause nightmares.[56] However, one study showed the treatment of cardiac failure with digoxin improved cognitive performance in 25% of patients treated (and in 23% of patients treated who did not have cardiac failure).[57] There are some case reports of amiodarone being associated with delirium.[58,59]

H_2 antagonists and proton pump inhibitors (PPIs)

Histamine-2 receptor antagonists (e.g. cimetidine, ranitidine, famotidine) are rarely used nowadays. Cimetidine causes several pharmacokinetic interactions, and ranitidine products have been recalled due to possible contamination with N-nitrosodimethylamine, identified as a potential risk factor in the development of certain cancers. Famotidine remains in use. CNS reactions to these drugs have been reported, especially with cimetidine.[60] A study looking at observational data on PPIs found an association between PPI use and incident dementia. This is supported by pharmacoepidemiological analyses on primary data and is in line with animal studies in which the use of PPIs increased the levels of β-amyloid in the brains of mice.[61] Randomised prospective clinical trials are needed to confirm this association. Many patients on PPIs have *Helicobacter pylori*-infected gastric mucosa. As *Helicobacter* has been reported to be associated with cognitive deterioration, this could be the mechanism behind the apparent link between PPI drugs and dementia. Furthermore, this association was not replicated in other studies.[62,63] Despite reports that PPIs are associated with an increased risk of developing dementia,[61,64] data collected in a large-scale real-world setting using linked national health data in the UK were unable to confirm this association. This suggests that previously reported links may be associated with confounders of people using PPIs, such as increased risk of cardiovascular disease and/or depression and their associated medications.[65]

Antibiotics

There are reports of many antibiotics being associated with delirium[66,67] but there is no consistent pattern of them causing cognitive impairment. Given the importance of treating infection in dementia the most appropriate antibiotic for the infection being treated should be used. Antituberculous therapy, particularly isoniazid, has attracted some case reports of adverse psychiatric reactions.[68]

Table 6.5 lists drugs that are recommended for use in dementia and those that should be avoided.

Table 6.5 Recommended drugs and drugs to avoid in dementia. Adapted with permission.[69]

Condition	Drug class or drug name	Drugs to avoid in dementia	Recommended drugs in dementia
Allergic conditions	Antihistamines	Chlorphenamine Promethazine Hydroxyzine Cyproheptadine Cyclizine (and other first-generation antihistamines)	Cetirizine Loratadine Fexofenadine (and other second-generation antihistamines)
Asthma/COPD	Bronchodilators		Beta agonists Inhaled anticholinergics (have not been reported to affect cognition) Theophylline
Constipation	Laxatives	No evidence to suggest that laxatives have any negative impact on cognitive function. Constipation itself may worsen cognition	
Diarrhoea	Loperamide	Low-potency anticholinergic. Not known to have effects on cognitive function, however may add to the anticholinergic cognitive burden if used in combination with other anticholinergics	
Hyperlipidaemia	Statins		All are safe but atorvastatin and pravastatin are less likely to cross the BBB.
Hypersalivation	Anticholinergics	Hyoscine hydrobromide	Pirenzepine Atropine (sublingually)
Hypertension	Antihypertensives	Beta blockers (avoidance may not always be possible)	Calcium channel blockers, angiotensin-converting enzyme inhibitors and angiotensin receptor blockers may all improve cognitive function.
Infections	Antibiotics	Delirium reported mostly with quinolone and macrolide antibiotics. But given the importance of treating infections, the most appropriate antibiotic for the infection should be used.	
Myasthenia gravis	Peripheral acetylcholinesterase inhibitors, e.g. neostigmine and pyridostigmine	May add to the cholinergic adverse effects of central acetylcholinesterase inhibitors (e.g. donepezil) in patients with dementia, e.g. increased risk of nausea/vomiting.	
Nausea/vomiting	Antiemetics	Cyclizine Metoclopramide Prochlorperazine	Domperidone (see main text for restrictions) Serotonin $5HT_3$ receptor antagonists

(*Continued*)

Table 6.5 *(Continued)*

Condition	Drug class or drug name	Drugs to avoid in dementia	Recommended drugs in dementia
Other GI conditions	Antispasmodics	Atropine sulphate Dicycloverine hydrochloride	Alverine, mebeverine, peppermint oil Hyoscine-n-butylbromide Propantheline bromide
Pain	Analgesics	Pethidine Pentazocine Dextropropoxyphene Codeine Tramadol Methadone	Paracetamol Oxycodone Buprenorphine Topical NSAIDs (where appropriate)
		Fentanyl patches (caution in opioid-naïve patients) Morphine (may be indicated in treatment-resistant pain or palliative care; use cautiously due to associated cognitive and other adverse effects)	
Urinary frequency	Anticholinergic drugs used in overactive bladder	Oxybutynin Tolterodine	Fesoterodine Darifenacin Trospium Solifenacin (use if others are not available; some reports of cognitive adverse effects)
		Data for fesoterodine are still lacking; it is non-selective, has high central anticholinergic activity but theoretically has very low ability to cross the BBB.	
Urinary retention	Alpha blockers	Not known to have effects on cognitive function.	

BBB, blood–brain barrier; COPD, chronic obstructive pulmonary disease; GI, gastrointestinal.

References

1. Sink KM, et al. Dual use of bladder anticholinergics and cholinesterase inhibitors: long-term functional and cognitive outcomes. *J Am Geriatr Soc* 2008; **56**:847–853.
2. Ruxton K, et al. Drugs with anticholinergic effects and cognitive impairment, falls and all-cause mortality in older adults: a systematic review and meta-analysis. *Br J Clin Pharmacol* 2015; **80**:209–220.
3. Sunderland T, et al. Anticholinergic sensitivity in patients with dementia of the Alzheimer type and age-matched controls. A dose-response study. *Arch Gen Psychiatry* 1987; **44**:418–426.
4. Fox C, et al. Anticholinergic medication use and cognitive impairment in the older population: the Medical Research Council Cognitive Function and Ageing Study. *J Am Geriatr Soc* 2011; **59**:1477–1483.
5. Bishara D, et al. The anticholinergic effect on cognition (AEC) scale – associations with mortality, hospitalisation and cognitive decline following dementia diagnosis. *Int J Geriatr Psychiatry* 2020; **35**:1069–1077.
6. Bishara D, et al. Anticholinergic effect on cognition (AEC) of drugs commonly used in older people. *Int J Geriatr Psychiatry* 2017; **32**:650–656.
7. Wagg A. The cognitive burden of anticholinergics in the elderly – implications for the treatment of overactive bladder. *Eur Urol Rev* 2012; **7**:42–49.
8. Pagoria D, et al. Antimuscarinic drugs: review of the cognitive impact when used to treat overactive bladder in elderly patients. *Curr Urol Rep* 2011; **12**:351–357.
9. Womack KB, et al. Tolterodine and memory: dry but forgetful. *Arch Neurol* 2003; **60**:771–773.
10. Tsao JW, et al. Transient memory impairment and hallucinations associated with tolterodine use. *N Engl J Med* 2003; **349**:2274–2275.

11. Edwards KR, et al. Risk of delirium with concomitant use of tolterodine and acetylcholinesterase inhibitors. *J Am Geriatr Soc* 2002; 50:1165–1166.

12. Kay G, et al. Differential effects of the antimuscarinic agents darifenacin and oxybutynin ER on memory in older subjects. *Eur Urol* 2006; 50:317–326.

13. Lipton RB, et al. Assessment of cognitive function of the elderly population: effects of darifenacin. *J Urol* 2005; 173:493–498.

14. Chancellor MB, et al. Blood-brain barrier permeation and efflux exclusion of anticholinergics used in the treatment of overactive bladder. *Drugs Aging* 2012; 29:259–273.

15. Park JW. The effect of solifenacin on cognitive function following stroke. *Dement Geriatr Cogn Dis Extra* 2013; 3:143–147.

16. Liabeuf S, et al. Trospium chloride for overactive bladder may induce central nervous system adverse events. *Eur Geriatr Med* 2014; 5:220–224.

17. Isik AT, et al. Trospium and cognition in patients with late onset Alzheimer disease. *J Nutr Health Aging* 2009; 13:672–676.

18. Geller EJ, et al. Effect of trospium chloride on cognitive function in women aged 50 and older: a randomized trial. *Female Pelvic Med Reconstr Surg* 2017; 23:118–123.

19. Heesakkers J, et al. Safety and tolerability of fesoterodine in older adult patients with overactive bladder. *Can Geriatr J* 2022; 25:72–78.

20. Wagg A. Fesoterodine fumarate for the treatment of overactive bladder in the elderly – a review of the latest clinical data. *Clin Investig* 2012; 2:825–833.

21. Yonguc T, et al. Randomized, controlled trial of fesoterodine fumarate for overactive bladder in Parkinson's disease. *World J Urol* 2020; 38:2013–2019.

22. Joint Formulary Committee. *British National Formulary (online)*. London: BMJ and Pharmaceutical Press; http://www.medicinescomplete.com.

23. Mahdy AM, et al. Histamine and antihistamines. *Anaesth Intens Care Med* 2011; 12:324–329.

24. Roy-Desruisseaux J, et al. Domperidone-induced tardive dyskinesia and withdrawal psychosis in an elderly woman with dementia. *Ann Pharmacother* 2011; 45:e51.

25. Medicines and Healthcare products Regulatory Agency. Domperidone: risks of cardiac side effects – indication restricted to nausea and vomiting, new contraindications, and reduced dose and duration of use. 2014; http://www.mhra.gov.uk/Safetyinformation/DrugSafetyUpdate/CON418518.

26. Bentley KR, et al. Therapeutic potential of serotonin 5-HT3 antagonists in neuropsychiatric disorders. *CNS Drugs* 1995; 3:363–392.

27. Gridelli C. Same old story? Do we need to modify our supportive care treatment of elderly cancer patients? Focus on antiemetics. *Drugs Aging* 2004; 21:825–832.

28. Flicker C, et al. Hypersensitivity to scopolamine in the elderly. *Psychopharmacology (Berl)* 1992; 107:437–441.

29. Ebert U, et al. Scopolamine model of dementia: electroencephalogram findings and cognitive performance. *Eur J Clin Invest* 1998; 28:944–949.

30. Sanofi. Summary of product characteristics. Buscopan 10 mg tablets. 2020 (last updated November 2021); https://www.medicines.org.uk/emc/medicine/30089.

31. Gupta P, et al. Potential adverse effects of bronchodilators in the treatment of airways obstruction in older people: recommendations for prescribing. *Drugs Aging* 2008; 25:415–443.

32. Ramsdell JW, et al. Effects of theophylline and ipratropium on cognition in elderly patients with chronic obstructive pulmonary disease. *Ann Allergy Asthma Immunol* 1996; 76:335–340.

33. Fritze J, et al. Pirenzepine for clozapine-induced hypersalivation. *Lancet* 1995; 346:1034.

34. Pohanka M. Acetylcholinesterase inhibitors: a patent review (2008 – present). *Expert Opin Ther Pat* 2012; 22:871–886.

35. Gray SL, et al. Drug-induced cognition disorders in the elderly: incidence, prevention and management. *Drug Saf* 1999; 21:101–122.

36. Bailey RB, et al. Chronic salicylate intoxication. A common cause of morbidity in the elderly. *J Am Geriatr Soc* 1989; 37:556–561.

37. Hoppmann RA, et al. Central nervous system side effects of nonsteroidal anti-inflammatory drugs. Aseptic meningitis, psychosis, and cognitive dysfunction. *Arch Intern Med* 1991; 151:1309–1313.

38. Wysenbeek AJ, et al. Assessment of cognitive function in elderly patients treated with naproxen. A prospective study. *Clin Exp Rheumatol* 1988; 6:399–400.

39. Bruce-Jones PN, et al. Indomethacin and cognitive function in healthy elderly volunteers. *Br J Clin Pharmacol* 1994; 38:45–51.

40. Barber JB, et al. Treatment of chronic non-malignant pain in the elderly: safety considerations. *Drug Saf* 2009; 32:457–474.

41. Ripamonti C, et al. CNS adverse effects of opioids in cancer patients. *CNS Drugs* 1997; 8:21–37.

42. Alagiakrishnan K, et al. An approach to drug induced delirium in the elderly. *Postgrad Med J* 2004; 80:388–393.

43. McLachlan AJ, et al. Clinical pharmacology of analgesic medicines in older people: impact of frailty and cognitive impairment. *Br J Clin Pharmacol* 2011; 71:351–364.

44. Dosa DM, et al. Frequency of long-acting opioid analgesic initiation in opioid-naive nursing home residents. *J Pain Symptom Manage* 2009; 38:515–521.

45. Tannenbaum C, et al. A systematic review of amnestic and non-amnestic mild cognitive impairment induced by anticholinergic, antihistamine, GABAergic and opioid drugs. *Drugs Aging* 2012; 29:639–658.

46. McGuinness B, et al. Statins for the treatment of dementia. *Cochrane Database Syst Rev* 2014; 7:CD007514.

47. Wagstaff LR, et al. Statin-associated memory loss: analysis of 60 case reports and review of the literature. *Pharmacotherapy* 2003; 23:871–880.

48. Zhou Z, et al. Effect of statin therapy on cognitive decline and incident dementia in older adults. *J Am Coll Cardiol* 2021; 77:3145–3156.

49. McGuinness B, et al. Statins for the prevention of dementia. *Cochrane Database Syst Rev* 2016; 1:CD003160.

50. Olmastroni E, et al. Statin use and risk of dementia or Alzheimer's disease: a systematic review and meta-analysis of observational studies. *Eur J Prev Cardiol* 2022; 29:804–814.

CHAPTER 6

51. Qiu C, et al. The age-dependent relation of blood pressure to cognitive function and dementia. *Lancet Neurol* 2005; **4**:487–499.

52. Wändell P, et al. Antihypertensive drugs and relevant cardiovascular pharmacotherapies and the risk of incident dementia in patients with atrial fibrillation. *Int J Cardiol* 2018; **272**:149–154.

53. Levi MN, et al. Antihypertensive classes, cognitive decline and incidence of dementia: a network meta-analysis. *J Hypertens* 2013; **31**:1073–1082.

54. Branco DR, et al. Direct oral anticoagulants vs vitamin K antagonist on dementia risk in atrial fibrillation: systematic review with meta-analysis. *J Thromb Thrombolysis* 2023; **56**:474–484.

55. Eisendrath SJ, et al. Toxic neuropsychiatric effects of digoxin at therapeutic serum concentrations. *Am J Psychiatry* 1987; **144**:506–507.

56. Brezis M, et al. Nightmares from digoxin. *Ann Intern Med* 1980; **93**:639–640.

57. Laudisio A, et al. Digoxin and cognitive performance in patients with heart failure: a cohort, pharmacoepidemiological survey. *Drugs Aging* 2009; **26**:103–112.

58. Athwal H, et al. Amiodarone-induced delirium. *Am J Geriatr Psychiatry* 2003; **11**:696–697.

59. Foley KT, et al. Separate episodes of delirium associated with levetiracetam and amiodarone treatment in an elderly woman. *Am J Geriatr Pharmacother* 2010; **8**:170–174.

60. Cantu TG, et al. Central nervous system reactions to histamine-2 receptor blockers. *Ann Intern Med* 1991; **114**:1027–1034.

61. Gomm W, et al. Association of proton pump inhibitors with risk of dementia: a pharmacoepidemiological claims data analysis. *JAMA Neurol* 2016; **73**:410–416.

62. Goldstein FC, et al. Proton pump inhibitors and risk of mild cognitive impairment and dementia. *J Am Geriatr Soc* 2017; **65**:1969–1974.

63. Lochhead P, et al. Association between proton pump inhibitor use and cognitive function in women. *Gastroenterology* 2017; **153**:971–979.e974.

64. Haenisch B, et al. Risk of dementia in elderly patients with the use of proton pump inhibitors. *Eur Arch Psychiatry Clin Neurosci* 2015; **265**:419–428.

65. Cooksey R, et al. Proton pump inhibitors and dementia risk: evidence from a cohort study using linked routinely collected national health data in Wales, UK. *PLoS One* 2020; **15**:e0237676.

66. Grahl JJ, et al. Antimicrobial exposure and the risk of delirium in critically ill patients. *Crit Care* 2018; **22**:337.

67. Bhattacharyya S, et al. Antibiotic-associated encephalopathy. *Neurology* 2016; **86**:963–971.

68. Kass JS, et al. Nervous system effects of antituberculosis therapy. *CNS Drugs* 2010; **24**:655–667.

69. Bishara D, et al. Safe prescribing of physical health medication in patients with dementia. *Int J Geriatr Psychiatry* 2014; **29**:1230–1241.

CHAPTER 6

Management of behavioural and psychological symptoms of dementia (BPSD)

Behavioural and psychological symptoms of dementia (BPSD) cover a range of difficulties including aggression, agitation, vocalisation, distress during care, disinhibition, hallucinations, delusions, apathy, low mood and anxiety.[1] Such symptoms occur in over 90% of patients to varying degrees.[2] Drug treatment of BPSD is not well supported by evidence[3] and many of the drugs used in BPSD have serious adverse effects.

Non-drug measures

Since the publication in the UK of *Time for Action*, a report which highlighted the risks of antipsychotic use in dementia,[4] there has been a drive to formulate and employ non-pharmacological treatment for BPSD. Systematic reviews have been completed,[5] new models of care developed[6,7] and guidance documents written.[8] The key themes include:

1. An individualised approach rather than the application of more generalised therapies.
2. Ensuring contributory physical factors are addressed as a first step. These factors include pain (see following section), infection, constipation and medication adverse effects (see 'Safer prescribing for physical conditions in dementia' earlier in this chapter).
3. The importance of understanding and reframing 'problem behaviours' as an expression of distress and unmet need.[6,7]
4. Use of life history, direct observation of care and data collection (e.g. sleep, pain and ABC charts) to uncover unmet needs and to inform treatment.[8]
5. Formulation meetings to develop a model of the factors contributing to the behaviour.
6. Clear care plans developed with carers to address unmet needs.
7. Care plans reviewed and adjusted according to effectiveness of the interventions tried.

Some structured psychosocial interventions for BPSD[9] are supported by research.[10] These can be useful to consider within an individualised care plan and are better if implemented by supporting caregivers. Behavioural management techniques and caregiver psychoeducation centred on an individual patient's behaviour have been found to be generally successful and the effects can last for months.[11]

A 2017 systematic review of systematic reviews[12] provided a comprehensive summary of the evidence for non-pharmacological interventions in BPSD. Among sensory stimulation interventions, the only convincingly effective intervention (reducing agitation and aggressive behaviour) was **music therapy**.[12,13] **Multicomponent interventions** that use a comprehensive, integrated multidisciplinary approach combining medical, psychiatric and nursing interventions may be more effective at reducing severe behavioural problems in nursing home patients.[12] **Animal-assisted therapy** has shown a significant reduction in BPSD, especially depression.[14] **Doll therapy** has been shown to reduce agitation, aggressiveness as well as dysphoria, wandering, apathy, professional caregiver burden and delirium.[15] **Increasing light exposure** and **bright light therapy** may be beneficial in BPSD and sundowning.[16,17] A systematic review suggested that aerobic exercise might be effective in reducing neuropsychiatric symptoms.[18] A 2020 Cochrane review of **aromatherapy** (13 studies with 708 participants) found no evidence that it is beneficial for people with dementia although there are many limitations to the existing data.[19]

Clinicians have limited time to develop non-drug interventions, but in essence they are no more than good clinical practice: taking a clear history to understand factors contributing to behaviours and drawing up a care plan to address these factors. Given drug therapy has such a limited evidence base in this area, there is a duty to do this before even considering prescribing.

Recommendation: The first-line treatments for BPSD are personalised, multicomponent non-drug measures, which involve working closely with caregivers.

Pharmacological measures

Analgesics

Pain in people with dementia may cause agitation and the treatment of pain may reduce agitation.[13,20] An RCT investigating the effects of a stepwise protocol of treatment with analgesics noted significant improvement in agitation, overall neuropsychiatric symptoms and pain. Most patients received only paracetamol (acetaminophen). Education of nursing staff on the link between pain and behaviour may be as effective as an algorithm-based pain management intervention.[21]

A Cochrane review investigated the efficacy and safety of opioids for agitation in people with dementia.[22] RCTs of opioids compared with placebo were assessed but there was insufficient evidence to establish any benefit.

Recommendation: The assessment and effective treatment of pain in people with BPSD are important. Even in people without overt pain, a trial of analgesics (usually paracetamol) may be worthwhile.

Antipsychotics

Antipsychotic drugs were once widely used in BPSD[23] but their use is now discouraged.[24,25] Their effect size is small,[26–29] tolerability is poor[29–31] and they increase mortality.[32] Despite this, antipsychotic medications have been the subject of the largest number of studies of any intervention for BPSD.

Typical antipsychotics (with the exception of haloperidol) show no efficacy in BPSD, but SGAs do have some efficacy. A comparative effectiveness review found the most effective antipsychotics include risperidone (psychosis, agitation, overall BPSD), olanzapine (agitation) and aripiprazole (overall BPSD). Though commonly used, quetiapine has failed to show effectiveness for BPSD, except at doses (100–200mg/day) that may not be well tolerated.[33]

A 2006 Cochrane review[34] of atypical antipsychotics for aggression and psychosis in AD concluded that risperidone and olanzapine can diminish aggression and that risperidone reduces psychotic symptoms. However, because of modest efficacy and significant increase in adverse effects, neither drug should be used to treat BPSD unless there is severe distress or a serious risk of physical harm to those living or working with the patient.

Brexpiprazole is a relatively newly introduced dopamine D_2 receptor partial agonist, like aripiprazole. It has a lower intrinsic activity at D_2 and D_3 than aripiprazole and so has a lower risk for akathisia and extrapyramidal side effects (EPSEs).[35] Brexpiprazole's efficacy and tolerability in the treatment of agitation in AD were investigated in a 12-week RCT. A dose of 2 or 3mg/day showed a statistically significant improvement versus placebo in agitation over 12 weeks and it was generally well tolerated.[36] Brexpiprazole is the only drug that is FDA approved for agitation associated with dementia due to AD.[37] It is not available in the UK.

Increased mortality with antipsychotics in dementia

Following analysis of published and unpublished data in 2004, warnings were issued in the UK and USA regarding increased mortality in patients with dementia taking certain atypical antipsychotics.[38–40] Warnings now apply to all antipsychotics[40,41] and a warning about a possible risk of cerebrovascular events has been added to product labelling for all antipsychotics when used in dementia.

Whether mortality risk varies between antipsychotics has been investigated in several studies.[42–45] In general, haloperidol led to an increased mortality whereas quetiapine users had a decreased risk. No clinically meaningful differences were observed for olanzapine, aripiprazole and ziprasidone[42] (or valproic acid[43]). The effects were strongest shortly after the start of treatment and remained after adjustment for dose. There was a dose–response relationship for all drugs except quetiapine[42] (the higher the dose, the greater the mortality risk).

In a 2019 network meta-analysis of 17 studies (5373 patients), no significant differences were found across measures of effectiveness and safety among aripiprazole, olanzapine, quetiapine and risperidone.[46,47]

> **Recommendation: Risperidone is licensed for persistent aggression in Alzheimer's disease. An alternative agent may be justified if risperidone is contraindicated, not tolerated or not effective. Effect is modest at best. When prescribed, regular review is recommended.**

Clinical information for antipsychotic use in dementia

Antipsychotics should not be used routinely to treat agitation and aggression in people with dementia.[48]

Risperidone and haloperidol are the only drugs licensed in the UK for the management of BPSD. Owing to the dangers of haloperidol, risperidone is the agent of choice. It is specifically indicated for short-term treatment (up to 6 weeks) of persistent aggression in moderate to severe AD unresponsive to non-pharmacological approaches and when there is a risk of harm to self or others.[49] Risperidone is licensed up to 1mg twice a day[50] although the optimal dose in dementia is 500mcg twice a day (1mg daily).[51]

Alternative antipsychotic drugs may be used (off-licence) if risperidone is contraindicated or not tolerated (e.g. because of extrapyramidal symptoms or hyperprolactinaemia). Olanzapine has some positive efficacy data for reducing aggression in dementia,[34] aripiprazole has shown modest efficacy for BPSD[47] and both are less likely to cause Parkinsonian effects. Quetiapine is often considered in patients with Parkinson's disease or DLB (at very small doses) because of its low propensity for causing movement disorders, however it was found to have limited efficacy in dementia so low-dose alternatives (including clozapine) may be required.[52] Always consider anticholinergic burden when selecting an antipsychotic drug in dementia (see 'Safer prescribing for physical conditions in dementia' earlier in this chapter).

Only prescribe antipsychotics after:

- Treating any physical illness, pain or constipation.
- Addressing sensory deficits (find and clean the person's glasses, get a battery for the hearing aid).
- Trying person-centred non-pharmacological options.
- Only use antipsychotics for psychosis or aggression. Other BPSD need different approaches.
- Assess if the antipsychotic drug is safe to use. Assess fall risk and risk factors for stroke.
- Discussing possible risks and benefits with carer (and patient if they have capacity).
- Clear documentation of the above points.[48]
- Review appropriateness of treatment regularly so that an ineffective drug is not continued unnecessarily.
- Monitor for adverse effects.

Guidance on the monitoring of antipsychotic use in dementia is limited. See *Appropriate Prescribing of Antipsychotic Medication in Dementia Toolkit* (https://www.england.nhs.uk/london/wp-content/uploads/sites/8/2022/10/Antipsychotic-Prescribing-Toolkit-for-Dementia.pdf).

Ideally, patients prescribed antipsychotics for longer than a few weeks (and who are not terminally ill) should have the following tests at **baseline**, at **3 months** and **annually** (or as appropriate), if possible, and if it does not lead to unnecessary distress.

1. Blood pressure and pulse.
2. Weight (ideally also monitor monthly for the first 3 months).
3. Blood tests:
   a. fasting glucose or HbA_{1c}
   b. urea and electrolytes (U&Es) including eGFR
   c. full blood count (FBC)
   d. lipids (if possible fasting)
   e. liver function tests (LFTs)
   f. prolactin levels.
4. ECG (repeat at between 4 weeks and 3 months or when clinically indicated).

- In-patients or physically frail patients may need more frequent physical health monitoring.
- Review of the antipsychotic drug needs to be done at 4–6 weeks (maybe earlier for in-patients), then at 3 months and then every 6 months if physically stable and there are no adverse effects. Consider stopping the antipsychotic at each review, where appropriate.

- Several deprescribing studies have shown that antipsychotics[53-55] (and other psychotropics)[55,56] can be deprescribed successfully (Table 6.6) as the reductions in psychotropic drug use did not negatively affect BPSD, while ADL improved.[55]

Table 6.6 Reduction or discontinuation regimen for antipsychotic drugs in BPSD – a guide.[57,58]

Antipsychotic	Usual dose range in dementia	Suggested regimen for reduction/discontinuation (generally over 4 weeks if possible)*
Amisulpride	25–50mg/day	Reduce by 12.5–25mg every 1–2 weeks (depending on dose) then stop
Aripiprazole	5–15mg/day	Reduce by 5mg every 1–2 weeks (depending on dose) then stop (if patient is on 5mg daily, reduce to 2.5mg for 2 weeks)
Haloperidol	Not recommended in older people with dementia (except in delirium) Reduce by 0.25–0.5mg every 1–2 weeks (depending on dose) then stop	
Olanzapine	2.5–10mg/day	Reduce by 2.5mg every 1–2 weeks (depending on dose) then stop
Quetiapine	12.5–300mg/day	For doses 12.5–100mg/day – reduce by 12.5–25mg every 1–2 weeks (depending on dose) then stop
		For doses >100–300mg/day – reduce by 25–50mg every 1–2 weeks (depending on dose) then stop
		If dose is 300mg/day – reduce to 150–200mg/day for 1 week then by 50mg/week then stop
Risperidone	0.25–2mg/day	Reduce by 0.25–0.5mg every 1–2 weeks (depending on dose) then stop

*Duration of taper should not normally exceed the duration of treatment.
NB If serious adverse effects occur, stop the antipsychotic drug immediately. BPSD, behavioural and psychological symptoms of dementia.

Other pharmacological agents in BPSD

Cognitive enhancers

Acetylcholinesterase inhibitors and memantine have a modest effect on BPSD.[13] According to a meta-analysis[59] and systematic review,[60] the effect of AChE-Is on BPSD is at least statistically significant. Overall, cholinesterase inhibitors are more effective for depression, dysphoria, apathy and anxiety than for agitation or aggression. Memantine can help to improve agitation, aggression and delusions.

> **Recommendation: AChE-Is or memantine can help with mild BPSD and are worth considering if a patient is not already on one of these drugs.**

Benzodiazepines

Benzodiazepines[61,62] are widely used but their use is poorly supported. Benzodiazepines increase the rate of cognitive decline,[61] risk of dementia,[63] risk of pneumonia[64] and *increase all-cause mortality*.[65] They may contribute to the increased frequency of falls and hip fractures[62,66] in older people.

> *Recommendation: Avoid benzodiazepines other than as a single use for emergency sedation.*

Antidepressants

Depression is a risk factor and consequence of AD. The prevalence of depression and AD comorbidity is estimated to be 30–50%.[67]

As with other BPSD, non-pharmacological approaches such as reminiscence, cognitive stimulation/rehabilitation, therapeutic approaches, music-based approaches and education/training have the potential to reduce symptoms of depression in dementia.[68] If you can, try simple measures to improve quality of life as the first-line intervention in mild to moderate depression in dementia.

The evidence for efficacy of antidepressants in BPSD is mixed and limited, showing that antidepressants are most helpful for treating agitation and less useful for depression, apathy, anxiety or psychosis in dementia.[33] **Citalopram** has the strongest evidence for efficacy in agitation, with the CitAD trial[69] showing that a high dose (30mg) of citalopram daily had a positive effect on agitation in dementia; unfortunately this study also confirmed a risk of QT prolongation with citalopram. The maximum dose of citalopram in older people is limited to 20mg a day because of the drug's effect on cardiac QT interval. Although there is less evidence, **escitalopram** may also be effective in BPSD. The evidence for efficacy of **sertraline** is mixed, though its cardiac safety is compelling.[33]

One Cochrane review of **trazodone** for agitation in dementia[70] found insufficient evidence from RCTs to support its use in dementia, but another Cochrane review found trazodone 50mg at bedtime was well tolerated and improved sleep for people with dementia and insomnia.[71] Additionally, trazodone 150–300mg/day was found effective in reducing BPSD in frontotemporal dementia.[72] Although **mirtazapine** is frequently used to treat older adults with depression, a pilot study showed no significant therapeutic effect of 15mg mirtazapine on Alzheimer's patients with sleep disorders and in fact found worsening of daytime sleep patterns.[73] A study of mirtazapine for agitation in dementia randomly assigned patients to receive either mirtazapine (titrated to 45mg) or placebo, and found no benefit of mirtazapine and a potentially higher mortality in patients who received it.[74] **Bupropion** has not been studied in controlled trials in dementia.[33]

Vortioxetine has multimodal activity and potential effects on cognitive function through its mechanisms on glutamate neurotransmission and neuroplasticity in the prefrontal cortex, which may be useful in dementia. In a 12-month open-label observational study of 108 patients with mild AD and depressive symptoms, vortioxetine had a beneficial effect on cognition and mood and was well tolerated.[75] However, a 12-week placebo-controlled RCT of 100 patients with AD and depression found no statistically significant difference between the two groups in terms of depressive symptoms, cognitive functions and ADL. The percentage of adverse events and drug discontinuation was similar between groups.[76] A possible explanation for the divergent results is that the second study included patients with more severe cognitive impairment and depressive symptoms. An open-label prospective study in patients with Parkinson's disease and major depression showed that vortioxetine was well tolerated and improved depressive symptoms as well as cognitive function, apathy, fatigue and quality of life 3 months after starting the drug.[77]

Tricyclic antidepressants are best avoided in patients with dementia. They can cause falls, via orthostatic hypotension, and worsen cognition owing to their anticholinergic adverse effect.[78]

While some studies have found that antidepressant use in older people may be associated with an increased risk of dementia,[79] it is important to keep in mind that previous studies have shown that late-life depression is associated with an increased risk for dementia. Hence any comparisons of antidepressant users with non-depressed non-users are subject to indication bias as the increased dementia risk could be due to depression, not the medication.

Recommendation: Although evidence is weak, use of antidepressants is justified in people with dementia who have clear symptoms of moderate or severe depression, especially if non-pharmacological approaches have been ineffective.

Mood stabilisers/antiseizure medications

Randomised controlled trials of mood stabilisers in BPSD have been completed for oxcarbazepine,[80] carbamazepine[81] and valproate.[82] Gabapentin, lamotrigine and topiramate have also been used.[83] Of the mood stabilisers, carbamazepine has the most robust evidence of efficacy in non-cognitive symptoms.[84] However, its serious adverse effects (especially Stevens-Johnson syndrome, ataxia and hyponatraemia) and its potential for drug interactions limit its use.

One RCT of valproate found it to be ineffective in controlling BPSD symptoms.[85] A Cochrane review of valproate for the treatment of agitation in dementia concluded that it was ineffective and associated with a higher rate of adverse effects, and possibly of serious ones.[86] Valproate does not delay emergence of agitation in dementia.[87] Literature reviews of anticonvulsants in non-cognitive symptoms of dementia found that valproate, oxcarbazepine and lithium showed low or no evidence of efficacy and that more RCTs are needed to strengthen the evidence for gabapentin, topiramate and lamotrigine.[84]

Preliminary low-grade evidence based on case series and case reviews suggests a possible benefit of gabapentin and pregabalin in patients with BPSD in AD. Evidence in frontotemporal dementia is lacking.[88] In a small case series, gabapentin reduced aggression among seven patients with vascular dementia or mixed vascular/AD, using daily doses ranging from 200 to 600mg daily. Three of the seven patients were able to discontinue antipsychotics after gabapentin initiation; thus, it may be useful in patients with cardiac conditions where antipsychotics are inappropriate. Caution should be noted about the use of gabapentin in DLB. Dramatic worsening of neuropsychiatric symptoms has been reported after its use to treat behavioural symptoms.[89] There is inadequate evidence to support the use of levetiracetam for BPSD, with concerns regarding tolerability.[90]

Although clearly beneficial in some patients, anticonvulsants/mood stabilisers cannot be recommended for routine use in the treatment of the neuropsychiatric symptoms in dementia at present.[83]

Recommendation: Limited evidence to support use; use may be justified where other treatments are contraindicated or ineffective. Valproate is best avoided.

CHAPTER 6

Management of sleep disturbances in dementia

Non-pharmacological management of sleep disturbances using established sleep hygiene methods should be the first-line treatment for insomnia in dementia.[91,92]

A 2020 Cochrane review[93] of pharmacotherapies for sleep disturbances in dementia found a distinct lack of evidence to guide decisions about drug treatment of sleep problems in dementia. There were no RCTs for the many widely prescribed drugs (including benzodiazepine and non-benzodiazepine hypnotics), despite considerable uncertainty about the balance of benefits and risks for these common treatments. The authors found no evidence for beneficial effects of **melatonin** (up to 10mg) or a melatonin receptor agonist. There was evidence of some beneficial effects on sleep outcomes from **trazodone** and **orexin antagonists** (**suvorexant** and **lemborexant**; two studies, n = 323) and no evidence of harmful effects in these small trials, although larger trials are needed.

Of note, melatonin (at 2mg and occasionally up to 10mg/day modified release) is used in patients with dementia with good effects. In one study, melatonin 9mg resulted in improvement in subjective sleep, reduction of sundowning behaviour and lack of decline in cognitive function testing over a period of 22–35 months. Several other case reports and small open-label trials described benefits on subjective sleep characteristics and cognitive function, but data quality is limiting.[94]

An expert review[92] also deduced that non-pharmacological interventions are generally preferred as the first-line approach to improve sleep-related symptoms in AD; however, when non-pharmacological interventions alone are insufficient, a range of pharmacological agents can be considered. Trazodone and melatonin are commonly used as adjunctive therapies, while Z-drugs including zopiclone and zolpidem are specifically employed to treat insomnia in patients with late-onset AD. Furthermore, dual orexin receptor antagonists have emerged and gained approval for improving sleep onset and maintenance in AD patients. The review proposed a stepwise algorithm for the management of sleep disturbances in AD.[92]

> **Recommendation: Despite limited evidence for the efficacy of melatonin, it is safe to use and may be justified in cases where benefits are seen. Non-pharmacological management of sleep disturbances should be tried first.**

Sedating antihistamines

Promethazine is frequently used in BPSD for its sedative effects. It has strong anticholinergic effects and readily penetrates the BBB, potentially causing significant cognitive impairment.[95]

> **Recommendation: Promethazine should be avoided.**

Miscellaneous agents[96,97]

A meta-analysis of RCTs for **Gingko biloba** (240mg daily, 22–24-week treatment) showed improvement in BPSD (except psychotic-like features) and in caregiver distress caused by such symptoms.[98]

Pimavanserin (inverse agonist and antagonist at $5HT_{2A}$ receptors) is approved by the FDA for the treatment of hallucinations and delusions associated with Parkinson's disease psychosis. One RCT evaluated its use for the treatment of psychosis in AD and showed improved psychotic symptoms when compared with placebo and a lower risk of relapse with continuation. Headache, constipation, urinary tract infection and asymptomatic QT prolongation occurred with pimavanserin.[99] It has also shown improvement of depressive symptoms in patients with Parkinson's disease.[100]

A recent phase III, randomised double-blind placebo-controlled multicentre study investigating the efficacy of **lumateperone** (a potent antagonist at $5HT_{2A}$ receptors, and a serotonin reuptake inhibitor) in reducing dementia-related agitation failed to show any benefit.[101]

Other agents being investigated for BPSD include **dextromethorphan/quinidine** (one RCT found it decreased agitation and was well tolerated),[102] **bupropion/dextromethorphan**[103] and **methylphenidate** (one RCT found it to be effective for apathy in AD in individuals who were not anxious or agitated).[103,104] **Prazosin** (a centrally acting $\alpha1$ adrenoceptor antagonist) appears to benefit individuals with dementia and agitation and aggression. When compared with other treatments for BPSD, the data for its use in BPSD are limited to just one good-quality RCT. Given these limitations, its routine use for the management of BPSD cannot be recommended at this time; however, it may be used when other medications (e.g. acetylcholinesterase inhibitors, memantine, antidepressants and/or atypical antipsychotics) have been ineffective or not tolerated.[47,105]

A Cochrane review (4 small studies, 110 participants) found low-certainty evidence suggesting there may be little or no clinically important effect of **cannabinoids** on overall BPSD assessed with the Neuropsychiatric Inventory.[106]

Electroconvulsive therapy (ECT)

Electroconvulsive therapy may have a place in the treatment of severe and refractory BPSD. A review (20 published reports, 172 individuals with dementia; 40% AD) found that over 90% of the individuals responded to ECT treatment. Adverse effects were infrequent, mild and transient. The most common adverse event noted was postictal confusion/memory impairment that was seen in approximately 15% of the individuals.[47]

However, ECT would not be recommended as a common intervention given limited evidence, and the considerable practical aspects of transporting patients to the ECT clinic and difficulty with obtaining consent.

> **Recommendation: There is insufficient evidence to recommend ECT use in BPSD. Caution: It can cause significant cognitive adverse effects.**

Summary

The evidence base available to guide treatment in this area is insufficient to allow specific recommendations on appropriate management and drug choice. The basic approach is to exclude physical illness and try non-drug measures before resorting to the use of psychotropics. When using pharmacological treatments, there should be clearly documented treatment aims and prescribing should cease if these aims are not met within a specified timeframe.

CHAPTER 6

References

1. National Institute for Health and Care Excellence. Dementia: assessment, management and support for people living with dementia and their carers. NICE Guidance [NG97]. 2018 (last checked September 2023, last accessed December 2023); https://www.nice.org.uk/guidance/ng97.

2. Steinberg M, et al. Point and 5-year period prevalence of neuropsychiatric symptoms in dementia: the Cache County Study. *Int J Geriatr Psychiatry* 2008; **23**:170–177.

3. Salzman C, et al. Elderly patients with dementia-related symptoms of severe agitation and aggression: consensus statement on treatment options, clinical trials methodology, and policy. *J Clin Psychiatry* 2008; **69**:889–898.

4. Department of Health. The use of antipsychotic medication for people with dementia: time for action. A report for the Minister of State for Care Services by Professor Sube Banerjee. 2009; https://psychrights.org/research/digest/nlps/banerjeereportongeriatricneurolepticuse.pdf.

5. Livingston G, et al. A systematic review of the clinical effectiveness and cost-effectiveness of sensory, psychological and behavioural interventions for managing agitation in older adults with dementia. *Health Technol Assess* 2014; **18**:1–226, v–vi.

6. Kales HC, et al. Assessment and management of behavioral and psychological symptoms of dementia. *BMJ* 2015; **350**:h369.

7. James IA. *Understanding Behaviour in Dementia That Challenges: A Guide to Assessment and Treatment.* London: Jessica Kingsley Publishers; 2011.

8. Brechin D, et al. British Psychological Society. Briefing paper. Alternatives to antipsychotic medication: psychological approaches in managing psychological and behavioural distress in people with dementia. 2013; https://explore.bps.org.uk/content/report-guideline/bpsrep.2013.inf207.

9. Douglas S, et al. Non-pharmacological interventions in dementia. *Adv Psychiatric Treat* 2004; **10**:171–177.

10. Ayalon L, et al. Effectiveness of nonpharmacological interventions for the management of neuropsychiatric symptoms in patients with dementia: a systematic review. *Arch Intern Med* 2006; **166**:2182–2188.

11. Livingston G, et al. Systematic review of psychological approaches to the management of neuropsychiatric symptoms of dementia. *Am J Psychiatry* 2005; **162**:1996–2021.

12. Abraha I, et al. Systematic review of systematic reviews of non-pharmacological interventions to treat behavioural disturbances in older patients with dementia. The SENATOR-OnTop series. *BMJ Open* 2017; **7**:e012759.

13. Dyer SM, et al. An overview of systematic reviews of pharmacological and non-pharmacological interventions for the treatment of behavioral and psychological symptoms of dementia. *Int Psychogeriatr* 2018; **30**:295–309.

14. Chen H, et al. Effects of animal-assisted therapy on patients with dementia: a systematic review and meta-analysis of randomized controlled trials. *Psychiatry Res* 2022; **314**:114619.

15. Santagata F, et al. The doll therapy as a first line treatment for behavioral and psychologic symptoms of dementia in nursing homes residents: a randomized, controlled study. *BMC Geriatr* 2021; **21**:545.

16. Guu TW, et al. Light, sleep-wake rhythm, and behavioural and psychological symptoms of dementia in care home patients: revisiting the sundowning syndrome. *Int J Geriatr Psychiatry* 2022; **37**:10.

17. Kolberg E, et al. The effects of bright light treatment on affective symptoms in people with dementia: a 24-week cluster randomized controlled trial. *BMC Psychiatry* 2021; **21**:377.

18. Steichele K, et al. The effects of exercise programs on cognition, activities of daily living, and neuropsychiatric symptoms in community-dwelling people with dementia – a systematic review. *Alzheimers Res Ther* 2022; **14**:97.

19. Ball EL, et al. Aromatherapy for dementia. *Cochrane Database Syst Rev* 2020; **8**:CD003150.

20. Husebo BS, et al. Efficacy of treating pain to reduce behavioural disturbances in residents of nursing homes with dementia: cluster randomised clinical trial. *BMJ* 2011; **343**:d4065.

21. Manietta C, et al. Algorithm-based pain management for people with dementia in nursing homes. *Cochrane Database Syst Rev* 2022; **4**:CD013339.

22. Brown R, et al. Opioids for agitation in dementia. *Cochrane Database Syst Rev* 2015; **5**:CD009705.

23. Lee PE, et al. Atypical antipsychotic drugs in the treatment of behavioural and psychological symptoms of dementia: systematic review. *BMJ* 2004; **329**:75.

24. Jeste DV, et al. Atypical antipsychotics in elderly patients with dementia or schizophrenia: review of recent literature. *Harv Rev Psychiatry* 2005; **13**:340–351.

25. Jeste DV, et al. ACNP White Paper: update on use of antipsychotic drugs in elderly persons with dementia. *Neuropsychopharmacology* 2008; **33**:957–970.

26. Aupperle P. Management of aggression, agitation, and psychosis in dementia: focus on atypical antipsychotics. *Am J Alzheimers Dis Other Demen* 2006; **21**:101–108.

27. Yury CA, et al. Meta-analysis of the effectiveness of atypical antipsychotics for the treatment of behavioural problems in persons with dementia. *Psychother Psychosom* 2007; **76**:213–218.

28. Deberdt WG, et al. Comparison of olanzapine and risperidone in the treatment of psychosis and associated behavioral disturbances in patients with dementia. *Am J Geriatr Psychiatry* 2005; **13**:722–730.

29. Schneider LS, et al. Efficacy and adverse effects of atypical antipsychotics for dementia: meta-analysis of randomized, placebo-controlled trials. *Am J Geriatr Psychiatry* 2006; **14**:191–210.

30. Anon. How safe are antipsychotics in dementia? *Drug Ther Bull* 2007; **45**:81–86.

31. Rosack J. Side-effect risk often tempers antipsychotic use for dementia. *Psychiatr News* 2006; **41**:1–38.

32. Schneider LS, et al. Risk of death with atypical antipsychotic drug treatment for dementia: meta-analysis of randomized placebo-controlled trials. *JAMA* 2005; **294**:1934–1943.

33. Bessey LJ, et al. Management of behavioral and psychological symptoms of dementia. *Curr Psychiatry Rep* 2019; **21**:66.

34. Ballard C, et al. The effectiveness of atypical antipsychotics for the treatment of aggression and psychosis in Alzheimer's disease (review). *Cochrane Database Syst Rev* 2006; **1**:CD003476.

35. Stahl SM. Mechanism of action of brexpiprazole: comparison with aripiprazole. *CNS Spectr* 2016; **21**:1–6.

36. Lee D, et al. Brexpiprazole for the treatment of agitation in Alzheimer dementia: a randomized clinical trial. *JAMA Neurol* 2023; **80**:1307–1316.

37. US Food and Drug Administration. FDA approves first drug to treat agitation symptoms associated with dementia due to Alzheimer's disease. 2023 (last accessed January 2024); https://www.fda.gov/news-events/press-announcements/fda-approves-first-drug-treat-agitation-symptoms-associated-dementia-due-alzheimers-disease.

38. Gov.UK. PhVWP assessment report: antipsychotics and cerebrovascular accident. 2005; https://www.gov.uk/government/publications/antipsychotic-medicines-licensed-products-uses-and-side-effects.

39. Duff G. Atypical antipsychotic drugs and stroke – Committee on Safety of Medicines. 2004; https://webarchive.nationalarchives.gov.uk/20141206131857/http://www.mhra.gov.uk/home/groups/pl-p/documents/websiteresources/con019488.pdf.

40. US Food and Drug Administration. Information on conventional antipsychotics – FDA alert [6/16/2008]. 2008; http://www.fda.gov/.

41. European Medicines Agency. CHMP assessment report on conventional antipsychotics. 2008; http://www.emea.europa.eu.

42. Huybrechts KF, et al. Differential risk of death in older residents in nursing homes prescribed specific antipsychotic drugs: population based cohort study. *BMJ* 2012; **344**:e977.

43. Kales HC, et al. Risk of mortality among individual antipsychotics in patients with dementia. *Am J Psychiatry* 2012; **169**:71–79.

44. Schmedt N, et al. Comparative risk of death in older adults treated with antipsychotics: a population-based cohort study. *Eur Neuropsychopharmacol* 2016; **26**:1390–1400.

45. Maust DT, et al. Antipsychotics, other psychotropics, and the risk of death in patients with dementia: number needed to harm. *JAMA Psychiatry* 2015; **72**:438–445.

46. Yunusa I, et al. Assessment of reported comparative effectiveness and safety of atypical antipsychotics in the treatment of behavioral and psychological symptoms of dementia: a network meta-analysis. *JAMA Network Open* 2019; **2**:e190828.

47. Tampi RR, et al. Prazosin for the management of behavioural and psychological symptoms of dementia. *Drugs Context* 2022; **11**;2022-3-3.

48. Corbett A, et al. Don't use antipsychotics routinely to treat agitation and aggression in people with dementia. *BMJ* 2014; **349**:g6420.

49. Janssen-Cilag Ltd. Summary of product characteristics. RISPERDAL CONSTA 25mg, 37.5mg, 50mg powder and solvent for prolonged-release suspension for injection. 2022 (last accessed December 2023); https://www.medicines.org.uk/emc/product/1690/smpc#gref.

50. Joint Formulary Committee. *British National Formulary (online)*. London: BMJ and Pharmaceutical Press; http://www.medicinescomplete.com.

51. Katz IR, et al. Comparison of risperidone and placebo for psychosis and behavioral disturbances associated with dementia: a randomized, double-blind trial. Risperidone Study Group. *J Clin Psychiatry* 1999; **60**:107–115.

52. Kyle K, et al. Treatment of psychosis in Parkinson's disease and dementia with Lewy bodies: a review. *Parkinsonism Relat Disord* 2020; **75**:55–62.

53. Brodaty H, et al. Antipsychotic deprescription for older adults in long-term care: the HALT Study. *J Am Med Dir Assoc* 2018; **19**:592–600.e597.

54. Ballard C, et al. The Dementia Antipsychotic Withdrawal Trial (DART-AD): long-term follow-up of a randomised placebo-controlled trial. *Lancet Neurol* 2009; **8**:151–157.

55. Gedde MH, et al. Less is more: the impact of deprescribing psychotropic drugs on behavioral and psychological symptoms and daily functioning in nursing home patients. results from the cluster-randomized controlled COSMOS Trial. *Am J Geriatr Psychiatry* 2021; **29**:304–315.

56. Cossette B, et al. Optimizing practices, use, care, and services-antipsychotics (OPUS-AP) in long-term care centers in Quebec, Canada: a successful scale-up. *J Am Med Dir Assoc* 2022; **23**:1084–1089.

57. NHS PrescQIPP. T7: reducing antipsychotic prescribing in dementia. 2014; https://www.prescqipp.info/our-resources/bulletins/t7-reducing-antipsychotic-prescribing-in-dementia/.

58. Bjerre LM, et al. Deprescribing antipsychotics for behavioural and psychological symptoms of dementia and insomnia: evidence-based clinical practice guideline. *Can Fam Physician* 2018; **64**:17–27.

59. Campbell N, et al. Impact of cholinesterase inhibitors on behavioral and psychological symptoms of Alzheimer's disease: a meta-analysis. *Clin Interv Aging* 2008; **3**:719–728.

60. Seibert M, et al. Efficacy and safety of pharmacotherapy for Alzheimer's disease and for behavioural and psychological symptoms of dementia in older patients with moderate and severe functional impairments: a systematic review of controlled trials. *Alzheimers Res Ther* 2021; **13**:131.

61. Verdoux H, et al. Is benzodiazepine use a risk factor for cognitive decline and dementia? A literature review of epidemiological studies. *Psychol Med* 2005; **35**:307–315.

62. Lagnaoui R, et al. Benzodiazepine utilization patterns in Alzheimer's disease patients. *Pharmacoepidemiol Drug Saf* 2003; **12**:511–515.

63. Billioti de Gage S, et al. Benzodiazepine use and risk of dementia: prospective population based study. *BMJ* 2012; **345**:e6231.

64. Taipale H, et al. Risk of pneumonia associated with incident benzodiazepine use among community-dwelling adults with Alzheimer disease. *CMAJ* 2017; **189**:e519–e525.

65. Palmaro A, et al. Benzodiazepines and risk of death: results from two large cohort studies in France and UK. *Eur Neuropsychopharmacol* 2015; **25**:1566–1577.

66. Chang CM, et al. Benzodiazepine and risk of hip fractures in older people: a nested case-control study in Taiwan. *Am J Geriatr Psychiatry* 2008; **16**:686–692.

67. Aboukhatwa M, et al. Antidepressants are a rational complementary therapy for the treatment of Alzheimer's disease. *Mol Neurodegener* 2010; 5:10.

68. Burley CV, et al. Nonpharmacological approaches reduce symptoms of depression in dementia: a systematic review and meta-analysis. *Ageing Res Rev* 2022; 79:101669.

69. Porsteinsson AP, et al. Effect of citalopram on agitation in Alzheimer disease: the CitAD randomized clinical trial. *JAMA* 2014; 311:682–691.

70. Martinon-Torres G, et al. Trazodone for agitation in dementia. *Cochrane Database Syst Rev* 2004; 4:CD004990.

71. McCleery J, et al. Pharmacotherapies for sleep disturbances in dementia. *Cochrane Database Syst Rev* 2016; 11:CD009178.

72. Trieu C, et al. Effectiveness of pharmacological interventions for symptoms of behavioral variant frontotemporal dementia: a systematic review. *Cogn Behav Neurol* 2020; 33:1–15.

73. Scoralick FM, et al. Mirtazapine does not improve sleep disorders in Alzheimer's disease: results from a double-blind, placebo-controlled pilot study. *Psychogeriatrics* 2017; 17:89–96.

74. Banerjee S, et al. Study of mirtazapine for agitated behaviours in dementia (SYMBAD): a randomised, double-blind, placebo-controlled trial. *Lancet* 2021; 398:1487–1497.

75. Cumbo E, et al. Treatment effects of vortioxetine on cognitive functions in mild Alzheimer's disease patients with depressive symptoms: a 12 month, open-label, observational study. *J Prev Alzheimers Dis* 2019; 6:192–197.

76. Jeong HW, et al. Vortioxetine treatment for depression in Alzheimer's disease: a randomized, double-blind, placebo-controlled study. *Clin Psychopharmacol Neurosci* 2022; 20:311–319.

77. Santos García D, et al. Vortioxetine improves depressive symptoms and cognition in Parkinson's disease patients with major depression: an open-label prospective study. *Brain Sci* 2022; 12:1466.

78. Ballard C, et al. Management of neuropsychiatric symptoms in people with dementia. *CNS Drugs* 2010; 24:729–739.

79. Wang YC, et al. Increased risk of dementia in patients with antidepressants: a meta-analysis of observational studies. *Behav Neurol* 2018; 2018:5315098.

80. Sommer OH, et al. Effect of oxcarbazepine in the treatment of agitation and aggression in severe dementia. *Dement Geriatr Cogn Disord* 2009; 27:155–163.

81. Tariot PN, et al. Efficacy and tolerability of carbamazepine for agitation and aggression in dementia. *Am J Psychiatry* 1998; 155:54–61.

82. Lonergan E, et al. Valproate preparations for agitation in dementia. *Cochrane Database Syst Rev* 2009; 3:CD003945.

83. Konovalov S, et al. Anticonvulsants for the treatment of behavioral and psychological symptoms of dementia: a literature review. *Int Psychogeriatr* 2008; 20:293–308.

84. Yeh YC, et al. Mood stabilizers for the treatment of behavioral and psychological symptoms of dementia: an update review. *Kaohsiung J Med Sci* 2012; 28:185–193.

85. Sival RC, et al. Sodium valproate in aggressive behaviour in dementia: a twelve-week open label follow-up study. *Int J Geriatr Psychiatry* 2004; 19:305–312.

86. Baillon SF, et al. Valproate preparations for agitation in dementia. *Cochrane Database Syst Rev* 2018; 10:CD003945.

87. Tariot PN, et al. Chronic divalproex sodium to attenuate agitation and clinical progression of Alzheimer disease. *Arch Gen Psychiatry* 2011; 68:853–861.

88. Supasitthumrong T, et al. Gabapentin and pregabalin to treat aggressivity in dementia: a systematic review and illustrative case report. *Br J Clin Pharmacol* 2019; 85:690–703.

89. Cooney C, et al. Use of low-dose gabapentin for aggressive behavior in vascular and mixed vascular/Alzheimer dementia. *J Neuropsychiatry Clin Neurosci* 2013; 25:120–125.

90. Gallagher D, et al. Antiepileptic drugs for the treatment of agitation and aggression in dementia: do they have a place in therapy? *Drugs* 2014; 74:1747–1755.

91. David R, et al. Non-pharmacologic management of sleep disturbance in Alzheimer's disease. *J Nutr Health Aging* 2010; 14:203–206.

92. Javed B, et al. Pharmacological and non-pharmacological treatment options for sleep disturbances in Alzheimer's disease. *Expert Rev Neurother* 2023; 23:501–514.

93. McCleery J, et al. Pharmacotherapies for sleep disturbances in dementia. *Cochrane Database Syst Rev* 2020; 11:CD009178.

94. Roland JP, et al. Impact of pharmacotherapy on insomnia in patients with Alzheimer's disease. *Drugs Aging* 2021; 38:951–966.

95. Bishara D, et al. Anticholinergic effect on cognition (AEC) of drugs commonly used in older people. *Int J Geriatr Psychiatry* 2017; 32:650–656.

96. Porsteinsson AP, et al. An update on the advancements in the treatment of agitation in Alzheimer's disease. *Expert Opin Pharmacother* 2017; 18:611–620.

97. Carrarini C, et al. Agitation and dementia: prevention and treatment strategies in acute and chronic conditions. *Front Neurol* 2021; 12:644317.

98. Savaskan E, et al. Treatment effects of Ginkgo biloba extract EGb 761® on the spectrum of behavioral and psychological symptoms of dementia: meta-analysis of randomized controlled trials. *Int Psychogeriatr* 2018; 30:285–293.

99. Tariot PN, et al. Trial of pimavanserin in dementia-related psychosis. *N Engl J Med* 2021; 385:309–319.

100. DeKarske D, et al. An open-label, 8-week study of safety and efficacy of pimavanserin treatment in adults with Parkinson's disease and depression. *J Parkinsons Dis* 2020; 10:1751–1761.

101. ClinicalTrials.gov. ITI-007 for the treatment of agitation in patients with dementia, including Alzheimer's disease [NCT02817906]. 2021; https://clinicaltrials.gov/study/NCT02817906.

102. Tampi RR, et al. Evidence for using dextromethorphan-quinidine for the treatment of agitation in dementia. *World J Psychiatry* 2020; **10**:29–33.

103. Ahmed M, et al. Current agents in development for treating behavioral and psychological symptoms associated with dementia. *Drugs Aging* 2019; **36**:589–605.

104. Lanctôt KL, et al. Heterogeneity of response to methylphenidate in apathetic patients in the ADMET 2 Trial. *Am J Geriatr Psychiatry* 2023; **31**:1077–1087.

105. Chen A, et al. The Psychopharmacology Algorithm Project at the Harvard South Shore Program: an update on management of behavioral and psychological symptoms in dementia. *Psychiatry Res* 2021; **295**:113641.

106. Bosnjak Kuharic D, et al. Cannabinoids for the treatment of dementia. *Cochrane Database Syst Rev* 2021; **9**:CD012820.

Management of inappropriate sexual behaviour in older adults

This section deals with sexual behaviours that are causing distress either to the person with dementia or to other people. Sexually inappropriate behaviours have been reported in between 1.8% and 25.9% of patients with neurocognitive disorders,[1] and in people with dementia the prevalence rate is 2–17%, occurring with about equal frequency in men and women.[2] Sexual symptoms are more prevalent in frontal lobe disorders (most commonly stroke and behavioural variant frontotemporal dementia) and in Parkinson's (adverse effects of dopaminergic drugs), but can occur in any dementia subtype.[1] These symptoms present a challenge for patients, carers and healthcare workers.

Assessment of the behaviours, the contexts in which they arise and their risks is essential. It is important to manage the environment and to educate and discuss the behaviour with carers and families. Behavioural measures are probably helpful, although no specific intervention has been shown to be effective in this area. Several classes of drug may help to control aberrant sexual behaviours, but owing to the lack of large-scale studies there is no gold standard treatment. No treatments are licensed for hypersexuality in this population and the medications used are all potentially harmful.[2]

A thorough history should be taken before starting any drug therapy to obtain the relevant medical, psychiatric, medication and sexual history. Changes in sexual behaviour can be caused by urinary or genital conditions, delirium or a medication side effect. Benzodiazepines, dopamine-receptor agonists (e.g. apomorphine, pramipexole, rotigotine) and L-dopa can cause hypersexuality.[2] Non-pharmacological treatment, such as distraction/diversion of the patient when inappropriate sexual behaviours occur,[1] is recommended as first-line therapy (Box 6.3). Antidepressants

---

Box 6.3 Non-pharmacological measures[1]

- Identify and treat medical causes for behaviour, e.g. urinary retention and genital disorders causing the patient to touch their genitals due to discomfort. Delirium can cause sexual disinhibition
- Identify and treat any psychiatric disorder that may cause inappropriate sexual behaviour, e.g. mania or depression
- If possible, stop or reduce dose of medication that may be causing the behaviour, e.g. benzodiazepines, dopamine agonists and high-dose L-dopa
- Prevention: fulfil the need for intimacy/connection in other ways such as having meals in groups, conversation among peers and activities such as walking or exercise
- Discussion with patient, caregivers and relatives to better understand the behaviour and explore attitudes to sexuality, which may inform therapy
- Distraction or diversion, redirect behaviour, engage patients in activities that involve the hands and reduce sexual stimulation (e.g. iPads, magazines, TV)
- Provide sensory and environmental stimulation (e.g. aromatherapy, music therapy, multisensory therapy, pet therapy).
- Behavioural/cognitive behavioural therapy if available (though evidence is limited)

have been recommended as the first line of pharmacological treatment after attempting non-pharmacological interventions. Several other categories of pharmacological interventions are listed in Table 6.7.

Management

To inform the management of inappropriate sexual behaviour, evaluation should include a medical history, physical examination, sexual history and medication review. The history should cover specifics of the demonstrated behaviour, such as potential precipitants and consequences including the frequencies of episodes, when and where they occur and with whom.[3] Sometimes normal sexual behaviour, such as a patient masturbating in their bedroom, can be labelled as 'disinhibition', particularly in care home settings. In these cases, a discussion with staff and relatives about simple measures (e.g. a care plan to allow the resident periods of privacy in their room at set times each day) can avoid normal behaviours being pathologised. Non-pharmacological treatments should be tried first to prevent unnecessary prescription of psychotropics.

Because of the complex nature of sexual disinhibition and varying origins of this behaviour, treatment will be most successful when tailored to the patient's specific presentation.[1] Studies on the pharmacological treatment of sexual disinhibition are limited and larger studies are necessary to establish a preferred medication regimen. In addition, there are few data available on treating these symptoms in women.[1] A systematic review[4] concluded that when treating patients with Alzheimer's disease, vascular dementia or unspecified dementia, serotonergic agents including SSRIs and TCAs are recommended as a first-line treatment, followed by antiandrogens as a second line, and luteinising hormone-releasing hormone agonists and oestrogens as a third line. A literature review[5] determined SSRIs to be the first line of treatment, antipsychotics to be the second line and hormonal modulators to be the third line (owing to cost and adverse effects).

Table 6.7 Pharmacological options in inappropriate sexual behaviour in older adults.[1,6-8]

Medication	Drug	Dose	Mechanism of action	Adverse effects	Cautions/additional information
Antiandrogens	Cyproterone acetate	Low dose 10mg/day[9] High dose 50–100mg/day[10] Cyproterone is licensed in the UK for hypersexuality in males: 50mg bd[11]	Reduction in serum testosterone level by inhibiting LH and FSH[1]	Gynaecomastia, galactorrhoea, elevated blood glucose, depression, osteoporosis[1]	Cyproterone acetate has been associated with risk of meningioma. Monitor patients for meningiomas and discontinue treatment if diagnosed. Surgical implantation of hormonal therapy to reduce male sex drive is subject to the conditions of Section 57 of the UK MHA and requires patient consent and a second medical opinion.[12]
	Medroxyprogesterone acetate (MPA)	Oral 5mg/day[7] Oral 100–400mg/day[13] IM 100–300mg/week every 2 weeks[14]	Reduction in testosterone[1]	Sedation, weight gain, hot flushes, depression, elevated blood glucose[1]	
	Finasteride (for men who have benign prostatic hyperplasia)	5mg/day[7]	Reduction in testosterone[1]	Gynaecomastia, testicular pain, depression[1]	
Antidepressants SSRIs usually first-line treatment	Citalopram	20mg/day[15]	Decreased libido and antiobsessive effects	Insomnia, somnolence, nausea, diarrhoea, headache, anorexia[1]	SSRIs cited as best first-line treatment
	Escitalopram	10–20mg/day			
	Paroxetine	20mg/day[16]			
	Clomipramine	150–175mg/day[16]	Decreased libido[1]	Postural hypotension, anticholinergic effects including constipation, dry mouth, urinary retention and memory impairment[1]	Anticholinergic activity less than ideal in this group of patients
	Trazodone	100–500mg/day[16]	Decreased libido[1]	Day-time sedation, orthostatic hypotension, priapism, falls and fractures, delirium[1]	
	Mirtazapine	30mg/day[16]	Unknown	Appetite increase, arthralgia, confusion, constipation, diarrhoea, dizziness, drowsiness, dry mouth, fatigue	

Anticonvulsants				
Gabapentin	300–1800mg/day[17]	Increased GABA[1]	GI upset, skin reactions, confusion, nystagmus, dizziness, drowsiness[6]	
Carbamazepine	200–800mg/day[16]	May help lower testosterone levels leading to decreased libido[1]	Dizziness, ataxia, drowsiness, diplopia, hyponatraemia, blood dyscrasias, severe skin reaction[6]	Potent enzyme inducer with many interactions
Oxcarbazepine	Starting dose 150mg/day, titrated by 150mg/day in two divided doses. Average effective dose 600–750mg/day in two divided doses[18]	May help lower testosterone levels leading to decreased libido[1]	Abdominal pain, alopecia, asthenia, ataxia, concentration impaired, depression, dizziness, drowsiness, hyponatraemia, nausea, nystagmus, skin reactions, vertigo, vision disorders, leucopenia	
Valproate	Dose not specified but 50–200mg/day has been used	Unknown	Abdominal pain, tremor, agitation, alopecia (regrowth may be curly), anaemia, confusion, deafness, diarrhoea, drowsiness, haemorrhage, hallucination, headache, hepatic disorders	Valproate causes serious harm in pregnancy and in children of men taking valproate (see Chapter 7).

(Continued)

Table 6.7 (Continued)

Medication	Drug	Dose	Mechanism of action	Adverse effects	Cautions/additional information
Antipsychotics	Haloperidol	1.5–3mg/day[16]	Blocks dopamine receptors to decrease libido[1]	Cognitive decline, extrapyramidal symptoms, sedation, gait disturbances, falls, tardive dyskinesia, delirium, QT prolongation, increases in UTI and respiratory infections[1]	Increased risk of stroke and mortality in dementia. Extrapyramidal symptoms First-line treatment in cases where patients present with pathological irritability or unstable mood[1]
	Olanzapine	2.5–15mg/day[7]		Arrhythmias, constipation, dizziness, drowsiness, dry mouth, erectile dysfunction, fatigue, galactorrhoea, gynaecomastia, hyperglycaemia, weight increase[11]	
	Quetiapine	25–75mg/day[16]		Appetite increased, asthenia, dysarthria, dyspepsia, dyspnoea, fever, headache, irritability, palpitations, peripheral oedema[11]	
	Zuclopenthixol	50mg IM monthly[6]		Tardive dyskinesia, delirium, QT prolongation, increases in UTI and respiratory infections, peripheral oedema, extrapyramidal effects[1]	
Beta blockers	Pindolol	5–40mg/day[6,16]	Decreased adrenergic drive[1]	Dizziness, sleep disturbance, headache, weakness, fatigue, GI upset	
Buspirone		10–60mg/day[16,19]	Unknown	Abdominal pain, cold sweat, confusion, depression, dizziness, drowsiness, dry mouth, laryngeal pain, movement disorders, musculoskeletal pain, paraesthesia, skin reactions, tachycardia	

Cimetidine		600–1600mg/day[14]	Antiandrogen actions[1]	Worsening cognition, dizziness, nausea, arthralgia, headache[1]	A small study (n = 20) on elderly patients exhibiting hypersexual behaviours with dementia. This study found that 14 patients improved with cimetidine alone while six patients improved with a combination of cimetidine with ketoconazole or spironolactone.[1]
Ketoconazole		100–200mg/day[20]	Antiandrogen actions[1]	Sedation, headache, rash, photosensitivity, pruritus, hepatotoxicity, GI upset[1]	
Gonadotropin and luteinising hormone-releasing hormone (GnRH and LHRH) agonists	Leuprolide	7.5mg IM monthly[6] Triptorelin is licensed in the UK for male hypersexuality: 11.25 mg IM every 12 weeks	Decrease testosterone and decrease libido[1]	Hot flushes, decreased erectile dysfunction[1]	Caution: risk factors for osteoporosis
L-tryptophan supplementation		Dose not specified	Increases 5HT synthesis in brain, stimulating 5HT release and function[1]	High blood glucose, increased risk of bladder cancer, eosinophilia-myalgia syndrome[1]	
Naltrexone		100–150mg/day[21]	Unknown	Abdominal pain, anxiety, appetite abnormal, arthralgia, asthenia, chest pain, dizziness, eye disorders, headache, hyperhidrosis, myalgia, nausea, palpitations, sexual dysfunction, skin reactions, sleep disorders, tachycardia, thirst	Naltrexone is used after establishing normal liver and kidney function tests.

(Continued)

Table 6.7 (Continued)

Medication	Drug	Dose	Mechanism of action	Adverse effects	Cautions/additional information
Oestrogens	Conjugated oestrogens	0.625mg once daily 0.05–0.1mg/day transdermal patch[8]	Decreased testosterone and decreased libido	Weight gain, gynaecomastia, venous thromboembolism, risk of cardiovascular adverse effects, fluid retention, GI effects[1]	
	Diethylstilbestrol	1mg once to twice daily[7]			
Rivastigmine		Up to 4.5mg bd (oral)[22]	Reduces behavioural symptoms by improving cognitive functioning[1]	Nausea, diarrhoea, urinary incontinence, syncope[1]	Conflicting evidence. Rivastigmine has been shown to help many patients with sexual disinhibition while donepezil may exacerbate these symptoms.[1]
		4.6–9.5mg/day (patch)			
Spironolactone		12.5[8]–75mg/day[20]	Antiandrogen actions[1]	Hyperkalaemia, gynaecomastia, GI ulcers[1]	

bd, twice a day; FSH, follicle-stimulating hormone; GABA, gamma-aminobutyric acid; GI, gastrointestinal; LH, luteinising hormone; MHA, Mental Health Act; UTI, urinary tract infection.

References

1. Sarangi A, et al. Treatment and management of sexual disinhibition in elderly patients with neurocognitive disorders. *Cureus* 2021; **13**:e18463.

2. Dégano P, et al. Hypersexuality in dementia. *Adv Psychiatr Treat* 2005; **11**:424–431.

3. Cipriani G, et al. Sexual disinhibition and dementia. *Psychogeriatrics* 2016; **16**:145–153.

4. Guay DRP. Inappropriate sexual behaviors in cognitively impaired older individuals. *Am J Geriatr Pharmacother* 2008; **6**:269–288.

5. Ibrahim C, et al. Hypersexuality in neurocognitive disorders in elderly people – a comprehensive review of the literature and case study. *Psychiatr Danub* 2014; **26** Suppl 1:36–40.

6. Tucker I. Management of inappropriate sexual behaviors in dementia: a literature review. *Int Psychogeriatr* 2010; **22**:683–692.

7. Kindrat A, et al. Pharmacologic management of inappropriate sexual behaviour in long-term care residents. *Can Fam Physician* 2023; **69**:687–689.

8. Joller P, et al. Approach to inappropriate sexual behaviour in people with dementia. *Can Fam Physician* 2013; **59**:255–260.

9. Haussermann P, et al. Low-dose cyproterone acetate treatment of sexual acting out in men with dementia. *Int Psychogeriatr* 2003; **15**:181–186.

10. Tavares A, et al. Cyproterone for treatment of hypersexuality in an elderly Huntington's disease patient. *Progr Neuropsychopharmacol Biol Psychiatry* 2008; **32**:1994–1995.

11. Joint Formulary Committee. *British National Formulary (online)*. London: BMJ and Pharmaceutical Press; http://www.medicinescomplete.com.

12. Department of Health. Code of practice: Mental Health Act 1983 (last updated October 2017); https://www.gov.uk/government/publications/code-of-practice-mental-health-act-1983#history.

13. Cross BS, et al. High-dose oral medroxyprogesterone for inappropriate hypersexuality in elderly men with dementia: a case series. *Ann Pharmacother* 2013; **47**:e1.

14. Ozkan B, et al. Pharmacotherapy for inappropriate sexual behaviors in dementia: a systematic review of literature. *Am J Alzheimers Dis Other Demen* 2008; **23**:344–354.

15. Mania I, et al. Citalopram treatment for inappropriate sexual behavior in a cognitively impaired patient. *Prim Care Companion J Clin Psychiatry* 2006; **8**:106.

16. De Giorgi R, et al. Treatment of inappropriate sexual behavior in dementia. *Curr Treat Options Neurol* 2016; **18**:41.

17. Alkhalil C, et al. Can gabapentin be a safe alternative to hormonal therapy in the treatment of inappropriate sexual behavior in demented patients? *Int Urol Nephrol* 2003; **35**:299–302.

18. Shua-Haim JR, et al. P1–446: safety and efficacy of oxcarbazepine in the treatment of hypersexuality in Alzheimer's disease patients residing in a special care unit in an assisted living facility. *Alzheimers Dement* 2006; **2**:S228–S229.

19. Plantier D, et al. Drugs for behavior disorders after traumatic brain injury: systematic review and expert consensus leading to French recommendations for good practice. *Ann Phys Rehabil Med* 2016; **59**:42–57.

20. Wiseman SV, et al. Hypersexuality in patients with dementia: possible response to cimetidine. *Neurology* 2000; **54**:2024.

21. Sultana T, et al. Compulsive sexual behavior and alcohol use disorder treated with naltrexone: a case report and literature review. *Cureus* 2022; **14**:e25804.

22. Canevelli M, et al. Rivastigmine in the treatment of hypersexuality in Alzheimer disease. *Alzheimer Dis Assoc Disord* 2013; **27**:287–288.

CHAPTER 6

Depression in older adults

The prevalence of most physical illnesses increases with age and physical problems such as cardiovascular disease, chronic pain, diabetes and Parkinson's disease are associated with a high risk of depressive illness.[1,2] The morbidity and mortality associated with depression are increased in older adults[3] as older people are more likely to be physically frail and therefore vulnerable to serious consequences from self-neglect (e.g. life-threatening dehydration or hypothermia) and immobility (e.g. venous stasis). Suicide is relatively more common in older people.[4] Mortality is reduced by effective treatment of depression.[5]

A meta-analysis of placebo-controlled and antidepressant-controlled studies found a response rate of 51% in older patients,[6] similar to that for the adult population.[7] There is a common perception that older patients do not respond as well or as quickly to antidepressants as their younger counterparts,[8] perhaps because of structural brain changes or higher rates of physical comorbidity.[9] It may be that biological age is more relevant than chronological age.[10] The presence of physical illness, as well as baseline anxiety and reduced executive functioning, is also associated with poorer treatment outcomes.[11] Nonetheless, even in older people, it may still be possible to identify non-responders as early as 4 weeks into treatment.[12,13]

A Cochrane review examined the efficacy and associated withdrawal rates of different classes of antidepressants in older people and found that SSRIs and tricyclics have similar efficacy, but TCAs are associated with higher withdrawal rates.[14] A 2022 population study found non-TCA antidepressants to have broadly similar effectiveness.[15] In the UK, NICE guidance for depression in adults recommends starting with an SSRI in the first instance (sertraline is commonly used first line in older people). When switching to another antidepressant, NICE recommends switching initially to a different SSRI or a better tolerated newer-generation antidepressant (this effectively indicates mirtazapine). Subsequently, an antidepressant of a different pharmacological class that may be less well tolerated is recommended, for example venlafaxine or lofepramine.[16] The OTIMUM trial[17] found that augmenting with aripiprazole or bupropion was better than switching to bupropion in 'treatment-resistant geriatric depression'.

Network meta-analysis suggests that quetiapine, duloxetine, agomelatine, imipramine and vortioxetine have the highest efficacy in major depressive disorder in older people, although individual data are somewhat inconsistent.[18] Two studies have found that, in older people who had recovered from an episode of depression and had received antidepressants for 2 years, over 60% relapsed within 2 years if antidepressant treatment was withdrawn.[19,20] Some of this relapse may have been a result of the speed and method of antidepressant discontinuation.[21] Deprescribing antidepressants in older people presents a particular conundrum. Effective treatment should usually be continued, especially if depression was severe or recurrent. Ineffective treatment (i.e. was never effective or has become ineffective) should usually be withdrawn owing to the risk of adverse effects and interaction with polypharmacy regimens.[22]

There is no ideal antidepressant in older people; all are associated with problems. TCAs are broadly considered to be agents of last resort owing to the increased risk of cardiac conduction abnormalities and because of anticholinergic effects. Although SSRIs are generally better tolerated than TCAs[14] they do, however, increase the risk of gastrointestinal bleeds, particularly in the very old and those with established risk factors such as a history of bleeds or who are on treatment with an NSAID, steroid or warfarin. The risk of other types of bleed such as haemorrhagic stroke may also be increased[23,24] (see Chapter 3). In older people, this increase in risk of stroke may persist after cessation of antidepressants.[25] Older people are also particularly prone to develop hyponatraemia[26] when starting SSRIs and most other antidepressants (see Chapter 3), as well as postural hypotension and falls[27] (the clinical consequences of which may be increased by SSRI-induced osteopenia[28]). TCAs may also increase fracture risk.[29]

Table 6.8 summarises the use of antidepressants in older adults.

Trazodone was once widely used in elderly populations[30] but sedation and postural hypotension may be dose limiting. It retains some utility in depression occurring in dementia.[31] **Agomelatine** is effective in older patients, is well tolerated and has not been linked to hyponatraemia.[32,33] Its use is limited by the need for frequent blood sampling to check LFTs. **Vortioxetine** and **duloxetine** have also been shown to be effective and reasonably well tolerated in the older person[34] but the caveats related to SSRIs are relevant here. A general practice database study found that, compared with SSRIs, 'other antidepressants' (**venlafaxine, mirtazapine**, etc.) were associated with a greater risk of a number of potentially serious adverse effects in the old (stroke/transient ischaemic attack [TIA], fracture, seizures, attempted suicide/self-harm) as well as increased all-cause mortality.[26] However, SSRIs showed the highest risk for falls and hyponatraemia. All classes of antidepressant were associated with an increased risk of a range of adverse outcomes compared with no use. The study was observational and so could not separate the effect of antidepressants from any increased risk inherent in the group of patients treated with these antidepressants. **Polysaturated fatty acids** (fish oils) may be helpful in mild to moderate depression (compared with placebo),[35] as may **memantine**.[36] Methylphenidate seems effective in older people[37] and may be useful where a rapid onset of action is required. There is some evidence that **esketamine** and **ketamine** are rapidly effective in people over 65 (without worsening cognition).[38,39]

The effect of antidepressants on cognition in later life is still debated – some studies find antidepressants to worsen cognitive outcomes,[40–42] others find no effect.[43] The choice of antidepressant may affect the risk – highly anticholinergic medicines undoubtedly worsen cognition and are known to increase the likelihood of developing dementia.[44] Depression in dementia is probably best treated by cognitive or physical therapies rather than antidepressants.[45] Antidepressants are of doubtful benefit.[45–48] The same might be said for their use in the treatment of MCI in older people.[49]

Ultimately, choice is determined by the individual clinical circumstances of each patient, particularly physical comorbidity and concomitant medication (both prescribed and 'over the counter').

CHAPTER 6

Table 6.8 Antidepressants and older people.

	Anticholinergic side effects (urinary retention, dry mouth, blurred vision, constipation)	Postural hypotension	Sedation	Weight gain	Safety in overdose	Other side effects	Drug interactions
Older tricyclics[50]	Moderate to severe with all TCAs All can also cause central anticholinergic effects (confusion, impaired cognition)	All can cause postural hypotension Dosage titration is required	Variable: from moderate with imipramine to profound with amitriptyline	All tricyclics can cause weight gain	All are toxic in overdose (seizures, cardiac arrhythmia)	Seizures, anticholinergic-induced cognitive impairment Increased risk of bleeds with serotonergic drugs	Mainly pharmacodynamic: increased sedation with benzodiazepines, increased hypotension with diuretics, increased constipation with other anticholinergic drugs, etc.
Lofepramine	Moderate, although constipation/sweating can be severe	Can be a problem but generally better tolerated than older tricyclics	Minimal	Few data, but lack of spontaneous reports may indicate less potential than older tricyclics	Relatively safe	Raised LFTs Less likely to cause hyponatraemia than other TCAs and SSRIs	
SSRIs[50,51]	Dry mouth with paroxetine – probably best avoided in older people	Unlikely, but an increased risk of falls is documented with SSRIs	Sometimes seen with paroxetine and fluvoxamine Unlikely with the other SSRIs	Paroxetine and possibly citalopram may cause weight gain Others are weight neutral	Safe with the possible exceptions of citalopram and escitalopram which have the greatest effect on QT. Still much less toxic than TCAs	GI effects and headaches, hyponatraemia, increased risk of bleeds in the older person (add gastroprotection if also on an NSAID or aspirin), orofacial dyskinesia with paroxetine, cognitive impairment,[41] interstitial lung disease[52,53]	Fluvoxamine, fluoxetine and paroxetine are potent inhibitors of several hepatic cytochrome enzymes (see Chapter 3). Sertraline is safer and citalopram, escitalopram and vortioxetine are safest.

Others[54,55]						
Minimal with mirtazapine, trazodone and venlafaxine* Can be observed with reboxetine* Duloxetine* – few effects Agomelatine has no anticholinergic potential	Venlafaxine and duloxetine can cause hypotension at lower doses, but usually increase BP at higher doses Occasional postural hypotension with trazodone Dizziness common with agomelatine	Mirtazapine, mianserin and trazodone are sedative with significant hangover in older people Venlafaxine, duloxetine have neutral effects Agomelatine aids sleep	Highest risk with mirtazapine, although older people are not particularly prone to weight gain Low incidence with agomelatine	Venlafaxine is more toxic in overdose than SSRIs, but safer than TCAs Others are relatively safe	Insomnia and hypokalaemia with reboxetine Nausea with venlafaxine and duloxetine Weight loss and nausea with duloxetine Possibly hepatotoxicity with agomelatine – monitor LFTs Cognitive impairment reported with trazodone[41] but may be no worse than other antidepressants[56] Interstitial lung disease with SNRIs[53]	Duloxetine inhibits CYP2D6 Moclobemide and venlafaxine inhibit CYP450 enzymes. Check for potential interactions. Reboxetine has a low interaction potential. Agomelatine should be avoided in patients who take potent CYP1A2 inhibitors.

*Noradrenergic drugs may produce 'anticholinergic' effects via norepinephrine reuptake inhibition.

GI, gastrointestinal; TCA, tricyclic antidepressant.

References

1. Katona C, et al. Impact of screening old people with physical illness for depression? *Lancet* 2000; **356**:91–92.
2. Lyketsos CG. Depression and diabetes: more on what the relationship might be. *Am J Psychiatry* 2010; **167**:496–497.
3. Gallo JJ, et al. Long term effect of depression care management on mortality in older adults: follow-up of cluster randomized clinical trial in primary care. *BMJ* 2013; **346**:f2570.
4. Naghavi M. Global, regional, and national burden of suicide mortality 1990 to 2016: systematic analysis for the Global Burden of Disease Study 2016. *BMJ* 2019; **364**:l94.
5. Ryan J, et al. Late-life depression and mortality: influence of gender and antidepressant use. *Br J Psychiatry* 2008; **192**:12–18.
6. Gutsmiedl K, et al. How well do elderly patients with major depressive disorder respond to antidepressants: a systematic review and single-group meta-analysis. *BMC Psychiatry* 2020; **20**:102.
7. Cipriani A, et al. Comparative efficacy and acceptability of 21 antidepressant drugs for the acute treatment of adults with major depressive disorder: a systematic review and network meta-analysis. *Lancet* 2018; **391**:1357–1366.
8. Paykel ES, et al. Residual symptoms after partial remission: an important outcome in depression. *Psychol Med* 1995; **25**:1171–1180.
9. Iosifescu DV, et al. Brain white-matter hyperintensities and treatment outcome in major depressive disorder. *Br J Psychiatry* 2006; **188**:180–185.
10. Brown PJ, et al. Biological age, not chronological age, is associated with late-life depression. *J Gerontol A Biol Sci Med Sci* 2018; **73**:1370–1376.
11. Tunvirachaisakul C, et al. Predictors of treatment outcome in depression in later life: a systematic review and meta-analysis. *J Affect Disord* 2018; **227**:164–182.
12. Zilcha-Mano S, et al. Early symptom trajectories as predictors of treatment outcome for citalopram versus placebo. *Am J Geriatr Psychiatry* 2017; **25**:654–661.
13. Mulsant BH, et al. What is the optimal duration of a short-term antidepressant trial when treating geriatric depression? *J Clin Psychopharmacol* 2006; **26**:113–120.
14. Mottram P, et al. Antidepressants for depressed elderly. *Cochrane Database Syst Rev* 2006; **1**:CD003491.
15. Hsu CW, et al. Comparative effectiveness of antidepressants on geriatric depression: real-world evidence from a population-based study. *J Affect Disord* 2022; **296**:609–615.
16. National Institute for Health and Care Excellence. Depression in adults: treatment and management. NICE Guideline [NG222]. 2022 (last accessed December 2023); https://www.nice.org.uk/guidance/ng222.
17. Lenze EJ, et al. Antidepressant augmentation versus switch in treatment-resistant geriatric depression. *N Engl J Med* 2023; **388**:1067–1079.
18. Krause M, et al. Efficacy and tolerability of pharmacological and non-pharmacological interventions in older patients with major depressive disorder: a systematic review, pairwise and network meta-analysis. *Eur Neuropsychopharmacol* 2019; **29**:1003–1022.
19. Flint AJ, et al. Recurrence of first-episode geriatric depression after discontinuation of maintenance antidepressants. *Am J Psychiatry* 1999; **156**:943–945.
20. Reynolds CF, III, et al. Maintenance treatment of major depression in old age. *N Engl J Med* 2006; **354**:1130–1138.
21. Horowitz MA, et al. Distinguishing relapse from antidepressant withdrawal: clinical practice and antidepressant discontinuation studies. *BJPsych Advances* 2022; **28**:297–311.
22. Romdhani A, et al. Discontinuation of antidepressants in older adults: a literature review. *Ther Clin Risk Manag* 2023; **19**:291–299.
23. Smoller JW, et al. Antidepressant use and risk of incident cardiovascular morbidity and mortality among postmenopausal women in the Women's Health Initiative study. *Arch Intern Med* 2009; **169**:2128–2139.
24. Laporte S, et al. Bleeding risk under selective serotonin reuptake inhibitor (SSRI) antidepressants: a meta-analysis of observational studies. *Pharmacol Res* 2017; **118**:19–32.
25. Ön BI, et al. Antidepressant use and stroke or mortality risk in the elderly. *Eur J Neurol* 2022; **29**:469–477.
26. Coupland C, et al. Antidepressant use and risk of adverse outcomes in older people: population based cohort study. *BMJ* 2011; **343**:d4551.
27. Haddad YK, et al. A comparative analysis of selective serotonin reuptake inhibitors and fall risk in older adults. *J Am Geriatr Soc* 2022; **70**:1450–1460.
28. Williams LJ, et al. Selective serotonin reuptake inhibitor use and bone mineral density in women with a history of depression. *Int Clin Psychopharmacol* 2008; **23**:84–87.
29. Power C, et al. Bones of contention: a comprehensive literature review of non-SSRI antidepressant use and bone health. *J Geriatr Psychiatry Neurol* 2019; **33**:340–352.
30. Fagiolini A, et al. Rediscovering trazodone for the treatment of major depressive disorder. *CNS Drugs* 2012; **26**:1033–1049.
31. Fagiolini A, et al. Trazodone in the management of major depression among elderly patients with dementia: a narrative review and clinical insights. *Neuropsychiatr Dis Treat* 2023; **19**:2817–2831.
32. Heun R, et al. The efficacy of agomelatine in elderly patients with recurrent major depressive disorder: a placebo-controlled study. *J Clin Psychiatry* 2013; **74**:587–594.
33. Laux G. The antidepressant efficacy of agomelatine in daily practice: Results of the non-interventional study VIVALDI. *Eur Psychiatry* 2011; **26 Suppl 1**:647.
34. Katona C, et al. A randomized, double-blind, placebo-controlled, duloxetine-referenced, fixed-dose study comparing the efficacy and safety of Lu AA21004 in elderly patients with major depressive disorder. *Int Clin Psychopharmacol* 2012; **27**:215–223.
35. Bae JH, et al. Systematic review and meta-analysis of omega-3-fatty acids in elderly patients with depression. *Nutr Res* 2018; **50**:1–9.
36. Hsu TW, et al. The efficacy and tolerability of memantine for depressive symptoms in major mental diseases: a systematic review and updated meta-analysis of double-blind randomized controlled trials. *J Affect Disord* 2022; **306**:182–189.

37. Smith KR, et al. Methylphenidate use in geriatric depression: a systematic review. *Int J Geriatr Psychiatry* 2021; **36**:1304–1312.

38. Ochs-Ross R, et al. Comparison of long-term efficacy and safety of esketamine nasal spray plus oral antidepressant in younger versus older patients with treatment-resistant depression: post-hoc analysis of SUSTAIN-2, a long-term open-label phase 3 safety and efficacy study. *Am J Geriatr Psychiatry* 2022; **30**:541–556.

39. Subramanian S, et al. Ketamine for depression in older adults. *Am J Geriatr Psychiatry* 2021; **29**:914–916.

40. Moraros J, et al. The association of antidepressant drug usage with cognitive impairment or dementia, including Alzheimer disease: a systematic review and meta-analysis. *Depress Anxiety* 2017; **34**:217–226.

41. Leng Y, et al. Antidepressant use and cognitive outcomes in very old women. *J Gerontol A Biol Sci Med Sci* 2018; **73**:1390–1395.

42. Chan JYC, et al. Depression and antidepressants as potential risk factors in dementia: a systematic review and meta-analysis of 18 longitudinal studies. *J Am Med Dir Assoc* 2019; **20**:279–286.e271.

43. Carriere I, et al. Antidepressant use and cognitive decline in community-dwelling elderly people – the Three-City Cohort. *BMC Med* 2017; **15**:81.

44. Wang YC, et al. Increased risk of dementia in patients with antidepressants: a meta-analysis of observational studies. *Behav Neurol* 2018; **2018**:5315098.

45. Watt JA, et al. Comparative efficacy of interventions for reducing symptoms of depression in people with dementia: systematic review and network meta-analysis. *BMJ* 2021; **372**:n532.

46. Jeong HW, et al. Vortioxetine treatment for depression in Alzheimer's disease: a randomized, double-blind, placebo-controlled study. *Clin Psychopharmacol Neurosci* 2022; **20**:311–319.

47. Leong C. Antidepressants for depression in patients with dementia: a review of the literature. *Consult Pharm* 2014; **29**:254–263.

48. Costello H, et al. Antidepressant medications in dementia: evidence and potential mechanisms of treatment-resistance. *Psychol Med* 2023; **53**:654–667.

49. Jin B, et al. Comparative efficacy and acceptability of treatments for depressive symptoms in cognitive impairment: a systematic review and Bayesian network meta-analysis. *Front Aging Neurosci* 2022; **14**:1037414.

50. Draper B, et al. Tolerability of selective serotonin reuptake inhibitors: issues relevant to the elderly. *Drugs Aging* 2008; **25**:501–519.

51. Bose A, et al. Escitalopram in the acute treatment of depressed patients aged 60 years or older. *Am J Geriatr Psychiatry* 2008; **16**:14–20.

52. Deidda A, et al. Interstitial lung disease induced by fluoxetine: systematic review of literature and analysis of Vigiaccess, Eudravigilance and a national pharmacovigilance database. *Pharmacol Res* 2017; **120**:294–301.

53. Rosenberg T, et al. The relationship of SSRI and SNRI usage with interstitial lung disease and bronchiectasis in an elderly population: a case-control study. *Clin Interv Aging* 2017; **12**:1977–1984.

54. Raskin J, et al. Safety and tolerability of duloxetine at 60 mg once daily in elderly patients with major depressive disorder. *J Clin Psychopharmacol* 2008; **28**:32–38.

55. Johnson EM, et al. Cardiovascular changes associated with venlafaxine in the treatment of late-life depression. *Am J Geriatr Psychiatry* 2006; **14**:796–802.

56. Gonçalo AMG, et al. The effects of trazodone on human cognition: a systematic review. *Eur J Clin Pharmacol* 2021; **77**:1623–1637.

Covert administration of medicines within food and drink

This section deals with covert medication administration within UK law only. Other countries may have different laws pertaining to this area, or indeed no laws or official guidance.[1]

In mental health settings it is common for patients to refuse medication. People with psychiatric disorders may lack capacity to make an informed choice about whether medication will be beneficial to them or not. In these cases, the clinical team may consider whether it would be in the patient's best interests to administer medication covertly. This practice is known as covert administration of medicines. Guidance from the Royal Pharmaceutical Society and Royal College of Nursing[2] and the Royal College of Psychiatrists[3] has been published in order to protect patients from the unlawful and inappropriate administration of medication in this way. In the UK, the legal framework for such interventions is either the Mental Capacity Act (MCA)[4] or, more rarely, the Mental Health Act (MHA).[5]

Assessment of mental capacity[4,6,7]

The assessment of capacity regarding medication is primarily a matter for the prescriber, usually a doctor treating the patient,[4,6] or less commonly a pharmacist or nurse. Nurses and allied health professionals who are not prescribers will also have to be mindful of their own codes of professional practice and should be satisfied that the doctor's assessment is reasonable. The assessment must be made in relation to the particular treatment proposed as part of a covert medication care plan. Capacity can vary over time and the assessment should be made at the time of the proposed treatment. The assessment should be documented in the patient's notes and recorded in the care plan. Assessment of capacity should be conducted in line with the MCA code of practice.

Guidance on covert administration

If a patient has the capacity to give a valid refusal to medication and is not detainable under the MHA, their refusal should be respected.

If a patient has the capacity to give a valid refusal and is either being treated under the MHA or is legally detainable under the Act, the provisions of the MHA with regard to treatment will apply (which are outside the scope of this chapter).

The administration of medicines to patients who lack the capacity to consent and who are unable to appreciate that they are taking medication (e.g. unconscious patients) should not need to be carried out covertly. However, some patients who lack the capacity to consent would be aware of receiving medication if they were not deceived into thinking otherwise,[7] for example a patient with moderate dementia who has no insight and does not believe they need to take medication but will take liquid medication if this is mixed with their tea without being aware of this. It is this group to whom this guidance applies.

Treatment may be given to people who lack capacity if the treatment is in the patient's best interests (Section 5, MCA[4]) and is proportionate to the harm to be avoided (Chapter 6.41, MCA Code of Practice[7]). So, there should be a clear expectation that the patient will benefit from covert administration, and that this will avoid significant harm (either mental or physical) to the patient or others. The treatment must be necessary to save the patient's life, to prevent deterioration in health or to ensure an improvement in physical or mental health.[4,7]

Covert administration must be the least restrictive option after trying all other options. An assessment should be carried out to understand why the person is refusing to take their medicines. Alternative methods of administration (e.g. liquid formulation) and trial of different approaches in nursing care (e.g. explaining to the patient about the medicines at the time they are administered or changing the time of administration to a time of day when the patient is more alert or less distressed) should be considered.[8]

The decision to administer medication covertly should not be made by a single individual but through discussion with the multidisciplinary team caring for the patient and the patient's relatives or informal carers. A Best Interests meeting should be held, except in urgent situations if the decision cannot wait, in which case a less formal decision can take place with a view to arranging a Best Interests meeting as soon as practicably possible. If it were determined at this meeting that the provision of covert medication would amount to a deprivation of liberty (where previously there was none), then an application for Deprivation of Liberty Safeguards (DoLS) authorisation should be made. Decisions regarding covert administration of medication should be carefully documented in the patient's medical records with a clear management plan, including details of how the covert medication plan will be reviewed. This documentation must be easily accessible on viewing the person's records and the decision should be subject to regular review.

It is not necessary to have a new Best Interests meeting each time there is a change in medication. However, when covert medication is first considered, healthcare professionals should consider what types of changes in medication may be anticipated in future and should agree on the thresholds of what changes may require a new Best Interests meeting. This management plan should be recorded in the patient's notes. If significant changes that could cause adverse effects are envisaged, then a new meeting should be held before changes are made.

In deciding how often capacity assessments should be repeated, clinicians should follow the guidance within the practical guide to the MCA.[6] If there is any evidence that the patient has regained capacity with regard to administration of their medication, an immediate capacity assessment must be done. Decisions in the patient's best interest can no longer be made if they are under a DoLS authorisation for reasons including the administration of medication covertly; this part of the DoLS authorisation will no longer be valid and covert administration of medication must cease immediately.

Case law[9,10] has dealt with the relationship between the use of covert medication and the need for a DoLS authorisation. A person is deprived of their liberty when they are under continuous supervision and control and are not free to leave. The administration of covert medication will only in itself lead to a deprivation of liberty where that covert medication affects the person's behaviour, mental health or it acts as a sedative to such an extent that it will deprive the person of their liberty. The use of covert medication within a care plan must be clearly identified within the DoLS assessment and authorisation.

CHAPTER 6

When considering covert use of psychiatric medication the following must be considered:[11]

1. If the patient meets the criteria for the MHA, this must be used in preference to the MCA.
2. The MCA might be used to provide authority for covert medication for physical health whether or not the patient is detained under the MHA. The MCA can be used as authority for covert use of psychiatric medication in patients not under the MHA if the medication is necessary to prevent deterioration or ensure an improvement in the patient's mental health and it is in the person's best interest to receive the drug. The usual procedures for covert medication, including documentation of capacity assessment, Best Interests meeting and pharmacist's review, should be followed.
3. Caution is needed in the use of medication that may sedate or reduce a patient's physical mobility, as use of such drugs may constitute a deprivation of liberty and require the patient to be under the DoLS framework. Documentation of whether the proposed use of a covert psychiatric drug constitutes a deprivation of liberty is important. Note that if a patient is found to lack capacity to consent to the admission and does not meet the criteria for detention under the MHA, DoLS should be used, so most in-patients who lack capacity to consent to medication will already be under the MHA or DoLS, although there may be some who can consent to admission but not to medication. However, even if the patient is already under the MHA or MCA as part of their admission, there still needs to be the same approach and considerations as documented here with regard to medication being given covertly.

Summary of process

The process for covert administration of medicines should include:

- The assurance that all efforts have been made to give medication openly in its normal form before considering covert administration.
- Assessment of capacity of the patient to make a decision regarding their treatment with medication. If the patient has capacity their wishes should be respected and covert medication not administered.
- A record of the examination of the patient's capacity must be made in the clinical notes, and evidence for incapacity documented.
- If the patient lacks capacity there should be a Best Interests meeting which should be attended by relevant health professionals and a person who can communicate the views and interests of the patient (family member, friend or independent mental capacity advocate). These meetings can be held virtually. If the patient has an attorney appointed under the MCA for health and welfare decisions then this person should be present at the meeting.
- Those attending the meeting should ascertain whether the patient has made an 'advance decision' refusing a particular medication or treatment which can be used to guide decision-making.

- The Best Interests meeting should consider whether a formal legal procedure such as the MHA or DoLS is appropriate. Discussion of the indications and use of this legislation in the context of covert medication is outside the scope of this guidance but specialist psychiatric and/or legal opinion should be sought in individual circumstances if necessary. However, the other considerations given here – including the involvement of pharmacy, the recording of medication being given covertly on the drug chart, the dispensing nurse ensuring the covert medication is taken by the patient and regular reviews – apply for all patients, whichever legal framework is being used to give medication covertly.
- Medication should not be administered covertly until a Best Interests meeting has been held. If the situation is urgent, it is acceptable for a less formal discussion to occur between carer/nursing staff, prescriber and family/advocate in order to make an urgent decision, but a formal meeting should be arranged as soon as possible.
- After the meeting, there should be clear documentation of the outcome of the meeting. If the decision is to use covert administration of medication, a check should be made with the pharmacy to determine whether the properties of the medications are likely to be affected by crushing and/or being mixed with food or drink.[12] The medication chart and electronic prescribing and medicines administration record should be amended to describe how the medication is to be administered.
- When the medication is administered in foodstuffs, it is the responsibility of the dispensing nurse to ensure that the medication is taken. This can be facilitated by direct observation or by nominating another member of the clinical team to observe the patient taking the medication.
- A plan should be made to review on a regular basis the need for continued covert administration of medicines.

Additional information

- For patients in care homes, the NICE guideline 'Managing medicines in care homes' should be referred to.[13,14] The basic principles of this NICE guidance are the same as the policy discussed in this section. Mental health practitioners have a duty to inform the care home manager if they suspect the correct procedures are not being followed as regards covert medication, and to discuss with their team leader possible safeguarding referral if the home manager does not act on their advice. The role of mental health teams supporting care homes is to support the care homes and prescriber (usually GP) in carrying out this guidance. For patients with complex mental health needs, it may be appropriate that they attend or contribute to the Best Interests meeting. However, it should be the prescriber (usually the GP), care home staff and care home pharmacist who manage the process.
- There are no specific restrictions to state that relatives or other informal carers cannot give medication covertly and in certain cases it may be acceptable as long as they have been advised to do so by a health professional (e.g. GP) and all standards of the policy have been met.

Figure 6.2 provides an algorithm for determining whether or not to administer medicines covertly.

CHAPTER 6

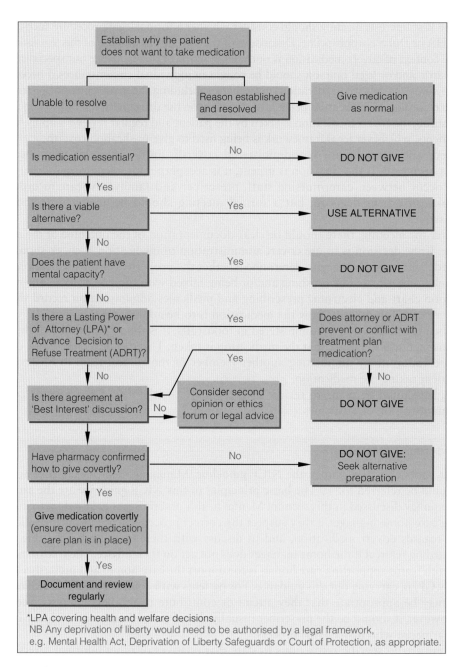

Figure 6.2 Flow chart for the use of covert medication.

References

1. Wikipedia. Covert medication. 2023; https://en.wikipedia.org/wiki/covert_medication.

2. Royal Pharmaceutical Society and Royal College of Nursing. Professional guidance on the administration of medicines in healthcare settings. 2019; https://www.rpharms.com/Portals/0/RPS%20document%20library/Open%20access/Professional%20standards/SSHM%20and%20Admin/Admin%20of%20Meds%20prof%20guidance.pdf?ver=2019-01-23-145026-567.

3. Royal College of Psychiatrists. College statement on covert administration of medicines. *Psychiatric Bull* 2004; **28**:385–386.

4. Office of Public Sector Information. Mental Capacity Act 2005 – Chapter 9. 2005; http://www.legislation.gov.uk/ukpga/2005/9/pdfs/ukpga_20050009_en.pdf.

5. The National Archives. Mental Health Act 2007. 2007; http://www.legislation.gov.uk/ukpga/2007/12/contents.

6. British Medical Association and the Law Society. *Assessment of Mental Capacity. A Practical Guide for Doctors and Lawyers*, 4th edn. London: Law Society Publishing; 2015.

7. Gov.uk. Office of the Public Guardian. Mental Capacity Act Code of Practice. 2013 (last updated October 2020); https://www.gov.uk/government/publications/mental-capacity-act-code-of-practice.

8. Care Quality Commission. Covert administration of medicines. 2020; https://www.cqc.org.uk/guidance-providers/adult-social-care/covert-administration-medicines.

9. Medication Training Company. Covert administration of medicines. Recent Court of Protection ruling on covert medication – 6th July 2016. 2016; https://medicationtraining.co.uk/covert-administration-medicines/.

10. Doughty Street Chambers. Covert medication of persons lacking capacity. What guidance is there? 2023; https://insights.doughtystreet.co.uk/post/102i743/covert-medication-of-persons-lacking-capacity-what-guidance-is-there.

11. Care Quality Commission. Brief guide: covert medication in mental health services. 2018 (reviewed 2019); https://www.cqc.org.uk/sites/default/files/20180406_9001398_briefguide-covert_medication_mental_health_v2.pdf.

12. Specialist Pharmacy Service. Covert administration of medicines in adults: pharmaceutical issues. 2022 (last updated June 2023); https://www.sps.nhs.uk/articles/covert-administration-of-medicines-in-adults-pharmaceutical-issues/.

13. National Institute for Health and Care Excellence. Managing medicines in care homes. Social Care Guideline [SC1]. 2014 (last updated 2020); https://www.nice.org.uk/guidance/sc1.

14. PrescQIPP. Bulletin 101. Best practice guidance in covert administration of medication. 2015; https://www.prescqipp.info/umbraco/surface/authorisedmediasurface/index?url=%2fmedia%2f1174%2fb101-covert-administration-21.pdf.

CHAPTER 6

A guide to medication doses of commonly used psychotropics in older adults, [1] / National Institute for Health and Care Excellence (NICE).

Drug	Specific indication/ additional notes	Starting dose	Usual maintenance dose	Maximum dose in elderly
Antidepressants				
Agomelatine	Depression Monitor LFTs Data suggest agomelatine is not effective in patients >75 years	25mg nocte	25–50mg daily	50mg nocte
Bupropion[2]	Depression	Immediate release tablets: 100mg bd[2] Sustained release tablets (SR): 150mg once daily[2] Extended-release tablets (XL): 150mg once daily[2]	May increase to 100mg tds after 3 days[2] May increase dose to 150mg SR twice daily after 3 days[2] May increase dose to 300mg XL once daily after at least 4 days[2]	300mg/day* Consider reduced dosage and/or dosage frequency in patients with a CrCl <90mL/min[2]
Bupropion and dextromethorphan[3]	Depression Each tablet contains 45mg dextromethorphan hydrobromide (equivalent to 32.98mg dextromethorphan base) in an immediate-release formulation and 105mg bupropion hydrochloride (equivalent to 91.14mg bupropion base) in an XL formulation.[3]	1 tablet mane[3]	1 tablet bd (at least 8 hours apart; dose can be increased to bd after 3 days)[3] Reduced dosage of 1 tablet mane is recommended for patients with moderate kidney impairment (eGFR 30–59mL/min/1.73m[2]), those known to be poor CYP2D6 metabolisers and when co-administered with strong CYP2D6 inhibitors. Concomitant use with strong CYP2B6 inducers should be avoided.	1 tablet bd[3]
Citalopram	Depression/anxiety disorder	10mg mane	10–20mg mane	20mg mane
Clomipramine	Depression/phobic and obsessional states	10mg nocte (dose increases should be cautious)	30–75mg daily[4] should be reached after about 10 days.	75mg daily[4]

Drug	Specific indication/ additional notes	Starting dose	Usual maintenance dose	Maximum dose in elderly
Desvenlafaxine[5]	Major depression No formal recommendations are available for dosing in older adults.[5] However, possible reduced renal clearance of desvenlafaxine should be considered when determining an appropriate dose.	50mg daily Dosage in renal impairment: CrCl 50–80mL/min: no dosage adjustment needed CrCl 30–50mL/min: 50mg daily is recommended daily and max. dose CrCl <30mL/min or ESRD: 50mg every other day is recommended daily and max. dose	50mg daily	Usual dose 50mg/day Max. dose 400mg daily[5] however no additional benefit was demonstrated at doses >50mg/day and adverse reactions and discontinuations were more frequent at higher doses.
Duloxetine	Depression/anxiety disorder	30mg daily*	60mg daily	120mg daily[6] (caution as limited data in elderly for this dose)
Escitalopram	Depression/anxiety disorder	5mg mane	5–10mg mane	10mg mane
Fluoxetine	Depression/anxiety disorder Caution as long half-life and inhibitor of several CYP enzymes	20mg mane	20mg mane	40mg mane usually (but 60mg can be used)
Lofepramine	Depression	35mg nocte*	70mg nocte*	140mg nocte or in divided doses* (occasionally 210mg nocte required)
Mirtazapine	Depression	7.5mg nocte or usually 15mg nocte*	15–30mg nocte	45mg nocte
Sertraline	Depression/anxiety disorder	25–50mg mane (25mg can be increased to 50mg mane after 1 week)	50–100mg mane*	100mg (occasionally up to 150mg mane)*
Trazodone	Depression	100mg daily in divided doses or as a single night time dose[7]	100–200mg daily*	300mg daily[7]

(Continued)

CHAPTER 6

Drug	Specific indication/additional notes	Starting dose	Usual maintenance dose	Maximum dose in elderly
	Agitation in dementia Avoid single doses >100mg	25mg bd*	25–100mg daily*	200mg daily* (in divided doses)
Venlafaxine	Depression/anxiety disorder Monitor BP on initiation	37.5mg mane (increased to 75mg XL mane after 1 week)*	75–150mg (XL) mane*	150mg daily (occasionally 225mg daily is necessary)*
Vortioxetine[8]	Major depressive disorder Vortioxetine is extensively metabolised in the liver, primarily by CYP2D6 and to a minor extent by CYP3A4/5 and CYP2C9. Co-administration of certain drugs may need to be avoided or dosage adjustments may be necessary; review drug interactions.	5mg daily	5–10mg daily	10mg daily Caution advised in ≥65 years with doses >10mg daily for which data are limited[8]

Antipsychotics[†]

Drug	Specific indication/additional notes	Starting dose	Usual maintenance dose	Maximum dose in elderly
Amisulpride	Chronic schizophrenia	50mg daily*	100–200mg daily*	400mg daily[9] (caution >200mg daily)*
	Late life psychosis	25–50mg daily*	50–100mg daily* (increase in 25mg steps)	200mg daily[10] (caution >100mg daily)*
	Agitation/psychosis in dementia Caution QTc prolongation	25mg nocte[11]	25–50mg daily[11]	50mg daily[11]
Aripiprazole	Schizophrenia, mania (oral)	5mg mane*	5-15mg daily*	20mg mane*
	Control of agitation (IM injection)	5.25mg*	5.25–9.75mg*	15mg daily* (combined oral + IM)
Brexpiprazole[12]	Schizophrenia[12] Metabolism is primarily mediated by CYP3A4 and CYP2D6. Co-administration of certain drugs may need to be avoided or dosage adjustments may be necessary.	0.5mg once daily	On day 5 may increase to 1mg once daily On day 8 may further increase to 2mg daily	4mg daily Max. 3mg/day if CrCl <60mL/min, including ESRD[12]

Drug	Specific indication/ additional notes	Starting dose	Usual maintenance dose	Maximum dose in elderly
			Further titration may be made weekly in 1mg increments based on response and tolerability. Recommended range: 2–4mg once daily[12]	
	Depression (adjunctive treatment)	0.5 once daily[12]	Target dose 2mg once daily. Titrate dosage at weekly intervals based on response and tolerability.[12]	3mg/day[12] Max. 2mg/day if CrCl <60mL/min, including ESRD[12]
	Agitation in Alzheimer's disease	0.5mg once daily[12]	On day 8 increase dose to 1mg once daily for an additional 7 days. On day 15 increase to 2mg po once daily, the recommended target dose. May increase to 3mg once daily after at least 14 more days based on clinical response and tolerability.[12]	3mg/day[12] Max. 2mg/day if CrCl <60mL/min, including ESRD[12]
Cariprazine[13]	Schizophrenia Cariprazine and its major active metabolites are highly protein bound and extensively metabolised by CYP3A4 and, to a lesser extent, by CYP2D6. Co-administration of certain drugs may need to be avoided or dosage adjustments may be necessary; review drug interactions.	1.5mg once daily[13]	May increase to 3mg once daily on day 2 Make further dose adjustments in 1.5mg increments based on response and tolerability.[13] Effective range: 1.5–6mg po once daily[14]	6mg/day[14]

(Continued)

CHAPTER 6

Drug	Specific indication/ additional notes	Starting dose	Usual maintenance dose	Maximum dose in elderly
	Mania or mixed episodes of bipolar disorder	1.5mg once daily[14]	May increase to 3mg once daily on day 2 Adjust dose by 1.5–3mg/day based on clinical response and tolerability Usual dose: 3–6mg/day[14]	6mg/day for acute mania[14]
	Bipolar depression and adjunctive treatment of major depressive disorder	1.5mg once daily[14]	May increase dose to 3mg/day after 2 weeks based on clinical response and tolerability[14]	3mg/day[14]
	BPSD	Dose not yet established[14]		
Clozapine	Schizophrenia	6.25–12.5mg daily,[15,16] increased by no more than 6.25–12.5mg once or twice a week[15]	50–100mg daily[15,16]	100mg daily[15,16]
	Parkinson's related psychosis	6.25mg daily[17]	25–37.5mg daily[17]	50mg daily[17]
	IM injection	The oral bioavailability of clozapine is about half that of the IM injection (e.g. 50mg daily of the IM injection is roughly equivalent to 100mg daily of the tablets/oral solution). After each injection has been given the patient must be observed every 15 minutes for the first 2 hours to check for excess sedation. NB If IM lorazepam is required, leave at least 1 HOUR between administration of IM clozapine and IM lorazepam.		
Iloperidone	No formal recommendations are available for dosing in older adults[18]			
Lumateperone[19]	Schizophrenia	42mg daily (equivalent to 60mg lumateperone tosylate) Dose titration not required	42mg daily	42mg daily
Lurasidone	Schizophrenia	37mg once daily (or 18.5mg daily when given with concomitant moderate CYP3A4 inhibitors, max. dose 74mg once daily)	18.5–111mg daily[20]	Limited data on higher doses used in older adults. No data are available in elderly people treated with 148mg. Caution should be exercised when treating patients ≥65 years of age with higher doses.[20]

Drug	Specific indication/ additional notes	Starting dose	Usual maintenance dose	Maximum dose in elderly
		Dosing for elderly with normal renal function (CrCl ≥80mL/min) is the same as for adults with normal renal function. In diminished renal function, dose adjustments may be required according to their renal function status.[20]		
Olanzapine	Schizophrenia	2.5mg nocte*	5–10mg daily*	15mg nocte[16]
	Agitation/psychosis in dementia	2.5mg nocte*	2.5–10mg daily*	10mg nocte* (optimal dose is 5mg daily)[16]
Olanzapine and samidorphan	No formal recommendations are available for dosing in older adults.[21]			
Pimavanserin[22,23]	Treatment of hallucinations and delusions associated with Parkinson's disease psychosis	34mg daily (or 10mg daily if co-administered with strong CYP3A4 inhibitors)	34mg daily (or 10mg daily if co-administered with strong CYP3A4 inhibitors)	34mg daily (or 10mg daily if co-administered with strong CYP3A4 inhibitors)
		Dose titration not required		Monitor patients for reduced efficacy if used concomitantly with strong CYP3A4 inducers.
Quetiapine	Schizophrenia	12.5–25mg daily[16]	75–125mg daily[15]	200–300mg daily[16]
	Agitation/psychosis in dementia	12.5–25mg daily*	50–100mg daily*	100–300mg daily[16]
Risperidone	Psychosis	0.5mg bd (0.25–0.5mg daily in some cases)[16]	1–2.5mg daily[15]	4mg daily
	Late-onset psychosis	0.5mg daily*	1mg daily*	2mg daily* (optimal dose is 1mg daily)
	Agitation/psychosis in dementia	0.25mg daily* or bd	0.5mg bd	2mg daily (optimal dose is 1mg daily)[16]

(Continued)

CHAPTER 6

Drug	Specific indication/ additional notes	Starting dose	Usual maintenance dose	Maximum dose in elderly
Haloperidol	Psychosis/mania associated with bipolar disorder/delirium	0.25–0.5mg daily[15]	1–3.5mg daily[15]	Caution >3.5mg – assess tolerability and ECG
	Agitation Avoid in older adults (except in delirium) owing to risk of QTc prolongation.	0.25–0.5mg daily*	0.5–1.5mg daily or bd	Max. 5mg/day (oral) Max. 5mg/day (IM) Doses >5mg/day should only be considered in patients who have tolerated higher doses and after reassessment of the patient's individual benefit–risk profile

Long-acting conventional antipsychotic drugs†

Drug	Specific indication/ additional notes	Starting dose	Usual maintenance dose	Maximum dose in elderly
Flupentixol decanoate		Test dose: 5–10mg	After at least 7 days of test dose: 10–20mg every 2–4 weeks* Dose increased gradually according to response and tolerability in steps of 5–10mg every 2 weeks*	40mg every 2 weeks* (extend frequency to every 3–4 weeks if EPSE develop) Occasionally up to 50 or 60mg every 2 weeks* may be used if tolerated
Fluphenazine decanoate	Caution – high risk of EPSE	Test dose: 6.25mg	After 4–7 days of test dose: 12.5–25mg every 2-4 weeks Dose increased gradually according to response and tolerability in steps of 12.5mg every 2–4 weeks*	50mg every 4 weeks*
Haloperidol decanoate	Risk of EPSE and QTc prolongation	No test dose 12.5–25mg every 4 weeks	12.5–25mg every 4 weeks	50mg every 4 weeks*
Pipotiazine palmitate		Test dose: 5–10mg	25–100mg every 4 weeks	100mg every 4 weeks*
Zuclopenthixol decanoate		Test dose: 25–50mg	After at least 7 days of test dose: 50–200mg every 2–4 weeks*	200mg every 2 weeks*

Drug	Specific indication/ additional notes	Starting dose	Usual maintenance dose	Maximum dose in elderly
Long-acting atypical antipsychotic drugs[†]				
Aripiprazole (long-acting injection[24])	One injection start No detectable effect of age on pharmacokinetics[24]	One injection of 400mg and continue treatment with oral dose 10–20mg/day for 14 days One injection of 300mg in frail individuals or poor metabolisers of CYP2D6 (and continue with prescribed oral dose for 14 days) One injection of 200mg used for patients known to be CYP2D6 poor metabolisers or concomitantly use a strong CYP3A4 inhibitor (and continue with prescribed oral dose for 14 days)	400mg monthly (reduce to 300mg/ month if adverse effects) 300mg monthly in frail individuals or poor metabolisers of CYP2D6	400mg monthly (reduce to 300mg/ month if adverse effects) 300mg monthly in frail individuals or poor metabolisers of CYP2D6
	Two injection start (two injection start not to be used in patients who are known to be CYP2D6 poor metabolisers and concomitantly use a strong CYP3A4 inhibitor)	Two separate injections of 400mg at separate injection sites along with one 10–20mg dose of oral aripiprazole Two injections of 300mg in frail individuals or poor metabolisers of CYP2D6 (along with one single dose of the previous prescribed dose of oral aripiprazole)	400mg monthly (reduce to 300mg/ month if adverse effects) 300mg monthly in frail individuals or poor metabolisers of CYP2D6	400mg monthly (reduce to 300mg/ month if adverse effects) 300mg monthly in frail individuals or poor metabolisers of CYP2D6

(Continued)

CHAPTER 6

Drug	Specific indication/ additional notes	Starting dose	Usual maintenance dose	Maximum dose in elderly
Olanzapine pamoate[25]	Has not been systematically studied in elderly patients (>65 years). Not recommended for treatment in the elderly population unless a well-tolerated and effective dose regimen using oral olanzapine has been established. A lower starting dose (150mg/4 weeks) is not routinely indicated but should be considered for those 65 and over when clinical factors warrant. Not recommended to be started in patients >75 years.			
Paliperidone palmitate	Dose based on renal function Because elderly patients may have diminished renal function, they are dosed as in mild renal impairment even if tests show normal renal function.*	Loading doses: day 1: 100mg day 8: 75mg (lower loading doses may be appropriate in some)*	25–100mg monthly*	100mg monthly*
Paliperidone palmitate 3-monthly injection	Dose based on renal function Because elderly patients may have diminished renal function, they are dosed as in mild renal impairment even if tests show normal renal function.*	If the last dose of 1-monthly paliperidone palmitate injectable is: 50mg 75mg 100mg	Initiate the 3-monthly injection at the following doses: 175mg 263mg 350mg (There is no equivalent dose for the 25mg dose of 1-monthly paliperidone palmitate injection).[26]	350mg 3-monthly*
Paliperidone palmitate 6-monthly injection[27]	Dose based on renal function Because elderly patients may have diminished renal function, they are dosed as in mild renal impairment even if tests show normal renal function.*	Patients adequately treated with 1-monthly paliperidone palmitate injection 100mg (preferably for 4 months or more) or 3-monthly paliperidone palmitate injection at 350mg (for at least one injection cycle) may be transitioned to 6-monthly paliperidone palmitate injection 700mg	700mg every 6 months* There are no equivalent doses of 6-monthly paliperidone palmitate for the 25, 50 or 75mg doses of 1-monthly injection, nor for the 175 or 263 mg 3-monthly injection.	700mg every 6 months*

Drug	Specific indication/ additional notes	Starting dose	Usual maintenance dose	Maximum dose in elderly
Risperidone long-acting injection	Monitor renal function	25mg every 2 weeks	25mg every 2 weeks	25mg every 2 weeks Consider 37.5mg every 2 weeks in patients treated with oral risperidone doses >4mg/day[28]
Mood stabilisers				
Carbamazepine	Bipolar disorder Caution – drug interactions Check LFTs, FBC and U&Es; consider checking plasma levels.	50mg bd or 100mg bd*	200–400mg/day*	600–800mg/day*
Lamotrigine	Bipolar disorder (titration as in young adults) Check for interactions and make appropriate dose alterations (see *BNF*).	25mg daily (monotherapy) 25mg on alternate days (if with valproate) 50mg daily (if with carbamazepine)	Increase by 25mg steps every 14 days Increase by 25mg steps every 14 days Increase by 50mg steps every 14 days	200mg/day* 100mg/day* 100mg bd*
Lithium carbonate modified release	Bipolar disorder Mania/depression Caution – drug interactions Check renal and thyroid function and regularly monitor plasma levels.	100–200mg nocte*	200–600mg daily*	600–1200mg daily (aim for plasma levels 0.4–0.7mmol/L in elderly)[29]
Sodium valproate	Bipolar disorder Check LFTs and consider checking plasma levels.	Sodium valproate: 100–200mg bd* Semi-sodium valproate: 250mg daily or bd*	Sodium valproate: 200–400mg bd* Semi-sodium valproate: 500mg to 1g daily*	Sodium valproate: 400mg bd* Semi-sodium valproate: 1g daily*
	Agitation in dementia (not licensed and not recommended) Check response, tolerability and plasma levels for guide.	Sodium valproate: 50mg bd (liquid) or 100mg bd*	Sodium valproate: 100–200mg bd*	Sodium valproate: 200mg bd*

(Continued)

CHAPTER 6

Drug	Specific indication/ additional notes	Starting dose	Usual maintenance dose	Maximum dose in elderly
Anxiolytics/hypnotics				
Clonazepam	Agitation	0.5mg daily	1–2mg/day*	4mg/day*
Daridorexant[30]	Insomnia Taken within 30 minutes before going to bed, with at least 7 hours remaining prior to planned awakening	25mg nocte	25–50mg nocte	50mg nocte
Diazepam	Agitation	1mg tds	1mg tds*	7.5–15mg/day in divided doses (for anxiety)
Lemborexant[31]	Insomnia	5mg nocte (take no more than once per night, immediately before bed)	5–10mg nocte	10mg nocte Elderly are at a higher risk of falls. Caution when using doses >5mg in patients ≥65 years old The maximum recommended dose is 5mg nocte when co-administered with weak CYP3A inhibitors or in moderate hepatic impairment (avoid in severe hepatic impairment).
Lorazepam	PRN only – avoid regular use due to short half-life and risk of dependence	0.5mg daily	0.5–2mg daily*	2mg/day
Melatonin	Insomnia – short-term use (up to 13 weeks)	2mg (modified release) once daily (1–2 hours before bedtime)	2mg once daily	Occasionally 10mg/day (modified release) has been used successfully in dementia
Pregabalin	Generalised anxiety disorder Dose adjustment based on renal function (see product information)[32]	Usually 25mg bd (increase by 25mg bd weekly) Up to 75mg bd (if healthy and normal renal function)	Usually 150mg daily* Up to 150mg bd (if healthy and normal renal function)	150–300mg/day*

Drug	Specific indication/additional notes	Starting dose	Usual maintenance dose	Maximum dose in elderly
Zolpidem	Insomnia (short-term use – up to 4 weeks)	5mg nocte	5mg nocte	5mg nocte
Zopiclone	Insomnia (short-term use – up to 4 weeks)	3.75mg nocte	3.75–7.5mg nocte	7.5mg nocte

Where no references were given the *British National Formulary (BNF)* October 2023[1] was used.

*There is no specific information available in the literature for these drug doses in elderly patients. The doses stated are a guide only. Where there are no data, the maximum doses are conservative and may be exceeded if the drug is well tolerated and following clinician's assessment.

†NB All antipsychotic drugs contain warnings for increased mortality in elderly patients with dementia.

bd, twice a day; BPSD, behavioural and psychological symptoms of dementia; CrCl, creatinine clearance; eGFR, estimated glomerular filtration rate; EPSE, extrapyramidal side effects; ESRD, end-stage renal disease; mane, in the morning; nocte, at night; po, by mouth; prn, as required; tds, three times a day.

References

1. Joint Formulary Committee. *British National Formulary (online)*. London: BMJ and Pharmaceutical Press; http://www.medicinescomplete.com.
2. Prescribers' Digital Reference (PDR) by Connective Rx®. Bupropion – drug summary. 2023 (last assessed October 2023); https://www.pdr.net/drug-summary/?drugLabelId=237.
3. Keam SJ. Dextromethorphan/bupropion: first approval. *CNS Drugs* 2022; **36**:1229–1238.
4. Mylan. Summary of product characteristics. Clomipramine 25mg capsules, hard. 2021 (last checked December 2023); https://www.medicines.org.uk/emc/medicine/33260.
5. Prescribers' Digital Reference (PDR) by Connective Rx®. Desvenlafaxine – drug summary. 2023 (last accessed October 2023); https://www.pdr.net/drug-summary/?drugLabelId=3333.
6. Eli Lilly and Company Ltd. Summary of product characteristics. Cymbalta 30mg, 60mg hard gastro-resistant capsules. 2023; https://www.medicines.org.uk/emc/medicine/15694.
7. Zentiva. Summary of product characteristics. Molipaxin 100mg/trazodone 100mg capsules. 2021 (last checked December 2023); https://www.medicines.org.uk/emc/medicine/26734.
8. Lundbeck Ltd. Summary of product characteristics. Brintellix 10mg film-coated tablets (vortioxetine). 2023; https://www.medicines.org.uk/emc/product/10441/smpc;%202022.
9. Muller MJ, et al. Amisulpride doses and plasma levels in different age groups of patients with schizophrenia or schizoaffective disorder. *J Psychopharmacol* 2009; **23**:278–286.
10. Psarros C, et al. Amisulpride for the treatment of very-late-onset schizophrenia-like psychosis. *Int J Geriatr Psychiatry* 2009; **24**:518–522.
11. Clark-Papasavas C, et al. Towards a therapeutic window of D2/3 occupancy for treatment of psychosis in Alzheimer's disease, with [18F] fallypride positron emission tomography. *Int J Geriatr Psychiatry* 2014; **29**:1001–1009.
12. Prescribers' Digital Reference (PDR) by Connective Rx®. Brexpiprazole – drug summary. 2023 (last accessed October 2023); https://www.pdr.net/drug-summary/?drugLabelId=3759.
13. Prescribers' Digital Reference (PDR) by Connective Rx®. Cariprazine – drug summary. 2023 (last accessed October 2023); https://www.pdr.net/drug-summary/?drugLabelId=3792.
14. Szatmári B, et al. Cariprazine safety in adolescents and the elderly: analyses of clinical study data. *Front Psychiatry* 2020; **11**:61.
15. Jeste DV, et al. Conventional vs. newer antipsychotics in elderly patients. *Am J Geriatr Psychiatry* 1999; **7**:70–76.
16. Karim S, et al. Treatment of psychosis in elderly people. *Adv Psychiatr Treat* 2005; **11**:286–296.
17. Parkinson Study Group. Low-dose clozapine for the treatment of drug-induced psychosis in Parkinson's disease. *N Engl J Med* 1999; **340**:757–763.
18. Caccia S, et al. New atypical antipsychotics for schizophrenia: iloperidone. *Drug Des Devel Ther* 2010; **4**:33–48.
19. Intra-Cellular Therapies, Inc. Highlights of prescribing information. CAPLYTA (lumateperone) capsules, for oral use. 2019; https://www.accessdata.fda.gov/drugsatfda_docs/label/2019/209500s000lbl.pdf.
20. CNX Therapeutics Ltd (formerly Sunovion Pharmaceuticals Europe). Summary of product characteristics. Latuda 18.5mg, 37mg and 74mg film-coated tablets. 2022 (last checked December 2023); https://www.medicines.org.uk/emc/product/3299/smpc.
21. Alkermes, Inc. Highlights of prescribing information. LYBALVI® (olanzapine and samidorphan) tablets, for oral use. 2023; https://www.lybalvi.com/lybalvi-prescribing-information.pdf.
22. ACADIA Pharmaceuticals, Inc. Highlights of prescribing information. Nuplazid (pimavanserin) tablets for oral use. 2016; https://www.accessdata.fda.gov/drugsatfda_docs/label/2016/207318lbl.pdf.
23. Prescribers' Digital Reference (PDR) by Connective Rx®. Pimavanserin – drug summary. 2023 (last accessed October 2023); https://www.pdr.net/drug-summary/?drugLabelId=3909#dosing-considerations.

24. Otsuka Pharmaceuticals (UK) Ltd. Summary of product characteristics. Abilify Maintena 300mg powder and solvent for prolonged-release suspension for injection in pre-filled syringe (aripiprazole). 2022 (last checked December 2023); https://www.medicines.org.uk/emc/product/12955/smpc%202022.
25. Eli Lily and Company Ltd. Summary of product characteristics. Zypadhera 210mg powder and solvent for prolonged release suspension for injection (olanzapine). 2023; https://www.medicines.org.uk/emc/product/6429/smpc.
26. Janssen-Cilag Ltd. Summary of product characteristics. TREVICTA 175mg, 263mg, 350mg, 525mg prolonged release suspension for injection (paliperidone). 2023; https://www.medicines.org.uk/emc/medicine/32050.
27. Janssen-Cilag Ltd. Summary of product characteristics. Byannli 700mg prolonged-release suspension for injection in pre-filled syringe (paliperidone). 2023; https://www.medicines.org.uk/emc/product/13307/smpc.
28. Janssen-Cilag Ltd. Summary of product characteristics. RISPERDAL CONSTA 25mg powder and solvent for prolonged-release suspension for intramuscular injection (risperidone). 2022 (last checked December 2023); https://www.medicines.org.uk/emc/medicine/9939.
29. Essential Pharma Ltd. Summary of product characteristics. Camcolit 400mg controlled release lithium carbonate. 2023; https://www.medicines.org.uk/emc/product/10829/smpc.
30. Idorsia Pharmaceuticals US, Inc. Highlights of prescribing information. QUVIVIQ (daridorexant) tablets, for oral use (controlled substance schedule pending). 2022 (last checked December 2023); https://www.accessdata.fda.gov/drugsatfda_docs/label/2022/214985s000lbl.pdf.
31. Eisai, Inc. Medication guide. DAYVIGO™ (lemborexant) tablets, for oral use (controlled substance schedule pending). 2019; https://www.accessdata.fda.gov/drugsatfda_docs/label/2019/212028s000lbl.pdf#page=21.
32. Upjohn UK Ltd. Summary of product characteristics. Lyrica (pregabalin) 25mg, 50mg, 75mg, 100mg, 150mg, 200mg, 225mg, 300mg capsules. 2023; https://www.medicines.org.uk/emc/product/10303/smpc.

Chapter 7

Prescribing in pregnancy and breastfeeding

Drug choice in pregnancy

A 'normal' outcome to pregnancy can never be guaranteed. The spontaneous abortion rate in confirmed early pregnancy is 10–20%, and the risk of major malformation in the newborn is 2–3% (approximately 1 in 40 pregnancies).[1] Lifestyle factors, such as smoking cigarettes, poor diet and drinking alcohol during pregnancy, can have adverse consequences for the fetus. Pre-pregnancy obesity increases the risk of neural tube defects and is associated with risk factors for the mother.

Psychiatric illness during pregnancy is an independent risk factor for congenital malformations, stillbirths and neonatal deaths[2] and perinatal mental disorders are associated with a broad range of negative child outcomes, many of which can persist into late adolescence.[3] Severe mental illness is also associated with increased risk of obstetric near misses (life-threatening obstetric complications).[4]

The safety of psychotropics in pregnancy cannot be clearly established because robust, prospective trials are unethical and long-term observational studies are challenging to undertake. Data are derived from database studies (many of which fail to control for confounders such as the impact of maternal mental illness, use of illicit drugs and alcohol, smoking, obesity and other medications), limited prospective data from teratology information centres and published case reports. For many drugs, the perceived association or otherwise with adverse outcomes changes over time, as more information is gathered and analysed.

The patient's view of risks and benefits has paramount importance and needs to be informed by up-to-date evidence. Clinicians should be aware of the importance of prescribing medication to women with a severe mental illness. Perinatal suicides are notable for being associated with lack of active treatment, specifically the lack of treatment with psychotropic medication.[5] The American College of Obstetricians and Gynecologists (ACOG) warns against withholding or discontinuing medications for mental health conditions because of pregnancy or lactation status alone.[6]

Box 7.1 provides a brief summary of the relevant issues and evidence available in early 2024.

The Maudsley® Prescribing Guidelines in Psychiatry, Fifteenth Edition. David M. Taylor, Thomas R. E. Barnes and Allan H. Young.
© 2025 David M. Taylor. Published 2025 by John Wiley & Sons Ltd.

Box 7.1 General principles of prescribing in pregnancy

In all women of child-bearing potential

- Always discuss the possibility of pregnancy – half of all pregnancies are unplanned[7]
- Avoid using drugs that are contraindicated during pregnancy (notably **valproate**, **topiramate** and **carbamazepine**). If use of these drugs is unavoidable then women should be made fully aware of their teratogenic properties even if not planning pregnancy. In addition, the prescriber should confirm the presence of an effective and stable long-term contraceptive plan

If mental illness is newly diagnosed in a pregnant woman

- Consider non-pharmacological interventions
- Try to avoid all drugs in the first trimester (when major organs are being formed) unless benefits clearly outweigh risks (i.e. if non-drug treatments are not effective/appropriate)
- Use an established drug and use the lowest effective dose
- Review current medication regimen to ensure there is a clear indication for each drug and that ineffective drugs are stopped

If a woman taking psychotopic drugs is planning a pregnancy

- Consideration should be given to discontinuing treatment if the woman is well and at low risk of relapse, after a careful review of her history
- Discontinuation of treatment for women with severe mental illness (SMI) and at a high risk of relapse is generally unwise but consideration should be given to switching to a low-risk drug. However, be aware that switching drugs may increase the risk of relapse. Any changes must be made with caution and considered in the context of the woman's illness history and previous response to treatment
- Drug-induced hyperprolactinaemia may prevent pregnancy. Consider switching to an alternative drug if hyperprolactinaemia occurs and a pregnancy is planned
- For women with SMI, pre-conception advice from a perinatal psychiatrist should be sought to ensure that women are aware of their risk of relapse in the perinatal period and are able to discuss a prospective perinatal care plan

If a woman taking psychotropic medication discovers that she is pregnant

- Abrupt discontinuation of treatment post-conception is unwise for women with SMI and at a high risk of relapse. Relapse may ultimately be more harmful to the mother and child than continued, effective drug therapy
- Consider continuing with current (effective) medication rather than switching, to minimise the risk of relapse and the number of drugs to which the fetus is exposed
- Valproate (if prescribed as a mood stabiliser) must be stopped immediately
- Early pregnancy can be associated with noticeable changes in mood, therefore it may be necessary to review the medication plan at this stage to ensure symptoms are well controlled

If the patient smokes (smoking is more common in pregnant women with psychiatric illness[8])

- Smoking has been associated with the greatest proportion of excess risk of poor pregnancy outcomes[9]
- Always encourage switching to nicotine replacement therapy. Referral to smoking cessation services is mandated by NICE in the UK
- Vaping is probably safer than tobacco smoking but is not without risk. Nicotine replacement is probably safer than vaping[10]
- Stopping smoking can increase plasma levels of certain drugs (e.g. clozapine)

In all pregnant women

- Ensure that parents are as involved as possible in all decisions
- Prescribe as few drugs as possible (both simultaneously and in sequence) and use the lowest effective dose
- Be prepared to adjust doses as pregnancy progresses and drug handling is altered. Dose increases are frequently required in the third trimester[11] when blood volume expands by around 30%. Plasma level monitoring may be helpful, where available. Hepatic enzyme activity also changes markedly during pregnancy. CYP2D6 activity is increased by almost 50% by the end of pregnancy while the activity of CYP1A2 is reduced by up to 70%[12]
- For patients with SMI, discuss with the patient a referral to specialist perinatal services
- Ensure adequate fetal screening by liaison with obstetric services
- Be aware of potential problems with individual drugs around the time of delivery
- Inform the obstetric team of psychotropic use and possible complications and where appropriate liaise with the neonatology team
- Monitor the neonate for withdrawal effects after birth
- Document all decisions (including the plan for medication)

Psychosis during pregnancy and postpartum

Pregnancy does not protect against psychotic relapse and psychosis during pregnancy predicts postpartum psychosis.[13] The incidence of postpartum psychosis is 0.1–0.25% in the general population (around 1–2 psychiatric hospitalisations per 1000 births). Women with bipolar disorder have an increased risk of postpartum psychosis with around one in five experiencing a psychotic relapse postpartum.[14] There is a high risk of relapse in women with a family history of postpartum psychosis or a personal history of postpartum psychosis.[15] The risk of postpartum psychosis for women with a previous episode of illness, a diagnosis of bipolar disorder type 1 or schizoaffective disorder, and genetic loading for postpartum psychosis, bipolar 1 or schizoaffective disorder, can be as high as 50%. The mental health of the mother in the perinatal period influences fetal well-being, obstetric outcome and child development. The risks of not treating psychosis include harm to the mother and harm to the fetus or neonate (ranging from neglect to infanticide).

First-generation antipsychotics

- Some specific malformations have been reported with individual agents. However, first-generation antipsychotics (FGAs) are unlikely to be major teratogens.[16]
- Most initial data originated from studies that included primarily women with hyperemesis gravidarum (a condition associated with an increased risk of congenital malformations) treated with low doses of phenothiazines. The modest increase in risk identified in some of these studies, along with the absence of clear clustering of congenital abnormalities, suggested that the condition being treated may be responsible rather than drug treatment.
- In a large American study including over a million women, no meaningful increase in the risk of major malformations or cardiac malformations was seen in 733 women prescribed an FGA.[17] A 2023 study of nearly 6.5 million women (6371 prescribed an FGA) in the USA and Nordic countries found that antipsychotics were not major

teratogens. In the same study, the authors reported an observed increased risk of cardiac malformations with (the rarely used) **chlorprothixene**, which the authors suggest should be viewed as a safety signal for further study.[18]

- There may be an association between **haloperidol** and limb defects (based on a small number of cases) but, if real, the risk is likely to be extremely low and it has not been replicated in larger studies.

- An increased risk of gestational diabetes[19] and possibly preterm birth[20] has been reported. A prospective study that included 284 women who took an FGA during pregnancy concluded that preterm birth and low birth weight were more common with FGAs than second-generation antipsychotics (SGAs) (or no antipsychotic exposure).[21] In addition to this, 20% of neonates exposed to an FGA in the last week of gestation experienced early somnolence and jitteriness.

- A higher risk of postpartum bleeding in vaginal delivery and a higher placenta to birth weight ratio has been reported.[22]

- Neonatal dyskinesia has been reported with FGAs.[23]

- Neonatal jaundice has been reported with **phenothiazines**.[24]

- An increased risk (greater in late pregnancy exposure) of neonatal withdrawal symptoms, neurological disorders and persistent pulmonary hypertension has been reported. The absolute risk is low, and the effects appear to be predominantly mild and transient.[25] Prolonged neonatal hospital stay after birth has been reported.[22]

Second-generation antipsychotics

- Some specific malformations have been reported with individual agents. However, SGAs are unlikely to be major teratogens.[16]

- In a large American study, no meaningful increase in the risk of major malformations or cardiac malformations was seen in 9258 women prescribed an SGA. In this same study a small increase in absolute risk of malformations was seen with **risperidone**. The authors suggested that this particular finding should be interpreted with caution and be seen as a possible safety signal that requires further investigation.[17] In a separate study of 214 women taking an SGA, the absolute risk of major malformation was estimated to be 1.4% (1.1% in the control group).[17] Another American study which analysed data from the National Birth Defects Prevention Study reported an association between SGA use in early pregnancy and conotruncal heart defects, tetralogy of Fallot, anorectal atresia/stenosis and gastroschisis. The study included over 22,000 cases and over 11,000 controls. Notably (and this may explain the findings in relation to SGAs), women exposed to SGAs were more likely to report pre-pregnancy obesity, illicit drug use, smoking and alcohol use and use of other psychiatric medications during pregnancy.[26] A 2023 study of nearly 6.5 million women (21,751 prescribed an SGA) in the USA and Nordic countries reported that antipsychotics were not major teratogens. In the same study there was an observed increased risk of oral clefts with **olanzapine** and gastroschisis and brain anomalies with all SGAs, which the authors suggested should be viewed only as safety signals for further study.[18]

- A prospective study of 561 women who took an SGA during pregnancy concluded that SGA exposure was associated with increased birth weight, a modestly increased risk of cardiac septal defects (possibly due to screening bias or co-exposure to selective serotonin reuptake inhibitors [SSRIs]) and, as with FGAs, withdrawal effects in 15% of neonates.[20]

- Available data do not suggest that **lurasidone** is a major teratogen.[27]
- **Olanzapine** has been associated with lower birth weight and increased risk of intensive care admission,[28] a large head circumference[29] and macrosomia[30] (the last of these is consistent with the reported increase in the risk of gestational diabetes[24,29,31,32]).
- Neonatal seizures may be more likely to occur with **clozapine**[31] than with other SGAs. There is a single case report of maternal overdose resulting in fetal death[24] and there are theoretical concerns about the risk of agranulocytosis in the fetus/neonate.[24] Overall, pharmacovigilance data do not indicate that clozapine is less safe in pregnancy than other antipsychotics.[33] Clozapine is included by the UK National Institute for Health and Care Excellence (NICE) in medications that may be prescribed in pregnancy. Lower mean adaptive behaviour scores have been reported in infants exposed to clozapine in utero compared with risperidone, quetiapine or olanzapine. A higher rate of disturbed sleep and lability were reported in clozapine-exposed infants in the same study.[34] On the balance of evidence available, clozapine should usually be continued during pregnancy. Clozapine plasma level monitoring may be beneficial,[35] especially if there are changes in smoking habits.
- An increased risk of gestational diabetes has been reported for SGAs[19] and possibly preterm birth,[20] low birth weight[36] and postpartum bleeding in vaginal delivery. The risk of gestational diabetes may be greatest with clozapine, olanzapine and quetiapine,[37] and **aripiprazole** may not be associated with an increased risk.[38] In a population-based study of over a million women, an increased risk of caesarean section, large for gestational age and preterm birth were reported in women prescribed an SGA compared with no antipsychotic. The risk of caesarean section and large for gestational age was higher with SGAs than with FGAs.[39] Maternal mental illness and lifestyle may also be important factors in the risk for gestational diabetes.[40,41] A lower risk with SGAs compared with FGAs has also been reported[19] and other studies did not report increased risk of metabolic complications.[36]
- An increased risk (greater in late pregnancy exposure) of neonatal withdrawal symptoms, neurological disorders and persistent pulmonary hypertension has been reported. The absolute risk is low, and the effects appear to be predominantly mild and transient.[37]
- **Quetiapine** has a relative low rate of placental passage.[42,43] One study of antipsychotic use in Finland showed a higher risk of increased postpartum bleeding in vaginal delivery, prolonged neonatal hospitalisation stay and a higher placenta to birth weight ratio with antipsychotics use. Quetiapine was the most commonly used antipsychotic in this study.[22]
- The manufacturers of **cariprazine** have advised against its use in pregnancy because of an increased risk of malformations noted in animal studies. It should probably be avoided.

Antipsychotic use and longer-term neurodevelopment

The effect of antipsychotics on longer-term neurodevelopment is unclear.[44] A small prospective case–control study reported that babies who were exposed to SGAs in utero had delayed cognitive, motor and social–emotional development at 2 and 6 months old but not at 12 months.[45] The clinical significance of this finding is unclear. No significant adverse effect on IQ or neurodevelopmental functioning was shown in a small study of school-aged children following exposure to antipsychotics during pregnancy.[46] A cohort study of 667,517 children did not show an association between maternal antipsychotic prescription and poorer standardised test performance in language and mathematics in schoolchildren.[47] Two large cohort studies have reported increased risk of attention deficit hyperactivity disorder (ADHD) and autism spectrum disorder (ASD) associated with maternal mental illness but not with prenatal antipsychotic exposure.[20,48] A smaller study reported no increased risk of psychiatric disorders in children born to women who continued antipsychotics in pregnancy.[49] A 2022 birth cohort study found antipsychotics to not be causally associated with neurodevelopmental disorders although there was a safety signal for aripiprazole, which requires further study.[50]

Recommendations for psychosis in pregnancy are outlined in Box 7.2.

Box 7.2 Recommendations – psychosis in pregnancy

- Overall, the data do not allow an assessment of relative risks associated with different agents and certainly do not confirm absolutely the safety of any particular drug. However, the high risk of adverse outcomes for the mother and child associated with untreated maternal illness should be noted
- Patients with a history of psychosis who are maintained on antipsychotic medication should be advised to discuss a planned pregnancy as early as possible
- Women should be supported to minimise the risks in pregnancy from smoking and alcohol and drug misuse. Women should be referred to appropriate services such as smoking cessation clinics and addictions services
- Drug-induced hyperprolactinaemia may prevent pregnancy. Consider switching to an alternative drug if hyperprolactinaemia occurs and a pregnancy is planned
- If a pregnant woman is stable on an antipsychotic and likely to relapse without medication, advise her to continue the antipsychotic.[51] Switching medication is generally not advised owing to the risk of relapse
- When initiating an antipsychotic consider using the antipsychotic that has previously worked best for the woman, after discussion of benefits and risks.[43] This may minimise fetal exposure by avoiding the need for higher doses and/or multiple drugs should relapse occur
- Be clear of the indication for each drug, use the lowest **effective** dose and prescribe as few drugs as possible both simultaneously and in sequence. Do not continue medication that is not effective
- Advise pregnant women taking antipsychotic medication about diet and monitor for excessive weight gain
- Women taking an antipsychotic during pregnancy should be monitored for gestational diabetes. In the UK, NICE recommends women are offered an oral glucose tolerance test
- In the UK, NICE recommends avoiding depot preparations in a woman who is planning a pregnancy, pregnant or considering breastfeeding, unless she is responding well to a depot and has a previous history of non-adherence with oral medication[51]
- The Australian Centre of Perinatal Excellence (COPE) recommends a 13- or 18–20-week ultrasound for women taking antipsychotics in the first trimester[52]
- Antipsychotic discontinuation symptoms can occur in the neonate (e.g. crying, agitation, increased suckling). This is thought to be a class effect.[53] When antipsychotics are taken in pregnancy it is recommended that the woman gives birth in a unit that has access to paediatric intensive care facilities.[21] Some centres used mixed (breast/bottle) feeding to minimise withdrawal symptoms
- Document all decisions

Depression during pregnancy and postpartum[54–56]

Approximately 10% of pregnant women develop or have a pre-existing depressive illness. Around a third of cases of postpartum depression begin before birth and there is a significant increase in new psychiatric episodes in the first 3 months after delivery. At least 80% of these are mood disorders, particularly severe depression. Women who have had a previous episode of depressive illness (postpartum or not) are at higher risk of further episodes during pregnancy and postpartum. The risk is highest in women with bipolar illness who are also at risk of mania or mixed affective episodes. There is some evidence that depression increases the risk of spontaneous abortion (miscarriage),[57] having a low birth weight or small for gestational age baby, or of preterm delivery, although effects are small.[3,58,59] The mental health of the mother influences fetal well-being, obstetric outcome and child development. The risks of not treating depression include harm to the mother through poor self-care, lack of obstetric care or self-harm and harm to the fetus or neonate (ranging from neglect to infanticide).

Antidepressants

Relapse rates are higher in those with a history of depression who discontinue medication compared with those who continue. One study found that 68% of women who were well on antidepressant treatment and stopped during pregnancy relapsed, compared with 26% who continued antidepressants.[54] Risk is likely to be highest for women with a history of severe and/or recurrent depression.[60] The rate of antidepressant withdrawal will also influence the risk of depressive relapse.

Available data do not suggest an association between prenatal antidepressant use and neurodevelopmental disorders (after controlling for maternal illness and other confounders).[61] There is also some evidence that successful antidepressant use can be beneficial for child behavioural outcomes. A Danish study found that adverse outcomes were relatively more likely in depressed women not taking antidepressants.[62] However, antidepressant exposure in pregnancy may be an important marker of the need for early screening and intervention.

Tricyclic antidepressants

- Fetal exposure to tricyclics (via the umbilicus and amniotic fluid) is high.[63,64]
- Tricyclic antidepressants (TCAs) have been widely used throughout pregnancy without apparent detriment to the fetus.[65–67]
- A weak association between **clomipramine** use and cardiovascular defects cannot be excluded[68] and the European summary of product characteristics (SPC) for Anafranil states: 'Neonates whose mothers had taken tricyclic antidepressants until delivery have developed dyspnoea, lethargy, colic, irritability, hypotension or hypertension, tremor or spasms, during the first few hours or days. Studies in animals have shown reproductive toxicity. **Anafranil** (i.e. branded clomipramine) is not recommended during pregnancy and in women of child-bearing potential not using contraception.' The labels for other TCAs also contain a caution about withdrawal effects in neonates. One case of neonatal QT prolongation and torsades de pointes has been reported following maternal **clomipramine** use[69] and one case of Timothy syndrome

(a disorder characterised by severe QT prolongation) in a newborn whose mother took **amitriptyline** in early pregnancy.[70]

- TCA use during pregnancy is associated with an increased risk of preterm delivery.[65,66,71]
- Use of TCAs in the third trimester is well known to produce neonatal withdrawal effects, such as agitation, irritability, seizures, respiratory distress and endocrine and metabolic disturbances.[65] These are usually mild and self-limiting.
- Little is known of the early developmental effects of prenatal exposure to tricyclics, although one small study detected no adverse consequences.[72] Limited data suggest in utero exposure to tricyclics has no effects on later development.[72,73] The authors of a study that reported an association between maternal antidepressant use and an increased risk of affective disorders in offspring[74] suggested the observed associations may be attributable to underlying parental psychopathology. There are no convincing data suggesting an association between prenatal antidepressant use and neurodevelopmental disorders[61] or ASD diagnoses or traits.[75]

Selective serotonin reuptake inhibitors (SSRIs)

- SSRIs appear not to be major teratogens.[65,67,76–78] An association between prenatal SSRI use and congenital heart defects has been reported, with some studies reporting a higher risk with **fluoxetine** and **paroxetine**.[79] However, other studies have found no association between any SSRI and an increased risk of cardiac septal defects[80–82] nor any other heart defects[83–87] and it is suggested that mood disorders alone may be the cause of any increased risk of congenital heart defects.[78]
- One database study reported that fetal alcohol disorders were 10 times more common in those exposed to SSRIs in utero than in controls,[88] and that alcohol use during pregnancy (which may be used as self-medication for depression) is associated with an increased risk of cardiac defects in the fetus.[68]
- **Sertraline** appears to result in the least placental exposure.[89]
- There may be a small increased risk of preterm birth and low birth weight and lower Apgar scores and admission to neonatal intensive care units with SSRIs.[78] Maternal depression itself increases these risks.[90,91] Poor neonatal adaptation (including withdrawal symptoms) has been reported and risk may be increased with prematurity[92] and increasing dose, and may be higher with other SSRIs than sertraline.[93]
- SSRIs may increase the risk for persistent pulmonary hypertension of the newborn. The absolute risk appears to be small and more modest than previously estimated.[94] The risk may exist only in late pregnancy exposure[95] and may be lower with sertraline.[96]
- Gestational hypertension, pre-eclampsia, placental abnormalities and postpartum haemorrhage have been reported with SSRI use. The risks appear to be small and it should be noted that maternal depression itself increases the risk of these outcomes.[78] The UK Medicines and Healthcare products Regulatory Agency (MHRA) advises that healthcare professionals need to be aware of the small increased risk of postpartum haemorrhage with SSRI/serotonin–noradrenaline reuptake inhibitor (SNRI) antidepressant use during the month before delivery.
- Data relating to neurodevelopmental outcome of fetal exposure to SSRIs are less than conclusive.[72,73,97–100] Depression itself may have more obvious adverse effects on development.[72,101] Some studies have reported a small increased risk of ASD.[102–104]

However, larger studies have either failed to show this association after accounting for maternal illness and other demographic confounders[75,105–107] or have found it to be no longer statistically significant.[108,109] A large cohort study in 2022 reported that antidepressant use in pregnancy itself does not appear to increase the risk of neurodevelopmental disorders in children.[61] There is no reliable evidence indicating an increased risk of ADHD.[91] Poorer cognitive and gross motor development[110] and problems with speech and language,[111–113] behaviour[114,115] and fine motor control have been reported[116] but it is not clear whether or not this is a result of confounding. Authors of two separate studies, one reporting an association between antidepressant exposure in pregnancy and increased risk in the offspring of affective disorders[74] and the other describing higher rates of emotional disorders and antidepressant medication prescriptions,[117] have suggested the observed associations may be attributable to underlying parental psychopathology rather than direct exposure in utero. A 2023 study reported changes in brain morphology associated with SSRI exposure during pregnancy, some of which persisted into adolescence. The study did not assess clinical outcomes in the children and as such the significance of these findings is unclear.[118]

Other antidepressants

- Despite a previous reported association between **venlafaxine** and increased risk of specific birth defects[111] including cardiac defects, anencephaly and cleft palate,[119] a 2022 meta-analysis concluded that available data do not indicate any SNRIs to be major teratogens.[120] An earlier observational study of 281 venlafaxine-exposed pregnancies did not find conclusive evidence that venlafaxine increased the risk of adverse pregnancy or fetal outcomes.[121] However, venlafaxine has been associated with neonatal withdrawal and poor neonatal adaptation syndrome,[122] babies being born small for gestational age[123] and postpartum haemorrhage.[124] The UK MHRA advises that healthcare professionals need to be aware of the small increased risk of postpartum haemorrhage with SSRI/SNRI antidepressant use during the month before delivery. SNRIs may be associated with an increased risk for persistent pulmonary hypertension of the newborn. The absolute risk appears to be low.[96]

- A large cohort study using propensity scores and several sensitivity analyses found **duloxetine** use in pregnancy may be associated with a small increase in the risk of postpartum hemorrhage,[124] and a case of suspected withdrawal syndrome in the newborn requiring hospitalisation has been reported.[125] However, no specific risks were identified with duloxetine in a study that prospectively followed 233 women through pregnancy and delivery.[126] A population-based observational study from Sweden and Denmark did not show an increased risk of major or minor congenital malformations or stillbirth with duloxetine.[127]

- **Trazodone, bupropion** (amfebutamone) and **mirtazapine** have few data supporting their safety.[122,128,129] A 2023 observational study did not find a significant difference in the risk of major congenital anomalies after first-trimester exposure to trazodone compared with SSRI exposure.[130] Available data suggest that both bupropion and mirtazapine are not associated with malformations but, like SSRIs, may be linked to an increased rate of spontaneous abortion;[131–133] however this might be attributable to underlying psychiatric disease. A 2022 Danish study did not observe an association between mirtazapine use and major congenital malformations, spontaneous abortion, stillbirth or neonatal death.[134]

■ First-trimester exposure to bupropion may be associated with a slightly elevated risk of ventricular septal defects.[135] Bupropion exposure in utero has been associated with an increased risk of ADHD in young children.[136,137] Rather limited data suggest the absence of teratogenic potential with **moclobemide**[138] and **reboxetine**.[139]

■ **Monamine oxidase inhibitors** should be avoided in pregnancy because of a suspected increased risk of congenital malformations and because of the risk of hypertensive crisis.[140]

■ There is no evidence to suggest that **electroconvulsive therapy** (**ECT**) causes harm to either the mother or fetus during pregnancy[141] although general anaesthesia is of course not without risks. NICE recommends ECT for pregnant women with severe depression, severe mixed affective states or mania, or catatonia, whose physical health or that of the fetus is at serious risk.

Box 7.3 summarises recommendations for treating depression in pregnancy.

Box 7.3 Recommendations – depression in pregnancy

■ Patients who are already receiving antidepressants and are at high risk of relapse are best maintained on the same antidepressant (assuming it is effective and well tolerated) during and after pregnancy
  ■ Those who develop a moderate to severe or severe depressive illness during pregnancy should be treated with antidepressant drugs. If initiating an antidepressant during pregnancy or for a woman considering pregnancy, previous response to treatment must be taken into account. The antidepressant which has previously proved to be effective should be considered. For previously untreated patients, sertraline may be considered. ACOG recommends selective serotonin reuptake inhibitors (SSRIs) first line (with serotonin–noradrenaline reuptake inhibitors [SNRIs] a reasonable alternative) and if there is no pharmacotherapy history, sertraline or escitalopram is a reasonable first-line medication. COPE recommends SSRIs first line
■ For moderate to severe perinatal depression with onset in the third trimester, ACOG recommends consideration of brexanolone
■ Screen for alcohol use and be vigilant for the development of hypertension and pre-eclampsia
■ Women who take SSRIs or SNRIs late in pregnancy may be at increased risk of postpartum haemorrhage
■ When taken in late pregnancy, SSRIs may increase the risk of persistent pulmonary hypertension of the newborn. The absolute risk is very low
■ The neonate may experience poor neonatal adaptation syndrome or discontinuation symptoms
■ NICE in the UK[142] advises additional monitoring of the newborn of women who have taken an SRRI or SNRI antidepressant during pregnancy

---

Bipolar illness during pregnancy and postpartum

The risk of relapse during pregnancy if mood-stabilising medication is discontinued is high[143] and the risk of relapse after delivery is hugely increased. The mental health of the mother influences fetal well-being, obstetric outcome and child development. The risks of not stabilising mood include harm to the mother through poor self-care, lack of obstetric care, the need for hospital admission and harm to the fetus or neonate (ranging from neglect to infanticide).

Mood stabilisers (non-antipsychotics)

- **Lithium** completely equilibrates across the placenta.[144] Lithium exposure during pregnancy has been associated with an increased risk of congenital anomalies.[145] The risk is higher in the first trimester[146] and may be greater at higher doses.[145] Although the overall risk of major malformations in infants exposed in utero has probably been overestimated in the past, lithium should be avoided in pregnancy if possible. However, if lithium is the best drug for the woman and the drug most likely to keep her well, she should be advised of the increased risk but supported to stay on lithium. If discontinuation is planned, slow discontinuation before conception is the preferred course of action[31,147] because abrupt discontinuation worsens the risk of relapse. The relapse rate postpartum may be as high as 70% in women who discontinued lithium before conception.[148]

- Lithium use during pregnancy has a well-known association with the cardiac malformation Ebstein's anomaly. However, more recent data suggest that the magnitude of the effect is much smaller than previously estimated.[149,150] Furthermore, a large surveillance study of 5.6 million births found an association of Ebstein's anomaly with maternal mental health problems generally rather than specifically with lithium.[151] The period of maximum risk to the fetus is 2–6 weeks after conception,[152] before many women know that they are pregnant. The risk of atrial and ventricular septal defects may also be increased.[28] If lithium is continued during pregnancy, high-resolution ultrasound and echocardiography should be performed in liaison with fetal medicine obstetric services.

- In the third trimester, the use of lithium may be problematic because of changing pharmacokinetics. An increasing dose of lithium is required to maintain the lithium level during pregnancy as total body water increases, but the requirements return abruptly to pre-pregnancy levels immediately after delivery.[153] Women taking lithium should deliver in hospital where fluid balance can be monitored and maintained.

- Lithium use in pregnancy has been associated with an increased risk of spontaneous preterm birth and large for gestational age neonates.[154] However, a large cohort study reported that lithium was not associated with placenta-mediated complications or preterm birth.[155] Lithium use may increase the risk of neonatal readmission within 4 weeks postpartum,[146] although a later study failed to replicate this finding.[156] Neonatal goitre, hypotonia, lethargy, cardiac arrhythmia, respiratory symptoms[157] and low Apgar scores[158] have been reported.

- Lithium probably does not affect neonatal brain development.[159]

- Most data relating to **carbamazepine**, **valproate** and **lamotrigine** come from studies in epilepsy, a condition associated with increased neonatal malformation. These data may not be precisely relevant to use in mental illness. Both carbamazepine and valproate have a clear causal link with increased risk of a variety of fetal abnormalities, particularly neural tube defects including spina bifida.[160] Both drugs should be avoided, and an antipsychotic prescribed instead. Valproate confers a higher risk (around 10% for major malformations) than carbamazepine[161-163] and should not be used in women of child-bearing age except where all other treatment has failed and when there is a long-term effective contraception plan. There is no evidence that folate protects against anticonvulsant-induced neural tube defects if given during pregnancy,[164] but it may do so if given prior to conception (the neural tube is essentially formed by 8 weeks of pregnancy[165] before many women realise they are pregnant). However, folate supplementation may be beneficial with regard to early neurodevelopment and so should always be offered.[164] Valproate monotherapy has also been associated with an increased relative risk of atrial septal defects, cleft palate, hypospadias, polydactyly and craniosynostosis, although absolute risks are low.[166] Valproate is also associated with a reduced head circumference in the neonate.[167]

- There appears to be a clear causal association between valproate use in pregnancy and motor and neurodevelopmental problems in exposed children. A review of studies by the European Medicines Agency showed that up to 40% of pre-school children exposed to valproate in utero experienced some form of developmental delay, including delayed walking and talking, memory problems, difficulty with speech and language and a lower intellectual ability. Poorer outcomes have been shown in language functioning, attention, memory, executive functioning and adaptive behaviour compared with carbamazepine and lamotrigine exposure. Lower IQs and an increased diagnosis rate of ASD are also reported.[168,169] Processing, working memory and learning deficits appear to be dose-related.[170] Decreased school performance has been associated with valproate use compared with children unexposed to anticonvulsants and with children exposed to lamotrigine.[171]

- Valproate use may increase risk of pre-eclampsia.[172]

- Where continued use of carbamazepine is deemed essential, low-dose (but effective) monotherapy is strongly recommended as the teratogenic effect is probably dose related.[173,174] Use of carbamazepine in the third trimester may necessitate maternal vitamin K.

- There is growing evidence that lamotrigine is safer in pregnancy than carbamazepine or valproate across a range of outcomes.[164,168,175–177] The risk of major malformations appears to be in the range reported for children not exposed to anticonvulsants.[178] Clearance of lamotrigine seems to increase radically during pregnancy[179,180] and then reduces postpartum[181] so frequent lamotrigine levels are necessary.

- Behaviour problems have been reported by parents of children exposed to lamotrigine in pregnancy.[182] Lamotrigine may be associated with an increased risk of autism.[183] However, available data suggest the effect of lamotrigine on neurodevelopment appears to not be significant.[184]

- Lower Apgar scores at birth have been reported with carbamazepine, valproate and **topiramate**. If an association exists, the absolute risk is low.[185]

- Major malformations,[186] specifically orofacial clefts, have been reported with topiramate.[187] The risk of oral clefts may be higher in women with epilepsy who use higher doses of the drug.[188] A large population study reported an increased risk of neurodevelopmental disorders, small for gestational age and congenital malformations[189] with prenatal topiramate exposure. Topiramate should not be used in pregnant women, and women of child-bearing age should take precautions to avoid getting pregnant.[190]

- The data for oxcarbazepine are not clear. A 2022 meta-analysis reported a small but not statistically significant increased risk of malformations in children exposed to **oxcarbazepine**.[191] Three studies in the same analysis reported an association with fetal/perinatal deaths. Because of some notable limitations in the studies incuded in this analysis, it is difficult to draw firm conclusions.

- Similarly, data for **pregabalin** are not clear.[192] However, based on a Nordic study[193] that showed a small increased risk of major malformations (compared with lamotrigine and duloxetine) the UK MHRA[194] and the manufacturers of pregabalin advise that women taking pregabalin be made aware of this risk and advised to use effective contraception.

■ A large cohort study reported that anticonvulsant mood stabilisers were not associated with placenta-mediated complications or preterm birth.[170]

Recommendations for the treatment of bipolar disorder in pregnancy are outlined in Box 7.4.

Box 7.4 Recommendations – bipolar disorder in pregnancy

■ For women who have had a long period without relapse, the possibility of switching to a safer drug (antipsychotic) or withdrawing treatment completely before conception and for at least the first trimester should be considered

■ For women with a severe mental illness, discuss referral to perinatal services for pre-conception advice

■ The risk of relapse both pre- and postpartum is very high if medication is discontinued abruptly

■ No mood stabiliser is clearly safe. In the UK, NICE recommends the use of mood-stabilising antipsychotics as a preferable alternative to continuation with a mood stabiliser

■ Women with severe illness or who are known to relapse quickly after discontinuation of a mood-stabilising agent should be advised to continue their medication, following discussion of the risks. (This advice does not apply to valproate.) NICE recommends that if a woman taking lithium becomes pregnant, consider stopping lithium gradually over 4 weeks if she is well. Explain to her that there is a risk of relapse, particularly in the postnatal period, if she has bipolar disorder. If a woman taking lithium becomes pregnant and is not well or is at high risk of relapse, consider switching gradually to an antipsychotic or stopping lithium and restarting it in the second trimester (if the woman is not planning to breastfeed and her symptoms have responded better to lithium than to other drugs in the past) or continuing with lithium if she is at high risk of relapse and an antipsychotic is unlikely to be effective. If lithium is considered essential in a woman planning pregnancy, the woman should be informed of the risk of fetal heart malformations when lithium is taken in the first trimester and the risk of toxicity in the baby if lithium is continued during breastfeeding. In the UK, NICE recommends checking the plasma lithium levels every 4 weeks, then weekly from the 36th week, and to adjust the dose to keep plasma lithium levels in the woman's therapeutic range, ensuring the woman maintains an adequate fluid balance. The woman should give birth in hospital and be monitored by the obstetric team when labour starts, including checking plasma lithium levels and fluid balance because of the risk of dehydration and lithium toxicity. Lithium should be stopped during labour and plasma lithium levels checked 12 hours after the mother's last dose. ACOG recommends that pregnant patients taking lithium in the first trimester receive a detailed ultrasound examination in the second trimester to evaluate the fetal anatomy with a particular focus on cardiac anatomy. COPE recommends a 13- or 18–20-week ultrasound for women taking lithium or anticonvulsants in the first trimester

■ Women prescribed lithium should undergo appropriate monitoring of the fetus in liaison with fetal medicine obstetric services to screen for Ebstein's anomaly

■ NICE, ACOG and COPE strongly advise against the use of valproate in pregnancy. Valproate should be discontinued before a woman becomes pregnant. Women taking valproate who are planning a pregnancy should be strongly advised to gradually stop the drug because of the high risk of fetal malformations and adverse neurodevelopmental outcomes after any exposure in pregnancy. COPE recommends once the decision to conceive is made to stop valproate over 2–4 weeks, while adding in high-dose folic acid (5mg/day), which should continue for the first trimester.[52] **In the UK, valproate may not be initiated in patients under 55 or continued in women of child-bearing potential unless two specialists agree and document that there is no other effective or tolerated treatment**[195]

- If valproate is the only drug that works for a particular woman, and this is seen as the only option for her during pregnancy, then the patient should be given a clear briefing of the risks and give written consent confirming that she understands the risk of malformations and developmental delays. Having said this, it is difficult to imagine any situation where the benefits of valproate outweigh the huge risks presented by using valproate in pregnancy
- NICE advises that carbamazepine not be offered to treat a mental health problem in women who are planning a pregnancy, pregnant or considering breastfeeding. NICE advises discussing the possibility of stopping carbamazepine if a woman is planning a pregnancy or becomes pregnant. If carbamazepine is used, prophylactic vitamin K should be administered to the mother and neonate after delivery. ACOG recommends against discontinuing mood stabilisers (except for valproate) during pregnancy due to the risk of recurrence or exacerbation of mood symptoms
- NICE advises if a woman is taking lamotrigine to check lamotrigine levels frequently during pregnancy and into the postnatal period because they vary substantially at these times
- In acute mania in pregnancy use an antipsychotic and, if ineffective, consider electroconvulsive therapy
- In bipolar depression during pregnancy use cognitive behavioural therapy for moderate depression and a selective serotonin reuptake inhibitor for more severe depression. Lamotrigine is also an option

Anxiety and insomnia during pregnancy and postpartum

Anxiety disorders and insomnia are commonly seen in pregnancy.[196] Preferred treatments are cognitive behavioural therapy (CBT) and sleep-hygiene measures, respectively.

Sedatives

- First-trimester exposure to **benzodiazepines** has been associated with specific malformations[197] such as oral clefts in newborns,[198] although other studies[198–202] have failed to confirm this association. Benzodiazepine use in pregnancy may be a marker for cardiac and total malformation risk.[203]
- Benzodiazepine use in pregnancy has been associated with caesarean delivery, spontaneous abortion, neonatal intensive care admission, neonatal ventilatory support, low birth weight, preterm delivery, small head circumference and small for gestational age babies.[199,204–208] Third-trimester use is commonly associated with neonatal difficulties (floppy baby syndrome).[209] A Taiwanese population-based study which accounted for confounding factors such as indication reported that benzodiazepine or Z drug use in early pregnancy was not associated with a substantial increase in the risk of stillbirth and preterm birth but there was an increased risk of small for gestational age. Exposure during late pregnancy was found to be associated with a substantially elevated risk of stillbirth and preterm birth.[210]
- Note that, in the UK, NICE advises that benzodiazepines are not offered to women in pregnancy and the postnatal period except for the short-term treatment of severe anxiety and agitation. It also suggests gradually stopping benzodiazepines in women who are planning a pregnancy, pregnant or considering breastfeeding.[51] ACOG recommends that benzodiazepines be avoided or prescribed sparingly as a treatment for perinatal anxiety.
- **Promethazine** has been used in hyperemesis gravidarum and appears not to be teratogenic, although data are limited.

- Hypnotic benzodiazepine receptor agonists (Z drugs) are probably not associated with an increased risk of congenital malformations,[211,212] but an increased risk of premature birth, low birth weight and small for gestational age has been reported.[211]
- **Zolpidem** may be associated with an increased likelihood of caesarean section.[213]
- Available data do not appear to show an association between in utero benzodiazepine and/or Z drug exposure and neurodevelopmental disorders.[214–216]

Attention deficit hyperactivity disorder (ADHD) in pregnancy

Methylphenidate and **amfetamines** are probably not major teratogens.[217,218] A small increased risk of cardiac malformations has been reported with methylphenidate but is not seen with amfetamines.[219] There may be a small increased risk of spontaneous abortion with methylphenidate and a small increased risk of premature birth and low birth weight with amfetamines.[218] **Modafinil** may be associated with an increased risk of congenital malformations (including congenital heart defects, hypospadias and orofacial clefts).[220,221] In the UK, the MHRA advises that modafinil should not be used during pregnancy.[220] Women of child-bearing age must understand the risk of taking modafinil in pregnancy and should be advised to use effective contraception during treatment with modafinil and for 2 months after discontinuing treatment.[220] Available data do not show an increased risk of neurodevelopmental disorders in children exposed to ADHD medications in utero.[222,223]

References

1. McElhatton PR. Pregnancy: (2) general principles of drug use in pregnancy. *Pharm J* 2003; 270:232–234.
2. Schneid-Kofman N, et al. Psychiatric illness and adverse pregnancy outcome. *Int J Gynaecol Obstet* 2008; 101:53–56.
3. Stein A, et al. Effects of perinatal mental disorders on the fetus and child. *Lancet* 2014; 384:1800–1819.
4. Easter A, et al. Obstetric near misses among women with serious mental illness: data linkage cohort study. *Br J Psychiatry* 2021; **219**: 494–500.
5. Khalifeh H, et al. Suicide in perinatal and non-perinatal women in contact with psychiatric services: 15 year findings from a UK national inquiry. *Lancet Psychiatry* 2016; 3:233–242.
6. Treatment and management of mental health conditions during pregnancy and postpartum: ACOG Clinical Practice Guideline No. 5. *Obstet Gynecol* 2023; **141**:1262–1288.
7. De La Rochebrochard E, et al. Children born after unplanned pregnancies and cognitive development at 3 years: social differentials in the United Kingdom Millennium Cohort. *Am J Epidemiol* 2013; 178:910–920.
8. Goodwin RD, et al. Mental disorders and nicotine dependence among pregnant women in the United States. *Obstet Gynecol* 2007; **109**:875–883.
9. Vigod SN, et al. Maternal schizophrenia and adverse birth outcomes: what mediates the risk? *Soc Psychiatry Psychiatr Epidemiol* 2020; 55:561–570.
10. Vilcassim MJR, et al. Electronic cigarette use during pregnancy: is it harmful? *Toxics* 2023; **11**:278.
11. Sit DK, et al. Changes in antidepressant metabolism and dosing across pregnancy and early postpartum. *J Clin Psychiatry* 2008; 69:652–658.
12. Ter Horst PG, et al. Pharmacological aspects of neonatal antidepressant withdrawal. *Obstet Gynecol Surv* 2008; 63:267–279.
13. Harlow BL, et al. Incidence of hospitalization for postpartum psychotic and bipolar episodes in women with and without prior prepregnancy or prenatal psychiatric hospitalizations. *Arch Gen Psychiatry* 2007; 64:42–48.
14. Wesseloo R, et al. Risk of postpartum relapse in bipolar disorder and postpartum psychosis: a systematic review and meta-analysis. *Am J Psychiatry* 2016; 173:117–127.
15. Jones I, et al. Bipolar disorder, affective psychosis, and schizophrenia in pregnancy and the post-partum period. *Lancet* 2014; 384:1789–1799.
16. Wang Z, et al. Prenatal exposure to antipsychotic agents and the risk of congenital malformations in children: a systematic review and meta-analysis. *Br J Clin Pharmacol* 2021; **87**:4101–4123.
17. Huybrechts KF, et al. Antipsychotic use in pregnancy and the risk for congenital malformations. *JAMA Psychiatry* 2016; 73:938–946.
18. Huybrechts KF, et al. Association of in utero antipsychotic medication exposure with risk of congenital malformations in Nordic countries and the US. *JAMA Psychiatry* 2023; 80:156–166.

CHAPTER 7

19. Kulkarni J, et al. The use of first and second-generation antipsychotic drugs and the potential to develop gestational diabetes mellitus among perinatal patients with psychosis. *Schizophr Res* 2023; **254**:22–26.

20. Wang Z, et al. Association between prenatal exposure to antipsychotics and attention-deficit/hyperactivity disorder, autism spectrum disorder, preterm birth, and small for gestational age. *JAMA Intern Med* 2021; **181**:1332–1340.

21. Habermann F, et al. Atypical antipsychotic drugs and pregnancy outcome: a prospective, cohort study. *J Clin Psychopharmacol* 2013; **33**:453–462.

22. Kananen A, et al. Quetiapine and other antipsychotic medications during pregnancy: a 15-year follow-up of a university hospital birth register. *Nord J Psychiatry* 2023; **77**:651–660.

23. Collins KO, et al. Maternal haloperidol therapy associated with dyskinesia in a newborn. *Am J Health Syst Pharm* 2003; **60**:2253–2255.

24. Gentile S. Antipsychotic therapy during early and late pregnancy. A systematic review. *Schizophr Bull* 2010; **36**:518–544.

25. Heinonen E, et al. Neonatal morbidity after fetal exposure to antipsychotics: a national register-based study. *BMJ Open* 2022; **12**:e061328.

26. Anderson KN, et al. Atypical antipsychotic use during pregnancy and birth defect risk: National Birth Defects Prevention Study, 1997–2011. *Schizophr Res* 2020; **215**:81–88.

27. Cohen LS, et al. Reproductive safety of lurasidone and quetiapine: update from the National Pregnancy Registry for Psychiatric Medications. *J Women's Health (Larchmt)* 2023; **32**:452–462.

28. Reis M, et al. Maternal use of antipsychotics in early pregnancy and delivery outcome. *J Clin Psychopharmacol* 2008; **28**:279–288.

29. Boden R, et al. Antipsychotics during pregnancy: relation to fetal and maternal metabolic effects. *Arch Gen Psychiatry* 2012; **69**:715–721.

30. Newham JJ, et al. Birth weight of infants after maternal exposure to typical and atypical antipsychotics: prospective comparison study. *Br J Psychiatry* 2008; **192**:333–337.

31. Ernst CL, et al. The reproductive safety profile of mood stabilizers, atypical antipsychotics, and broad-spectrum psychotropics. *J Clin Psychiatry* 2002; **63** Suppl 4:42–55.

32. McKenna K, et al. Pregnancy outcome of women using atypical antipsychotic drugs: a prospective comparative study. *J Clin Psychiatry* 2005; **66**:444–449.

33. Beex-Oosterhuis MM, et al. Safety of clozapine use during pregnancy: analysis of international pharmacovigilance data. *Pharmacoepidemiol Drug Saf* 2020; **29**:725–735.

34. Shao P, et al. Effects of clozapine and other atypical antipsychotics on infants development who were exposed to as fetus: a post-hoc analysis. *PLoS One* 2015; **10**:e0123373.

35. Nguyen T, et al. Obstetric and neonatal outcomes of clozapine exposure in pregnancy: a consecutive case series. *Arch Women's Ment Health* 2020; **23**:441–445.

36. Lin HY, et al. Antipsychotic use in early pregnancy and the risk of maternal and neonatal complications. *Mayo Clin Proc* 2022; **97**:2086–2096.

37. Heinonen E, et al. Antipsychotic use during pregnancy and risk for gestational diabetes: a national register-based cohort study in Sweden. *CNS Drugs* 2022; **36**:529–539.

38. Galbally M, et al. Aripiprazole and pregnancy: a retrospective, multicentre study. *J Affect Disord* 2018; **238**:593–596.

39. Ellfolk M, et al. Second-generation antipsychotics and pregnancy complications. *Eur J Clin Pharmacol* 2020; **76**:107–115.

40. Galbally M, et al. The association between gestational diabetes mellitus, antipsychotics and severe mental illness in pregnancy: a multicentre study. *Aust N Z J Obstet Gynaecol* 2020; **60**:63–69.

41. Uguz F. Antipsychotic use during pregnancy and the risk of gestational diabetes mellitus: a systematic review. *J Clin Psychopharmacol* 2019; **39**:162–167.

42. Schoretsanitis G, et al. Excretion of antipsychotics into the amniotic fluid, umbilical cord blood, and breast milk: a systematic critical review and combined analysis. *Ther Drug Monit* 2020; **42**:245–254.

43. McAllister-Williams RH, et al. British Association for Psychopharmacology consensus guidance on the use of psychotropic medication preconception, in pregnancy and postpartum 2017. *J Psychopharmacol* 2017; **31**:519–552.

44. Gentile S, et al. Neurodevelopmental outcomes in infants exposed in utero to antipsychotics: a systematic review of published data. *CNS Spectr* 2017; **22**:273–281.

45. Peng M, et al. Effects of prenatal exposure to atypical antipsychotics on postnatal development and growth of infants: a case-controlled, prospective study. *Psychopharmacology (Berl)* 2013; **228**:577–584.

46. Schrijver L, et al. Neurodevelopment in school-aged children after intrauterine exposure to antipsychotics. *Acta Psychiatr Scand* 2023; **147**:43–53.

47. Liu X, et al. Association of maternal antipsychotic prescription during pregnancy with standardized test scores of schoolchildren in Denmark. *JAMA Intern Med* 2022; **182**:1035–1043.

48. Hálfdánarson Ó, et al. Antipsychotic use in pregnancy and risk of attention/deficit-hyperactivity disorder and autism spectrum disorder: a Nordic cohort study. *Evid Based Ment Health* 2022; **25**:54–62.

49. Momen NC, et al. In utero exposure to antipsychotic medication and psychiatric outcomes in the offspring. *Neuropsychopharmacology* 2022; **47**:759–766.

50. Straub L, et al. Association of antipsychotic drug exposure in pregnancy with risk of neurodevelopmental disorders: a national birth cohort study. *JAMA Intern Med* 2022; **182**:522–533.

51. National Institute for Health and Care Excellence. Antenatal and postnatal mental health: clinical management and service guidance. Clinical Guidance [CG192]. 2014 (last updated February 2020, last accessed March 2024); https://www.nice.org.uk/guidance/cg192.

52. Centre of Perinatal Excellence (COPE). National Perinatal Mental Health Guideline. 2023; https://www.cope.org.au/health-professionals/review-of-new-perinatal-mental-health-guidelines/.

53. European Medicines Agency. Antipsychotics – risk of extrapyramidal effects and withdrawal symptoms in newborns after exposure during pregnancy. Pharmacovigilance Working Party, July 2011 plenary meeting. Issue 1107. 2011; http://www.ema.europa.eu/docs/en_GB/document_library/Report/2011/07/WC500109581.pdf.

54. Cohen LS, et al. Relapse of major depression during pregnancy in women who maintain or discontinue antidepressant treatment. *JAMA* 2006; **295**:499–507.

55. Munk-Olsen T, et al. New parents and mental disorders: a population-based register study. *JAMA* 2006; **296**:2582–2589.

56. Mahon PB, et al. Genome-wide linkage and follow-up association study of postpartum mood symptoms. *Am J Psychiatry* 2009; **166**:1229–1237.

57. Smith S, et al. Association between antidepressant use during pregnancy and miscarriage: a systematic review and meta-analysis. *BMJ Open* 2024; **14**:e074600.

58. Engelstad HJ, et al. Perinatal outcomes of pregnancies complicated by maternal depression with or without selective serotonin reuptake inhibitor therapy. *Neonatology* 2014; **105**:149–154.

59. Yonkers KA, et al. The management of depression during pregnancy: a report from the American Psychiatric Association and the American College of Obstetricians and Gynecologists. *Gen Hosp Psychiatry* 2009; **31**:403–413.

60. Yonkers KA, et al. Does antidepressant use attenuate the risk of a major depressive episode in pregnancy? *Epidemiology* 2011; **22**:848–854.

61. Suarez EA, et al. Association of antidepressant use during pregnancy with risk of neurodevelopmental disorders in children. *JAMA Intern Med* 2022; **182**:1149–1160.

62. Grzeskowiak LE, et al. Antidepressant use in late gestation and risk of postpartum haemorrhage: a retrospective cohort study. *BJOG* 2016; **123**:1929–1936.

63. Loughhead AM, et al. Placental passage of tricyclic antidepressants. *Biol Psychiatry* 2006; **59**:287–290.

64. Loughhead AM, et al. Antidepressants in amniotic fluid: another route of fetal exposure. *Am J Psychiatry* 2006; **163**:145–147.

65. Davis RL, et al. Risks of congenital malformations and perinatal events among infants exposed to antidepressant medications during pregnancy. *Pharmacoepidemiol Drug Saf* 2007; **16**:1086–1094.

66. Kallen B. Neonate characteristics after maternal use of antidepressants in late pregnancy. *Arch Pediatr Adolesc Med* 2004; **158**:312–316.

67. Ban L, et al. Maternal depression, antidepressant prescriptions, and congenital anomaly risk in offspring: a population-based cohort study. *BJOG* 2014; **121**:1471–1481.

68. Gentile S. Tricyclic antidepressants in pregnancy and puerperium. *Expert Opin Drug Saf* 2014; **13**:207–225.

69. Fukushima N, et al. A neonatal prolonged QT syndrome due to maternal use of oral tricyclic antidepressants. *Eur J Pediatr* 2016; **175**:1129–1132.

70. Corona-Rivera JR, et al. Unusual retrospective prenatal findings in a male newborn with Timothy syndrome type 1. *Eur J Med Genet* 2015; **58**:332–335.

71. Maschi S, et al. Neonatal outcome following pregnancy exposure to antidepressants: a prospective controlled cohort study. *BJOG* 2008; **115**:283–289.

72. Nulman I, et al. Child development following exposure to tricyclic antidepressants or fluoxetine throughout fetal life: a prospective, controlled study. *Am J Psychiatry* 2002; **159**:1889–1895.

73. Nulman I, et al. Neurodevelopment of children exposed in utero to antidepressant drugs. *N Engl J Med* 1997; **336**:258–262.

74. Rommel AS, et al. Long-term prenatal effects of antidepressant use on the risk of affective disorders in the offspring: a register-based cohort study. *Neuropsychopharmacology* 2021; **46**:1518–1525.

75. Brennan PA, et al. Prenatal antidepressant exposures and autism spectrum disorder or traits: a retrospective, multi-cohort study. *Res Child Adolesc Psychopathol* 2023; **51**:513–527.

76. Ramos E, et al. Duration of antidepressant use during pregnancy and risk of major congenital malformations. *Br J Psychiatry* 2008; **192**:344–350.

77. Gentile S. Selective serotonin reuptake inhibitor exposure during early pregnancy and the risk of birth defects. *Acta Psychiatr Scand* 2011; **123**:266–275.

78. Lebin LG, et al. Selective serotonin reuptake inhibitors (SSRIs) in pregnancy: an updated review on risks to mother, fetus, and child. *Curr Psychiatry Rep* 2022; **24**:687–695.

79. Reefhuis J, et al. Specific SSRIs and birth defects: Bayesian analysis to interpret new data in the context of previous reports. *BMJ* 2015; **351**:h3190.

80. Alwan S, et al. Use of selective serotonin-reuptake inhibitors in pregnancy and the risk of birth defects. *N Engl J Med* 2007; **356**:2684–2692.

81. Margulis AV, et al. Use of selective serotonin reuptake inhibitors in pregnancy and cardiac malformations: a propensity-score matched cohort in CPRD. *Pharmacoepidemiol Drug Saf* 2013; **22**:942–951.

82. Riggin L, et al. The fetal safety of fluoxetine: a systematic review and meta-analysis. *J Obstet Gynaecol Can* 2013; **35**:362–369.

83. Anderson KN, et al. Maternal use of specific antidepressant medications during early pregnancy and the risk of selected birth defects. *JAMA Psychiatry* 2020; **77**:1246–1255.

84. Furu K, et al. Selective serotonin reuptake inhibitors and venlafaxine in early pregnancy and risk of birth defects: population based cohort study and sibling design. *BMJ* 2015; **350**:h1798.

85. Petersen I, et al. Selective serotonin reuptake inhibitors and congenital heart anomalies: comparative cohort studies of women treated before and during pregnancy and their children. *J Clin Psychiatry* 2016; **77**:e36–e42.

86. Wang S, et al. Selective serotonin reuptake inhibitors (SSRIs) and the risk of congenital heart defects: a meta-analysis of prospective cohort studies. *J Am Heart Assoc* 2015; **4**:e001681.

87. Ansah DA, et al. A prospective study evaluating the effects of SSRI exposure on cardiac size and function in newborns. *Neonatology* 2019; **115**:320–327.

88. Malm H, et al. Selective serotonin reuptake inhibitors and risk for major congenital anomalies. *Obstet Gynecol* 2011; **118**:111–120.

89. Hendrick V, et al. Placental passage of antidepressant medications. *Am J Psychiatry* 2003; **160**:993–996.

CHAPTER 7

90. Vlenterie R, et al. Associations between maternal depression, antidepressant use during pregnancy, and adverse pregnancy outcomes: an individual participant data meta-analysis. *Obstet Gynecol* 2021; **138**:633–646.

91. Desaunay P, et al. Benefits and risks of antidepressant drugs during pregnancy: a systematic review of meta-analyses. *Paediatr Drugs* 2023; **25**:247–265.

92. Yang A, et al. Neonatal discontinuation syndrome in serotonergic antidepressant-exposed neonates. *J Clin Psychiatry* 2017; **78**:605–611.

93. Cornet MC, et al. Maternal treatment with selective serotonin reuptake inhibitors during pregnancy and delayed neonatal adaptation: a population-based cohort study. *Arch Dis Child Fetal Neonatal Ed* 2024; **109**:294–300.

94. Huybrechts KF, et al. Antidepressant use late in pregnancy and risk of persistent pulmonary hypertension of the newborn. *JAMA* 2015; **313**:2142–2151.

95. Byatt N, et al. Exposure to selective serotonin reuptake inhibitors in late pregnancy increases the risk of persistent pulmonary hypertension of the newborn, but the absolute risk is low. *Evid Based Nurs* 2015; **18**:15–16.

96. Masarwa R, et al. Prenatal exposure to selective serotonin reuptake inhibitors and serotonin norepinephrine reuptake inhibitors and risk for persistent pulmonary hypertension of the newborn: a systematic review, meta-analysis, and network meta-analysis. *Am J Obstet Gynecol* 2019; **220**:57.e1–57.e13.

97. Gentile S. SSRIs in pregnancy and lactation: emphasis on neurodevelopmental outcome. *CNS Drugs* 2005; **19**:623–633.

98. Casper RC, et al. Follow-up of children of depressed mothers exposed or not exposed to antidepressant drugs during pregnancy. *J Pediatr* 2003; **142**:402–408.

99. Hermansen TK, et al. Prenatal SSRI exposure: effects on later child development. *Child Neuropsychol* 2015; **21**:543–569.

100. Kaplan YC, et al. Maternal SSRI discontinuation, use, psychiatric disorder and the risk of autism in children: a meta-analysis of cohort studies. *Br J Clin Pharmacol* 2017; **83**:2798–2806.

101. Ames JL, et al. Maternal psychiatric conditions, treatment with selective serotonin reuptake inhibitors, and neurodevelopmental disorders. *Biol Psychiatry* 2021; **90**:253–262.

102. Boukhris T, et al. Antidepressant use in pregnancy and the risk of attention deficit with or without hyperactivity disorder in children. *Paediatr Perinat Epidemiol* 2017; **31**:363–373.

103. Croen LA, et al. Antidepressant use during pregnancy and childhood autism spectrum disorders. *Arch Gen Psychiatry* 2011; **68**:1104–1112.

104. Healy D, et al. Links between serotonin reuptake inhibition during pregnancy and neurodevelopmental delay/spectrum disorders: a systematic review of epidemiological and physiological evidence. *Int J Risk Saf Med* 2016; **28**:125–141.

105. Brown HK, et al. Association between serotonergic antidepressant use during pregnancy and autism spectrum disorder in children. *JAMA* 2017; **317**:1544–1552.

106. Sujan AC, et al. Associations of maternal antidepressant use during the first trimester of pregnancy with preterm birth, small for gestational age, autism spectrum disorder, and attention-deficit/hyperactivity disorder in offspring. *JAMA* 2017; **317**:1553–1562.

107. Castro VM, et al. Absence of evidence for increase in risk for autism or attention-deficit hyperactivity disorder following antidepressant exposure during pregnancy: a replication study. *Transl Psychiatry* 2016; **6**:e708.

108. Clements CC, et al. Prenatal antidepressant exposure is associated with risk for attention-deficit hyperactivity disorder but not autism spectrum disorder in a large health system. *Mol Psychiatry* 2015; **20**:727–734.

109. Brown HK, et al. The association between antenatal exposure to selective serotonin reuptake inhibitors and autism: a systematic review and meta-analysis. *J Clin Psychiatry* 2017; **78**:e48–e58.

110. Van der Veere CN, et al. Intra-uterine exposure to selective serotonin reuptake inhibitors (SSRIs), maternal psychopathology, and neurodevelopment at age 2.5years – results from the prospective cohort SMOK study. *Early Hum Dev* 2020; **147**:105075.

111. Brown AS, et al. Association of selective serotonin reuptake inhibitor exposure during pregnancy with speech, scholastic, and motor disorders in offspring. *JAMA Psychiatry* 2016; **73**:1163–1170.

112. Skurtveit S, et al. Prenatal exposure to antidepressants and language competence at age three: results from a large population-based pregnancy cohort in Norway. *BJOG* 2014; **121**:1621–1631.

113. Handal M, et al. Prenatal exposure to folic acid and antidepressants and language development: a population-based cohort study. *J Clin Psychopharmacol* 2016; **36**:333–339.

114. Hanley GE, et al. Prenatal exposure to serotonin reuptake inhibitor antidepressants and childhood behavior. *Pediatr Res* 2015; **78**:174–180.

115. Johnson KC, et al. Preschool outcomes following prenatal serotonin reuptake inhibitor exposure: differences in language and behavior, but not cognitive function. *J Clin Psychiatry* 2016; **77**:e176–e182.

116. Partridge MC, et al. Fine motor differences and prenatal serotonin reuptake inhibitors exposure. *J Pediatr* 2016; **175**:144–149.e141.

117. Bliddal M, et al. Prenatal antidepressant exposure and emotional disorders until age 22: a Danish register study. *Child Adolesc Psychiatry Ment Health* 2023; **17**:73.

118. Koc D, et al. Prenatal antidepressant exposure and offspring brain morphologic trajectory. *JAMA Psychiatry* 2023; **80**:1208–1217.

119. Polen KN, et al. Association between reported venlafaxine use in early pregnancy and birth defects, national birth defects prevention study, 1997–2007. *Birth Defects Res A Clin Mol Teratol* 2013; **97**:28–35.

120. Lou ZQ, et al. Exposure to selective noradrenalin reuptake inhibitors during the first trimester of pregnancy and risk of congenital malformations: a meta-analysis of cohort studies. *Psychiatry Res* 2022; **316**:114756.

121. Richardson JL, et al. Pregnancy outcomes following maternal venlafaxine use: a prospective observational comparative cohort study. *Reprod Toxicol* 2019; **84**:108–113.

122. Gentile S. The safety of newer antidepressants in pregnancy and breastfeeding. *Drug Saf* 2005; **28**:137–152.

123. Ramos E, et al. Association between antidepressant use during pregnancy and infants born small for gestational age. *Can J Psychiatry* 2010; **55**:643–652.

124. Huybrechts KF, et al. Maternal and fetal outcomes following exposure to duloxetine in pregnancy: cohort study. *BMJ* 2020; **368**:m237.

125. Abdy NA, et al. Duloxetine withdrawal syndrome in a newborn. *Clin Pediatr (Phila)* 2013; **52**:976–977.

126. Hoog SL, et al. Duloxetine and pregnancy outcomes: safety surveillance findings. *Int J Med Sci* 2013; **10**:413–419.

127. Ankarfeldt MZ, et al. Exposure to duloxetine during pregnancy and risk of congenital malformations and stillbirth: a nationwide cohort study in Denmark and Sweden. *PLoS Med* 2021; **18**:e1003851.

128. Einarson A, et al. A multicentre prospective controlled study to determine the safety of trazodone and nefazodone use during pregnancy. *Can J Psychiatry* 2003; **48**:106–110.

129. Rohde A, et al. Mirtazapine (Remergil) for treatment resistant hyperemesis gravidarum: rescue of a twin pregnancy. *Arch Gynecol Obstet* 2003; **268**:219–221.

130. Dao K, et al. Reproductive safety of trazodone after maternal exposure in early pregnancy: a comparative ENTIS cohort study. *J Clin Psychopharmacol* 2023; **43**:12–19.

131. Djulus J, et al. Exposure to mirtazapine during pregnancy: a prospective, comparative study of birth outcomes. *J Clin Psychiatry* 2006; **67**:1280–1284.

132. Cole JA, et al. Bupropion in pregnancy and the prevalence of congenital malformations. *Pharmacoepidemiol Drug Saf* 2007; **16**:474–484.

133. Smit M, et al. Mirtazapine in pregnancy and lactation – a systematic review. *Eur Neuropsychopharmacol* 2016; **26**:126–135.

134. Ostenfeld A, et al. Mirtazapine exposure in pregnancy and fetal safety: a nationwide cohort study. *Acta Psychiatr Scand* 2022; **145**:557–567.

135. Louik C, et al. First-trimester exposure to bupropion and risk of cardiac malformations. *Pharmacoepidemiol Drug Saf* 2014; **23**:1066–1075.

136. Figueroa R. Use of antidepressants during pregnancy and risk of attention-deficit/hyperactivity disorder in the offspring. *J Dev Behav Pediatr* 2010; **31**:641–648.

137. Forsberg L, et al. School performance at age 16 in children exposed to antiepileptic drugs in utero – a population-based study. *Epilepsia* 2010; **52**:364–369.

138. Rybakowski JK. Moclobemide in pregnancy. *Pharmacopsychiatry* 2001; **34**:82–83.

139. Pharmacia Ltd. Erdronax: use on pregnancy, renally and hepatically impaired patients. Personal communication, 2003.

140. Hendrick V, et al. Management of major depression during pregnancy. *Am J Psychiatry* 2002; **159**:1667–1673.

141. Miller LJ. Use of electroconvulsive therapy during pregnancy. *Hosp Community Psychiatry* 1994; **45**:444–450.

142. National Institute for Care and Health Excellence. Intrapartum care. NICE Guideline [NG235]. 2023 (last checked March 2024); https://www.nice.org.uk/guidance/ng235/chapter/Recommendations#care-of-the-newborn-baby.

143. Taylor CL, et al. Predictors of severe relapse in pregnant women with psychotic or bipolar disorders. *J Psychiatr Res* 2018; **104**:100–107.

144. Newport DJ, et al. Lithium placental passage and obstetrical outcome: implications for clinical management during late pregnancy. *Am J Psychiatry* 2005; **162**:2162–2170.

145. Fornaro M, et al. Lithium exposure during pregnancy and the postpartum period: a systematic review and meta-analysis of safety and efficacy outcomes. *Am J Psychiatry* 2020; **177**:76–92.

146. Munk-Olsen T, et al. Maternal and infant outcomes associated with lithium use in pregnancy: an international collaborative meta-analysis of six cohort studies. *Lancet Psychiatry* 2018; **5**:644–652.

147. Dodd S, et al. The pharmacology of bipolar disorder during pregnancy and breastfeeding. *Exp Opin Drug Saf* 2004; **3**:221–229.

148. Viguera AC, et al. Risk of recurrence of bipolar disorder in pregnant and nonpregnant women after discontinuing lithium maintenance. *Am J Psychiatry* 2000; **157**:179–184.

149. Diav-Citrin O, et al. Pregnancy outcome following in utero exposure to lithium: a prospective, comparative, observational study. *Am J Psychiatry* 2014; **171**:785–794.

150. McKnight RF, et al. Lithium toxicity profile: a systematic review and meta-analysis. *Lancet* 2012; **379**:721–728.

151. Boyle B, et al. The changing epidemiology of Ebstein's anomaly and its relationship with maternal mental health conditions: a European registry-based study. *Cardiol Young* 2017; **27**:677–685.

152. Yonkers KA, et al. Lithium during pregnancy: drug effects and therapeutic implications. *CNS Drugs* 1998; **4**:269.

153. Blake LD, et al. Lithium toxicity and the parturient: case report and literature review. *Int J Obstet Anesth* 2008; **17**:164–169.

154. Hastie R, et al. Maternal lithium use and the risk of adverse pregnancy and neonatal outcomes: a Swedish population-based cohort study. *BMC Med* 2021; **19**:291.

155. Cohen JM, et al. Anticonvulsant mood stabilizer and lithium use and risk of adverse pregnancy outcomes. *J Clin Psychiatry* 2019; **80**:18m12572.

156. Schonewille NN, et al. Neonatal admission after lithium use in pregnant women with bipolar disorders: a retrospective cohort study. *Int J Bipolar Disord* 2023; **11**:24.

157. Torfs M, et al. Early postnatal outcome and care after in utero exposure to lithium: a single center analysis of a Belgian tertiary university hospital. *Int J Environ Res Public Health* 2022; **19**:10111.

158. Sagué-Vilavella M, et al. Obstetric outcomes regarding the use of lithium in pregnant women with bipolar disorders: a prospective cohort study. *Arch Womens Ment Health* 2022; **25**:729–737.

159. Poels EMP, et al. Brain development after intrauterine exposure to lithium: a magnetic resonance imaging study in school-age children. *Bipolar Disord* 2023; **25**:181–190.

160. James L, et al. Informing patients of the teratogenic potential of mood stabilising drugs: a case note review of the practice of psychiatrists. *J Psychopharmacol* 2007; **21**:815–819.

161. Wide K, et al. Major malformations in infants exposed to antiepileptic drugs in utero, with emphasis on carbamazepine and valproic acid: a nation-wide, population-based register study. *Acta Paediatr* 2004; **93**:174–176.

CHAPTER 7

162. Wyszynski DF, et al. Increased rate of major malformations in offspring exposed to valproate during pregnancy. *Neurology* 2005; **64**:961–965.

163. Weston J, et al. Monotherapy treatment of epilepsy in pregnancy: congenital malformation outcomes in the child. *Cochrane Database Syst Rev* 2016; **11**:CD010224.

164. Campbell E, et al. Malformation risks of antiepileptic drug monotherapies in pregnancy: updated results from the UK and Ireland Epilepsy and Pregnancy Registers. *J Neurol Neurosurg Psychiatry* 2014; **85**:1029–1034.

165. Bestwick JP, et al. Prevention of neural tube defects: a cross-sectional study of the uptake of folic acid supplementation in nearly half a million women. *PLoS One* 2014; **9**:e89354.

166. Jentink J, et al. Valproic acid monotherapy in pregnancy and major congenital malformations. *N Engl J Med* 2010; **362**:2185–2193.

167. Tomson T, et al. Teratogenic effects of antiepileptic drugs. *Lancet Neurol* 2012; **11**:803–813.

168. Bromley R, et al. Treatment for epilepsy in pregnancy: neurodevelopmental outcomes in the child. *Cochrane Database Syst Rev* 2014; **10**:CD010236.

169. Bromley RL, et al. Fetal antiepileptic drug exposure and cognitive outcomes. *Seizure* 2017; **44**:225–231.

170. Cohen MJ, et al. Fetal antiepileptic drug exposure and learning and memory functioning at 6 years of age: the NEAD prospective observational study. *Epilepsy Behav* 2019; **92**:154–164.

171. Elkjær LS, et al. Association between prenatal valproate exposure and performance on standardized language and mathematics tests in school-aged children. *JAMA Neurol* 2018; **75**:663–671.

172. Danielsson KC, et al. Hypertensive pregnancy complications in women with epilepsy and antiepileptic drugs: a population-based cohort study of first pregnancies in Norway. *BMJ Open* 2018; **8**:e020998.

173. Vajda FJ, et al. Critical relationship between sodium valproate dose and human teratogenicity: results of the Australian register of antiepileptic drugs in pregnancy. *J Clin Neurosci* 2004; **11**:854–858.

174. Vajda FJ, et al. Maternal valproate dosage and foetal malformations. *Acta Neurol Scand* 2005; **112**:137–143.

175. Tomson T, et al. Dose-dependent risk of malformations with antiepileptic drugs: an analysis of data from the EURAP epilepsy and pregnancy registry. *Lancet Neurol* 2011; **10**:609–617.

176. Molgaard-Nielsen D, et al. Newer-generation antiepileptic drugs and the risk of major birth defects. *JAMA* 2011; **305**:1996–2002.

177. Vajda FJE, et al. Antiepileptic drugs and foetal malformation: analysis of 20 years of data in a pregnancy register. *Seizure* 2019; **65**:6–11.

178. Tomson T, et al. Comparative risk of major congenital malformations with eight different antiepileptic drugs: a prospective cohort study of the EURAP registry. *Lancet Neurol* 2018; **17**:530–538.

179. De Haan GJ, et al. Gestation-induced changes in lamotrigine pharmacokinetics: a monotherapy study. *Neurology* 2004; **63**:571–573.

180. Karanam A, et al. Lamotrigine clearance increases by 5 weeks gestational age: relationship to estradiol concentrations and gestational age. *Ann Neurol* 2018; **84**:556–563.

181. Clark CT, et al. Lamotrigine dosing for pregnant patients with bipolar disorder. *Am J Psychiatry* 2013; **170**:1240–1247.

182. Huber-Mollema Y, et al. Neurocognition after prenatal levetiracetam, lamotrigine, carbamazepine or valproate exposure. *J Neurol* 2020; **267**:1724–1736.

183. Veroniki AA, et al. Comparative safety of antiepileptic drugs for neurological development in children exposed during pregnancy and breast feeding: a systematic review and network meta-analysis. *BMJ Open* 2017; **7**:e017248.

184. Knight R, et al. Neurodevelopmental outcomes in children exposed to newer antiseizure medications: a systematic review. *Epilepsia* 2021; **62**:1765–1779.

185. Christensen J, et al. Apgar-score in children prenatally exposed to antiepileptic drugs: a population-based cohort study. *BMJ Open* 2015; **5**:e007425.

186. Cohen JM, et al. Comparative safety of antiseizure medication monotherapy for major malformations. *Ann Neurol* 2023; **93**:551–562.

187. Bromley RL, et al. Cognition in school-age children exposed to levetiracetam, topiramate, or sodium valproate. *Neurology* 2016; **87**:1943–1953.

188. Hernandez-Diaz S, et al. Topiramate use early in pregnancy and the risk of oral clefts: a pregnancy cohort study. *Neurology* 2018; **90**:e342–e351.

189. Bjørk MH, et al. Association of prenatal exposure to antiseizure medication with risk of autism and intellectual disability. *JAMA Neurol* 2022; **79**:672–681.

190. European Medicines Agency. Topiramate. New measures to avoid topiramate exposure in pregnancy. 2023; https://www.ema.europa.eu/en/medicines/human/referrals/topiramate.

191. Athar F, et al. Adverse fetal and neonatal outcomes following in-utero exposure to oxcarbazepine: a systematic review and meta-analysis. *Br J Clin Pharmacol* 2022; **88**:3600–3609.

192. Richardson JL, et al. A critical appraisal of controlled studies investigating malformation risks following pregabalin use in early pregnancy. *Br J Clin Pharmacol* 2023; **89**:630–640.

193. Dudukina E, et al. Prenatal exposure to pregabalin, birth outcomes and neurodevelopment – a population-based cohort study in four Nordic countries. *Drug Saf* 2023; **46**:661–675.

194. Medicines and Healthcare products Regulatory Agency. Pregabalin and risks in pregnancy. 2022; https://www.gov.uk/government/publications/pregabalin-and-risks-in-pregnancy.

195. Medicines and Healthcare products Regulatory Agency. Valproate: review of safety data and expert advice on management of risks. 2023; https://www.gov.uk/government/publications/valproate-review-of-safety-data-and-expert-advice-on-management-of-risks.

196. Ross LE, et al. Anxiety disorders during pregnancy and the postpartum period: a systematic review. *J Clin Psychiatry* 2006; **67**:1285–1298.

197. Noh Y, et al. First-trimester exposure to benzodiazepines and risk of congenital malformations in offspring: a population-based cohort study in South Korea. *PLoS Med* 2022; **19**:e1003945.

198. Dolovich LR, et al. Benzodiazepine use in pregnancy and major malformations or oral cleft: meta-analysis of cohort and case-control studies. *BMJ* 1998; **317**:839–843.

199. Wikner BN, et al. Use of benzodiazepines and benzodiazepine receptor agonists during pregnancy: neonatal outcome and congenital malformations. *Pharmacoepidemiol Drug Saf* 2007; **16**:1203–1210.

200. Reis M, et al. Combined use of selective serotonin reuptake inhibitors and sedatives/hypnotics during pregnancy: risk of relatively severe congenital malformations or cardiac defects. A register study. *BMJ Open* 2013; **3**(2):e002166.

201. Tinker SC, et al. Use of benzodiazepine medications during pregnancy and potential risk for birth defects, National Birth Defects Prevention Study, 1997–2011. *Birth Defects Res* 2019; **111**:613–620.

202. Grigoriadis S, et al. Benzodiazepine use during pregnancy alone or in combination with an antidepressant and congenital malformations: systematic review and meta-analysis. *J Clin Psychiatry* 2019; **80**:18r12412.

203. Andrade C. Gestational exposure to benzodiazepines, 2: the risk of congenital malformations examined through the prism of compatibility intervals. *J Clin Psychiatry* 2019; **80**:19f13081.

204. Calderon-Margalit R, et al. Risk of preterm delivery and other adverse perinatal outcomes in relation to maternal use of psychotropic medications during pregnancy. *Am J Obstet Gynecol* 2009; **201**:579–578.

205. Okun ML, et al. A review of sleep-promoting medications used in pregnancy. *Am J Obstet Gynecol* 2015; **212**:428–441.

206. Yonkers KA, et al. Maternal antidepressant use and pregnancy outcomes. *JAMA* 2017; **318**:665–666.

207. Freeman MP, et al. Obstetrical and neonatal outcomes after benzodiazepine exposure during pregnancy: results from a prospective registry of women with psychiatric disorders. *Gen Hosp Psychiatry* 2018; **53**:73–79.

208. Sheehy O, et al. Association between incident exposure to benzodiazepines in early pregnancy and risk of spontaneous abortion. *JAMA Psychiatry* 2019; **76**:948–957.

209. McElhatton PR. The effects of benzodiazepine use during pregnancy and lactation. *Reprod Toxicol* 1994; **8**:461–475.

210. Meng LC, et al. Association between maternal benzodiazepine or Z-hypnotic use in early pregnancy and the risk of stillbirth, preterm birth, and small for gestational age: a nationwide, population-based cohort study in Taiwan. *Lancet Psychiatry* 2023; **10**:499–508.

211. Grigoriadis S, et al. Hypnotic benzodiazepine receptor agonist exposure during pregnancy and the risk of congenital malformations and other adverse pregnancy outcomes: a systematic review and meta-analysis. *Acta Psychiatr Scand* 2022; **146**:312–324.

212. Wikner BN, et al. Are hypnotic benzodiazepine receptor agonists teratogenic in humans? *J Clin Psychopharmacol* 2011; **31**:356–359.

213. Wang LH, et al. Increased risk of adverse pregnancy outcomes in women receiving zolpidem during pregnancy. *Clin Pharmacol Ther* 2010; **88**:369–374.

214. Chen VC, et al. Association of prenatal exposure to benzodiazepines with development of autism spectrum and attention-deficit/hyperactivity disorders. *JAMA Network Open* 2022; **5**:e2243282.

215. Sundbakk LM, et al. Association of prenatal exposure to benzodiazepines and Z-hypnotics with risk of attention-deficit/hyperactivity disorder in childhood. *JAMA Network Open* 2022; **5**:e2246889.

216. Chan AYL, et al. Maternal benzodiazepines and Z-drugs use during pregnancy and adverse birth and neurodevelopmental outcomes in offspring: a population-based cohort study. *Psychother Psychosom* 2023; **92**:113–123.

217. Pottegard A, et al. First-trimester exposure to methylphenidate: a population-based cohort study. *J Clin Psychiatry* 2014; **75**:e88–e93.

218. Ornoy A, et al. Neurotropic drugs in pregnancy and lactation from the point of view of the clinical teratologist. *Curr Neuropharmacol* 2021; **19**:1792–1793.

219. Huybrechts KF, et al. Association between methylphenidate and amphetamine use in pregnancy and risk of congenital malformations: a cohort study from the International Pregnancy Safety Study Consortium. *JAMA Psychiatry* 2018; **75**:167–175.

220. Gov.UK. Modafinil (Provigil): increased risk of congenital malformations if used during pregnancy. 2020; https://www.gov.uk/drug-safety-update/modafinil-provigil-increased-risk-of-congenital-malformations-if-used-during-pregnancy?utm_source=e-shot&utm_medium=email&utm_campaign=DSU_November2020split1.

221. Damkier P, et al. First-trimester pregnancy exposure to modafinil and risk of congenital malformations. *JAMA* 2020; **323**:374–376.

222. Bang Madsen K, et al. In utero exposure to ADHD medication and long-term offspring outcomes. *Mol Psychiatry* 2023; **28**:1739–1746.

223. Suarez EA, et al. Prescription stimulant use during pregnancy and risk of neurodevelopmental disorders in children. *JAMA Psychiatry* 2024; **81**:477–488.

Drug choice in breastfeeding

The long-term benefits of breastfeeding on a child's physical health and cognitive development are well known. Women are generally encouraged to breastfeed for at least 6 months. One factor that may influence a mother's decision to breastfeed is the safety of a drug taken while breastfeeding. With some notable exceptions, most psychotropic drugs should be continued in breastfeeding women because of the benefits of breastfeeding and the lack of evidence of harm for most drugs. However, current evidence suggests that for a few drugs the woman should be advised not to breastfeed if such medications are the best and only option for her care.

Data on the safety of psychotropic medication in breastfeeding are largely derived from small studies or case reports and case series. Reported infant and neonatal outcomes in most cases are limited to short-term acute adverse effects. Long-term safety cannot therefore be guaranteed for the psychotropics mentioned here. The information presented must be interpreted with caution with respect to the limits of the data from which it is derived and the need for such information to be regularly updated.

There are two distinct clinical scenarios. In the first, the mother will have been taking the psychotropic drug(s) during pregnancy and often up until birth. In these people, the same psychotropic(s) should be continued during breastfeeding to mitigate withdrawal symptoms in the neonate (but see exceptions later). In the second, the mother is newly prescribed a psychotropic after the child has been born but wishes to breastfeed. Decisions in this scenario are rather more complex and the reader is referred to the tables in this section.

Infant exposure

All psychotropics are excreted in breast milk to varying degrees. The most direct measure of infant exposure is, of course, infant plasma levels but these data are rarely available. Instead, many publications report only drug concentrations in breast milk and in maternal plasma. Maternal plasma levels of antipsychotics may be a useful estimate of infant exposure.[1] Breast milk drug concentrations can be used to estimate the daily infant dose (by assuming a milk intake of 150mL/kg/day). The infant weight-adjusted dose when expressed as a proportion of the maternal weight-adjusted dose is known as the relative infant dose (RID). The RID should be used as a guide only, as values are estimates and these estimates vary widely in the literature for individual drugs.

Drugs with an RID below 10% are usually regarded as safe in breastfeeding. Where measured, infant plasma levels below 10% of average maternal plasma levels have also been proposed as being safe in breastfeeding.[2]

General principles of prescribing psychotropics in breastfeeding

- The safety of individual drugs in breastfeeding should be taken into account when prescribing psychotropic medication for women considering pregnancy.
- Discussions about the safety of drugs in breastfeeding should be held as early as possible – ideally before conception or early in pregnancy. Decisions about the use of drugs in pregnancy should include the discussion about breastfeeding. Switching drugs at the end of pregnancy or in the days after birth is not advisable because of the high risk of relapse.

- Where a mother has taken a particular psychotropic during pregnancy and until delivery, continuation with the drug while breastfeeding will usually be appropriate (but see notable exceptions later), as this may minimise withdrawal symptoms in the infant.
- In each case the benefits of breastfeeding to the mother and infant must be weighed against the risk of drug exposure in the infant. Consider the infant's general health and gestational age at birth.[3]
- It is usually inappropriate to stop breastfeeding unless the currently prescribed drug is absolutely contraindicated in breastfeeding. As treatment of maternal mental illness is the priority, in such cases treatment should not be withheld but the mother should be advised to bottle feed with formula milk.
- When *initiating* a drug postpartum it is:
  - important to consider the mother's previous response to treatment
  - best to avoid a psychotropic with high reported infant plasma levels or a high RID
  - important to consider the half-lives of the drugs: drugs with a long half-life can accumulate in breast milk and the infant.
- Neonates and infants do not have the same capacity for drug clearance as adults. Premature infants and infants with renal, hepatic, cardiac or neurological impairment are at a greater risk from exposure to drugs.
- Infants should be monitored for any specific adverse effects of the drugs as well as for abnormalities in feeding patterns and growth and development.
- Infant plasma levels should be monitored if adverse effects are noted or toxicity is suspected.
- Women receiving sedating medication should be strongly advised to not breastfeed in bed as they may fall asleep and roll onto the baby, with a potential risk of hypoxia to the baby.
- Sedation may affect women's ability to interact with their children. Women receiving sedating drugs should be monitored for this effect.
- Wherever possible:
  - use the lowest effective dose
  - avoid polypharmacy
  - continue the regimen prescribed during pregnancy.

Table 7.1 outlines recommendations for treatment with psychotropics in breastfeeding.

Antidepressants in breastfeeding

Table 7.2 provides information on individual drugs in breastfeeding based on available published data in late 2023. Manufacturers' formal advice on drugs in breastfeeding is available in the formal product literature or European Public Assessment Report for individual drugs. Table 7.2 does not include this advice (which is often uninformative), but instead uses primary reference sources. It is worth repeating that it is usually advisable to continue the antidepressant prescribed during pregnancy. Switching drugs postpartum for the purpose of breastfeeding is usually not sensible. Table 7.2 should be used as a guide when initiating treatment postpartum. In each case previous response (and lack of response) to treatment must be considered.

CHAPTER 7

Table 7.1 Summary of recommendations.

It is usually advisable to continue whichever drug has been used during pregnancy. When initiating a drug postpartum, previous response and tolerability should be considered

Drug group	Recommended drugs
Antidepressants	When initiating an antidepressant postpartum, sertraline may be considered. Other drugs may be used. See Table 7.2.
Antipsychotics	**Women taking clozapine should be advised against breastfeeding and clozapine should be continued** When initiating an antipsychotic postpartum, olanzapine or quetiapine may be considered. Other drugs may be used. See Table 7.3.
Mood stabilisers	**Women taking lithium should be advised against breastfeeding and lithium should be continued** When initiating a mood stabiliser postpartum, a mood-stabilising antipsychotic such as olanzapine or quetiapine may be considered. Other drugs may be used. See Table 7.4.
Sedatives	Best avoided. Use a drug with a short half-life. See Table 7.5.

Antipsychotics in breastfeeding

Table 7.3 provides information on individual drugs in breastfeeding based on available published data in mid-2024. Manufacturers' formal advice on drugs in breastfeeding is available in the SPC or European Public Assessment Report for individual drugs. Table 7.3 does not include this advice (which is often uninformative), but instead uses primary reference sources. It is usually advisable to continue the antipsychotic prescribed during pregnancy. Switching drugs postpartum for the purpose of breastfeeding is usually not sensible. The exception to this is clozapine; clozapine should continue but breastfeeding should be avoided. Table 7.3 should be used as a guide when initiating treatment postpartum. In each case the previous response (and lack of response) to treatment must be considered.

Mood stabilisers in breastfeeding

Table 7.4 provides information on individual drugs in breastfeeding based on available published data in mid-2024. Manufacturers' formal advice on drugs in breastfeeding is available in the SPC or European Public Assessment Report for individual drugs. Table 7.4 does not include this advice (which is often uninformative), but instead uses primary reference sources. It is usually advisable to continue the mood stabiliser prescribed during pregnancy. Switching drugs postpartum for the purpose of breastfeeding is usually not sensible. The exception to this is lithium. Lithium should be continued but breastfeeding should not be permitted. Table 7.4 should be used as a guide when initiating treatment postpartum. In each case the previous response (and lack of response) to treatment must be considered.

Hypnotics in breastfeeding

Table 7.5 provides information on individual drugs in breastfeeding based on available published data in mid-2024. Manufacturers' formal advice on drugs in breastfeeding is available in the SPC or European Public Assessment Report for individual drugs. Table 7.5 does not include this advice (which is often uninformative), but instead uses primary reference sources.

Table 7.2 Antidepressants in breastfeeding.

Drug	Infant plasma concentrations	Relative infant dose (RID)	Reported acute adverse effects in infant	Reported developmental effects in infant
Agomelatine[4,5]	Not assessed	Not available	None reported but not studied	None reported but not studied
Brexanolone[6]	Not assessed	1–2%	None reported but not studied	None reported but not studied
Bupropion[5,7–14]	Undetectable or low	0.2–2%	Two reports of seizure-like activity in 6-month-olds. In one of the cases the infant experienced sleep disturbance, severe emesis and somnolence. The infant plasma levels were below the level required for quantification. The mother was also taking escitalopram.	None reported but not studied
Citalopram[2,5,12,15–24]	Undetectable to up to 10% of maternal plasma levels Higher than for fluvoxamine, sertraline, paroxetine and escitalopram, but lower than for fluoxetine	3.56–5.37%[5]	Sleep disturbance (which resolved on halving maternal dose), colic, decreased feeding, irritability and restlessness One case of irregular breathing, sleep disorder and hypo- and hypertonia; the Infant was exposed to citalopram in utero. Symptoms were attributed to withdrawal syndrome despite the mother continuing citalopram postpartum.	None reported In a study of 78 infants of mothers taking an SSRI or venlafaxine, no difference in weight was noted at 6 months compared with the 'normative' weight. In a study of 11 infants, normal neurodevelopment was observed up to 1 year. One of the children was unable to walk at 1 year, However, neurological status of the child was deemed normal 6 months later.
Duloxetine[5,12,25–28]	<1% of maternal plasma levels	<1%	Dizziness, nausea and fatigue	None reported but not assessed

(*Continued*)

Table 7.2 (Continued)

Drug	Infant plasma concentrations	Relative infant dose (RID)	Reported acute adverse effects in infant	Reported developmental effects in infant
Escitalopram[5,12,14,29–34]	Undetectable or low	3–8.3%	Necrotising enterocolitis in 5-day-old infant (necessitating intensive care admission and intravenous antibiotic treatment). Infant was exposed to escitalopram in utero. Symptoms were lethargy, decreased oral intake and blood in the stools. Seizure-like activity, sleep disturbance, severe emesis and somnolence in 6-month-old. Mother was also taking bupropion.	None reported but not studied
Fluoxetine[2,5,12,15,24,35–46]	Variable: can be >10% of maternal plasma levels. Highest reported levels of SSRIs	1.6–14.6%	Colic, excessive crying, decreased sleep, diarrhoea, vomiting, somnolence, decreased feeding, hypotonia, moaning, grunting and hyperactivity One case of seizure activity at 3 weeks, 4 months and then 5 months. Mother was also taking carbamazepine. One case of tachypnoea, jitteriness, irritability, fever and compensated metabolic acidosis. Infant plasma levels were in the adult therapeutic range. The authors diagnosed serotonin syndrome. Mother was taking fluoxetine 60mg.	Normal weight gain and neurological development have been reported for many infants. One retrospective study found lower growth curves compared with non-exposed infants. One case of a reduction in platelet serotonin
Fluvoxamine[5,12,15,47–54]	Undetectable to up to half the maternal plasma level	1–2%	Neonatal jaundice, severe diarrhoea, mild vomiting, decreased sleep and agitation	None reported In a study of 78 infants of mothers taking an SSRI or venlafaxine, no difference in weight was noted at 6 months compared with the 'normative' weight.
MAOIs[55,56]	No published data available at the time of writing	Isoniazid = 1.2–18%	None reported	None reported but not assessed

Drug	Infant serum level	Milk:plasma	Adverse effects in infant	Developmental/other outcomes
Mianserin[5,57]	Not assessed	Not assessed	None reported	None reported but not studied
Mirtazapine[5,12,58,59]	Undetectable or low. There was one case of higher mirtazapine plasma levels. Elimination rates may differ between individual infants	0.5–4.4%	In a study of 54 infants exposed to mirtazapine in utero, the incidence of poor neonatal adaptation syndrome was significantly diminished in those who were breastfed.	None reported. In a study of eight infants, weights for three were observed to be between the 10th to 25th percentiles; all three were noted to also have a low birth weight.
Moclobemide[5,60,61]	Low	3.4%	None reported	None reported but not studied
Paroxetine[2,5,12,15,24,39,47,62–71]	Undetectable or low	0.5–2.8%	Vomiting and irritability which were attributed to severe hyponatraemia. In a study of 72 infants, adverse effects were noted in nine infants. Insomnia, restlessness and constant crying were most commonly reported.	None reported. In a study of 78 infants of mothers taking an SSRI or venlafaxine, no difference in weight was noted at 6 months compared with the 'normative' weight. Breastfed infants of 27 women taking paroxetine reached the usual developmental milestones at 3, 6 and 12 months, similar to a control group.
Reboxetine[5,12,72]	Undetectable or low	1–3%	None reported	In a study of four infants, three reached normal milestones. The fourth had developmental problems thought not to be related to reboxetine.
Sertraline[5,12,24,39,66,73–81]	Undetectable or low. There was one report of an unusually high infant serum level (half maternal serum level). The infant was reported to be 'clinically thriving'	0.5–3%	Serotonergic overstimulation reported in preterm infant also exposed to sertraline in utero. Symptoms included hyperthermia, shivering, myoclonus, tremor, irritability, high-pitched crying, decreased suckling reflex and reactivity. Withdrawal symptoms (agitation, restlessness, insomnia and an enhanced startle reaction) developed in a breastfed neonate, after abrupt withdrawal of maternal sertraline. The neonate was exposed to sertraline in utero.	None reported. In a study of 78 infants of mothers taking an SSRI or venlafaxine, no difference in weight was noted at 6 months compared with the 'normative' weight.

(Continued)

Table 7.2 (Continued)

Drug	Infant plasma concentrations	Relative infant dose (RID)	Reported acute adverse effects in infant	Reported developmental effects in infant
Trazodone[5,82,83]	Not assessed	2.8%	None reported	None reported
Tricyclic antidepressants (TCAs)[5,15,84–92]	Undetectable or low	Nortriptyline Amitriptyline } 1–3% Clomipramine	Adverse effects have not been reported in infants exposed to nortriptyline, clomipramine, imipramine, dosulepin and desipramine through breast milk. Severe sedation and poor feeding reported with amitriptyline Poor suckling, muscle hypotonia, drowsiness and respiratory depression reported with doxepin	None reported A study of 15 children did not show a negative outcome in regard to cognitive development in breastfed children 3–5 years postpartum.
Venlafaxine[5,12,24,39,66,93–100]	Undetectable to up to 37% of maternal plasma levels	6–9% (>10% reported in one case)[101]	Lethargy, jitteriness, rapid breathing, poor suckling and dehydration in an infant also exposed in utero. Symptoms subsided over a week on breastfeeding. Authors suggested that breastfeeding may have helped manage infant withdrawal symptoms postpartum.	None reported In a study of 78 infants of mothers taking an SSRI or venlafaxine, no difference in weight was noted at 6 months compared with the 'normative' weight.
Vortioxetine	1.1 –1.7%[102]	1.1–1.8%	None reported	None reported but not studied

MAOI, monoamine oxidase inhibitor; SSRI, selective serotonin reuptake inhibitor.

Table 7.3 Antipsychotics in breastfeeding.

Drug	Infant plasma concentration	Estimated daily infant dose as proportion of maternal dose (RID)	Acute adverse effects in infant	Developmental effects in infant
Amisulpride[5,96,103-105]	10.5% of maternal plasma concentration*	4.7–10.7%	None reported	None reported
Aripiprazole[5,106-111] (may lead to reduced milk supply)[112,113]	4% of maternal plasma concentration*	0.9–8.3%	None reported	None reported
Asenapine	No published data available at the time of writing			
Brexpiprazole (may lead to reduced milk supply)[112]	No published data available at the time of writing			
Butyrophenones[5,15,39,84,104,114-117]	Not reported	Haloperidol = 0.2–12%	One case of hypersomnia, poor feeding and slowing in motor movements. Mother was also taking risperidone. The effects were noted when haloperidol dose was increased.	Delayed development was noted in three infants exposed to a combination of haloperidol and chlorpromazine in breast milk. Normal development has also been reported.
Cariprazine	No published data available at the time of writing			
Clozapine[5,15,39,84,115,118-121] **NB avoid**	6.5% of maternal plasma concentration*	1.4%	Sedation, agranulocytosis, decreased sucking reflex, irritability, seizures and cardiovascular instability	There is one report of delayed speech acquisition. The infant was also exposed to clozapine in utero.
Iloperidone	No published data available at the time of writing			
Lurasidone	No published data available at the time of writing			

(Continued)

Table 7.3 (Continued)

Drug	Infant plasma concentration	Estimated daily infant dose as proportion of maternal dose (RID)	Acute adverse effects in infant	Developmental effects in infant
Lumateperone	Published data not available			
Olanzapine[5,15,39,104,122–134]	Undetectable or low One case of plasma levels decreasing over 5 months. The authors proposed that an infant's capacity to metabolise olanzapine 'developed rapidly' around the age of 4 months	1.0–1.6%	Somnolence, drowsiness, irritability, tremor, insomnia, lethargy, poor suckling and shaking One case of jaundice and sedation. Infant was exposed in utero and had cardiomegaly.	One case of lower developmental age than chronological age. Mother was taking additional psychotropic medication. One case of speech delay and one of motor developmental delay Two cases of failure to gain weight Normal development has also been reported.
Paliperidone	No specific data available (see risperidone)			
Phenothiazines[5,15,84,114–116]	Variable	Chlorpromazine = 0.3%	Lethargy	Delayed development in three infants exposed to a combination of chlorpromazine and haloperidol
Pimavanserin	No published data available at the time of writing			
Quetiapine[5,97,131,135–144]	Undetectable	0.09–0.1%	Excessive sleep. Mother was also taking mirtazapine and a benzodiazepine.	In a small study of quetiapine augmentation of maternal antidepressant, there were two cases of mild developmental delays, thought not to be related to quetiapine.

Drug		RID	Infant adverse effects (breastfeeding)	
Risperidone[5,117,145-149]	Risperidone undetectable 9-hydoxyrisperidone low	Risperidone = 2.8–9.1% 9-hydoxyrisperidone = 3.46–4.7%	One case of hypersomnia, poor feeding and slowing in motor movements. Mother was also taking haloperidol. The effects were noted when haloperidol dose was increased.	None reported
Sertindole	No published data available at the time of writing			
Sulpiride[5,150-154]	Not reported	2.7–20.7%	None reported	None reported but not assessed
Thioxanthenes[5,15,116,155-157]	Not reported	Zuclopenthixol = 0.4–0.9% Flupentixol = 0.7–1.75%	None reported	None reported for flupentixol Not assessed for zuclopenthixol
Ziprasidone[5,23,116,158]	Not reported	0.07–1.2%	None reported	None reported

*A proportion of the drug detected may have been due to placental transfer following in utero exposure. RID, relative infant dose.

Table 7.4 Mood stabilisers in breastfeeding.

Drug	Infant plasma concentration	Estimated daily infant dose as proportion of maternal dose (RID)	Acute adverse effects in infant	Developmental effects in infant
Carbamazepine[5,15,159–169]	Generally low although one report of an infant plasma level within adult therapeutic range	1.1–7.3%	Adverse effects have not been reported for a number of infants. One case of cholestatic hepatitis, one of transient hepatic dysfunction with hyperbilirubinaemia and elevated GGT. Adverse effects in the first case resolved after discontinuation of breastfeeding and the second resolved despite continued feeding. One case of seizure-like activity, drowsiness, irritability and high-pitched crying. Mother was taking multiple agents. Poor suckling, poor feeding and two cases of hyperexcitability	None reported A prospective study of children of women with epilepsy found no adverse development at ages 6–36 months. The study assessed outcomes in children exposed to anticonvulsants in utero who were subsequently breastfed compared with those who were not. A study of 199 infants exposed to antiepileptic medications in utero and through breast milk failed to show a difference in IQ between breastfed and non-breastfed infants at the age of 3 years. A study of 181 children concluded that IQ was not adversely affected by anticonvulsant exposure through breast milk.
Lamotrigine[5,162,167,170–181]	Up to 48% of maternal plasma levels[182] In Australia, the Centre for Perinatal Excellence (COPE) recommends close monitoring of the infant and a specialist neonatologist consultation where possible[3]	9.2–18.3%	No adverse effects have been reported in a number of infants. Seven cases of thrombocytosis One case of a severe cyanotic episode (preceded by mild episodes of apnoea) requiring resuscitation. Neonatal serum concentration was in the upper therapeutic range. The infant was exposed in utero and the mother was taking a high dose (850mg/day). One case of normocytic normochromic anaemia and asymptomatic neutropenia.[183] Three cases of rash. In one case the rash was attributed to eczema, and to soy allergy in another. The third case resolved spontaneously.	No abnormalities reported A prospective study of children of women with epilepsy found that breastfeeding while taking an anticonvulsant was not associated with adverse development of infants at ages 6–36 months. The study assessed outcomes in children exposed to anticonvulsants in utero who were subsequently breastfed compared with those who were not. A study of 199 infants exposed to antiepileptic medications during breastfeeding failed to show a difference in IQ between breastfed and non-breastfed infants at the age of 3 years. The infants were exposed to antiepileptic medications in utero. A study of 181 children concluded that IQ was not adversely affected by anticonvulsant exposure in breast milk.

Drug	Level in milk	RID	Reported adverse effects	Comments
Lithium[184] **NB avoid**	Up to 57% of maternal plasma levels	12–30.1%	Early feeding problems, increased urea, raised creatinine and non-specific signs of toxicity One case of elevated TSH. In utero exposure. One case of cyanosis, lethargy, hypothermia, hypotonia and a heart murmur. In utero exposure No adverse effects have been reported in others.	None reported
Topiramate[185,186]	Undetectable to 20% of maternal plasma levels	3–35%	Diarrhoea	None reported but not assessed
Valproate[5,15,159–162,167,187,188]	<2% of maternal plasma levels	1.4–1.7%	Thrombocytopenia and anaemia which reversed on stopping breastfeeding. In utero exposure	A prospective study of children of women with epilepsy found that breastfeeding while taking an anticonvulsant was not associated with adverse development of infants at ages 6–36 months. The study assessed outcomes in children exposed to anticonvulsants in utero who were subsequently breastfed compared with those who were not. A study of 199 infants exposed to antiepileptic medications during breastfeeding failed to show a difference in IQ between breastfed and non-breastfed infants at the age of 3 years. The infants were exposed to antiepileptic medications in utero. A study of 181 children concluded that IQ was not adversely affected by anticonvulsant exposure through breast milk.

GGT, gamma-glutamyl transferase; RID, relative infant dose; TSH, thyroid-stimulating hormone.

Table 7.5 Hypnotics in breastfeeding.

Drug	Infant plasma concentration	Estimated daily infant dose as proportion of maternal dose (RID)	Acute adverse effects in infant	Developmental effects in infant
Benzodiazepines[5,15,39,189-196]	Clonazepam: undetectable to 10% of maternal plasma levels[197]	Clonazepam = 2.8% Diazepam = 0.88-7.1% Lorazepam = 2.6-2.9% Oxazepam = 0.28-1%	Sedation, lethargy, weight loss and mild jaundice One case of persistent apnoea with clonazepam Restlessness and mild drowsiness with alprazolam In a telephone survey of 124 women two reported CNS depression in their breastfeeding neonates. One of the children was exposed to benzodiazepines in utero. No adverse effects have been reported in others.	None reported but not studied
Promethazine	No published data available at the time of writing			
Zopiclone, zolpidem and zaleplon[5,198-200]	Zolpidem: undetectable[201] Zopiclone and zaleplon: not reported	Zaleplon = 1.5% Zopiclone = 1.5% Zolpidem = 0.02-0.18%	None reported	None reported but not studied

RID, relative infant dose.

Stimulants in breastfeeding

Table 7.6 provides information on individual drugs in breastfeeding based on available published data in mid-2024. Manufacturers' formal advice on drugs in breastfeeding is available in the SPC or European Public Assessment Report for individual drugs. Table 7.6 does not include this advice (which is often uninformative), but instead uses primary reference sources. It is usually advisable to continue the drug prescribed during pregnancy. Switching drugs postpartum for the purpose of breastfeeding is usually not sensible. Table 7.6 should be used as a guide when initiating treatment postpartum. In each case the previous response (and lack of response) to treatment must be considered.

Table 7.6 Stimulants in breastfeeding.

Drug	Infant plasma concentration	Estimated daily infant dose as proportion of maternal dose (RID)	Acute adverse effects in infant	Developmental effects in infant
Atomoxetine	No published data available at the time of writing			
Dexamfetamine[202]	Undetectable to 14% of maternal plasma level	2.4–10.6%	None reported	None reported but not assessed
Lisdexamfetamine	No published data available at the time of writing			
Methylphenidate[28,203–205]	Undetectable	0.16–0.7%	None reported	None reported
Modafinil[206,207]	Armodafinil = 1.5%[208] Modafinil not reported	Armodafinil = 4.85%[208] Modafinil = 5.3%	None reported	None reported but not assessed

RID, relative infant dose.

References

1. Schoretsanitis G, et al. Excretion of antipsychotics into the amniotic fluid, umbilical cord blood, and breast milk: a systematic critical review and combined analysis. *Ther Drug Monit* 2020; **42**:245–254.
2. Weissman AM, et al. Pooled analysis of antidepressant levels in lactating mothers, breast milk, and nursing infants. *Am J Psychiatry* 2004; **161**:1066–1078.
3. COPE (Centre of Perinatal Excellence). 2023 National Perinatal Mental Health Guideline. 2023; https://www.cope.org.au/health-professionals/review-of-new-perinatal-mental-health-guidelines/.
4. Schmidt FM, et al. Agomelatine in breast milk. *Int J Neuropsychopharmacol* 2013; **16**:497–499.
5. Hale TW, et al. *Medications and Mothers' Milk*, 20th edn. New York: Springer Publishing Company; 2023.
6. Hoffmann E, et al. Brexanolone injection administration to lactating women: breast milk allopregnanolone levels [30J]. *Obstet Gynecol* 2019; **133**:115S.
7. Briggs GG, et al. Excretion of bupropion in breast milk. *Ann Pharmacother* 1993; **27**:431–433.
8. Chaudron LH, et al. Bupropion and breastfeeding: a case of a possible infant seizure. *J Clin Psychiatry* 2004; **65**:881–882.
9. Nonacs RM, et al. Bupropion SR for the treatment of postpartum depression: a pilot study. *Int J Neuropsychopharmacol* 2005; **8**:445–449.
10. Haas JS, et al. Bupropion in breast milk: an exposure assessment for potential treatment to prevent post-partum tobacco use. *Tob Control* 2004; **13**:52–56.
11. Baab SW, et al. Serum bupropion levels in 2 breastfeeding mother-infant pairs. *J Clin Psychiatry* 2002; **63**:910–911.

12. Berle JO, et al. Antidepressant use during breastfeeding. *Curr Womens Health Rev* 2011; 7:28–34.

13. Davis MF, et al. Bupropion levels in breast milk for 4 mother-infant pairs: more answers to lingering questions. *J Clin Psychiatry* 2009; 70:297–298.

14. Neuman G, et al. Bupropion and escitalopram during lactation. *Ann Pharmacother* 2014; 48:928–931.

15. Burt VK, et al. The use of psychotropic medications during breast-feeding. *Am J Psychiatry* 2001; 158:1001–1009.

16. Lee A, et al. Frequency of infant adverse events that are associated with citalopram use during breast-feeding. *Am J Obstet Gynecol* 2004; 190:218–221.

17. Heikkinen T, et al. Citalopram in pregnancy and lactation. *Clin Pharmacol Ther* 2002; 72:184–191.

18. Jensen PN, et al. Citalopram and desmethylcitalopram concentrations in breast milk and in serum of mother and infant. *Ther Drug Monit* 1997; 19:236–239.

19. Spigset O, et al. Excretion of citalopram in breast milk. *Br J Clin Pharmacol* 1997; 44:295–298.

20. Rampono J, et al. Citalopram and demethylcitalopram in human milk; distribution, excretion and effects in breast fed infants. *Br J Clin Pharmacol* 2000; 50:263–268.

21. Schmidt K, et al. Citalopram and breast-feeding: serum concentration and side effects in the infant. *Biol Psychiatry* 2000; 47:164–165.

22. Franssen EJ, et al. Citalopram serum and milk levels in mother and infant during lactation. *Ther Drug Monit* 2006; 28:2–4.

23. Werremeyer A. Ziprasidone and citalopram use in pregnancy and lactation in a woman with psychotic depression. *Am J Psychiatry* 2009; 166:1298.

24. Hendrick V, et al. Weight gain in breastfed infants of mothers taking antidepressant medications. *J Clin Psychiatry* 2003; 64:410–412.

25. Boyce PM, et al. Duloxetine transfer across the placenta during pregnancy and into milk during lactation. *Arch Women's Ment Health* 2011; 14:169–172.

26. Briggs GG, et al. Use of duloxetine in pregnancy and lactation. *Ann Pharmacother* 2009; 43:1898–1902.

27. Lobo ED, et al. Pharmacokinetics of duloxetine in breast milk and plasma of healthy postpartum women. *Clin Pharmacokinet* 2008; 47:103–109.

28. Collin-Lévesque L, et al. Infant exposure to methylphenidate and duloxetine during lactation. *Breastfeed Med* 2018; 13:221–225.

29. Gentile S. Escitalopram late in pregnancy and while breast-feeding (Letter). *Ann Pharmacother* 2006; 40:1696–1697.

30. Castberg I, et al. Excretion of escitalopram in breast milk. *J Clin Psychopharmacol* 2006; 26:536–538.

31. Rampono J, et al. Transfer of escitalopram and its metabolite demethylescitalopram into breastmilk. *Br J Clin Pharmacol* 2006; 62:316–322.

32. Potts AL, et al. Necrotizing enterocolitis associated with in utero and breast milk exposure to the selective serotonin reuptake inhibitor, escitalopram. *J Perinatol* 2007; 27:120–122.

33. Ilett KF, et al. Estimation of infant dose and assessment of breastfeeding safety for escitalopram use in postnatal depression. *Ther Drug Monit* 2005; 27:248.

34. Bellantuono C, et al. The safety of escitalopram during pregnancy and breastfeeding: a comprehensive review. *Hum Psychopharmacol* 2012; 27:534–539.

35. Yoshida K, et al. Fluoxetine in breast-milk and developmental outcome of breast-fed infants. *Br J Psychiatry* 1998; 172:175–178.

36. Lester BM, et al. Possible association between fluoxetine hydrochloride and colic in an infant. *J Am Acad Child Adolesc Psychiatry* 1993; 32:1253–1255.

37. Hendrick V, et al. Fluoxetine and norfluoxetine concentrations in nursing infants and breast milk. *Biol Psychiatry* 2001; 50:775–782.

38. Hale TW, et al. Fluoxetine toxicity in a breastfed infant. *Clin Pediatr* 2001; 40:681–684.

39. Malone K, et al. Antidepressants, antipsychotics, benzodiazepines, and the breastfeeding dyad. *Perspect Psychiatr Care* 2004; 40:73–85.

40. Heikkinen T, et al. Pharmacokinetics of fluoxetine and norfluoxetine in pregnancy and lactation. *Clin Pharmacol Ther* 2003; 73:330–337.

41. Epperson CN, et al. Maternal fluoxetine treatment in the postpartum period: effects on platelet serotonin and plasma drug levels in breast-feeding mother-infant pairs. *Pediatrics* 2003; 112:e425.

42. Taddio A, et al. Excretion of fluoxetine and its metabolite, norfluoxetine, in human breast milk. *J Clin Pharmacol* 1996; 36:42–47.

43. Brent NB, et al. Fluoxetine and carbamazepine concentrations in a nursing mother/infant pair. *Clin Pediatr (Phila)* 1998; 37:41–44.

44. Kristensen JH, et al. Distribution and excretion of fluoxetine and norfluoxetine in human milk. *Br J Clin Pharmacol* 1999; 48:521–527.

45. Burch KJ, et al. Fluoxetine/norfluoxetine concentrations in human milk. *Pediatrics* 1992; 89:676–677.

46. Morris R, et al. Serotonin syndrome in a breast-fed neonate. *BMJ Case Rep* 2015; 2015:bcr2015209418.

47. Hendrick V, et al. Use of sertraline, paroxetine and fluvoxamine by nursing women. *Br J Psychiatry* 2001; 179:163–166.

48. Piontek CM, et al. Serum fluvoxamine levels in breastfed infants. *J Clin Psychiatry* 2001; 62:111–113.

49. Yoshida K, et al. Fluvoxamine in breast-milk and infant development. *Br J Clin Pharmacol* 1997; 44:210–211.

50. Hagg S, et al. Excretion of fluvoxamine into breast milk. *Br J Clin Pharmacol* 2000; 49:286–288.

51. Arnold LM, et al. Fluvoxamine concentrations in breast milk and in maternal and infant sera. *J Clin Psychopharmacol* 2000; 20:491–492.

52. Kristensen JH, et al. The amount of fluvoxamine in milk is unlikely to be a cause of adverse effects in breastfed infants. *J Hum Lact* 2002; 18:139–143.

53. Wright S, et al. Excretion of fluvoxamine in breast milk. *Br J Clin Pharmacol* 1991; 31:209.

54. Uguz F. Gastrointestinal side effects in the baby of a breastfeeding woman treated with low-dose fluvoxamine. *J Hum Lact* 2015; 31:371–373.

55. Snider DE, Jr, et al. Should women taking antituberculosis drugs breast-feed? *Arch Intern Med* 1984; 144:589–590.

56. Singh N, et al. Transfer of isoniazid from circulation to breast milk in lactating women on chronic therapy for tuberculosis. *Br J Clin Pharmacol* 2008; 65:418–422.

57. Buist A, et al. Mianserin in breast milk (Letter). *Br J Clin Pharmacol* 1993; 36:133–134.

58. Smit M, et al. Mirtazapine in pregnancy and lactation: data from a case series. *J Clin Psychopharmacol* 2015; 35:163–167.
59. Smit M, et al. Mirtazapine in pregnancy and lactation – a systematic review. *Eur Neuropsychopharmacol* 2016; 26:126–135.
60. Buist A, et al. Plasma and human milk concentrations of moclobemide in nursing mothers. *Hum Psychopharmacol* 1998; 13:579–582.
61. Pons G, et al. Moclobemide excretion in human breast milk. *Br J Clin Pharmacol* 1990; 29:27–31.
62. Begg EJ, et al. Paroxetine in human milk. *Br J Clin Pharmacol* 1999; 48:142–147.
63. Stowe ZN, et al. Paroxetine in human breast milk and nursing infants. *Am J Psychiatry* 2000; 157:185–189.
64. Misri S, et al. Paroxetine levels in postpartum depressed women, breast milk, and infant serum. *J Clin Psychiatry* 2000; 61:828–832.
65. Ohman R, et al. Excretion of paroxetine into breast milk. *J Clin Psychiatry* 1999; 60:519–523.
66. Berle JO, et al. Breastfeeding during maternal antidepressant treatment with serotonin reuptake inhibitors: infant exposure, clinical symptoms, and cytochrome p450 genotypes. *J Clin Psychiatry* 2004; 65:1228–1234.
67. Merlob P, et al. Paroxetine during breast-feeding: infant weight gain and maternal adherence to counsel. *Eur J Pediatr* 2004; 163:135–139.
68. Abdul Aziz A, et al. Severe paroxetine induced hyponatremia in a breast fed infant. *J Bahrain Med Soc* 2004; 16:195–198.
69. Hendrick V, et al. Paroxetine use during breast-feeding. *J Clin Psychopharmacol* 2000; 20:587–589.
70. Spigset O, et al. Paroxetine level in breast milk. *J Clin Psychiatry* 1996; 57:39.
71. Uguz F, et al. Short-term safety of paroxetine and sertraline in breastfed infants: a retrospective cohort study from a university hospital. *Breastfeed Med* 2016; 11:487–489.
72. Hackett LP, et al. Transfer of reboxetine into breastmilk, its plasma concentrations and lack of adverse effects in the breastfed infant. *Eur J Clin Pharmacol* 2006; 62:633–638.
73. Llewellyn A, et al. Psychotropic medications in lactation. *J Clin Psychiatry* 1998; 59 Suppl 2:41–52.
74. Mammen OK, et al. Sertraline and norsertraline levels in three breastfed infants. *J Clin Psychiatry* 1997; 58:100–103.
75. Altshuler LL, et al. Breastfeeding and sertraline: a 24-hour analysis. *J Clin Psychiatry* 1995; 56:243–245.
76. Dodd S, et al. Sertraline analysis in the plasma of breast-fed infants. *Aust N Z J Psychiatry* 2001; 35:545–546.
77. Dodd S, et al. Sertraline in paired blood plasma and breast-milk samples from nursing mothers. *Hum Psychopharmacol* 2000; 15:161–264.
78. Epperson N, et al. Maternal sertraline treatment and serotonin transport in breast-feeding mother-infant pairs. *Am J Psychiatry* 2001; 158:1631–1637.
79. Stowe ZN, et al. The pharmacokinetics of sertraline excretion into human breast milk: determinants of infant serum concentrations. *J Clin Psychiatry* 2003; 64:73–80.
80. Muller MJ, et al. Serotonergic overstimulation in a preterm infant after sertraline intake via breastmilk. *Breastfeed Med* 2013; 8:327–329.
81. Wisner KL, et al. Serum sertraline and N-desmethylsertraline levels in breast-feeding mother-infant pairs. *Am J Psychiatry* 1998; 155:690–692.
82. Verbeeck RK, et al. Excretion of trazodone in breast milk. *Br J Clin Pharmacol* 1986; 22:367–370.
83. Saito J, et al. Trazodone levels in maternal serum, cord blood, breast milk, and neonatal serum. *Breastfeed Med* 2021; 16:922–925.
84. Yoshida K, et al. Psychotropic drugs in mothers' milk: a comprehensive review of assay methods, pharmacokinetics and of safety of breastfeeding. *J Psychopharmacol* 1999; 13:64–80.
85. Misri S, et al. Benefits and risks to mother and infant of drug treatment for postnatal depression. *Drug Saf* 2002; 25:903–911.
86. Yoshida K, et al. Investigation of pharmacokinetics and of possible adverse effects in infants exposed to tricyclic antidepressants in breastmilk. *J Affect Disord* 1997; 43:225–237.
87. Frey OR, et al. Adverse effects in a newborn infant breast-fed by a mother treated with doxepin. *Ann Pharmacother* 1999; 33:690–693.
88. Ilett KF, et al. The excretion of dothiepin and its primary metabolites in breast milk. *Br J Clin Pharmacol* 1992; 33:635–639.
89. Kemp J, et al. Excretion of doxepin and N-desmethyldoxepin in human milk. *Br J Clin Pharmacol* 1985; 20:497–499.
90. Buist A, et al. Effect of exposure to dothiepin and northiaden in breast milk on child development. *Br J Psychiatry* 1995; 167:370–373.
91. Khachman D, et al. Clomipramine in breast milk: a case study (article in French). *J Pharm Clin* 2007; 28:33–38.
92. Uguz F. Poor feeding and severe sedation in a newborn nursed by a mother on a low dose of amitriptyline. *Breastfeed Med* 2017; 12:67–68.
93. Koren G, et al. Can venlafaxine in breast milk attenuate the norepinephrine and serotonin reuptake neonatal withdrawal syndrome. *J Obstet Gynaecol Can* 2006; 28:299–302.
94. Ilett KF, et al. Distribution of venlafaxine and its O-desmethyl metabolite in human milk and their effects in breastfed infants. *Br J Clin Pharmacol* 2002; 53:17–22.
95. Newport DJ, et al. Venlafaxine in human breast milk and nursing infant plasma: determination of exposure. *J Clin Psychiatry* 2009; 70:1304–1310.
96. Ilett KF, et al. Assessment of infant dose through milk in a lactating woman taking amisulpride and desvenlafaxine for treatment-resistant depression. *Ther Drug Monit* 2010; 32:704–707.
97. Misri S, et al. Quetiapine augmentation in lactation: a series of case reports. *J Clin Psychopharmacol* 2006; 26:508–511.
98. Hendrick V, et al. Venlafaxine and breast-feeding. *Am J Psychiatry* 2001; 158:2089–2090.
99. Rampono J, et al. Estimation of desvenlafaxine transfer into milk and infant exposure during its use in lactating women with postnatal depression. *Arch Womens Ment Health* 2011; 14:49–53.
100. Ilett KF, et al. Distribution and excretion of venlafaxine and O-desmethylvenlafaxine in human milk. *Br J Clin Pharmacol* 1998; 45:459–462.
101. Baldelli S, et al. Passage of venlafaxine in human milk during 12 months of lactation: a case report. *Ther Drug Monit* 2022; 44:707–708.

102. Marshall K, et al. Transfer of the serotonin modulator vortioxetine into human milk: a case series. *Breastfeed Med* 2021; **16**:843–845.

103. Teoh S, et al. Estimation of rac-amisulpride transfer into milk and of infant dose via milk during its use in a lactating woman with bipolar disorder and schizophrenia. *Breastfeed Med* 2010; **6**:85–88.

104. Uguz F. Breastfed infants exposed to combined antipsychotics: two case reports. *Am J Ther* 2016; **23**:e1962–e1964.

105. O'Halloran SJ, et al. A liquid chromatography-tandem mass spectrometry method for quantifying amisulpride in human plasma and breast milk, applied to measuring drug transfer to a fully breast-fed neonate. *Ther Drug Monit* 2016; **38**:493–498.

106. Schlotterbeck P, et al. Aripiprazole in human milk. *Int J Neuropsychopharmacol* 2007; **10**:433.

107. Lutz UC, et al. Aripiprazole in pregnancy and lactation: a case report. *J Clin Psychopharmacol* 2010; **30**:204–205.

108. Watanabe N, et al. Perinatal use of aripiprazole: a case report. *J Clin Psychopharmacol* 2011; **31**:377–379.

109. Mendhekar DN, et al. Aripiprazole use in a pregnant schizoaffective woman. *Bipolar Disord* 2006; **8**:299–300.

110. Nordeng H, et al. Transfer of aripiprazole to breast milk: a case report. *J Clin Psychopharmacol* 2014; **34**:272–275.

111. Frew JR. Psychopharmacology of bipolar I disorder during lactation: a case report of the use of lithium and aripiprazole in a nursing mother. *Arch Womens Ment Health* 2015; **18**:135–136.

112. Naughton S, et al. Aripiprazole, brexpiprazole, and cariprazine can affect milk supply: advice to breastfeeding mothers. *Australas Psychiatry* 2023; **31**:201–204.

113. Sahoo MK, et al. Safety profile of aripiprazole during pregnancy and lactation: report of 2 cases. *Turk Psikiyatri derg* = Turkish journal of psychiatry 2023; **34**:133–135.

114. Yoshida K, et al. Breast-feeding and psychotropic drugs. *Int Rev Psychiatry* 1996; **8**:117–124.

115. Patton SW, et al. Antipsychotic medication during pregnancy and lactation in women with schizophrenia: evaluating the risk. *Can J Psychiatry* 2002; **47**:959–965.

116. Klinger G, et al. Antipsychotic drugs and breastfeeding. *Pediatr Endocrinol Rev* 2013; **10**:308–317.

117. Uguz F. Adverse events in a breastfed infant exposed to risperidone and haloperidol. *Breastfeed Med* 2019; **14**:683–684.

118. Mendhekar DN. Possible delayed speech acquisition with clozapine therapy during pregnancy and lactation. *J Neuropsychiatry Clin Neurosci* 2007; **19**:196–197.

119. Barnas C, et al. Clozapine concentrations in maternal and fetal plasma, amniotic fluid, and breast milk. *Am J Psychiatry* 1994; **151**:945.

120. Shao P, et al. Effects of clozapine and other atypical antipsychotics on infants development who were exposed to as fetus: a post-hoc analysis. *PLoS One* 2015; **10**:e0123373.

121. Imaz ML, et al. Clozapine use during pregnancy and lactation: a case-series report. *Front Pharmacol* 2018; **9**:264.

122. Goldstein DJ, et al. Olanzapine-exposed pregnancies and lactation: early experience. *J Clin Psychopharmacol* 2000; **20**:399–403.

123. Croke S, et al. Olanzapine excretion in human breast milk: estimation of infant exposure. *Int J Neuropsychopharmacol* 2002; **5**:243–247.

124. Gardiner SJ, et al. Transfer of olanzapine into breast milk, calculation of infant drug dose, and effect on breast-fed infants. *Am J Psychiatry* 2003; **160**:1428–1431.

125. Ambresin G, et al. Olanzapine excretion into breast milk: a case report. *J Clin Psychopharmacol* 2004; **24**:93–95.

126. Lutz UC, et al. Olanzapine treatment during breast feeding: a case report. *Ther Drug Monit* 2008; **30**:399–401.

127. Whitworth A, et al. Olanzapine and breast-feeding: changes of plasma concentrations of olanzapine in a breast-fed infant over a period of 5 months. *J Psychopharmacol* 2010; **24**:121–123.

128. Eli Lilly and Company Ltd. Personal correspondence: olanzapine use in pregnant or nursing women. 2011.

129. Gilad O, et al. Outcome of infants exposed to olanzapine during breastfeeding. *Breastfeed Med* 2010; **6**:55–58.

130. Goldstein DJ, et al. Olanzapine use during breast-feeding. *Schizophr Res* 2002; 53 Suppl 1:185.

131. Aydin B, et al. Olanzapine and quetiapine use during breastfeeding: excretion into breast milk and safe breastfeeding strategy. *J Clin Psychopharmacol* 2015; **35**:206–208.

132. Stiegler A, et al. Olanzapine treatment during pregnancy and breastfeeding: a chance for women with psychotic illness? *Psychopharmacology (Berl)* 2014; **231**:3067–3069.

133. Var L, et al. Management of postpartum manic episode without cessation of breastfeeding: a longitudinal follow up of drug excretion into breast milk. *Eur Neuropsychopharmacol* 2013; 23 Suppl 1:S382.

134. Manouilenko I, et al. Long-acting olanzapine injection during pregnancy and breastfeeding: a case report. *Arch Womens Ment Health* 2018; **21**:587–589.

135. Lee A, et al. Excretion of quetiapine in breast milk. *Am J Psychiatry* 2004; **161**:1715–1716.

136. Gentile S. Quetiapine-fluvoxamine combination during pregnancy and while breastfeeding (Letter). *Arch Womens Ment Health* 2006; **9**:158–159.

137. Seppala J. Quetiapine (Seroquel) is effective and well tolerated in the treatment of psychotic depression during breast feeding. *Eur Neuropsychopharmacol* 2004; 7 Suppl 1:S245.

138. Kruninger U, et al. Pregnancy and lactation under treatment with quetiapine. *Psychiatr Prax* 2007; 34 Suppl 1:S75–S76.

139. Ritz S. Quetiapine monotherapy in post-partum onset bipolar disorder with a mixed affective state. *Eur Neuropsychopharmacol* 2005; 15 Suppl 3:S407.

140. Rampono J, et al. Quetiapine and breast feeding. *Ann Pharmacother* 2007; **41**:711–714.

141. Tanoshima R, et al. Quetiapine in human breast milk – population PK analysis of milk levels and simulated infant exposure. *J Popul Ther Clin Pharmacol* 2012; **19**:e259–e298.

142. Yazdani-Brojeni P, et al. Quetiapine in human milk and simulation-based assessment of infant exposure. *Clin Pharmacol Ther* 2010; 87 Suppl 1:S3–S4.

143. Var L, et al. Management of postpartum manic episode without cessation of breastfeeding: a longitudinal follow up of drug excretion into breast milk. *Eur Neuropsychopharmacol* 2013; 23 Suppl 2:S382.

CHAPTER 7

144. Van Boekholt AA, et al. Quetiapine concentrations during exclusive breastfeeding and maternal quetiapine use. *Ann Pharmacother* 2015; **49**:743–744.

145. Hill RC, et al. Risperidone distribution and excretion into human milk: case report and estimated infant exposure during breast-feeding. *J Clin Psychopharmacol* 2000; **20**:285–286.

146. Aichhorn W, et al. Risperidone and breast-feeding. *J Psychopharmacol* 2005; **19**:211–213.

147. Ilett KF, et al. Transfer of risperidone and 9-hydroxyrisperidone into human milk. *Ann Pharmacother* 2004; **38**:273–276.

148. Ratnayake T, et al. No complications with risperidone treatment before and throughout pregnancy and during the nursing period. *J Clin Psychiatry* 2002; **63**:76–77.

149. Weggelaar NM, et al. A case report of risperidone distribution and excretion into human milk: how to give good advice if you have not enough data available. *J Clin Psychopharmacol* 2011; **31**:129–131.

150. Ylikorkala O, et al. Treatment of inadequate lactation with oral sulpiride and buccal oxytocin. *Obstet Gynecol* 1984; **63**:57–60.

151. Ylikorkala O, et al. Sulpiride improves inadequate lactation. *BMJ* 1982; **285**:249–251.

152. Aono T, et al. Augmentation of puerperal lactation by oral administration of sulpiride. *J Clin Endocrinol Metab* 1970; **48**:478–482.

153. Polatti F. Sulpiride isomers and milk secretion in puerperium. *Clin Exp Obstet Gynecol* 1982; **9**:144–147.

154. Aono T, et al. Effect of sulpiride on poor puerperal lactation. *Am J Obstet Gynecol* 1982; **143**:927–932.

155. Matheson I, et al. Milk concentrations of flupenthixol, nortriptyline and zuclopenthixol and between-breast differences in two patients. *Eur J Clin Pharmacol* 1988; **35**:217–220.

156. Kirk L, et al. Concentrations of Cis(Z)-flupentixol in maternal serum, amniotic fluid, umbilical cord serum, and milk. *Psychopharmacology (Berl)* 1980; **72**:107–108.

157. Aes-Jorgensen T, et al. Zuclopenthixol levels in serum and breast milk. *Psychopharmacology (Berl)* 1986; **90**:417–418.

158. Schlotterbeck P, et al. Low concentration of ziprasidone in human milk: a case report. *Int J Neuropsychopharmacol* 2009; **12**:437–438.

159. Chaudron LH, et al. Mood stabilizers during breastfeeding: a review. *J Clin Psychiatry* 2000; **61**:79–90.

160. Wisner KL, et al. Serum levels of valproate and carbamazepine in breastfeeding mother-infant pairs. *J Clin Psychopharmacol* 1998; **18**:167–169.

161. Ernst CL, et al. The reproductive safety profile of mood stabilizers, atypical antipsychotics, and broad-spectrum psychotropics. *J Clin Psychiatry* 2002; **63** Suppl 4:42–55.

162. Meador KJ, et al. Effects of breastfeeding in children of women taking antiepileptic drugs. *Neurology* 2010; **75**:1954–1960.

163. Zhao M, et al. [A case report of monitoring on carbamazepine in breast feeding woman]. *Beijing Da Xue Xue Bao* 2010; **42**:602–603.

164. Froescher W, et al. Carbamazepine levels in breast milk. *Ther Drug Monit* 1984; **6**:266–271.

165. Frey B, et al. Transient cholestatic hepatitis in a neonate associated with carbamazepine exposure during pregnancy and breast-feeding. *Eur J Pediatr* 1990; **150**:136–138.

166. Merlob P, et al. Transient hepatic dysfunction in an infant of an epileptic mother treated with carbamazepine during pregnancy and breast-feeding. *Ann Pharmacother* 1992; **26**:1563–1565.

167. Veiby G, et al. Early child development and exposure to antiepileptic drugs prenatally and through breastfeeding: a prospective cohort study on children of women with epilepsy. *JAMA Neurol* 2013; **70**:1367–1374.

168. Pynnonen S, et al. Carbamazepine and mother's milk (Letter). *Lancet* 1975; **2**:563.

169. Meador KJ, et al. Breastfeeding in children of women taking antiepileptic drugs: cognitive outcomes at age 6 years. *JAMA Pediatr* 2014; **168**:729–736.

170. Ohman I, et al. Lamotrigine in pregnancy: pharmacokinetics during delivery, in the neonate, and during lactation. *Epilepsia* 2000; **41**:709–713.

171. Liporace J, et al. Concerns regarding lamotrigine and breast-feeding. *Epilepsy Behav* 2004; **5**:102–105.

172. Gentile S. Lamotrigine in pregnancy and lactation (Letter). *Arch Womens Ment Health* 2005; **8**:57–58.

173. Page-Sharp M, et al. Transfer of lamotrigine into breast milk (Letter). *Ann Pharmacother* 2006; **40**:1470–1471.

174. Rambeck B, et al. Concentrations of lamotrigine in a mother on lamotrigine treatment and her newborn child. *Eur J Clin Pharmacol* 1997; **51**:481–484.

175. Tomson T, et al. Lamotrigine in pregnancy and lactation: a case report. *Epilepsia* 1997; **38**:1039–1041.

176. Newport DJ, et al. Lamotrigine in breast milk and nursing infants: determination of exposure. *Pediatrics* 2008; **122**:e223–e231.

177. Fotopoulou C, et al. Prospectively assessed changes in lamotrigine-concentration in women with epilepsy during pregnancy, lactation and the neonatal period. *Epilepsy Res* 2009; **85**:60–64.

178. Nordmo E, et al. Severe apnea in an infant exposed to lamotrigine in breast milk. *Ann Pharmacother* 2009; **43**:1893–1897.

179. Wakil L, et al. Neonatal outcomes with the use of lamotrigine for bipolar disorder in pregnancy and breastfeeding: a case series and review of the literature. *Psychopharmacol Bull* 2009; **42**:91–98.

180. Birnbaum AK, et al. Antiepileptic drug exposure in infants of breastfeeding mothers with epilepsy. *JAMA Neurol* 2020; **77**:441–450.

181. Kacirova I, et al. A short communication: lamotrigine levels in milk, mothers, and breastfed infants during the first postnatal month. *Ther Drug Monit* 2019; **41**:401–404.

182. Kacirova I, et al. Monitoring of lamotrigine concentrations in mothers, colostrum, and breastfed newborns during the early postpartum period. *Biomed Pharmacother* 2022; **151**:113167.

183. Bedussi F, et al. Normocytic normochromic anaemia and asymptomatic neutropenia in a 40-day-old infant breastfed by an epileptic mother treated with lamotrigine: infant's adverse drug reaction. *J Paediatr Child Health* 2018; **54**:104–105.

184. Newmark RL, et al. Risk-benefit assessment of infant exposure to lithium through breast milk: a systematic review of the literature. *Int Rev Psychiatry* 2019; **31**:295–304.

185. Westergren T, et al. Probable topiramate-induced diarrhea in a 2-month-old breast-fed child – a case report. *Epilepsy Behav Case Rep* 2014; 2:22–23.

186. Gentile S. Topiramate in pregnancy and breastfeeding. *Clin Drug Investig* 2009; 29:139–141.

187. Piontek CM, et al. Serum valproate levels in 6 breastfeeding mother-infant pairs. *J Clin Psychiatry* 2000; 61:170–172.

188. Bjornsson E. Hepatotoxicity associated with antiepileptic drugs. *Acta Neurol Scand* 2008; 118:281–290.

189. Spigset O, et al. Excretion of psychotropic drugs into breast milk: pharmacokinetic overview and therapeutic implications. *CNS Drugs* 1998; 9:111–134.

190. Hagg S, et al. Anticonvulsant use during lactation. *Drug Saf* 2000; 22:425–440.

191. Iqbal MM, et al. Effects of commonly used benzodiazepines on the fetus, the neonate, and the nursing infant. *Psychiatr Serv* 2002; 53:39–49.

192. Buist A, et al. Breastfeeding and the use of psychotropic medication: a review. *J Affect Disord* 1990; 19:197–206.

193. Fisher JB, et al. Neonatal apnea associated with maternal clonazepam therapy: a case report. *Obstet Gynecol* 1985; 66:34S–35S.

194. Davanzo R, et al. Benzodiazepine e allattamento materno. *Med Bambino* 2008; 27:109–114.

195. Kelly LE, et al. Neonatal benzodiazepines exposure during breastfeeding. *J Pediatr* 2012; 161:448–451.

196. Birnbaum CS, et al. Serum concentrations of antidepressants and benzodiazepines in nursing infants: a case series. *Pediatrics* 1999; 104:e11.

197. Tomson T, et al. Breastfeeding while on treatment with antiseizure medications: a systematic review from the ILAE Women Task Force. *Epileptic Disord* 2022; 24:1020–1032.

198. Darwish M, et al. Rapid disappearance of zaleplon from breast milk after oral administration to lactating women. *J Clin Pharmacol* 1999; 39:670–674.

199. Pons G, et al. Excretion of psychoactive drugs into breast milk. Pharmacokinetic principles and recommendations. *Clin Pharmacokinet* 1994; 27:270–289.

200. Matheson I, et al. The excretion of zopiclone into breast milk. *Br J Clin Pharmacol* 1990; 30:267–271.

201. Saito J, et al. Presence of hypnotics in the cord blood and breast milk, with no adverse effects in the infant: a case report. *Breastfeed Med* 2022; 17:349–352.

202. Ilett KF, et al. Transfer of dexamphetamine into breast milk during treatment for attention deficit hyperactivity disorder. *Br J Clin Pharmacol* 2007; 63:371–375.

203. Hackett LP, et al. Methylphenidate and breast-feeding. *Ann Pharmacother* 2006; 40:1890–1891.

204. Bolea-Alamanac BM, et al. Methylphenidate use in pregnancy and lactation: a systematic review of evidence. *Br J Clin Pharmacol* 2014; 77:96–101.

205. Marchese M, et al. Is it safe to breastfeed while taking methylphenidate? *Can Fam Physician* 2015; 61:765–766.

206. Aurora S, et al. Evaluating transfer of modafinil into human milk during lactation: a case report. *J Clin Sleep Med* 2018; 14:2087–2089.

207. Calvo-Ferrandiz E, et al. Narcolepsy with cataplexy and pregnancy: a case-control study. *J Sleep Res* 2018; 27:268–272.

208. Leggett C, et al. Infant exposure to armodafinil through human milk following maternal use of modafinil. *J Hum Lact* 2023; 39:218–222.

Prescribing in hepatic and renal impairment

Hepatic impairment

Patients with hepatic impairment may have the following:

- **Reduced capacity to metabolise** biological waste products, dietary proteins and foreign substances such as drugs. Clinical consequences include hepatic encephalopathy and increased dose-related adverse effects from drugs.
- **Reduced ability to synthesise** plasma proteins and vitamin K-dependent clotting factors. Clinical consequences include hypoalbuminaemia, leading in extreme cases to ascites. Increased toxicity from highly protein-bound drugs should be anticipated. There is also an increased risk of bleeding from gastrointestinal irritant drugs and with selective serotonin reuptake inhibitors (SSRIs).
- **Reduced hepatic blood flow.** Clinical consequences include oesophageal varices and elevated plasma levels of drugs that are subject to first-pass metabolism.

General principles of prescribing in hepatic impairment

Liver function tests (LFTs) are a poor marker of hepatic metabolising capacity. Many patients with chronic liver disease are asymptomatic or have fluctuating clinical symptoms. LFTs help evaluate hepatic damage but tell us little about hepatic function.

There are few clinical studies relating to the use of psychotropic drugs in people with hepatic disease. The following principles should be adhered to:

1. Prescribe as **few drugs** as possible.
2. Use **lower starting doses**, particularly of drugs that are highly protein bound. Tricyclic antidepressants (TCAs), SSRIs (except citalopram), trazodone and

The Maudsley® Prescribing Guidelines in Psychiatry, Fifteenth Edition. David M. Taylor, Thomas R. E. Barnes and Allan H. Young.
© 2025 David M. Taylor. Published 2025 by John Wiley & Sons Ltd.

antipsychotics may have increased free plasma levels, at least initially. This will not be reflected in measured (total) plasma levels. Use lower doses of drugs known to be subject to extensive first-pass metabolism. Examples include TCAs and haloperidol.

3. **Be cautious with drugs that are extensively hepatically metabolised** (most psychotropic drugs). Lower doses may be required. Exceptions are sulpiride, amisulpride, lithium and gabapentin, which all undergo no or minimal hepatic metabolism.

4. **Leave longer intervals between dosage increases.** The half-life of most drugs is prolonged in hepatic impairment and the duration of action is longer. Accumulation is more likely. Time to steady state is prolonged.

5. If albumin is reduced, consider the implications for drugs that are **highly protein bound,** and **if ascites is present, consider the increased volume of distribution for water-soluble drugs.**

6. **Avoid medicines with a very long half-life** or those that need to be metabolised to render them active (**pro-drugs**).

7. Always **monitor carefully for adverse effects,** which may be delayed.

8. **Avoid drugs that are very sedative** because of the risk of precipitating hepatic encephalopathy.

9. **Avoid drugs that are very constipating** because of the risk of precipitating hepatic encephalopathy.

10. **Avoid drugs that are known to be hepatotoxic** in their own right (e.g. monoamine oxidase inhibitors [MAOIs], chlorpromazine). Pre-existing liver disease does not increase the risk of drug-induced hepatotoxicity, but it may be more catastrophic if it does occur.

11. **Choose a low-risk drug** (see the tables in this section) and **monitor LFTs** weekly, at least initially. If LFTs deteriorate after a new drug is introduced, consider switching to another drug. Note that cross-hepatotoxicity between drugs is possible, especially if they are structurally related.[1]

These rules should always be observed in severe liver disease (low albumin, increased clotting time, ascites, jaundice, encephalopathy, etc.). The information here and following should be interpreted in the context of the patient's clinical presentation.

Antipsychotics in hepatic impairment[2]

One-third of patients who are prescribed antipsychotic medication have at least one abnormal LFT and in 4% at least one LFT is elevated three times above the upper limit of normal.[3] Transaminases are most often affected and this generally occurs within 1–6 weeks of treatment initiation.[3] Only rarely does clinically significant hepatic damage result.[3] Later in the treatment, the development of metabolic syndrome (obesity, insulin resistance) may be linked to the emergence of non-alcoholic fatty liver disease.[4,5]

Table 8.1 summarises antipsychotic medications used in hepatic impairment.

Table 8.1 Antipsychotics in hepatic impairment.

Drug	Comments
Amisulpride[6–8]	Predominantly renally excreted, so dosage reduction should not be necessary as long as renal function is normal. Uncommonly associated with rises in transaminases and rarely hepatocellular injury.[9]
Aripiprazole[6,7,10,11]	Extensively hepatically metabolised. Limited data that hepatic impairment has minimal effect on pharmacokinetics. Manufacturer states no dosage reduction required in mild to moderate hepatic impairment, but caution required in severe impairment. Small number of reports of hepatotoxicity, increased LFTs, hepatitis and jaundice.[3,9,12–14]
Asenapine[6,7,11]	Hepatically metabolised. Manufacturer advises to avoid use in severe hepatic disease (sevenfold increase in asenapine exposure). No dose adjustment required in mild to moderate disease,[15] but be aware of the possibility of increased plasma levels in patients with moderate impairment. Transient, asymptomatic rises in transaminases, AST and ALT are common, especially early in treatment. Single case report of mild cholestatic liver injury that resolved on stopping treatment.[16]
Brexpiprazole[7,17]	Little information. Use no more than 3mg/day (schizophrenia) or 2mg/day (depression or agitation in Alzheimer's disease) in moderate or severe hepatic failure. Long half-life (~90 hours).
Cariprazine[7,18]	Occasional, non-clinically relevant increases in ALT and AST. No dosage adjustment is required in patients with mild or moderate hepatic failure; not advised in severe hepatic disease (has not been evaluated). Long half-life (~2–4 days). Hepatitis has been reported.
Clozapine[1,6,7,19,20]	Very sedative and constipating. Contraindicated in active liver disease (associated with nausea, anorexia or jaundice), progressive liver disease or hepatic failure. In less severe disease, start with 12.5mg and increase slowly, using plasma levels to gauge metabolising capacity and guide dosage adjustment. More frequently associated with changes in liver enzymes than other antipsychotics. Transient elevations in AST, ALT and GGT to over twice the normal range occur in up to a third of people, resolving spontaneously in 6–12 weeks.[21] Clozapine-induced hepatitis, jaundice, cholestasis and liver failure have been reported. Clozapine should be discontinued if these develop. Successful rechallenge following hepatitis has been described.[22,23]
Flupentixol/ zuclopenthixol[6,7,24,25]	Both are extensively hepatically metabolised. Abnormal LFTs and (rarely) jaundice have been reported with flupentixol.[6] Small, transient elevations in transaminases, cholestatic hepatitis and jaundice[6] have been reported in some patients treated with zuclopenthixol. One report of flupentixol-induced hepatitis.[26] No other literature reports of use or harm.[27] Reduce doses by 50% in patients with compromised hepatic function. Depot preparations are best avoided, as altered pharmacokinetics will make dosage adjustment difficult and adverse effects from accumulation more likely.
Haloperidol[6]	Extensively hepatically metabolised. Halve initial doses, adjust dose with smaller increments and at longer intervals. Transient and asymptomatic elevations in LFTs reported in 20% of patients.[28] Isolated reports of cholestasis, acute hepatic failure, hepatitis and abnormal LFTs.[6,7]
Iloperidone[7,11,29]	Hepatically metabolised. Reduce dose in moderate impairment (twofold increase in active metabolites) and avoid completely in severe hepatic impairment (no studies done). No dose reduction necessary in mild impairment. Infrequent reports of cholelithiasis.
Lumateperone[30,31]	Hepatically metabolised to active metabolites. No dose adjustment required in mild impairment. Increased exposure to lumateperone in moderate and severe impairment; manufacturer recommends dose of 21mg daily. Increases in transaminases reported in licensing trials.

(Continued)

CHAPTER 8

Table 8.1 (*Continued*)

Drug	Comments
Lurasidone[6,7,11]	Hepatically metabolised. No dose adjustment is required in mild hepatic impairment. Manufacturer recommends a starting dose of 18.5mg (20mg) in moderate or severe hepatic impairment, and a maximum dose of 74mg (80mg)/day in moderate impairment (1.7-fold increase in exposure) and of 37mg (40mg)/day in severe impairment (threefold increase in exposure). Increases in ALT reported infrequently.
Olanzapine[1,6,7,11]	Although extensively hepatically metabolised, the pharmacokinetics of olanzapine seem to change little in severe hepatic impairment. It is sedative and anticholinergic (can cause constipation) so caution is advised. Start with 5mg/day in moderate or severe impairment and consider using plasma levels to guide dosage (aim for 20–40mcg/L). Dose-related, transient, asymptomatic elevations in ALT and AST are very common in physically healthy adults, particularly early in treatment. Along with clozapine, more often associated with drug-induced liver injury than other antipsychotics.[32,33]
Paliperidone[6,7,11]	Mainly excreted unchanged so no dosage adjustment required for mild to moderate impairment. May be a good choice for patients with pre-existing hepatic disease.[34–37] However, no data are available with respect to severe hepatic impairment, so caution required. Rises in transaminases and GGT reported, and some cases of jaundice and hepatic steatosis.[38] One case report of hepatotoxicity with risperidone that did not remit on switching to paliperidone – it is possible that paliperidone may cause hepatotoxicity.[39]
Phenothiazines[6,7,32]	All cause sedation and constipation. Transient abnormalities in LFTs reported. Associated with cholestasis and some reports of fulminant hepatic cirrhosis. Best avoided completely in hepatic impairment, some phenothiazines are actively contraindicated. Chlorpromazine is particularly hepatotoxic and is also associated with rare cases of immune-mediated obstructive jaundice which may progress to liver disease.
Pimavanserin[7]	Active metabolite has a very long half-life (200 hours) but hepatic impairment does not appear to affect plasma concentrations. Manufacturer advises that no dose adjustment is required. No reports of hepatotoxicity.
Quetiapine[6,7,11,40]	Extensively hepatically metabolised but short half-life. Clearance reduced by a mean of 30% in hepatic impairment so start at 25mg/day (IR preparation) or 50mg/day (XL preparation) and increase in 25–50mg/day increments. Can cause sedation and constipation. Transient rises in AST, ALT and GGT reported, as well as jaundice and hepatitis.[41] Severe hepatic toxicity probably more common with quetiapine (1.65% of patients) than other SGAs.[41] Several cases of fatal hepatic failure and of hepatocellular damage reported. A number of studies describe safe use in patients with alcohol dependence.[42–44]
Risperidone[1,6,7,11]	Extensively hepatically metabolised and highly protein bound. Those with severe impairment should start at 0.5mg bd and increase by 0.5mg bd at a maximum rate of weekly for doses above 1.5mg bd. Risperidone Consta can be started at 12.5mg, or 25mg every 2 weeks if 2mg daily oral dosing has been tolerated. Okedi should be started at 75mg, after confirming tolerability of 3mg oral risperidone. Perseris can be given at 90mg monthly if 3mg oral risperidone is tolerated, and Uzedy at 50mg monthly if 2mg oral is tolerated. Transient, asymptomatic elevations in LFTs, cholestatic hepatitis, jaundice and rare cases of hepatic failure have been reported. Cross-hepatotoxicity with paliperidone has been reported.[39] Steatohepatitis may arise as a result of weight gain.[45]
Sulpiride[6,7]	Almost completely renally excreted with a low potential to cause sedation or constipation. Dosage reduction should not be required. Rises in hepatic enzymes are common. Isolated case reports of cholestatic jaundice and primary biliary cirrhosis.

ALT, alanine aminotransferase; AST, aspartate aminotransferase; bd, twice a day; GGT, gamma-glutamyl transferase.

Antidepressants in hepatic impairment[2]

Of those treated with antidepressants, 0.5–3% develop asymptomatic mild elevation of hepatic transaminases.[46] Onset is normally between several days and 6 months of treatment initiation and the elderly are more vulnerable.[46] Frank, clinically significant liver damage however is rare and mostly idiosyncratic (unpredictable and not related to dose). Cross-toxicity within class has been described.[46]

Table 8.2 lists antidepressants commonly used in hepatic impairment.

Table 8.2 Antidepressants in hepatic impairment.

Drug	Comments
Agomelatine[6,7,46–48]	Liver injury including hepatic failure, liver enzyme increases more than 10 x ULN, and hepatitis reported, most commonly in first months of treatment. Contraindicated in hepatic impairment, including cirrhosis and active liver disease. Dose-related increase in transaminases reported; perform LFTs at baseline, 3, 6, 12 and 24 weeks during initiation and at each dose increase, and thereafter where clinically indicated. Stop treatment if transaminases rise more than 3 x ULN. Use cautiously where other risk factors for hepatic disease are present. Under current monitoring restrictions, risk of liver injury is no higher than for other antidepressants.[49,50] Almost all reactions are reversible on stopping agomelatine.[47]
Brexanolone[7,28]	No dose adjustment required in hepatic impairment. Does not appear to be hepatotoxic, although experience is limited.
Citalopram[7,51,52]	Hepatically metabolised and accumulates in chronic dosing. Dosage reduction required in renal impairment because of the extended half-life of citalopram in renal impairment which results in steady-state concentrations at a given dose to be about twice as high as those found in patients with normal renal function. Greater risk of QT interval prolongation because of higher drug exposure. Restrict the maximum daily dose to 20mg in hepatic impairment. Exercise caution due to the increased risk of bleeding seen with all SSRIs.
Duloxetine[6,7,53–57]	Hepatically metabolised. Clearance markedly reduced even in mild impairment. Reports of hepatocellular injury (liver enzyme increases more than 10 x ULN) and, less commonly, jaundice. Hepatic failure, sometimes fatal, has been reported. Contraindicated in hepatic impairment.
Escitalopram[7,58,59]	Hepatically metabolised and accumulates in chronic dosing. Longer half-life and 60% higher exposure in mild to moderate impairment. Initiate the dose at 5mg daily for the first 2 weeks, maximum dose 10mg daily. Careful dose titration in severe hepatic impairment. Be aware of increased risk of bleeding and QT prolongation.
Fluoxetine[6,7,60–64]	Extensively hepatically metabolised with a long half-life (further increased in hepatic insufficiency). Kinetic studies demonstrate accumulation in compensated cirrhosis. Dose reduction (of at least 50%) or alternate-day dosing is recommended. Attainment of steady state is delayed. Asymptomatic increases in LFTs found in 0.5% of healthy adults. Rare cases of hepatitis reported.
Fluvoxamine[7,28,65]	Hepatically metabolised and accumulates in chronic dosing. Dose adjustments are necessary in hepatic impairment. Low risk of hepatotoxicity. Raised LFTs rarely reported and do not require dose change or fluvoxamine discontinuation. Be mindful of increased risk of bleeding.
Levomilnacipran, milnacipran[7,28]	No dose adjustment required in hepatic impairment, although the manufacturers of milnacipran advise avoiding in chronic liver disease, alcohol use or severe hepatic dysfunction. Increased liver enzymes have been reported, and hepatitis with milnacipran. Discontinue use if jaundice or liver dysfunction occurs.

(Continued)

Table 8.2 (*Continued*)

Drug	Comments
MAOIs[6,7,66]	Rare cases of fatal hepatic necrosis, hepatotoxicity and jaundice with phenelzine. Rarely hepatitis is reported with tranylcypromine, and one isolated case of fatal hepatotoxicity with moclobemide. Doses of moclobemide should be reduced to half or one-third in hepatic impairment. Selegiline has not been associated with liver injury, although one study reported serum enzyme elevations in 41% of patients (other studies found no changes). Transdermal doses do not need to be adjusted in mild or moderate impairment (no data for severe impairment).[67] Selegiline orodispersible tablets should be started at 1.25mg/day in mild to moderate impairment and are contraindicated in severe disease. Non-selective MAOIs are contraindicated in patients with hepatic impairment.
Mirtazapine[6,7,68]	Hepatically metabolised and sedative. 50% dose reduction recommended based on kinetic data. Mild, asymptomatic increases in LFTs seen in healthy adults (ALT >3 times the upper limit of normal in 2%). Few cases of cholestatic and hepatocellular damage reported. Has been used safely in patients with primary biliary cholangitis.[69]
Paroxetine[70–72]	Hepatically metabolised and accumulates in chronic dosing. Dose adjustments are necessary in hepatic impairment. Raised LFTs and rare cases of hepatitis, with or without jaundice, including chronic active hepatitis, have been reported. Paroxetine has demonstrated mild to moderate antipruritic effects in cholestatic pruritus. Be aware of increased risk of bleeding.
Reboxetine[6,7,73]	50% reduction in starting dose advised. Does not seem to be associated with hepatotoxicity.
Sertraline[7,28,72,74]	Hepatically metabolised and accumulates in chronic dosing. Use a low or less frequent dose in mild hepatic impairment. Avoid in patients with moderate (Child–Pugh score 7–10) or severe hepatic impairment (Child–Pugh score 10–15). Rare instances of acute liver injury, with or without jaundice, have been described. Sertraline is used in the management of cholestatic pruritus. Be aware of increased risk of bleeding.
Tricyclics[6,7,75]	All are hepatically metabolised, highly protein bound and will accumulate. They vary in their propensity to cause sedation and constipation. All are associated with raised LFTs and rare cases of hepatitis. Sedative TCAs such as trimipramine, imipramine, dothiepin (dosulepin) and amitriptyline are best avoided.
Venlafaxine/ desvenlafaxine[6,7,76,77]	Dosage reduction of 50% advised in mild and moderate hepatic impairment. Rare cases of hepatitis reported.
Vilazodone[7]	No dose adjustment required in hepatic impairment. Does not appear to affect liver enzymes and no cases of hepatotoxicity, but data are limited, and all other SSRIs have been linked to liver toxicity.
Vortioxetine[6,78,79]	Extensively metabolised in the liver. Little experience in hepatic impairment, but pharmacokinetic studies suggest no dose reduction is required. Does not seem to be associated with hepatotoxicity, but experience is limited and all other SSRIs are implicated in rare instances of liver toxicity.

ALT, alanine aminotransferase; LFTs, liver function tests; MAOIs, monoamine oxidase inhibitors; TCAs, tricyclic antidepressants; ULN, upper limit of normal.

Mood stabilisers in hepatic impairment[6,7,80]

Recommendations for the use of mood-stabilising medications in hepatic impairment are summarised in Table 8.3.

Table 8.3 Mood stabilisers in hepatic impairment.

Drug	Comments
Carbamazepine[6,7,80]	Extensively hepatically metabolised and potent inducer of CYP450 enzymes (this can cause modest elevations in gamma-glutamyl transferase and alkaline phosphatase, which in themselves are not an indication for stopping[6]). In chronic stable disease, caution is advised. Associated with hepatitis, cholangitis, cholestatic and hepatocellular jaundice, and hepatic failure (rare). Adverse hepatic effects are most common in the first 2 months of treatment.[80] Hepatocellular damage is often associated with a poor outcome. Vulnerability to carbamazepine-induced hepatic damage may be genetically determined.[80] Avoid use in acute liver disease. In chronic liver disease reduce starting dose by 50%[7] and titrate up slowly, using plasma levels to guide dosage. Stop if liver function tests (LFTs) deteriorate.
Lamotrigine[28]	Manufacturers advise 50% reduction in initial dose, dose escalation and maintenance dose in moderate hepatic impairment and 75% reduction of these parameters in severe hepatic impairment. Discontinue if there is lamotrigine-induced rash (which can be serious). Elevated LFTs and hepatitis reported. Women, children and patients taking valproate appear to be at increased risk of lamotrigine-related hepatotoxicity.
Lithium[7]	Not metabolised so dosage reduction not required as long as renal function is normal. Use serum levels to guide dosage and monitor more frequently if ascites status changes (volume of distribution will change). Asymptomatic and transient LFT abnormalities reported in small proportion of patients on long-term therapy.[28] One case of ascites and one of hyperbilirubinaemia reported over many decades of lithium use worldwide.
Valproate[81]	Highly protein bound and hepatically metabolised. Reduce doses and closely monitor LFTs in hepatic impairment. Use plasma levels (measure free levels; total concentrations may appear to be normal) to guide dosage. Contraindicated in severe and/or active hepatic impairment or family history of severe impairment. Impairment of usual metabolic pathway can lead to generation of hepatotoxic metabolites via alternative pathway. Risk of liver toxicity is increased in people with hepatic insufficiency if salicylates are used concomitantly. Associated with elevated LFTs and serious hepatotoxicity including fulminant hepatic failure (sometimes fatal). Mitochondrial disease, learning disability, polypharmacy, metabolic disorders and underlying hepatic disease may be risk factors. Particularly hepatotoxic in very young children. The greatest risk is in the first 3 months of treatment.

Stimulants in hepatic impairment[6,7,82]

Recommendations for the use of stimulant medications in hepatic impairment are outlined in Table 8.4.

Table 8.4 Stimulants in hepatic impairment.

Drug	Comments
Atomoxetine[83]	Reduce initial and target dose by 50% in moderate impairment, and by 75% in severe impairment. Very rare reports of liver toxicity, manifested by elevated hepatic enzymes, and raised bilirubin with jaundice. Manufacturer states 'discontinue in patients with jaundice or laboratory evidence of liver injury, and do not restart'.
Dexamfetamine/ lisdexamfetamine[84,85]	Little experience in liver disease. Manufacturers recommend cautious dose titration. Very rarely associated with abnormal liver function, two case reports of hepatotoxicity.[86,87]
Methylphenidate[88]	Mild and transient elevations in liver enzymes have been reported. Rare reports of liver dysfunction and hypersensitivity reactions. Limited experience in liver disease.

Sedatives in hepatic impairment

Table 8.5 summarises recommended sedatives in hepatic impairment.

Table 8.5 Sedatives in hepatic impairment.

Drug	Comments
Benzodiazepines	Extensively hepatically metabolised. Prolonged duration of effect particularly for drugs with active metabolites (diazepam, midazolam, clonazepam). Lorazepam, oxazepam and temazepam do not have active metabolites and are preferred. Lorazepam is considered the best tolerated in advanced liver disease[28] and is commonly used in alcohol withdrawal. Liver enzyme elevations are uncommon and liver injury very rare.[28]
Melatonin[7,89]	Complex handling of melatonin in liver impairment. Reduced clearance and prolonged half-life contribute to higher circulating levels of endogenous melatonin in daytime hours; negative feedback and accumulation of toxic products results in reduced endogenous production. Relevance to dosing of exogenous melatonin is unclear, although toxicity of melatonin is minimal. Manufacturer advises avoiding in moderate or severe liver disease. Rarely associated with changes in liver function tests (LFTs).
Promethazine[7]	Extensive hepatic metabolism. Manufacturers advise caution in liver impairment. Jaundice reported with high doses. Despite widespread use, no reports of LFT abnormalities or toxicity with lower doses.[28]
Z drugs[7,90,91]	Hepatically metabolised, but all have a relatively short half-life. Reduce initial doses in mild to moderate impairment (use zopiclone 3.75mg, zolpidem 5mg, zaleplon 5mg). Avoid in severe impairment. Manufacturers warn that benzodiazepines as a class may precipitate encephalopathy. Zaleplon is subject to significant first-pass metabolism and zolpidem plasma concentrations and half-life are significantly increased in hepatic impairment. These agents should be used with caution.[92] Although zopiclone has the longer half-life, this may not be clinically relevant except in severe disease.[90] Zopiclone and zaleplon have not been associated with hepatotoxicity. There are rare reports of abnormal LFTs and a single case of liver injury with zolpidem.[28] There is one case of acute liver injury with eszopiclone (a zopiclone isomer).[93]

Other psychotropics in hepatic impairment

Table 8.6 gives a summary of other psychotropics recommended in hepatic impairment.

Table 8.6 Other psychotropics in hepatic impairment.

Drug	Comments
Bremelanotide[7]	No dose adjustment required in mild to moderate hepatic impairment. Use with caution in severe impairment; adverse effects more likely.[30] One case of acute hepatitis reported.
Deutetrabenazine[6,28]	Not studied in hepatic impairment but, based on experience with tetrabenazine, use is contraindicated. Limited information available but clinically relevant hepatotoxicity not reported. Occasional asymptomatic rises in ALT.
Gabapentin	Largely renally excreted but occasional cases of liver toxicity reported.[94,95]
Lemborexant, daridorexant, suvorexant[7,30]	No dose adjustments in mild or moderate impairment required for suvorexant. For lemorexant and daridorexant, no dose adjustment in mild impairment (risk of increased somnolence). In moderate impairment, starting and maximum dose of 5mg for lemborexant, 25mg for daridorexant. None is recommended in severe impairment. Little experience but hepatotoxicity not reported.[96]
Pitolisant[6,30]	Extensively hepatically metabolised. No dose adjustment in mild impairment. In moderate impairment the half-life is doubled; daily dose can be increased 2 weeks after initiation, daily maximum 17.8mg. Manufacturers recommend monitoring patients with hepatic impairment for increased QTc. Contraindicated in severe impairment. Hepatic enzyme increases are uncommon. No reports of liver injury.
Pregabalin	Not metabolised and largely renally excreted.[97] Rare cases of hepatotoxicity.[98,99]
Solriamfetol[6]	Not metabolised. No known problems in liver impairment, no reports of liver injury.
Valbenazine[7,28]	Hepatically metabolised pro-drug of α-dihydrotetrabenazine. Unlike deutetrabenazine, valbenazine is not contraindicated in liver disease, but maximum dose of 40mg in moderate to severe impairment. Few data, but no reports of clinically relevant liver injury other than a single report of reactivation of pre-existing hepatitis C.

ALT, alanine aminotransferase.

Summary of recommended psychotropics in hepatic impairment

Table 8.7 gives an outline of the drug groups of psychotropics recommended for use in hepatic impairment.

Table 8.7 Psychotropic drug groups in hepatic impairment.

Drug group	Recommended drugs
Antipsychotics	**Sulpiride/amisulpride**: no dosage reduction required if renal function is normal **Paliperidone**: if depot required.
Antidepressants	**Paroxetine, sertraline, citalopram, escitalopram or vortioxetine**: start at low dose. Titrate slowly (if required) as above.
Mood stabilisers	**Lithium**: use plasma levels to guide dosage. Care needed if ascites status changes.
Sedatives	**Lorazepam, oxazepam, temazepam**: short half-life with no active metabolites. Use low doses with caution, as sedative drugs used in severe disease can precipitate hepatic encephalopathy. **Zopiclone**: 3.75mg with care in moderate hepatic impairment.

CHAPTER 8

Drug-induced hepatic damage

Hy's rule is defined as alanine aminotransferase (ALT) more than three times the upper limit of normal combined with serum bilirubin more than two times the upper limit of normal. This is recommended by the US Food and Drug Administration (FDA) to assess the hepatotoxicity of new drugs.[80]

Drug-induced hepatic damage can be due to:

- Direct dose-related hepatotoxicity (type 1 adverse drug reaction). A small number of drugs fall into this category (e.g. paracetamol, alcohol).
- Hypersensitivity reactions (type 2 adverse drug reaction). These can present with rash, fever and eosinophilia. Almost all drugs have been associated with cases of hepatotoxicity; the frequency varies.

Almost any type of liver damage can occur, ranging from mild transient asymptomatic increases in LFTs to fulminant hepatic failure. See Tables 8.1–8.6 for details of the hepatotoxic potential of individual drugs.

Risk factors for drug-induced hepatotoxicity include:[100]

- Increasing age.
- Female gender.
- Alcohol consumption.
- Co-prescription of enzyme-inducing drugs.
- Genetic predisposition.
- Obesity.
- Pre-existing liver disease (small effect).

When interpreting LFTs, remember that:[101]

- About 12% of the healthy adult population have one LFT outside (above or below) the normal reference range.
- Up to 10% of patients with clinically significant hepatic disease have normal LFTs.
- Individual LFTs lack specificity for the liver, but more than one abnormal test greatly increases the likelihood of liver pathology.
- The absolute values of LFTs are a poor indicator of disease severity.

When monitoring LFTs consider the following:

- Ideally LFTs should be measured before treatment starts so that 'baseline' values are available.
- LFT elevations of over two times the upper limit of the normal reference range are rarely clinically significant.
- Most drug-related LFT elevations occur early in treatment (first month) and are transient. They may indicate adaptation of the liver to the drug rather than damage per se. Transient LFT elevations may also occur during periods of weight gain.[102]
- If LFTs are persistently elevated more than threefold, continuing to rise or accompanied by clinical symptoms, the suspected drugs should be withdrawn.
- When tracking change, >20% change in liver enzymes is required to exclude biological or analytical variation.

References

1. Slim M, et al. Hepatic safety of atypical antipsychotics: current evidence and future directions. *Drug Saf* 2016; 39:925–943.
2. Todorović Vukotić N, et al. Antidepressants- and antipsychotics-induced hepatotoxicity. *Arch Toxicol* 2021; 95:767–789.
3. Marwick KF, et al. Antipsychotics and abnormal liver function tests: systematic review. *Clin Neuropharmacol* 2012; 35:244–253.
4. Morlán-Coarasa MJ, et al. Incidence of non-alcoholic fatty liver disease and metabolic dysfunction in first episode schizophrenia and related psychotic disorders: a 3-year prospective randomized interventional study. *Psychopharmacology (Berl)* 2016; 233:3947–3952.
5. Baeza I, et al. One-year prospective study of liver function tests in children and adolescents on second-generation antipsychotics: is there a link with metabolic syndrome? *J Child Adolesc Psychopharmacol* 2018; 28:463–473.
6. Datapharm Communications Ltd. Electronic Medicines Compendium. 2023; https://www.medicines.org.uk/emc.
7. IBM Watson Health. IBM Micromedex Solutions. 2024; https://www.ibm.com/watson-health/about/micromedex.
8. Zeiss R, et al. Drug-associated liver injury related to antipsychotics: exploratory analysis of pharmacovigilance data. *J Clin Psychopharmacol* 2022; 42:440–444.
9. Nikogosyan G, et al. Acute aripiprazole-associated liver injury. *J Clin Psychopharmacol* 2021; 41:344–346.
10. Mallikaarjun S, et al. Effects of hepatic or renal impairment on the pharmacokinetics of aripiprazole. *Clin Pharmacokinet* 2008; 47:533–542.
11. Preskorn SH. Clinically important differences in the pharmacokinetics of the ten newer 'atypical' antipsychotics: Part 3. Effects of renal and hepatic impairment. *J Psychiatr Pract* 2012; 18:430–437.
12. Chico G, et al. Clinical vignettes 482 aripiprazole causes cholelithiasis and hepatitis: a rare finding. *Am J Gastroenterol* 2005; 100:S164.
13. Kornischka J, et al. Acute drug-induced hepatitis during aripiprazole monotherapy: a case report. *J Pharmacovigil* 2016; 4:1000201.
14. Castanheira L, et al. Aripiprazole-induced hepatitis: a case report. *Clin Psychopharmacol Neurosci* 2019; 17:551–555.
15. Peeters P, et al. Asenapine pharmacokinetics in hepatic and renal impairment. *Clin Pharmacokinet* 2011; 50:471–481.
16. Schultz K, et al. A case of pseudo-Stauffer's syndrome related to asenapine use. *Schizophr Res* 2015; 169:500–501.
17. Parikh NB, et al. Clinical role of brexpiprazole in depression and schizophrenia. *Ther Clin Risk Manag* 2017; 13:299–306.
18. Cutler AJ, et al. Evaluation of the long-term safety and tolerability of cariprazine in patients with schizophrenia: results from a 1-year open-label study. *CNS Spectr* 2018; 23:39–50.
19. Brown CA, et al. Clozapine toxicity and hepatitis. *J Clin Psychopharmacol* 2013; 33:570–571.
20. Tucker P. Liver toxicity with clozapine. *Aust NZ J Psychiatry* 2013; 47:975–976.
21. Gaertner HJ, et al. Side effects of clozapine. *Psychopharmacology (Berl)* 1989; 99 Suppl:S97–100.
22. Lally J, et al. Hepatitis, interstitial nephritis, and pancreatitis in association with clozapine treatment: a systematic review of case series and reports. *J Clin Psychopharmacol* 2018; 38:520–527.
23. Takács A, et al. Clozapine rechallenge in a patient with clozapine-induced hepatitis. *Australas Psychiatry* 2019; 27:535.
24. Amdisen A, et al. Zuclopenthixol acetate in viscoleo – a new drug formulation. An open Nordic multicentre study of zuclopenthixol acetate in Viscoleo in patients with acute psychoses including mania and exacerbation of chronic psychoses. *Acta Psychiatr Scand* 1987; 75:99–107.
25. Wistedt B, et al. Zuclopenthixol decanoate and haloperidol decanoate in chronic schizophrenia: a double-blind multicentre study. *Acta Psychiatr Scand* 1991; 84:14–21.
26. Demuth N, et al. [Flupentixol-induced acute hepatitis]. *Gastroenterol Clin Biol* 1999; 23:152–153.
27. Nolen WA, et al. Disturbances of liver function of long acting neuroleptic drugs. *Pharmakopsychiatr Neuropsychopharmakol* 1978; 11:199–204.
28. LiverTox. *Clinical and Research Information on Drug-induced Liver Injury.* Bethesda, MD: National Institute of Diabetes and Digestive and Kidney Diseases; 2012.
29. Vanda Pharmaceuticals Inc. FANAPT® (iloperidone) tablets 1mg, 2mg, 4mg, 6mg, 8mg, 10mg, 12mg indication and important safety information. 2021; http://www.fanapt.com/product/pi/pdf/fanapt.pdf.
30. US Food and Drug Administration. Drugs@FDA: FDA-approved drugs. 2023; https://www.accessdata.fda.gov/scripts/cder/daf.
31. Greenwood J, et al. Lumateperone: a novel antipsychotic for schizophrenia. *Ann Pharmacother* 2021; 55:98–104.
32. Druschky K, et al. Severe drug-induced liver injury in patients under treatment with antipsychotic drugs: data from the AMSP study. *World J Biol Psychiatry* 2021; 22:373–386.
33. Gunther M, et al. Antipsychotic safety in liver disease: a narrative review and practical guide for the clinician. *J Acad Consult Liaison Psychiatry* 2023; 64:73–82.
34. Amatniek J, et al. Safety of paliperidone extended-release in patients with schizophrenia or schizoaffective disorder and hepatic disease. *Clin Schizophr Relat Psychoses* 2014; 8:8–20.
35. Macaluso M, et al. Pharmacokinetic drug evaluation of paliperidone in the treatment of schizoaffective disorder. *Expert Opin Drug Metab Toxicol* 2017; 13:871–879.
36. Chang CH, et al. Paliperidone is associated with reduced risk of severe hepatic outcome in patients with schizophrenia and viral hepatitis: a nationwide population-based cohort study. *Psychiatry Res* 2019; 281:112597.
37. Vats A, et al. Treatment of patients with schizophrenia and comorbid chronic hepatitis with paliperidone: a systematic review. *Cureus* 2023; 15:e34234.
38. Braude MR, et al. Liver disease prevalence and severity in people with serious mental illness: a cross-sectional analysis using non-invasive diagnostic tools. *Hepatol Int* 2021; 15:812–820.
39. Khorassani F, et al. Risperidone- and paliperidone-induced hepatotoxicity: case report and review of literature. *Am J Health Syst Pharm* 2020; 77:1578–1584.
40. Das A, et al. Liver injury associated with quetiapine: an illustrative case report. *J Clin Psychopharmacol* 2017; 37:623–625.

CHAPTER 8

41. Ko S, et al. Investigation of hepatic adverse events due to quetiapine by using the common data model. *Pharmacoepidemiol Drug Saf* 2023; **32**:1341–1349.

42. Monnelly EP, et al. Quetiapine for treatment of alcohol dependence. *J Clin Psychopharmacol* 2004; **24**:532–535.

43. Brown ES, et al. A randomized, double-blind, placebo-controlled trial of quetiapine in patients with bipolar disorder, mixed or depressed phase, and alcohol dependence. *Alcohol Clin Exp Res* 2014; **38**:2113–2118.

44. Vatsalya V, et al. Safety assessment of liver injury with quetiapine fumarate XR management in very heavy drinking alcohol-dependent patients. *Clin Drug Investig* 2016; **36**:935–944.

45. Holtmann M, et al. Risperidone-associated steatohepatitis and excessive weight-gain. *Pharmacopsychiatry* 2003; **36**:206–207.

46. Voican CS, et al. Antidepressant-induced liver injury: a review for clinicians. *Am J Psychiatry* 2014; **171**:404–415.

47. Freiesleben SD, et al. A systematic review of agomelatine-induced liver injury. *J Mol Psychiatry* 2015; **3**:4.

48. Gahr M, et al. Safety and tolerability of agomelatine: focus on hepatotoxicity. *Curr Drug Metab* 2014; **15**:694–702.

49. Billioti de Gage S, et al. Antidepressants and hepatotoxicity: a cohort study among 5 million individuals registered in the French National Health Insurance Database. *CNS Drugs* 2018; **32**:673–684.

50. Pladevall-Vila M, et al. Risk of acute liver injury in agomelatine and other antidepressant users in four European countries: a cohort and nested case-control study using automated health data sources. *CNS Drugs* 2019; **33**:383–395.

51. Lundbeck Limited. Summary of product characteristics. Citalopram 20mg film-coated tablets. 2023; https://www.medicines.org.uk/emc/product/992/smpc.

52. Lopez-Torres E, et al. Hepatotoxicity related to citalopram (Letter). *Am J Psychiatry* 2004; **161**:923–924.

53. Hanje AJ, et al. Case report: fulminant hepatic failure involving duloxetine hydrochloride. *Clin Gastroenterol Hepatol* 2006; **4**:912–917.

54. Vuppalanchi R, et al. Duloxetine hepatotoxicity: a case-series from the drug-induced liver injury network. *Aliment Pharmacol Ther* 2010; **32**:1174–1183.

55. Lin ND, et al. Hepatic outcomes among adults taking duloxetine: a retrospective cohort study in a US health care claims database. *BMC Gastroenterol* 2015; **15**:134.

56. McIntyre RS, et al. The hepatic safety profile of duloxetine: a review. *Expert Opin Drug Metab Toxicol* 2008; **4**:281–285.

57. Bunchorntavakul C, et al. Drug hepatotoxicity: newer agents. *Clin Liver Dis* 2017; **21**:115–134.

58. Lundbeck Limited. Summary of product characteristics. Escitalopram 10mg film-coated tablets. 2023; https://www.medicines.org.uk/emc/product/7718/smpc.

59. Rao N. The clinical pharmacokinetics of escitalopram. *Clin Pharmacokinet* 2007; **46**:281–290.

60. Schenker S, et al. Fluoxetine disposition and elimination in cirrhosis. *Clin Pharmacol Ther* 1988; **44**:353–359.

61. Cai Q, et al. Acute hepatitis due to fluoxetine therapy. *Mayo Clin Proc* 1999; **74**:692–694.

62. Friedenberg FK, et al. Hepatitis secondary to fluoxetine treatment. *Am J Psychiatry* 1996; **153**:580.

63. Johnston DE, et al. Chronic hepatitis related to use of fluoxetine. *Am J Gastroenterol* 1997; **92**:1225–1226.

64. Hale AS. New antidepressants: use in high-risk patients. *J Clin Psychiatry* 1993; **54** Suppl:61–70.

65. Mylan. Summary of product characteristics. Fluvoxamine 100mg film-coated tablets. 2023; https://www.medicines.org.uk/emc/product/6603/smpc.

66. Stoeckel K, et al. Absorption and disposition of moclobemide in patients with advanced age or reduced liver or kidney function. *Acta Psychiatr Scand Suppl* 1990; **360**:94–97.

67. Mylan Specialty LP. Highlights of prescribing information. EMSAM® (selegiline transdermal system) 2014; https://www.accessdata.fda.gov/drugsatfda_docs/label/2014/021336s005s010,021708s000lbl.pdf.

68. Thomas E, et al. Mirtazapine-induced steatosis. *Int J Clin Pharmacol Ther* 2017; **55**:630–632.

69. Shaheen AA, et al. The impact of depression and antidepressant usage on primary biliary cholangitis clinical outcomes. *PLoS One* 2018; **13**:e0194839.

70. Sandoz Limited. Summary of product characteristics. Paroxetine 20mg tablets. 2024; https://www.medicines.org.uk/emc/product/4168/smpc.

71. Colakoglu O, et al. Toxic hepatitis associated with paroxetine. *Int J Clin Pract* 2005; **59**:861–862.

72. Düll MM, et al. Evaluation and management of pruritus in primary biliary cholangitis. *Clin Liver Dis* 2022; **26**:727–745.

73. Tran A, et al. Pharmacokinetics of reboxetine in volunteers with hepatic impairment. *Clin Drug Investig* 2000; **19**:473–477.

74. Mylan. Summary of product characteristics. Setraline 100mg tablets. 2023; https://www.medicines.org.uk/emc/product/10586/smpc.

75. Committee on Safety of Medicines. Lofepramine (Gamanil) and abnormal blood tests of liver function. *Curr Problems* 1988; **23**:371.

76. Archer DF, et al. Cardiovascular, cerebrovascular, and hepatic safety of desvenlafaxine for 1 year in women with vasomotor symptoms associated with menopause. *Menopause* 2013; **20**:47–56.

77. Baird-Bellaire S, et al. An open-label, single-dose, parallel-group study of the effects of chronic hepatic impairment on the safety and pharmacokinetics of desvenlafaxine. *Clin Ther* 2013; **35**:782–794.

78. Ryan PB, et al. Atypical antipsychotics and the risks of acute kidney injury and related outcomes among older adults: a replication analysis and an evaluation of adapted confounding control strategies. *Drugs Aging* 2017; **34**:211–219.

79. Chen G, et al. Vortioxetine: clinical pharmacokinetics and drug interactions. *Clin Pharmacokinet* 2018; **57**:673–686.

80. Bjornsson E. Hepatotoxicity associated with antiepileptic drugs. *Acta Neurol Scand* 2008; **118**:281–290.

81. Guo HL, et al. Valproic acid and the liver injury in patients with epilepsy: an update. *Curr Pharm Des* 2019; **25**:343–351.

82. Panei P, et al. Safety of psychotropic drug prescribed for attention-deficit/hyperactivity disorder in Italy. *Adv Drug Reaction Bull* 2010; **260**:999–1002.

83. Reed VA, et al. The safety of atomoxetine for the treatment of children and adolescents with attention-deficit/hyperactivity disorder: a comprehensive review of over a decade of research. *CNS Drugs* 2016; **30**:603–628.

84. Shire Pharmaceuticals Limited. Summary of product characteristics. Elvanse 20mg, 30mg, 40mg, 50mg, 60mg, 70mg hard capsules. 2023; https://www.medicines.org.uk/emc/search?q=%22Elvanse%22.

85. Medice UK Ltd. Summary of product characteristics. Amfexa 5mg, 10mg, 20mg tablets. 2023; https://www.medicines.org.uk/emc/search?q=amfexa.

86. Vanga RR, et al. Adderall induced acute liver injury: a rare case and review of the literature. *Case Rep Gastrointest Med* 2013; **2013**:902892.

87. Hood B, et al. Eosinophilic hepatitis in an adolescent during lisdexamfetamine dimesylate treatment for ADHD. *Pediatrics* 2010; **125**:e1510–1513.

88. Tong HY, et al. Liver transplant in a patient under methylphenidate therapy: a case report and review of the literature. *Case Rep Pediatr* 2015; **2015**:437298.

89. Flynn Pharma Ltd. Summary of product characteristics. Circadin 2mg prolonged-release tablets. 2021; https://www.medicines.org.uk/emc/product/2809/smpc.

90. SANOFI. Summary of product characteristics. Zimovane 7.5mg and 3.75mg LS film-coated tablets. 2023; https://www.medicines.org.uk/emc/product/2855/smpc.

91. Zentiva. Summary of product characteristics. Zolpidem tartrate 5mg, 10mg tablets. 2021; https://www.medicines.org.uk/emc/search?q=zolpidem.

92. Gunja N. The clinical and forensic toxicology of Z-drugs. *J Med Toxicol* 2013; **9**:155–162.

93. Wu T, et al. Case report of acute liver injury caused by the eszopiclone in a patient with chronic liver disease. *Medicine (Baltimore)* 2021; **100**:e26243.

94. Jackson CD, et al. Hold the gaba: a case of gabapentin-induced hepatotoxicity. *Cureus* 2018; **10**:e2269.

95. Chahal J, et al. Gabapentin-induced liver toxicity. *Am J Ther* 2022; **29**:e751–e752.

96. Kärppä M, et al. Long-term efficacy and tolerability of lemborexant compared with placebo in adults with insomnia disorder: results from the phase 3 randomized clinical trial SUNRISE 2. *Sleep* 2020; **43**:zsaa123.

97. Upjohn UK Limited. Summary of product characteristics. Lyrica (pregabalin) 25mg, 50mg, 75mg, 100mg, 150mg, 200mg, 225mg, 300mg capsules. 2024; https://www.medicines.org.uk/emc/product/10303/smpc.

98. Sendra JM, et al. Pregabalin-induced hepatotoxicity. *Ann Pharmacother* 2011; **45**:e32.

99. Düzenli T, et al. Pregabaline as a rare cause of hepatotoxicity. *Pain Med* 2017; **18**:1407–1408.

100. Grattagliano I, et al. Biochemical mechanisms in drug-induced liver injury: certainties and doubts. *World J Gastroenterol* 2009; **15**:4865–4876.

101. Rosalki SB, et al. Liver function profiles and their interpretation. *Br J Hosp Med* 1994; **51**:181–186.

102. Rettenbacher MA, et al. Association between antipsychotic-induced elevation of liver enzymes and weight gain: a prospective study. *J Clin Psychopharmacol* 2006; **26**:500–503.

CHAPTER 8

Renal impairment

Using drugs in patients with renal impairment needs careful consideration. This is partly because some drugs are nephrotoxic but principally because the pharmacokinetics (absorption, distribution, metabolism, excretion) of drugs are altered in renal impairment. In particular, **patients with renal impairment have a reduced capacity to excrete drugs and their metabolites.**

General principles of prescribing in renal impairment

- **Estimate the excretory capacity of the kidney.** Laboratories usually report renal function based on the estimated glomerular filtration rate (eGFR). This is derived from either the Chronic Kidney Disease Epidemiology Collaboration (CKD-EPI) formula or the Modification of Diet in Renal Disease (MDRD) formula. The CKD-EPI formula is more accurate than the MDRD and is preferred, but note that these estimates are still less than perfect when compared with directly measured GFR.[1]
- **Check proteinuria** by measuring urinary albumin and calculate the albumin : creatinine ratio. This is because proteinuria is a significant risk factor for progression to end stage disease.[1]
- For **most drugs and most adult patients of average build and height**, eGFR (calculated using the CKD-EPI formula, Box 8.1) can be used to determine dose adjustments.
- For **nephrotoxic drugs, elderly patients (75 years and over) and patients at both extremes of muscle mass (body mass index [BMI] <18 or >40kg/m²)**, calculate creatinine clearance (CrCl) to determine dose adjustments. In addition, the Medicines Healthcare products Regulatory Agency (MHRA) advises that CrCl should be used as an estimate of renal function for direct-acting oral anticoagulants (DOACs) and drugs with a narrow therapeutic index that are mainly renally excreted (e.g. lithium) (UK Kidney Association, https://ukkidney.org). The Cockroft and Gault equation should be used to calculate CrCl (Box 8.2).

Box 8.1 Chronic Kidney Disease Epidemiology Collaboration (CKD-EPI) formula

This replaces the previously used modification of diet in renal disease (MDRD) equation[2] although some pathology departments still use MDRD.

$$GFR = 141 \times \min (S_{cr}/k, 1)^{\alpha} \times \max (S_{cr}/k, 1)^{-1.209} \times 0.993^{Age} \times 1.018 \text{ [if female]} \times 1.159 \text{ [if black]}$$

Where S_{cr} is serum creatinine in mg/dL
κ is 0.7 for females and 0.9 for males
α is -0.329 for females and -0.411 for males
min indicates the minimum of S_{cr}/κ or 1
max indicates the maximum of S_{cr}/κ or 1

- Online calculator available at https://www.kidney.org/professionals/kdoqi/gfr_calculator

Box 8.2 Cockroft and Gault equation*

$$CrCl\,(ml/min) = \frac{F\,(140 - age\,(in\ years)) \times ideal\ body\ weight\,(kg)}{Serum\ creatinine\,(\mu mol/L)}$$

Where F = 1.23 (men) and 1.04 (women)

Ideal body weight should be used for patients at extremes of body weight or else the result of the calculation is a poor estimate

For men, ideal body weight (kg) = 50kg + 2.3kg per inch over 5 feet
For women, ideal body weight (kg) = 45.5kg + 2.3kg per inch over 5 feet

- Online calculator available at https://www.nuh.nhs.uk/staff-area/antibiotics/creatinine-clearance-calculator

* This equation is not accurate if plasma creatinine is unstable (e.g. acute renal failure), in obesity, in pregnant women, in children or in diseases causing the production of abnormal amounts of creatinine. It has only been validated in white patients. Creatinine clearance is not the same as GFR and is relatively less representative of GFR in severe renal failure.

Stage of renal impairment

Figure 8.1 indicates how to classify the stage of renal impairment.[2]

<table>
<tr><td colspan="4" rowspan="4"></td><td colspan="3">ACR categories (mg/mmol)
Description and range</td></tr>
<tr><td>A1</td><td>A2</td><td>A3</td></tr>
<tr><td>Normal to mildly increased</td><td>Moderately increased</td><td>Severely increased</td></tr>
<tr><td><3</td><td>3–30</td><td>>30</td></tr>
<tr><td rowspan="6">GFR categories (mL/min/1.73m²)
Description and range</td><td>G1</td><td>Normal and high</td><td>≥90</td><td rowspan="2">No CKD in the absence of markers of kidney damage</td><td colspan="2">Manage in primary care according to recommendations</td></tr>
<tr><td>G2</td><td>Mild reduction related to normal range for a young adult</td><td>60–89</td><td rowspan="3">Refer for specialist assessment if the person has:
• a sustained decrease in GFR of 25% or more and a change in GFR category or sustained decrease in GFR of 15 mL/min/1.73 m² or more within 12 months
• hypertension that remains poorly controlled despite the use of at least 4 antihypertensive drugs at therapeutic doses (see also 'Hypertension' NICE clinical guideline 127)
• known or suspected rare or genetic causes of CKD
• suspected renal artery stenosis</td><td rowspan="3">Refer for specialist assessment if the person has any of the criteria in A2, or:
• ACR 70mg/mmol or more, unless known to be caused by diabetes and already appropriately treated
• haematuria</td></tr>
<tr><td>G3a</td><td>Mild–moderate reduction</td><td>45–59</td><td></td></tr>
<tr><td>G3b</td><td>Moderate–severe reduction</td><td>30–44</td><td></td></tr>
<tr><td>G4</td><td>Severe reduction</td><td>15–29</td><td colspan="3" rowspan="2">Refer for specialist assessment</td></tr>
<tr><td>G5</td><td>Kidney failure</td><td><15</td></tr>
</table>

Figure 8.1 Classification of renal impairment. ACR, albumin : creatinine ratio; CKD, chronic kidney disease; GFR, glomerular filtration rate.

Notes

- **Monitor decline in renal function over a considerable period** as a 30% change over 2 years is associated with a fivefold increase in risk of end stage renal disease. Chronic kidney disease (CKD) progression is often non-linear.[1]
- **Monitor risk of moving from CKD stage 3–5 (eGFR 10–59) to dialysis/transplantation using the Tangri score at** https://qxmd.com/calculate/calculator_125/kidney-failure-risk-equation-8-variable. The four (age, sex, eGFR, urine albumin : creatinine ratio) and eight (previous four items plus serum calcium, phosphorus, bicarbonate, albumin) variable equations accurately predict the 2- and 5-year probability of treated kidney failure (dialysis or transplantation) for a potential patient with CKD stage 3–5.[3]
- In general, renal function significantly affects overall drug elimination so the amount of drug excreted unchanged in urine should be 30% or more of the dose.[4]
- **Older adults (>65 years) should be assumed to have at least mild renal impairment.** Their serum creatinine may not be raised because they have a smaller muscle mass.
- **Avoid drugs that are nephrotoxic** (e.g. lithium, non-steroidal anti-inflammatory drugs) where renal reserve is limited.
- **Be cautious when using drugs that are extensively renally cleared** (e.g. sulpiride, amisulpride, lithium).
- Elimination of drugs metabolised hepatically can be reduced in kidney disease possibly by inhibition of enzymatic activity caused by uraemia.[5]
- **Start at a low dose and increase slowly** because, in renal impairment, the half-life of a drug and the time for it to reach steady state (amount absorbed is the same as cleared when the drug is given continuously) are often prolonged. Plasma level monitoring may be useful for some drugs.
- **Try to avoid long-acting drugs** (e.g. depot preparations). Their dose and frequency cannot be easily adjusted should renal function change.
- **Prescribe as few drugs as possible.** Patients with renal failure take many medications requiring regular review. Interactions and adverse effects can be avoided if fewer drugs are used.
- **Monitor patient for adverse effects.** Patients with renal impairment are more likely to experience adverse effects and they may take longer to develop than in healthy patients. Adverse effects such as sedation, confusion and postural hypotension can be more common.
- **Be cautious when using drugs with anticholinergic effects,** since they may cause urinary retention.
- There are **few clinical studies** of the use of psychotropic drugs in people with renal impairment. Advice about drug use in renal impairment is often based on knowledge of the drug's pharmacokinetics in healthy patients.
- **The effect of renal replacement therapies (e.g. dialysis) on drugs is difficult to predict.** See Tables 8.8–8.14. Seek specialist advice.
- **Try to avoid drugs known to prolong the QTc interval.** In established renal failure electrolyte changes are common so it is probably best to avoid antipsychotics with the greatest risk of QTc prolongation (see section on ECG changes – QT prolongation in Chapter 1).
- **Monitor weight carefully.** Weight gain predisposes to diabetes which can contribute to rhabdomyolysis[6] and renal failure. Psychotropic medications commonly cause weight gain.

CHAPTER 8

- Be vigilant for serotonin syndrome with antidepressants, dystonias and neuroleptic malignant syndrome (NMS) with antipsychotics. The resulting rhabdomyolysis can cause renal failure. There are case reports of rhabdomyolysis occurring with antipsychotics without other symptoms of NMS.[7–9]
- **Depression is common in CKD** but evidence for effectiveness of antidepressants in this condition is lacking.[10,11] In CKD starting some antidepressants at a higher versus lower dose reduces mortality risk.[12] Depression is poorly treated in patients on haemodialysis.[13] In common with other chronic physical illnesses, depression in end stage renal disease may be associated with increased mortality,[14–16] and the degree of risk may be linked to the severity of the depression.[17] Non-drug treatment such as cognitive behavioural therapy, exercise or relaxation techniques probably reduces depressive symptoms for adults on dialysis.[18] SSRIs are associated with hip fracture in patients on haemodialysis (adjusted odds ratio 1.25; 95% confidence interval [CI] 1.17, 1.35).[19]
- **Both schizophrenia and bipolar disorder are associated with an increased risk of CKD.**[20,21]
- **Antipsychotics (e.g. olanzapine, quetiapine) may be associated with acute kidney injury**[22] possibly via their effects on blood pressure and urinary retention but studies are conflicting.[23]
- **Mood-stabilising anticonvulsants used in bipolar disorder are associated with an increased rate of CKD.**[21]

Table 8.8 Antipsychotic medications in renal impairment.

Drug	Comments
Amisulpride[24–27]	Primarily renally excreted. 50% excreted unchanged in urine. Limited experience in renal disease, one study in Chinese patients showing more than twofold increase in AUC, trough and peak plasma concentrations with GFR 30mL/min.[28] Manufacturer states no data with doses of >50mg but recommends following dosing: 50% of dose if GFR 30–60mL/min; 33% of dose if GFR is 10–30mL/min; no recommendations for GFR <10mL/min so **best avoided in established renal failure.**
Aripiprazole[24,25,27,29–32]	Less than 1% of unchanged aripiprazole renally excreted. Manufacturer states no dose adjustment required in renal failure as pharmacokinetics are similar in healthy and severely renally diseased patients. There is one case report of safe use of oral aripiprazole 5mg in an 83-year-old man having haemodialysis. Avoid depot formulation where possible although there is a case report of aripiprazole 400mg depot use in a 64-year-old man on haemodialysis.
Asenapine[25,27,33]	Extensively hepatically metabolised. Manufacturer states no dose adjustment required for patients with renal impairment but no experience with use if GFR <15mL/min. A 5mg single-dose study suggests that no dose adjustment is needed with any degree of renal impairment.
Chlorpromazine[24,27,34–36]	Less than 1% excreted unchanged in urine. Caution required in severe impairment because of the risk of accumulation. No dose adjustment required for GFR >10mL/min. For GFR <10mL/min, start with small doses and monitor for anticholinergic, sedative and hypotensive adverse effects.

(Continued)

CHAPTER 8

Table 8.8 (*Continued*)

Drug	Comments
Clozapine[25,27,37–41]	Contraindicated by manufacturer in severe renal disease, but only trace amounts of unchanged clozapine are excreted in urine. No dose adjustment required in GFR >10mL/min, titrate cautiously in very severe impairment. Nocturnal enuresis and urinary retention are common adverse effects. Anticholinergic, sedative and hypotensive adverse effects are more frequent in patients with renal disease. May cause and aggravate diabetes, a common cause of renal disease. Rare case reports of interstitial nephritis and acute renal failure, but also successful continuation after renal transplantation.[42]
Flupentixol[24,25,27]	Negligible renal excretion of unchanged flupentixol. Dosing: GFR 10–50mL/min dose as in normal renal function; GFR <10mL/min start with quarter to half of normal dose and titrate slowly. May cause hypotension and sedation in renal impairment and can accumulate. Manufacturer advises caution in renal failure because of increased cerebral sensitivity to antipsychotics. Avoid depot preparations in renal impairment.
Haloperidol[8,24,25,27,43,44]	Less than 1% excreted unchanged in the urine. Manufacturer advises caution in renal failure. Dosing: GFR 10–50mL/min dose as in normal renal function; GFR <10mL/min start with a lower dose as can accumulate with repeated dosing. A case report of haloperidol use in renal failure suggests starting at a low dose and increasing slowly. Has been used to treat uraemia-associated nausea in renal failure. Avoid depot preparations in renal impairment.
Lumateperone[45,46]	<1% excreted unchanged in urine. Manufacturer advises no dose adjustment needed in renal impairment.
Lurasidone[24]	9% excreted unchanged in the urine. Serum concentrations are increased by 1.5-, 1.9- and 2.0-fold in mild, moderate and severe impairment, respectively. Manufacturer advises a starting dose of 18.75mg (20mg) and maximum dose of 74mg (80mg) per day if GFR <50mL/min. Avoid in GFR <15mL/min unless benefits outweigh risks (no data to support use). Renal failure has been reported rarely.
Olanzapine[7,25,27,34,44,47]	57% of olanzapine is excreted mainly as metabolites (7% excreted unchanged) in urine. Dosing: UK manufacturers recommend GFR <50mL/min initially 5mg daily and titrate as necessary. Avoid long-acting preparations in renal impairment unless the oral dose is well tolerated and effective. UK manufacturer recommends a lower long-acting injection starting dose of 150mg, 4-weekly in patients with renal impairment. US manufacturers state that no dose adjustment is required for oral or depot preparation. May cause and aggravate diabetes, a common cause of renal disease. Hypothermia has been reported when used in renal failure.
Paliperidone[25,27,34]	Paliperidone is a metabolite of risperidone. 59% excreted unchanged in urine. Dosing: GFR 50–80mL/min, 3mg daily and increase according to response to max. of 6mg daily; GFR 10–50mL/min, 3mg alternate days (or 1.5mg daily) increasing to 3mg daily according to response. Use with caution as clearance is reduced by 71% in severe kidney disease. Manufacturer contraindicates oral form if GFR <10mL/min due to lack of experience, and monthly, 3-monthly and 6-monthly depot preparations if GFR <50mL/min (reduced loading and maintenance doses if GFR >50mL/min). Two case reports of successful paliperidone monthly injection use in patients with renal failure undergoing haemodialysis.[48,49]

Table 8.8 *(Continued)*

Drug	Comments
Pimavanserin[45,50]	<1% excreted unchanged in urine. Manufacturer states no dose adjustment needed in GFR ≥30mL/min but advises to avoid if GFR <30mL/min due to lack of data.
Pimozide[24,25,27]	<1% of pimozide excreted unchanged in the urine; dose reductions not usually needed in renal impairment. Dosing: GFR 10–50mL/min dose as in normal renal function; GFR <10mL/min start at a low dose and increase according to response. Manufacturer cautions in renal failure.
Quetiapine[24,25,27,51–53]	<5% of quetiapine excreted unchanged in the urine. Plasma clearance reduced by an average of 25% in patients with a GFR <30mL/min but manufacturer states no dose adjustment is necessary. Case reports (thrombotic thrombocytopenic purpura, DRESS and non-NMS rhabdomyolysis) resulting in acute renal failure with quetiapine have been published.
Risperidone[24,25,27,44,54–57]	Clearance of risperidone and the active metabolite of risperidone (9-OH-) is reduced by 60% in patients with moderate to severe renal disease. Dosing: GFR <50mL/min 0.5mg twice daily for at least 1 week then increasing by 0.5mg twice daily to 1–2mg bd. The long-acting injection should only be used after titration with oral risperidone as described above. If 2mg orally is tolerated, 25mg intramuscularly every 2 weeks (Risperdal Consta®) can be administered. Manufacturers of the Okedi® monthly injection do not recommend use in GFR <60mL/min. Risvan® 75mg monthly or Perseris™ (subcutaneous) 90mg monthly can be used if 3mg oral is tolerated. Uzedy™ can be given 50mg monthly if 2mg oral is tolerated. There are two case reports of successful use of risperidone long-acting injection in haemodialysis at a dose of 50mg 2 weekly in one patient and 37.5mg then 25mg in an older adult. Another describes the successful use of risperidone in a child with steroid-induced psychosis and nephrotic syndrome.
Sulpiride[6,24,25,27,58]	Almost totally renally excreted, with 95% excreted in urine and faeces as unchanged sulpiride. Dosing regimen: GFR 30–60mL/min give 70% of normal dose; GFR 10–30mL/min give 50% of normal dose; GFR <10mL/min give 34% of normal dose. Alternately, the dosing interval can be prolonged by a factor of 1.5, 2 and 3, respectively. There is a case report of renal failure with sulpiride due to diabetic coma and rhabdomyolysis. **Probably best avoided in renal impairment**.
Trifluoperazine[27]	Less than 1% excreted unchanged in the urine. Dose GFR <10–50mL/min as for normal renal function – start with a low dose. Very limited data.
Ziprasidone[24,44,59,60]	<1% renally excreted unchanged. No dose adjustment needed for GFR >10mL/min but care needed with using the injection as it contains a renally eliminated excipient (cyclodextrin sodium). Case report of 80mg twice daily dose used in a patient on haemodialysis who then developed agranulocytosis.[61]
Zuclopenthixol[24,27]	10–20% of unchanged drug and metabolites excreted unchanged in urine. Manufacturer cautions use in renal disease as can accumulate. Dosing: 10–50mL/min dose as in normal renal function; GFR <10mL/min start with 50% of the dose and titrate slowly. Avoid both intramuscular preparations (acetate and decanoate) in renal impairment. If use is essential, follow the same dosing guidance as for oral.

AUC, area under the curve; bd, twice a day; DRESS, drug reaction with eosinophilia and systemic symptoms; GFR, glomerular filtration rate.

CHAPTER 8

Table 8.9 Antidepressants in renal impairment.[10]

Drug	Comments
Agomelatine[25]	Negligible renal excretion of unchanged agomelatine. No data on use in renal disease. Manufacturer says pharmacokinetics unchanged in small study of 25mg dose in severe renal impairment but cautions use in moderate or severe renal disease. A growing number of studies demonstrate nephroprotective effects in rats.
Amitriptyline[24,25,27,36,44,62–64]	<2% excreted unchanged in urine; no dose adjustment needed in renal failure. Dose as in normal renal function but start at a low dose and increase slowly. Monitor patient for urinary retention, confusion, sedation and postural hypotension. Has been used to treat pain in those with renal disease. Associated with acute kidney injury.[64]
Brexanolone[45,65]	<1% excreted unchanged in urine. Manufacturer states no dosage adjustment is recommended in patients with GFR 15–60mL/min; avoid use in patients with GFR of <15mL/min because of the potential accumulation of the injection solubilising agent, betadex sulfobutyl ether sodium.
Bupropion[24,25,27,36,44,66–68] (amfebutamone)	0.5% excreted unchanged in urine but in patients with renal impairment, plasma concentrations are higher, elimination half-life is longer and oral clearance is significantly lower. Metabolites may accumulate, increasing the risk of seizures. In renal impairment, reduce dose to 150mg once daily and/or reduce frequency of dosing. A single-dose study in haemodialysis patients (stage 5 disease) recommended a dose of 150mg every 3 days. Has been used to treat sexual dysfunction in mild to moderately depressed patients with chronic kidney disease.
Citalopram[24,25,27,44,69–75]	<13% of citalopram excreted unchanged in urine. Single-dose studies in mild and moderate renal impairment show no change in the pharmacokinetics of citalopram. Dosing is as for normal renal function; however, use with caution if GFR <10mL/min due to reduced clearance. The manufacturer does not advise use if GFR <20mL/min. Renal failure has been reported with citalopram overdose. Citalopram can treat depression in chronic renal failure and improve quality of life but use of citalopram (or escitalopram) is associated with a higher risk of sudden cardiac death vs other SSRIs (fluoxetine, fluvoxamine, paroxetine, sertraline) when used in patients on haemodialysis (adjusted hazard ratio 1.18; 95%CI 1.05, 1.31). Concurrent PPI use may increase the risk in haemodialysis;[76] minimising the serum-to-dialystate potassium gradient may attenuate it.[77] A case report of hyponatraemia has been reported in a renal transplant patient on citalopram.
Clomipramine[25,27,34,36,78]	2% of unchanged clomipramine excreted in urine. Dosing: GFR 20–50mL/min dose as for normal renal function; GFR <20mL/min, effects unknown, start at a low dose and monitor patient for urinary retention, confusion, sedation and postural hypotension as accumulation can occur. There is a case report of clomipramine-induced interstitial nephritis and reversible acute renal failure.
Desvenlafaxine[10,34,79,80]	45% of desvenlafaxine excreted unchanged in urine. Manufacturer recommends GFR 30–50mL/min 50mg/day; GFR <30mL/min 25mg/day or 50mg on alternate days. Half-life is prolonged and desvenlafaxine accumulates as GFR decreases. Urinary retention, delay when starting to pass urine and proteinuria have been reported as adverse effects.
Dosulepin[27,34,81] (dothiepin)	56% of mainly active metabolites renally excreted. They have a long half-life and may accumulate, resulting in excessive sedation. Dosing: GFR 20–50mL/min dose as for normal renal function; GFR <20mL/min start with a small dose and titrate to response. Monitor patient for urinary retention, confusion, sedation and postural hypotension.
Doxepin[25,27,34,36,82]	<1% excreted unchanged in urine. Dosing: GFR 10–50mL/min as in normal renal function but monitor patient for urinary retention, confusion, sedation and postural hypotension; GFR <10mL/min start with a small dose and increase slowly. Manufacturer advises using with caution. Haemolytic anaemia with renal failure has been reported with doxepin. Used topically to treat pruritis in chronic renal failure.

Table 8.9 *(Continued)*

Drug	Comments
Duloxetine[27,34,83–85]	<1% excreted unchanged in urine. Manufacturer states no dose adjustment is necessary for GFR >30mL/min; however, starting at a low dose and increasing slowly are advised. Duloxetine is contraindicated in patients with a GFR <30mL/min as it can accumulate in chronic kidney disease. Two case reports of acute renal failure with duloxetine have been reported. Serotonin syndrome was reported in a patient with chronic kidney disease on trazodone and duloxetine.[86]
Escitalopram[27,34,75,87–89]	8% excreted unchanged in urine. The manufacturer states dosage adjustment is not necessary in patients with mild or moderate renal impairment, but caution is advised if GFR <30mL/min so start with a low dose and increase slowly. A case study of reversible renal tubular defects and another of renal failure have been reported with escitalopram. One study says effective vs placebo in end stage renal disease. Use of escitalopram (or citalopram) is associated with a higher risk of sudden cardiac death vs other SSRIs (fluoxetine, fluvoxamine, paroxetine, sertraline) when used in patients on haemodialysis (adjusted hazard ratio 1.18; 95%CI 1.05, 1.31). Concurrent PPI use may increase the risk in haemodialysis;[76] minimising the serum-to-dialystate potassium gradient may attenuate it.[77]
Fluoxetine[11,25,27,34,36,44,90–93]	2.5–5% of fluoxetine and 10% of the active metabolite norfluoxetine are excreted unchanged in urine. Dosing: GFR 20–50mL/min dose as normal renal function; GFR <20mL/min consider using a low dose or on alternate days and increase according to response. Plasma levels after 2 months' treatment with 20mg (in patients on dialysis with GFR <10mL/min) are similar to those with normal renal function. Efficacy studies of fluoxetine in depression and renal disease are conflicting. One small placebo-controlled study of fluoxetine in patients on chronic dialysis found no significant differences in depression scores between the two groups after 8 weeks of treatment. Another found fluoxetine effective. A case series (n = 4) of once-weekly fluoxetine 90mg or 180mg use in depressed patients on haemodialysis describes efficacious use with better tolerability at 90mg dose.
Fluvoxamine[27,34,36,44,94]	2% excreted unchanged in urine. Renal impairment does not appear to affect the pharmacokinetics of fluvoxamine, but the UK manufacturer recommends starting at a low dose. Acute renal failure has been reported. Variations in albumin levels might affect serum concentrations of fluvoxamine in haemodialysis.
Imipramine[25,27,34,36,62]	<5% excreted unchanged in urine. No specific dose adjustment necessary in renal impairment. Monitor patient for urinary retention, confusion, sedation and postural hypotension. Renal impairment with imipramine has been reported and manufacturer advises caution in severe renal impairment. Renal damage reported rarely.
Lofepramine[25,27,34,95]	There is little information about the use of lofepramine in renal impairment. <5% excreted unchanged in urine. Dosing: GFR 10–50mL/min dose as in normal renal function; GFR <10mL/min start with a small dose and titrate slowly. Manufacturer contraindicates in severe renal impairment.
Mirtazapine[25,27,34,96]	75% excreted unchanged in urine. Clearance is reduced by 30% in patients with GFR of 11–39mL/min and by 50% in patients with GFR <10mL/min. Dosing advice: GFR 10–40mL/min dose as for normal renal function but monitor for adverse effects; GFR <10mL/min start at a low dose and monitor closely. Mirtazapine has been used to treat pruritis caused by renal failure[97] and appetite loss in chronic kidney disease.[98,99] Rarely associated with kidney calculus formation.
Moclobemide[25,27,34,100,101]	<1% of parent drug excreted unchanged in urine; an active metabolite was found to be raised in patients with renal impairment but this does not appear to be clinically significant. Dose adjustments are not required in renal impairment.

CHAPTER 8

(Continued)

Table 8.9 (*Continued*)

Drug	Comments
Nortriptyline[27,34,36,44,62,102]	<5% excreted unchanged in urine. If GFR 10–50mL/min dose as in normal renal function; if GFR <10mL/min start at a low dose. Plasma level monitoring recommended at doses of >100mg/day, as plasma concentrations of active metabolites are raised in renal impairment. Worsening of GFR in elderly patients has also been reported.
Paroxetine[25,27,34,36,103–106]	<2% of oral dose excreted unchanged in urine. Single-dose studies show increased plasma concentrations of paroxetine when GFR <30mL/min. Dosing advice differs: GFR 30–50mL/min dose as normal renal function; GFR <10–30mL/min start at 10mg/day (other source says start at 20mg) and increase dose according to response in 10mg increments/week, max. dose 40mg/day. Extended release paroxetine should be started at 12.5mg/day in severe renal impairment, max. dose 50mg/day in depression or panic disorder, 37.5mg/day in social anxiety disorder. Paroxetine 10mg daily has been used to treat depression in patients on haemodialysis. Rarely associated with Fanconi syndrome and acute renal failure.
Phenelzine[27,34]	Approximately 1% excreted unchanged in urine. No dose adjustment required in renal failure.
Reboxetine[25,27,34,107,108]	Approximately 10% of unchanged drug excreted unchanged in urine. Dosing: GFR <80mL/min, 2mg twice daily, adjusting dose according to response. Half-life is prolonged and plasma concentration increased as renal function decreases.
Sertraline[25,27,34,36,109–113]	<0.2% of unchanged sertraline excreted in urine. Pharmacokinetics in renal impairment are unchanged in single-dose studies but no published data on multiple dosing. Dosing is as for normal renal function. Sertraline has been used to treat dialysis-associated hypotension[114] and uraemic pruritis;[115] however acute renal failure has been reported so it should be used with caution. Overall, studies of sertraline in patients with depression and chronic kidney disease fail to show efficacy. The CAST study, an RCT of sertraline (median dose 150mg) vs placebo in chronic non-dialysis-dependent kidney disease, found no difference in change in depressive symptoms.[113] The ASCEND trial of sertraline vs CBT in patients on haemodialysis with depression found no significant differences between sertraline (to 200mg) and CBT in response and remission rates but QIDS-C depression scores at 12 weeks were lower for sertraline than CBT.[116] Another small RCT (ASSertID study) in patients with depression on haemodialysis reported no difference between sertraline and placebo.[117] Has been associated with serotonin syndrome when used in patents on haemodialysis. Case report of neutropenia when used in end stage renal disease.[118] May reduce CRP in patients on haemodialysis with depression[119] and a high CRP may predict response to sertraline (not placebo) in depression with chronic kidney disease.[120]
Trazodone[25,27,34,121]	<5% excreted unchanged in urine but care needed as approximately 70% of active metabolite also excreted. Dosing: GFR 20–50mL/min dose as normal renal function; GFR <20mL/min start with small dose and increase gradually; serotonin syndrome reported in a patient with chronic kidney disease on trazodone and duloxetine.[86] Has been trialled (unsuccessfully) for insomnia in haemodialysis, incidence of adverse events was higher with trazodone vs placebo.[122] Long-term use may be associated with an increased risk of chronic kidney disease.[123]
Trimipramine[27,34,36,62,124,125]	No dose reduction required in renal impairment; however, elevated urea, acute renal failure and interstitial nephritis have been reported. As with all tricyclic antidepressants in renal impairment, monitor patient for urinary retention, confusion, sedation and postural hypotension.

Table 8.9 (*Continued*)

Drug	Comments
Venlafaxine[25,34,36,126–128]	1–10% excreted unchanged in urine (30% as the active metabolite). Clearance is decreased and half-life prolonged in renal impairment. Dosing: GFR 30–90mL/min reduce by 25–50%; GFR <30mL/min reduce dose by at least 50%, consider alternate day dosing. Rhabdomyolyisis[129] and renal failure have been reported rarely with venlafaxine. Has been used to treat peripheral diabetic neuropathy in haemodialysis patients. High doses may cause hypertension.
Vortioxetine[25,130]	Negligible amounts are excreted unchanged in urine. Manufacturer advises that no dose adjustment is needed in renal impairment and end stage disease but advises caution due to a lack of data.

CBT, cognitive behavioural therapy; CRP, C-reactive protein; GFR, glomerular filtration rate; PPIs, proton pump inhibitors.

Table 8.10 Mood stabilisers in renal impairment.

Drug	Comments
Carbamazepine[25,27,34,131–134]	2–3% of dose excreted unchanged in urine. Dose reduction not necessary in renal disease, although cases of renal failure, tubular necrosis and tubulointerstitial nephritis have been reported rarely and metabolites may accumulate. Can cause Stevens–Johnson syndrome and toxic epidermal necrolysis, which may result in acute renal failure. Maintenance therapy in bipolar disorder is associated with an increased rate of chronic kidney disease.[21]
Lamotrigine[25,27,34,135–139]	<10% of lamotrigine excreted unchanged in urine. Single-dose studies in renal failure show pharmacokinetics are little affected; however, inactive metabolites can accumulate (effects unknown) and half-life can be prolonged. Renal failure and interstitial nephritis have also been reported. Dosing: GFR <10–50mL/min use cautiously, start with a low dose, increase slowly and monitor closely. One source suggests in GFR <10mL/min use 100mg every other day.
Lithium[25,27,34,36,140,141]	Lithium is nephrotoxic and contraindicated in severe renal impairment; 95% excreted unchanged in urine. Long-term treatment may result in impaired renal function in about a quarter of patients[142] ('creatinine creep'), permanent changes in kidney histology, microcysts, oncocytoma and collecting duct renal carcinoma, nephrogenic diabetes insipidus, nephrotic syndrome and both reversible and irreversible kidney damage.[143,144] However shorter studies in younger populations do not show declining GFR[145] or the development of end stage renal disease.[21,146,147] These differences may be due to methodology, improved monitoring and targeting recommended maintenance serum levels (0.6–0.8mmol/L in BPAD). Prevent nephrotoxicity by using once daily dosing, tightly adhering to recommended plasma levels, avoiding intoxication, assertively treating comorbidities and actively monitoring kidney function. Collaboration is vital between psychiatrist, nephrologist and patient in decision-making if chronic kidney disease occurs.[148] Risk factors for lithium-induced nephrotoxicity include increasing age, duration of treatment, cumulative dose, lower initial eGFR, female gender, hypertension and diabetes, concomitant nephrotoxic drugs, nephrogenic diabetes insipidus and previous lithium toxicity.[149] If lithium is used in renal impairment, toxicity is more likely and lithium toxicity increases the risk of renal impairment. Renal damage is more likely with chronic toxicity than acute. The manufacturer contraindicates lithium in severe renal impairment. Dosing: GFR 10–50mL/min avoid or reduce dose (50–75% of normal dose) and monitor levels; GFR <10mL/min avoid if possible, however if used it is essential to reduce dose (25–50% of normal dose). Lithium can be used successfully during haemodialysis.[150]

CHAPTER 8

Table 8.10 (Continued)

Drug	Comments
Valproate[25,27,34,151–155]	Approximately 2% excreted unchanged. Dose adjustment usually not required in renal impairment; however free valproate levels may be increased. Renal impairment, interstitial nephritis, Fanconi syndrome, renal tubular acidosis and renal failure have been reported. Risk factors for renal tubular dysfunction include being bedbound and low serum carnitine and phosphorus levels.[156] Dose as in normal renal function, however in severe impairment (GFR <10mL/min) it may be necessary to alter doses according to free (unbound) valproate levels. Possibly less likely than lithium to cause chronic kidney disease in patients with bipolar disorder[157,158] but data are conflicting.[159]

BPAD, bipolar affective disorder; eGFR, estimated glomerular filtration rate; GFR, glomerular filtration rate.

Table 8.11 Anxiolytics and hypnotics in renal impairment.

Drug	Comments
Buspirone[25,27,34,36]	<1% excreted unchanged; however, active metabolite is renally excreted. Dosing advice contradictory, suggests GFR 20–50mL/min start at a low dose and give twice daily; GFR <20mL/min avoid if possible due to accumulation of active metabolites; if essential, reduce dose by 25–50% if patient is anuric. Manufacturer contraindicates in severe renal impairment (GFR <20mL/min).
Chlordiazepoxide[25,27,36]	1–2% excreted unchanged but chlordiazepoxide has a long-acting active metabolite that can accumulate. Dosing: GFR 10–50mL/min dose as normal renal function; GFR <10mL/min reduce dose by 50%. Monitor for excessive sedation. Manufacturer cautions in chronic renal disease. Long-term use may be associated with an increased risk of CKD.[123]
Clomethiazole[25,27,34,160] (chlormethiazole)	0.1–5% of drug excreted unchanged in urine. Dose as in normal renal function but monitor for excessive sedation. Manufacturer recommends caution in renal disease.
Clonazepam[25,27,34,161]	<0.5% of clonazepam excreted unchanged in urine. Dose adjustment not required in impaired renal function; however with long-term administration, active metabolites may accumulate so start at a low dose and increase according to response. Monitor for excessive sedation. Has been used for insomnia in patients on haemodialysis. Long-term use may be associated with an increased risk of CKD.[123]
Diazepam[27,34,36,162]	<0.5% is excreted unchanged. Dosing: GFR 20–50mL/min dose as in normal renal function; GFR <20mL/min use small doses and titrate to response. Long-acting, active metabolites accumulate in renal impairment; monitor patients for excessive sedation and encephalopathy. One case of interstitial nephritis with diazepam has been reported in a patient with chronic renal failure. Long-term use may be associated with an increased risk of CKD.[123]
Eszopiclone[163]	<10% excreted unchanged in urine. No dose adjustment is needed in renal impairment.
Gabapentin	100% excreted unchanged in urine, clearance is reduced in renal impairment resulting in higher plasma concentrations and longer elimination half-lives.[164] As expected this may result in toxicity in renal impairment if doses are not reduced.[165] Acute renal failure has been reported,[166] as has myoclonus,[167] altered mental status, fall and fracture when used in patients on haemodialysis for restless legs, itch and neuropathic pain.[168,169] Has been used to treat pruritis, muscle cramps and restless legs syndrome in haemodialysis patients in RCTs.[170–172] Dosing advice differs: GFR 15–60mL/min start low and increase according to response; GFR <15mL/min 300mg alternate days[36,166] or 100mg at night then increase according to tolerability[27,173] but check for toxicity as described above. Manufacturer has table of very specific dosing in renal impairment in SMPC.[166]

Table 8.11 (*Continued*)

Drug	Comments
Lemborexant,[45,174] suvorexant, daridorexant	<1% excreted unchanged in urine. Manufacturers state no dose adjustment needed in renal impairment. Exposure to lemborexant may increase during severe renal impairment with a potential increased risk of somnolence.[175]
Lorazepam[25,27,34,36,176–181]	<1% excreted unchanged in urine, dose as in normal renal function but carefully according to response as some may need lower doses. Monitor for excessive sedation. Impaired elimination reported in two patients with severe renal impairment and also reports of propylene glycol in lorazepam injection causing renal impairment and acute tubular necrosis. However, lorazepam injection has been successfully used to treat catatonia in two patients with renal failure, and it is the drug of choice in status epilepticus for patients with renal disease.[182]
Melatonin	<1% excreted unchanged in urine. Manufacturers state limited information on use in renal impairment, but numerous studies suggest melatonin may be renoprotective in acute kidney injury and chronic renal disease[183,184] and beneficial for sleep in haemodialysis patients.[185,186] Dose as for normal renal function but monitor for oversedation in severe impairment.
Nitrazepam[25,27]	<5% excreted unchanged in urine. Dosing: GFR 10–50mL/min dose as in normal renal function; GFR <10mL/min start with small dose and increase slowly. Manufacturer advises reducing dose in renal impairment. Monitor patient for sedation and unsteadiness. Long-term use may be associated with an increased risk of CKD.[123]
Pregabalin	Up to 99% excreted unchanged in urine. Acute renal failure reported.[187] Associated with altered mental status and falls when used in patients on haemodialysis[168] and myoclonus.[188] Case report of seizure on abrupt cessation in patient with CKD.[189] Used to treat uraemic pruritis and neuropathic pain in patients on haemodialysis[190–192] and restless legs syndrome in CKD.[193] Dosing advice differs; titrate dosing by tolerability and response for all GFRs; initial dose for GFR 30–60mL/min 75mg daily and max. 300mg daily; GFR 15–30mL/min 25–50mg daily and max. 150mg daily; GFR <15mL/min 25mg daily and max. 75mg daily. Manufacturer has table of very specific dosing in renal impairment in SMPC.[187]
Oxazepam[27,34,36,194]	<1% excreted unchanged in urine. Dose adjustment may be needed in severe renal impairment. Oxazepam may take longer to reach steady state in patients with renal impairment. Dosing: GFR 10–50mL/min dose as in normal renal function; GFR <10mL/min start at a low dose and increase according to response. Monitor for excessive sedation.
Promethazine[25,27,34,36,195]	Dose reduction usually not necessary; however, promethazine has a long half-life so monitor for excessive sedative effects in patients with renal impairment. Manufacturer advises caution in renal impairment. There is a case report of interstitial nephritis in a patient who was a poor metaboliser of promethazine.
Temazepam[25,27,34,36]	<2% excreted unchanged in urine. In renal impairment the inactive metabolite can accumulate. Monitor for excessive sedative effects. Dosing: GFR 20–50mL/min dose as normal renal function; GFR <20mL/min dose as in normal renal function but start with 5mg.
Zolpidem[25,27,34,161,196]	Clearance moderately reduced in renal impairment. No dose adjustment required in renal impairment. Zolpidem 1mg has been used to treat insomnia in patients on haemodialysis. One trial of use as a sleep aid in haemodialysis patients with pruritus.[197] Associated with acute pyelonephritis in women.[198] Long-term use may be associated with an increased risk of CKD.[123]
Zopiclone[25,27,34,199,200]	<5% excreted unchanged in urine. Manufacturer states no accumulation of zopiclone in renal impairment but suggests starting at 3.75mg. Dosing: GFR <10mL/min start with lower dose. Interstitial nephritis reported rarely. Long-term use may be associated with an increased risk of CKD.[123]

CKD, chronic kidney disease; GFR, glomerular filtration rate; SMPC, summary of product characteristics.

CHAPTER 8

Table 8.12 Anti-dementia drugs in renal impairment.

Drug	Comments
Donepezil[25,27,201–203]	17% excreted unchanged in urine. Dosing is as in normal renal function for GFR ≤10–50mL/min. Manufacturer states that clearance not affected by renal impairment. Single-dose studies find similar pharmacokinetics in moderate and severe renal impairment compared with healthy controls. Has been used at a dose of 3mg/day in an elderly patient with Alzheimer's dementia on dialysis. Single case of rhabdomyolysis causing acute renal failure[204] and one of donepezil-induced parkinsonism in end stage renal disease.[205]
Galantamine[25,27]	18–22% excreted unchanged in urine. Dose as in normal renal function for GFR 9–50mL/min and at GFR <9mL/min start at a low dose and increase slowly. Maximum 16mg/day in moderate impairment. Manufacturer contraindicates use in GFR <9mL/min. Plasma levels may be increased in patients with moderate and severe renal impairment.
Memantine[25,34,206]	Manufacturers recommend a 10mg immediate release dose if GFR 5–29mL/min; 10mg daily for 7 days then increased to 20mg daily if tolerated for GFR 30–49mL/min; no dose adjustment required for GFR >50mL/min. Extended release dose is 14mg daily for GFR 5–29mL/min. Renal tubular acidosis, severe urinary tract infections and alkalisation of urine (e.g. by drastic dietary changes, such as switching from carnivore to vegetarian diet) can increase plasma levels of memantine. Acute renal failure has been reported, and one case of encephalopathy in chronic kidney disease.[207]
Rivastigmine[25,27]	0% excreted unchanged in urine but manufacturer states caution is required for patients with renal disease because of an increased risk of adverse effects. Dosing advice for GFR <50mL/min start at a low dose and gradually increase. Steady-state plasma concentrations are not affected by renal function.[208]

GFR, glomerular filtration rate.

Table 8.13 Other psychotropic drugs in renal impairment.

Drug	Comments
Bremelanotide[45,209]	64.8% excreted unchanged in urine. Manufacturer states GFR 30–89mL/min no dosage adjustment necessary; caution for GFR <30mL/min as increased adverse effects (nausea and vomiting). Exposure is increased in renal impairment. Case report of Melotan II (bremelanotide is a variation of Melotan II) and rhabdomyolysis and renal dysfunction.[210]
Deutetrabenazine[211]	No clinical studies in renal impairment. Data limited, no specific dosing advice.
Pitolisant[45,212]	<2% excreted unchanged in urine. Dosing: GFR 15–59mL/min 8.9mg daily, increase after 7 days to max. 17.8mg once daily;[213] GFR <15mL/min not recommended.[213] Peak concentrations and exposure increased in all stages of renal impairment.
Solriamfetol[45,214]	95% excreted unchanged in urine. Dosing: GFR 60–89mL/min no dose adjustment is required; GFR 30–59mL/min 37.5mg once daily, increased to max. of 75mg once daily after 5 days; GFR 15–29mL/min 37.5mg once daily; GFR <15mL/min not recommended. In moderate or severe renal impairment risk of increased blood pressure and heart rate because of the prolonged half-life. Increased exposure and $t_{1/2}$ in all stages of renal impairment particularly end stage renal disease.[215]
Valbenazine[45]	<2% excreted unchanged in urine. No adjustment is necessary. Urinary retention reported as adverse effect in clinical trials.

GFR, glomerular filtration rate.

Table 8.14 Attention deficit hyperactivity disorder (ADHD) drugs in renal impairment.

Drug	Comments
Atomoxetine[24,216]	No dose adjustment required. Atomoxetine may exacerbate hypertension in patients with end stage renal disease.
Dexamfetamine[24,217]	30–40% excreted unchanged in normal urine pH (renal elimination is decreased under alkaline conditions, increased under acidic conditions). Limited data in renal disease, manufacturers state that peak plasma levels could be higher and elimination prolonged. For the transdermal patch: GFR 15–30mL/min max. dose 13.5mg/9 hours; GFR <15mL/min max. dose 9mg/9 hours. For oral dosing: start at low doses and increase cautiously.
Lisdexamfetamine[24,218]	Reduced clearance in patients with severe renal insufficiency. GFR 15–30mL/min max. dose 50mg/day; GFR <15mL/min max. dose 30mg/day.[219]
Methylphenidate[24,220]	<1% excreted unchanged in urine. Limited data in renal disease, but pharmacokinetics suggest dose adjustment is unlikely to be necessary. Two case reports (one in a patient undergoing peritoneal dialysis) suggest no change in clearance of methylphenidate in end stage renal disease.[221] One case report of use in polycystic kidney disease.[222]

GFR, glomerular filtration rate.

Summary of recommended psychotropics in renal impairment

Where renal function declines while on existing drug treatment, rule out existing drugs as a cause of reduced function and continue at a dose suggested in Tables 8.9–8.14. Where new drug treatment is required follow the suggestions in Table 8.15.

Table 8.15 Recommended psychotropics in renal impairment.

Drug group	Recommended drugs
Antipsychotics	No agent clearly preferred to another, however: ■ Avoid sulpiride and amisulpride ■ Avoid highly anticholinergic agents because they can contribute to urinary retention ■ First-generation antipsychotic – suggest **haloperidol** 2–6mg a day ■ Second-generation antipsychotic – suggest **olanzapine** 5mg a day
Antidepressants[223]	No agent clearly preferred to another, however reasonable choices are: ■ **Sertraline** but poor efficacy data in renal disease ■ **Citalopram** (NB QTc-prolonging effects and greater risk of sudden death in those on haemodialysis vs other selective serotonin reuptake inhibitors) ■ **Fluoxetine** but consider long half-life and need for alternate day dosing at lower GFRs
Mood stabilisers	No agent clearly preferred to another, however: ■ Avoid lithium if possible ■ Suggest start one of the following at a low dose and increase slowly, monitor for adverse effects: **valproate** or **lamotrigine**
Anxiolytics and hypnotics	No agent clearly preferred to another, however: ■ Excessive sedation is more likely to occur in patients with renal impairment, so monitor all patients carefully ■ **Lorazepam** and **zopiclone** are suggested as reasonable choices
Anti-dementia drugs	No agent clearly preferred to another, however: ■ **Rivastigmine** is a reasonable choice

GFR, glomerular filtration rate.

CHAPTER 8

References

1. National Institute for Health and Care Excellence. Chronic kidney disease: assessment and management NICE Guideline [NG203]. 2021 (last checked May 2024); https://www.nice.org.uk/guidance/ng203.
2. Levey AS, et al. A new equation to estimate glomerular filtration rate. *Ann Intern Med* 2009; **150**:604–612.
3. Tangri N, et al. A predictive model for progression of chronic kidney disease to kidney failure. *JAMA* 2011; **305**:1553–1559.
4. Brater DC. Measurement of renal function during drug development. *Br J Clin Pharmacol* 2002; **54**:87–95.
5. Chinnadurai R, et al. Impact of chronic kidney disease on the drugs eliminated predominantly through a non-renal route: a proof of concept study with citalopram. *Nephrol Dial Transplant* 2019; **34**:gfz103.SP268.
6. Toprak O, et al. New-onset type II diabetes mellitus, hyperosmolar non-ketotic coma, rhabdomyolysis and acute renal failure in a patient treated with sulpiride. *Nephrol Dial Transplant* 2005; **20**:662–663.
7. Baumgart U, et al. Olanzapine-induced acute rhabdomyolysis—a case report. *Pharmacopsychiatry* 2005; **38**:36–37.
8. Marsh SJ, et al. Rhabdomyolysis and acute renal failure during high-dose haloperidol therapy. *Ren Fail* 1995; **17**:475–478.
9. Smith RP, et al. Quetiapine overdose and severe rhabdomyolysis. *J Clin Psychopharmacol* 2004; **24**:343.
10. Nagler EV, et al. Antidepressants for depression in stage 3–5 chronic kidney disease: a systematic review of pharmacokinetics, efficacy and safety with recommendations by European Renal Best Practice (ERBP). *Nephrol Dial Transplant* 2012; **27**:3736–3745.
11. Palmer SC, et al. Antidepressants for treating depression in adults with end-stage kidney disease treated with dialysis. *Cochrane Database Syst Rev* 2016; **5**:CD004541.
12. Dev V, et al. Higher anti-depressant dose and major adverse outcomes in moderate chronic kidney disease: a retrospective population-based study. *BMC Nephrol* 2014; **15**:79.
13. Guirguis A, et al. Antidepressant usage in haemodialysis patients: evidence of sub-optimal practice patterns. *J Ren Care* 2020; **46**:124–132.
14. Farrokhi F, et al. Association between depression and mortality in patients receiving long-term dialysis: a systematic review and meta-analysis. *Am J Kidney Dis* 2014; **63**:623–635.
15. Lopes AA, et al. Depression as a predictor of mortality and hospitalization among hemodialysis patients in the United States and Europe. *Kidney Int* 2002; **62**:199–207.
16. Wu PH, et al. Depression amongst patients commencing maintenance dialysis is associated with increased risk of death and severe infections: a nationwide cohort study. *PLoS One* 2019; **14**:e0218335.
17. Saglimbene V, et al. Depression and all-cause and cardiovascular mortality in patients on haemodialysis: a multinational cohort study. *Nephrol Dial Transplant* 2017; **32**:377–384.
18. Natale P, et al. Psychosocial interventions for preventing and treating depression in dialysis patients. *Cochrane Database Syst Rev* 2019; **12**:CD004542.
19. Vangala C, et al. Selective serotonin reuptake inhibitor use and hip fracture risk among patients on hemodialysis. *Am J Kidney Dis* 2020; **75**:351–360.
20. Tzeng NS, et al. Is schizophrenia associated with an increased risk of chronic kidney disease? A nationwide matched-cohort study. *BMJ Open* 2015; **5**:e006777.
21. Kessing LV, et al. Use of lithium and anticonvulsants and the rate of chronic kidney disease: a nationwide population-based study. *JAMA Psychiatry* 2015; **72**:1182–1191.
22. Jiang Y, et al. A retrospective cohort study of acute kidney injury risk associated with antipsychotics. *CNS Drugs* 2017; **31**:319–326.
23. Ryan PB, et al. Atypical antipsychotics and the risks of acute kidney injury and related outcomes among older adults: a replication analysis and an evaluation of adapted confounding control strategies. *Drugs Aging* 2017; **34**:211–219.
24. IBM Watson Health. IBM Micromedex solutions. 2024 (accessed May 2024); https://www.ibm.com/watson-health/about/micromedex.
25. EMC. Summaries of product characteristics. 2024; https://www.medicines.org.uk/emc.
26. Noble S, et al. Amisulpride: a review of its clinical potential in dysthymia. *CNS Drugs* 1999; **12**:471–483.
27. Taylor & Francis Group. Renal drug database. 2024 (accessed May 2024); https://renaldrugdatabase.com.
28. Li A, et al. Population pharmacokinetics of amisulpride in Chinese patients with schizophrenia with external validation: the impact of renal function. *Front Pharmacol* 2023; **14**:1215065.
29. Aragona M. Tolerability and efficacy of aripiprazole in a case of psychotic anorexia nervosa comorbid with epilepsy and chronic renal failure. *Eat Weight Disord* 2007; **12**:e54–e57.
30. Mallikaarjun S, et al. Effects of hepatic or renal impairment on the pharmacokinetics of aripiprazole. *Clin Pharmacokinet* 2008; **47**:533–542.
31. Tzeng NS, et al. Delusional parasitosis in a patient with brain atrophy and renal failure treated with aripiprazole: case report. *Prog Neuropsychopharmacol Biol Psychiatry* 2010; **34**:1148–1149.
32. De Donatis D, et al. Serum aripiprazole concentrations prehemodialysis and posthemodialysis in a schizophrenic patient with chronic renal failure: a case report. *J Clin Psychopharmacol* 2020; **40**:200–202.
33. Peeters P, et al. Asenapine pharmacokinetics in hepatic and renal impairment. *Clin Pharmacokinet* 2011; **50**:471–481.
34. Merative US L.P. Micromedex. 2024 (accessed May 2024); https://www.micromedexsolutions.com/home/dispatch.
35. Fabre J, et al. Influence of renal insufficiency on the excretion of chloroquine, phenobarbital, phenothiazines and methacycline. *Helv Med Acta* 1967; **33**:307–316.
36. Aronoff GR, et al. *Drug Prescribing in Renal Failure: Dosing Guidelines for Adults and Children*, 5th edn. Philadelphia: American College of Physicians; 2007.
37. Fraser D, et al. An unexpected and serious complication of treatment with the atypical antipsychotic drug clozapine. *Clin Nephrol* 2000; **54**:78–80.
38. Au AF, et al. Clozapine-induced acute interstitial nephritis. *Am J Psychiatry* 2004; **161**:1501.

39. Elias TJ, et al. Clozapine-induced acute interstitial nephritis. *Lancet* 1999; **354**:1180–1181.
40. Siddiqui BK, et al. Simultaneous allergic interstitial nephritis and cardiomyopathy in a patient on clozapine. *NDT Plus* 2008; **1**:55–56.
41. Davis EAK, et al. Clozapine-associated renal failure: a case report and literature review. *Ment Health Clin* 2019; **9**:124–127.
42. Lim AM, et al. Clozapine, immunosuppressants and renal transplantation. *Asian J Psychiatr* 2016; **23**:118.
43. Lobeck F, et al. Haloperidol concentrations in an elderly patient with moderate chronic renal failure. *J Geriatric Drug Ther* 1986; **1**:91–97.
44. Cohen LM, et al. Update on psychotropic medication use in renal disease. *Psychosomatics* 2004; **45**:34–48.
45. Lendac Data Systems Ltd. Drugdex systems. 2024 (accessed May 2024); https://www.drugdiscoveryonline.com/doc/drugdex-system-0001.
46. Intra-Cellular Therapies Inc. Highlights of prescribing information. Caplyta (lumateperone) capsules for oral use. 2019 (last accessed May 2024); https://www.accessdata.fda.gov/drugsatfda_docs/label/2019/209500s000lbl.pdf.
47. Kansagra A, et al. Prolonged hypothermia due to olanzapine in the setting of renal failure: a case report and review of the literature. *Ther Adv Psychopharmacol* 2013; **3**:335–339.
48. Samalin L, et al. Interest of clozapine and paliperidone palmitate plasma concentrations to monitor treatment in schizophrenic patients on chronic hemodialysis. *Schizophr Res* 2015; **166**:351–352.
49. Lin JH, et al. Long-acting injectable paliperidone palmitate in a haemodialysis patient with schizophrenia. *Aust NZ J Psychiatry* 2021; **55**:829–830.
50. ACADIA Pharmaceuticals Inc. Highlights of prescribing information. Nuplazid (pimavanserin) tablets for oral use. 2016 (last accessed May 2024); https://www.accessdata.fda.gov/drugsatfda_docs/label/2016/207318lbl.pdf.
51. Thyrum PT, et al. Single-dose pharmacokinetics of quetiapine in subjects with renal or hepatic impairment. *Prog Neuropsychopharmacol Biol Psychiatry* 2000; **24**:521–533.
52. Huynh M, et al. Thrombotic thrombocytopenic purpura associated with quetiapine. *Ann Pharmacother* 2005; **39**:1346–1348.
53. Torroba Sanz B, et al. Permanent renal sequelae secondary to drug reaction with eosinophilia and systemic symptoms (DRESS) syndrome induced by quetiapine. *Eur J Hosp Pharm* 2020; **5**:285–288.
54. Snoeck E, et al. Influence of age, renal and liver impairment on the pharmacokinetics of risperidone in man. *Psychopharmacology (Berl)* 1995; **122**:223–229.
55. Herguner S, et al. Steroid-induced psychosis in an adolescent: treatment and prophylaxis with risperidone. *Turk J Pediatr* 2006; **48**:244–247.
56. Batalla A, et al. Antipsychotic treatment in a patient with schizophrenia undergoing hemodialysis. *J Clin Psychopharmacol* 2010; **30**:92–94.
57. Tourtellotte R, et al. Use of therapeutic drug monitoring of risperidone microspheres long-acting injection in hemodialysis: a case report. *Ment Health Clin* 2019; **9**:404–407.
58. Bressolle F, et al. Pharmacokinetics of sulpiride after intravenous administration in patients with impaired renal function. *Clin Pharmacokinet* 1989; **17**:367–373.
59. Aweeka F, et al. The pharmacokinetics of ziprasidone in subjects with normal and impaired renal function. *Br J Clin Pharmacol* 2000; **49**:27S–33S.
60. Roerig. Highlights of prescribing information: GEODON® (ziprasidone HCl) capsules; GEODON® (ziprasidone mesylate) injection for intramuscular use. 2021 (last accessed May 2024); http://labeling.pfizer.com/ShowLabeling.aspx?id=584.
61. Iskandar JW, et al. Transient agranulocytosis associated with ziprasidone in a 45-year-old man on hemodialysis. *J Clin Psychopharmacol* 2015; **35**:347–348.
62. Lieberman JA, et al. Tricyclic antidepressant and metabolite levels in chronic renal failure. *Clin Pharmacol Ther* 1985; **37**:301–307.
63. Murphy EJ. Acute pain management pharmacology for the patient with concurrent renal or hepatic disease. *Anaesth Intensive Care* 2005; **33**:311–322.
64. Chen TY, et al. Amitriptyline-induced acute kidney injury and acute hepatitis: a case report. *Am J Ther* 2021; **28**:e256–e258.
65. Sage Therapeutics Inc. Highlights of prescribing information. Zulresso (brexanolone) injection for intravenous use [controlled substance schedule pending]. 2019 (last checked May 2024); https://www.accessdata.fda.gov/drugsatfda_docs/label/2019/211371lbl.pdf.
66. Turpeinen M, et al. Effect of renal impairment on the pharmacokinetics of bupropion and its metabolites. *Br J Clin Pharmacol* 2007; **64**:165–173.
67. Worrall SP, et al. Pharmacokinetics of bupropion and its metabolites in haemodialysis patients who smoke. A single dose study. *Nephron Clin Pract* 2004; **97**:c83–c89.
68. Ghoreishi A, et al. Bupropion as a treatment for sexual dysfunction among chronic kidney disease patients. *Acta Med Iran* 2019; **57**:320–327.
69. Joffe P, et al. Single-dose pharmacokinetics of citalopram in patients with moderate renal insufficiency or hepatic cirrhosis compared with healthy subjects. *Eur J Clin Pharmacol* 1998; **54**:237–242.
70. Kalender B, et al. Antidepressant treatment increases quality of life in patients with chronic renal failure. *Ren Fail* 2007; **29**:817–822.
71. Kelly CA, et al. Adult respiratory distress syndrome and renal failure associated with citalopram overdose. *Hum Exp Toxicol* 2003; **22**:103–105.
72. Spigset O, et al. Citalopram pharmacokinetics in patients with chronic renal failure and the effect of haemodialysis. *Eur J Clin Pharmacol* 2000; **56**:699–703.
73. Hosseini SH, et al. Citalopram versus psychological training for depression and anxiety symptoms in hemodialysis patients. *Iran J Kidney Dis* 2012; **6**:446–451.
74. Sran H, et al. Confusion after starting citalopram in a renal transplant patient. *BMJ Case Rep* 2013; **2013**:bcr2013010511.
75. Assimon MM, et al. Comparative cardiac safety of selective serotonin reuptake inhibitors among individuals receiving maintenance hemodialysis. *J Am Soc Nephrol* 2019; **30**:611–623.

CHAPTER 8

76. Assimon MM, et al. Proton pump inhibitors may enhance the risk of citalopram- and escitalopram-associated sudden cardiac death among patients receiving hemodialysis. *Pharmacoepidemiol Drug Saf* 2022; 31:670–679.
77. Assimon MM, et al. The modifying effect of the serum-to-dialysate potassium gradient on the cardiovascular safety of SSRIs in the hemodialysis population: a pharmacoepidemiologic study. *Nephrol Dial Transplant* 2022; 37:2241–2252.
78. Onishi A, et al. Reversible acute renal failure associated with clomipramine-induced interstitial nephritis. *Clin Exp Nephrol* 2007; 11:241–243.
79. Wyeth Pharmaceuticals Inc. Highlights of prescribing information. PRISTIQ® (desvenlafaxine) extended-release tablets, for oral use. 2023 (last checked May 2024); http://labeling.pfizer.com/showlabeling.aspx?id=497%20.
80. Nichols AI, et al. The pharmacokinetics and safety of desvenlafaxine in subjects with chronic renal impairment. *Int J Clin Pharmacol Ther* 2011; 49:3–13.
81. Rees JA. Clinical interpretation of pharmacokinetic data on dothiepin hydrochloride (Dosulepin, Prothiaden). *J Int Med Res* 1981; 9:98–102.
82. Swarna SS, et al. Pruritus associated with chronic kidney disease: a comprehensive literature review. *Cureus* 2019; 11:e5256.
83. Lobo ED, et al. Effects of varying degrees of renal impairment on the pharmacokinetics of duloxetine: analysis of a single-dose phase I study and pooled steady-state data from phase II/III trials. *Clin Pharmacokinet* 2010; 49:311–321.
84. Ho NV, et al. Duloxetine-induced multi-system organ failure: a case report. Poster presented at American Geriatrics Society Annual Meeting, May 11–15, 2011, National Harbor, Maryland; 2011.
85. Nguyen T, et al. Duloxetine uses in patients with kidney disease: different recommendations from the United States versus Europe and Canada. *Am J Ther* 2019; 26:e516–e519.
86. Uong C, et al. Poster 91. Serotonin syndrome in chronic kidney disease patient after given a dose of duloxetine while on trazodone: a case report. *PM&R* 2014; 6 Suppl:S214–S215.
87. Miriyala K, et al. Renal failure in a depressed adolescent on escitalopram. *J Child Adolesc Psychopharmacol* 2008; 18:405–408.
88. Adiga GU, et al. Renal tubular defects from antidepressant use in an older adult: an uncommon but reversible adverse drug effect. *Clin Drug Invest* 2006; 26:607–610.
89. Yazici AE, et al. Efficacy and tolerability of escitalopram in depressed patients with end stage renal disease: an open placebo-controlled study. *Bull Clin Psychopharmacol* 2012; 22:23–30.
90. Bergstrom RF, et al. The effects of renal and hepatic disease on the pharmacokinetics, renal tolerance, and risk-benefit profile of fluoxetine. *Int Clin Psychopharmacol* 1993; 8:261–266.
91. Blumenfield M, et al. Fluoxetine in depressed patients on dialysis. *Int J Psychiatry Med* 1997; 27:71–80.
92. Levy NB, et al. Fluoxetine in depressed patients with renal failure and in depressed patients with normal kidney function. *Gen Hosp Psychiatry* 1996; 18:8–13.
93. Kauffman KM, et al. Higher dose weekly fluoxetine in hemodialysis patients: a case series report. *Int J Psychiatry Med* 2021; 56:3–13.
94. Constantino JL, et al. Pharmacokinetics of antidepressants in patients undergoing hemodialysis: a narrative literature review. *Braz J Psychiatry* 2019; 41:441–446.
95. Lancaster SG, et al. Lofepramine. A review of its pharmacodynamic and pharmacokinetic properties, and therapeutic efficacy in depressive illness. *Drugs* 1989; 37:123–140.
96. Davis MP, et al. Mirtazapine for pruritus. *J Pain Symptom Manage* 2003; 25:288–291.
97. Fawaz B, et al. Defining the role of mirtazapine in the treatment of refractory pruritus. *J Dermatolog Treat* 2021; 32:132–136.
98. Liles AM, et al. Appetite stimulants for treatment of protein energy wasting of chronic kidney disease. *Nephrol Nurs J* 2021; 48:267–273.
99. Shibata K, et al. SP704 The effect of mirtazapine in dialysis patient with appetite loss. *Nephrol Dial Transplant* 2015; 30 Suppl 3:iii611.
100. Schoerlin MP, et al. Disposition kinetics of moclobemide, a new MAO-A inhibitor, in subjects with impaired renal function. *J Clin Pharmacol* 1990; 30:272–284.
101. Stoeckel K, et al. Absorption and disposition of moclobemide in patients with advanced age or reduced liver or kidney function. *Acta Psychiatr Scand Suppl* 1990; 360:94–97.
102. Pollock BG, et al. Metabolic and physiologic consequences of nortriptyline treatment in the elderly. *Psychopharmacol Bull* 1994; 30:145–150.
103. Doyle GD, et al. The pharmacokinetics of paroxetine in renal impairment. *Acta Psychiatr Scand Suppl* 1989; 350:89–90.
104. Ishii T, et al. A rare case of combined syndrome of inappropriate antidiuretic hormone secretion and Fanconi syndrome in an elderly woman. *Am J Kidney Dis* 2006; 48:155–158.
105. Kaye CM, et al. A review of the metabolism and pharmacokinetics of paroxetine in man. *Acta Psychiatr Scand Suppl* 1989; 350:60–75.
106. Koo JR, et al. Treatment of depression and effect of antidepression treatment on nutritional status in chronic hemodialysis patients. *Am J Med Sci* 2005; 329:1–5.
107. Coulomb F, et al. Pharmacokinetics of single-dose reboxetine in volunteers with renal insufficiency. *J Clin Pharmacol* 2000; 40:482–487.
108. Dostert P, et al. Review of the pharmacokinetics and metabolism of reboxetine, a selective noradrenaline reuptake inhibitor. *Eur Neuropsychopharmacol* 1997; 7 Suppl 1:S23–S35.
109. Brewster UC, et al. Addition of sertraline to other therapies to reduce dialysis-associated hypotension. *Nephrology (Carlton)* 2003; 8:296–301.
110. Chan KY, et al. Use of sertraline for antihistamine-refractory uremic pruritus in renal palliative care patients. *J Palliat Med* 2013; 16:966–970.
111. Chander WP, et al. Serotonin syndrome in maintenance haemodialysis patients following sertraline treatment for depression. *J Indian Med Assoc* 2011; 109:36–37.
112. Jain N, et al. Rationale and design of the Chronic Kidney Disease Antidepressant Sertraline Trial (CAST). *Contemp Clin Trials* 2013; 34:136–144.

113. Hedayati SS, et al. Effect of sertraline on depressive symptoms in patients with chronic kidney disease without dialysis dependence: the CAST randomized clinical trial. *JAMA* 2017; **318**:1876–1890.

114. Razeghi E, et al. A randomized crossover clinical trial of sertraline for intradialytic hypotension. *Iran J Kidney Dis* 2015; **9**:323–330.

115. Elsayed MM, et al. The effectiveness of sertraline in alleviating uremic pruritus in hemodialysis patients: a randomized clinical trial. *BMC Nephrol* 2023; **24**:155.

116. Mehrotra R, et al. Comparative efficacy of therapies for treatment of depression for patients undergoing maintenance hemodialysis: a randomized clinical trial. *Ann Intern Med* 2019; **170**:369–379.

117. Friedli K, et al. Sertraline versus placebo in patients with major depressive disorder undergoing hemodialysis: a randomized, controlled feasibility trial. *Clin J Am Soc Nephrol* 2017; **12**:280–286.

118. Chien CW, et al. Sertraline-induced neutropenia and fatigue in a patient with end-stage renal disease. *Am J Ther* 2020; **29**:e101–e103.

119. Zahed NS, et al. Impact of sertraline on serum concentration of CRP in hemodialysis patients with depression. *J Ren Injury Prevent* 2017; **6**:65–69.

120. Gregg LP, et al. Inflammation and response to sertraline treatment in patients with CKD and major depression. *Am J Kidney Dis* 2020; **75**:457–460.

121. Catanese B, et al. A comparative study of trazodone serum concentrations in patients with normal or impaired renal function. *Boll Chim Farm* 1978; **117**:424–427.

122. Mehrotra R, et al. Effectiveness of existing insomnia therapies for patients undergoing hemodialysis: a randomized clinical trial. *Ann Intern Med* 2024; **177**:177–188.

123. Liao CY, et al. Taking sleeping pills and the risk of chronic kidney disease: a nationwide population-based retrospective cohort study. *Front Pharmacol* 2021; **11**:524113.

124. Leighton JD, et al. Trimipramine-induced acute renal failure (Letter). *NZ Med J* 1986; **99**:248.

125. Simpson GM, et al. A preliminary study of trimipramine in chronic schizophrenia. *Curr Ther Res Clin Exp* 1966; **99**:248.

126. Troy SM, et al. The effect of renal disease on the disposition of venlafaxine. *Clin Pharmacol Ther* 1994; **56**:14–21.

127. Guldiken S, et al. Complete relief of pain in acute painful diabetic neuropathy of rapid glycaemic control (insulin neuritis) with venlafaxine HCL. *Diabetes Nutr Metab* 2004; **17**:247–249.

128. Pascale P, et al. Severe rhabdomyolysis following venlafaxine overdose. *Ther Drug Monit* 2005; **27**:562–564.

129. Ren J, et al. Venlafaxine-associated rhabdomyolysis: a literature review. *J Clin Psychopharmacol* 2024; **44**:297–301.

130. Takeda Pharmaceuticals America Inc. Highlights of prescribing information. BRINTELLIX (vortioxetine) tablets 2023 (last accessed May 2024); www.us.brintellix.com.

131. Hegarty J, et al. Carbamazepine-induced acute granulomatous interstitial nephritis. *Clin Nephrol* 2002; **57**:310–313.

132. Tutor-Crespo MJ, et al. Relative proportions of serum carbamazepine and its pharmacologically active 10,11-epoxy derivative: effect of polytherapy and renal insufficiency. *Ups J Med Sci* 2008; **113**:171–180.

133. Verrotti A, et al. Renal tubular function in patients receiving anticonvulsant therapy: a long-term study. *Epilepsia* 2000; **41**:1432–1435.

134. Hung CC, et al. Acute renal failure and its risk factors in Stevens-Johnson syndrome and toxic epidermal necrolysis. *Am J Nephrol* 2009; **29**:633–638.

135. Fervenza FC, et al. Acute granulomatous interstitial nephritis and colitis in anticonvulsant hypersensitivity syndrome associated with lamotrigine treatment. *Am J Kidney Dis* 2000; **36**:1034–1040.

136. Fillastre JP, et al. Pharmacokinetics of lamotrigine in patients with renal impairment: influence of haemodialysis. *Drugs Exp Clin Res* 1993; **19**:25–32.

137. Schaub JE, et al. Multisystem adverse reaction to lamotrigine. *Lancet* 1994; **344**:481.

138. Wootton R, et al. Comparison of the pharmacokinetics of lamotrigine in patients with chronic renal failure and healthy volunteers. *Br J Clin Pharmacol* 1997; **43**:23–27.

139. Bansal AD, et al. Use of antiepileptic drugs in patients with chronic kidney disease and end stage renal disease. *Semin Dial* 2015; **28**:404–412.

140. Gitlin M. Lithium and the kidney: an updated review. *Drug Saf* 1999; **20**:231–243.

141. Lepkifker E, et al. Renal insufficiency in long-term lithium treatment. *J Clin Psychiatry* 2004; **65**:850–856.

142. Schoretsanitis G, et al. Prevalence of impaired kidney function in patients with long-term lithium treatment: a systematic review and meta-analysis. *Bipolar Disord* 2022; **24**:264–274.

143. McKnight RF, et al. Lithium toxicity profile: a systematic review and meta-analysis. *Lancet* 2012; **379**:721–728.

144. Shine B, et al. Long-term effects of lithium on renal, thyroid, and parathyroid function: a retrospective analysis of laboratory data. *Lancet* 2015; **386**:461–468.

145. Clos S, et al. Long-term effect of lithium maintenance therapy on estimated glomerular filtration rate in patients with affective disorders: a population-based cohort study. *Lancet Psychiatry* 2015; **2**:1075–1083.

146. Kessing LV, et al. Lithium versus anticonvulsants and the risk of physical disorders – results from a comprehensive long-term nation-wide population-based study emulating a target trial. *Eur Neuropsychopharmacol* 2024; **84**:48–56.

147. Bosi A, et al. Absolute and relative risks of kidney outcomes associated with lithium vs valproate use in Sweden. *JAMA Network Open* 2023; **6**:e2322056.

148. Schoot TS, et al. Systematic review and practical guideline for the prevention and management of the renal side effects of lithium therapy. *Eur Neuropsychopharmacol* 2020; **31**:16–32.

149. Davis J, et al. Lithium and nephrotoxicity: a literature review of approaches to clinical management and risk stratification. *BMC Nephrol* 2018; **19**:305.

150. Kuiper WJ, et al. Concurrent lithium and haemodialysis treatment: clinical recommendations based on the literature and a multicentre survey. *Bipolar Disord* 2024; **26**:335–347.

151. Smith GC, et al. Anticonvulsants as a cause of Fanconi syndrome. *Nephrol Dial Transplant* 1995; **10**:543–545.
152. Fukuda Y, et al. Immunologically mediated chronic tubulo-interstitial nephritis caused by valproate therapy. *Nephron* 1996; **72**:328–329.
153. Watanabe T, et al. Secondary renal Fanconi syndrome caused by valproate therapy. *Pediatr Nephrol* 2005; **20**:814–817.
154. Tanaka H, et al. Distal type of renal tubular acidosis after anti-epileptic therapy in a girl with infantile spasms. *Clin Exp Nephrol* 1999; 3:311–313.
155. Rahman MH, et al. Acute hemolysis with acute renal failure in a patient with valproic acid poisoning treated with charcoal hemoperfusion. *Hemodial Int* 2006; **10**:256–259.
156. Koga S, et al. Risk factors for sodium valproate-induced renal tubular dysfunction. *Clin Exp Nephrol* 2018; **22**:420–425.
157. Hayes JF, et al. Adverse renal, endocrine, hepatic, and metabolic events during maintenance mood stabilizer treatment for bipolar disorder: a population-based cohort study. *PLoS Med* 2016; **13**:e1002058.
158. Damba JJ, et al. Psychotropic drugs and adverse kidney effects: a systematic review of the past decade of research. *CNS Drugs* 2022; **36**:1049–1077.
159. Kessing LV, et al. Continuation of lithium after a diagnosis of chronic kidney disease. *Acta Psychiatr Scand* 2017; **136**:615–622.
160. Pentikainen PJ, et al. Pharmacokinetics of chlormethiazole in healthy volunteers and patients with cirrhosis of the liver. *Eur J Clin Pharmacol* 1980; **17**:275–284.
161. Dashti-Khavidaki S, et al. Comparing effects of clonazepam and zolpidem on sleep quality of patients on maintenance hemodialysis. *Iran J Kidney Dis* 2011; 5:404–409.
162. Sadjadi SA, et al. Allergic interstitial nephritis due to diazepam. *Arch Intern Med* 1987; **147**:579.
163. Sunovion Pharmaceuticals Inc. Highlights of prescribing information. LUNESTA® (eszopiclone) tablets, for oral use. 2014 (last accessed May 2024); https://www.accessdata.fda.gov/drugsatfda_docs/label/2014/021476s030lbl.pdf.
164. Blum RA, et al. Pharmacokinetics of gabapentin in subjects with various degrees of renal function. *Clin Pharmacol Ther* 1994; **56**:154–159.
165. Miller A, et al. Gabapentin toxicity in renal failure: the importance of dose adjustment. *Pain Med* 2009; **10**:190–192.
166. Upjohn UK Limited. Summary of product characteristics. Neurontin (gabapentin) 600mg film-coated tablets. 2023 (last accessed May 2024); https://www.medicines.org.uk/emc/product/3197/smpc.
167. Yeddi A, et al. Myoclonus and altered mental status induced by single dose of gabapentin in a patient with end-stage renal disease: a case report and literature review. *Am J Ther* 2019; **26**:e768–e770.
168. Ishida JH, et al. Gabapentin and pregabalin use and association with adverse outcomes among hemodialysis patients. *J Am Soc Nephrol* 2018; **29**:1970–1978.
169. Gobo-Oliveira M, et al. Gabapentin versus dexchlorpheniramine as treatment for uremic pruritus: a randomised controlled trial. *Eur J Dermatol* 2018; **28**:488–495.
170. Gunal AI, et al. Gabapentin therapy for pruritus in haemodialysis patients: a randomized, placebo-controlled, double-blind trial. *Nephrol Dial Transplant* 2004; **19**:3137–3139.
171. Beladi Mousavi SS, et al. The effect of gabapentin on muscle cramps during hemodialysis: a double-blind clinical trial. *Saudi J Kidney Dis Transpl* 2015; **26**:1142–1148.
172. Razazian N, et al. Gabapentin versus levodopa-c for the treatment of restless legs syndrome in hemodialysis patients: a randomized clinical trial. *Saudi J Kidney Dis Transpl* 2015; **26**:271–278.
173. Rossi GM, et al. Randomized trial of two after-dialysis gabapentin regimens for severe uremic pruritus in hemodialysis patients. *Intern Emerg Med* 2019; **14**:1341–1346.
174. Eisai Inc. Highlights of prescribing information. Dayvigo (lemborexant) tablets for oral use [controlled substance schedule pending]. 2019 (last accessed May 2024); https://www.accessdata.fda.gov/drugsatfda_docs/label/2019/212028s000lbl.pdf.
175. Landry I, et al. Effect of severe renal impairment on pharmacokinetics, safety, and tolerability of lemborexant. *Pharmacol Res Perspect* 2021; **9**:e00734.
176. Huang CE, et al. Intramuscular lorazepam in catatonia in patients with acute renal failure: a report of two cases. *Chang Gung Med J* 2010; 33:106–109.
177. Reynolds HN, et al. Hyperlactatemia, increased osmolar gap, and renal dysfunction during continuous lorazepam infusion. *Crit Care Med* 2000; **28**:1631–1634.
178. Verbeeck RK, et al. Impaired elimination of lorazepam following subchronic administration in two patients with renal failure. *Br J Clin Pharmacol* 1981; **12**:749–751.
179. Yaucher NE, et al. Propylene glycol-associated renal toxicity from lorazepam infusion. *Pharmacotherapy* 2003; **23**:1094–1099.
180. Zar T, et al. Acute kidney injury, hyperosmolality and metabolic acidosis associated with lorazepam. *Nat Clin Pract Nephrol* 2007; **3**:515–520.
181. Hayman M, et al. Acute tubular necrosis associated with propylene glycol from concomitant administration of intravenous lorazepam and trimethoprim-sulfamethoxazole. *Pharmacotherapy* 2003; **23**:1190–1194.
182. Mastroianni G, et al. Management of status epilepticus in patients with liver or kidney disease: a narrative review. *Expert Rev Neurother* 2021; **21**:1251–1264.
183. Markowska M, et al. Melatonin treatment in kidney diseases. *Cells* 2023; **12**:838.
184. Yang J, et al. Effects of melatonin against acute kidney injury: a systematic review and meta-analysis. *Int Immunopharmacol* 2023; **120**:110372.
185. Aperis G, et al. The role of melatonin in patients with chronic kidney disease undergoing haemodialysis. *J Ren Care* 2012; **38**:86–92.
186. Russcher M, et al. The role of melatonin treatment in chronic kidney disease. *Front Biosci (Landmark Ed)* 2012; **17**:2644–2656.
187. Upjohn UK Limited. Lyrica (pregabalin) 25mg, 50mg, 75mg, 100mg, 150mg, 200mg, 225mg and 300mg hard capsules. 2024 (last accessed May 2024); https://www.medicines.org.uk/emc/product/10303/smpc.

188. Desai A, et al. Gabapentin or pregabalin induced myoclonus: a case series and literature review. *J Clin Neurosci* 2019; **61**:225–234.

189. Du YT, et al. Seizure induced by sudden cessation of pregabalin in a patient with chronic kidney disease. *BMJ Case Rep* 2017; **2017**:bcr2016219158.

190. Foroutan N, et al. Comparison of pregabalin with doxepin in the management of uremic pruritus: a randomized single blind clinical trial. *Hemodial Int* 2017; **21**:63–71.

191. Otsuki T, et al. Efficacy and safety of pregabalin for the treatment of neuropathic pain in patients undergoing hemodialysis. *Clin Drug Investig* 2017; **37**:95–102.

192. Khan NJ, et al. Comparing the efficacy and safety of pregabalin vs gabapentin in uremic pruritus in patients of chronic kidney injury undergoing haemodialysis. *J Ayub Med Coll Abbottabad* 2022; **34**:524–527.

193. Safarpour Y, et al. Restless legs syndrome in chronic kidney disease – a systematic review. *Tremor Other Hyperkinet Mov (NY)* 2023; **13**:10.

194. Murray TG, et al. Renal disease, age, and oxazepam kinetics. *Clin Pharmacol Ther* 1981; **30**:805–809.

195. Leung N, et al. Acute kidney injury in patients with inactive cytochrome P450 polymorphisms. *Ren Fail* 2009; **31**:749–752.

196. Drover DR. Comparative pharmacokinetics and pharmacodynamics of short-acting hypnosedatives: zaleplon, zolpidem and zopiclone. *Clin Pharmacokinet* 2004; **43**:227–238.

197. Rehman IU, et al. Effectiveness and safety profiling of zolpidem and acupressure in CKD associated pruritus: an interventional study. *Medicine (Baltimore)* 2021; **100**:e25995.

198. Hsu FG, et al. Use of zolpidem and risk of acute pyelonephritis in women: a population-based case-control study in Taiwan. *J Clin Pharmacol* 2017; **57**:376–381.

199. Goa KL, et al. Zopiclone. A review of its pharmacodynamic and pharmacokinetic properties and therapeutic efficacy as an hypnotic. *Drugs* 1986; **32**:48–65.

200. Hussain N, et al. Zopiclone-induced acute interstitial nephritis. *Am J Kidney Dis* 2003; **41**:E17.

201. Suwata J, et al. New acetylcholinesterase inhibitor (donepezil) treatment for Alzheimer's disease in a chronic dialysis patient. *Nephron* 2002; **91**:330–332.

202. Nagy CF, et al. Steady-state pharmacokinetics and safety of donepezil HCl in subjects with moderately impaired renal function. *Br J Clin Pharmacol* 2004; **58** Suppl 1:18–24.

203. Tiseo PJ, et al. An evaluation of the pharmacokinetics of donepezil HCl in patients with moderately to severely impaired renal function. *Br J Clin Pharmacol* 1998; **46** Suppl 1:56–60.

204. Sahin OZ, et al. A rare case of acute renal failure secondary to rhabdomyolysis probably induced by donepezil. *Case Rep Nephrol* 2014; **2014**:214359.

205. Wang HM, et al. Letter to the editor: Donepezil-induced parkinsonism in end-stage renal disease. *Neurol Sci* 2021; **42**:4809–4812.

206. Periclou A, et al. Pharmacokinetic study of memantine in healthy and renally impaired subjects. *Clin Pharmacol Ther* 2006; **79**:134–143.

207. Prasad P, et al. Memantine induced encephalopathy in chronic kidney disease: a case report. *Postgrad Med J* 2023; **99**:498–499.

208. Lefevre G, et al. Effects of renal impairment on steady-state plasma concentrations of rivastigmine: a population pharmacokinetic analysis of capsule and patch formulations in patients with Alzheimer's disease. *Drugs Aging* 2016; **33**:725–736.

209. AMAG Pharmaceutical Inc. Highlights of prescribing information. Vyleesi (bremelanotide injection) for subcutaneous use. 2019 (last accessed May 2024); https://www.accessdata.fda.gov/drugsatfda_docs/label/2019/210557s000lbl.pdf.

210. Nelson ME, et al. Melanotan II injection resulting in systemic toxicity and rhabdomyolysis. *Clin Toxicol (Phila)* 2012; **50**:1169–1173.

211. Teva Pharmaceuticals USA Inc. Highlights of prescribing information. Austedo (deutetrabenazine) tablets for oral use. 2017 (last accessed May 2024); https://www.accessdata.fda.gov/drugsatfda_docs/label/2017/209885lbl.pdf.

212. Lincoln Medical Limited. Wakix 4.5mg/18mg film-coated tablets. 2023 (last accessed May 2024); https://www.medicines.org.uk/emc/product/7402.

213. Bioprojet Pharma. Highlights of prescribing information. Wakix (pitolisant) tablets for oral use. 2019 (last accessed May 2024); https://www.accessdata.fda.gov/drugsatfda_docs/label/2019/211150s000lbl.pdf.

214. Atnahs Pharma UK Ltd. Sunosi (solriamfetol) 75mg and 140mg film-coated tablets. 2023 (last accessed May 2024); https://www.medicines.org.uk/emc/product/14978/pil#gref.

215. Zomorodi K, et al. Single-dose pharmacokinetics and safety of solriamfetol in participants with normal or impaired renal function and with end-stage renal disease requiring hemodialysis. *J Clin Pharmacol* 2019; **59**:1120–1129.

216. Genus Pharmaceuticals. Summary of product characteristics. Atomoxetine 40 mg hard capsules. 2020 (last accessed April 2024); https://www.medicines.org.uk/emc/product/11126/smpc.

217. Medice UK Ltd. Summary of product characteristics. Amfexa 5mg, 10mg, 20mg tablets. 2023 (last accessed May 2024); https://www.medicines.org.uk/emc/search?q=amfexa.

218. Takeda UK Limited. Summary of product characteristics. Elvanse 20mg, 30mg, 40mg, 50mg, 60mg and 70mg capsules, hard (lisdexafetamine). 2023 (last accessed May 2024); https://www.medicines.org.uk/emc/product/14091/smpc.

219. Ermer J, et al. A single-dose, open-label study of the pharmacokinetics, safety, and tolerability of lisdexamfetamine dimesylate in individuals with normal and impaired renal function. *Ther Drug Monit* 2016; **38**:546–555.

220. Janssen-Cilag Ltd. Summary of product characteristics. Concerta XL 18 mg, 27 mg, 36 mg, 54 mg prolonged-release tablets. 2023 (last accessed April 2024); https://www.medicines.org.uk/emc/product/6872/smpc.

221. Stiebel VG. Methylphenidate plasma levels in depressed patients with renal failure. *Psychosomatics* 1994; **35**:498–500.

222. Kasahara S, et al. Case report: guanfacine and methylphenidate improved chronic lower back pain in autosomal dominant polycystic kidney disease with comorbid attention deficit hyperactivity disorder and autism spectrum disorder. *Front Pediatr* 2023; **11**:1283823.

223. Gregg LP, et al. Pharmacologic and psychological interventions for depression treatment in patients with kidney disease. *Curr Opin Nephrol Hypertens* 2020; **29**:457–464.

CHAPTER 8

Chapter 9

Drug treatment of other psychiatric conditions

Borderline personality disorder (BPD)

Borderline personality disorder (BPD) is common in psychiatric settings, affecting 2% of individuals living in the community,[1] over 10% of community mental health patients and 20% of in-patients.[2] People diagnosed with BPD on average have higher prevalence of a wide range of other comorbid mental health conditions including mood disorders (both unipolar and bipolar affective disorder), anxiety disorders, eating disorders, post-traumatic stress disorder (PTSD) and substance use disorders. Concurrent mental health conditions will affect successful treatment of BPD and should be treated prior to BPD, according to usual guidance for the particular condition, irrespective of any coexisting BPD diagnosis. More than 75% of people with BPD attempt suicide with 2–5% of patients dying from suicide.[2,3]

A high proportion of people with BPD are prescribed psychotropic drugs, often in polypharmacy regimens.[4] A survey of prescribing practice in England found that over 90% of patients with BPD had been prescribed psychotropic medication, most commonly antidepressants or antipsychotics, particularly for affective instability.[5] Individuals with BPD appear to be just as likely to be prescribed antipsychotics, antidepressants and mood stabilisers, whether or not they have a clear and documented comorbid diagnosis of schizophrenia, depression or bipolar disorder.[4,5] This suggests that medicines are sometimes prescribed for the treatment of BPD per se (for which there is very limited support) rather than for specific comorbid conditions. No medicine is specifically licensed for the treatment of BPD, or indeed any aspect of BPD. Psychological treatments such as Dialectical Behaviour Therapy (DBT) have garnered much better evidence – a Cochrane review noted 75 randomised controlled trials (RCTs) of psychological treatments in 2020[6] and a 2023 network meta-analysis included 43 studies.[7]

The Maudsley® Prescribing Guidelines in Psychiatry, Fifteenth Edition. David M. Taylor, Thomas R. E. Barnes and Allan H. Young.
© 2025 David M. Taylor. Published 2025 by John Wiley & Sons Ltd.

In 2009 the UK National Institute for Health and Care Excellence (NICE)[8] recommended that:

- Drug treatment should not be used routinely for BPD or for the individual symptoms or behaviour associated with the disorder (e.g. repeated self-harm, marked emotional instability, risk-taking behaviour and transient psychotic symptoms).
- Drug treatment may be considered in the overall treatment of comorbid conditions.
- Short-term use of sedative medication may be considered as part of the overall treatment plan for people with BPD in a crisis. The duration of treatment should be agreed with the patient but should be no longer than 1 week.

Owing to changes in the latest revision of ICD-11, which now defines all personality disorders as a single condition classified by severity, the current UK NICE guidelines are under review.[8] A number of systematic reviews have been completed since the initial publication of the NICE guideline, concluding that evidence does not support the use of medicines alone, although when coupled with psychotherapy significant improvements in mood and behaviour can be anticipated.[9,10]

A 2022 Cochrane review[11] concluded that medication has little or no effect on BPD symptom severity, self-harm, suicide-related outcomes and psychosocial functioning compared with placebo but may slightly reduce interpersonal problems. However, the evidence considered by the Cochrane review was rated as very low or low certainty and reporting on adverse events was poor and mostly non-standardised. It is clear that further research of good quality is required in this area.

Drug treatments of BPD

Antipsychotics

A systematic review of RCTs evaluating the efficacy of second-generation antipsychotics (SGAs) in a number of aspects of BPD found that there was no overall improvement in BPD or in functioning.[10] A beneficial effect of **aripiprazole** on anger and of **quetiapine** on aggression were shown, but a number of trials were rated as having moderate or high risk of bias and most of the evidence was deemed to be of low certainty.[10] **Olanzapine** may have the best supported effectiveness in treating some BPD symptoms, along with depressive and anxiety symptoms, although it has not been shown to improve self-harm or aggression.[10] Furthermore, olanzapine's propensity for inducing metabolic syndrome means that patients must be fully informed of the risks of this before commencing off-label treatment with this agent and it should only be considered an option of 'last resort' for individuals with distressing symptoms that cannot be managed psychologically. Quetiapine is perhaps the most widely used antipsychotic in BPD. Its use is supported by small studies that reported modest improvement in a number of symptoms, but not impulsivity.[12,13]

In general, SGAs appear to improve general psychopathology, although this may be a reflection of improvement in comorbid conditions. There is some evidence to support the use of **clozapine** to improve psychotic symptoms, aggression, impulsivity, self-harming behaviour and overall functioning (with associated reduced hospital use) in those with severe treatment-refractory BPD, high suicide risk and frequent hospitalisations.[9,14] A placebo-controlled RCT of **lumateperone** is underway at the time of writing.[15]

Antidepressants

Several open studies and small RCTs have investigated the use of selective serotonin reuptake inhibitors (SSRIs), serotonin–noradrenaline reuptake inhibitors (SNRIs) and flupentixol in BPD. **Fluoxetine** has been noted to improve symptoms of BPD including impulsivity, self-harm, anger and mood instability, but one RCT comparing DBT or supportive therapy alone or in combination with fluoxetine showed higher rates of suicide attempts in those given fluoxetine.[16] **Duloxetine** has been reported to improve overall psychopathology, depression, impulsivity and affective dysregulation[17] and **venlafaxine** reduced somatic symptoms and self-injurious behaviour.[18] In an open study, antidepressant doses of **flupentixol** showed significant improvements in general psychopathology and impulsivity symptoms but no further studies have been published to confirm this effect.[9,19] Lastly, in a large database review of patients with BPD, **bupropion** decreased the risk of psychiatric re-hospitalisation.[20] Overall, evidence supporting the use of antidepressants is weak and any beneficial effects are modest at best.

Mood stabilisers and anticonvulsants

There is some evidence in BPD that **valproate** and **topiramate** may improve anger.[10] Valproate may reduce aggression and irritability and **gabapentin** may improve anxiety, affective instability and depressive symptoms.[9] Obviously, given the risk of teratogenicity associated with valproate, it should never be prescribed to people of child-bearing age. **Lithium** is licensed for the control of aggressive behaviour or intentional self-harm, although its use in BPD has declined owing to concerns over long-term toxicity.[21] Small studies have suggested **lamotrigine** may improve anger and reduce aggression, impulsivity and affective lability, though a large RCT found it had no effect at all on any symptom domain.[9,10] **Carbamazepine**[9] and **mifepristone** are likewise ineffective.[22]

Lisdexamfetamine and methylphenidate

In a large database review of patients with BPD, **lisdexamfetamine** and **methylphenidate** decreased the risk of all hospitalisations, death and psychiatric re-hospitalisation.[20] This probably reflects prescribing for attention deficit hyperactivity disorder (ADHD) in the context of BPD.

Memantine

An RCT of 33 subjects found adjunctive **memantine** 20mg a day to be more effective than placebo and well tolerated. More trials are needed.[9]

Opioid antagonists

Very limited evidence supports the efficacy of **naltrexone** in reducing dissociative symptoms, but there have been no definitive trials supporting the effectiveness of naltrexone in the treatment of patients with BPD.[9]

Ketamine

A small RCT investigating the effects of one infusion of **ketamine** (vs midazolam) found more improvement in socio-occupational functioning in the ketamine group at day 14.[23] However, the apparent improvement in BPD may well reflect changes in underlying mood rather than change in BPD psychopathology. In treatment-resistant depression with comorbid BPD, ketamine was shown significantly to improve both depressive and borderline symptoms.[24] A case report of BPD and treatment-resistant depression that was managed with citalopram and esketamine nasal spray resulted in improvement in depression, anxiety and behavioural symptoms.[25] Clearly, further studies are required.

Omega-3 fatty acids

A 2021 meta-analysis concluded that marine omega-3 fatty acids improve symptoms of BPD, particularly impulsive behaviour and affective dysregulation, and that they could be considered as an add-on therapy.[26]

Botulinum toxin

In an RCT comparing glabellar botulinum toxin with acupuncture, both groups showed significant reductions in symptoms, but findings did not support the superiority of any particular treatment.[27]

Management of crisis

Medications are often used during periods of crisis when symptoms can be severe, distressing and potentially life-threatening. In BPD these symptoms can be expected to fluctuate.[28] Consequently, pharmacological therapy may then be required intermittently, and with each episode the decision to prescribe needs to be informed by a careful consideration of the relative harms and benefits of medication. It is generally easy to see when treatment is required, but much more difficult to decide when modest gains are worthwhile and whether or not continuation is likely to be necessary. The use of psychotropic drugs is not without harm, so treatment should always take the form of a rigorously evaluated short-term trial.

In the UK, NICE[8] recommends that during periods of crisis, time-limited treatment with a sedative drug may be helpful. The anticipated side effect profile and potential toxicity in overdose should guide choice. For example, benzodiazepines (particularly short-acting drugs) can cause disinhibition in this group of patients,[29] ultimately compounding problems. Sedative antipsychotics can cause extrapyramidal side effects (EPSEs) and/or considerable weight gain, and tricyclic antidepressants are particularly toxic in overdose. A sedative antihistamine such as **promethazine** (25–50mg) is usually well tolerated and may be a helpful short-term treatment when used as part of a coordinated care plan (although there is no study evidence to support this assumption). Its adverse effects (dry mouth, constipation), deleterious effects on sleep architecture and lack of clear anxiolytic effects militate against longer-term use.

References

1. Winsper C, et al. The prevalence of personality disorders in the community: a global systematic review and meta-analysis. *Br J Psychiatry* 2020; **216**:69–78.
2. Leichsenring F, et al. Borderline personality disorder: a review. *JAMA* 2023; **329**:670–679.
3. Pascual JC, et al. Pharmacological management of borderline personality disorder and common comorbidities. *CNS Drugs* 2023; **37**:489–497.
4. Riffer F, et al. Psychopharmacological treatment of patients with borderline personality disorder: comparing data from routine clinical care with recommended guidelines. *Int J Psychiatry Clin Pract* 2019; **23**:178–188.
5. Paton C, et al. The use of psychotropic medication in patients with emotionally unstable personality disorder under the care of UK mental health services. *J Clin Psychiatry* 2015; **76**:e512–e518.
6. Storebø OJ, et al. Psychological therapies for people with borderline personality disorder. *Cochrane Database Syst Rev* 2020; **5**:CD012955.
7. Setkowski K, et al. Which psychotherapy is most effective and acceptable in the treatment of adults with a (sub)clinical borderline personality disorder? A systematic review and network meta-analysis. *Psychol Med* 2023; **53**:3261–3280.
8. National Institute for Clinical Excellence. Borderline personality disorder: recognition and management. Clinical Guideline [CG78]. 2009 (last checked April 2022, last accessed January 2024); https://www.nice.org.uk/guidance/CG78.
9. Del Casale A, et al. Current clinical psychopharmacology in borderline personality disorder. *Curr Neuropharmacol* 2021; **19**:1760–1779.
10. Gartlehner G, et al. Pharmacological treatments for borderline personality disorder: a systematic review and meta-analysis. *CNS Drugs* 2021; **35**:1053–1067.
11. Stoffers-Winterling JM, et al. Pharmacological interventions for people with borderline personality disorder. *Cochrane Database Syst Rev* 2022; **11**:CD012956.
12. ClinicalTrials.gov. Seroquel extended release (XR) for the management of borderline personality disorder (BPD). NCT00880919. 2017; https://clinicaltrials.gov/study/NCT00880919?tab=results.
13. Black DW, et al. Comparison of low and moderate dosages of extended-release quetiapine in borderline personality disorder: a randomized, double-blind, placebo-controlled trial. *Am J Psychiatry* 2014; **171**:1174–1182.
14. Han J, et al. A systematic review of the role of clozapine for severe borderline personality disorder. *Psychopharmacology (Berl)* 2023; **240**:2015–2031.
15. ClinicalTrials.gov. Caplyta in borderline personality disorder. NCT05356013. 2023; https://clinicaltrials.gov/study/NCT05356013?cond=Borderline%20Personality%20Disorder&page=2&rank=11.
16. ClinicalTrials.gov. Treating suicidal behavior and self-mutilation in people with borderline personality disorder. NCT00533117. 2024; https://clinicaltrials.gov/ct2/show/results/NCT00533117.
17. Bellino S, et al. Efficacy and tolerability of duloxetine in the treatment of patients with borderline personality disorder: a pilot study. *J Psychopharmacol* 2010; **24**:333–339.
18. Markovitz PJ, et al. Venlafaxine in the treatment of borderline personality disorder. *Psychopharmacol Bull* 1995; **31**:773–777.
19. Kutcher S, et al. The successful pharmacological treatment of adolescents and young adults with borderline personality disorder: a preliminary open trial of flupenthixol. *J Psychiatry Neurosci* 1995; **20**:113–118.
20. Lieslehto J, et al. Association of pharmacological treatments and real-world outcomes in borderline personality disorder. *Acta Psychiatr Scand* 2023; **147**:603–613.
21. Essential Pharma Ltd. Summary of product characteristics. Camcolit 400mg prolonged release lithium carbonate. 2023; https://www.medicines.org.uk/emc/product/10829/smpc.
22. ClinicalTrials.gov. Preliminary trial of the effect of glucocorticoid receptor antagonist on borderline personality disorder (BPD). NCT01212588. 2019; https://clinicaltrials.gov/ct2/show/NCT01212588.
23. Fineberg SK, et al. A pilot randomized controlled trial of ketamine in borderline personality disorder. *Neuropsychopharmacology* 2023; **48**:991–999.
24. Danayan K, et al. Real world effectiveness of repeated ketamine infusions for treatment-resistant depression with comorbid borderline personality disorder. *Psychiatry Res* 2023; **323**:115133.
25. Nandan NK, et al. 'Esketamine' in borderline personality disorder: a look beyond suicidality. *Cureus* 2022; **14**:e24632.
26. Karaszewska DM, et al. Marine omega-3 fatty acid supplementation for borderline personality disorder: a meta-analysis. *J Clin Psychiatry* 2021; **82**:20r13613.
27. Wollmer MA, et al. Clinical effects of glabellar botulinum toxin injections on borderline personality disorder: a randomized controlled trial. *J Psychopharmacol* 2022; **36**:159–169.
28. Links PS, et al. Prospective follow-up study of borderline personality disorder: prognosis, prediction of outcome, and axis II comorbidity. *Can J Psychiatry* 1998; **43**:265–270.
29. Gardner DL, et al. Alprazolam-induced dyscontrol in borderline personality disorder. *Am J Psychiatry* 1985; **142**:98–100.

Eating disorders

The incidence of eating disorders continues to increase.[1] Lifetime risk of any eating disorder is 8.4% in women and 2.2% in men.[2] Those with eating disorders may misuse medication and substances to manage their weight (e.g. laxatives, diuretics, ADHD stimulants, slimming pills, semaglutide and caffeine).[3,4] Other psychiatric conditions (particularly anxiety, depression and obsessive compulsive disorder [OCD]) often coexist with eating disorders, and this may in part explain the benefit sometimes seen with medication. Any medicine prescribed should be accompanied by close monitoring to check for possible adverse reactions, and the timing of medicine administration should be considered in the context of purging.

Anorexia nervosa (AN)

General guidance

Medicines have limited efficacy in AN and none is currently licensed for this condition.[5] Prompt weight restoration to a safe weight, family therapy and structured psychotherapy are the main interventions.[6,7] The aim of (physical) treatment is to improve nutritional health through re-feeding and there is very limited evidence to support the use of any pharmacological interventions other than those used to correct metabolic deficiencies. Medicines may be used to treat comorbid conditions which should be managed according to usual guidance for the particular condition. These may need to be treated before addressing AN, depending on the severity.[6]

Weight restoration

Medicines have a limited role in weight restoration.[8–10] **Olanzapine** has shown a positive effect on weight in AN in seven RCTs.[11] One of these[12] showed that 87.5% of patients given olanzapine achieved weight restoration (vs 55.6% on placebo), although olanzapine use was limited by poor tolerance and low patient acceptability. There is also some non-RCT evidence to support the use of **aripiprazole**.[13,14] One RCT with **risperidone** showed no benefit on weight.[15] Early data for **quetiapine** were encouraging[16] but were not replicated in a later RCT.[17]

A 2023 review and guideline concluded that amitriptyline, clomipramine, fluoxetine, citalopram and sertraline do not restore weight and are not recommended.[15] Two case reports with **mirtazapine** suggest it may improve weight[18,19] although a small case–control study was negative.[20]

Benzodiazepines or antihistamines (e.g. promethazine) are not usually recommended for the promotion of weight gain.[6]

Metreleptin, a recombinant human leptin analogue, shows some promise with five cases reported of weight gain and improvement in hyperactivity and psychological symptoms associated with eating disorders.[15]

Dronabinol, a synthetic cannabinoid agonist, has some limited evidence supporting significant weight gain,[21] but in the absence of any improvements in symptoms or psychological features. Adverse effects (particularly dysphoria) are common, and this may limit its usefulness.

Treatment of psychological symptoms

Antidepressants

A Cochrane review found no evidence from four placebo-controlled trials that antidepressants improved eating disorder or associated psychopathology.[22] It has been suggested that neurochemical abnormalities in starvation may partially explain this non-response.[22] Co-prescribing nutritional supplementation (including tryptophan) with fluoxetine has not been shown to increase efficacy.[23] In the UK, NICE found little evidence to support the use of antidepressants.[6] Naturalistic studies suggest an important risk of switch to mania.[24]

Since 2021 case studies in adults with AN have shown that **ketamine** reduces depression scores and suicidality while improving psychological features of eating disorders.[25,26] **Psilocybin** is hypothesised to alleviate neurobiological and behavioural features associated with AN, and several trials are underway.[27]

Other psychotropic medicines

Antipsychotics, benzodiazepines or antihistamines (e.g. promethazine) are often used to reduce the high levels of anxiety associated with AN. A 2023 expert guideline noted that a number of RCTs suggest olanzapine may reduce agitation, pre-meal anxiety and obsessional or abnormal beliefs, while there is relatively limited evidence that aripiprazole reduces eating-specific anxiety and one RCT with risperidone showed no benefit for body image or psychological symptoms.[15] Quetiapine may improve psychological symptoms but there are few data.[16] If antipsychotics are used, only prolactin-sparing antipsychotics should be considered owing to the risk of osteoporosis (i.e. avoid risperidone, amisulpride and sulpiride).

Many other medications[15] have been investigated in small placebo-controlled trials of varying quality and success. These include lithium, zinc, naltrexone and cyproheptadine. None is currently widely used in practice. Case reports[15] have shown a potential role for valproate and growth hormone-releasing peptide-2. Relamorelin (a ghrelin agonist), oxytocin, growth hormone and testosterone are probably not effective.[15] An RCT is to be conducted to assess short-chain fatty acids (acetate, propionate, butyrate) in AN.[28]

Healthcare professionals should be aware of the risk of medicines that prolong the QT interval. All patients with a diagnosis of AN should have an alert placed in their prescribing record noting that they are at increased risk of arrhythmias secondary to electrolyte disturbances and potential cardiac complications associated with inadequate nutrition. Electrocardiogram (ECG) monitoring should be undertaken if the prescription of any medicine that may compromise cardiac functioning is essential.[6]

Treatment of physical aspects

Vitamins and minerals

Treatment with a multivitamin and multimineral supplement in oral form is recommended during both in-patient and out-patient weight restoration.[6] Vitamin D supplementation may also be required.[29]

Electrolytes

Electrolyte disturbances (e.g. hypokalaemia) may be asymptomatic and develop slowly. Life-threatening medical complications can result. Caution is required because electrolyte disturbances often resolve with re-feeding, but rapid correction may be hazardous and result in re-feeding-precipitated hypophosphataemia. Oral supplementation is used to prevent serious sequelae rather than to restore normal levels. If supplements are used, urea and electrolytes (U&Es), bicarbonate, calcium, phosphorus and magnesium need to be monitored and an ECG needs to be performed.[30]

Osteoporosis

Bone loss is an important complication of AN with serious consequences. There is limited and conflicting evidence regarding the use of oestrogen, dehydroepiandrosterone (DHEA), combined oral contraceptives and bisphosphonates to improve bone density in AN. For those who have long-term low body weight and low bone mineral density, 17β-estradiol (with cyclic progesterone) or oestrogen (in young women aged 13–17 years) and bisphosphonates (for women over 18 years) can be used. Antipsychotics that raise prolactin levels can further increase the risk of bone loss and osteoporosis[6] and should be avoided.

Relapse prevention

A 2018 review suggested that fluoxetine, citalopram, sertraline or mirtazapine may have a role to play in relapse prevention and improving symptoms in weight-restored patients.[31] Evidence for this is very weak and since this review an RCT of fluoxetine has been published showing no effect.[32] SSRIs can sometimes elevate prolactin so monitoring is recommended.

Comorbid disorders

Second-generation antidepressants are often used to treat comorbid major depression, anxiety and OCD. However, caution is necessary because depressive symptoms that are a consequence of self-starvation are only likely to improve with weight restoration. As weight loss is a frequent side effect of bupropion, this antidepressant is contraindicated for the treatment of comorbid depression in AN.[33] Mania and psychosis occurring in the context of AN is probably best treated with olanzapine, and bipolar depression with olanzapine plus fluoxetine.[33]

Bulimia nervosa (BN) and binge eating disorder (BED)

Medicines should not be offered as the sole treatment for BN or BED.[6] Fluoxetine is the only SSRI to hold a product licence for BN, and adults with BN and BED may be offered a trial of fluoxetine. The effective dose of fluoxetine is 60mg daily.[34] Patients should be informed that fluoxetine can reduce the frequency of binge eating and purging but long-term effects are unknown.[35] Early response (at 3 weeks) is a strong predictor of response overall.[36] Sertraline has also shown a reduction in binge eating and purging in both BN and BED, whereas citalopram showed improvement only in BED.[15]

Antidepressants may sometimes be used for the treatment of BN in adolescents, but they are not licensed for this age group and there is little evidence for this practice. They should not be considered as a first-line treatment in adolescent BN.[6]

There is some reasonable evidence that topiramate[15] reduces the frequency of binge eating although topiramate is contraindicated in pregnancy and in women of childbearing potential (if not using a highly effective method of contraception). There is rather limited evidence for the usefulness of aripiprazole, bupropion, duloxetine, reboxetine, lamotrigine, liraglutide, methylphenidate, zonisamide and sodium oxybate in BN/BED or both.[15] Bupropion is not recommended due to a high risk of seizures in BN.[15] Acamprosate[37] also has limited evidence in BED.

Systematic reviews[35,38] confirm the modest efficacy of SSRIs and also suggest benefit for lisdexamfetamine (based on one high-quality RCT[39]). Lisdexamfetamine is approved for BED in the USA.[40] Some limited evidence supports the use of a slow-release combination of phentermine and topiramate, however this combination was refused marketing author-isation owing to serious adverse effects.[15] The noradrenaline/dopamine reuptake inhibitor dasotraline may also be effective[41] but its development appears to have ceased in 2020.

Comorbid depression

Depression is a frequent comorbidity in BN and BED. Citalopram has been shown to be more effective than fluoxetine for depressive symptoms in BN patients.[42] As weight gain is a frequent side effect of mirtazapine, this antidepressant should be avoided or used with caution for the treatment of comorbid depression in BED.[33]

Other atypical eating disorders

There have been very few useful studies of the use of medicines to treat atypical eating disorders other than AN, BN and BED.[6,43] Evidence for avoidant restrictive food intake disorder based on case reports/series and chart reviews suggests some benefit for mir-tazapine, SSRIs (fluoxetine, sertraline), olanzapine and cyproheptadine.[15] In the absence of evidence to guide the management of other atypical eating disorders (also known as 'eating disorders not otherwise specified'), it is recommended that the clinician consid-ers following the guidance of the eating disorder that most closely resembles the indi-vidual patient's eating disorder (Box 9.1).[6]

Box 9.1 Summary of UK NICE guidance on eating disorders[6]

Anorexia nervosa

- Psychological interventions are the treatments of choice and should be accompanied by psychoedu-cation and monitoring of the patient's weight, mental and physical health and any risk factors
- Do not offer medication as the sole treatment for anorexia nervosa

Bulimia nervosa

- An evidence-based self-help programme or cognitive behaviour therapy for bulimia nervosa should be the first choice of treatment followed by other psychological therapies
- A trial of fluoxetine may be offered in combination with other treatments. Do not offer medication as the sole treatment for bulimia nervosa

Binge eating disorder

- An evidence-based self-help programme of cognitive behavioural therapy for binge eating disorder should be the first choice of treatment followed by cognitive behavioural therapy
- A trial of a selective serotonin reuptake inhibitor can be considered in combination with other treatments. Do not offer medication as the sole treatment for binge eating disorder
- Lisdexamfetamine is also an option

References

1. Martínez-González L, et al. Incidence of anorexia nervosa in women: a systematic review and meta-analysis. *Int J Environ Res Public Health* 2020; **17**:3824.
2. Galmiche M, et al. Prevalence of eating disorders over the 2000–2018 period: a systematic literature review. *Am J Clin Nutr* 2019; **109**:1402–1413.
3. Nitsch A, et al. Medical complications of bulimia nervosa. *Cleve Clin J Med* 2021; **88**:333–343.
4. Chiappini S, et al. Exploring the nexus of binge eating disorder (BED), new psychoactive substances (NPS), and misuse of pharmaceuticals: charting a path forward. *Expert Opin Pharmacother* 2023; **24**:1915–1918.
5. Frank GKW. Pharmacotherapeutic strategies for the treatment of anorexia nervosa – too much for one drug? *Expert Opin Pharmacother* 2020; **21**:1045–1058.
6. National Institute for Health and Care Excellence. Eating disorders: recognition and treatment. NICE Guideline [NG69]. 2017 (last updated March 2020); https://www.nice.org.uk/guidance/ng69.
7. American Psychiatric Association. Treatment of patients with eating disorders, third edition. *Am J Psychiatry* 2006; **163**:4–54.
8. Frank B, et al. Antipsychotic effects on anthropometric outcomes in anorexia nervosa: a retrospective chart review of hospitalized children and adolescents. *J Eat Disord* 2023; **11**:151.
9. Costandache GI, et al. An overview of the treatment of eating disorders in adults and adolescents: pharmacology and psychotherapy. *Postep Psychiatr Neurol* 2023; **32**:40–48.
10. Bauschka M, et al. Atypical antipsychotic use does not impact weight gain for individuals with extreme anorexia nervosa: a retrospective case-control study. *J Eat Disord* 2023; **11**:215.
11. Thorey S, et al. Efficacy and tolerance of second-generation antipsychotics in anorexia nervosa: a systematic scoping review. *PLoS One* 2023; **18**:e0278189.
12. Bissada H, et al. Olanzapine in the treatment of low body weight and obsessive thinking in women with anorexia nervosa: a randomized, double-blind, placebo-controlled trial. *Am J Psychiatry* 2008; **165**:1281–1288.
13. Tahıllıoğlu A, et al. Is aripiprazole a key to unlock anorexia nervosa? A case series. *Clin Case Rep* 2020; **8**:2827–2834.
14. Frank GK, et al. The partial dopamine D2 receptor agonist aripiprazole is associated with weight gain in adolescent anorexia nervosa. *Int J Eat Disord* 2017; **50**:447–450.
15. Himmerich H, et al. World Federation of Societies of Biological Psychiatry (WFSBP) guidelines update 2023 on the pharmacological treatment of eating disorders. *World J Biol Psychiatry* 2023; 1–64.
16. Court A, et al. Investigating the effectiveness, safety and tolerability of quetiapine in the treatment of anorexia nervosa in young people: a pilot study. *J Psychiatr Res* 2010; **44**:1027–1034.
17. Powers PS, et al. Double-blind placebo-controlled trial of quetiapine in anorexia nervosa. *Eur Eat Disord Rev* 2012; **20**:331–334.
18. Naguy A, et al. An adolescent male with anorexia nervosa favorably responded to mirtazapine. *Am J Ther* 2018; **25**:e675–e676.
19. Safer DL, et al. Use of mirtazapine in an adult with refractory anorexia nervosa and comorbid depression: a case report. *Int J Eat Disord* 2011; **44**:178–181.
20. Hrdlicka M, et al. Mirtazapine in the treatment of adolescent anorexia nervosa. Case-control study. *Eur Child Adolesc Psychiatry* 2008; **17**:187–189.
21. Andries A, et al. Dronabinol in severe, enduring anorexia nervosa: a randomized controlled trial. *Int J Eat Disord* 2014; **47**:18–23.
22. Claudino AM, et al. Antidepressants for anorexia nervosa. *Cochrane Database Syst Rev* 2006; **1**:CD004365.
23. Barbarich NC, et al. Use of nutritional supplements to increase the efficacy of fluoxetine in the treatment of anorexia nervosa. *Int J Eat Disord* 2004; **35**:10–15.
24. Rossi G, et al. Pharmacological treatment of anorexia nervosa: a retrospective study in preadolescents and adolescents. *Clin Pediatr (Phila)* 2007; **46**:806–811.
25. Keeler JL, et al. Ketamine as a treatment for anorexia nervosa: a narrative review. *Nutrients* 2021; **13**:4158.
26. Keeler JL, et al. Case report: intramuscular ketamine or intranasal esketamine as a treatment in four patients with major depressive disorder and comorbid anorexia nervosa. *Front Psychiatry* 2023; **14**:1181447.
27. Keeler JL, et al. Novel treatments for anorexia nervosa: insights from neuroplasticity research. *Eur Eat Disord Rev* 2024; **32**:1069–1084.
28. Quagebeur R, et al. The role of short-chain fatty acids (SCFAs) in regulating stress responses, eating behavior, and nutritional state in anorexia nervosa: protocol for a randomized controlled trial. *J Eat Disord* 2023; **11**:191.
29. Nagata JM, et al. Assessment of vitamin D among male adolescents and young adults hospitalized with eating disorders. *J Eat Disord* 2022; **10**:104.
30. Royal College of Psychiatrists. Medical emergencies in eating disorders (MEED). Guidance on recognition and management. College Report [CR233]. 2022; https://www.rcpsych.ac.uk/improving-care/campaigning-for-better-mental-health-policy/college-reports/2022-college-reports/cr233.
31. Marvanova M, et al. Role of antidepressants in the treatment of adults with anorexia nervosa. *Ment Health Clin* 2018; **8**:127–137.
32. Walsh BT, et al. Time course of relapse following acute treatment for anorexia nervosa. *Am J Psychiatry* 2021; **178**:848–853.
33. Himmerich H, et al. Pharmacological treatment of eating disorders, comorbid mental health problems, malnutrition and physical health consequences. *Pharmacol Ther* 2020; **217**:107667.
34. Bacaltchuk J, et al. Antidepressants versus placebo for people with bulimia nervosa. *Cochrane Database Syst Rev* 2003; **4**:CD003391.
35. Ghaderi A, et al. Psychological, pharmacological, and combined treatments for binge eating disorder: a systematic review and meta-analysis. *Peer J* 2018; **6**:e5113.
36. Sysko R, et al. Early response to antidepressant treatment in bulimia nervosa. *Psychol Med* 2010; **40**:999–1005.

37. McElroy SL, et al. Acamprosate in the treatment of binge eating disorder: a placebo-controlled trial. *Int J Eat Disord* 2011; **44**:81–90.

38. Hilbert A, et al. Meta-analysis on the long-term effectiveness of psychological and medical treatments for binge-eating disorder. *Int J Eat Disord* 2020; **53**:1353–1376.

39. McElroy SL, et al. Efficacy and safety of lisdexamfetamine for treatment of adults with moderate to severe binge-eating disorder: a randomized clinical trial. *JAMA Psychiatry* 2015; **72**:235–246.

40. Citrome L. Lisdexamfetamine for binge eating disorder in adults: a systematic review of the efficacy and safety profile for this newly approved indication – what is the number needed to treat, number needed to harm and likelihood to be helped or harmed? *Int J Clin Pract* 2015; **69**:410–421.

41. Grilo CM, et al. Efficacy and safety of dasotraline in adults with binge-eating disorder: a randomized, placebo-controlled, fixed-dose clinical trial. *CNS Spectr* 2021; **26**:481–490.

42. Leombruni P, et al. Citalopram versus fluoxetine for the treatment of patients with bulimia nervosa: a single-blind randomized controlled trial. *Adv Ther* 2006; **23**:481–494.

43. Leombruni P, et al. A 12 to 24 weeks pilot study of sertraline treatment in obese women binge eaters. *Hum Psychopharmacol* 2006; **21**:181–188.

Attention deficit hyperactivity disorder (ADHD) in adults

While globally ADHD may still be under-recognised and under-treated, rates of ADHD diagnoses and psychostimulant use have been rapidly rising over the past two decades in many countries, including the UK.[1-3] Increased awareness about this often life-long and disabling condition has also fuelled societal debates on 'pathologising' a condition that many interpret as indissoluble from their identity, with relevant implications on the appropriateness of potentially life-long pharmacological treatment.

A first-time diagnosis of ADHD in an adult is compatible with both ICD-11 and DSM-5 and should only be made after a comprehensive assessment by a healthcare professional with training and expertise in diagnosing and managing ADHD. Whenever possible, this should include information from other informants and from adults who knew the patient as a child. It is recommended to establish the symptoms and impairments of ADHD using a validated diagnostic interview assessment such as the Diagnostic Interview for ADHD in Adults (DIVA-5), based on the DSM-5 adult ADHD criteria.[4] Evaluation of innovative technology in addition to routine clinical assessment to diagnose ADHD and evaluate different treatments is underway.[5]

People with untreated ADHD might have poorer long-term outcomes in several life domains compared with people without ADHD and people with treated ADHD.[6] However, assumptions of efficacy, tolerability or better functional outcomes from long-term ADHD medication use are currently unsubstantiated due to the scarcity of data from randomised placebo-controlled trials of ADHD treatment lasting more than 52 weeks. Short-term trials have consistently found that ADHD medications improved inattentiveness and restlessness more than quality-of-life measures. There is inadequate direct comparative evidence to guide clinical practice on choice of ADHD medications or augmentation regimens. Moreover, the strength of the evidence for efficacy of the most frequently used pharmacological treatments for ADHD in adults is 'low' or 'very low'.[7-9]

To some extent, adult ADHD clinical guidelines and consensus documents do not reflect this uncertainty and recommend medications as first-line treatment in adults with ADHD whose symptom severity cannot be sufficiently reduced by environmental modifications. Daily intake of ADHD medication is usually advised, although ad hoc trial periods of stopping medication, medication off-days or reducing the dose should be considered to minimise any possible adverse outcomes.

Doubts remain about the long-term cardiovascular effects of stimulant drugs. A 2022 meta-analysis suggested no adverse effect, but a 2024 population study found increased (and dose-related) risk of cardiovascular disease.[10,11] Clinicians should regularly and consistently monitor cardiovascular signs and symptoms throughout the course of treatment.

A healthcare professional with training and expertise in managing ADHD should review ADHD medication at least once a year and discuss with the person (and their family and carers as appropriate) whether medication should be continued.[12] Additional considerations in adults (as opposed to children) include a diagnosis of bipolar or psychosis (ADHD medication may worsen these conditions[13]) and the need to reduce the opportunity for diversion or misuse (**prescribe modified-release [MR] preparations or non-stimulants**).

Medications for the treatment of adult ADHD belong to two broad categories:

1. Psychostimulants (i.e. methylphenidate, dexamfetamine, lisdexamfetamine [Controlled Drugs in most countries]).
2. Non-stimulants[14] (i.e. atomoxetine or other non-controlled drugs).

The enhancement of dopaminergic and noradrenergic neurotransmission in the prefrontal cortex is the probable mechanism of ADHD drugs.[15] Evidence largely supports amfetamines in adults as the preferred first-choice medication for the short-term treatment of ADHD, followed by methylphenidate preparations.[16] Lisdexamfetamine or methylphenidate is considered first-line choice of medication in adults.[12] Lisdexamfetamine is associated with improved outcomes in persons with ADHD and co-occurring amfetamine or methamfetamine use disorders.[17] Atomoxetine might be an appropriate alternative for patients who did not tolerate or have contraindications to stimulants, or in cases of concern of medication misuse or diversion. Stimulant medication response may lessen over longer durations of treatment in a significant percentage of patients.[18]

MR stimulant preparations are generally preferred to immediate-release (IR) tablets because of the higher liability to tolerance, misuse and diversion (for recreational use, cognitive enhancement or appetite suppression) of IR stimulant preparations, and the convenience of a once-daily intake (compared with twice or three times daily).

It is possible that several formulations will need to be tried before one is found that suits an individual. While all long-acting methylphenidate preparations include an IR component as well as an MR component, the biphasic release profiles of these products are not equivalent and contain different IR/MR proportions. The different time–action profiles provided by long-acting formulations facilitate individualisation of ADHD treatment. Transferring to another formulation can result in changes in symptom management at key time periods during the day.

Patient preference should guide clinicians' decisions on any medication change, which, during worldwide ADHD medication supply disruptions at the time of writing, is frequently the only alternative to discontinuation.

For adults with ADHD and drug or alcohol addiction disorders, there should be close liaison between the professional considering prescribing ADHD medication and an addiction specialist. As with any prescription of controlled substances, the clinician must weigh the risk of misuse/diversion against the stimulant's potential therapeutic benefit.[19]

In the UK, atomoxetine, lisdexamfetamine and two MR capsule formulations of methylphenidate (Medikinet XL, Ritalin XL) are licensed for first-time use in adults with ADHD, while most MR tablet formulations of methylphenidate are licensed for children and for continued treatment when initiated before the age of 18 years. In some cases, starting drug-naïve adults with ADHD on formulations prescribed off-licence might be appropriate.

Guanfacine is also effective and well tolerated in adults. A 2023 meta-analysis of 12 studies showed a response rate of around 60% (placebo 30%).[20] Viloxazine also appears to be effective[21] as is bupropion[22] but data are limited compared with guanfacine.

Prescribers should be familiar with the national and international requirements of Controlled Drug legislation governing the prescription and supply of stimulants.[23,24] Generally, for Controlled Drugs or medicines that are liable to abuse, overuse or misuse or when there is a risk of addiction and monitoring is important, prescribing should be considered only when it is possible to access relevant information from the patient's medical records.[25]

Box 9.2 summarises UK NICE guidelines and Table 9.1 lists the advantages and disadvantages of different medications for the treatment of ADHD in adults. See Chapter 5 for details of products available in the UK (see also local and national prescribing information).

Box 9.2 Summary of NICE guidance for the treatment of ADHD in adults[12]

- Drug treatment should only be initiated by a specialist and only after comprehensive assessment of mental and physical health and social influences
- Medication for ADHD should be offered to adults if their ADHD symptoms are still causing a significant impairment in at least one domain after environmental modifications have been implemented and reviewed
- Non-pharmacological options (supportive therapy, cognitive behavioural therapy, regular reviews) can be considered depending on choice, difficulties with adherence or intolerable adverse effects. Combination of medication with non-pharmacological options can also be considered in partial response to medication treatment
- Methylphenidate or lisdexamfetamine is recommended for use in adults with ADHD as first-line treatment. Switching between the two could be considered after a 6-week trial of an adequate dose with suboptimal response
- Atomoxetine could be offered to adults if:
  - they cannot tolerate lisdexamfetamine or methylphenidate, or
  - their symptoms have not responded to separate 6-week trials of lisdexamfetamine and methylphenidate, having considered alternative preparations and adequate doses
- Monitoring should include measurement of weight, blood pressure and heart rate
- For atomoxetine, monitoring for symptoms of liver dysfunction and suicidal thinking is advised
- An ECG is not needed before starting stimulants, atomoxetine or guanfacine if cardiovascular history and examination are normal and the person is not on medicine that poses an increased cardiovascular risk

---

Table 9.1 The advantages and disadvantages of medications indicated for treating ADHD in adults.

Drug group	Drug	Advantages	Disadvantages	
ADHD stimulants	Immediate release: ■ Methylphenidate ■ Dexamfetamine	Quick onset of effect Allows for flexible dosing regimens, or during initial titration to determine correct dosing levels	May be associated with euphoric effects, misuse/diversion and adverse effects	Higher effect size compared with non-stimulants
	Modified or prolonged release: ■ Lisdexamfetamine ■ Methylphenidate	Convenient once-daily regimen Less risk of misuse and diversion compared with IR stimulants	Less flexible dose titration and regimen compared with IR stimulants In the UK some preparations are not licensed for initiation in adults. Caution when switching between apparently bioequivalent preparations owing to differences in dosing frequency, requirements for administration with food, differences in the MR component and overall clinical effect Tablet and capsule preparations might be difficult to swallow.	Generally well tolerated and safe short term

Table 9.1 (*Continued*)

Drug group	Drug	Advantages	Disadvantages
Non-stimulants	Atomoxetine (NE reuptake inhibitor)	Not Controlled Drugs – less restrictive prescribing regulations Can help when stimulants are not indicated or not tolerated (e.g. tic disorders, active substance use disorders, others)	Require weeks to attain full effect Higher risk of interactions (metabolised by CYP2D6) and effect variability due to genotype – might require dose adjustments[26] Lower effect size than stimulants
	Guanfacine (α2A-adrenoceptor agonist)	Might be considered by specialists in case of refractory ADHD or as an alternative to stimulants	In many countries off-label (unlicensed) for ADHD in adults Off-label prescribing may restrict opportunities to transfer to primary care.
	Viloxazine (5HT- and NE-modulating agent)		USA only
	Bupropion (dopamine and NE reuptake inhibitor)		Limited evidence base

5HT, 5-hydroxytryptamine; NE, norepinephrine.

References

1. Raman SR, et al. Trends in attention-deficit hyperactivity disorder medication use: a retrospective observational study using population-based databases. *Lancet Psychiatry* 2018; 5:824–835.
2. Piper BJ, et al. Trends in use of prescription stimulants in the United States and Territories, 2006 to 2016. *PLoS One* 2018; 13:e0206100.
3. NHS Business Services Authority. Medicines used in mental health – England – 2015/16 to 2022/23. 2023; https://www.nhsbsa.nhs.uk/statistical-collections/medicines-used-mental-health-england/medicines-used-mental-health-england-201516-202223.
4. DIVA Foundation. DIVA-5: Diagnostic Interview for ADHD in adults (DIVA). 2019 (last accessed December 2023); https://www.divacenter.eu/DIVA.aspx?id=461.
5. National Institute for Health and Care Excellence. QbTest for the assessment of attention deficit hyperactivity disorder (ADHD). Medtech Innovation Briefing [MIB318]. 2023; https://www.nice.org.uk/advice/mib318.
6. Shaw M, et al. A systematic review and analysis of long-term outcomes in attention deficit hyperactivity disorder: effects of treatment and non-treatment. *BMC Med* 2012; 10:99.
7. Boesen K, et al. Extended-release methylphenidate for attention deficit hyperactivity disorder (ADHD) in adults. *Cochrane Database Syst Rev* 2022; 2:CD012857.
8. Cândido RCF, et al. Immediate-release methylphenidate for attention deficit hyperactivity disorder (ADHD) in adults. *Cochrane Database Syst Rev* 2021; 1:CD013011.
9. Castells X, et al. Amphetamines for attention deficit hyperactivity disorder (ADHD) in adults. *Cochrane Database Syst Rev* 2018; 8:CD007813.
10. Zhang L, et al. Risk of cardiovascular diseases associated with medications used in attention-deficit/hyperactivity disorder: a systematic review and meta-analysis. *JAMA Network Open* 2022; 5:e2243597.
11. Zhang L, et al. Attention-deficit/hyperactivity disorder medications and long-term risk of cardiovascular diseases. *JAMA Psychiatry* 2024; 81:178–187.
12. National Institute for Health and Care Excellence. Attention deficit hyperactivity disorder: diagnosis and management. NICE Guideline [NG87]. 2018 (last updated September 2019, last accessed December 2023); https://www.nice.org.uk/guidance/NG87.
13. Viktorin A, et al. The risk of treatment-emergent mania with methylphenidate in bipolar disorder. *Am J Psychiatry* 2017; 174:341–348.
14. Radonjić NV, et al. Nonstimulant medications for attention-deficit/hyperactivity disorder (ADHD) in adults: systematic review and meta-analysis. *CNS Drugs* 2023; 37:381–397.

15. Bolea-Alamañac B, et al. Evidence-based guidelines for the pharmacological management of attention deficit hyperactivity disorder: update on recommendations from the British Association for Psychopharmacology. *J Psychopharmacol* 2014; **28**:179–203.

16. Cortese S, et al. Comparative efficacy and tolerability of medications for attention-deficit hyperactivity disorder in children, adolescents, and adults: a systematic review and network meta-analysis. *Lancet* Psychiatry 2018; **5**:727–738.

17. Heikkinen M, et al. Association of pharmacological treatments and hospitalization and death in individuals with amphetamine use disorders in a Swedish nationwide cohort of 13 965 patients. *JAMA Psychiatry* 2023; **80**:31–39.

18. Cunill R, et al. Efficacy, safety and variability in pharmacotherapy for adults with attention deficit hyperactivity disorder: a meta-analysis and meta-regression in over 9000 patients. *Psychopharmacology (Berl)* 2016; **233**:187–197.

19. Crunelle CL, et al. International consensus statement on screening, diagnosis and treatment of substance use disorder patients with comorbid attention deficit/hyperactivity disorder. *Eur Addict Res* 2018; **24**:43–51.

20. Yu S, et al. Guanfacine for the treatment of attention-deficit hyperactivity disorder: an updated systematic review and meta-analysis. *J Child Adolesc Psychopharmacol* 2023; **33**:40–50.

21. Nasser A, et al. A phase III, randomized, double-blind, placebo-controlled trial assessing the efficacy and safety of viloxazine extended-release capsules in adults with attention-deficit/hyperactivity disorder. *CNS Drugs* 2022; **36**:897–915.

22. Verbeeck W, et al. Bupropion for attention deficit hyperactivity disorder (ADHD) in adults. *Cochrane Database Syst Rev* 2017; **10**:CD009504.

23. National Institute for Health and Care Excellence. Controlled drugs: safe use and management. NICE Guideline [NG46]. 2016 (last checked December 2023); https://www.nice.org.uk/guidance/ng46/chapter/context.

24. Gallagher CT, et al. Doctor or drug dealer? International legal provisions for the legitimate handling of drugs of abuse. *Drug Sci Policy Law* 2020; **6**:2050324519900070.

25. General Medical Council. Controlled drugs and other medicines where additional safeguards are needed. 2021; https://www.gmc-uk.org/ethical-guidance/ethical-guidance-for-doctors/good-practice-in-prescribing-and-managing-medicines-and-devices/controlled-drugs-and-other-medicines-where-additional-safeguards-are-needed.

26. Clinical Pharmacogenetics Implementation Consortium (CPIC). CPIC® guideline for atomoxetine based on CYP2D6 genotype. 2019 (last checked December 2023); https://cpicpgx.org/guidelines/cpic-guideline-for-atomoxetine-based-on-cyp2d6-genotype/.

Chapter 10

Drug treatment of psychiatric symptoms occurring in the context of other conditions

Prescribing in human immunodeficiency virus (HIV)

People living with human immunodeficiency virus (PLWH) may experience symptoms of mental illness because of a variety of factors (Box 10.1). In practice, several of these factors may coexist within an individual.[1]

Box 10.1 Factors contributing to the development of psychiatric symptoms in people living with HIV

- Primary (or pre-existing) psychiatric disorders
- Neurobiological changes caused by HIV in the CNS
- Other infections or CNS tumours
- Antiretroviral drugs and other medical treatments
- Alcohol or substance misuse (particularly crystal methamfetamine and GHB/GBL)
- Adverse psychosocial factors (e.g. stigma, social isolation)
- Awareness of a chronic disease requiring strict adherence to medication

CNS, central nervous system; GHB/GBL, gamma hydroxybutyrate/gamma butyrolactone.

When prescribing psychotropics, the following principles should be adhered to:

- Start with a low dose and titrate according to tolerability and response.
- Select the simplest dosing regimen possible. (Remember that the patient's drug regimen is likely to be complex already.)
- Select an agent with the fewest adverse effects. Consider drug interactions, medical comorbidities and any ongoing substance misuse.
- Ensure that management is conducted in close co-operation with the HIV specialists and the rest of the multidisciplinary team.

The Maudsley® Prescribing Guidelines in Psychiatry, Fifteenth Edition. David M. Taylor, Thomas R. E. Barnes and Allan H. Young.
© 2025 David M. Taylor. Published 2025 by John Wiley & Sons Ltd.

Although most psychotropic agents are thought to be safe in PLWH, definitive data are lacking in many cases. PLWH may be more sensitive to higher doses, adverse effects and to interactions.[2] Patients with advanced HIV disease are particularly more likely to suffer exaggerated adverse reactions to psychotropic medication.

HIV treatment advances and mental health

Treatment of HIV infection has evolved in recent years to include long-acting injectable antiretroviral therapy (ART) (e.g. cabotegravir/rilpivirine)[3] aiming to improve adherence to and persistence with treatment.[3] Ensuring continuous ART is crucial for a number of reasons including the fact that inflammation associated with untreated HIV can worsen pre-existing cognitive decline in people with psychosis. Successful treatment with ART is associated with a lower risk of mental health disorders.[4] In those at high risk of psychiatric relapse and poor compliance with medicines, long-acting injections of both antipsychotics and antiretrovirals are available and could be used concurrently.

Psychotic illness

For most PLWH and comorbid psychosis, treatment is similar to that used in people without HIV[5] but with some specific considerations. PLWH are more susceptible to extrapyramidal side effects (EPSEs) because HIV, a neurotropic virus, enters the brain and replicates in the basal ganglia leading to dopaminergic neuronal loss.[6] In addition to this, both HIV and ART are implicated in metabolic abnormalities, hyperlipidaemia, weight gain and insulin resistance.[7]

Use of second-generation antipsychotics (SGAs) in PLWH has been shown to increase the cardiovascular risk and metabolic complications compared with those not on SGAs.[8] Likewise, QT interval prolongation can be a complication of HIV progression, HIV comorbidities and use of antiretrovirals as well as antipsychotics.[9] Pharmacokinetic interactions should be considered and are discussed further in this section. SGAs are clearly first-line options for the treatment of psychosis in PLWH although close physical health monitoring is essential, as is the use of preventative measures if required.

Clozapine is a treatment option in PLWH[10-12] and comorbid treatment-resistant schizophrenia. Haematological abnormalities, including leukopenia, neutropenia, lymphopenia, thrombocytopenia and anaemias, are frequent complications of HIV[13] as well as ART. Clozapine treatment may be erroneously interrupted if these are considered as clozapine-induced, with detrimental consequences for the treatment of both HIV and psychosis. The safe and effective management of the additive haematological, metabolic and cardiovascular effects of clozapine and ART and complex pharmacokinetic interactions require the close collaboration of specialist medical teams and pharmacists. Clozapine may also be helpful in the treatment of individuals with HIV-associated psychosis with drug-induced parkinsonism.[14]

Depression

Depression is the most common mental health disorder in PLWH, with prevalence estimated to be between 14% and 78%.[1] Depressive symptoms can be a consequence of HIV infection or ART or of a pre-existing disorder. Untreated depression in PLWH is associated with reduced viral suppression and faster HIV illness progression.[15] Antidepressants are more effective than placebo in the treatment of depression in PLWH[16] and may improve adherence to ART.[17] Selective serotonin reuptake inhibitors (SSRIs) are preferred as first-line agents. Escitalopram/citalopram[18,19] probably have lower risk of pharmacokinetic interactions, although one study found no difference between the efficacy of escitalopram and placebo, possibly because of a large placebo response.[20] Electrocardiogram (ECG) monitoring is recommended when citalopram/escitalopram is co-administered with ART that prolongs the QT interval.[9,21] Mirtazapine is effective[22,23] and may be beneficial in coexisting HIV wasting and depression[24] or in reducing methamfetamine use among active users.[25] The serotonin–noradrenaline reuptake inhibitors (SNRIs) duloxetine and venlafaxine were found to be as effective as SSRIs for depressive symptoms in PLWH.[26] Bupropion was effective with similar tolerability to SSRIs in a 6-week open-label study in a small number of HIV-positive, depressed out-patients.[27]

The adverse effect burden of tricyclic antidepressants (TCAs) may limit efficacy and compliance, although their use may be appropriate, particularly in patients troubled with insomnia, irritable bowel disease or painful neuropathy related to HIV or ART. Constipation and dry mouth are frequently reported in PLWH on TCAs.[16] Monoamine oxidase inhibitors (MAOIs) are not recommended in PLWH.

Bipolar affective disorder

Mania in PLWH can be primary (pre-existing bipolar affective disorder) or, rarely, secondary ('HIV mania' associated with late-stage HIV infection). Treatment of bipolar disorder in HIV is similar to that in the general population.[27] Lithium is renally excreted and so cytochrome P450 (CYP) interactions are unlikely. However, its use can be problematic in renal impairment, something which is often seen in PLWH. Lithium may be used cautiously in PLWH for primary bipolar disorder with close monitoring to avoid development of toxicity. Carbamazepine should be avoided because of significant drug interactions with ART and the risk of blood dyscrasias.[28] Valproate is a known teratogen and should not be used in women of childbearing age.[29] Its use is also best avoided with other hepatotoxic drugs (e.g. nevirapine, rifampicin)[28] and where there is infection involving the liver (e.g. hepatitis C, mycobacterium avium complex[30]). Mood-stabilising antipsychotics such as risperidone, quetiapine, aripiprazole and olanzapine may be preferred.

Secondary mania ('HIV mania')

Secondary mania may infrequently be seen in advanced illness in the context of HIV-associated neurocognitive disorders or central nervous system (CNS) opportunistic infections. The primary aim is to identify and treat the potential underlying cause (infections, substance misuse, alcohol withdrawal, metabolic abnormalities). Secondary mania may respond to quetiapine, olanzapine, aripiprazole or ziprasidone[31] but their efficacy has not been demonstrated in clinical trials.

Anxiety disorders

Anxiety disorders, including generalised anxiety disorder, obsessive compulsive disorder, panic disorder and post-traumatic stress disorder (PTSD), are highly prevalent in PLWH.[32] Treatment follows standard guidelines for the management of anxiety disorders, with

SSRIs being the first-line options. Benzodiazepines may have some utility in the acute treatment of anxiety but require caution because of potential misuse, possible drug interactions and a higher risk of sedative and neurocognitive adverse effects in PLWH.[33] Lorazepam is metabolised by non-CYP pathways, and so has a lower risk of interactions. Clonazepam has no active metabolites and so it may be a preferred short-term option for PLWH.[34,35] Buspirone may also be helpful.[34]

HIV-associated neurocognitive disorders (HAND)

HAND encompasses three sub-disorders, ranging from the more common asymptomatic neurocognitive impairment (ANI) to a mild neurocognitive disorder (MND) and the more severe but less common HIV-associated dementia (HAD). Screening for cognitive impairment is recommended in PLWH using scales such as the MoCA or the three-item Cognitive Concerns Questionnaire.[36] In 2023, the International HIV-Cognition Working Group published recommendations to better define the cognitive impairment in HIV.[37]

Treatment involves the use of ART with high CNS penetration effectiveness (e.g. raltegravir), aiming to achieve therapeutic levels in the CNS with minimal drug-related neurotoxicity. Cognitive rehabilitation is an essential treatment component. Effective treatment of depression is essential as is management of substance use disorders and physical health comorbidities. Psychostimulants, modafinil, memantine, lithium and valproate have been studied but there is currently no licensed treatment for HAND.[38]

Delirium

Delirium in HIV can be difficult to differentiate from HAND, although onset of delirium is more acute and its severity may fluctuate. Organic causes should be identified and treated. Antipsychotics are probably not effective in treating delirium and so should only be used as a last resort in severe cases and when non-pharmacological measures fail.[27] Early studies document the efficacy of haloperidol, but the lowest possible dose should be used given the high incidence of EPSEs, particularly in those with advanced HIV (e.g. doses used in delirium in palliative care may be considered).[27] Benzodiazepines should be used cautiously as they may worsen delirium except when alcohol or benzodiazepine withdrawal is the precipitating factor.[27]

Substance use disorders

Substance use disorders are highly prevalent in PLWH. Commonly used substances include alcohol, stimulants (including cocaine and methamfetamine), benzodiazepines, opioids and cannabinoids. The potential for interactions between drug use and prescribed medicines should be considered. Treatment should be offered to PLWH with comorbid substance use disorders. Naltrexone is safe and effective for alcohol relapse prevention in PLWH,[39] while acamprosate has not been studied in this population and has a high tablet burden. Methadone and buprenorphine are possible evidence-based options for opioid use disorder but care is required with ART drug interactions.[27,40]

Interactions between antiretroviral drugs and psychotropics

Pharmacokinetic interactions between antiretroviral drugs and psychotropics occur frequently and can be clinically significant. Potential interactions should be investigated for all patients receiving antiretrovirals and psychotropics concomitantly and include current prescribed medication, alternative/herbal treatments, recreational drugs and other non-prescribed medicines. Interactions are numerous and complex. Readers are directed to regularly updated online resources for information about individual pharmacokinetic interactions such as www.hiv-druginteractions.org (also available as an app).

Pharmacodynamic interactions may also occur, usually through overlapping adverse effects. Potential pharmacodynamic interactions are shown in Table 10.1.

Table 10.1 Potential pharmacodynamic interactions with antiretrovirals.[40,41]

Potential adverse effect	Implicated antiretroviral drug(s)[21,42,43]	Implications for psychotropic prescribing
Bone marrow suppression	Zidovudine (anaemia, neutropenia)	Concurrent use with certain psychotropics (e.g. clozapine) may increase the risk of myelosuppression/neutropenia
Bone mineral density (BMD) reduction	Tenofovir disoproxil fumarate (TDF) (tenofovir alafenamide has smaller decline of BMD) NNRTIs, PIs, INSTIs: decreases in BMD following any regimen	May compound the reductions in BMD possible with prolactin elevating antipsychotics
Creatine kinase (CK) elevations	Dolutegravir, emtricitabine, raltegravir	May be important to acknowledge associated link if diagnosis of NMS is being considered
ECG changes	Efavirenz, rilpivirine, saquinavir/ritonavir: QT prolongation Atazanavir, lopinavir saquinavir: PR prolongation	May increase risk of arrhythmias associated with certain psychotropic drugs
Cardiovascular effects	Abacavir, darunavir/ritonavir, lopinavir/ritonavir	Cardiovascular events (e.g. myocardial infarction) occurred in some cohorts
Renal effects	TDF (risk increased if used with ritonavir) Tenofovir alafenamide: less impact on renal function versus TDF Atazanavir (kidney stones, tubo-interstitial nephritis)	Proteinuria, hypophosphataemia, glycosuria, hypokalaemia, renal tubular
Gastrointestinal disturbances	Atazanavir, darunavir, dolutegravir, didanosine, elvitegravir/cobicistat, fosamprenavir, indinavir, lopinavir, nelfinavir, raltegravir, saquinavir, tipranavir, zidovudine	May compound gastrointestinal disturbances associated with certain psychotropics (e.g. SSRIs)

(Continued)

Table 10.1 (*Continued*)

Potential adverse effect	Implicated antiretroviral drug(s)[21,42,43]	Implications for psychotropic prescribing
Seizure(s)	Darunavir, efavirenz, maraviroc, ritonavir, saquinavir, zidovudine	May increase seizure risk associated with certain psychotropic drugs (e.g. clozapine)
Metabolic abnormalities such as hypertriglyceridaemia, hypercholesterolaemia, insulin resistance, hyperglycaemia and hyperlactataemia	All combination antiretroviral therapy Raltegravir, elvitegravir, dolutegravir: greater risk of weight gain	May compound risk of metabolic adverse effects associated with certain psychotropic drugs (particularly SGAs)

INSTIs, integrase strand transfer inhibitors; NMS, neuroleptic malignant syndrome; NNRTIs, non-nucleoside reverse transcriptase inhibitors; PIs, protease inhibitors.

Adverse psychiatric effects of antiretroviral drugs

Psychiatric adverse events have been reported with most antiretroviral drugs, but a causal relationship remains uncertain for many. Efavirenz has been most commonly implicated, and HIV guidelines suggest avoiding its use in patients with psychiatric comorbidity.

Table 10.2 summarises the most important psychiatric adverse effects of antiretroviral drugs. Note that this is not an exhaustive list and readers are directed to the summaries of product characteristics/product labelling for greater detail.

Table 10.2 Summary of psychiatric adverse drug reactions (ADRs) with antiretroviral drugs.[21,40–45]

Drug	Adverse psychiatric effects/comments
Nucleoside reverse transcriptase inhibitors	
Abacavir	Depression, anxiety, nightmares, labile mood, mania, psychosis. Very few cases reported. In all reported cases, the patient rapidly returned to baseline after discontinuing drug.
Didanosine	Lethargy, nervousness, anxiety, confusion, sleep disturbance, mood disorders, psychosis, mania. Very rare.
Emtricitabine	Confusion, irritability, insomnia
Tenofovir alafenamide	Insomnia
Zidovudine	Sleep disturbance, vivid dreams, agitation, mania, depression, psychosis, delirium. Psychiatric ADRs are usually dose-related. Onset varies widely, from <24 hours to 7 months.
Non-nucleoside reverse transcriptase inhibitors	
Efavirenz	Somnolence, insomnia, abnormal dreams, impaired concentration, depression, psychosis, suicidal ideation. Symptoms usually subside or diminish after 2–4 weeks. However, subtler long-term neuropsychiatric effects may occur. Can exacerbate psychiatric symptoms; avoid in patients with a history of psychiatric illness.

Table 10.2 (Continued)

Drug	Adverse psychiatric effects/comments
Etravirine	Sleep disturbance
Nevirapine	Visual hallucinations, persecutory delusions, mood changes, nightmares and vivid dreams, depression. A handful of cases have been reported. Onset of symptoms was within the first couple of weeks. Symptoms all resolved on discontinuation of nevirapine.
Rilpivirine	Depression, suicidality, sleep disturbances. A similar adverse effect profile to efavirenz but a lower incidence of each event. May exacerbate psychiatric symptoms; consider avoiding in patients with a history of psychiatric illness.
Integrase strand transfer inhibitors	
Dolutegravir, elvitegravir, raltegravir	Insomnia, depression, suicidal ideation (particularly with dolutegravir and symptoms may appear within first months of treatment)
Bictegravir	Depression incidence similar to dolutegravir (though suicidality greater for dolutegravir) but further data required
Cabotegravir	Limited data but incidence appears low – also long acting and so effects may be prolonged

A 2023 systematic review concluded that dolutegravir-based regimens led to higher discontinuation rates due to neuropsychiatric adverse effects compared with those treated with bictegravir, emtricitabine and tenofovir alafenamide. Antiretroviral regimen choice should evidently take into account the individual's risk factors for developing neuropsychiatric adverse effects.[46]

References

1. Hoare J, et al. Global systematic review of common mental health disorders in adults living with HIV. *Curr HIV/AIDS Rep* 2021; **18**:569–580.
2. Hill L, et al. Pharmacotherapy considerations in patients with HIV and psychiatric disorders: focus on antidepressants and antipsychotics. *Ann Pharmacother* 2013; **47**:75–89.
3. Wang W, et al. Safety and efficacy of long-acting injectable agents for HIV-1: systematic review and meta-analysis. *JMIR Public Health Surveill* 2023; **9**:e46767.
4. Ba DM, et al. Human immunodeficiency virus (HIV) treatment with antiretroviral therapy mitigates the high risk of mental health disorders associated with HIV infection in the US population. *Open Forum Infect Dis* 2023; **10**:ofad555.
5. Cohen M, et al. *Comprehensive Textbook of AIDS Psychiatry: A Paradigm for Integrated Care*. Oxford: Oxford University Press; 2017.
6. Amod F, et al. A review of movement disorders in persons living with HIV. *Parkinsonism Relat Disord* 2023; **114**:105774.
7. Ergin HE, et al. HIV, antiretroviral therapy and metabolic alterations: a review. *Cureus* 2020; **12**:e8059.
8. Ferrara M, et al. The concomitant use of second-generation antipsychotics and long-term antiretroviral therapy may be associated with increased cardiovascular risk. *Psychiatry Res* 2014; **218**:201–208.
9. Liu J, et al. QT prolongation in HIV-positive patients: review article. *Indian Heart J* 2019; **71**:434–439.
10. Nejad SH, et al. Clozapine use in HIV-infected schizophrenia patients: a case-based discussion and review. *Psychosomatics* 2009; **50**:626–632.
11. Sanz-Cortés S, et al. A case report of schizophrenia and HIV: HAART in association with clozapine. *J Psychiatric Intensive Care* 2009; **5**:47–49.
12. Whiskey E, et al. Clozapine, HIV and neutropenia: a case report. *Ther Adv Psychopharmacol* 2018; **8**:365–369.
13. Duguma N, et al. Hematological parameters abnormalities and associated factors in HIV-positive adults before and after highly active antiretroviral treatment in Goba Referral Hospital, southeast Ethiopia: a cross-sectional study. *SAGE Open Med* 2021; **9**:20503121211020175.
14. Lera G, et al. Pilot study with clozapine in patients with HIV-associated psychosis and drug-induced parkinsonism. *Mov Disord* 1999; **14**:128–131.
15. Lesko CR, et al. Depression and HIV viral nonsuppression among people engaged in HIV care in an urban clinic, 2014–2019. *AIDS* 2021; **35**:2017–2024.

16. Eshun-Wilson I, et al. Antidepressants for depression in adults with HIV infection. *Cochrane Database Syst Rev* 2018; 1:CD008525.

17. Gokhale RH, et al. Depression prevalence, antidepressant treatment status, and association with sustained HIV viral suppression among adults living with HIV in care in the United States, 2009–2014. *AIDS Behav* 2019; 23:3452–3459.

18. Currier MB, et al. Citalopram treatment of major depressive disorder in Hispanic HIV and AIDS patients: a prospective study. *Psychosomatics* 2004; 45:210–216.

19. Freudenreich O, et al. Psychiatric treatment of persons with HIV/AIDS: an HIV-psychiatry consensus survey of current practices. *Psychosomatics* 2010; 51:480–488.

20. Hoare J, et al. Escitalopram treatment of depression in human immunodeficiency virus/acquired immunodeficiency syndrome: a randomized, double-blind, placebo-controlled study. *J Nerv Ment Dis* 2014; 202:133–137.

21. European AIDS Clinical Society. Guidelines version 10.1 October 2020. 2020 (last accessed May 2024); https://www.eacsociety.org/media/guidelines-10.1_finaljan2021_1.pdf.

22. Patel S, et al. Escitalopram and mirtazapine for the treatment of depression in HIV patients: a randomized controlled open label trial. *ASEAN J Psychiatry* 2013; 14:3139.

23. Elliott AJ, et al. Mirtazapine for depression in patients with human immunodeficiency virus. *J Clin Psychopharmacol* 2000; 20:265–267.

24. Badowski M, et al. Pharmacologic management of human immunodeficiency virus wasting syndrome. *Pharmacotherapy* 2014; 34:868–881.

25. Coffin PO, et al. Effects of mirtazapine for methamphetamine use disorder among cisgender men and transgender women who have sex with men: a placebo-controlled randomized clinical trial. *JAMA Psychiatry* 2020; 77:246–255.

26. Mills JC, et al. Comparative effectiveness of dual-action versus single-action antidepressants for the treatment of depression in people living with HIV/AIDS. *J Affect Disord* 2017; 215:179–186.

27. Hirsch CH, et al. HIV-associated neurocognitive disorders and delirium. In: Bourgeois JA, Cohen MAA, Makurumidze G (eds.) *HIV Psychiatry: A Practical Guide for Clinicians*. Cham: Springer Nature; 2022:181–233.

28. Gallego L, et al. Psychopharmacological treatments in HIV patients under antiretroviral therapy. *AIDS Rev* 2012; 14:101–111.

29. Medicines and Healthcare Products Regulatory Agency. New valproate safety measures apply from 31 January 2024; https://www.gov.uk/government/news/new-valproate-safety-measures-apply-from-31-january.

30. Pieper AA, et al. Depression, mania, and schizophrenia in HIV-infected patients. 2021 (last accessed May 2024); https://pro.uptodatefree.ir/Show/4864.

31. Spiegel DR, et al. The successful treatment of mania due to acquired immunodeficiency syndrome using ziprasidone: a case series. *J Neuropsychiatry Clin Neurosci* 2010; 22:111–114.

32. Armoon B, et al. HIV related stigma associated with social support, alcohol use disorders, depression, anxiety, and suicidal ideation among people living with HIV: a systematic review and meta-analysis. *Int J Ment Health Syst* 2022; 16:17.

33. Saloner R, et al. Benzodiazepine use is associated with an increased risk of neurocognitive impairment in people living with HIV. *J Acquir Immune Defic Syndr* 2019; 82:475–482.

34. Brogan K, et al. Management of common psychiatric conditions in the HIV-positive population. *Curr HIV/AIDS Rep* 2009; 6:108–115.

35. Bourgeois J, et al. *HIV Psychiatry*. Cham: Springer; 2022.

36. Wang Y, et al. Global prevalence and burden of HIV-associated neurocognitive disorder. *Neurology* 2020; 95:e2610–e2621.

37. Nightingale S, et al. Cognitive impairment in people living with HIV: consensus recommendations for a new approach. *Nat Rev Neurol* 2023; 19:424–433.

38. Elendu C, et al. HIV-related neurocognitive disorders: diagnosis, treatment, and mental health implications: a review. *Medicine (Baltimore)* 2023; 102:e35652.

39. Farhadian N, et al. Effectiveness of naltrexone treatment for alcohol use disorders in HIV: a systematic review. *Subst Abuse Treat Prev Policy* 2020; 15:24.

40. Panel on Antiretroviral Guidelines for Adults and Adolescents. Guidelines for the use of antiretroviral agents in adults and adolescents with HIV. Department of Health and Human Services. 2024 (last accessed May 2024); https://clinicalinfo.hiv.gov/sites/default/files/guidelines/documents/adult-adolescent-arv/guidelines-adult-adolescent-arv.pdf.

41. Waters L, et al. BHIVA guidelines on antiretroviral treatment for adults living with HIV-1 2022. *HIV Med* 2022; 23 Suppl 5:3–115.

42. Panel on Antiretroviral Guidelines for Adults and Adolescents. Guidelines for the use of antiretroviral agents in adults and adolescents living with HIV. Department of Health and Human Services. 2017 (last accessed August 2024); https://clinicalinfo.hiv.gov/en/guidelines/hiv-clinical-guidelines-adult-and-adolescent-arv/whats-new.

43. World Health Organization. Consolidated guidelines on the use of antiretroviral drugs for treating and preventing HIV infection: recommendations for a public health approach, 2nd edn. 2016; http://www.who.int/hiv/pub/arv/arv-2016/en.

44. Parker C. Psychiatric effects of drugs for other disorders. *Medicine* 2016; 44:768–774.

45. Préta LH, et al. Association of depression and suicidal behaviour reporting with HIV integrase inhibitors: a global pharmacovigilance study. *J Antimicrob Chemother* 2023; 78:1944–1947.

46. Pérez-Valero I, et al. Real-world discontinuations due to neuropsychiatric symptoms in people living with HIV treated with second-generation integrase inhibitors: a systematic review. *Expert Rev Anti Infect Ther* 2023; 21:655–665.

Epilepsy

Psychiatric comorbidities in epilepsy

People with epilepsy (PWE) have an elevated prevalence of several psychiatric disorders including depression (13–37%), anxiety (20%) and psychosis (5%).[1,2] Suicide is three-fold higher in PWE compared with the general population[3] and is an important cause of premature mortality.[4] The link between epilepsy and mental illness is bidirectional as patients with depression, anxiety and psychosis have an increased risk of developing new-onset epilepsy.[5,6] Suicide attempts are also associated with the development of epilepsy.[7] This bidirectional relationship might be explained by a common underlying pathology between mental illness and epilepsy. Disturbances in neurotransmission, neuroinflammation and the hypothalamic–pituitary–adrenal (HPA) axis have all been suggested[8] to be the shared pathology.

Interictal psychiatric disorders (with symptoms occurring independently of seizures) are likely to require treatment with psychotropics.[9–11] When prescribing psychotropics to people with epilepsy, the following general principles[12,13] should be adhered to:

- First, rule out other possible causes of psychiatric symptoms (both peri-ictal and iatrogenic – Table 10.3).
- Optimise the treatment of epilepsy (ideally before prescribing psychotropics).
- Consider using psychotropics with known antiseizure properties (e.g. antiseizure medications in bipolar disorder).
- Check for interactions with antiseizure medications.
- Start with a low dose and titrate according to tolerability and response (proconvulsive effects are dose-related).
- If seizures do occur, consider changing the psychotropic drug or optimising the antiseizure medication.

Table 10.3 Possible causes of psychiatric symptoms in people with epilepsy (PWE) and their management.[5]

Cause of symptoms	Description	Management
Interictal psychiatric disorders	Symptoms occurring independently of seizures. Although common in PWE, other causes and relatedness to seizures should be ruled out first.	Likely to require treatment with psychotropics. See Table 10.5 for more information about the use of specific psychotropics in PWE.
Peri-ictal symptoms	PWE may experience psychiatric symptoms that are temporally related to seizures.	All peri-ictal psychiatric symptoms (pre-ictal, postictal and ictal) are initially treated by optimising antiseizure medications.[12] Peri-ictal depressive symptoms do not appear to respond to treatment with antidepressants.[14,15]
Pre-ictal symptoms	Typically presents as a dysphoric mood preceding a seizure by a period of 30 minutes to hours to 2 or 3 days.	
Postictal symptoms	Typically presents between several hours to 7 days following a seizure (depression, anxiety, suicidal ideation and psychosis reported) PWE and interictal psychiatric disorders may experience worsening of symptoms previously in remission (breakthrough symptoms).	Postictal psychosis can remit spontaneously or respond to treatment with low doses of antipsychotics.[16] Short-term symptomatic treatment with a benzodiazepine or antipsychotic is recommended for up to 3 months.[17] Taper off carefully after symptom resolution.[15]
Ictal symptoms	May present as ictal fear/panic (most commonly), depressive symptoms or, rarely, psychosis.	There is no evidence that psychotropics can prevent ictal symptoms.[18]

(Continued)

Table 10.3 *(Continued)*

Cause of symptoms	Description	Management
Para-ictal episodes 'forced normalisation' (psychiatric symptoms emerging as a result of a reduction in seizure frequency)	Psychotic or, less commonly, severe affective symptoms following seizure remission in PWE Rapid medication titration schedules, rapid seizure control, previously medication-resistant epilepsy, and temporal lobe epilepsy may be risk factors.[16]	A decision should be made on how to proceed with antiseizure medications and psychotropics through a process of shared decision-making with carers.[15] Symptomatic treatment with antipsychotics or antidepressants may be indicated.
Iatrogenic psychiatric symptoms	Changes in treatments for seizures could result in psychiatric symptoms as a result of: Starting antiseizure medications with known negative psychotropic properties (particularly in those with a psychiatric history). Stopping antiseizure medications with beneficial psychotropic properties (e.g. mood stabilisation). Starting antiseizure medications with enzyme-inducing properties in people stable on psychotropics. Surgery for epilepsy: de novo postsurgical episodes of depression, anxiety and, rarely, psychosis have been reported. Exacerbation of pre-existing conditions more common.	Symptoms are managed by resolving the underlying cause in the first instance. Consider switching antiseizure medications with known negative psychotropic properties to better tolerated antiseizure medications (see Table 10.4). Antiseizure medications can lower folate levels which may affect mood. Folate levels should be checked and low levels remedied if necessary. If changing antiseizure medications is not suitable, antidepressants can be considered for iatrogenic depressive symptoms.[19] Postsurgical neuropsychiatric symptoms may be treated successfully with psychotropics.[18]

Psychiatric side effects of antiseizure medications

Virtually all antiseizure medications are known to have psychotropic effects. These effects can be both helpful and unhelpful. The adverse and beneficial psychiatric side effects of antiseizure medications are summarised in Table 10.4.

Table 10.4 Adverse and beneficial psychiatric side effects of antiseizure medications.[5,20,21]

Antiseizure medication	Adverse psychiatric symptoms	Psychiatric benefits
Barbiturates, primidone	Behavioural disturbance/ADHD symptoms, depression, cognitive impairment	Anxiolytic, hypnotic
Benzodiazepines		
Brivaracetam	Depression, aggression, rage, suicidality	None reported
Carbamazepine, eslicarbazepine, oxcarbazepine	Insomnia	Mood stabilising, anti-manic

Table 10.4 *(Continued)*

Antiseizure medication	Adverse psychiatric symptoms	Psychiatric benefits
Ethosuximide	Behavioural disturbance, depression, psychosis	None reported
Felbamate	Anxiety, depression	None reported
Gabapentin, pregabalin	Depression and anxiety on cessation	Anxiolytic
Lacosamide	None reported	None reported
Lamotrigine	Anxiogenic in some. Behavioural disturbance in cognitive impairment	Antidepressant, mood stabilising
Levetiracetam	Anxiety, behavioural disturbance, depression, suicidality	None confirmed
Perampanel	Behavioural disturbance, depression, psychosis	None reported
Phenytoin	Behavioural disturbance, depression	Anti-manic
Rufinamide	Anxiety, insomnia	None reported
Tiagabine	Behavioural disturbance, depression	Anxiolytic
Topiramate	Anxiety, behavioural disturbance, depression, psychosis	Unclear. Possible anti-manic/antipsychotic
Valproate	Behavioural disturbance (at high doses in children)	Mood stabilising, anti-manic, anti-panic
Vigabatrin	Behavioural disturbance/ADHD symptoms, depression, psychosis	None reported
Zonisamide	Behavioural disturbance, depression	None confirmed

Interactions of antiseizure medications[22]

Pharmacokinetic interactions

Important pharmacokinetic interactions occur in both directions between antiseizure medications and psychotropics, primarily mediated through cytochrome enzymes.[9,23] Psychotropics with enzyme-inhibiting effects (e.g. fluoxetine, fluvoxamine, paroxetine and, at higher doses, sertraline) may increase antiseizure plasma levels. This is especially relevant to antiseizure medications with a narrow therapeutic index (e.g. carbamazepine and phenytoin). Plasma levels should be monitored, and dosage adjustment may be required. Citalopram and escitalopram are very weak inhibitors of CYP1A2 and CYP2D6, and so may be preferred in some cases.

Some antiseizure medications are potent enzyme inducers (e.g. phenytoin, carbamazepine, phenobarbital, primidone) and others are weak inducers (e.g. oxcarbazepine at doses $\geq$900mg/day, topiramate at doses $\geq$400mg/day). These drugs can lower plasma levels of many psychotropics, leading to treatment failure.

Pharmacodynamic interactions[14]

Adverse effects with antiseizure medications that may overlap with psychotropic adverse effects include:

- Weight gain: caused by some antiseizure medications (e.g. carbamazepine, gabapentin, pregabalin, valproate).
- Sexual adverse effects: with phenobarbital and primidone but possible with all enzyme-inducing antiseizure medications.
- Hyponatraemia: with carbamazepine and oxcarbazepine (note, if severe, can provoke seizures).
- Osteoporosis and osteopenia: reported with long-term use of enzyme-inducing antiseizure medications.
- Blood dyscrasias: reported with valproate, carbamazepine[11] and especially with felbamate.

Psychotropics and the risk of seizures in people with epilepsy

In the general population, the annual incidence of unprovoked seizures is about 50 per 100,000 persons.[24,25] It is notable that the incidence of unprovoked seizures in the placebo arms of randomised controlled trials of antidepressants and antipsychotics is approximately 15-fold higher, suggesting that both depression and psychosis are risk factors for seizures.[26] A bidirectional relationship between epilepsy and several psychiatric illnesses has been demonstrated, whereby not only do PWE have a higher risk of developing a psychiatric illness, but people with psychiatric illness have a higher risk of developing epilepsy.[5,6] This bidirectional relationship exists for depression, anxiety, psychosis and suicidality.[5-7] Thus, the occurrence of seizures may, in some cases, be the expression of the natural progression of a psychiatric illness and be unrelated to the use of psychotropics.

Reports of seizures associated with psychotropics must factor in this bidirectional relationship between psychiatric illness and epilepsy. For example, although observational studies have reported an association between antidepressant treatment and seizures,[27] a similar association is also found with non-drug treatments for depression (counselling, for example).[28] These findings are consistent with depression itself being the main risk factor for seizures. In fact, one analysis of controlled studies with psychotropics showed that the incidence of seizures was substantially lower among patients receiving most antidepressants (e.g. SSRIs) in comparison with those randomised to placebo.[26] Nonetheless, definitive data are lacking in PWE[29,30] and certain psychotropics have a dose-related risk of seizures within usual dose ranges. Most can cause seizures in overdose. Note also that almost all antidepressants and antipsychotics have been associated with hyponatraemia (see sections on hyponatraemia in Chapters 1 and 3) and seizures may occur if this is severe.[18,31] General guidance on the safety of psychotropics in PWE is summarised in Table 10.5.

Electroconvulsive therapy (ECT) has anticonvulsive properties and is worth considering in the treatment of depression in patients with unstable epilepsy.[9,18,23] ECT does not appear to cause or worsen epilepsy.[18,32]

Table 10.5 Psychotropics in epilepsy.

Safety in epilepsy	Drug	Comments
Antidepressants		
Low risk – good choices[33]	SSRIs	Recommended in PWE.[15,19] SSRIs may be anticonvulsant at therapeutic doses[14] but proconvulsant in overdose.[34] SSRIs with the lowest risk of interactions with antiseizure medications are generally preferred (citalopram/escitalopram, followed by sertraline).[15,19,35,36] Escitalopram is preferred over citalopram in PWE (lower risk of seizures in overdose).[37] Others have low risk of seizures (e.g. fluoxetine[37]) but drug interactions with antiseizure medications should be considered.[15,19] Fluoxetine may be less likely to provoke seizures in older people than escitalopram or citalopram.[38] Some evidence that sertraline is safe and effective in PWE.[39]
	Mirtazapine	Recommended in PWE.[19,40] Not known to be proconvulsive.[26]
	Duloxetine	Recommended for PWE.[12,19] Risk of seizures is probably negligible.[37,38]
Probably low risk – use with caution (limited evidence)	Agomelatine	Not known to be proconvulsive.[41] Anticonvulsant in animal models.[37]
	MAOIs	Not known to be proconvulsive at therapeutic doses.[37] Low risk of seizures in overdose.[18]
	Moclobemide	Not known to be proconvulsive.[37] Anticonvulsant in animal models.[37]
	Reboxetine	Small open-label study suggests no problems in PWE.[42]
	Vortioxetine	Not known to be proconvulsive.[37,43] One report of successful use of vortioxetine in three PWE.[44]
Moderate risk – care required	Lithium	Low risk of seizures.[37] Anticonvulsant in animal models.[37] However, limited data showing both increases and decreases in seizures frequency in PWE.[37] At standard plasma levels lithium is probably not proconvulsive.[45] For bipolar, consider anticonvulsant mood stabilisers.[46]
	Trazodone	Limited data suggest some risk of seizures.[37,47]
	Venlafaxine	Effective in PWE[12] and has been recommended[19] but mixed evidence on seizure risk.[37]
	Vilazodone	Limited data. Seizure exacerbation in a patient with epilepsy has been reported.[37]
Higher risk – avoid (proconvulsive at therapeutic doses[14])	Amoxapine	Several reports of seizures at therapeutic doses[47]
	Bupropion	Dose-related risk of seizures (particularly with immediate-release formulations).[37] Risk is less with slow-release formulations at doses under 300mg/day.[37] At least one study found no increased risk with bupropion.[48]
	Maprotiline	Several reports of seizures at therapeutic doses.[47]
	TCAs	Most TCAs are epileptogenic at higher doses (particularly clomipramine and amitriptyline[11,26,47]). Doxepin possibly lower risk (one small study in PWE).[37] SNRIs are preferred over TCAs in PWE[18]

(Continued)

Table 10.5 *(Continued)*

Safety in epilepsy	Drug	Comments
Antipsychotics		
Low risk – good choices	Amisulpride/sulpiride	Considered to be safe in PWE.[49] Renally excreted, so low risk of pharmacokinetic interactions with antiseizure medications. Seizures uncommon in overdose.[50]
	Aripiprazole	Rarely lowers seizure threshold.[5] Incidence of seizures similar to placebo in RCTs.[26]
	Ziprasidone	
	High-potency FGAs	e.g. fluphenazine, haloperidol, trifluoperazine, flupentixol. Low risk of lowering the seizure threshold.[5]
	Risperidone	Unlikely to lower the seizure threshold.[5] Incidence of seizures similar to placebo in RCTs.[26] Has been recommended for PWE.[35,51] Evidence of safety in a case series of adolescents with epilepsy.[52]
Probably low risk – use with caution (limited evidence)	Asenapine	Seizure rate similar to placebo in RCTs.[53] Data and clinical experience of use in PWE is extremely limited.
	Brexpiprazole	
	Cariprazine	
	Lurasidone	
Moderate risk – care required	Olanzapine	Olanzapine and quetiapine both associated with seizures in RCTs.[26] Overall risk of reducing the seizure threshold is considered to be low[5] and olanzapine has been recommended by some for PWE.[35] Data relating to olanzapine are difficult to interpret. EEG changes are seen in some but not all studies[54] and it has been reported to be both anticonvulsant[55] and proconvulsant.[56] Quetiapine has a high risk of drug interaction in PWE.[51]
	Quetiapine	
Higher risk – care required	Clozapine	Most proconvulsive antipsychotic.[35] However, has been used successfully in PWE stable on antiseizure medications without worsening seizures[57] and even in treatment-resistant epilepsy.[58] Note, should not be used with carbamazepine (risk of blood dyscrasias and reduced clozapine levels). Lamotrigine is the antiseizure medication of choice.
Higher risk – avoid	Low-potency FGAs (e.g. chlorpromazine)	Best avoided in PWE.[34] Doses of chlorpromazine above 1g/day have a 9% incidence of seizures.
	Loxapine	Highest rate of seizures among the FGAs.[59]
	Depot antipsychotics	None of the depot preparations currently available is thought to be epileptogenic, however the kinetics of depots are complex (seizures may be delayed). If seizures do occur, the offending drug may not be easily withdrawn. Depots should be used with extreme care.
	Zotepine	Has established dose-related proconvulsive effect[50]
Drugs for ADHD		
Low risk	Methylphenidate	Three RCTs support safety and efficacy in children with epilepsy at therapeutic doses (0.3–1mg/kg/day).[11] Two single-dose RCTs and one open-label extension study demonstrated no effect on seizures in adults.[60,61] A large case–control study found an increased rate of seizures after the start of methylphenidate but not in the longer term.[62] This is difficult to interpret but suggests caution would be appropriate. May be a higher risk of seizures at higher doses.[63]

Table 10.5 *(Continued)*

Safety in epilepsy	Drug	Comments
Probably low risk[64,65] – use with caution (limited data)	Amfetamines	Data are limited to one small retrospective study in PWE.[11] No patients who had well-controlled epilepsy experienced an increase in seizure frequency.[66] Dexamfetamine was historically used as an adjunctive antiseizure agent.[67]
	Atomoxetine	Data are limited to one small retrospective study in PWE.[11] Discontinuation rates were high (though none due to seizure exacerbation[68]). Seizure rate similar to placebo for patients without epilepsy.[69]
Low risk	Acetylcholinesterase inhibitors: donepezil/ rivastigmine/ galantamine	No increased risk of seizures has been observed.[70]

This table contains information about the proconvulsive effects of antidepressants and antipsychotics when used in therapeutic doses. See Chapter 13 for information about supratherapeutic doses.
EEG, electroencephalogram; MAOIs, monoamine oxidase inhibitors; PWE, people with epilepsy; TCAs, tricyclic antidepressants.

Epilepsy and driving

In the UK, people with epilepsy may not drive a car if they have had a seizure while awake in the previous year. However, they may be eligible to drive if seizures occur only during sleep and this has been an established nocturnal pattern for at least 3 years. The consequences of inducing seizure with antidepressants or antipsychotics can therefore be significant. For further information see https://www.gov.uk/epilepsy-and-driving. Other countries have different rules, but most require a seizure-free period of between 6 and 36 months.[71]

References

1. Scott AJ, et al. Anxiety and depressive disorders in people with epilepsy: a meta-analysis. *Epilepsia* 2017; **58**:973–982.
2. Clancy MJ, et al. The prevalence of psychosis in epilepsy; a systematic review and meta-analysis. *BMC Psychiatry* 2014; **14**:75.
3. Wang H, et al. Suicidality and epilepsy: a systematic review and meta-analysis. *Front Psychiatry* 2023; **14**:1097516.
4. Thurman DJ, et al. The burden of premature mortality of epilepsy in high-income countries: a systematic review from the Mortality Task Force of the International League Against Epilepsy. *Epilepsia* 2017; **58**:17–26.
5. Kanner AM. Management of psychiatric and neurological comorbidities in epilepsy. *Nat Rev Neurol* 2016; **12**:106–116.
6. Hesdorffer DC. Comorbidity between neurological illness and psychiatric disorders. *CNS Spectr* 2016; **21**:230–238.
7. Hesdorffer DC, et al. Occurrence and recurrence of attempted suicide among people with epilepsy. *JAMA Psychiatry* 2016; **73**:80–86.
8. Kanner AM. Can neurochemical changes of mood disorders explain the increase risk of epilepsy or its worse seizure control? *Neurochem Res* 2017; **42**:2071–2076.
9. Curran S, et al. Selecting an antidepressant for use in a patient with epilepsy. Safety considerations. *Drug Saf* 1998; **18**:125–133.
10. Blumer D, et al. Treatment of the interictal psychoses. *J Clin Psychiatry* 2000; **61**:110–122.
11. Mula M. The pharmacological management of psychiatric comorbidities in patients with epilepsy. *Pharmacol Res* 2016; **107**:147–153.
12. Elger CE, et al. Diagnosing and treating depression in epilepsy. *Seizure* 2017; **44**:184–193.
13. Anbarasan D. Psychoactive medications and seizures—challenges and pitfalls. *Neurol Rep* 2016; **9**:24–27.
14. Kanner AM. Most antidepressant drugs are safe for patients with epilepsy at therapeutic doses: a review of the evidence. *Epilepsy Behav* 2016; **61**:282–286.
15. Kerr MP, et al. International consensus clinical practice statements for the treatment of neuropsychiatric conditions associated with epilepsy. *Epilepsia* 2011; **52**:2133–2138.
16. Josephson CB, et al. Psychiatric comorbidities in epilepsy. *Int Rev Psychiatry* 2017; **29**:409–424.
17. Maguire M, et al. Epilepsy and psychosis: a practical approach. *Pract Neurol* 2018; **18**:106–114.
18. Mula M. *Neuropsychiatric Symptoms of Epilepsy*. Basel: Springer International Publishing; 2016.
19. Villanueva V, et al. Proposed recommendations for the management of depression in adults with epilepsy: an expert consensus. *Neurol Ther* 2023; **12**:479–503.

20. Schmidt D, et al. Drug treatment of epilepsy in adults. *BMJ* 2014; **348**:g254.
21. Piedad J, et al. Beneficial and adverse psychotropic effects of antiepileptic drugs in patients with epilepsy: a summary of prevalence, underlying mechanisms and data limitations. *CNS Drugs* 2012; **26**:319–335.
22. Spina E, et al. Clinically significant pharmacokinetic drug interactions of antiepileptic drugs with new antidepressants and new antipsychotics. *Pharmacol Res* 2016; **106**:72–86.
23. Harden CL, et al. Mood disorders in patients with epilepsy: epidemiology and management. *CNS Drugs* 2002; **16**:291–302.
24. Ngugi AK, et al. Incidence of epilepsy: a systematic review and meta-analysis. *Neurology* 2011; **77**:1005–1012.
25. Wigglesworth S, et al. The incidence and prevalence of epilepsy in the United Kingdom 2013–2018: a retrospective cohort study of UK primary care data. *Seizure* 2023; **105**:37–42.
26. Alper K, et al. Seizure incidence in psychopharmacological clinical trials: an analysis of Food and Drug Administration (FDA) summary basis of approval reports. *Biol Psychiatry* 2007; **62**:345–354.
27. Wu CS, et al. Seizure risk associated with antidepressant treatment among patients with depressive disorders: a population-based case-crossover study. *J Clin Psychiatry* 2017; **78**:e1226–e1232.
28. Josephson CB, et al. Association of depression and treated depression with epilepsy and seizure outcomes: a multicohort analysis. *JAMA Neurol* 2017; **74**:533–539.
29. Farooq S, et al. Interventions for psychotic symptoms concomitant with epilepsy. *Cochrane Database Syst Rev* 2015; **12**:CD006118.
30. Maguire MJ, et al. Antidepressants for people with epilepsy and depression. *Cochrane Database Syst Rev* 2014; **4**:CD010682.
31. Maramattom BV. Duloxetine-induced syndrome of inappropriate antidiuretic hormone secretion and seizures. *Neurology* 2006; **66**:773–774.
32. Ray AK. Does electroconvulsive therapy cause epilepsy? *J ECT* 2013; **29**:201–205.
33. Tallarico M, et al. Antidepressant drugs for seizures and epilepsy: where do we stand? *Curr Neuropharmacol* 2023; **21**:1691–1713.
34. Steinert T, et al. [Epileptic seizures during treatment with antidepressants and neuroleptics]. *Fortschr Neurol Psychiatr* 2011; **79**:138–143.
35. Mula M. Epilepsy and psychiatric comorbidities: drug selection. *Curr Treat Options Neurol* 2017; **19**:44.
36. National Institute for Health and Care Excellence. Depression in adults with a chronic physical health problem: recognition and management. Clinical Guidance [CG91] 2009 (last updated and checked May 2024); http://www.nice.org.uk/CG91.
37. Steinert T, et al. Epileptic seizures under antidepressive drug treatment: systematic review. *Pharmacopsychiatry* 2018; **51**:121–135.
38. Finkelstein Y, et al. Second-generation anti-depressants and risk of new-onset seizures in the elderly. *Clin Toxicol (Phila)* 2018; **56**:1179–1184.
39. Gilliam FG, et al. A trial of sertraline or cognitive behavior therapy for depression in epilepsy. *Ann Neurol* 2019; **86**:552–560.
40. Craig DP, et al. Risk of seizures with antidepressants: what is the evidence? *Drug Ther Bull* 2020; **58**:137–140.
41. Servier Laboratories Limited. Summary of product characteristics. Valdoxan (agomelatine). 2021 (last accessed May 2024); https://www.medicines.org.uk/emc/medicine/21830.
42. Kuhn KU, et al. Antidepressive treatment in patients with temporal lobe epilepsy and major depression: a prospective study with three different antidepressants. *Epilepsy Behav* 2003; **4**:674–679.
43. Lundbeck Limited. Summary of product characteristics. Brintellix (vortioxetine) tablets 5, 10 and 20mg. 2024 (last checked May 2024); https://www.medicines.org.uk/emc/medicine/30904.
44. Siwek M, et al. Case report: vortioxetine in the treatment of depressive symptoms in patients with epilepsy – case series. *Front Pharmacol* 2022; **13**:852042.
45. Bojja SL, et al. What is the role of lithium in epilepsy? *Curr Neuropharmacol* 2022; **20**:1850–1864.
46. Knott S, et al. Epilepsy and bipolar disorder. *Epilepsy Behav* 2015; **52**:267–274.
47. Johannessen Landmark C, et al. Proconvulsant effects of antidepressants – what is the current evidence? *Epilepsy Behav* 2016; **61**:287–291.
48. Chu C-S, et al. Antidepressant drugs use and epilepsy risk: a nationwide nested case-control study. *Epilepsy Behav* 2023; **140**:109102.
49. Elnazer H, et al. Managing aggression in epilepsy. *BJPsych Advances* 2017; **23**:253.
50. Steinert T, et al. Seizures. In: Manu P, Flanagan RJ, Donaldson K, eds. *Life-threatening Effects of Antipsychotic Drugs*. San Diego, CA: Academic Press; 2016:207–222.
51. Agrawal N, et al. Treatment of psychoses in patients with epilepsy: an update. *Ther Adv Psychopharmacol* 2019; **9**:2045125319862968.
52. Gonzalez-Heydrich J, et al. No seizure exacerbation from risperidone in youth with comorbid epilepsy and psychiatric disorders: a case series. *J Child Adolesc Psychopharmacol* 2004; **14**:295–310.
53. IBM Watson Health. IBM micromedex solutions. 2024; https://www.ibm.com/watson-health/about/micromedex.
54. Jackson A, et al. EEG changes in patients on antipsychotic therapy: a systematic review. *Epilepsy Behav* 2019; **95**:1–9.
55. Qiu X, et al. Antiepileptic effect of olanzapine in epilepsy patients with atypical depressive comorbidity. *Epileptic Disord* 2018; **20**:225–231.
56. Mansoor M, et al. Generalised tonic-clonic seizures on the subtherapeutic dose of olanzapine. *BMJ Case Rep* 2019; **12**:e230018.
57. Langosch JM, et al. Epilepsy, psychosis and clozapine. *Hum Psychopharmacol* 2002; **17**:115–119.
58. Jette Pomerleau V, et al. Clozapine safety and efficacy for interictal psychotic disorder in pharmacoresistant epilepsy. *Cogn Behav Neurol* 2017; **30**:73–76.
59. Habibi M, et al. The impact of psychoactive drugs on seizures and antiepileptic drugs. *Curr Neurol Neurosci Rep* 2016; **16**:71.
60. Adams J, et al. Methylphenidate, cognition, and epilepsy: a 1-month open-label trial. *Epilepsia* 2017; **58**:2124–2132.
61. Adams J, et al. Methylphenidate, cognition, and epilepsy: a double-blind, placebo-controlled, single-dose study. *Neurology* 2017; **88**:470–476.

62. Man KKC, et al. Association between methylphenidate treatment and risk of seizure: a population-based, self-controlled case-series study. *Lancet Child Adolesc Health* 2020; **4**:435–443.

63. Eaton C, et al. Stimulant and non-stimulant drug therapy for people with attention deficit hyperactivity disorder and epilepsy. *Cochrane Database Syst Rev* 2022; **7**:CD013136.

64. Besag F, et al. Psychiatric and behavioural disorders in children with epilepsy (ILAE Task Force Report): epilepsy and ADHD. *Epileptic Disord* 2016; **18**:S8–S15.

65. Besag F, et al. Psychiatric and behavioural disorders in children with epilepsy (ILAE Task Force Report): when should pharmacotherapy for psychiatric/behavioural disorders in children with epilepsy be prescribed? *Epileptic Disord* 2016; **18**:S77–S86.

66. Gonzalez-Heydrich J, et al. Comparing stimulant effects in youth with ADHD symptoms and epilepsy. *Epilepsy Behav* 2014; **36**:102–107.

67. Schubert R. Attention deficit disorder and epilepsy. *Pediatr Neurol* 2005; **32**:1–10.

68. Torres A, et al. Tolerability of atomoxetine for treatment of pediatric attention-deficit/hyperactivity disorder in the context of epilepsy. *Epilepsy Behav* 2011; **20**:95–102.

69. Williams AE, et al. Epilepsy and attention-deficit hyperactivity disorder: links, risks, and challenges. *Neuropsychiatr Dis Treat* 2016; **12**:287–296.

70. Ha J, et al. Association of cognitive enhancers and incident seizure risk in dementia: a population-based study. *BMC Geriatr* 2022; **22**:480.

71. Ooi WW, et al. International regulations for automobile driving and epilepsy. *J Travel Med* 2006; **7**:1–4.

22q11.2 deletion syndrome

Clinical features

22q11.2 deletion syndrome (22q11.2DS), the most common microdeletion syndrome in humans, is a multisystem disorder with a heterogenous presentation which varies greatly in severity between affected individuals.[1] Prevalence is estimated at 1 in 2148 live births.[1,2] The syndrome has been known by many names (including velocardiofacial syndrome and DiGeorge syndrome) in part because of its broad phenotypic range of clinical features (Table 10.6).

Table 10.6 Selected clinical features and risks in people with 22q11.2 deletion syndrome.[1,3]

	Clinical risks
Cognitive and adaptive functioning	Intellectual disabilities Deficits in adaptive functioning
Endocrinological	Hypocalcaemia and hypoparathyroidism Hypomagnesaemia Thyroid disease (usually hypothyroidism) Obesity and type 2 diabetes mellitus
Gastroenterology	General gastrointestinal symptoms (constipation, dysphagia) GERD Fatty liver
Psychiatric disorders	Anxiety Psychosis Autism spectrum disorder ADHD
Cardiovascular	Congenital cardiac defects Hypertension, arrhythmia, heart failure, aortic root dilation
Genitourinary	Congenital anomalies, renal cysts, renal failure Menstrual disorders (e.g. dysmenorrhoea)
Neurology	Seizures, often secondary (e.g. to hypocalcaemia) Early-onset Parkinson's disease Other motor disorders (e.g. dystonia, myoclonus)
Sleep	Sleep pattern disruptions Obstructive sleep apnoea
Haematology	Mild to moderate thrombocytopenia, mild cytopenias Immune thrombocytopenia Impaired haemostasis (e.g. epistaxis, menorrhagia)

GERD, gastro-esophageal reflux disease.

Psychiatric disorders in people with 22q11.2DS

Around 60% of people with 22q11.2DS meet diagnostic criteria for some type of psychiatric disorder during their lives.[4] Children with 22q11.2DS have an elevated prevalence of anxiety, attention deficit hyperactivity disorder (ADHD) and autism spectrum disorders.[2] Anxiety disorders are profoundly increased in adults, with about 2–3 times the expected population prevalence.[1] Schizophrenia is diagnosed in approximately one in every four to five adults with 22q11.2DS.[1]

Box 10.2 summarises the general principles of prescribing in 22q11.2DS. Few studies have evaluated the safety and efficacy of psychotropics in people with 22q11.2DS. However, standard pharmacological (and non-pharmacological) treatments for ADHD, anxiety, mood disorders and schizophrenia appear to be effective and treatment protocols used in the general population should be followed.[1,5] Current evidence and opinion on the treatment of psychiatric disorders in people with 22q11.2DS are summarised in Table 10.7.

Box 10.2 General principles of prescribing in 22q11.2 deletion syndrome[6,7]

- 22q11.2DS confers an increased risk of treatable psychiatric disorders
- Standard pharmacological treatment protocols should be followed
- Consider the individual patient comorbidities and clinical features (Table 10.6) that may increase the propensity to adverse effects from psychotropics (e.g. arrhythmias, seizures, weight gain, EPSEs)
- Endocrine abnormalities (e.g. hypoparathyroidism and hypothyroidism) should be corrected before starting psychotropics because they can mimic psychiatric symptoms and complicate treatment with psychotropics[4,5]

DS, deletion syndrome; EPSEs, extrapyramidal side effects.

Table 10.7 Management of psychiatric disorders in people with 22q11.2 deletion syndrome.[8]

Psychiatric disorder	Treatments
ADHD	There is a theoretical risk of psychosis with psychostimulants in people with 22q11.2DS but standard treatment protocols are advised.[4] In those with congenital heart disease, cardiology advice should be sought before initiating stimulant medications.[9]
	Three studies support the efficacy of methylphenidate in children with 22q11.2DS.[4,10] Treatment was generally well tolerated. A comprehensive cardiovascular assessment before and during treatment is recommended.
Depression and anxiety	Both depression and anxiety appear to respond favourably to SSRIs.[4] Further management after treatment failure follows standard protocols. Caution should be exercised with drugs that lower the seizure threshold (e.g. bupropion).[7]
Obsessive compulsive disorder	One study of four people with OCD and 22q11.2DS found a mean rate of improvement of 35% in symptom score after treatment with fluoxetine (30–60mg/day). Treatment was well tolerated.[11]

(Continued)

Table 10.7 (*Continued*)

Psychiatric disorder	Treatments
Schizophrenia	Standard treatment protocols are generally recommended.[1,5] People with 22q11.2DS may be more susceptible to seizures and EPSEs with antipsychotics.[7,8] EPSEs must be distinguished from motor problems that may be a direct effect of the 22q11.2DS (diagnosis of Parkinson's disease may be delayed if misattributed to antipsychotics).[7] Specialist neurological opinion and neuroimaging have been recommended to distinguish Parkinson's disease from antipsychotic-induced parkinsonism.[6] There is a significantly elevated risk of obesity in 22q11.2DS so metabolic adverse effects should be closely monitored.[12] Those with cardiac abnormalities have an increased risk of QTc prolongation.[8] Close ECG monitoring is recommended.[8] Antipsychotics with a low effect on the QT interval are preferred[8] (note that hypocalcaemia can also prolong the QT interval[7]). Low starting doses and slow dose titrations are recommended.[8] Case reports have described the successful use of various antipsychotics, with remission of psychosis in 41% of published reports.[6] Treatment resistance has been described in 19% of case series and 8% of case reports (although treatment failure was due to adverse effects rather than inefficacy in some).[6]
	Clozapine was found to be effective in one retrospective study of 20 patients with 22q11.2DS.[4] Compared with matched controls, lower doses were needed (a median of 250mg/day vs 450mg/day). However, half of the 22q11.2DS group experienced at least one serious adverse effect from clozapine, primarily seizures, but also myocarditis and neutropenia. Several case reports further support the efficacy of clozapine at low doses (median of 200mg/day) for people with 22q11.2DS, while highlighting the risk of both seizures (generalised or myoclonic) and thrombocytopenia.[12]
	Overall, clozapine appears to have demonstrable efficacy at lower than usual doses, but the risk of rare serious adverse events appears to be relatively high.[4] Adjunctive anticonvulsants should be considered[12] to mitigate the increased seizure risk when prescribing clozapine.[1] Several authors advocate the use of lower starting doses and slower titrations.[6]
	Seizures with other antipsychotics: investigate low calcium and magnesium levels in all cases and ensure adequate treatment.[13] Adjunctive anticonvulsants can be considered[1] although they should not be prescribed routinely as many do not experience seizures.[6]
	Other agents: drugs that act directly against catecholamine excess may also be effective. Metyrosine, used as a monotherapy or as an adjunctive agent, was found to be effective in 22 of 29 patients in one study.[14] An additional positive case report has been published[15] but there are no further recent studies. There is a single case study where methyldopa was used successfully.[16]

DS, deletion syndrome; EPSEs, extrapyramidal side effects; OCD, obsessive compulsive disorder.

References

1. Boot E, et al. Updated clinical practice recommendations for managing adults with 22q11.2 deletion syndrome. *Genet Med* 2023; **25**:100344.
2. McDonald-McGinn DM, et al. 22q11.2 deletion syndrome. *Nat Rev Dis Primers* 2015; **1**:15071.
3. Bayat M, et al. Neurological manifestation of 22q11.2 deletion syndrome. *Neurol Sci* 2022; **43**:1695–1700.
4. Mosheva M, et al. Effectiveness and side effects of psychopharmacotherapy in individuals with 22q11.2 deletion syndrome with comorbid psychiatric disorders: a systematic review. *Eur Child Adolesc Psychiatry* 2020; **29**:1035–1048.
5. Fung WL, et al. Practical guidelines for managing adults with 22q11.2 deletion syndrome. *Genet Med* 2015; **17**:599–609.
6. Tanham M, et al. The effectiveness and tolerability of pharmacotherapy for psychosis in 22q11.2 deletion syndrome: a systematic review. *Aust NZ J Psychiatry* 2024; **58**:393–403.
7. Van L, et al. Mental health in adults with 22q11. 2 deletion syndrome. In: McDonald-McGinn DM, ed. *The Chromosome 22q11. 2 Deletion Syndrome*. London: Academic Press; 2022:322–337.
8. Baker K, et al. Psychiatric illness. Consensus document on 22q11 deletion syndrome (22q11DS) MaxAppeal. 2017; https://www.maxappeal.org.uk/library-consensus-document.
9. Chung LM, et al. Safety of stimulant medications for attention deficit hyperactivity disorder in paediatric congenital heart disease. *J Paediatr Child Health* 2023; **59**:580–588.

10. Maeder J, et al. Selective effects of methylphenidate on attention and inhibition in 22q11.2 deletion syndrome: results from a clinical trial. *Int J Neuropsychopharmacol* 2022; **25**:215–225.

11. Gothelf D, et al. Obsessive-compulsive disorder in patients with velocardiofacial (22q11 deletion) syndrome. *Am J Med Genet B Neuropsychiatr Genet* 2004; **126b**:99–105.

12. De Boer J, et al. Adverse effects of antipsychotic medication in patients with 22q11.2 deletion syndrome: a systematic review. *Am J Med Genet A* 2019; **179**:2292–2306.

13. Bassett AS, et al. Practical guidelines for managing patients with 22q11.2 deletion syndrome. *J Pediatr* 2011; **159**:332–339.

14. Faedda GL, et al. 4.19 Treatment of velo-cardio-facial syndrome-related psychosis with metyrosine. *J Am Acad Child Adolesc Psychiatry* 2016; **55**:S169.

15. Engebretsen MH, et al. Metyrosine treatment in a woman with chromosome 22q11.2 deletion syndrome and psychosis: a case study. *Int J Dev Disabil* 2019; **65**:116–121.

16. O'Hanlon JF, et al. Replacement of antipsychotic and antiepileptic medication by L-alpha-methyldopa in a woman with velocardiofacial syndrome. *Int Clin Psychopharmacol* 2003; **18**:117–119.

Learning disabilities

General considerations[1]

Prescribing psychotropic medications for people with learning disabilities (LD) is a challenging and controversial area of psychiatric practice.[2,3] There are concerns that psychotropic drugs of all kinds (antipsychotics, antidepressants, benzodiazepines [both regular and as required] and antiepileptics as mood stabilisers) are overprescribed with poor review and assessment of their benefit. The LD field is notable in having only a small therapeutics research base of its own, with particular ethical and practical considerations regarding how emotional and behavioural disturbances are classified and treated. Although prescribing for individuals with mild or borderline intellectual impairment may be undertaken by mainstream mental health services, the assessment and treatment of behavioural and emotional disorders in people with more marked (or, as in the case of autism, atypical) patterns of significant cognitive impairment should be undertaken in the first instance by, or at least in consultation with, specialist clinicians.

The term 'dual diagnosis' in this context refers to the co-occurrence of an identifiable psychiatric disorder (mental illness, personality disorder) and LD. 'Diagnostic overshadowing' is the misattribution of emotional or behavioural problems to LD itself rather than a comorbid condition. LD is an important risk factor for all psychiatric disorders (including dementia, particularly for individuals with Down's syndrome).[4] Where it is possible to diagnose a mental illness using conventional or modified criteria then drug treatment in the first instance should, in general, be similar to that in the population at large. Most treatment guidelines are increasingly stating their intended applicability to people with LD.

Mental illness may present in unusual ways in LD, for example depression as self-injurious behaviour, or persecutory ideation as complaints of being 'picked on'. Conversely, behaviours such as self-talk may be normal in some individuals but mistakenly identified as a disorder such as psychosis. In general, diagnosis becomes increasingly complex with increasing severity of disability and associated communication impairment.

Comorbid autistic spectrum disorder has special assessment considerations and in its own right is an important risk factor for psychiatric disorder, in particular anxiety and depression, bipolar spectrum disorder, severe obsessional behaviour, anger disorders and psychosis-like episodes that may not meet criteria for schizophrenia but nonetheless require treatment. Autistic traits are common among patients using LD services. Guidance on the treatment of mental health problems in autism can be found in Chapter 5.

Key practice areas

Capacity and consent

It is uncommon for patients in LD services (who often represent a subpopulation of those identified with special educational needs in childhood) to have sufficient understanding of their treatment in order to be able to take truly informed decisions. There is inevitably an increased onus on the clinician to bear the weight of decision-making. The patient's decision-making capacity, depending on the severity of intellectual impairment, may be improved through appropriate verbal and written communication. The involvement of carers in this process is generally essential.

Physical comorbidity, especially epilepsy

Epilepsy is over-represented in LD populations, becoming more prevalent as severity increases, with approximately one-third of affected individuals developing a seizure disorder by early adulthood. Special consideration is needed when considering the use of medications that may lower seizure threshold or interact with drugs used for epilepsy.

Assessment of care environments

Behavioural and emotional disturbance may sometimes be a reflection of problems or failings in the care environment. Different staff in a care home may have different thresholds of tolerance (or make different attributions) for these difficulties which can lead to varied reports of their significance and impact. Allowing for a period of prospective assessment and using simple assessment tools (e.g. simple ABC or sleep charts) can be very helpful to the clinician in making judgements about recommending medication. If medication is used in a care home, staff may need special education in its use and anticipated adverse effects and, for 'as required' medications, clear guidelines for its use. This may make it difficult to initiate certain treatments in the community.

Adverse effect sensitivity

It is widely thought that people with LD are especially sensitive to adverse effects of psychotropics and more at risk of long-term effects such as the metabolic syndrome. However, we only know of one study that has given support to this view. A cohort study extracting information from a large UK primary care database compared the incidence of EPSEs of antipsychotics in adults with LD with that in adults without LD. The incidence of EPSEs was 30% higher in people with LD than in those without LD.[5] It is good practice to start at lower doses and increase more slowly than might be usual in general psychiatric practice. Notable adverse effects include worsening of seizures, sedation, extrapyramidal reactions (including with risperidone at normal doses, especially in individuals who already have mobility problems), problems with swallowing (with clozapine and other antipsychotics) and worsening of cognitive function with anticholinergic medications (see Chapter 6).

Psychological interventions

In the absence of an identifiable mental illness (including atypical presentations) with clear treatment implications, psychological interventions such as functional behavioural analysis should be considered as first-line intervention for all but the most serious or intractable presentations of behavioural disturbance (Table 10.8). In studies where it has been possible to infer the severity of challenging behaviour, treatment response is generally associated with more severe problems at baseline.

Table 10.8 Some notes on currently and historically used medications for behaviour disorder.

Drug class	Clinical applications	Notes
Antipsychotics[6]	Use in psychosis with LD is justified Used across a broad range of behavioural disturbances[7] May be useful for aggression and irritability	The most widely used[8,9] yet most controversial medication for behavioural problems.[10,11] Although an RCT[12] casts doubt on their efficacy for this indication the study was not without its problems and there is a significant body of other evidence supporting their use, including a number of small RCTs in children with LD. Discontinuation studies in long-term treatment commonly (but not always) show re-emergence of problem behaviours. NICE suggests considering slow withdrawal of antipsychotics in all those who do not have psychotic symptoms.[13] The UK STOMP programme promotes deprescribing of antipsychotics.[14] It has been successful, but antipsychotics are often replaced by other psychotropics.[15] A 2022 analysis of UK NHS data suggests antidepressants now replace antipsychotics as the most widely prescribed psychotropic.[16] Before the advent of SGAs the best evidence was for **haloperidol**[17] in the context of autism and for zuclopenthixol for behavioural disturbance.[18] **Zuclopenthixol** may reduce aggression and challenging behaviour.[19] Among SGAs the best evidence is for **risperidone**[20,21] at low dose (0.5–2mcg) for aggression and mood instability, particularly with associated autism though also in non-autistic cases. **Aripiprazole** has a US FDA licence for behavioural disturbance in young people with autism.[22,23] Some evidence to support **olanzapine**[24] and case reports of **clozapine**[25] for very severe cases of aggression, though not widely used and unlikely to be used outside highly specialist (in-patient) settings. In 2015, Cochrane uncovered 38 case reports and chart reviews but found no RCT evidence for the use of clozapine in psychosis in LD.[26] Results for **quetiapine** are modest at best.[27]
SSRIs	Helpful for severe anxiety and obsessionality in autistic spectrum disorder. Use here is off-licence unless an additional diagnosis of anxiety disorder or OCD is made Also used as a first-line alternative to antipsychotics for aggression and impulsivity	Commonly used in combination with antipsychotics though limited evidence base for combination treatment. Effectiveness in absence of mood or anxiety spectrum disorder is unclear, however, and a 2013 Cochrane review was pessimistic[28] about the evidence for their effectiveness for behaviour disorder in autistic children (who may be at heightened risk of adverse effects) though a little more encouraging for use in adults. Some good evidence for fluoxetine in OCD in LD/autism although the drop-out rate is high.[29] Generally, quality of trials is poor and effects may be exaggerated by use in less severe cases.[30] Caution needed because of the risk of precipitation of hypomania in this population.[31] As with antipsychotics, there are major concerns about overprescribing.[32] **Venlafaxine** is probably not effective.[33]

Table 10.8 (*Continued*)

Drug class	Clinical applications	Notes
Anticonvulsants[34]	Aggression and self-injury	Some uncontrolled studies supporting **sodium valproate**[35] in LD populations though evidence is not strong and research findings are contradictory. However, valproate remains best supported of the anticonvulsants for mood lability and aggression, partly because of positive studies in non-LD groups.[36]
		Limited studies of **lamotrigine**, mostly in children, suggest no effect, at least in autism and in the absence of affective instability.[27]
		Data for **carbamazepine** also unconvincing, but it is still widely used.[37]
Lithium[38]	Licensed for the treatment of self-injurious behaviour and aggression	Some RCT evidence[39] for LD but there have been no studies in this population for many years,[3] although there has been one fairly recent positive RCT for its use in aggression in adolescents without developmental impairment.[40] Experience suggests it can be very helpful in individual cases where other treatments have failed and is possibly underused, though adverse effects can be problematic.
		Perhaps best considered where there is a sub-syndromal or non-specific 'affective component'. Some authorities suggest that, on close examination, challenging behaviour may occur in the context of very rapid cycling bipolar disorder in some individuals with severe and profound LD and that the diagnosis is easily missed.
		Some RCT evidence that short-term use is reasonably well tolerated (at 6mg/kg).[41]
Methylphenidate	Effective in ADHD associated with LD	NICE[13] conducted a meta-analysis and found clear benefit for methylphenidate (and risperidone and clonidine) in ADHD in the context of LD. Insomnia is common.
Naltrexone[42]	Has been used for severe self-injurious behaviour[43]	Evidence not strong and results are inconsistent. Use may still be an option in severe and intractable cases. One case of successful treatment of kleptomania.[44] Overall, clinical use has declined of late.[45]

FDA, Food and Drug Administration; LD, learning disability; OCD, obsessive compulsive disorder.

References

1. Deb S. The use of medications for the management of problem (challenging) behaviours in adults who have intellectual disabilities. University of Hertfordshire. 2012 (revised 2018, last accessed July 2024); https://www.intellectualdisability.info/mental-health/articles/the-use-of-medications-for-the-management-of-problem-behaviours-in-adults-who-have-intellectual-disabilities.
2. Sheehan R, et al. Psychotropic prescribing in people with intellectual disability and challenging behaviour. *BMJ* 2017; **358**:j3896.
3. Ji NY, et al. Pharmacotherapy for mental health problems in people with intellectual disability. *Curr Opin Psychiatry* 2016; **29**:103–125.
4. Cooper SA, et al. Mental ill-health in adults with intellectual disabilities: prevalence and associated factors. *Br J Psychiatry* 2007; **190**:27–35.
5. Sheehan R, et al. Movement side effects of antipsychotic drugs in adults with and without intellectual disability: UK population-based cohort study. *BMJ Open* 2017; **7**:e017406.
6. Antochi R, et al. Psychopharmacological treatments in persons with dual diagnosis of psychiatric disorders and developmental disabilities. *Postgrad Med J* 2003; **79**:139–146.

7. Lunsky Y, et al. Antipsychotic use with and without comorbid psychiatric diagnosis among adults with intellectual and developmental disabilities. *Can J Psychiatry* 2017; **63**:361–369.

8. Deb S, et al. Characteristics and the trajectory of psychotropic medication use in general and antipsychotics in particular among adults with an intellectual disability who exhibit aggressive behaviour. *J Intellect Disabil Res* 2015; **59**:11–25.

9. Sheehan R, et al. Mental illness, challenging behaviour, and psychotropic drug prescribing in people with intellectual disability: UK population based cohort study. *BMJ* 2015; **351**:h4326.

10. Deb S, et al. The effectiveness of antipsychotic medication in the management of behaviour problems in adults with intellectual disabilities. *J Intellect Disabil Res* 2007; **51**:766–777.

11. Roy D, et al. Pharmacologic management of aggression in adults with intellectual disability. *J Intellect Disabil Res* 2013; **1**:28–43.

12. Tyrer P, et al. Risperidone, haloperidol, and placebo in the treatment of aggressive challenging behaviour in patients with intellectual disability: a randomised controlled trial. *Lancet* 2008; **371**:57–63.

13. National Institute of Health and Care Excellence. Mental health problems in people with learning disabilities: prevention, assessment and management. NICE Guideline [NG54]. 2016 (last checked November 2020, last accessed March 2024); https://www.nice.org.uk/Guidance/NG54.

14. Shankar R, et al. Stopping, rationalising or optimising antipsychotic drug treatment in people with intellectual disability and/or autism. *Drug Ther Bull* 2019; **57**:10–13.

15. Deb S, et al. UK psychiatrists' experience of withdrawal of antipsychotics prescribed for challenging behaviours in adults with intellectual disabilities and/or autism. *Br J Psych Open* 2020; **6**:e112.

16. Branford D, et al. Antidepressant prescribing for adult people with an intellectual disability living in England. *Br J Psychiatry* 2022; **221**:488–493.

17. Malone RP, et al. The role of antipsychotics in the management of behavioural symptoms in children and adolescents with autism. *Drugs* 2009; **69**:535–548.

18. Malt UF, et al. Effectiveness of zuclopenthixol compared with haloperidol in the treatment of behavioural disturbances in learning disabled patients. *Br J Psychiatry* 1995; **166**:374–377.

19. Hassler F, et al. Treatment of aggressive behavior problems in boys with intellectual disabilities using zuclopenthixol. *J Child Adolesc Psychopharmacol* 2014; **24**:579–581.

20. Nagaraj R, et al. Risperidone in children with autism: randomized, placebo-controlled, double-blind study. *J Child Neurol* 2006; **21**:450–455.

21. Pandina GJ, et al. Risperidone improves behavioral symptoms in children with autism in a randomized, double-blind, placebo-controlled trial. *J Autism Dev Disord* 2007; **37**:367–373.

22. Owen R, et al. Aripiprazole in the treatment of irritability in children and adolescents with autistic disorder. *Pediatrics* 2009; **124**:1533–1540.

23. Marcus RN, et al. A placebo-controlled, fixed-dose study of aripiprazole in children and adolescents with irritability associated with autistic disorder. *J Am Acad Child Adolesc Psychiatry* 2009; **48**:1110–1119.

24. Fido A, et al. Olanzapine in the treatment of behavioral problems associated with autism: an open-label trial in Kuwait. *Med Princ Pract* 2008; **17**:415–418.

25. Zuddas A, et al. Clinical effects of clozapine on autistic disorder. *Am J Psychiatry* 1996; **153**:738.

26. Ayub M, et al. Clozapine for psychotic disorders in adults with intellectual disabilities. *Cochrane Database Syst Rev* 2015; **9**:CD010625.

27. Stigler KA, et al. Pharmacotherapy of irritability in pervasive developmental disorders. *Child Adolesc Psychiatr Clin N Am* 2008; **17**:739–752.

28. Williams K, et al. Selective serotonin reuptake inhibitors (SSRIs) for autism spectrum disorders (ASD). *Cochrane Database Syst Rev* 2013; **8**:CD004677.

29. Reddihough DS, et al. Effect of fluoxetine on obsessive-compulsive behaviors in children and adolescents with autism spectrum disorders: a randomized clinical trial. *JAMA* 2019; **322**:1561–1569.

30. Myers SM. Citalopram not effective for repetitive behaviour in autistic spectrum disorders. *Evid Based Ment Health* 2010; **13**:22.

31. Cook Jr, EH, et al. Fluoxetine treatment of children and adults with autistic disorder and mental retardation. *J Am Acad Child Adolesc Psychiatry* 1992; **31**:739–745.

32. Oswald DP, et al. Medication use among children with autism spectrum disorders. *J Child Adolesc Psychopharmacol* 2007; **17**:348–355.

33. Carminati GG, et al. Using venlafaxine to treat behavioral disorders in patients with autism spectrum disorder. *Prog Neuropsychopharmacol Biol Psychiatry* 2016; **65**:85–95.

34. Deb S, et al. The effectiveness of mood stabilizers and antiepileptic medication for the management of behaviour problems in adults with intellectual disability: a systematic review. *J Intellect Disabil Res* 2008; **52**:107–113.

35. Ruedrich S, et al. Effect of divalproex sodium on aggression and self-injurious behaviour in adults with intellectual disability: a retrospective review. *J Intellect Disabil Res* 1999; **43 Pt 2**:105–111.

36. Donovan SJ, et al. Divalproex treatment for youth with explosive temper and mood lability: a double-blind, placebo-controlled crossover design. *Am J Psychiatry* 2000; **157**:818–820.

37. Unwin GL, et al. Use of medication for the management of behavior problems among adults with intellectual disabilities: a clinicians' consensus survey. *Am J Ment Retard* 2008; **113**:19–31.

38. Pary RJ. Towards defining adequate lithium trials for individuals with mental retardation and mental illness. *Am J Ment Retard* 1991; **95**:681–691.

39. Craft M, et al. Lithium in the treatment of aggression in mentally handicapped patients. A double-blind trial. *Br J Psychiatry* 1987; **150**:685–689.

40. Malone RP, et al. A double-blind placebo-controlled study of lithium in hospitalized aggressive children and adolescents with conduct disorder. *Arch Gen Psychiatry* 2000; **57**:649–654.

41. Yuan J, et al. Lithium treatment is safe in children with intellectual disability. *Front Mol Neurosci* 2018; **11**:425.

42. Campbell M, et al. Naltrexone in autistic children: an acute open dose range tolerance trial. *J Am Acad Child Adolesc Psychiatry* 1989; **28**:200–206.

43. Barrett RP, et al. Effects of naloxone and naltrexone on self-injury: a double-blind, placebo-controlled analysis. *Am J Ment Retard* 1989; **93**:644–651.

44. Mouaffak F, et al. Kleptomania treated with naltrexone in a patient with intellectual disability. *J Psychiatry Neurosci* 2020; **45**:71–72.

45. Sabus A, et al. Management of self-injurious behaviors in children with neurodevelopmental disorders: a pharmacotherapy overview. *Pharmacotherapy* 2019; **39**:645–664.

Huntington's disease

Huntington's disease (HD) is a genetic neurodegenerative disease with an estimated prevalence of 4.88 individuals per 100,000 worldwide, and a higher incidence in Europe and North America.[1] The mutant Huntington protein causes neuronal dysfunction and death through several mechanisms, resulting in a triad of motor, cognitive and neuropsychiatric symptoms.[2] There are currently no disease-modifying treatments[3,4] so symptomatic therapies are used to improve quality of life (Box 10.3).

Box 10.3 General principles of pharmacological symptom management in Huntington's disease[5,6]

- Tailor management to the needs of the individual patient (treatment is typically initiated when symptoms become bothersome, interfering or socially stigmatising)
- Check whether existing medications are causing or exacerbating symptoms before commencing new treatments
- Prioritise treatment to target the most troublesome symptoms first, with consideration of comorbid features
- Balance therapeutic benefit with the potential for adverse effects
- Start with a low dose and titrate according to tolerability and response (patients are relatively more sensitive to cognitive and motor adverse effects which may also be difficult to distinguish from disease progression)
- Regularly follow up with patients to address changes in treatment (because symptomology evolves with disease progression)

There are few controlled studies to guide practice in this area,[3] although some direction can be drawn from published expert opinion and clinical experience. A summary of the available literature is given in this section. Readers are directed to the reports cited for details of dosage regimens and further information about tolerability. Clinicians who treat patients with HD are encouraged to publish reports of both positive and negative outcomes to increase the primary literature base.

Motor symptoms

Motor disturbances follow a biphasic course – an initial hyperkinetic phase with prominent chorea which tends to plateau over time, and a later hypokinetic phase characterised by bradykinesia, dystonia, balance and gait disturbance.[7] With regard to chorea, the goal of treatment is not to obliterate movements but to reduce their severity to achieve better tolerability.[5] Treatment pathways are available to guide management.[8] First-line treatments include tetrabenazine (licensed) or SGAs (unlicensed) (Table 10.9).[8] Monotherapy is preferred to prevent an increased risk of adverse effects and complicating the management of non-motor symptoms.[8]

Table 10.9 Evidence and experience regarding the pharmacological treatment of motor symptoms in Huntington's disease (HD).

Symptoms	Treatment
Chorea	**Tetrabenazine**: unlike antipsychotics, tetrabenazine's effectiveness is well established.[2,3,8] However, adverse effects including sedation, depression and parkinsonism may limit its clinical benefit. In clinical practice, many prefer to use tetrabenazine first line in patients without depressive symptoms and suicidal behaviour.[8] Compliance with a multiple daily dosing regimen (e.g. three times a day) is needed.
	Other VMAT2 inhibitors: deutetrabenazine and valbenazine are licensed in the USA for the treatment of chorea in HD.[2,4,9] Where available, they may be preferred over tetrabenazine owing to an improved pharmacokinetic and adverse effect profile,[2,9] although direct comparisons are lacking.[4]
	Antipsychotics: considered first-line treatment in clinical practice, particularly in the presence of depression, aggression, psychosis or when poor drug compliance is suspected[5,8,10] despite a lack of data from RCTs.[2] SGAs such as aripiprazole, risperidone or olanzapine are used most commonly.[8,11] Potentially limiting adverse effects include dyskinesia, parkinsonism and metabolic syndrome.[5] FGAs have been used successfully but are less popular in clinical practice because of the risk of EPSEs.[10] LAI antipsychotics have been used in some published case reports, in cases of non-compliance or motor fluctuations with oral antipsychotics.[12] For severe chorea, antipsychotics and VMAT2 inhibitors have been used in combination.[8] Note that VMAT2 inhibitors have the potential for QT prolongation, as do most antipsychotics.
Hypokinetic rigidity	Levodopa may provide partial and temporary relief of symptoms.[8] Note the potential for such drugs to exacerbate behavioural disturbances. Rigidity may be caused/worsened by antipsychotics or tetrabenazine; dose reduction or discontinuation should be considered in the first instance, after weighing any derived benefits against symptom severity.[8] Positive case reports exist for amantadine and dopamine agonists (although guidelines do not make recommendations on their use).[8]
Myoclonus	Valproate or clonazepam has been suggested, used alone or combination.[8] Levetiracetam is a therapeutic alternative.[8]
Dystonia	Low-dose tetrabenazine has been suggested[11] and a 2022 review concluded that deutetrabenazine is likely also to be effective.[2] Botulinum toxin injections have been suggested for focal dystonia;[8] clonazepam or baclofen has been suggested for non-focal dystonia.[5]

EPSEs, extrapyramidal side effects; LAI, long-acting injectable; VMAT2, vesicular monoamine transporter 2.

Mental and behavioural symptoms

A wide variety of mental and behavioural symptoms occur in HD, including anxiety, depression, suicidality, preservation, disinhibition, irritability, apathy and, rarely, psychosis.[13] Mental and behavioural symptoms can emerge before motor disturbances and reduce quality of life substantially.[13] In comparison with other HD features, psychiatric symptoms are perhaps the most amenable to pharmacotherapy.[6] In general, psychiatric treatment choices are selected as they would be in other conditions[5] although patients are relatively more sensitive to adverse effects.[5] The most commonly prescribed psychotropics are summarised in Tables 10.10 and 10.11 (mostly based on low-quality evidence).[13]

CHAPTER 10

Table 10.10 Pharmacological treatment of mental and behavioural symptoms in Huntington's disease (HD).

Symptoms	Treatment
Anxiety	Reported 16.7–24% lifetime prevalence in HD.[13] There are no RCTs to guide choice; however, olanzapine 5mg/day substantially improved anxiety symptoms in one small open-label pilot study.[13] SSRIs and SNRIs have been suggested as first-line treatment.[5,8] Some guidelines have recommended considering SGAs (quetiapine[8], risperidone or olanzapine) for anxiety associated with personality or behavioural disturbances[14] or when other treatments fail.[8] Anxiolytics such as benzodiazepines or buspirone may also be useful.[11,14]
Depression	Reported 30–70% prevalence in HD.[15] Treatment is typically required because depression is linked to a lower quality of life in HD and increases the risk of suicide.[13,15] There are almost no RCTs to guide choice.[11,16] However, most experts agree that depression in HD responds well to antidepressants. SSRIs are the preferred first-line treatment[5,8] but this is based on a less than perfect literature base.[17]
	SSRIs: two controlled trials examined the effects of fluoxetine and citalopram in non-depressed patients with HD. Despite excluding depressed patients, both showed near significant improvements in depressive symptoms.[16] Note that VMAT2 inhibitors are metabolised by CYP2D6; so inhibitors of this enzyme (e.g. fluoxetine, paroxetine) are predicted to increase exposure to active metabolites.
	SNRIs: venlafaxine was effective in an uncontrolled study;[16] however, one in five developed adverse effects such as nausea and irritability.[13]
	TCAs: beneficial effects reported in some cases[18] but generally their use should be avoided or limited. Anticholinergic properties of TCAs may worsen hyperkinesias and cognition.[11,18] Toxicity in overdose may also make them less suitable choices (suicidality is increased in HD[13]).
	Others: Mirtazapine was used successfully in one case report of severe depression.[5] In a case registry study it was one of the most frequently prescribed treatments for depression in HD.[13] Bupropion and SSRIs were found to be superior to SNRIs in one analysis of an observational study.[19] Lithium produced improvements in suicidality in a small case series[16] but experience is very limited, and tolerability may be poor. MAOIs have been used in earlier case studies;[18] a lack of recent experience and important interactions with VMAT2 inhibitors make these less suitable. ECT can be used safely and effectively and may be considered in life-threatening cases.[8,20]
Obsessive compulsive behaviours or perseveration	There are no RCTs.[21] International consensus supports the use of SSRIs first line;[8] use of clomipramine is also supported[13] but tolerability may be poor. Case studies document the successful use of fluoxetine, paroxetine and sertraline.[5] One study of two patients with perseveration and aggression reported beneficial effects with buspirone.[13] For ideational perseveration, consensus also supports the use of olanzapine or risperidone (particularly if associated with irritability).[8]
Irritability or agitation[22]	Reported prevalence of 38–73% in HD. Initial management is non-pharmacological (e.g. by addressing possible triggers such as pain or akathisia and using behavioural/psychological approaches). No medications are approved specifically, but expert consensus supports the use of SSRIs as preferred first-line agents, with antipsychotics being the next most favoured alternative monotherapy. Clinical features influence treatment choice. For example, SGAs (e.g. olanzapine, risperidone, quetiapine) may be preferred in the presence of chorea, acute irritability, aggression or impulsivity. Benzodiazepines are a widely used adjunctive therapy. Guidelines have also recommended mirtazapine or mianserin in patients not benefitting from maximum doses of SSRIs, especially in those with a comorbid sleep disorder. In cases non-responsive to antidepressants and/or antipsychotics, adjunctive mood stabilisers have also been recommended.[8] The effect of dextromethorphan/quinidine for irritability in HD is, at the time of writing, being studied in a phase III RCT.[4]
	Aggressive behaviours: a wide variety of psychotropics have been used with reported beneficial effects (e.g. antipsychotics, lithium, valproate, propranolol, medroxyprogesterone, SSRIs, buspirone).[18,23] Antipsychotics have been used most commonly. The evidence base is too limited to make specific treatment recommendations[23] but low-dose antipsychotics can be considered.[5] ECT was helpful in a few case reports of agitation refractory to pharmacotherapy.[20]

Table 10.10 (*Continued*)

Symptoms	Treatment
Apathy	Common in HD and appears to worsen with disease progression.[13] Some sedative medications (e.g. antipsychotics, benzodiazepines, tetrabenazine) may contribute, so dose reduction or withdrawal should be considered.[8] In one small open study of 16 participants, cariprazine was associated with improvements in apathy, depressive symptoms and cognitive test scores.[11] Bupropion was studied in one multicentre RCT and found to be ineffective.[11] Other agents, including methylphenidate, atomoxetine, modafinil, amantadine and bromocriptine, have been trialled with little success.[13]
Psychosis	One of the least prevalent psychiatric manifestations of HD, perhaps because of the use of antidopaminergics for motor symptoms.[13] There are no RCTs to guide choice[11] – treatment is empirical. Note that antipsychotic drugs may exacerbate any underlying movement disorder. VMAT2 inhibitors may have antipsychotic activity[24] but they are not drugs of choice for psychosis in HD. **SGAs**: olanzapine and risperidone are used most frequently.[13] Low starting doses are recommended.[5] Case reports support the efficacy of risperidone, quetiapine, aripiprazole and amisulpride.[18] Clozapine may be considered in refractory cases[6,18] or akinetic forms of HD with debilitating parkinsonian symptoms.[8,11] **FGAs**: used less frequently due to the risk of dystonia and parkinsonism; however, haloperidol has been used when chorea is also problematic to the patient.[18]

MAOIs, monoamine oxidase inhibitors; TCAs, tricyclic antidepressants; VMAT2, vesicular monoamine transporter 2.

Table 10.11 Summary of treatments for mental state and behavioural changes in Huntington's disease.[6,8,13]

Symptoms	Most commonly prescribed pharmacological treatments	Alternatives
Anxiety	SSRIs, mirtazapine, pregabalin, venlafaxine	Olanzapine, risperidone, quetiapine, benzodiazepines, propranolol, buspirone
Depression or suicidality	SSRIs, bupropion, mirtazapine, venlafaxine	TCAs; ECT in refractory cases
Obsessive compulsive behaviours	SSRIs	Clomipramine
Irritability or agitation	SSRIs, SGAs (olanzapine, risperidone, sulpiride), tiapride, benzodiazepines	Anticonvulsants (lamotrigine, carbamazepine, valproate), TCAs, buspirone, propranolol; consider trial of an analgesic
Apathy	None	None
Psychosis	Olanzapine, risperidone, haloperidol, sulpiride, tiapride, LAI antipsychotics	Clozapine, quetiapine

LAI, long-acting injectable; TCAs, tricyclic antidepressants.

Cognitive symptoms

Cognitive disturbances may emerge many years before motor disturbances.[7] The progression of cognitive decline is gradual[25] and dementia is inevitable in late stages. Although a wide variety of agents have been studied,[2,11] none has become established treatment and the benefit of most remains unclear.[26] There is insufficient evidence to support the use of acetylcholinesterase inhibitors[27] and no evidence to support any other medications to treat dementia in HD.[11,28]

References

1. Medina A, et al. Prevalence and incidence of Huntington's disease: an updated systematic review and meta-analysis. *Mov Disord* 2022; 37:2327–2335.
2. Ferreira JJ, et al. An MDS evidence-based review on treatments for Huntington's disease. *Mov Disord* 2022; 37:25–35.
3. Mestre T, et al. Therapeutic interventions for disease progression in Huntington's disease. *Cochrane Database Syst Rev* 2009; 2009:CD006455.
4. Van de Roovaart HJ, et al. Huntington's disease drug development: a phase 3 pipeline analysis. *Pharmaceuticals (Basel)* 2023; 16:1513.
5. Killoran A, et al. Current therapeutic options for Huntington's disease: good clinical practice versus evidence-based approaches? *Mov Disord* 2014; 29:1404–1413.
6. Anderson KE, et al. Clinical management of neuropsychiatric symptoms of Huntington disease: expert-based consensus guidelines on agitation, anxiety, apathy, psychosis and sleep disorders. *J Huntingtons Dis* 2018; 7:355–366.
7. McColgan P, et al. Huntington's disease: a clinical review. *Eur J Neurol* 2018; 25:24–34.
8. Bachoud-Lévi AC, et al. International guidelines for the treatment of Huntington's disease. *Front Neurol* 2019; 10:710.
9. Furr Stimming E, et al. Safety and efficacy of valbenazine for the treatment of chorea associated with Huntington's disease (KINECT-HD): a phase 3, randomised, double-blind, placebo-controlled trial. *Lancet Neurol* 2023; 22:494–504.
10. Unti E, et al. Antipsychotic drugs in Huntington's disease. *Expert Rev Neurother* 2017; 17:227–237.
11. Saft C, et al. Symptomatic treatment options for Huntington's disease (guidelines of the German Neurological Society). *Neurol Res Pract* 2023; 5:61.
12. Javelot H, et al. Benefit of long-acting paliperidone in Huntington's disease: a case report. *Int Clin Psychopharmacol* 2021; 36:101–103.
13. Eddy CM, et al. Changes in mental state and behaviour in Huntington's disease. *Lancet Psychiatry* 2016; 3:1079–1086.
14. Desamericq G, et al. Guidelines for clinical pharmacological practices in Huntington's disease. *Rev Neurol (Paris)* 2016; 172:423–432.
15. Jellinger KA. The pathobiology of depression in Huntington's disease: an unresolved puzzle. *J Neural Transm* 2024; doi: 10.1007/s00702-024-02750-w.
16. Moulton CD, et al. Systematic review of pharmacological treatments for depressive symptoms in Huntington's disease. *Mov Disord* 2014; 29:1556–1561.
17. Zadegan SA, et al. Treatment of depression in Huntington's disease: a systematic review. *J Neuropsychiatry Clin Neurosci* 2024; doi: 10.1176/appi.neuropsych.20230120.
18. van Duijn E. Medical treatment of behavioral manifestations of Huntington disease. *Handb Clin Neurol* 2017; 144:129–139.
19. McLauchlan DJ, et al. Different depression: motivational anhedonia governs antidepressant efficacy in Huntington's disease. *Brain Commun* 2022; 4:fcac278.
20. Yahya A, et al. Electroconvulsive therapy in Huntington's disease. *Prog Neurol Psychiatry* 2021; 25:33–38.
21. Oosterloo M, et al. Obsessive-compulsive and perseverative behaviors in Huntington's disease. *J Huntingtons Dis* 2019; 8:1–7.
22. Karagas NE, et al. Irritability in Huntington's disease. *J Huntingtons Dis* 2020; 9:107–113.
23. Fisher CA, et al. Aggression in Huntington's disease: a systematic review of rates of aggression and treatment methods. *J Huntingtons Dis* 2014; 3:319–332.
24. Connolly A, et al. Meta-analysis and systematic review of vesicular monoamine transporter (VMAT-2) inhibitors in schizophrenia and psychosis. *Psychopharmacology (Berl)* 2024; 241:225–241.
25. Ross CA, et al. Huntington disease: natural history, biomarkers and prospects for therapeutics. *Nat Rev Neurol* 2014; 10:204–216.
26. Van der Vaart T, et al. Treatment of cognitive deficits in genetic disorders: a systematic review of clinical trials of diet and drug treatments. *JAMA Neurol* 2015; 72:1052–1060.
27. Li Y, et al. Cholinesterase inhibitors for rarer dementias associated with neurological conditions. *Cochrane Database Syst Rev* 2015; 3:CD009444.
28. O'Brien JT, et al. Clinical practice with anti-dementia drugs: a revised (third) consensus statement from the British Association for Psychopharmacology. *J Psychopharmacol* 2017; 31:147–168.

Multiple sclerosis

Individuals with multiple sclerosis (MS) experience a variety of psychiatric and neuro-logical disorders. These include depression, anxiety, pathological laughter and crying (pseudobulbar affect, PBA), mania, euphoria, psychosis, bipolar disorder, fatigue and cognitive impairment. Psychiatric disorders result from a variety of factors – the psychological impact of MS diagnosis and its prognosis, perceived lack of social support or unhelpful coping styles, increased stress, iatrogenic effects of treatments used with MS and MS-related inflammation and damage to neuronal pathways.[1]

Depression

In people with MS, depression is common with a point prevalence of 14–31%[2,3] and lifetime prevalence of up to 50%.[4,5] Suicide rates are 2–7.5 times higher than the general population[6] and suicidality is seen in more than a fifth of people with MS.[7] Depression in MS is often associated with fatigue and pain, although the relationship direction is unclear.[8] Overlapping symptoms of depression, PBA and MS can complicate diagnosis and so co-operation between neurologists and psychiatrists is essential to ensure optimal treatment. Depression in MS may result from structural changes in the brain related to MS pathology and, as such, it may differ fundamentally from non-MS depression.[9,10] Suggested treatments are described in Table 10.12.

Table 10.12 Recommendations for treatment for depression in multiple sclerosis (MS).

Step	Intervention
1	Screen for depression with PHQ-9 HADS/BDI[11]/CES-D.[12] Exclude or treat any organic causes. Consider iatrogenic effects of medications as potential cause of depression. Ensure there is no past history of mania or bipolar disorder. People with mild depression should be considered for CBT[13] or self-help.[14]
2	Guidelines recommend SSRIs as first-line treatment[12,15,16] but have been criticised for the dearth of MS-specific data.[17] Sertraline was as effective as CBT in one trial[18] but paroxetine was equivalent to placebo in another.[19] Fluoxetine was effective in MS-related depression in a small case series.[20] For those with comorbid pain, consideration should be given to treating with an SNRI such as duloxetine[21] or venlafaxine.[22] One RCT of desipramine showed it was more effective than placebo but tricyclics in general are often poorly tolerated.[23] In 2011, a Cochrane review was not convinced by many of the studies cited here,[24] but there is little reason to suppose that antidepressants are any less effective in depression associated with physical illness.[25] In 2023, bupropion was shown to be effective in a small RCT.[26] Vortioxetine may also improve both depression and anxiety.[27] CBT is the most appropriate psychological intervention with best efficacy in comparison with supportive therapy or usual care, and should be used in conjunction with medication for those who are moderately to severely depressed.[18,28,29] Mindfulness training may also help.[30] Omega-3 fatty acids are ineffective.[31] Because of reduced tolerability of adverse effects in this patient group, medications should be titrated from an initial half dose. Many MS patients are prescribed low-dose TCAs for pain/bladder disturbance, so SSRIs should be used with caution and patients should be observed for serotonin syndrome.
3	If SSRIs are not tolerated or there is no response, there are limited data that moclobemide is effective and well tolerated.[32,33] There are no published trials on venlafaxine, duloxetine and mirtazapine but these are used widely. Mirtazapine may worsen fatigue, at least initially. Venlafaxine and duloxetine are used for pain management in MS.[34]
4	ECT could be considered for people who are actively suicidal or severely depressed and at high risk, but it may trigger an exacerbation of MS symptoms, although some studies suggest that no neurological disturbance occurs.[35]

CBT, cognitive behaviour therapy; TCAs, tricyclic antidepressants.

Anxiety

Anxiety affects many people with MS, with a point prevalence of up to 50%[36] and lifetime incidence of 35–37%.[37] Elevated rates in comparison with the general population are seen for generalised anxiety disorder, panic disorder, obsessive compulsive disorder[37] and social anxiety. The uncertainty of prognosis is a major cause of anxiety in MS.[38] There are no published trials for the drug treatment of anxiety in MS, but SSRIs can be used and, in non-responsive cases, venlafaxine might be considered (based on practice in non-MS patients). Bupropion may also be effective.[26]

Benzodiazepines may be used for acute and severe anxiety but only for a maximum of 4 weeks and should not be prescribed in the long term. Buspirone and beta-blockers could also be considered although there is no demonstrated efficacy in MS. Pregabalin is also licensed for anxiety and may be useful in this population group especially where pain relief is required.[39,40] People with MS may also respond to cognitive behaviour therapy (CBT). Generally, treatment is as for non-MS anxiety disorders.

Pseudobulbar affect

Around 25% of individuals with MS experience pathological laughing or crying or other incongruence of affect.[41] It is more common in the advanced stages of the disease and is associated with cognitive impairment.[37] There have been a few open-label trials recommending the use of small doses of TCAs such as amitriptyline or SSRIs such as fluoxetine[42,43] in MS. Citalopram,[44] nortriptyline[45] and sertraline[46] have been investigated in people with post-stroke pathological laughing or crying and have shown reasonable efficacy and rapid response. Valproic acid may be effective.[47] The combination of dextromethorphan and low-dose quinidine (DMq) is effective.[48] Dextromethorphan plus fluoxetine may show similar effects.[49] In these combinations, dextromethorphan (an analgesic and cough suppressant) is the active ingredient and quinidine/fluoxetine the metabolic inhibitor. DMq is approved by the US Food and Drug Administration (FDA) as Nuedexta and once held approval in the EU but is not marketed there.

Bipolar disorder

The lifetime prevalence of bipolar disorder in MS is just less than 10%.[50] Lithium can cause diuresis and thus lead to increased difficulties with tolerance in people with MS-related bladder disorder. Mania accompanied by psychosis could be treated with low-dose antipsychotics such as risperidone, olanzapine[51] or ziprasidone.[52] Patients requiring psychiatric treatment for steroid-induced mania with psychosis have been shown to respond to olanzapine.[53]

Psychosis

Psychosis is relatively uncommon compared with other psychiatric disorders.[52] A 2015 meta-analysis estimated the prevalence of psychosis to be 4.3%.[1] In a very few cases, psychosis is the presenting complaint of MS.[54] There have been few published trials, but risperidone or clozapine has been recommended because of the low risk of extrapyramidal symptoms.[55] On this basis, olanzapine, aripiprazole and quetiapine might also, in theory at least, be possible options. ECT has been used in refractory cases.[56] Risperidone, quetiapine, olanzapine and, particularly, clozapine may have beneficial immunomodulatory properties.[57]

Psychosis may rarely be the presentation of an MS relapse in which case steroids may be beneficial but would need to be given under close supervision. Note also the small risk of psychotic reactions in patients receiving tetrahydrocannabinol (THC)-containing formulations.[58,59]

Cognitive impairment

Cognitive impairment occurs in at least 40–65% of people with MS. Some of the medications commonly prescribed can worsen cognition, such as tizanidine, diazepam and gabapentin.[60] Although there are no published trials, evidence from clinical case studies suggests that the treatment of sleep difficulties, depression and fatigue can enhance cognitive function.[60] There have been two small trials with donepezil for people with mild to moderate cognitive impairment showing moderate efficacy.[61,62] A larger study found no effect.[63] Similarly, data supporting the use of memantine are weak.[64] Overall, no treatment has proven worthwhile efficacy[65] and disease-modifying agents offer greater promise.[66]

Fatigue

Fatigue is a common symptom in MS, with up to 80% of people affected.[67] The aetiology of fatigue is unclear but there have been suggestions that disruption of neuronal networks,[68] depression or psychological reactions,[55] sleep disturbances, inflammation[69] or medication may play a role in its development. Pharmacological and non-pharmacological strategies[67] should be used in a treatment strategy.

Non-pharmacological strategies include reviewing history for any possible contributing factors, assessment and treatment of underlying depression if present, medication, pacing activities and appropriate exercise. One trial suggests that CBT reduces fatigue scores.[70]

Pharmacological strategies include the use of amantadine[71] or modafinil. In the UK, National Institute for Health and Care Excellence (NICE) guidelines suggest no medicine should be used routinely but that amantadine could have a small benefit and should be offered.[72] A Cochrane review of amantadine in people with MS suggested that the quality and outcomes of the amantadine trials are inconsistent and that therefore efficacy remains unclear.[71] A meta-analysis of 11 RCTs found supporting data for amantadine[73] and a later (2020) meta-analysis confirmed its value.[74]

Modafinil has mixed results in clinical trials, but a meta-analysis of five RCTs[75] found clear benefit. Despite doubts over its efficacy, modafinil is widely used in MS.[76]

A 2023 meta-analysis of five studies suggested benefit for vitamin D supplementation.[77]

References

1. Marrie RA, et al. The incidence and prevalence of psychiatric disorders in multiple sclerosis: a systematic review. *Mult Scler* 2015; **21**:305–317.

2. Gottberg K, et al. A population-based study of depressive symptoms in multiple sclerosis in Stockholm county: association with functioning and sense of coherence. *J Neurol Neurosurg Psychiatry* 2007; **78**:60–65.

3. Boeschoten RE, et al. Prevalence of depression and anxiety in multiple sclerosis: a systematic review and meta-analysis. *J Neurol Sci* 2017; **372**:331–341.

4. Patten SB, et al. Depression in multiple sclerosis. *Int Rev Psychiatry* 2017; **29**:463–472.

5. Kalb R, et al. Depression and suicidality in multiple sclerosis: red flags, management strategies, and ethical considerations. *Curr Neurol Neurosci Rep* 2019; **19**:77.

6. Sadovnick AD, et al. Cause of death in patients attending multiple sclerosis clinics. *Neurology* 1991; **41**:1193–1196.

7. Strupp J, et al. Risk factors for suicidal ideation in patients feeling severely affected by multiple sclerosis. *J Palliat Med* 2016; **19**:523–528.

8. Sparaco M, et al. Psychiatric disorders in multiple sclerosis. *J Neurol* 2021; **268**:45–60.

9. Corallo F, et al. A complex relation between depression and multiple sclerosis: a descriptive review. *Neurol Sci* 2019; **40**:1551–1558.

10. Menculini G, et al. Psychiatric symptoms in multiple sclerosis: a biological perspective on synaptic and network dysfunction. *J Neurol Neurosurg Psychiatry* 2023; **94**:389–395.

11. Moran PJ, et al. The validity of Beck Depression Inventory and Hamilton Rating Scale for Depression items in the assessment of depression among patients with multiple sclerosis. *J Behav Med* 2005; **28**:35–41.

12. Pandya R, et al. Predictive value of the CES-D in detecting depression among candidates for disease-modifying multiple sclerosis treatment. *Psychosomatics* 2005; **46**:131–134.

13. Minden SL, et al. Evidence-based guideline: assessment and management of psychiatric disorders in individuals with MS: report of the Guideline Development Subcommittee of the American Academy of Neurology. *Neurology* 2014; **82**:174–181.

14. Rickards H. Depression in neurological disorders: Parkinson's disease, multiple sclerosis, and stroke. *J Neurol Neurosurg Psychiatry* 2005; **76** Suppl 1:i48–i52.

15. Silveira C, et al. Neuropsychiatric symptoms of multiple sclerosis: state of the art. *Psychiatry Investig* 2019; **16**:877–888.

16. Patten SB. Current perspectives on co-morbid depression and multiple sclerosis. *Expert Rev Neurother* 2020; **20**:867–874.

17. McIntosh GE, et al. Clinical practice guidelines for the detection and treatment of depression in multiple sclerosis: a systematic review. *Neurol Clin Pract* 2023; **13**:e200154.

18. Mohr DC, et al. Comparative outcomes for individual cognitive-behavior therapy, supportive-expressive group psychotherapy, and sertraline for the treatment of depression in multiple sclerosis. *J Consult Clin Psychol* 2001; **69**:942–949.

19. Ehde DM, et al. Efficacy of paroxetine in treating major depressive disorder in persons with multiple sclerosis. *Gen Hosp Psychiatry* 2008; **30**:40–48.

20. Flax JW, et al. Effect of fluoxetine on patients with multiple sclerosis. *Am J Psychiatry* 1991; **148**:1603.

21. Vollmer TL, et al. A randomized, double-blind, placebo-controlled trial of duloxetine for the treatment of pain in patients with multiple sclerosis. *Pain Pract* 2014; **14**:732–744.

22. Hilty DM, et al. Psychopharmacology for neurologists: principles, algorithms, and other resources. *Continuum* 2006; **12**:33–46.

23. Barak Y, et al. Treatment of depression in patients with multiple sclerosis. *Neurologist* 1998; **4**:99–104.

24. Koch MW, et al. Pharmacologic treatment of depression in multiple sclerosis. *Cochrane Database Syst Rev* 2011; **2**:CD007295.

25. Taylor D, et al. Pharmacological interventions for people with depression and chronic physical health problems: systematic review and meta-analyses of safety and efficacy. *Br J Psychiatry* 2011; **198**:179–188.

26. Baghbanian SM, et al. The effects of bupropion on sexual dysfunction in female patients with multiple sclerosis: a double-blind randomized clinical trial. *Mult Scler Relat Disord* 2023; **69**:104399.

27. Gil-Sanchez A, et al. Effects of vortioxetine on cognition and fatigue in patients with multiple sclerosis and depression: a case series study. *CNS Neurol Disord Drug Targets* 2024; **23**:395–401.

28. Siegert RJ, et al. Depression in multiple sclerosis: a review. *J Neurol Neurosurg Psychiatry* 2005; **76**:469–475.

29. Larcombe NA, et al. An evaluation of cognitive-behaviour therapy for depression in patients with multiple sclerosis. *Br J Psychiatry* 1984; **145**:366–371.

30. Grossman P, et al. MS quality of life, depression, and fatigue improve after mindfulness training: a randomized trial. *Neurology* 2010; **75**:1141–1149.

31. Shinto L, et al. Omega-3 fatty acids for depression in multiple sclerosis: a randomized pilot study. *PLoS One* 2016; **11**:e0147195.

32. Schiffer RB, et al. Antidepressant pharmacotherapy of depression associated with multiple sclerosis. *Am J Psychiatry* 1990; **147**:1493–1497.

33. Barak Y, et al. Moclobemide treatment in multiple sclerosis patients with comorbid depression: an open-label safety trial. *J Neuropsychiatry Clin Neurosci* 1999; **11**:271–273.

34. Shkodina AD, et al. Pharmacological and non-pharmacological approaches for the management of neuropathic pain in multiple sclerosis. *CNS Drugs* 2024; **38**:205–224.

35. Rasmussen KG, et al. Electroconvulsive therapy in patients with multiple sclerosis. *J ECT* 2007; **23**:179–180.

36. Jones KH, et al. A large-scale study of anxiety and depression in people with multiple sclerosis: a survey via the web portal of the UK MS Register. *PLoS One* 2012; **7**:e41910.

37. Korostil M, et al. Anxiety disorders and their clinical correlates in multiple sclerosis patients. *Mult Scler* 2007; **13**:67–72.

38. Butler E, et al. 'It's the unknown' – understanding anxiety: from the perspective of people with multiple sclerosis. *Psychol Health* 2019; **34**:368–383.

39. Solaro C, et al. Pregabalin for treating paroxysmal painful symptoms in multiple sclerosis: a pilot study. *J Neurol* 2009; **256**:1773–1774.

40. Bittner S, et al. [Pregabalin and gabapentin in multiple sclerosis: clinical experiences and therapeutic implications]. *Nervenarzt* 2011; **82**:1273–1280.

41. Nabizadeh F, et al. Pseudobulbar affect in neurodegenerative diseases: a systematic review and meta-analysis. *J Clin Neurosci* 2022; **100**:100–107.

42. Feinstein A, et al. The effects of anxiety on psychiatric morbidity in patients with multiple sclerosis. *Mult Scler* 1999; **5**:323–326.

43. Feinstein A, et al. Prevalence and neurobehavioral correlates of pathological laughing and crying in multiple sclerosis. *Arch Neurol* 1997; **54**:1116–1121.

44. Andersen G, et al. Citalopram for post-stroke pathological crying. *Lancet* 1993; **342**:837–839.

45. Robinson RG, et al. Pathological laughing and crying following stroke: validation of a measurement scale and a double-blind treatment study. *Am J Psychiatry* 1993; **150**:286–293.

46. Burns A, et al. Sertraline in stroke-associated lability of mood. *Int J Geriatr Psychiatry* 1999; **14**:681–685.

47. Johnson B, et al. Crying and suicidal, but not depressed. Pseudobulbar affect in multiple sclerosis successfully treated with valproic acid: case report and literature review. *Palliat Support Care* 2015; **13**:1797–1801.

48. Pioro EP, et al. Dextromethorphan plus ultra low-dose quinidine reduces pseudobulbar affect. *Ann Neurol* 2010; **68**:693–702.

49. McGrane I, et al. Treatment of pseudobulbar affect with fluoxetine and dextromethorphan in a woman with multiple sclerosis. *Ann Pharmacother* 2017; **51**:1035–1036.

50. Joseph B, et al. Prevalence of bipolar disorder in multiple sclerosis: a systematic review and meta-analysis. *Evid Based Ment Health* 2021; **24**:88–94.

51. Patten SB, et al. Biopsychosocial correlates of lifetime major depression in a multiple sclerosis population. *Mult Scler* 2000; **6**:115–120.

52. Davids E, et al. Antipsychotic treatment of psychosis associated with multiple sclerosis. *Prog Neuropsychopharmacol Biol Psychiatry* 2004; **28**:743–744.

53. Budur K, et al. Olanzapine for corticosteroid-induced mood disorders. *Psychosomatics* 2003; **44**:353.

54. Camara-Lemarroy CR, et al. The varieties of psychosis in multiple sclerosis: a systematic review of cases. *Mult Scler Relat Disord* 2017; **12**:9–14.

55. Jefferies K. The neuropsychiatry of multiple sclerosis. *Adv Psychiatric Treat* 2006; **12**:214–220.

56. Narita Z, et al. Possible effects of electroconvulsive therapy on refractory psychosis in primary progressive multiple sclerosis: a case report. *Neuropsychopharmacol Rep* 2018; **38**:92–94.

57. Stamoula E, et al. Atypical antipsychotics in multiple sclerosis: a review of their in vivo immunomodulatory effects. *Mult Scler Relat Disord* 2022; **58**:103522.

58. Aragona M, et al. Psychopathological and cognitive effects of therapeutic cannabinoids in multiple sclerosis: a double-blind, placebo-controlled, crossover study. *Clin Neuropharmacol* 2009; **32**:41–47.

59. Black N, et al. Cannabinoids for the treatment of mental disorders and symptoms of mental disorders: a systematic review and meta-analysis. *Lancet Psychiatry* 2019; **6**:995–1010.

60. Pierson SH, et al. Treatment of cognitive impairment in multiple sclerosis. *Behav Neurol* 2006; **17**:53–67.

61. Krupp LB, et al. Donepezil improved memory in multiple sclerosis in a randomized clinical trial. *Neurology* 2004; **63**:1579–1585.

62. Greene YM, et al. A 12-week, open trial of donepezil hydrochloride in patients with multiple sclerosis and associated cognitive impairments. *J Clin Psychopharmacol* 2000; **20**:350–356.

63. Krupp LB, et al. Multicenter randomized clinical trial of donepezil for memory impairment in multiple sclerosis. *Neurology* 2011; **76**:1500–1507.

64. Lovera JF, et al. Memantine for cognitive impairment in multiple sclerosis: a randomized placebo-controlled trial. *Mult Scler* 2010; **16**:715–723.

65. Chen MH, et al. Cognitive efficacy of pharmacologic treatments in multiple sclerosis: a systematic review. *CNS Drugs* 2020; **34**:599–628.

66. Patti F. Treatment of cognitive impairment in patients with multiple sclerosis. *Expert Opin Investig Drugs* 2012; **21**:1679–1699.

67. Bakshi R. Fatigue associated with multiple sclerosis: diagnosis, impact and management. *Mult Scler* 2003; **9**:219–227.

68. Sepulcre J, et al. Fatigue in multiple sclerosis is associated with the disruption of frontal and parietal pathways. *Mult Scler* 2009; **15**:337–344.

69. Ormstad H, et al. Chronic fatigue and depression due to multiple sclerosis: immune-inflammatory pathways, tryptophan catabolites and the gut-brain axis as possible shared pathways. *Mult Scler Relat Disord* 2020; **46**:102533.

70. Van KK, et al. A randomized controlled trial of cognitive behavior therapy for multiple sclerosis fatigue. *Psychosom Med* 2008; **70**:205–213.

71. Pucci E, et al. Amantadine for fatigue in multiple sclerosis. *Cochrane Database Syst Rev* 2007; **1**:CD002818.

72. National Institute for Health and Care Excellence. Multiple sclerosis in adults: management. NICE guideline [NG220]. 2022 (last checked May 2024); https://www.nice.org.uk/guidance/ng220.

73. Yang TT, et al. Pharmacological treatments for fatigue in patients with multiple sclerosis: a systematic review and meta-analysis. *J Neurol Sci* 2017; **380**:256–261.

74. Perez DQ, et al. Efficacy and safety of amantadine for the treatment of fatigue in multiple sclerosis: a systematic review and meta-analysis. *Neurodegener Dis Manag* 2020; **10**:383–395.

75. Shangyan H, et al. Meta-analysis of the efficacy of modafinil versus placebo in the treatment of multiple sclerosis fatigue. *Mult Scler Relat Disord* 2018; **19**:85–89.

76. Davies M, et al. Safety profile of modafinil across a range of prescribing indications, including off-label use, in a primary care setting in England: results of a modified prescription-event monitoring study. *Drug Saf* 2013; **36**:237–246.

77. López-Muñoz P, et al. Effect of vitamin D supplementation on fatigue in multiple sclerosis: a systematic review and meta-analysis. *Nutrients* 2023; **15**:2861.

Parkinson's disease

Psychiatric comorbidity is common in Parkinson's disease (PD). Approximately 25% of PD patients will suffer from major depression, a further 25% from milder forms of depression, 25% from anxiety spectrum disorders and 25% from psychosis.[1-3] The risk of developing dementia is 3.5–6-fold higher, depending on definition, than in age- and gender-matched controls.[4] Depression and anxiety often precede PD diagnosis. Anti-parkinsonian treatment is likely to increase psychiatric comorbidity. Indeed treatment-linked prolonged cognitive processing may be a harbinger of more disabling morbidity, like deficits in attention, multitasking and difficulties in sequencing and planning.[5] While depression and anxiety can occur at any time in the course of PD, psychosis, dementia and delirium are more prevalent in the later stages of the illness. Close co-operation between the psychiatrist and prescriber of anti-parkinsonian medication is often required to optimise treatment for this group of patients.

Depression

Depression in PD predicts greater cognitive decline, deterioration in functioning and progression of motor symptoms,[6] possibly reflecting more advanced and widespread neurodegeneration involving a variety of neurotransmitter pathways[7] and/or inability/disinclination to seek or comply with remedial therapies. Depression may also occur after the withdrawal of dopamine agonists.[8] Similarly, cyclical mood changes follow the on/off fluctuations associated with the levodopa dosage cycle. Suggested treatments are described in Table 10.13.

Table 10.13 Recommendations for treatment of depression in Parkinson's disease (PD).

Step	Intervention
1	Exclude/treat organic causes such as hypothyroidism (the prevalence of which is relatively high in PD[6]).
2	**SSRIs** are considered to be first-line treatment although the effect size is modest.[9-11] Some patients may experience a worsening of motor symptoms,[12,13] in particular tremor. Sertraline is the preferred SSRI in PD.[14] Care must be taken when combining SSRIs with selegiline (or rasagiline), as the risk of serotonin syndrome is increased.[6] The SNRIs venlafaxine[15] and duloxetine[16] also appear to have some effect although venlafaxine may modestly worsen motor symptoms.[15] **TCAs** are generally poorly tolerated because of their anticholinergic (can worsen cognitive problems and constipation) and alpha-blocking effects (can worsen symptoms of autonomic dysfunction). A 2022 network meta-analysis[17] showed that dopamine agonists and SSRIs have the highest efficacy and acceptability. Limited evidence supports the safe and effective use of **agomelatine**,[18,19] **bupropion**[20] and **vortioxetine**.[21]
3	Consider augmentation with dopamine agonists/releasers such as **pramiprexole**.[22] Note though that these drugs increase the risk of impulse control disorders.[23,24] They have also rarely been associated with the development of psychosis.[25] Dopamine agonists are effective antidepressants when used as a single agent.[26]
4	Consider **ECT**. Depression and motor symptoms generally respond well[6] but the risk of inducing delirium is high,[27] particularly in patients with pre-existing cognitive impairment.
5	Follow the algorithm for treatment-resistant depression (see 'Drug treatment of depression' in Chapter 3) from this point. Be aware of the increased propensity for adverse effects and drug interactions in this patient group.

TCAs, tricyclic antidepressants.

Psychosis

Psychosis in PD is often characterised by visual hallucinations.[28] Auditory hallucinations and delusions occur far less frequently,[29] and usually in younger patients.[30] Psychosis and dementia frequently coexist. Having one predicts the development of the other.[31] Sleep disorders are also an established risk factor for the development of psychosis.[32]

The exact aetiology of PD psychosis is poorly understood. In the majority of patients, psychotic symptoms are thought to be secondary to dopaminergic medication rather than part of PD itself. Psychosis secondary to medication may be determined at least in part through polymorphisms of the ACE gene.[33] From the limited data available, anticholinergics and dopamine agonists seem to be associated with a higher risk of inducing psychosis than levodopa or catechol-O-methyltransferase (COMT) inhibitors.[29,34] Psychosis is a major contributor to caregiver distress and a risk factor for institutionalisation and early death.[31] Suggested treatments are described in Table 10.14.

Table 10.14 Recommendations for treatment of psychosis in Parkinson's disease (PD).

Step	Intervention
1	Exclude organic causes (delirium).
2	Optimise the environment to maximise orientation and minimise problems due to poor caregiver–patient interactions.
3	If the patient has insight and hallucinations are infrequent and not troubling, do not treat.
4	Consider reducing or stopping anticholinergics and dopamine agonists. Monitor for signs of motor deterioration. Be prepared to restart/increase the dose of these drugs again to achieve the best balance between psychosis and mobility.
5	Consider an atypical antipsychotic. The efficacy of **clozapine** (see step 7) is unequivocally supported by placebo-controlled RCTs.[28] In contrast, there are several negative placebo-controlled trials for **quetiapine** and olanzapine.[28] Low-dose quetiapine (25–200mg a day) is the least badly tolerated and may have marginal efficacy.[35] It is probably reasonable to try quetiapine[36] before clozapine but the success rate is minimal. **Olanzapine, ziprasidone** and **aripiprazole** are likely to all have greater adverse effects on motor function than quetiapine and have no proven therapeutic effect. Risperidone and conventional antipsychotics should be avoided completely.
	All antipsychotics may be relatively less effective in managing psychotic symptoms in patients with dementia, and such patients may be more prone to developing motor and cognitive adverse effects.[37] Antipsychotics have been associated with an increased risk of vascular events in the elderly. In PD all antipsychotics are linked to increased mortality[38] although the effect of clozapine is not known.
6	Consider a **cholinesterase inhibitor**, particularly if the patient has comorbid dementia.[39] Cholinesterase inhibitors may also reduce the risk of falls.[40] Early use of these drugs does not prevent or reduce episodes of psychosis although there is some benefit on cognition.[41,42]
7	Try **clozapine**. Clozapine is highly effective in PD psychosis but widely underused.[43] It also has useful anti-tremor properties equivalent to benztropine.[44] A 2023 European study[45] reported that only 1% of PD psychosis patients received clozapine (72% received quetiapine).
	Start at 6.25mg – usual dose 25–35mg/day.[28,46] Usually safe but neuroleptic malignant syndrome has been reported.[47] Monitor as for clozapine in schizophrenia. Older people are more prone to develop serious blood dyscrasia. A case of aplastic anaemia has been reported.[48] Overall, clozapine is safer than other antipsychotics in PD psychosis.[49]
8	Consider **ECT**.[50] Psychotic and motor symptoms usually respond well[51] but the risk of inducing delirium is high,[27] particularly in patients with pre-existing cognitive impairment.

Pimavanserin

Pimavanserin is a 5-HT2A receptor inverse agonist available in the USA and some other countries. It is effective in PD psychosis but has no dopamine receptor activity and does not worsen PD movement disorder or seem to increase mortality.[52,53] It is more effective and better tolerated than **quetiapine**[54] and **olanzapine**.[35] Its therapeutic effects seem to increase with the age of the patient.[55]

Pimavanserin and clozapine are the only drugs unreservedly recommended for PD psychosis.[56] A network meta-analysis suggested only these two drugs had efficacy in PD, while having minimal effect on motor function.[49] Clozapine may be effective in pimavanserin non-responders.[57]

Cholinesterase inhibitors

Cholinesterase inhibitors have been shown to improve cognition, delusions and hallucinations in patients with Lewy body dementia (which has many similarities to PD). Motor function may deteriorate.[58,59] Improvements in cognitive functioning are modest.[60–62] A Cochrane review and some large RCTs[61,63,64] concluded that there is evidence that cholinesterase inhibitors lead to improvements in global functioning, cognition, behavioural disturbance and activities of daily living in PD. Again, motor function may deteriorate[64,65] with particular increase in tremor.[62] Evidence for memantine is mixed.[66,67] Discontinuation of anticholinergic drugs should improve cognition and psychosis – PD patients often have a very high anticholinergic burden, some of this unrelated to the treatment of PD itself.[68] Where confounding by indication is removed (where dementia risk could be better explained by indication than a medicine), the classes of medicine with anti-cholinergic properties indicated in dementia are reduced somewhat.[69] RCTs are needed to compare deprescribing of maintenance medicines with their continuation in diseases with dementia.[5]

Other treatments

Many patients with PD use complementary therapies, some of which may be modestly beneficial; see Zesiewicz et al.[70] Caffeine (and perhaps nicotine)[71] may offer a protective effect against the development of PD and also modestly improve motor function in established disease.[72]

Box 10.4 summarises the treatment of PD.

Box 10.4 Simplified summary of treatment in Parkinson's disease	
Depression in PD	Sertraline is first choice. Venlafaxine and duloxetine are next option. Consider agomelatine or bupropion. Pramipexole is an option in those not already on a dopamine agonist.
Psychosis in PD	Try low-dose quetiapine but withdraw if ineffective. Clozapine is the drug of choice for PD psychosis. Pimavanserin may be used where available. Electroconvulsive therapy is a last resort.

References

1. Hely MA, et al. The Sydney multicenter study of Parkinson's disease: the inevitability of dementia at 20 years. *Mov Disord* 2008; 23:837–844.

2. Riedel O, et al. Frequency of dementia, depression, and other neuropsychiatric symptoms in 1,449 outpatients with Parkinson's disease. *J Neurol* 2010; 257:1073–1082.

3. Reijnders JS, et al. A systematic review of prevalence studies of depression in Parkinson's disease. *Mov Disord* 2008; 23:183–189.

4. Åström DO, et al. High risk of developing dementia in Parkinson's disease: a Swedish registry-based study. *Sci Rep* 2022; 12:16759.

5. Wang W, et al. Bradyphrenia and tachyphrenia in idiopathic parkinsonism appear, in part, iatrogenic: an observational study with systematic review background. *J Clin Med* 2023; 12:6499.

6. McDonald WM, et al. Prevalence, etiology, and treatment of depression in Parkinson's disease. *Biol Psychiatry* 2003; 54:363–375.

7. Cong S, et al. Prevalence and clinical aspects of depression in Parkinson's disease: a systematic review and meta-analysis of 129 studies. *Neurosci Biobehav Rev* 2022; 141:104749.

8. Rabinak CA, et al. Dopamine agonist withdrawal syndrome in Parkinson disease. *Arch Neurol* 2010; 67:58–63.

9. Rocha FL, et al. Antidepressants for depression in Parkinson's disease: systematic review and meta-analysis. *J Psychopharmacol* 2013; 27:417–423.

10. Liu J, et al. Comparative efficacy and acceptability of antidepressants in Parkinson's disease: a network meta-analysis. *PLoS One* 2013; 8:e76651.

11. Troeung L, et al. A meta-analysis of randomised placebo-controlled treatment trials for depression and anxiety in Parkinson's disease. *PLoS One* 2013; 8:e79510.

12. Gony M, et al. Risk of serious extrapyramidal symptoms in patients with Parkinson's disease receiving antidepressant drugs: a pharmacoepidemiologic study comparing serotonin reuptake inhibitors and other antidepressant drugs. *Clin Neuropharmacol* 2003; 26:142–145.

13. Kulisevsky J, et al. Motor changes during sertraline treatment in depressed patients with Parkinson's disease. *Eur J Neurol* 2008; 15:953–959.

14. Agüera-Ortiz L, et al. Focus on depression in Parkinson's disease: a Delphi consensus of experts in psychiatry, neurology, and geriatrics. *Parkinsons Dis* 2021; 2021:6621991.

15. Richard IH, et al. A randomized, double-blind, placebo-controlled trial of antidepressants in Parkinson disease. *Neurology* 2012; 78:1229–1236.

16. Bonuccelli U, et al. A non-comparative assessment of tolerability and efficacy of duloxetine in the treatment of depressed patients with Parkinson's disease. *Expert Opin Pharmacother* 2012; 13:2269–2280.

17. Wang XL, et al. Comparative efficacy and acceptability of drug treatments for Parkinson's disease with depression: a systematic review with network meta-analysis. *Eur J Pharmacol* 2022; 927:175070.

18. Avila A, et al. Agomelatine for depression in Parkinson disease: additional effect on sleep and motor dysfunction. *J Clin Psychopharmacol* 2015; 35:719–723.

19. De Berardis D, et al. Agomelatine treatment of major depressive disorder in Parkinson's disease: a case series. *J Neuropsychiatry Clin Neurosci* 2013; 25:343–345.

20. Vismara M, et al. Clinical uses of bupropion in patients with Parkinson's disease and comorbid depressive or neuropsychiatric symptoms: a scoping review. *BMC Neurol* 2022; 22:169.

21. Santos García D, et al. Vortioxetine improves depressive symptoms and cognition in Parkinson's disease patients with major depression: an open-label prospective study. *Brain Sci* 2022; 12:1466.

22. Barone P, et al. Pramipexole versus sertraline in the treatment of depression in Parkinson's disease: a national multicenter parallel-group randomized study. *J Neurol* 2006; 253:601–607.

23. Antonini A, et al. A reassessment of risks and benefits of dopamine agonists in Parkinson's disease. *Lancet Neurol* 2009; 8:929–937.

24. Weintraub D, et al. Impulse control disorders in Parkinson disease: a cross-sectional study of 3090 patients. *Arch Neurol* 2010; 67:589–595.

25. Li CT, et al. Pramipexole-induced psychosis in Parkinson's disease. *Psychiatry Clin Neurosci* 2008; 62:245.

26. Ziaei E, et al. Comparison of pramipexole and citalopram in the treatment of depression in Parkinson's disease: a randomized parallel-group trial. *J Res Med Sci* 2022; 27:55.

27. Figiel GS, et al. ECT-induced delirium in depressed patients with Parkinson's disease. *J Neuropsychiatry Clin Neurosci* 1991; 3:405–411.

28. Friedman JH. Parkinson's disease psychosis 2010: a review article. *Parkinsonism Relat Disord* 2010; 16:553–560.

29. Ismail MS, et al. A reality test: How well do we understand psychosis in Parkinson's disease? *J Neuropsychiatry Clin Neurosci* 2004; 16:8–18.

30. Kiziltan G, et al. Relationship between age and subtypes of psychotic symptoms in Parkinson's disease. *J Neurol* 2007; 254:448–452.

31. Factor SA, et al. Longitudinal outcome of Parkinson's disease patients with psychosis. *Neurology* 2003; 60:1756–1761.

32. Reich SG, et al. Ten most commonly asked questions about the psychiatric aspects of Parkinson's disease. *Neurologist* 2003; 9:50–56.

33. Lin JJ, et al. Genetic polymorphism of the angiotensin converting enzyme and L-dopa-induced adverse effects in Parkinson's disease. *J Neurol Sci* 2007; 252:130–134.

34. Stowe RL, et al. Dopamine agonist therapy in early Parkinson's disease. *Cochrane Database Syst Rev* 2008; 2:CD006564.

35. Yunusa I, et al. Comparative efficacy, safety, and acceptability of pimavanserin and other atypical antipsychotics for Parkinson's disease psychosis: systematic review and network meta-analysis. *J Geriatr Psychiatry Neurol* 2023; 36:417–432.

36. Divac N, et al. The efficacy and safety of antipsychotic medications in the treatment of psychosis in patients with Parkinson's disease. *Behav Neurol* 2016; 2016:4938154.

37. Prohorov T, et al. The effect of quetiapine in psychotic Parkinsonian patients with and without dementia. An open-labeled study utilizing a structured interview. *J Neurol* 2006; **253**:171–175.

38. Weintraub D, et al. Association of antipsychotic use with mortality risk in patients with Parkinson disease. *JAMA Neurol* 2016; **73**:535–541.

39. D'Angremont E, et al. Cholinesterase inhibitors for treatment of psychotic symptoms in Alzheimer disease and Parkinson disease: a meta-analysis. *JAMA Neurol* 2023; **180**:813–823.

40. Chung KA, et al. Effects of a central cholinesterase inhibitor on reducing falls in Parkinson disease. *Neurology* 2010; **75**:1263–1269.

41. Sawada H, et al. Early use of donepezil against psychosis and cognitive decline in Parkinson's disease: a randomised controlled trial for 2 years. *J Neurol Neurosurg Psychiatry* 2018; **89**:1332–1340.

42. Van Mierlo TJM, et al. Rivastigmine for minor visual hallucinations in Parkinson's disease: a randomized controlled trial with 24 months follow-up. *Brain Behav* 2021; **11**:e2257.

43. Friedman JH. Clozapine is severely underused in Parkinson's disease patients. *Mov Disord Clin Pract* 2022; **9**:1021–1024.

44. Friedman JH, et al. Benztropine versus clozapine for the treatment of tremor in Parkinson's disease. *Neurology* 1997; **48**:1077–1081.

45. Pirttilä A, et al. Hospitalization and the risk of initiation of antipsychotics in persons with Parkinson's disease. *J Am Med Dir Assoc* 2023; **24**:1290–1296.e4.

46. Pintor L, et al. Ziprasidone versus clozapine in the treatment of psychotic symptoms in Parkinson disease: a randomized open clinical trial. *Clin Neuropharmacol* 2012; **35**:61–66.

47. Mesquita J, et al. Fatal neuroleptic malignant syndrome induced by clozapine in Parkinson's psychosis. *J Neuropsychiatry Clin Neurosci* 2014; **26**:E34.

48. Ziegenbein M, et al. Clozapine-induced aplastic anemia in a patient with Parkinson's disease. *Can J Psychiatry* 2003; **48**:352.

49. Iketani R, et al. Efficacy and safety of atypical antipsychotics for psychosis in Parkinson's disease: a systematic review and Bayesian network meta-analysis. *Parkinsonism Relat Disord* 2020; **78**:82–90.

50. Factor SA, et al. Combined clozapine and electroconvulsive therapy for the treatment of drug-induced psychosis in Parkinson's disease. *J Neuropsychiatry Clin Neurosci* 1995; **7**:304–307.

51. Martin BA. ECT for Parkinson's? *CMAJ* 2003; **168**:1391–1392.

52. Sarva H, et al. Evidence for the use of pimavanserin in the treatment of Parkinson's disease psychosis. *Ther Adv Neurol Disord* 2016; **9**:462–473.

53. Rissardo JP, et al. Pimavanserin and Parkinson's disease psychosis: a narrative review. *Brain Sci* 2022; **12**:1286.

54. Alipour-Haris G, et al. Comparison of pimavanserin versus quetiapine for hospitalization and mortality risk among medicare beneficiaries with Parkinson's disease psychosis. *Mov Disord Clin Pract* 2023; **10**:406–414.

55. Mansuri Z, et al. Pimavanserin in the treatment of Parkinson's disease psychosis: meta-analysis and meta-regression of randomized clinical trials. *Innov Clin Neurosci* 2022; **19**:46–51.

56. Wilby KJ, et al. Evidence-based review of pharmacotherapy used for Parkinson's disease psychosis. *Ann Pharmacother* 2017; **51**:682–695.

57. Thames BH, et al. Clozapine: efficacy for Parkinson disease psychosis in patients refractory to pimavanserin. *Parkinsonism Relat Disord* 2023; **109**:105356.

58. Richard IH, et al. Rivastigmine-induced worsening of motor function and mood in a patient with Parkinson's disease. *Mov Disord* 2001; **16** Suppl 1:33–34.

59. McKeith I, et al. Efficacy of rivastigmine in dementia with Lewy bodies: a randomised, double-blind, placebo-controlled international study. *Lancet* 2000; **356**:2031–2036.

60. Emre M, et al. Rivastigmine for dementia associated with Parkinson's disease. *N Engl J Med* 2004; **351**:2509–2518.

61. Aarsland D, et al. Donepezil for cognitive impairment in Parkinson's disease: a randomised controlled study. *J Neurol Neurosurg Psychiatry* 2002; **72**:708–712.

62. Pagano G, et al. Cholinesterase inhibitors for Parkinson's disease: a systematic review and meta-analysis. *J Neurol Neurosurg Psychiatry* 2015; **86**:767–773.

63. Rolinski M, et al. Cholinesterase inhibitors for dementia with Lewy bodies, Parkinson's disease dementia and cognitive impairment in Parkinson's disease. *Cochrane Database Syst Rev* 2012; **3**:CD006504.

64. Dubois B, et al. Donepezil in Parkinson's disease dementia: a randomized, double-blind efficacy and safety study. *Mov Disord* 2012; **27**:1230–1238.

65. Connolly BS, et al. Pharmacological treatment of Parkinson disease: a review. *JAMA* 2014; **311**:1670–1683.

66. Emre M, et al. Memantine for patients with Parkinson's disease dementia or dementia with Lewy bodies: a randomised, double-blind, placebo-controlled trial. *Lancet Neurol* 2010; **9**:969–977.

67. Seppi K, et al. The Movement Disorder Society evidence-based medicine review update: treatments for the non-motor symptoms of Parkinson's disease. *Mov Disord* 2011; **26** Suppl 3:S42–S80.

68. Nawaz H, et al. Anticholinergic medication burden in Parkinson's disease outpatients. *J Parkinsons Dis* 2022; **12**:599–606.

69. Mur J, et al. Association between anticholinergic burden and dementia in UK Biobank. *Alzheimers Dement (NY)* 2022; **8**: e12290.

70. Zesiewicz TA, et al. Potential influences of complementary therapy on motor and non-motor complications in Parkinson's disease. *CNS Drugs* 2009; **23**:817–835.

71. Biswas S, et al. Study of the effects of nicotine and caffeine for the treatment of Parkinson's disease. *Appl Biochem Biotechnol* 2023; **195**:639–654.

72. Postuma RB, et al. Caffeine for treatment of Parkinson disease: a randomized controlled trial. *Neurology* 2012; **79**:651–658.

Atrial fibrillation

Atrial fibrillation (AF) is the most common cardiac arrhythmia. It particularly affects older people but may occur in an important proportion of people aged less than 40 years. Risk factors include anxiety, obesity, diabetes, hypertension, long-standing aerobic exercise and high alcohol consumption.[1-3] AF itself is not usually life-threatening but stasis of blood in the atria during fibrillation predisposes to clot formation and substantially increases the risk of stroke.[4] The use of warfarin or direct-acting oral anticoagulants is therefore essential.[3]

AF can be defined as 'lone' or **paroxysmal** (occurring infrequently, and spontaneously reverting to sinus rhythm), **persistent** (repeated and prolonged [>1 week] episodes usually, if temporarily, responsive to treatment) or **permanent** (unresponsive). Risk of stroke is increased in all three conditions.[3]

Treatment may involve DC conversion, rhythm control (usually flecainide, propafenone or amiodarone) or rate control (with diltiazem, verapamil or sotalol). With rhythm control the aim is to maintain sinus rhythm, although this is not always achieved. With rate control, AF is allowed to continue but ventricular response is controlled and the ventricles are filled passively. Many people with paroxysmal or persistent AF can be effectively cured of the condition by catheter or cryoablation of aberrant electrical pathways,[5,6] now a routine and effective procedure.[7]

AF is commonly encountered in psychiatry not least because of the high rates of obesity, diabetes and alcohol misuse seen in mental health patients. The onset of AF also provokes prescription of antidepressants, anxiolytics and hypnotics.[8]

When considering the use of psychotropics several factors need to be taken into account:

- Interactions between psychotropics and anticoagulant therapy.
- Arrhythmogenicity of psychotropics prescribed. AF usually results from cardiovascular disease, and drugs affecting cardiac ion channels may increase mortality in these patients, especially those with ischaemic disease.[9,10] Drugs that prolong the QT interval may also increase the risk of incident AF[11] although their effect on established AF is not known.
- Effect on ventricular rate: some drugs induce reflex tachycardia via postural hypotension, others (clozapine, quetiapine) directly increase heart rate.
- Reported association between individual psychotropics and AF (Table 10.15).
- Risk of interaction with co-prescribed antiarrhythmics or rate-controlling drugs.
- Whether AF is paroxysmal (aim to avoid precipitating AF), persistent (aim to avoid prolonging AF) or permanent (aim to avoid increasing ventricular rate).

Table 10.15 Recommendations for using psychotropics in atrial fibrillation (AF).

Condition	Suggested drugs	Drugs to avoid
Schizophrenia/ schizoaffective disorder The condition itself may be associated with an increased risk of AF[12] One case–control study suggested antipsychotics increase risk of AF by 17%[13]	In paroxysmal or persistent AF, **cariprazine**, **brexpiprazole** or **lurasidone** may be appropriate choices. In permanent AF with rate control, drug choice is less crucial but probably best to avoid drugs with potent effects on the ECG (ziprasidone, pimozide, etc.) and those that increase heart rate. All antipsychotics appear to increase the risk of bleeding when combined with DOACs in AF.[14]	AF reported with clozapine,[15,16] olanzapine,[17,18] aripiprazole[19,20] and paliperidone.[21] Causation not clearly established but avoid use in lone, paroxysmal or persistent AF. Avoid QT-prolonging drugs in ischaemic heart disease (see section on QT prolongation in Chapter 1). Association of antipsychotics with AF[13] may be linked to metabolic disturbance[22] although some studies suggest no link between antipsychotics and AF.[23]
Bipolar disorder	**Valproate** **Lithium** **Carbamazepine**	Mood stabilisers appear not to affect risk of AF. Valproate may cause AV conduction block.[24] One case of AF following lithium overdose[25] and one in chronic toxicity.[26]
Depression Untreated depression predicts recurrence of AF[27] Presence of AF increases risk of depression and anxiety[28]	**SSRIs** but beware interaction with warfarin and other anticoagulants[29] as severe bleeding risk is increased.[30] Animal studies suggest an antiarrhythmic effect for SSRIs.[31,32] **Paroxetine** improved paroxysmal AF in a series of non-depressed patients.[33] **Venlafaxine** does not directly affect atrial conduction[34] and may cardiovert paroxysmal AF.[35] One study suggested no increased risk of bleeding when combined with DOACs,[36] another suggested a particular risk of bleeding when SNRIs are combined with apixaban.[37] Mirtazapine and trazodone may increase bleeding risk when combined with DOACs in AF.[37] AF incidence falls after starting antidepressant treatment.[38,39] No evidence that **agomelatine** affects cardiac conduction or clotting.	Avoid tricyclics in coronary disease.[40] Tricyclics may provoke AF[41,42] but do not increase risk of haemorrhage when combined with warfarin[29] or DOACs.[37] One database study suggested antidepressants in general do not increase risk of AF[43] although another suggested both depression and antidepressant use are linked to incident AF.[44]

Table 10.15 (Continued)

Condition	Suggested drugs	Drugs to avoid
Anxiety disorders (anxiety symptoms increase risk of AF)[45]	**Benzodiazepines** (although a 2022 cohort study found a hugely increased risk of incident AF in benzodiazepine users[46]) **SSRIs** (see above)	Tricyclics (see above) Several reported cases of pregabalin- and gabapentin-associated AF[47,48] and one cohort study suggested increased risk of AF[49] with both drugs Promethazine may increase the risk of being hospitalised with AF[50]
Alzheimer's disease	**Acetylcholinesterase inhibitors** (but beware bradycardic effects in patients with paroxysmal 'vagal' AF [paroxysmal AF provoked by low heart rate]) **Rivastigmine** has least interaction potential **Memantine** may be able to prevent and terminate AF[51]	Avoid cholinesterase inhibitors in paroxysmal 'vagal' AF

AV, atrioventricular; DOACs, direct-acting oral anticoagulants.

References

1. Chen LY, et al. Epidemiology of atrial fibrillation: a current perspective. *Heart Rhythm* 2007; 4:S1–S6.
2. Tully PJ, et al. Anxiety, depression, and stress as risk factors for atrial fibrillation after cardiac surgery. *Heart Lung* 2011; 40:4–11.
3. National Institute for Health and Care Excellence. Atrial fibrillation: diagnosis and management. NICE guideline [NG196]. 2021 (last accessed August 2024); https://www.nice.org.uk/guidance/ng196.
4. Lakshminarayan K, et al. Clinical epidemiology of atrial fibrillation and related cerebrovascular events in the United States. *Neurologist* 2008; 14:143–150.
5. Rodgers M, et al. Curative catheter ablation in atrial fibrillation and typical atrial flutter: systematic review and economic evaluation. *Health Technol Assess* 2008; 12:iii–iv, xi–xiii, 1–198.
6. Latchamsetty R, et al. Catheter ablation of atrial fibrillation. *Cardiol Clin* 2014; 32:551–561.
7. Saglietto A, et al. Impact of atrial fibrillation catheter ablation on mortality, stroke, and heart failure hospitalizations: a meta-analysis. *J Cardiovasc Electrophysiol* 2020; 31:1040–1047.
8. Hagengaard L, et al. Incident atrial fibrillation and risk of psychoactive drug redemptions and psychiatric hospital contacts: a Danish Nationwide Register-based Follow-up Study. *Eur Heart J Qual Care Clin Outcomes* 2021; 7:76–82.
9. Cardiac Arrhythmia Suppression Trial (CAST) Investigators. Effect of the antiarrhythmic agent moricizine on survival after myocardial infarction. *N Engl J Med* 1992; 327:227–233.
10. Epstein AE, et al. Mortality following ventricular arrhythmia suppression by encainide, flecainide, and moricizine after myocardial infarction. The original design concept of the Cardiac Arrhythmia Suppression Trial (CAST). *JAMA* 1993; 270:2451–2455.
11. Zhang N, et al. Prolonged corrected QT interval in predicting atrial fibrillation: a systematic review and meta-analysis. *Pacing Clin Electrophysiol* 2018; 41:321–327.
12. Emul M, et al. P wave and QT changes among inpatients with schizophrenia after parenteral ziprasidone administration. *Pharmacol Res* 2009; 60:369–372.
13. Chou RH, et al. Antipsychotic treatment is associated with risk of atrial fibrillation: a nationwide nested case-control study. *Int J Cardiol* 2017; 227:134–140.
14. Chen CM, et al. Major bleeding risk in atrial fibrillation patients co-medicated with non-vitamin K oral anticoagulants and antipsychotics. *Front Pharmacol* 2022; 13:819878.
15. Cam B, et al. [Clozapine and olanzapine associated atrial fibrillation: a case report]. *Turk Psikiyatri Dergisi* 2015; 26:221–226.
16. Low Jr, RA, et al. Clozapine induced atrial fibrillation. *J Clin Psychopharmacol* 1998; 18:170.
17. Waters BM, et al. Olanzapine-associated new-onset atrial fibrillation. *J Clin Psychopharmacol* 2008; 28:354–355.
18. Yaylaci S, et al. Atrial fibrillation due to olanzapine overdose. *Clin Toxicol (Phila)* 2011; 49:440.

19. D'Urso G, et al. Aripiprazole-induced atrial fibrillation in a patient with concomitant risk factors. *Exp Clin Psychopharmacol* 2018; **26**:509–513.

20. Stefatos A, et al. Atrial fibrillation and injected aripiprazole: a case report. *Innov Clin Neurosci* 2018; **15**:43–45.

21. Schneider RA, et al. Apparent seizure and atrial fibrillation associated with paliperidone. *Am J Health Syst Pharm* 2008; **65**:2122–2125.

22. Zeng J, et al. Metabolic disorder caused by antipsychotic treatment may facilitate the development of atrial fibrillation. *Int J Cardiol* 2017; **239**:14.

23. Polcwiartek C, et al. Electrocardiogram characteristics and their association with psychotropic drugs among patients with schizophrenia. *Schizophr Bull* 2020; **46**:354–362.

24. Davutoglu V, et al. Valproic acid as a cause of transient atrio-ventricular conduction block episodes. *J Atr Fibrillation* 2017; **9**:1520.

25. Kalcik MDM, et al. Acute atrial fibrillation as an unusual form of cardiotoxicity in chronic lithium overdose. *J Atr Fibrillation* 2014; **6**:1009.

26. Acharya S, et al. Lithium-induced cardiotoxicity: a rare clinical entity. *Cureus* 2020; **12**:e7286.

27. Lange HW, et al. Depressive symptoms predict recurrence of atrial fibrillation after cardioversion. *J Psychosom Res* 2007; **63**:509–513.

28. Patel D, et al. A systematic review of depression and anxiety in patients with atrial fibrillation: the mind-heart link. *Cardiovasc Psychiatry Neurol* 2013; **2013**:159850.

29. Quinn GR, et al. Effect of selective serotonin reuptake inhibitors on bleeding risk in patients with atrial fibrillation taking warfarin. *Am J Cardiol* 2014; **114**:583–586.

30. Komen JJ, et al. Concomitant anticoagulant and antidepressant therapy in atrial fibrillation patients and risk of stroke and bleeding. *Clin Pharmacol Ther* 2020; **107**:287–294.

31. Pousti A, et al. Effect of sertraline on ouabain-induced arrhythmia in isolated guinea-pig atria. *Depress Anxiety* 2009; **26**:E106–E110.

32. Pousti A, et al. Effect of citalopram on ouabain-induced arrhythmia in isolated guinea-pig atria. *Hum Psychopharmacol* 2003; **18**:121–124.

33. Shirayama T, et al. Usefulness of paroxetine in depressed men with paroxysmal atrial fibrillation. *Am J Cardiol* 2006; **97**:1749–1751.

34. Emul M, et al. The influences of depression and venlafaxine use at therapeutic doses on atrial conduction. *J Psychopharmacol* 2009; **23**:163–167.

35. Finch SJ, et al. Cardioversion of persistent atrial arrhythmia after treatment with venlafaxine in successful management of major depression and posttraumatic stress disorder. *Psychosomatics* 2006; **47**:533–536.

36. Shao IY, et al. Association of type of antidepressant initiation with bleeding risk in atrial fibrillation patients taking oral anticoagulants. *Drugs Real World Outcomes* 2021; **8**:383–391.

37. Chang KH, et al. Major bleeding risk in patients with non-valvular atrial fibrillation concurrently taking direct oral anticoagulants and antidepressants. *Front Aging Neurosci* 2022; **14**:791285.

38. Andrade C. Antidepressants and atrial fibrillation: the importance of resourceful statistical approaches to address confounding by indication. *J Clin Psychiatry* 2019; **80**:19f12729.

39. Fenger-Grøn M, et al. Depression, antidepressants, and the risk of non-valvular atrial fibrillation: a nationwide Danish matched cohort study. *Eur J Prev Cardiol* 2019; **26**:187–195.

40. Taylor D. Antidepressant drugs and cardiovascular pathology: a clinical overview of effectiveness and safety. *Acta Psychiatr Scand* 2008; **118**:434–442.

41. Moorehead CN, et al. Imipramine-induced auricular fibrillation. *Am J Psychiatry* 1965; **122**:216–217.

42. Rosen BH. Case report of auricular fibrillation following the use of imipramine (Tofranil). *J Mt Sinai Hosp NY* 1960; **27**:609–611.

43. Lapi F, et al. The use of antidepressants and the risk of chronic atrial fibrillation. *J Clin Pharmacol* 2015; **55**:423–430.

44. Fu Y, et al. Association of depression, antidepressants with atrial fibrillation risk: a systemic review and meta-analysis. *Front Cardiovasc Med* 2022; **9**:897622.

45. Eaker ED, et al. Tension and anxiety and the prediction of the 10-year incidence of coronary heart disease, atrial fibrillation, and total mortality: the Framingham Offspring Study. *Psychosom Med* 2005; **67**:692–696.

46. Hu X, et al. Hypnotics use is associated with elevated incident atrial fibrillation: a propensity-score matched analysis of cohort study. *J Pers Med* 2022; **12**:1645.

47. Chilkoti G, et al. Could pregabalin premedication predispose to perioperative atrial fibrillation in patients with sepsis? *Saudi J Anaesth* 2014; 8 Suppl 1:S115–S116.

48. Park SH, et al. Atrial fibrillation induced by gabapentin: a case report. *J Med Case Rep* 2023; **17**:236.

49. Ortiz de Landaluce L, et al. Gabapentin and pregabalin and risk of atrial fibrillation in the elderly: a population-based cohort study in an electronic prescription database. *Drug Saf* 2018; **41**:1325–1331.

50. Sessa M, et al. The risk of fractures, acute myocardial infarction, atrial fibrillation and ventricular arrhythmia in geriatric patients exposed to promethazine. *Expert Opin Drug Saf* 2020; **19**:349–357.

51. Xie D, et al. Memantine targets glutamate receptors in atrial cardiomyocytes to prevent and treat atrial fibrillation. *Cell Discov* 2022; **8**:76.

Bariatric surgery

Psychiatric illness is relatively common in patients who have undergone bariatric surgery.[1] Over a third of those seeking bariatric surgery are prescribed psychotropics.[2] Bariatric surgery can be associated with clinically important changes in drug pharmacokinetics, although it is difficult to predict exactly how psychotropics will be affected because of interindividual differences and rather limited data. There is clearly a need for close treatment monitoring and the ongoing monitoring of symptoms after bariatric surgery.[3]

Surgical procedures can be classified as:

- **Predominantly restrictive:** sleeve gastrectomy and gastric banding.
- **Predominantly malabsorptive:** biliopancreatic diversion and jejunoileal bypass.
- **Mixed restrictive/malabsorptive:** Roux-en-Y gastric bypass (RYGB) and gastric reduction duodenal switch (GRDS).

Absorption following bariatric surgery is drug-specific and shows high variability among individuals. It can be affected by many factors including route of administration, dosage form, patient-specific factors, pharmacokinetic/pharmacodynamic considerations and type of surgery; it can be temporary or permanent.[4,5] Malabsorptive procedures (including RYGB and GRDS) have a relatively greater potential to alter drug absorption. Most data are derived from studies of patients undergoing RYGB. It is not clear how these data relate to the consequences of other procedures.

Pharmacokinetic changes following bariatric surgery

All procedures may alter the following:

- Tablet disintegration and dissolution times via changes in gastric pH and mixing.
- Area for drug absorption (reduced gastric and/or functional intestinal surface area).
- Rate of absorption via changes in the gastric emptying rate.
- Drug distribution via loss of adipose tissue (especially lipid-soluble drugs) and altered protein binding.
- Drug metabolism owing to improvements in hepatic function after weight loss.
- Drug excretion via changes in renal function after weight loss.

Malabsorptive surgical procedures may further lead to:

- Changes in the availability of certain enzymes and transporters.
- Altered lipophilic drug solubilisation (bypassing proximal small intestine bile salts).
- Reduced intestinal wall drug metabolism via decreased intestinal length.

Medication formulations[5,6]

Any formulation that prolongs drug disintegration or dissolution can potentially impair drug absorption following bariatric surgery. Switching to immediate-release formulations before surgery is generally recommended. Orodispersible and liquid preparations do not go through a disintegration phase, and may be preferred if reduced absorption from solid tablets is suspected.[7] Very large tablets (e.g. over 10mm in diameter) should be avoided as passage may be impeded by restrictive procedures.

Antidepressants

Table 10.16 summarises the use of antidepressants in bariatric surgery.

Table 10.16 Antidepressants in bariatric surgery.

Medication	Specific evidence and considerations
SSRIs[4,8,9]	Evidence demonstrates that plasma levels may be significantly reduced following RYGB or sleeve gastrectomy. The concentration of SSRIs may drop initially and then rebound within a few months; dose adjustments occurring in the immediate postoperative period might be temporary. Malabsorption has been implicated in cases of discontinuation symptoms and loss of efficacy. Sertraline and vortioxetine absorption appear to be the most affected and fluoxetine the least.
SNRIs[9–11]	Suggest avoid duloxetine owing to significant reduction in levels and risk of discontinuation syndrome. The absorption of venlafaxine MR capsules seems not to be altered by RYGB
Mirtazapine[9,12–14]	Plasma levels may be significantly reduced following RYGB or sleeve gastrectomy. Dose increase is often needed. Increased appetite and weight gain are possible.
TCAs[15,16]	Single case report suggests therapeutic plasma levels can be achieved within usual dose range after RYGB. Plasma levels may be increased after significant weight loss. Consider monitoring levels and reducing dose.
Agomelatine	No data available on absorption after bariatric surgery. Follow general recommendations.
Dextromethorphan and bupropion	There are no studies of the combined formulation after bariatric surgery No pharmacokinetic changes after bariatric surgery were reported for dextromethorphan liquid in the short or long term.[5,17] In an in vitro model bupropion was found to have a significantly higher dissolution after RYGB which may lead to increased bioavailability.[18]
Esketamine nasal spray[19]	Primarily absorbed via nasal mucosa. Problems after bariatric surgery are not expected.

General summary

- Antidepressants are the best-studied psychotropics in the bariatric population. Current evidence suggests that antidepressant absorption is reduced after surgery (though studies are mostly limited to SSRIs after RYGB).
- Signs of reduced absorption may include the rapid development of discontinuation symptoms and later loss of efficacy. Patients should be made aware of discontinuation symptoms and signs of relapse and seek medical advice if they occur.
- Patients require close monitoring as those at risk of reduced absorption cannot be reliably predicted.
- The risk of gastric bleeds with bariatric surgery will probably be increased by serotonergic antidepressants.

MR, modified release; RYGB, Roux-en-Y gastric bypass; TCAs, tricyclic antidepressants.

Antipsychotics

Table 10.17 summarises the use of antipsychotics in bariatric surgery.

Table 10.17 Antipsychotics in bariatric surgery.

Medication	Specific evidence and considerations
Aripiprazole[20]	One case report of subtherapeutic levels post RYGB using aripiprazole tablets that became therapeutic on switching to suspension. Available as an LAI.
Asenapine[21]	Primarily absorbed via oral mucosa. Problems after bariatric surgery are not expected One case report of successful use after RYGB.
Brexpiprazole	No data available on absorption after bariatric surgery
Cariprazine	No data available on absorption after bariatric surgery The absorption of oral contraceptives may be reduced after bariatric surgery.[22] Therefore, to ensure highly effective contraception for women prescribed cariprazine, non-oral methods are recommended.
Clozapine[23–25]	Two case reports of relapse after RYGB[26] Take drug plasma levels before surgery and regularly monitor after. Constipation is common after surgery; the manufacturer recommends close monitoring and active treatment. Check smoking status (quitting before surgery is encouraged); adjust dose accordingly.
Haloperidol[27]	Single case report suggests levels after RYGB are similar to those generally reported in the literature.
Iloperidone	No data available on absorption after bariatric surgery
Lumateperone	No data available on absorption after bariatric surgery
Lurasidone	Risk of reduced absorption with reduced or inconsistent calorific intake perioperatively. Must be taken with food for absorption (350kcal). One case report of relapse following GRDS. Significant reduction in bioavailability and peak serum concentration.[28] One case report post-RYGB showed significant reduction in plasma concentration with no worsening of psychotic symptoms.[29] Consider switching to alternatives before surgery.
Olanzapine	One report of reduction in dose-adjusted drug concentration following bariatric surgery[30] One case report following RYGB of continued efficacy with no dose adjustment required[31] In an in vitro model olanzapine was found to have a significantly lower dissolution after RYGB which may lead to decreased bioavailability.[32] Follow general recommendations.
Quetiapine[7,30,33]	Dose-adjusted concentrations decreased following bariatric surgery. Switching to immediate-release preparation and dividing doses above 300mg has been recommended.
Risperidone[34]	Consider switching stable patients to an equivalent dose of paliperidone LAI. Risperidone LAI has been used successfully when oral treatment was not tolerated after bariatric surgery.
Ziprasidone[35]	Must be taken with food for absorption (500kcal); risk of reduced absorption with reduced/inconsistent calorific intake perioperatively. Consider switching to alternatives before surgery.

(Continued)

Table 10.17 (*Continued*)

General summary

- Antipsychotics are not well studied in bariatric surgery. Data are limited to case reports or theoretical concerns.
- Monitor for decreased efficacy. Adjust dose accordingly or consider switching to another antipsychotic.
- Depot antipsychotics avoid the risk of reduced absorption after surgery. Given the limited data on pharmacokinetic changes after surgery and interindividual variability, routinely switching to depot antipsychotics before surgery may not be justified.[7] However, depot preparations remain an option for those stabilised on treatment available as a depot or in patients demonstrating signs of reduced bioavailability after surgery.
- Bariatric surgery may contribute additional cardiac stressors to patients with QT prolongation.[36] ECG monitoring before and after surgery is recommended.

GRDS, gastric reduction duodenal switch; LAI, long-acting injection; RYGB, Roux-en-Y gastric bypass.

Mood stabilisers

Table 10.18 summarises the use of mood stabilisers in bariatric surgery.

Table 10.18 Mood stabilisers in bariatric surgery.

Medication	Summary of evidence and considerations
Carbamazepine	Carbamazepine CR levels have been observed to both increase and decrease following bariatric surgery.[37] In a case series of eight following sleeve gastrectomy, levels were found to be reduced in half the cases, with two resulting in deterioration of previously well-controlled illness. One case had increased levels.[38] Single case report of agranulocytosis possibly related to increased plasma levels after sleeve gastrectomy.[38] Baseline plasma carbamazepine levels, FBC, renal function and LFTs with ongoing monitoring recommended.[38]
Lamotrigine[38]	Increased, decreased or unchanged lamotrigine levels after bariatric surgery are all possible; monitor for adverse effects and loss of efficacy.
Lithium[39,40] (see below)	Cases of lithium toxicity following RYGB and sleeve gastrectomy have been reported. Switch to an equivalent dose of lithium citrate solution in divided doses. In the preoperative period, plasma levels may be affected by prescribed dietary changes. In the postoperative period, plasma levels may be affected by malabsorption (mainly absorbed via small intestine), fluid shifts and weight loss (lithium clearance increased in obesity).
Valproate[7,41,42]	Single case report suggests that absorption may be significantly reduced after malabsorptive procedures; no data on restrictive procedures. Dose reductions may be necessary after weight loss (plasma levels related to body weight). Switch to liquid preparation before surgery or if malabsorption suspected on enteric-coated tablets. Avoid CR preparations. Baseline plasma valproate levels, FBC and LFTs with ongoing monitoring recommended. Monitor for clinical signs of poor tolerability, possibly occurring at normal plasma levels.

General summary

- The literature on mood stabilisers after bariatric surgery is limited to a few case reports; the use of lithium requires particular care owing to its narrow therapeutic index.
- The absorption of oral contraceptives may be reduced after bariatric surgery.[22] In patients prescribed teratogenic mood stabilisers, non-oral methods of contraception are recommended.

CR, controlled release; FBC, full blood count; LFTs, liver function tests; RYGB, Roux-en-Y gastric bypass.

Lithium around the time of bariatric surgery

The continued use of lithium throughout the perioperative phases of bariatric surgery requires particularly close monitoring. The following guidance is based on available case reports and expert opinion.[40]

- Monitor lithium plasma levels preoperatively and perform a scale-based clinical assessment of mood.
- Educate the patient preoperatively on the importance of drinking 2.5–3 litres of fluid per day (including liquid meal replacement).
- Postoperatively assess for toxicity by monitoring lithium plasma levels and renal function weekly for 6 weeks (as fluid intake gradually increases), 2-weekly for 6 months and monthly thereafter. Resume usual lithium monitoring 1 year post-bariatric surgery.
- If plasma levels increase by >25% or approach 1.2mmol/L consider decreasing the lithium dose.
- Withhold lithium if signs of toxicity are present and review the dose.
- To prevent dehydration, counsel the patient to alert their physician or psychiatrist in case of any changes in food or fluid intake or severe vomiting.
- Monitor mental state periodically, using formal rating scales if possible.

Other medicines

Table 10.19 summarises the use of other medicines in bariatric surgery.

Table 10.19 Miscellaneous agents in bariatric surgery.

Medication	Summary of evidence and considerations
Antimuscarinics	No data available on absorption after bariatric surgery
Benzodiazepines[43–46]	Bioavailability probably unaffected, shorter time to peak concentration
Lisdexamfetamine[47]	A single-dose case–control study found no significant differences in lisdexamfetamine and active metabolite d-amfetamine following RYGB compared to non-surgical controls. Due to potential for interindividual differences, monitor for adverse effects and loss of efficacy.
Methadone[48]	Substantial increase in bioavailability after sleeve gastrectomy in one case report, possibly related increased rate of gastric emptying; consider plasma level and QT monitoring
Methylphenidate[49,50]	Conflicting limited data; one case report of reduced treatment efficacy after RYGB that resolved after switching to transdermal patch suggesting reduced oral bioavailability; another reported signs of toxicity
Modafinil	No data available on absorption after bariatric surgery
Orexin antagonists	No data available on absorption after bariatric surgery
Pregabalin[17]	Increased levels shortly after surgery and decreased values in the long term post-surgery; monitor for adverse effects and loss of efficacy
Solriamfetol	No data available on absorption after bariatric surgery
Zolpidem	In an in vitro model found to have non-significant lower dissolution after RYGB.[32] Food delays the onset of effect; take on an empty stomach.[51]

RYGB, Roux-en-Y gastric bypass.

General recommendations

Box 10.5 outlines the general recommendations for prescribing in bariatric surgery, while Box 10.6 summarises the strategies used in patients who show signs of reduced bioavailability.

Box 10.5 General recommendations for prescribing in bariatric surgery[7,14]

Before surgery	**After surgery (0–6 weeks)**	**After surgery (>6 weeks after)**
■ Do not routinely increase doses; clinically relevant malabsorption cannot be reliably predicted ■ Assess mental state before surgery using validated scales and consider measuring baseline drug plasma levels ■ Switch modified-release/enteric-coated preparations to immediate-release tablets or to liquid preparations	■ Assess mental state using validated scales ■ Closely monitor for signs of adverse effects and drug malabsorption (symptom re-emergence, discontinuation symptoms) ■ Regularly monitor drug plasma levels if clinically indicated ■ If malabsorption suspected consider the recommended strategies ■ If medication toxicity suspected withhold and reassess dose	■ Continue regular monitoring for the first year postoperatively using validated scales, although frequency can be reduced if stable ■ Monitor for an increase in adverse effects, especially if doses were increased in the acute postoperative period ■ Consider returning to pre-surgical treatment regimen after 1 year (depending on clinical history)

Box 10.6 General management strategies for patients demonstrating signs of reduced bioavailability

- Consider non-oral routes of administration where available (e.g. depots for patients stable on antipsychotics)
- Dividing doses may improve malabsorption related to a reduced stomach capacity after surgery
- Switching modified/prolonged/delayed-release to immediate-release formulations
- Switching solid tablets to liquid or orodispersible preparations to bypass disintegration phase
- Switching large tablets to smaller ones
- In cases where doses have been increased to account for reduced bioavailability, monitor for emergent adverse effects as bioavailability may normalise over time

---

Psychotropics with a risk of weight gain after bariatric surgery

Around 70% of patients regain a significant amount of weight (more than 10% of lowest postoperative weight) within 5 years of bariatric surgery.[52] There has been conflicting information on how psychotropics affect weight loss outcomes after surgery. One study reported no significant differences in total weight loss 1 year post-surgery between those on psychotropics and those not.[2] Another reported that treatment with antidepressants, particularly SNRIs and TCAs, was associated with reduced weight loss after gastric bypass surgery[53] and another found that those on obesogenic medications lost statistically significantly less excess weight than controls.[54] Medicines with a high risk of weight gain should be avoided where possible. Binge eating disorder, problematic alcohol use and depressive symptoms are associated with postoperative weight gain.[52]

Alcohol[55,56]

Gastric bypass surgery is associated with accelerated alcohol absorption, higher maximum alcohol concentrations and a longer time to elimination. There is also an increased risk of alcohol misuse disorders after gastric bypass. Data are less clear for sleeve gastrectomy and there is no evidence that gastric banding leads to any changes.

Wider considerations[14,57]

Despite severe mental illness often being considered a contraindication for bariatric surgery it has been shown to be effective in those with schizophrenia and bipolar affective disorder. Because of the variability of pharmacokinetic changes of psychiatric medicines, it is important to monitor patients closely for adverse effects and loss of efficacy, and medicines should be adjusted accordingly if required. Significant improvements in mental health are well documented following surgery, however deterioration can also occur. Depression and/or eating disorders may persist, re-emerge or newly develop and there is an increased risk of self-harm, suicide, alcohol disorder and opioid misuse following bariatric surgery.

References

1. Dawes AJ, et al. Mental health conditions among patients seeking and undergoing bariatric surgery: a meta-analysis. *JAMA* 2016; **315**:150–163.
2. Hawkins M, et al. Psychiatric medication use and weight outcomes one year after bariatric surgery. *Psychosomatics* 2020; **61**:56–63.
3. Gondek W. Psychiatric suitability assessment for bariatric surgery. In: Sockalingam S, Hawa R, eds. *Psychiatric Care in Severe Obesity: An Interdisciplinary Guide to Integrated Care.* Cham: Springer International Publishing; 2017:173–186.
4. Lorico S, et al. Medication management and pharmacokinetic changes after bariatric surgery. *Can Fam Physician* 2020; **66**:409–416.
5. Alalwan AA, et al. Drug absorption in bariatric surgery patients: a narrative review. *Health Sci Rep* 2022; **5**:e605.
6. Girolamo T, et al. Bariatric surgery and medicines: from first principles to practice. *Aust Prescr* 2022; **45**:162–166.
7. Bingham KS, et al. Psychopharmacology in bariatric surgery patients. In: Sockalingam S, Hawa R, eds. *Psychiatric Care in Severe Obesity: An Interdisciplinary Guide to Integrated Care.* Cham: Springer International Publishing; 2017:313–333.
8. Pasi P, et al. Plasma concentrations of SSRI/SNRI after bariatric surgery and the effects on depressive symptoms. *Front Psychiatry* 2023; **14**:1132112.
9. Maass D, et al. Changes in serum concentration of antidepressants after bariatric surgery and recommendations for postbariatric surgery antidepressant therapy. *J Acad Consult Liaison Psychiatry* 2024; **65**:261–270.
10. Roerig JL, et al. A comparison of duloxetine plasma levels in postbariatric surgery patients versus matched nonsurgical control subjects. *J Clin Psychopharmacol* 2013; **33**:479–484.
11. Hamad GG, et al. The effect of gastric bypass on the pharmacokinetics of serotonin reuptake inhibitors. *Am J Psychiatry* 2012; **169**:256–263.
12. Teixeira FV, et al. Mirtazapine (Remeron) as treatment for non-mechanical vomiting after gastric bypass. *Obes Surg* 2005; **15**:707–709.
13. Huerta S, et al. Intractable nausea and vomiting following Roux-en-Y gastric bypass: role of mirtazapine. *Obes Surg* 2006; **16**:1399.
14. Coughlin JW, et al. Psychotropic medications in metabolic and bariatric surgery: research updates and clinical considerations. *Curr Psychiatry Rep* 2022; **24**:89–98.
15. Broyles JE, et al. Nortriptyline absorption in short bowel syndrome. *J Parenter Enteral Nutr* 1990; **14**:326–327.
16. Jobson K, et al. Weight loss and a concomitant change in plasma tricyclic levels. *Am J Psychiatry* 1978; **135**:237–238.
17. Lau C, et al. Impact of bariatric surgery in the short and long term: a need for time-dependent dosing of drugs. *Obes Surg* 2023; **33**:3266–3302.
18. Konstantinidou SK, et al. The effects of bariatric surgery on pharmacokinetics of drugs: a review of current evidence. *Curr Nutr Rep* 2023; **12**:695–708.
19. Jannsen-Cilag Ltd. Summary of product characteristics. Spravato 28mg nasal spray, solution. 2024 (last accessed August 2024); https://www.medicines.org.uk/emc/product/10977/smpc.
20. Kuzin M, et al. Switching from aripiprazole tablets to oral suspension in a patient with Roux-en-Y gastric bypass: a case report. *J Clin Psychopharmacol* 2023; **43**:300–302.
21. Tabaac BJ, et al. Pica patient, status post gastric bypass, improves with change in medication regimen. *Ther Adv Psychopharmacol* 2015; **5**:38–42.
22. Merhi ZO. Challenging oral contraception after weight loss by bariatric surgery. *Gynecol Obstet Investig* 2007; **64**:100–102.

23. Kaltsounis J, et al. Intravenous valproate treatment of severe manic symptoms after gastric bypass surgery: a case report. *Psychosomatics* 2000; **41**:454–456.

24. Afshar S, et al. The effects of bariatric procedures on bowel habit. *Obes Surg* 2016; **26**:2348–2354.

25. Leyden Delta BV. Summary of product characteristics. Zaponex 100mg tablets. 2020 (last accessed August 2024); https://www.medicines.org.uk/emc/product/7715/smpc.

26. Mahgoub Y, et al. Schizoaffective exacerbation in a Roux-en-Y gastric bypass patient maintained on clozapine. *Prim Care Companion CNS Disord* 2019; **21**:19l02462.

27. Fuller AK, et al. Haloperidol pharmacokinetics following gastric bypass surgery. *J Clin Psychopharmacol* 1986; **6**:376–378.

28. Ward HB, et al. Lurasidone malabsorption following bariatric surgery: a case report. *J Psychiatr Pract* 2019; **25**:313–317.

29. McGrane IR, et al. Roux-en-Y gastric bypass and antipsychotic therapeutic drug monitoring: two cases. *J Pharm Pract* 2021; **34**:503–506.

30. Wallerstedt SM, et al. Serum concentrations of antidepressants, antipsychotics, and antiepileptics over the bariatric surgery procedure. *Eur J Clin Pharmacol* 2021; **77**:1875–1885.

31. Brito ME, et al. Patients with schizophrenia undergoing gastric bypass surgery: a case series study. *Obes Surg* 2020; **30**:3813–3821.

32. Seaman JS, et al. Dissolution of common psychiatric medications in a Roux-en-Y gastric bypass model. *Psychosomatics* 2005; **46**:250–253.

33. Miller AD, et al. Medication and nutrient administration considerations after bariatric surgery. *Am J Health Syst Pharm* 2006; **63**:1852–1857.

34. Brietzke E, et al. Long-acting injectable risperidone in a bipolar patient submitted to bariatric surgery and intolerant to conventional mood stabilizers. *Psychiatry Clin Neurosci* 2011; **65**:205.

35. Gandelman K, et al. The impact of calories and fat content of meals on oral ziprasidone absorption: a randomized, open-label, crossover trial. *J Clin Psychiatry* 2009; **70**:58–62.

36. Woodard G, et al. Cardiac arrest during laparoscopic Roux-en-Y gastric bypass in a bariatric patient with drug-associated long QT syndrome. *Obes Surg* 2011; **21**:134–137.

37. Triplett JD, et al. The effect of weight reduction surgery on the efficacy and tolerability of epilepsy pharmacotherapy. *Epilepsy Behav* 2021; **124**:108307.

38. Porat D, et al. Carbamazepine therapy after bariatric surgery: eight sleeve gastrectomy cases and review of the literature. 2022; **32**:3481–3486.

39. Bingham KS, et al. Perioperative lithium use in bariatric surgery: a case series and literature review. *Psychosomatics* 2016; **57**:638–644.

40. Ayub S, et al. Lithium toxicity following Roux-en-Y gastric bypass: mini review and illustrative case. *Ment Health Clin* 2022; **12**:214–218.

41. Dahan A, et al. Lithium toxicity with severe bradycardia post sleeve gastrectomy: a case report and review of the literature. *Obes Surg* 2019; **29**:735–738.

42. Brown CS, et al. Antiseizure medication use in gastric bypass patients and other post-surgical malabsorptive states. *Epilepsy Behav Rep* 2021; **16**:100439.

43. Tandra S, et al. Pharmacokinetic and pharmacodynamic alterations in the Roux-en-Y gastric bypass recipients. *Ann Surg* 2013; **258**:262–269.

44. Chan LN, et al. Proximal Roux-en-Y gastric bypass alters drug absorption pattern but not systemic exposure of CYP3A4 and P-glycoprotein substrates. *Pharmacotherapy* 2015; **35**:361–369.

45. Brill MJ, et al. The pharmacokinetics of the CYP3A substrate midazolam in morbidly obese patients before and one year after bariatric surgery. *Pharm Res* 2015; **32**:3927–3936.

46. Ochs HR, et al. Diazepam absorption: effects of age, sex, and Billroth gastrectomy. *Dig Dis Sci* 1982; **27**:225–230.

47. Steffen KJ, et al. Lisdexamfetamine pharmacokinetic comparison between patients who underwent Roux-en-Y gastric bypass and nonsurgical controls. *Obes Surg* 2021; **31**:4289–4294.

48. Strømmen M, et al. Bioavailability of methadone after sleeve gastrectomy: a planned case observation. *Clin Ther* 2016; **38**:1532–1536.

49. Azran C, et al. Impaired oral absorption of methylphenidate after Roux-en-Y gastric bypass. *Surg Obes Relat Dis* 2017; **13**:1245–1247.

50. Ludvigsson M, et al. Methylphenidate toxicity after Roux-en-Y gastric bypass. *Surg Obes Relat Dis* 2016; **12**:e55–e57.

51. Greenblatt DJ, et al. Influence of food on pharmacokinetics of zolpidem from fast dissolving sublingual zolpidem tartrate tablets. *J Clin Pharmacol* 2013; **53**:1194–1198.

52. Noria SF, et al. Weight regain after bariatric surgery: scope of the problem, causes, prevention, and treatment. *Curr Diab Rep* 2023; **23**:31–42.

53. Plaeke P, et al. Postoperative continuation of antidepressant therapy is associated with reduced short-term weight loss following Roux-en-Y gastric bypass surgery. *Langenbecks Arch Surg* 2019; **404**:621–631.

54. Leggett CB, et al. The effects of provider-prescribed obesogenic drugs on post-laparoscopic sleeve gastrectomy outcomes: a retrospective cohort study. *Int J Obes* 2019; **43**:1154–1163.

55. Ivezaj V, et al. Changes in alcohol use after metabolic and bariatric surgery: predictors and mechanisms. *Curr Psychiatry Rep* 2019; **21**:85.

56. Parikh M, et al. ASMBS position statement on alcohol use before and after bariatric surgery. *Surg Obes Relat Dis* 2016; **12**:225–230.

57. Stogios N, et al. Antipsychotic-induced weight gain in severe mental illness: risk factors and special considerations. *Curr Psychiatry Rep* 2023; **25**:707–721.

Menopause

The menopause transition is a phase in a woman's reproductive life where ovarian function declines, menstruation stops and production of the female reproductive hormones oestrogen, progesterone and testosterone significantly declines. The menopause signifies a date in time 12 months after a women's last menstrual period (LMP). The normal age range for the menopause is 45–55 years. The perimenopause is the phase leading up to a women's LMP characterised by erratic ovarian function and fluctuations in hormones. Perimenopausal symptoms typically arise 2–7 years prior to the LMP. About 75% of women experience menopausal symptoms (Table 10.20), 25% of women experience severe menopausal symptoms and 20% of women experience lifelong symptoms.[1,2] Symptoms associated with the menopause should be considered in women older than 40. However, women may experience an early menopause before 45 years of age, or premature ovarian insufficiency (POI) below 40 years of age, so symptoms may present earlier.

Table 10.20 Menopause symptoms.

Vasomotor	Physical	Genitourinary	Psychological
Hot flushes/flashes	Sleep disturbance	Urinary frequency	Anxiety
Night sweats	Muscular aches and pains	Nocturia	Low mood
Excessive sweating	Period changes – flow, duration, frequency	Vaginal dryness/irritation	Loss of motivation
Cold chills	Headaches/migraines	Vulval itching and	Mood swings
	Weight gain	irritation	Tearfulness
	Tinnitus	Frequent UTIs	Increased PMS
	Breast tenderness	Low libido	Poor concentration
	Heart palpitations	Loss of sexual pleasure	and focus
	Acne	Vaginal discomfort	Brain fog
	Fatigue and low energy		Poor word-finding
			and short-term
			memory
			Irritability

PMS, premenstrual syndrome; UTIs, urinary tract infections.

Diagnosis

Clinical diagnosis using the Greene Climacteric questionnaire is sufficient in most women older than 40 years presenting with typical symptoms. In women younger than 45 years, two raised follicle-stimulating hormone (FSH) levels >30mIU/mL, taken 6 weeks apart, tested on days 2–5 of the menstrual cycle may help confirm a diagnosis if clinical symptoms are not conclusive.[1,3]

Psychological symptoms of the menopause

Depression and anxiety

The impact of the menopause on mental well-being is significant. Suicidal ideation is present in around 6% of women experiencing menopause-related psychological symptoms. There is a 2–5-fold increase in the risk of depression during the perimenopause.[4] Hormone replacement therapy (HRT) is first-line treatment for menopausal insomnia, anxiety and depression.[1]

Psychosis

The decline in production of protective oestrogens is thought to be the reason that women show an increased risk of psychosis later in life (particularly at menopause) that is not observed in men, with one study suggesting that first hospital admission rates for psychosis are twice as high in women (21%) than in men (10%) after the age of 40.

Pharmacodynamics

Oestrogen is thought to have complex effects on dopamine transmission and receptor sensitivity, as well as antipsychotic binding. Human positron emission tomography (PET) studies have revealed that women have more D2 receptors in the brain compared with men. As oestrogen is thought to enhance antipsychotic binding affinity to these receptors, declining oestrogen levels in menopause serve to reduce antipsychotic activity.[5-7] Consequently, many women require higher doses of antipsychotic medication after menopause to maintain previous effect.[8]

Pharmacokinetics

Gender variations in the pharmacokinetics of psychotropic drugs are often not considered but may play an important role in drug efficacy and adverse effects. Factors such as gastrointestinal transit time, drug distribution of lipophilic drugs (e.g. antipsychotics) and drug elimination can vary with age and with hormonal changes seen during and after menopause.[9] Oestrogen and progesterone can decrease levels of glycoproteins responsible for binding to antipsychotic drugs. Declining levels of these hormones may therefore result in less free drug entering the brain.[9] Oestrogens are also thought to influence the activity and expression of some of the enzymes responsible for the hepatic metabolism of antipsychotics, i.e. oestrogens can induce and inhibit CYP isoenzymes (Table 10.21).[9]

Alternative treatments and drug interactions

Polypharmacy in menopausal women is common, with many women using alternative treatments (such as herbal remedies) to address menopausal symptoms. It is important that drug interactions are ruled out when prescribing antipsychotic medication.[10] The use of several medications, for example for sleep, pain and depression, may also affect protein binding of concurrent antipsychotics leading to changes in the ability for certain drugs to enter the brain.[5]

Table 10.21 Summary of antipsychotic/oestrogen interactions.[5,8,11]

Isoenzyme	Substrates	Effect of oestrogen on enzyme activity	Recommendations
CYP1A2	Clozapine, olanzapine	Inhibits	Oestrogen is thought to inhibit/reduce CYP1A2 activity and thus doses of antipsychotics that are mainly metabolised by this isoenzyme may need to be increased at menopause.
			Extra care should be given to antipsychotic dosing in menopausal women who smoke.
CYP3A4	Aripiprazole, quetiapine, lurasidone	Induces	Women generally have a higher expression of CYP3A4 enzyme than men, and menopause may cause reduced expression of this enzyme. High levels of oestrogen in pregnancy are thought to increase the metabolism via CYP3A4, further suggesting that oestrogen (and progesterone) play a role in rate of hepatic drug metabolism. Lower doses of CYP3A4-metabolised antipsychotics may be required in menopause, particularly if onset of menopause causes an increase in adverse effects.
CYP2D6	Aripiprazole, haloperidol, risperidone, zuclopenthixol	Possibly induces	CYP2D6 activity is generally higher in women than men. The clinical relevance of increased activity may be small, particularly as there may be genetic variations in the CYP2D6 gene. Some evidence suggests that doses of aripiprazole may require lowering at menopause (this may also be because it is metabolised by CYP3A4).
CYP2C19	Clozapine (minor route)	Possibly inhibits	Females reportedly have a 40% lower enzyme activity than men. This difference is thought to be most pronounced from 18 to 40 years (generally prior to onset of menopause). As stated previously, clozapine doses may need to be higher in menopausal women, however this needs to be balanced against risk of adverse effects. More regular therapeutic drug monitoring may be required.

Long-acting injections (LAIs)

Switching to an antipsychotic depot may improve levels of drugs that are mainly hepatically metabolised by CYP enzymes, as first-pass metabolism is avoided.[6] The use of antipsychotic depot injections should be considered if oral medications appear to lose efficacy in menopause.[10] Longer dosage intervals for LAIs may be beneficial in menopause as older women tend to eliminate drugs more slowly than their male counterparts.[12]

Risk of adverse effects

Increasing age coupled with oestrogen loss in menopause can make women more vulnerable to antipsychotic-related adverse effects. Older women are more vulnerable to QTc prolongation and motor symptoms (parkinsonism, akathisia and tardive dyskinesia) and therefore it is best to avoid antipsychotic drugs that may worsen these adverse effects.[8] Increased adiposity in menopause may be associated with a heightened risk for adverse effects such as insulin resistance, diabetes, sleep apnoea, cardiovascular disease and hypertriglyceridaemia.[13]

Prolactin levels

Persistently high prolactin levels may cause hypo-oestrogenic states and subsequently induce iatrogenic menopause.[12] This may worsen psychotic symptoms and cognition[5] as well as further increase the risk of osteoporosis in an already vulnerable group.[8,13] There is some evidence to suggest that high prolactin levels can also increase the risk of breast cancer.[13] Genitourinary problems and sexual dysfunction (including diminished libido) are issues that can be troublesome due to menopause and can be further worsened by hyperprolactinaemia.[12] It is important to note that hormones other than prolactin and oestrogen (e.g. progesterone) may play a potentially key role when considering antipsychotic use in menopause, although further research is required in this area.[5]

Oestrogen augmentation for psychosis

Treatment with adjunct oestrogenic medications may be beneficial in helping to relieve menopausal symptoms as well as improving psychotic symptoms and increasing the efficacy of antipsychotic drugs.[8] Recent meta-analyses have shown that selective oestrogen receptor modulators (SERMs) such as raloxifene (60–120mg/day) are a safe and effective adjunct for treating schizophrenia in menopausal women.[14] Raloxifene may be more suitable for long-term use than HRT as it has oestrogenic effects on the brain and bone tissue but anti-oestrogenic effects on other tissues such as the breast and uterus (therefore reducing the risk of breast and uterine cancer).[8,15] Both HRT and SERMs may increase the risk of venous thromboembolism (VTE)[16] and so potential risks and benefits of using these drugs as oestrogen-augmenting agents should be balanced individually, for example oestrogen replacement therapy may not be appropriate for those with a history of thromboembolic conditions.[8]

The preferred options for treating menopausal women with antipsychotic medications are summarised in Box 10.7.

Box 10.7 Summary of preferred antipsychotic options for menopausal women[8,12]

First option(s): aripiprazole, lurasidone
Second option(s): olanzapine, quetiapine, clozapine
Avoid where possible: amisulpride, risperidone, paliperidone and FGAs
Monitor: weight, bone mineral density, blood pressure, blood glucose, cholesterol and prolactin levels (especially if using prolactin-raising antipsychotics); therapeutic drug monitoring – due to hormonal fluctuations[17]

- Consider augmentation with raloxifene or HRT at an early stage, i.e. at the beginning of menopause/perimenopausal stage, where appropriate[15,18]
- If the efficacy of previously effective antipsychotic doses wanes at menopause, review the drug dose
- Be mindful of the risk of dose-related adverse effects such as weight gain and cardiovascular and cerebrovascular events[6]
- Switching to prolactin-sparing medications can benefit both mental and physical health[13]
- Consider adding anti-diabetic drugs (where appropriate) such as metformin which may help to prevent excess weight gain[19]
- Consider using LAIs as an option if oral medication becomes ineffective[6]

HRT, hormone replacement therapy; LAIs, long-acting injections.

Elderly care

Genitourinary symptoms of menopause (GSM) may be a factor in agitation and aggression in elderly care. Consider vaginal atrophy and localised vaginal oestrogen or ospemifene use in women presenting with GSM symptoms, recurrent urinary tract infections, recurrent candida, urinary leakage and vaginal discomfort.[20,21]

Use of HRT

For most women, HRT is a very safe and effective first-line option for treatment of menopausal symptoms, reducing osteoporosis and cardiovascular disease risk,[21-23] although there are some contraindications and precautions to its use (Table 10.22).

Table 10.22 Summary of the risks of using hormone replacement therapy (HRT).

Contraindications to HRT use	Precautions for HRT use	Risks
Oestrogen-dependent malignant tumours	Symptomatic fibroids	Endometrial hyperplasia and cancer
Undiagnosed vaginal bleeding	Untreated hypertension	Clot risk – dependent on type of HRT
Pregnancy	Migraine with aura – clot risk	Breast cancer risk – small increased risk for women over 50 years. Use patient counselling aided by WHC
Active liver disease with abnormal LFTs	Epilepsy – lamotrigine interaction	Irregular bleeding – see Table 10.25
Active or recent thromboembolic disorder (angina/MI)	Endometriosis – choice of HRT important	Adverse effects – see Table 10.25
Active or idiopathic VTE untreated	VTE/stroke – choice of HRT important	
Untreated endometrial hyperplasia	Heart disease – choice of HRT important	

MI, myocardial infarction; VTE, venous thromboembolism; WHC, Women's Health Concern.

Treatment options

1 Perimenopause: sequential combined HRT (oestrogen + progesterone cover in luteal phase for 12–14 days of cycle) ± localised vaginal oestrogen, and testosterone (Table 10.23).
2 Post menopause: continuous combined HRT (oestrogen + progesterone) ± local vaginal oestrogen, and testosterone (Table 10.23).

Combined HRT – oestrogen and progesterone – is required in all women except those who have had a total hysterectomy who may have oestrogen-only treatment. Oral oestrogen imposes a small increase in thrombus risk and therefore transdermal oestrogen is preferred when there is an increased risk of VTE or stroke.[1,23]

Table 10.23 Hormone replacement therapy (HRT) products and regimens.

Estradiol	Progesterone
Sequential combined HRT – perimenopause (prescribe by brand name)	
Patch: 25–100mcg twice weekly	Micronised progesterone 200mg on, days 15–28 of cycle
Estradiol gel 0.6mg/g: 1–4 pumps daily	Progesterone 200mg on, days 15–28 of cycle
Estradiol gel sachets: 0.5–1.5mg daily	Medroxyprogesterone acetate 10mg od, days 16–27 of cycle
Estradiol 1.53mg/spray: 1–3 sprays daily	Levonorgestrel 52mg IUD
Estradiol hemihydrate/valerate tablets: 1–2mg daily	

Combined products:

- Estradiol hemihydrate 50mcg/24h and norethisterone acetate 11.2mg combined patch, used for 14/28 days, and estradiol 50mcg patch used for 14/28 days. Applied twice weekly
- Estradiol 1mg/2mg with dydrogesterone 10mg tablets – calendar pack one daily
- Estradiol 1mg/2mg with norethisterone 1mg tablets – calendar pack one daily

Continuous combined HRT – post menopause (prescribe by brand name)

Estradiol patch: 25–100mcg twice weekly	Micronised progesterone 100mg on
Estradiol gel 0.6mg/g: 1–4 pumps daily	Progesterone 100mg on
Estradiol gel sachets: 0.5–1.5mg daily	Medroxyprogesterone acetate 2.5–5mg od
Estradiol 1.53mg/spray: 1–3 sprays daily	Levonorgestrel 52mg IUD
Estradiol hemihydrate/valerate tablets: 1–2mg daily	

Combined products:

- Estradiol hemihydrate 50mcg/24h and norethisterone acetate 11.2mg combined patch, applied twice weekly
- Estradiol 0.5/1mg with 2.5/5mg dydrogesterone tablets: 1 od
- Estradiol 2mg with 1mg norethisterone tablets: 1 od

IUD, intrauterine device; od, once a day; on, every night.

Local treatment options with GSM

Additional topical treatment options when GSM symptoms are prominent are given in Table 10.24.

Table 10.24 Topical vaginal oestrogen or GSM treatment.

Drug	Dose
Estradiol 10mcg vaginal tablets	One pv daily for 14 days and then twice weekly
Estriol 0.03mg pessary	One pv daily for 21 days and then twice weekly
Estriol 1mg cream	1 applicator daily for 4 weeks and then twice weekly
Prasterone 6.5mg pessary	One daily
Ospemifene 60mg oral	One daily with food

GSM, genitorurinary symptoms of menopause; pv, per vagina.

Starting treatment

Start HRT at 25–50mcg estradiol patch dose equivalents (1mg estradiol tablet/1–2 pumps estradiol 0.6mg/g gel). Increase after 6–8 weeks if symptomatic. Higher doses of estradiol may require additional progesterone for endometrial protection.[24] HRT is not a contraceptive.

Management of adverse effects

Table 10.25 outlines the management of the possible adverse effects of HRT.

Table 10.25 Management of adverse effects of hormone replacement therapy (HRT).

Adverse effect	Comments
Breast tenderness Bloating Spotting	Common within first 3–6 months, or on dose adjustment, normally transient.
Headaches Nausea	Common in first 3 months of starting or dose increase. May need slower titration.
Mood swings Increase in PMS symptoms Increased anxiety/agitation	Often common when starting for first month, then transient. Consider progesterone intolerance if beyond 1 month or severe.
Irregular bleeding	Common for the first 3 months. Refer for investigation if after 4–6 months it has not settled or patient has been on HRT for a while and it is a new presentation.

PMS, premenstrual syndrome.

References

1. National Institute for Health and Care Excellence. Menopause: diagnosis and management. NICE guideline [NG23]. 2015 (last updated December 2019, last checked December 2023); https://www.nice.org.uk/guidance/ng23.
2. Avis NE, et al. Duration of menopausal vasomotor symptoms over the menopause transition. *JAMA Intern Med* 2015; **175**:531–539.
3. Greene JG. Constructing a standard climacteric scale. *Maturitas* 1998; **29**:25–31.
4. El Khoudary SR, et al. The menopause transition and women's health at midlife: a progress report from the Study of Women's Health Across the Nation (SWAN). *Menopause* 2019; **26**:1213–1227.
5. González-Rodríguez A, et al. The association between hormones and antipsychotic use: a focus on postpartum and menopausal women. *Ther Adv Psychopharmacol* 2019; **9**:2045125319859973.
6. González-Rodríguez A, et al. The effect of menopause on antipsychotic response. *Brain Sci* 2022; **12**:1342.
7. Brand BA, et al. Estrogens in schizophrenia: progress, current challenges and opportunities. *Curr Opin Psychiatry* 2021; **34**:228–237.
8. Brand BA, et al. Antipsychotic medication for women with schizophrenia spectrum disorders. *Psychol Med* 2022; **52**:649–663.
9. Seeman MV. Men and women respond differently to antipsychotic drugs. *Neuropharmacology* 2020; **163**:107631.
10. Seeman MV. Treating schizophrenia at the time of menopause. *Maturitas* 2012; **72**:117–120.
11. Choi SY, et al. Isoform-specific regulation of cytochromes P450 expression by estradiol and progesterone. *Drug Metab Dispos* 2013; **41**:263–269.
12. Lange B, et al. How gender affects the pharmacotherapeutic approach to treating psychosis – a systematic review. *Expert Opin Pharmacother* 2017; **18**:351–362.
13. Brand BA, et al. Towards better care for women with schizophrenia-spectrum disorders. *Lancet Psychiatry* 2022; **9**:330–336.
14. Li Z, et al. Estradiol and raloxifene as adjunctive treatment for women with schizophrenia: a meta-analysis of randomized, double-blind, placebo-controlled trials. *Acta Psychiatr Scand* 2023; **147**:360–372.
15. Sommer IE, et al. Women with schizophrenia-spectrum disorders after menopause: a vulnerable group for relapse. *Schizophr Bull* 2022; **49**:136–143.

16. González-Rodríguez A, et al. Women with schizophrenia over the life span: health promotion, treatment and outcomes. *Int J Environ Res Public Health* 2020; **17**:5594.

17. Brand BA, et al. Evidence-based recommendations for the pharmacological treatment of women with schizophrenia spectrum disorders. *Curr Psychiatry Rep* 2023; **25**:723–733.

18. Culbert KM, et al. Risk for midlife psychosis in women: critical gaps and opportunities in exploring perimenopause and ovarian hormones as mechanisms of risk. *Psychol Med* 2022; **52**:1612–1620.

19. Seeman MV. Selecting the right treatment plan for schizophrenia in postmenopausal women: an update of the literature. *Expert Rev Neurother* 2023; **23**:515–523.

20. Hamoda H, et al. The British Menopause Society and Women's Health Concern 2020 recommendations on hormone replacement therapy in menopausal women. *Post Reprod Health* 2020; **26**:181–209.

21. Chakrabarti R, et al. Prescribing hormone replacement therapy: key considerations for primary care physicians. *Br J Gen Pract* 2023; **73**:330–332.

22. Weiss SR, et al. A randomized controlled trial of four doses of transdermal estradiol for preventing postmenopausal bone loss. Transdermal Estradiol Investigator Group. *Obstet Gynecol* 1999; **94**:330–336.

23. Boardman HM, et al. Hormone therapy for preventing cardiovascular disease in post-menopausal women. *Cochrane Database Syst Rev* 2015; **2015**:CD002229.

24. British Menopause Society (BMS). Progestogens and endometrial protection. BMS consensus statement. 2021; https://thebms.org.uk/wp-content/uploads/2021/10/14-BMS-TfC-Progestogens-and-endometrial-protection-01H.pdf.

Chapter 11

Pharmacokinetics

Plasma level monitoring of psychotropic drugs

The measurement of blood or plasma drug concentrations is widely known as therapeutic drug monitoring or TDM. It is often used in psychiatry but not always well used. The interpretation of drug concentrations (drug 'levels') is a complex process that requires a thorough understanding of pharmacokinetics. Some principles are outlined here.

First-order pharmacokinetics

The metabolism and excretion of most drugs follow first-order elimination kinetics. The key feature of this model is that clearance of a drug is constant when expressed in volume per unit time – usually L/h. The mass of drug cleared (metabolised or excreted) increases as blood concentration increases. For example, if clearance of a drug is 10L/h and the concentration is 5mg/L then 50mg ($10 \times 50mg$) will be cleared in an hour. If the concentration increases to 10mg/L then 100mg will be cleared in an hour. The concept of first-order pharmacokinetics is important to the understanding of steady state.

Steady state

Repeated dosing of any drug that is not completely removed within the dosing interval will inevitably lead to accumulation. That is, the second dose will add to what remains of the first and the third dose will add to what remains of the first and second doses. As the drug concentration in the blood increases, the mass of the drug cleared will also rise, according to first-order principles. Eventually, a point is reached where blood levels remain stable within a specific peak-to-trough range – this is steady state. It is important

The Maudsley® Prescribing Guidelines in Psychiatry, Fifteenth Edition. David M. Taylor, Thomas R. E. Barnes and Allan H. Young.
© 2025 David M. Taylor. Published 2025 by John Wiley & Sons Ltd.

to know when a drug is or is not at steady state but there are two concepts connected to steady state that are often misunderstood.

- **Time to reach steady state follows a logarithmic pattern**
  The time taken to reach steady state is dependent on the drug half-life – the time taken for concentration to fall by 50%. This table shows the rise to steady state.

Number of half-lives	% of steady state reached
2	75%
3	87.5%
4	94%
5	97%

Most people know the adage that it takes four to five half-lives to reach steady state. In fact, three half-lives are sufficient for an approximation of steady state concentrations.

- **Steady state is not always related to therapeutic activity**
  Blood levels at steady state are determined by dose and drug half-life. The concentration at which therapeutic activity occurs is fixed (see later) and, during therapeutic dosing, is often exceeded before steady state is reached. Loading doses are sometimes used to achieve therapeutic concentrations as quickly as possible. Loading doses do not hasten the achievement of steady state levels.

Timing of sampling

Sampling time is vitally important for many but not all drugs. If the recommended sampling time is, say, 12 hours post-dose, then the sample should be taken 11–13 hours post-dose if possible; 10–14 hours post-dose, if absolutely necessary. A study of clozapine samples taken 1 and 2 hours before and after the 12-hour scheduled sample time showed a mean variation of clozapine blood concentration of less than 10%, but some individuals' levels varied by over 50%.[1] So, if a sample is not taken within 1–2 hours of the required time, it has the potential to mislead rather than inform. Always try to take samples as close to the scheduled time as possible. Obviously, if toxicity is suspected, take a sample straightaway, ignoring any scheduled timings.

For trough or 'pre-dose' samples, take the blood sample immediately before the next dose is due. Do not, under any circumstances, withhold the next dose for more than 1 or possibly 2 hours until the sample is taken. Withholding for longer than this will inevitably give a misleading result (it will give a lower result than that ever seen in the usual, regular dosing), and this may lead to an inappropriate dose increase. Sampling time is less critical with drugs with a long half-life (e.g. olanzapine, aripiprazole) but, as an absolute minimum, prescribers should always record the time of sampling and time of last dose. This cannot be emphasised enough, and is worth repeating in bold. **Always record the time of sampling and the time of the last dose.**

Interpretation of results

Is there a target range of plasma levels? If so, then plasma levels (from samples taken at the right time) will usefully guide dosing. If there is not an accepted target range, plasma levels can only indicate adherence or potential toxicity. However, if the sample is being used to check compliance, then bear in mind that a plasma level of zero indicates only that the drug has not been taken in the past several days. Plasma levels above zero may indicate erratic compliance, full compliance or even long-standing non-compliance disguised by recent taking of prescribed doses. Note also that target ranges have their limitations – patients may respond to lower levels than the quoted range and tolerate levels above the range. Also, ranges quoted by different laboratories vary sometimes widely, often without explanation. This is discussed further later.

The basic rule for sample level interpretation is to act upon assay results only in conjunction with reliable clinical observation ('*treat the patient, not the level*'). For example, if a patient is responding adequately to a drug but has a plasma level below the accepted target range, then the dose should not normally be increased. If a patient has intolerable adverse effects but a plasma level within the target range, then a dose decrease may be appropriate.

Where a plasma level result is substantially different from previous results, a repeat sample is usually advised. Check the dose, the timing of dose and recent compliance but ensure, in particular, the correct timing of the sample, or at the very least that the timing of sampling is known. Many anomalous results are the consequence of changes in sample timing.

Target ranges

In psychiatry, target ranges for psychotropic drug concentrations should be treated with some caution. Establishing a range of concentrations associated with response is made difficult by the presence in trials of non-responders (who show no response whatever the blood concentration) and by the presence of placebo responders and spontaneous remitters (who respond at any blood concentration). Establishing a target range based on adverse effects is made difficult by the development of tolerance over time. Thus, most studies aimed at determining target ranges have as much 'noise' as 'signal' and results ultimately represent broad approximations.

Interestingly, drug concentrations associated with response in clinical practice show a fairly close correlation to published target ranges.[2] The lower quartile (25th percentile) of drug concentrations is usually close to the lower end of the target range and the upper quartile (75th percentile) is around the value of, but usually less than, the upper limit. Broadly speaking, this means that around 25% of patients respond below the target range and up to 25% tolerate blood concentrations above the target range.

The simplicity of published target ranges disguises considerable complexity. For most drugs, the concentration at which therapeutic activity appears is fairly constant across a population. This is called the therapeutic threshold – above it, full effect is seen, but below it, activity is lost. A good example here is risperidone where the threshold concentration of active moiety is 20mcg/L. Risperidone and paliperidone could reasonably be considered to have a target concentration rather than a target range of concentrations. This concept of a therapeutic threshold is supported by neuroimaging studies. A concentration of 20mcg/L of active moiety is associated with a dopamine occupancy of 65–70%[3] – the degree of pharmacological activity associated with response for most antipsychotics.[4] Increasing dopamine occupancy above this level does not improve efficacy or likelihood of response but does make adverse effects more likely.[3]

Clozapine is completely different. For clozapine, the target range represents concentrations *usually* associated with both response and good tolerability. However, perhaps 10% of responders will improve with clozapine concentrations below the target range and as many as 20% of responders will only respond at concentrations above the target range. There is also a so-called point of futility – the concentration above which no additional responders will be uncovered. Responders to clozapine will have blood concentrations between 250 and 1000mcg/L[5] – a much wider range than the accepted target range. Unlike risperidone and many other drugs, the threshold concentration is not fixed across populations.

This subject is eloquently covered in much more detail in *The Clinical Use of Antipsychotic Plasma Levels* by Jonathan Meyer and Stephen Stahl (Cambridge University Press, 2021).

Table 11.1 discusses the interpretation of sample results for various drugs.

Table 11.1 Interpreting sample results for drugs with established target ranges.

Drug	Target range	Sample timing	Time to steady state	Comments
Amisulpride	200–320mcg/L 20–60mcg/L (elderly)	Trough	3 days	See text
Aripiprazole	100–210mcg/L	Trough	15–16 days	See text
Carbamazepine[6–8]	>7mg/L Bipolar disorder	Trough	2 weeks	Carbamazepine induces its own metabolism. Time to steady state dependent on auto-induction
Clozapine	350–600mcg/L	Trough	2–3 days	See text
Lamotrigine[9–11]	Not established but suggest **2.5–15mg/L**	Trough	5 days Auto-induction is thought to occur, so time to steady state may be longer	Some debate over utility of lamotrigine levels, especially in bipolar disorder. In treatment-resistant unipolar depression, plasma levels of above 12.7μmol/L (3.3mg/L) are associated with response.[12,13] Toxicity may be increased above 15mg/L but is normally well tolerated
Lithium[14–18]	**0.6–1.0mmol/L** (0.4mmol may be sufficient for some patients/indications; >1.0mmol/L required for mania)	12 hours	5 days post-dose	Well-established target range, albeit derived from ancient data sources. A fairly recent study[19] suggested 0.6mmol/L was the minimum level for a prophylactic effect

Table 11.1 (*Continued*)

Drug	Target range	Sample timing	Time to steady state	Comments
Olanzapine	20–40mcg/L	12 hours	1 week	See text
Paliperidone[20]	20–60mcg/L (9-OH risperidone)	Trough	2–3 days oral 2 months depot	Target range is the same as that established for risperidone.[21] As with risperidone, routine plasma level monitoring is not recommended.
Phenytoin[7]	10–20mg/L	Trough	Variable	Follows zero-order kinetics. Free levels may be useful in some circumstances.
Quetiapine	Around 50–100mcg/L?	Trough?	2–3 days oral	Target range poorly defined. Plasma level monitoring not recommended. See text.
Risperidone	20–60mcg/L (active moiety – risperidone + 9-OH risperidone)	Trough	**2–3 days oral** 6–8 weeks injection	Routine plasma level monitoring is not recommended. See text.
Tricyclics[22]	Nortriptyline **50–150mcg/L** Amitriptyline **100–200mcg/L**	Trough	2–3 days	Rarely used and of dubious benefit. Use ECG to assess toxicity.
Valproate[6,7,23–25]	**50–100mg/L** Epilepsy and bipolar	Trough	2–3 days	Some doubt over value of levels in epilepsy and in bipolar disorder. Some evidence that, in mania, levels up to 125mg/L are tolerated and more effective than lower concentrations. Valproate plasma levels are linearly related to plasma ammonia.[26]

Amisulpride

Amisulpride plasma levels are closely related to dose with insufficient variation to make routine plasma level monitoring prudent. Higher levels observed in women[27–29] seem to have little significant clinical implication for either therapeutic response or adverse effects. A (trough) threshold for clinical response has been suggested to be approximately 100mcg/L[30] and mean levels of 367mcg/L[29] have been noted in responders. Adverse effects (notably extrapyramidal side effects [EPSEs]) occur at mean levels of 336mcg/L,[27] 377mcg/L[30] and 395mcg/L.[28] A plasma level threshold of below 320mcg/L has been found to predict avoidance of EPSEs.[30] One review[31] has suggested an approximate range of **200–320mcg/L** for optimal clinical response and avoidance of adverse effects but a more recent consensus statement[32] suggested a target range of **100–320mcg/L**. A dose of 200mg a day is sufficient to give a blood level of 100mcg/L[33] so this lower threshold is probably too low for a reliable therapeutic effect. In older patients with psychosis, studies suggest plasma concentrations of **20–60mcg/L** may give optimal D_2 occupancy and clinical response.[34,35]

In practice, only a minority of treated patients have 'therapeutic' plasma levels (probably because of poor adherence[36]) so plasma monitoring may be of some benefit. However, amisulpride plasma level monitoring is rarely undertaken and few laboratories offer amisulpride assays. The dose–response relationship is sufficiently robust (in trials, at least) to obviate the need for plasma sampling within the licensed dose range (although in older patients, doses of 50–100mg a day may be sufficient) and adverse effects are usually well managed by dose adjustment alone. Plasma level monitoring is best reserved for those in whom clinical response is poor, adherence is questioned or in whom drug interactions or physical illness may make adverse effects more likely.

Aripiprazole

Plasma level monitoring of aripiprazole is sometimes undertaken in practice. The dose–response relationship for aripiprazole is well established with a plateau in clinical response and D_2 dopamine occupancy seen in doses above approximately 10mg/day.[37] Plasma levels of aripiprazole, its metabolite and the total moiety (parent plus metabolite) strongly relate linearly to dose, making it possible to predict, with some certainty, an approximate plasma level for a given dose.[38] Target plasma level ranges for optimal clinical response have been suggested as 146–254mcg/L[39] and 150–300mcg/L,[40] with adverse effects more frequent above 210mcg/L.[40] Inter-individual variation in aripiprazole plasma levels has been observed but not fully investigated, although gender appears to have little influence.[41,42] Age, metabolic enzyme genotype and interacting medications seem likely causes of variation.[40–43] A putative range of between **150 and 210mcg/L**[38] has been suggested as a target for patients taking aripiprazole and these are broadly the concentrations seen in patients receiving depot aripiprazole at 300 and 400mg monthly.[44] Some authorities suggest a lower threshold for clinical effect of 100mcg/L[32] – a plasma level usually afforded by an oral dose of 10mg a day[33,45] and around the minimum level reached during treatment with 2-monthly depot.[46]

Clozapine

Clozapine plasma levels are broadly related to daily dose[47] but there is sufficient variation to make impossible any precise prediction of plasma level. Plasma levels are generally lower in younger patients, males[48] and smokers[49] and higher in Asians.[50] Much lower doses of clozapine are required in East Asians,[51,52] Indians[53] and Bangladeshis.[54] The prevalence of clozapine poor metabolisers is also higher in East Asians.[55,56] A series of algorithms has been developed for the approximate prediction of clozapine levels according to patient factors and these are recommended.[57] Dose prediction using genetic analysis is more accurate that algorithm prediction.[58] Neither method can account for other influences on clozapine plasma levels such as changes in adherence, inflammation[59] and infection.[60,61]

The plasma level threshold for acute response to clozapine has been suggested to be 200mcg/L,[62] 350mcg/L,[63–65] 370mcg/L,[66] 420mcg/L,[67] 504mcg/L[68] and 550mcg/L.[69] Limited data suggest a level of at least 200mcg/L is required to prevent relapse.[70] Substantial variation in clozapine plasma level may also predict relapse.[71] Changes in

CHAPTER 11

an individual's clozapine plasma levels are common with a tendency for concentrations to slightly decrease over time,[72] although one study suggests a decrease only in norclozapine concentrations.[73]

Despite these somewhat varied estimates of response threshold, plasma levels can be useful in optimising treatment. In those not responding to clozapine, the dose should be adjusted to give plasma levels in the range **350–600mcg/L** (a range reflecting a consensus of the above findings[32]). Those not tolerating clozapine may benefit from a reduction to a dose giving plasma levels in this range. An upper limit to the clozapine target range has not been defined. Any upper limit must take into account two components: the level above which no therapeutic advantage is gained and the level at which toxicity/tolerability is unacceptable. Plasma levels do seem to predict EEG changes[74,75] and seizures occur more frequently in patients with levels above 1000mcg/L,[76] so levels should probably be kept well below this. Other non-neurological clozapine-related adverse effects also seem to be plasma-level related[77] as might be expected. An upper limit of concentrations around 600–800mcg/L has been proposed,[78] although a level of 1000mcg/L may be the point of futility.[79,80]

Placing an upper limit on the target range for clozapine levels may discourage potentially worthwhile dose increases within the licensed dose range. Before plasma levels were widely used, clozapine was sometimes given in doses up to 900mg/day, with valproate being added when the dose reached 600mg/day. It remains unclear whether using these high doses can benefit patients with plasma levels already above the accepted threshold. Nonetheless, it is prudent to use an antiseizure agent as prophylaxis against seizures and myoclonus when plasma levels are above 600mcg/L (a level based more on repeated recommendation than on being a clear evidence-based threshold[78]) and certainly when levels approach 1000μmcg/L.

Norclozapine is the major metabolite of clozapine. The ratio of clozapine to norclozapine averages 1.25 in populations[81] but may differ markedly for individuals.[82] In chronic dosing, the ratio should remain the same for a given patient. A decrease in ratio may suggest enzyme induction, an increase suggests enzyme inhibition, a non-trough sample or recent missed doses. Time of sampling radically alters the clozapine/norclozapine ratio as clozapine is relatively high in early samples and norclozapine is higher in late samples.[1] Clozapine metabolism may become saturated at higher doses: the ratio of clozapine to norclozapine increases with increasing plasma levels, suggesting saturation.[83–85] The effect of fluvoxamine also suggests that metabolism via CYP1A2 to norclozapine can be overwhelmed.[86]

Ultimately, changes in the clozapine/norclozapine ratio may be impossible to interpret. A systematic review concluded that knowledge of clozapine/norclozapine ratio had no clinical utility.[87]

Olanzapine

Plasma levels of olanzapine are linearly related to daily dose[88] but there is substantial variation,[89] with higher levels seen in women,[68] non-smokers[90] and those on enzyme-inhibiting drugs.[90,91] With once-daily dosing, the threshold level for response in schizophrenia has been suggested to be 9.3mcg/L (trough sample),[92] 23.2mcg/L (12-hour post-dose sample)[68] and 23mcg/L at a mean of 13.5 hours post-dose.[93] There is evidence to suggest that levels greater than around 40mcg/L (12-hour sampling) produce no further therapeutic benefit than lower levels.[94] Severe toxicity is uncommon but may be associated with levels above 100mcg/L, and death is occasionally seen at levels above 160mcg/L[95] (albeit when other drugs or physical factors are relevant). A target range for therapeutic use of **20–40mcg/L** (12-hour post-dose sample) has been proposed[96] for schizophrenia; the range for mania is probably similar.[97] This target range was for a time widened to **20–80mcg/L**[98,99] but the reasons for this were not clear. A 2023 systematic review suggests a target range of **20–40mcg/L** for 12-hour samples.[100]

Significant weight gain seems most likely to occur in those with plasma levels above 20mcg/L.[101] Constipation, dry mouth and tachycardia also seem to be related to plasma level.[102]

In practice, the dose of olanzapine should be largely governed by response and tolerability. However, a survey of UK sample assay results suggested that around 20% of patients on 20mg a day will have sub-therapeutic plasma levels and more than 40% have levels above 40mcg/L.[103] Plasma level determinations might then be useful for those suspected of non-adherence, those showing poor tolerability or those not responding to the maximum licensed dose. Where there is poor response and plasma levels are below 20mcg/L, dose may then be adjusted to give 12-hour plasma levels of 20–40mcg/L; where there is good response and poor tolerability, the dose should be tentatively reduced to give plasma levels below 40mcg/L. Changes in dose give proportionate changes in plasma levels.[104] A case might be made to increase the dose to give blood levels in the range 40–80mcg/L but only where no other options remain.

Quetiapine

Doses of quetiapine are weakly related to trough plasma samples.[105] Mean levels reported within the dose range 150–800mg/day vary from 27 to 387mcg/L,[106–111] although the highest and lowest levels are not necessarily found at the lowest and highest doses. Age, gender and co-medication may contribute to the significant inter-individual variance observed in TDM studies, with female gender,[111,112] older age[110,111] and CYP3A4-inhibiting drugs[106,110,111] likely to increase quetiapine concentration. Reports of these effects are conflicting[112] and not sufficient to support the routine use of plasma level monitoring based on these factors alone. Despite the substantial variation in plasma levels at each dose, there is insufficient evidence to suggest a target therapeutic range to aim for (although a target range of 100–500mcg/L has been proposed[113]), thus plasma level monitoring is likely to have little value. Moreover, the metabolites of quetiapine have major therapeutic effects and their concentrations are only loosely associated with parent drug levels.[114]

Most current reports of quetiapine concentration associations are derived from the analysis of trough samples. Because of the short half-life of quetiapine, trough levels tend to drop to within a relatively small range regardless of dose and previous peak level. Peak plasma levels may be more closely related to dose and clinical response,[105] although monitoring of such is not currently justified in the absence of an established peak plasma target range. Interestingly, a study of quetiapine in patients with borderline personality disorder or drug-induced psychosis showed a linear relationship between response and 12-hour plasma levels.[112] Peak to trough variation is greater for immediate-release formulations (roughly a maximum of 4000mcg/L to zero) than for slow-release preparations (roughly a maximum of 3000mcg/L to around 100mcg/L).[45]

Quetiapine has an established dose–response relationship, and appears to be well tolerated at doses well beyond the licensed dose range.[115] In practice, dose adjustment should be based on patient response and tolerability.

Risperidone

The therapeutic range for risperidone is generally agreed to be **20–60mcg/L** of the active moiety (risperidone + 9-OH-risperidone)[98,116,117] although other ranges (25–150mcg/L and 25–80mcg/L) have been proposed.[118] Plasma levels of 20–60mcg/L are usually afforded by oral doses of between 3mg and 6mg a day.[116,119–121] Occupancy of striatal dopamine D_2 receptors has been shown to be around 65% (the minimum required for acute therapeutic effect) at plasma levels of approximately 20mcg/L.[117,122]

Limited data for paliperidone palmitate 1-monthly long-acting injection (LAI) suggest that standard loading doses give plasma levels of 25–45mcg/L; while at steady state, plasma levels ranged from 10 to 25mcg/L for 100mg/month and 15 to 35mcg/L for 150mg/month.[123] Plasma concentrations may gradually rise in the first year of treatment to around 35mcg/L (mean dose 138mg/month)[124] and remain stable thereafter.[125] For the 3-monthly injection, steady state plasma concentrations range from 30 to 55mcg/L for 525mg every 3 months, 25 to 55mcg/L for 350mg every 3 months and 20 to 35mcg/L for 263mg every 3 months.[126,127] Six-monthly paliperidone, available as 700 and 1000mg injections, provides similar plasma concentrations to those achieved by the corresponding doses of 3-monthly injections.[128]

Plasma concentrations of risperidone ISM® remain above 20mcg/L throughout the dosing interval.[129]

Target ranges for other psychotropics

The target ranges listed in Table 11.2 have somewhat dubious usefulness and, in some cases, merely represent the range of values seen in clinical use. Assays for these drugs are likely to be available only in specialist units.

Table 11.2 Target ranges for other psychotropics.[32,98,130]

	Target range (mcg/L)
Antipsychotics	
Asenapine	1–5
Brexpiprazole	40–140
Cariprazine	10–20
Chlorpromazine	30–300
Flupentixol	0.5–5 (cis-isomer)
Fluphenazine	1–10
Haloperidol	1–10

(Continued)

Table 11.2 (*Continued*)

	Target range (mcg/L)
Iloperidone	5–10
Lurasidone	15–40
Melperone	30–100
Sulpiride	200–1000
Ziprasidone	50–200
Zuclopenthixol	4–50
Antidepressants	
Agomelatine	7–300
Citalopram	50–110
Desvenlafaxine	100–400
Dosulepin	45–100
Duloxetine	30–120
Escitalopram	15–80
Fluoxetine (+ norfluoxetine)	120–500
Fluvoxamine	60–230
Levomilnacipran	80–120
Mianserin	15–70
Milnacipram	100–150
Mirtazapine	30–80
Moclobemide	300–1000
Paroxetine	20–65
Reboxetine	60–350
Sertraline	10–150
Trazodone	700–1000
Venlafaxine (+ O-desmethylvenlafaxine)	100–400
Vilazodone	30–70
Vortioxetine	15–60

References

1. Jakobsen MI, et al. The significance of sampling time in therapeutic drug monitoring of clozapine. *Acta Psychiatr Scand* 2017; **135**:159–169.
2. Hiemke C. Concentration-effect relationships of psychoactive drugs and the problem to calculate therapeutic reference ranges. *Ther Drug Monit* 2019; **41**:174–179.
3. Hart XM, et al. Update lessons from positron emission tomography imaging Part I: a systematic critical review on therapeutic plasma concentrations of antipsychotics. *Ther Drug Monit* 2024; **46**:16–32.
4. Kapur S, et al. Relationship between dopamine D2 occupancy, clinical response, and side effects: a double-blind PET study of first-episode schizophrenia. *Am J Psychiatry* 2000; **157**:514–520.
5. Kronig MH, et al. Plasma clozapine levels and clinical response for treatment-refractory schizophrenic patients. *Am J Psychiatry* 1995; **152**:179–182.
6. Taylor D, et al. Doses of carbamazepine and valproate in bipolar affective disorder. *Psychiatric Bulletin* 1997; **21**:221–223.
7. Eadie MJ. Anticonvulsant drugs. *Drugs* 1984; **27**:328–363.
8. Chbili C, et al. Relationships between pharmacokinetic parameters of carbamazepine and therapeutic response in patients with bipolar disease. *Ann Biol Clin (Paris)* 2014; **72**:453–459.
9. Cohen AF, et al. Lamotrigine, a new anticonvulsant: pharmacokinetics in normal humans. *Clin Pharmacol Ther* 1987; **42**:535–541.
10. Kilpatrick ES, et al. Concentration-effect and concentration-toxicity relations with lamotrigine: a prospective study. *Epilepsia* 1996; **37**:534–538.
11. Johannessen SI, et al. Therapeutic drug monitoring of the newer antiepileptic drugs. *Ther Drug Monit* 2003; **25**:347–363.
12. Kagawa S, et al. Relationship between plasma concentrations of lamotrigine and its early therapeutic effect of lamotrigine augmentation therapy in treatment-resistant depressive disorder. *Ther Drug Monit* 2014; **36**:730–733.
13. Nakamura A, et al. Prediction of an optimal dose of lamotrigine for augmentation therapy in treatment-resistant depressive disorder from plasma lamotrigine concentration at week 2. *Ther Drug Monit* 2016; **38**:379–382.
14. Schou M. Forty years of lithium treatment. *Arch Gen Psychiatry* 1997; **54**:9–13.
15. Anon. Using lithium safely. *Drug Ther Bull* 1999; **37**:22–24.
16. Nicholson J, et al. Monitoring patients on lithium – a good practice guideline. *Psychiatric Bulletin* 2002; **26**:348–351.
17. National Institute for Health and Care Excellence. Bipolar disorder: assessment and management. Clinical guideline [CG185]. 2014 (last updated December 2023, last accessed August 2024); https://www.nice.org.uk/guidance/cg185.
18. Severus WE, et al. What is the optimal serum lithium level in the long-term treatment of bipolar disorder – a review? *Bipolar Disord* 2008; **10**:231–237.
19. Nolen WA, et al. The association of the effect of lithium in the maintenance treatment of bipolar disorder with lithium plasma levels: a post hoc analysis of a double-blind study comparing switching to lithium or placebo in patients who responded to quetiapine (Trial 144). *Bipolar Disord* 2013; **15**:100–109.
20. Nazirizadeh Y, et al. Serum concentrations of paliperidone versus risperidone and clinical effects. *Eur J Clin Pharmacol* 2010; **66**:797–803.
21. Schoretsanitis G, et al. A systematic review and combined analysis of therapeutic drug monitoring studies for oral paliperidone. *Expert Rev Clin Pharmacol* 2018; **11**:625–639.
22. Taylor D, et al. Plasma levels of tricyclics and related antidepressants: are they necessary or useful? *Psychiatric Bulletin* 1995; **19**:548–550.
23. Perucca E. Pharmacological and therapeutic properties of valproate. *CNS Drugs* 2002; **16**:695–714.
24. Allen MH, et al. Linear relationship of valproate serum concentration to response and optimal serum levels for acute mania. *Am J Psychiatry* 2006; **163**:272–275.
25. Bowden CL, et al. Relation of serum valproate concentration to response in mania. *Am J Psychiatry* 1996; **153**:765–770.
26. Vazquez M, et al. Hyperammonemia associated with valproic acid concentrations. *Biomed Res Int* 2014; **2014**:217269.
27. Muller MJ, et al. Amisulpride doses and plasma levels in different age groups of patients with schizophrenia or schizoaffective disorder. *J Psychopharmacol* 2008; **23**:278–286.
28. Muller MJ, et al. Gender aspects in the clinical treatment of schizophrenic inpatients with amisulpride: a therapeutic drug monitoring study. *Pharmacopsychiatry* 2006; **39**:41–46.
29. Bergemann N, et al. Plasma amisulpride levels in schizophrenia or schizoaffective disorder. *Eur Neuropsychopharmacol* 2004; **14**:245–250.
30. Muller MJ, et al. Therapeutic drug monitoring for optimizing amisulpride therapy in patients with schizophrenia. *J Psychiatr Res* 2007; **41**:673–679.
31. Sparshatt A, et al. Amisulpride – dose, plasma concentration, occupancy and response: implications for therapeutic drug monitoring. *Acta Psychiatr Scand* 2009; **120**:416–428.
32. Schoretsanitis G, et al. TDM in psychiatry and neurology: a comprehensive summary of the consensus guidelines for therapeutic drug monitoring in neuropsychopharmacology, update 2017; a tool for clinicians. *World J Biol Psychiatry* 2018; **19**:162–174.
33. Jönsson AK, et al. A compilation of serum concentrations of 12 antipsychotic drugs in a therapeutic drug monitoring setting. *Ther Drug Monit* 2019; **41**:348–356.
34. Reeves S, et al. Therapeutic window of dopamine D2/3 receptor occupancy to treat psychosis in Alzheimer's disease. *Brain* 2017; **140**:1117–1127.
35. Reeves S, et al. Therapeutic D2/3 receptor occupancies and response with low amisulpride blood concentrations in very late-onset schizophrenia-like psychosis (VLOSLP). *Int J Geriatr Psychiatry* 2018; **33**:396–404.
36. Bowskill SV, et al. Plasma amisulpride in relation to prescribed dose, clozapine augmentation, and other factors: data from a therapeutic drug monitoring service, 2002–2010. *Hum Psychopharmacol* 2012; **27**:507–513.
37. Mace S, et al. Aripiprazole: dose-response relationship in schizophrenia and schizoaffective disorder. *CNS Drugs* 2008; **23**:773–780.

CHAPTER 11

38. Sparshatt A, et al. A systematic review of aripiprazole – dose, plasma concentration, receptor occupancy and response: implications for therapeutic drug monitoring. *J Clin Psychiatry* 2010; **71**:1447–1456.

39. Kirschbaum KM, et al. Therapeutic monitoring of aripiprazole by HPLC with column-switching and spectrophotometric detection. *Clin Chem* 2005; **51**:1718–1721.

40. Kirschbaum KM, et al. Serum levels of aripiprazole and dehydroaripiprazole, clinical response and side effects. *World J Biol Psychiatry* 2008; **9**:212–218.

41. Molden E, et al. Pharmacokinetic variability of aripiprazole and the active metabolite dehydroaripiprazole in psychiatric patients. *Ther Drug Monit* 2006; **28**:744–749.

42. Bachmann CJ, et al. Large variability of aripiprazole and dehydroaripiprazole serum concentrations in adolescent patients with schizophrenia. *Ther Drug Monit* 2008; **30**:462–466.

43. Hendset M, et al. Impact of the CYP2D6 genotype on steady-state serum concentrations of aripiprazole and dehydroaripiprazole. *Eur J Clin Pharmacol* 2007; **63**:1147–1151.

44. Mallikaarjun S, et al. Pharmacokinetics, tolerability and safety of aripiprazole once-monthly in adult schizophrenia: an open-label, parallel-arm, multiple-dose study. *Schizophr Res* 2013; **150**:281–288.

45. Korell J, et al. Determination of plasma concentration reference ranges for oral aripiprazole, olanzapine, and quetiapine. *Eur J Clin Pharmacol* 2018; **74**:593–599.

46. Harlin M, et al. Aripiprazole plasma concentrations delivered from two 2-month long-acting injectable formulations: an indirect comparison. *Neuropsychiatr Dis Treat* 2023; **19**:1409–1416.

47. Haring C, et al. Influence of patient-related variables on clozapine plasma levels. *Am J Psychiatry* 1990; **147**:1471–1475.

48. Haring C, et al. Dose-related plasma levels of clozapine: influence of smoking behaviour, sex and age. *Psychopharmacology* 1989; **99** Suppl:S38–S40.

49. Taylor D. Pharmacokinetic interactions involving clozapine. *Br J Psychiatry* 1997; **171**:109–112.

50. Ng CH, et al. An inter-ethnic comparison study of clozapine dosage, clinical response and plasma levels. *Int Clin Psychopharmacol* 2005; **20**:163–168.

51. Ruan CJ, et al. Clozapine metabolism in East Asians and Caucasians: a pilot exploration of the prevalence of poor metabolizers and a systematic review. *J Clin Psychopharmacol* 2019; **39**:135–144.

52. De Leon J, et al. Do Asian patients require only half of the clozapine dose prescribed for Caucasians? A critical overview. *Indian J Psychol Med* 2020; **42**:4–10.

53. Suhas S, et al. Do Indian patients with schizophrenia need half the recommended clozapine dose to achieve therapeutic serum level? An exploratory study. *Schizophr Res* 2020; **222**:195–201.

54. Bhattacharya R, et al. Clozapine prescribing: comparison of clozapine dosage and plasma levels between white British and Bangladeshi patients. *BJPsych Bull* 2021; **45**:22–27.

55. Ruan CJ, et al. Exploring the prevalence of clozapine phenotypic poor metabolizers in 4 Asian samples: they ranged between 2% and 13. *J Clin Psychopharmacol* 2019; **39**:644–648.

56. De Leon J, et al. Using therapeutic drug monitoring to personalize clozapine dosing in Asians. *Asia Pac Psychiatry* 2020; **12**:e12384.

57. Rostami-Hodjegan A, et al. Influence of dose, cigarette smoking, age, sex, and metabolic activity on plasma clozapine concentrations: a predictive model and nomograms to aid clozapine dose adjustment and to assess compliance in individual patients. *J Clin Psychopharmacol* 2004; **24**:70–78.

58. Taylor D, et al. Predicting clozapine dose required to achieve a therapeutic plasma concentration – a comparison of a population algorithm and three algorithms based on gene variant models. *J Psychopharmacol* 2023; **37**:1030–1039.

59. Haack MJ, et al. Toxic rise of clozapine plasma concentrations in relation to inflammation. *Eur Neuropsychopharmacol* 2003; **13**:381–385.

60. De Leon J, et al. Serious respiratory infections can increase clozapine levels and contribute to side effects: a case report. *Prog Neuropsychopharmacol Biol Psychiatry* 2003; **27**:1059–1063.

61. Espnes KA, et al. A puzzling case of increased serum clozapine levels in a patient with inflammation and infection. *Ther Drug Monit* 2012; **34**:489–492.

62. VanderZwaag C, et al. Response of patients with treatment-refractory schizophrenia to clozapine within three serum level ranges. *Am J Psychiatry* 1996; **153**:1579–1584.

63. Perry PJ, et al. Clozapine and norclozapine plasma concentrations and clinical response of treatment refractory schizophrenic patients. *Am J Psychiatry* 1991; **148**:231–235.

64. Miller DD. Effect of phenytoin on plasma clozapine concentrations in two patients. *J Clin Psychiatry* 1991; **52**:23–25.

65. Spina E, et al. Relationship between plasma concentrations of clozapine and norclozapine and therapeutic response in patients with schizophrenia resistant to conventional neuroleptics. *Psychopharmacology* 2000; **148**:83–89.

66. Hasegawa M, et al. Relationship between clinical efficacy and clozapine concentrations in plasma in schizophrenia: effect of smoking. *J Clin Psychopharmacol* 1993; **13**:383–390.

67. Potkin SG, et al. Plasma clozapine concentrations predict clinical response in treatment-resistant schizophrenia. *J Clin Psychiatry* 1994; **55** Suppl B:133–136.

68. Perry PJ. Therapeutic drug monitoring of antipsychotics. *Psychopharmacol Bull* 2001; **35**:19–29.

69. Llorca PM, et al. Effectiveness of clozapine in neuroleptic-resistant schizophrenia: clinical response and plasma concentrations. *J Psychiatry Neurosci* 2002; **27**:30–37.

70. Xiang YQ, et al. Serum concentrations of clozapine and norclozapine in the prediction of relapse of patients with schizophrenia. *Schizophr Res* 2006; **83**:201–210.

71. Stieffenhofer V, et al. Clozapine plasma level monitoring for prediction of rehospitalization schizophrenic outpatients. *Pharmacopsychiatry* 2011; **44**:55–59.

72. Lee J, et al. Quantifying intraindividual variations in plasma clozapine levels: a population pharmacokinetic approach. *J Clin Psychiatry* 2016; **77**:681–687.

73. Turrion MC, et al. Intra-individual variation of clozapine and norclozapine plasma levels in clinical practice. *Rev Psiquiatr Salud Ment* 2020; **13**:31–35.

74. Khan AY, et al. Examining concentration-dependent toxicity of clozapine: role of therapeutic drug monitoring. *J Psychiatr Pract* 2005; **11**:289–301.

75. Varma S, et al. Clozapine-related EEG changes and seizures: dose and plasma-level relationships. *Ther Adv Psychopharmacol* 2011; **1**:47–66.

76. Greenwood-Smith C, et al. Serum clozapine levels: a review of their clinical utility. *J Psychopharmacol* 2003; **17**:234–238.

77. Yusufi B, et al. Prevalence and nature of side effects during clozapine maintenance treatment and the relationship with clozapine dose and plasma concentration. *Int Clin Psychopharmacol* 2007; **22**:238–243.

78. Remington G, et al. Clozapine and therapeutic drug monitoring: is there sufficient evidence for an upper threshold? *Psychopharmacology (Berl)* 2013; **225**:505–518.

79. Bogers J, et al. Feasibility and effect of increasing clozapine plasma levels in long-stay patients with treatment-resistant schizophrenia. *J Clin Psychopharmacol* 2023; **43**:97–105.

80. Northwood K, et al. Optimising plasma clozapine levels to improve treatment response: an individual patient data meta-analysis and receiver operating characteristic curve analysis. *Br J Psychiatry* 2023; **222**:241–245.

81. Couchman L, et al. Plasma clozapine, norclozapine, and the clozapine:norclozapine ratio in relation to prescribed dose and other factors: data from a therapeutic drug monitoring service, 1993–2007. *Ther Drug Monit* 2010; **32**:438–447.

82. Wickramarachchi P, et al. Biological variation in clozapine and metabolite reporting during therapeutic drug monitoring. *Clin Chim Acta* 2022; **531**:183–187.

83. Volpicelli SA, et al. Determination of clozapine, norclozapine, and clozapine-N-oxide in serum by liquid chromatography. *Clin Chem* 1993; **39**:1656–1659.

84. Guitton C, et al. Clozapine and metabolite concentrations during treatment of patients with chronic schizophrenia. *J Clin Pharmacol* 1999; **39**:721–728.

85. Palego L, et al. Clozapine, norclozapine plasma levels, their sum and ratio in 50 psychotic patients: influence of patient-related variables. *Prog Neuropsychopharmacol Biol Psychiatry* 2002; **26**:473–480.

86. Wang CY, et al. The differential effects of steady-state fluvoxamine on the pharmacokinetics of olanzapine and clozapine in healthy volunteers. *J Clin Pharmacol* 2004; **44**:785–792.

87. Schoretsanitis G, et al. A comprehensive review of the clinical utility of and a combined analysis of the clozapine/norclozapine ratio in therapeutic drug monitoring for adult patients. *Expert Rev Clin Pharmacol* 2019; **12**:603–621.

88. Bishara D, et al. Olanzapine: a systematic review and meta-regression of the relationships between dose, plasma concentration, receptor occupancy, and response. *J Clin Psychopharmacol* 2013; **33**:329–335.

89. Aravagiri M, et al. Plasma level monitoring of olanzapine in patients with schizophrenia: determination by high-performance liquid chromatography with electrochemical detection. *Ther Drug Monit* 1997; **19**:307–313.

90. Gex-Fabry M, et al. Therapeutic drug monitoring of olanzapine: the combined effect of age, gender, smoking, and comedication. *Ther Drug Monit* 2003; **25**:46–53.

91. Bergemann N, et al. Olanzapine plasma concentration, average daily dose, and interaction with co-medication in schizophrenic patients. *Pharmacopsychiatry* 2004; **37**:63–68.

92. Perry PJ, et al. Olanzapine plasma concentrations and clinical response in acutely ill schizophrenic patients. *J Clin Psychopharmacol* 1997; **17**:472–477.

93. Fellows L, et al. Investigation of target plasma concentration–effect relationships for olanzapine in schizophrenia. *Ther Drug Monit* 2003; **25**:682–689.

94. Mauri MC, et al. Clinical outcome and olanzapine plasma levels in acute schizophrenia. *Eur Psychiatry* 2005; **20**:55–60.

95. Rao ML, et al. Olanzapine: pharmacology, pharmacokinetics and therapeutic drug monitoring. *Fortschr Neurol Psychiatr* 2001; **69**:510–517.

96. Robertson MD, et al. Olanzapine concentrations in clinical serum and postmortem blood specimens – when does therapeutic become toxic? *J Forensic Sci* 2000; **45**:418–421.

97. Bech P, et al. Olanzapine plasma level in relation to antimanic effect in the acute therapy of manic states. *Nord J Psychiatry* 2006; **60**:181–182.

98. Schoretsanitis G, et al. Blood levels to optimize antipsychotic treatment in clinical practice: a joint consensus statement of the American Society of Clinical Psychopharmacology and the Therapeutic Drug Monitoring Task Force of the Arbeitsgemeinschaft für Neuropsychopharmakologie und Pharmakopsychiatrie. *J Clin Psychiatry* 2020; **81**:19cs13169.

99. Noel C. A review of a recently published guidelines' 'strong recommendation' for therapeutic drug monitoring of olanzapine, haloperidol, perphenazine, and fluphenazine. *Ment Health Clin* 2019; **9**:287–293.

100. Wesner K, et al. Therapeutic reference range for olanzapine in schizophrenia: systematic review on blood concentrations, clinical effects, and dopamine receptor occupancy. *J Clin Psychiatry* 2023; **84**:22r14626.

101. Perry PJ, et al. The association of weight gain and olanzapine plasma concentrations. *J Clin Psychopharmacol* 2005; **25**:250–254.

102. Kelly DL, et al. Plasma concentrations of high-dose olanzapine in a double-blind crossover study. *Hum Psychopharmacol* 2006; **21**:393–398.

103. Patel MX, et al. Plasma olanzapine in relation to prescribed dose and other factors: data from a therapeutic drug monitoring service, 1999–2009. *J Clin Psychopharmacol* 2011; **31**:411–417.

104. Tsuboi T, et al. Predicting plasma olanzapine concentration following a change in dosage: a population pharmacokinetic study. *Pharmacopsychiatry* 2015; **48**:286–291.

105. Sparshatt A, et al. Relationship between daily dose, plasma concentrations, dopamine receptor occupancy, and clinical response to quetiapine: a review. *J Clin Psychiatry* 2011; **72**:1108–1123.

106. Hasselstrom J, et al. Quetiapine serum concentrations in psychiatric patients: the influence of comedication. *Ther Drug Monit* 2004; **26**:486–491.

107. Winter HR, et al. Steady-state pharmacokinetic, safety, and tolerability profiles of quetiapine, norquetiapine, and other quetiapine metabolites in pediatric and adult patients with psychotic disorders. *J Child Adolesc Psychopharmacol* 2008; **18**:81–98.

108. Li KY, et al. Multiple dose pharmacokinetics of quetiapine and some of its metabolites in Chinese suffering from schizophrenia. *Acta Pharmacol Sin* 2004; **25**:390–394.

109. McConville BJ, et al. Pharmacokinetics, tolerability, and clinical effectiveness of quetiapine fumarate: an open-label trial in adolescents with psychotic disorders. *J Clin Psychiatry* 2000; **61**:252–260.

110. Castberg I, et al. Quetiapine and drug interactions: evidence from a routine therapeutic drug monitoring service. *J Clin Psychiatry* 2007; **68**:1540–1545.

111. Aichhorn W, et al. Influence of age, gender, body weight and valproate comedication on quetiapine plasma concentrations. *Int Clin Psychopharmacol* 2006; **21**:81–85.

112. Mauri MC, et al. Two weeks' quetiapine treatment for schizophrenia, drug-induced psychosis and borderline personality disorder: a naturalistic study with drug plasma levels. *Expert Opin Pharmacother* 2007; **8**:2207–2213.

113. Patteet L, et al. Therapeutic drug monitoring of common antipsychotics. *Ther Drug Monit* 2012; **34**:629–651.

114. Fisher DS, et al. Plasma concentrations of quetiapine, N-desalkylquetiapine, o-desalkylquetiapine, 7-hydroxyquetiapine, and quetiapine sulfoxide in relation to quetiapine dose, formulation, and other factors. *Ther Drug Monit* 2012; **34**:415–421.

115. Sparshatt A, et al. Quetiapine: dose-response relationship in schizophrenia. *CNS Drugs* 2008; **22**:49–68.

116. Olesen OV, et al. Serum concentrations and side effects in psychiatric patients during risperidone therapy. *Ther Drug Monit* 1998; **20**:380–384.

117. Remington G, et al. A PET study evaluating dopamine D2 receptor occupancy for long-acting injectable risperidone. *Am J Psychiatry* 2006; **163**:396–401.

118. Seto K, et al. Risperidone in schizophrenia: is there a role for therapeutic drug monitoring? *Ther Drug Monit* 2011; **33**:275–283.

119. Lane HY, et al. Risperidone in acutely exacerbated schizophrenia: dosing strategies and plasma levels. *J Clin Psychiatry* 2000; **61**:209–214.

120. Taylor D. Risperidone long-acting injection in practice – more questions than answers? *Acta Psychiatr Scand* 2006; **114**:1–2.

121. Nyberg S, et al. Suggested minimal effective dose of risperidone based on PET-measured D2 and 5-HT2A receptor occupancy in schizophrenic patients. *Am J Psychiatry* 1999; **156**:869–875.

122. Uchida H, et al. Predicting dopamine D receptor occupancy from plasma levels of antipsychotic drugs: a systematic review and pooled analysis. *J Clin Psychopharmacol* 2011; **31**:318–325.

123. Pandina GJ, et al. A randomized, placebo-controlled study to assess the efficacy and safety of 3 doses of paliperidone palmitate in adults with acutely exacerbated schizophrenia. *J Clin Psychopharmacol* 2010; **30**:235–244.

124. Mauri MC, et al. Paliperidone long-acting plasma level monitoring and a new method of evaluation of clinical stability. *Pharmacopsychiatry* 2017; **50**:145–151.

125. Paletta S, et al. Two years of maintenance therapy with paliperidone long-acting in schizophrenia and schizoaffective disorder: a study with plasma levels. *Eur Neuropsychopharmacol* 2016; **26**:S556–S557.

126. Berwaerts J, et al. Efficacy and safety of the 3-month formulation of paliperidone palmitate vs placebo for relapse prevention of schizophrenia: a randomized clinical trial. *JAMA Psychiatry* 2015; **72**:830–839.

127. Magnusson MO, et al. Dosing and switching strategies for paliperidone palmitate 3-month formulation in patients with schizophrenia based on population pharmacokinetic modeling and simulation, and clinical trial data. *CNS Drugs* 2017; **31**:273–288.

128. T'Jollyn H, et al. Model-informed clinical development of once-every-6-month injection of paliperidone palmitate in patients with schizophrenia: a pharmacometric bridging approach (Part I). *Eur J Drug Metab Pharmacokinet* 2024; **49**:477–489.

129. Álamo C. Risperidone ISM as a new option in the clinical management of schizophrenia: a narrative review. *Adv Ther* 2022; **39**:4875–4891.

130. Biso L, et al. Therapeutic drug monitoring in psychiatry: enhancing treatment precision and patient outcomes. *Pharmaceuticals (Basel)* 2024; **17**:642.

Interpreting postmortem blood concentrations

Much is known about the distribution of drugs in the body during life but relatively little about these same parameters after death. A great many drugs are subject to post-mortem distribution changes but, for obvious practical reasons, research into the mechanisms and extent of these effects is very limited. The best that can be said is that a drug *plasma* concentration measured during life may be very different from the concentration measured at some time after death (usually in *whole blood* from the femoral artery).

A number of processes are responsible for these changes. In life, active mechanisms serve to concentrate some drugs in certain organs or tissues. After death, passive diffusion occurs as cell membranes break down and this will mean that postmortem blood samples will, for some drugs, show higher concentrations than were seen during life. This is known as postmortem redistribution (PMR). In addition, central blood vessels surrounding major organs often demonstrate much higher drug concentrations than relatively distant peripheral samples.[1] PMR and other processes are temperature- and time-dependent so time since death and conditions of storage are important determinants of blood concentration changes.[2] PMR tends to be greater with drugs with a large volume of distribution (i.e. those for which tissue concentrations in life vastly exceed blood concentrations) especially when given over a long period during life.

Other processes of importance[3] include the postmortem synthesis of certain compounds. For example, the body is able to generate gamma-hydroxybutyrate. Trauma may allow the introduction of yeasts that metabolise glucose to alcohol. Another phenomenon is the degradation of drugs by bacteria (e.g. clonazepam and nitrazepam) or fungi. Also, the metabolism of some drugs (cocaine, for example) appears to continue after death (although this may be simple chemical instability of the parent compound).

All of the processes described here contribute to an overall direction of change of concentration postmortem. Antidepressant concentrations tend to increase in postmortem samples whereas those of benzodiazepines invariably decrease.[4] Mirtazapine concentrations also appear to decrease.[5,6] Antipsychotic concentrations both increase and decrease depending on the drug.[4] Thus, when an isolated postmortem concentration is considered (i.e. one which cannot be compared with a concentration measured in life), it can only be said that the in-life concentration would have been higher or lower.[7]

Table 11.3 lists some of the factors relevant to drug concentration changes after death and the possible consequences of these processes. Generally speaking, an isolated postmortem blood concentration cannot be sensibly interpreted. Even where in-life levels are available, for most drugs in most circumstances, interpretation of blood levels after death is near impossible. High postmortem concentrations should certainly not be taken, in the absence of other evidence, to indicate death by overdose, for example. Two valuable reference sources for interpretation of postmortem sample analysis are the systematic reviews of Ketola and Kriikku[8] and Ketola and Ojanperä.[9] Expert advice should always be sought when considering the role of medication in a death.[10]

Table 11.3 Factors affecting postmortem blood concentrations.

Factor	Examples	Consequences
Redistribution of drug from tissues to blood compartment	Most drugs with large volume of distribution, e.g. clozapine,[11,12] olanzapine,[13] methadone,[14] SSRIs,[15] TCAs, mirtazapine,[16] lithium[17] May not occur to any significant effect with risperidone,[4,18] aripiprazole[19] or quetiapine[4,19]	Postmortem levels up to 10× higher than in-life levels, sometimes higher still[9]
Uneven distribution of drugs in the blood compartment and in organs (i.e. site of blood collection affects concentration)	Most drugs,[8,20] e.g. clozapine, TCAs, SSRIs, duloxetine,[21] benzodiazepines, quetiapine[22]	Concentrations may vary several-fold according to site of collection at postmortem, e.g. femoral blood vs heart blood
Decay of drugs in postmortem tissue (usually by bacterial degradation)	Not widely studied but known to occur with olanzapine, risperidone[23] and some benzodiazepines. Fungi can metabolise amitriptyline, mirtazapine and zolpidem.[24,25]	Postmortem levels may be lower than in-life levels
Postmortem metabolism/ degradation	Cocaine metabolised/degraded postmortem. Many other drugs are unstable in postmortem samples. Yeasts may produce ethanol following trauma.[3]	Postmortem levels may be lower (cocaine) or higher (alcohol) than in-life levels

TCAs, tricyclic antidepressants.

References

1. Ferner RE. Post-mortem clinical pharmacology. *Br J Clin Pharmacol* 2008; **66**:430–443.
2. Flanagan RJ, et al. Analytical toxicology: guidelines for sample collection postmortem. *Toxicol Rev* 2005; **24**:63–71.
3. Kennedy MC. Post-mortem drug concentrations. *Intern Med J* 2010; **40**:183–187.
4. Mantinieks D, et al. Postmortem drug redistribution: a compilation of postmortem/antemortem drug concentration ratios. *J Anal Toxicol* 2021; **45**:368–377.
5. Brockbals L, et al. Time- and site-dependent postmortem redistribution of antidepressants and neuroleptics in blood and alternative matrices. *J Anal Toxicol* 2021; **45**:356–367.
6. Brockbals L, et al. Postmortem metabolomics: strategies to assess time-dependent postmortem changes of diazepam, nordiazepam, morphine, codeine, mirtazapine and citalopram. *Metabolites* 2021; **11**:643.
7. Maskell PD. Just say no to postmortem drug dose calculations. *J Forensic Sci* 2021; **66**:1862–1870.
8. Ketola RA, et al. Drug concentrations in post-mortem specimens. *Drug Test Anal* 2019; **11**:1338–1357.
9. Ketola RA, et al. Summary statistics for drug concentrations in post-mortem femoral blood representing all causes of death. *Drug Test Anal* 2019; **11**:1326–1337.
10. Flanagan RJ. Poisoning: fact or fiction? *Med Leg J* 2012; **80**:127–148.
11. Flanagan RJ, et al. Effect of post-mortem changes on peripheral and central whole blood and tissue clozapine and norclozapine concentrations in the domestic pig (Sus scrofa). *Forensic Sci Int* 2003; **132**:9–17.
12. Flanagan RJ, et al. Suspected clozapine poisoning in the UK/Eire, 1992–2003. *Forensic Sci Int* 2005; **155**:91–99.
13. Saar E, et al. The time-dependant post-mortem redistribution of antipsychotic drugs. *Forensic Sci Int* 2012; **222**:223–227.
14. Caplehorn JR, et al. Methadone dose and post-mortem blood concentration. *Drug Alcohol Rev* 2002; **21**:329–333.
15. Lewis RJ, et al. Paroxetine in postmortem fluids and tissues from nine aviation accident victims. *J Anal Toxicol* 2015; **39**:637–641.
16. Launiainen T, et al. Drug concentrations in post-mortem femoral blood compared with therapeutic concentrations in plasma. *Drug Test Anal* 2014; **6**:308–316.
17. Soderberg C, et al. Reference values of lithium in postmortem femoral blood. *Forensic Sci Int* 2017; **277**:207–214.
18. Linnet K, et al. Postmortem femoral blood concentrations of risperidone. *J Anal Toxicol* 2014; **38**:57–60.
19. Skov L, et al. Postmortem femoral blood reference concentrations of aripiprazole, chlorprothixene, and quetiapine. *J Anal Toxicol* 2015; **39**:41–44.
20. Rodda KE, et al. The redistribution of selected psychiatric drugs in post-mortem cases. *Forensic Sci Int* 2006; **164**:235–239.
21. Scanlon KA, et al. Comprehensive duloxetine analysis in a fatal overdose. *J Anal Toxicol* 2016; **40**:167–170.
22. Breivik H, et al. Post mortem tissue distribution of quetiapine in forensic autopsies. *Forensic Sci Int* 2020; **315**:110413.
23. Butzbach DM, et al. Bacterial degradation of risperidone and paliperidone in decomposing blood. *J Forensic Sci* 2013; **58**:90–100.
24. Martinez-Ramirez JA, et al. Search for fungi-specific metabolites of four model drugs in postmortem blood as potential indicators of postmortem fungal metabolism. *Forensic Sci Int* 2016; **262**:173–178.
25. Martinez-Ramirez JA, et al. Studies on drug metabolism by fungi colonizing decomposing human cadavers. Part II: biotransformation of five model drugs by fungi isolated from post-mortem material. *Drug Test Anal* 2015; **7**:265–279.

Acting on clozapine plasma concentration results

In most developed countries, clozapine blood concentration monitoring is widely used. Table 11.4 gives some general advice about actions that should be taken when clozapine levels are within a certain range. The ranges shown are somewhat arbitrary and convenient – the concentration at which a particular patient might respond cannot be known without a trial of clozapine. Most adverse effects are linearly or exponentially related to dose or plasma level. That is, there is no step-change in the risk of seizures, for example, at a particular dose or plasma concentration.[1] The same is broadly true of therapeutic effects. The likelihood of response in an individual increases from concentrations below the accepted therapeutic range up to around 1000mcg/L.[2-4] Table 11.4 should be considered more an aid to decision-making rather than a rigorous, unbending evidence-based instruction. Note also the effect of tolerance to adverse effects – many patients have a significant adverse effect burden before therapeutic concentrations are reached,[5] reducing over time as tolerance develops.

Table 11.4 Recommended actions in response to clozapine concentrations.*

Plasma concentration	Response status	Tolerability status	Suggested action
<350mcg/L	Poor	Poor	Increase dose very slowly to give level of 350mcg/L
	Poor	Good	Increase dose to give level of 350mcg/L
	Good	Poor	Maintain dose. Consider cautious dose reduction if tolerability does not improve.
	Good	Good	Continue to monitor. No action required.
350–500mcg/L	Poor	Poor	Increase dose slowly, according to tolerability, to give level of >500mcg/L. Consider prophylactic anticonvulsant.[†] If no improvement, consider augmentation.
	Poor	Good	Increase dose slowly, according to tolerability, to give level of >500mcg/L (up to 1000mcg/mL if tolerated). Consider prophylactic anticonvulsant.[†] If no improvement, consider augmentation.
	Good	Poor	Maintain dose to see if tolerability improves. Consider cautious dose reduction to give plasma level of around 350mcg/L.
	Good	Good	Continue to monitor. No action required.
500–1000mcg/L	Poor	Poor	Consider use of prophylactic antiseizure drug.[†] Consider augmentation. Attempt dose reduction if augmentation successful.
	Poor	Good	Consider use of prophylactic antiseizure drug.[†] Slowly increase dose (up towards 1000mcg/mL if tolerated). Also consider augmentation.
	Good	Poor	Attempt slow dose reduction to give plasma level of 350–500mcg/L unless there is known non-response at lower level. If this is the case, maintain dose and consider adding anticonvulsant.[†] Optimise treatment of adverse effects.
	Good	Good	Consider use of prophylactic antiseizure drug.[†] Maintain dose if good tolerability continues.

(Continued)

CHAPTER 11

Table 11.4 *(Continued)*

Plasma concentration	Response status	Tolerability status	Suggested action
>1000mcg/L	Poor	Poor	Add antiseizure drug. Attempt augmentation. Reduce dose to give level of <1000mcg/L. Consider abandoning clozapine treatment.
	Poor	Good	Add antiseizure drug. Attempt augmentation. If augmentation successful, reduce dose to give level <1000mcg/L. If unsuccessful, consider abandoning clozapine treatment.
	Good	Poor	Add antiseizure drug. Attempt slow dose reduction to give plasma level <1000mcg/L.
	Good	Good	Add antiseizure drug. Monitor closely; attempt dose reduction only if tolerability declines.

Notes

Poor response No response or unsatisfactory response to clozapine. For example, not sufficiently well to be discharged.

Good response Obvious positive changes related to use of clozapine. Patient likely to be suitable for discharge to either supported or unsupported care in the community.

Poor tolerability Dose constrained by adverse effects such as tachycardia, sedation, hypersalivation, hypotension, etc. (see Chapter 1 for suggestions of treatment for adverse effects).

Good tolerability Patient tolerates treatment well and there are no signs of serious toxicity.

Augmentation Adding another antipsychotic or mood stabiliser (see Chapter 1).

In all situations, ensure adequate treatment for clozapine-induced constipation. Constipation is dose-related. Ensure regular bowel movements and record bowel function. Stimulant laxatives such as senna are required (see Chapter 1).

Seizures are dose- and plasma level-dependent. Suitable antiseizure agents are valproate, lamotrigine and, rarely, topiramate. Use lamotrigine if response is poor; valproate if affective symptoms are present (see Chapter 2). Note that use of valproate increases risk of neutropenia with clozapine.[6] Both valproate and topiramate are contraindicated in women of child-bearing age.

*This table applies to results for patients on a stable clozapine dose with confirmed good adherence.
†Antiseizure drugs should usually be used in patients whose plasma level exceeds 600mcg/L, unless EEG is normal, and in those with lower plasma levels who experience clozapine-induced seizures.

References

1. Varma S, et al. Clozapine-related EEG changes and seizures: dose and plasma-level relationships. *Ther Adv Psychopharmacol* 2011; 1:47–66.
2. Northwood K, et al. Optimising plasma clozapine levels to improve treatment response: an individual patient data meta-analysis and receiver operating characteristic curve analysis. *Br J Psychiatry* 2023; 222:241–245.
3. Tralongo F, et al. Association between clozapine plasma concentrations and treatment response: a systematic review, meta-analysis and individual participant data meta-analysis. *Clin Pharmacokinet* 2023; 62:807–818.
4. Bogers J, et al. Feasibility and effect of increasing clozapine plasma levels in long-stay patients with treatment-resistant schizophrenia. *J Clin Psychopharmacol* 2023; 43:97–105.
5. Yusufi B, et al. Prevalence and nature of side effects during clozapine maintenance treatment and the relationship with clozapine dose and plasma concentration. *Int Clin Psychopharmacol* 2007; 22:238–243.
6. Malik S, et al. Sodium valproate and clozapine induced neutropenia: a case control study using register data. *Schizophr Res* 2018; 195:267–273.

CHAPTER 11

Psychotropic drugs and cytochrome (CYP) function

Information on the effect of drugs on CYP function helps predict or confirm suspected interactions that may not have been uncovered in regulatory trials or in clinical use.

In addition to the effect of co-administered drugs on CYP function, genetic polymorphism associated with some enzymes may also account for inter-individual variations in the metabolism of certain drugs. Genetic variation influences both likelihood of response and tolerability (see later in this section for more information on genetic variation).[1,2]

The effects of polymorphism and pharmacokinetic interaction are difficult to predict because some drugs are metabolised by more than one enzyme and an alternative pathway(s) may compensate if other enzyme pathways are inhibited. A further complication is that CYPs are active in sites other than the liver (e.g. gut, brain). The effect of psychotropics on brain CYPs can be markedly different from hepatic CYPs.[3]

The function of CYPs is not the only consideration. P-glycoprotein (P-gp) is a drug transporter protein found in the gut wall. P-gp can eject (active process) drugs that diffuse (passive process) across the gut wall. P-gp is also found in testes and in the blood–brain barrier. Drugs that inhibit P-gp are anticipated to increase the uptake of other drugs (that are substrates for P-gp), and drugs that induce P-gp are anticipated to reduce the uptake of other drugs (that are substrates for P-gp). Many drugs that are substrates for CYP3A4 have also been found to be substrates for P-gp.

Uridine diphosphate (UDP)-glucuronosyltransferase (UGT) has been identified as an enzyme that is responsible for phase II (conjugation) reactions. Valproate is a potent inhibitor of UGT, hence its interaction with lamotrigine, a drug which is primarily metabolised by UGT. UGT enzymes are also involved in the metabolism of lumateperone, olanzapine, topiramate and trifluoperazine.

In Table 11.5, drugs highlighted in **bold** indicate:

- Predominant metabolic enzyme pathway, or
- Predominant enzyme activity (inhibition or induction).

Drugs annotated with * are known to be a minor metabolic enzyme pathway or activity (i.e. not demonstrated to be clinically significant). Drugs in normal font (not bold and without *) indicate metabolic enzyme pathway(s) or activity where significance is unclear or unknown.

Table 11.5 does not include details of the effects of non-psychotropics on CYP function.

Table 11.5 Effects of psychotropics on CYP function.

CYP1A2

Substrates	Inhibitors	Inducers
Agomelatine	**Asenapine**[4]	**'Barbiturates'**
Amitriptyline*	**Fluvoxamine**	**Carbamazepine**
Bupropion*	Iloperidone	Modafinil*
Caffeine	Levomepromazine	**Phenobarbital**
Chlorpromazine	Melatonin[5]	Phenytoin
Clomipramine*	Moclobemide	
Clozapine	Perphenazine	
Duloxetine		
Fluphenazine		
Fluvoxamine		
Haloperidol		
Imipramine*		
Levomepromazine		
Lumateperone		
Melatonin		
Mirtazapine*		
Olanzapine		
Perphenazine		
Pimozide*		
Ramelteon		
Zolpidem*		

CYP2A6

Substrates	Inhibitors	Inducers
Bupropion*	Tranylcypromine	Phenobarbital
Caffeine		
Nicotine		

CYP2B6

Substrates	Inhibitors	Inducers
Bupropion	Fluoxetine*	Carbamazepine*
Methadone*	Fluvoxamine	Modafinil*
Nicotine	Memantine	Phenobarbital
Sertraline*	Paroxetine*	Phenytoin
	Sertraline*	

CYP2B7

Substrates	Inhibitors	Inducers
Buprenorphine*	Not known	Not known

Table 11.5 (*Continued*)

CYP2C8

Substrates	Inhibitors	Inducers
Lumateperone Zopiclone*	Not known	Not known

CYP2C9

Substrates	Inhibitors	Inducers
Agomelatine* Amitriptyline Bupropion* Doxepin Fluoxetine* **Lamotrigine** Phenobarbital Phenytoin Sertraline* **Valproate**	Fluoxetine* Fluvoxamine Modafinil Valproate	Carbamazepine SJW

CYP2C19

Substrates	Inhibitors	Inducers
Agomelatine* Amitriptyline Atomoxetine Carbamazepine* Citalopram Clomipramine* Diazepam **Escitalopram** Fluoxetine* Imipramine* Melatonin Methadone Moclobemide Phenytoin Sertraline* Suvorexant Trimipramine* Valproate	Escitalopram* **Fluoxetine** Fluvoxamine Iloperidone Melatonin[5] Moclobemide Modafinil Topiramate	Carbamazepine SJW

(*Continued*)

Table 11.5 (*Continued*)

CYP2D6

Substrates	Inhibitors	Inducers
'Amfetamines'	Amitriptyline	Not known
Amitriptyline	Asenapine⁴	
Aripiprazole	Bupropion	
Atomoxetine	Chlorpromazine	
Brexpiprazole	Citalopram*	
Cariprazine	Clomipramine	
Chlorpromazine	Clozapine	
Citalopram	Doxepin	
Clomipramine	Duloxetine	
Clozapine*	Escitalopram	
Deutetrabenazine	Fluoxetine	
Donepezil*	Fluphenazine	
Doxepin	Fluvoxamine*	
Duloxetine	Haloperidol	
Escitalopram	Iloperidone	
Fluoxetine	Levomepromazine	
Fluphenazine	Methadone*	
Fluvoxamine	Moclobemide	
Galantamine	Paroxetine	
Haloperidol	Perphenazine	
Iloperidone	Reboxetine*	
Imipramine	Risperidone	
Methadone*	Sertraline*	
Mianserin	Venlafaxine*	
Mirtazapine*	Ziprasidone*	
Moclobemide		
Nortriptyline		
Olanzapine		
Paroxetine		
Perphenazine		
Pimavanserin		
Pimozide*		
Quetiapine*		
Risperidone		
Sertindole		
Sertraline		
Trazodone*		
Trimipramine		
Valbenazine		
Venlafaxine		
Vortioxetine		
Zuclopenthixol		

CYP2E1

Substrates	Inhibitors	Inducers
Bupropion	Disulfiram	Ethanol
Ethanol	Paracetamol	

Table 11.5 (*Continued*)

CYP3A4

Substrates	Inhibitors	Inducers
Alfentanyl	Atomoxetine*	**Asenapine?**
Alprazolam	**Fluoxetine**	**Carbamazepine**
Amitriptyline	Fluvoxamine	Clozapine[6]
Aripiprazole	Iloperidone	Levomepromazine[6]
Blonaserin	Levomepromazine	**Modafinil**
Brexipiprazole	**Paroxetine**	**Phenobarbital**
Buprenorphine	Perphenazine	'and probably
Bupropion*	Reboxetine*	other barbituates'
Buspirone	Ziprasidone*	**Phenytoin**
Carbamazepine		**SJW**
Cariprazine		Topiramate
Chlorpromazine		
Citalopram		
Clomipramine*		
Clonazepam		
Clozapine*		
Diazepam		
Donepezil		
Dosulepin		
Escitalopram*		
Fentanyl		
Fluoxetine*		
?**Flurazepam**		
Galantamine		
Haloperidol		
Imipramine		
Lemborexant		
Levomepromazine		
Lumateperone		
Lurasidone		
Methadone		
Midazolam		
Mirtazapine		
Modafinil		
Nitrazepam		
Paliperidone		
Perphenazine		
Pimavanserin		
Pimozide		
Quetiapine		
Reboxetine		
Risperidone*		
Sertindole		
Sertraline*		
Suvorexant		
Trazodone		
Trimipramine*		
Valbenazine		
Venlafaxine		
Vilazodone		
Zaleplon		
Ziprasidone		
Zolpidem		
Zopiclone		
Zuclopenthixol		

Note: information on CYP function is derived from individual SPCs and US labelling (accessed August 2024), from systematic reviews[7,8] and the Flockhart table.[9]

SJW, St John's wort; SPC, summary of product characteristics.

Genetics of cytochrome function

The function of CYPs is under genetic control. Each individual's CYP function is determined by heredity and is often, but not always, linked to ethnicity. Phenotypes are usually described as poor metabolisers, intermediate metabolisers, normal metabolisers and rapid or ultrarapid metabolisers. Table 11.6 gives the approximate distribution of phenotypes across nine ethnicities. Awareness of differences in phenotype frequencies can help predict and understand drug metabolism differences. As an example, CYP1A2 ultrarapid metaboliser phenotypes are most often seen in African Americans and so we might expect a higher rate of clozapine failure (or at least low plasma levels) in this population.

Table 11.6 Estimated phenotype frequency by ancestry for CYP1A2, CYP2D6, CYP2C19, CYP2C9 and CYP3A4.[10-22]

Genotype-predicted phenotypes	African[10,11]	African American[12,13]	European ancestry + North American[14]	Near Eastern	East Asian	South/Central Asian	Americas	Latino[15]	Oceanian
CYP1A2									
Ultrarapid metaboliser	10–20%	15–30%	1–4%	5–10%	1–5%	3–8%	5–10%	7–12%	5–10%
Normal metaboliser	55–70%	50–60%	70–80%	65–75%	65–75%	60–70%	60–70%	65–75%	65–75%
Intermediate metaboliser	10–20%	10–15%	10–15%	10–15%	10–20%	10–15%	10–15%	10–15%	10–15%
Poor metaboliser	5–10%	5–10%	5–10%	5–10%	10–15%	10–15%	5–10%	5–10%	5–10%
CYP2D6									
Ultrarapid metaboliser	4%	5%	3%	10%	1%	2%	6%	4%	20%
Normal metaboliser	43%	56%	51%	55%	52%	62%	64%	59%	67%
Intermediate metaboliser	44%	36%	39%	30%	39%	30%	24%	29%	10%
Poor metaboliser	2%	2%	7%	2%	1%	2%	2%	3%	0%
CYP2C19									
Ultrarapid metaboliser	3%	4%	5%	4%	0%	3%	1%	3%	0%
Rapid metaboliser	19%	24%	27%	26%	3%	19%	14%	24%	2%
Normal metaboliser	30%	33%	40%	45%	38%	30%	63%	53%	4%
Intermediate metaboliser	36%	31%	26%	24%	46%	41%	21%	19%	37%
Likely intermediate metaboliser	4%	3%	0%	0%	0%	0%	0%	0%	0%
Poor metaboliser	6%	4%	2%	2%	13%	8%	2%	1%	57%
Likely poor metaboliser	1%	1%	0%	0%	0%	0%	0%	0%	0%
CYP2C9									
Normal metaboliser	73%	76%	63%	61%	84%	60%	83%	75%	91%

(Continued)

Table 11.6 (*Continued*)

Genotype-predicted phenotypes	African[10,11]	African American[12,13]	European ancestry + North American[14]	Near Eastern	East Asian	South/Central Asian	Americas	Latino[15]	Oceanian
Intermediate metaboliser	26%	24%	35%	36%	15%	36%	16%	25%	9%
Poor metaboliser	1%	1%	3%	3%	1%	4%	0%	1%	0%
CYP3A4									
Ultrarapid metaboliser	7–15%	10–15%	1–5%	5–10%	1–4%	2–6%	4–9%	3–8%	4–10%
Normal metaboliser	50–65%	55–70%	65–75%	60–70%	60–75%	60–70%	55–65%	60–70%	60–70%
Intermediate metaboliser	15–25%	10–20%	15–20%	15–20%	15–25%	15–20%	15–20%	15–20%	15–20%
Poor metaboliser	5–10%	5–10%	5–10%	5–10%	5–10%	5–10%	5–10%	5–10%	5–10%

References

1. Baldacci A, et al. Pharmacogenetic guidelines for psychotropic drugs: optimizing prescriptions in clinical practice. *Pharmaceutics* 2023; **15**:2540.
2. Cojocaru A, et al. The implications of cytochrome P450 2D6/CYP2D6 polymorphism in the therapeutic response of atypical antipsychotics in adolescents with psychosis – a prospective study. *Biomedicines* 2024; **12**:494.
3. Daniel WA, et al. The mechanisms of interactions of psychotropic drugs with liver and brain cytochrome P450 and their significance for drug effect and drug-drug interactions. *Biochem Pharmacol* 2022; **199**:115006.
4. Wójcikowski J, et al. In vitro inhibition of human cytochrome P450 enzymes by the novel atypical antipsychotic drug asenapine: a prediction of possible drug-drug interactions. *Pharmacol Rep* 2020; **72**:612–621.
5. Matura JM, et al. Dietary supplements, cytochrome metabolism, and pharmacogenetic considerations. *Ir J Med Sci* 2022; **191**:2357–2365.
6. Danek PJ, et al. Levomepromazine and clozapine induce the main human cytochrome P450 drug metabolizing enzyme CYP3A4. *Pharmacol Rep* 2021; **73**:303–308.
7. Hart XM, et al. Optimisation of pharmacotherapy in psychiatry through therapeutic drug monitoring, molecular brain imaging and pharmacogenetic tests: focus on antipsychotics. *World J Biol Psychiatry* 2024:1–123.
8. Schoretsanitis G, et al. TDM in psychiatry and neurology: a comprehensive summary of the consensus guidelines for therapeutic drug monitoring in neuropsychopharmacology, update 2017; a tool for clinicians. *World J Biol Psychiatry* 2018; **19**:162–174.
9. Indiana University School of Medicine. Drug Interactions Flockhart Table™ 2024 (last accessed August 2024); https://drug-interactions.medicine.iu.edu/MainTable.aspx.
10. Masimirembwa CM, et al. Genetic polymorphism of drug metabolising enzymes in African populations: implications for the use of neuroleptics and antidepressants. *Brain Res Bull* 1997; **44**:561–571.
11. Aklillu E, et al. Genetic polymorphism of CYP1A2 in Ethiopians affecting induction and expression: characterization of novel haplotypes with single-nucleotide polymorphisms in intron 1. *Mol Pharmacol* 2003; **64**:659.
12. Muscat JE, et al. Comparison of CYP1A2 and NAT2 phenotypes between black and white smokers. *Biochem Pharmacol* 2008; **76**:929–937.
13. Wrighton SA, et al. The human hepatic cytochromes P450 involved in drug metabolism. *Crit Rev Toxicol* 1992; **22**:1–21.
14. Rasmussen BB, et al. The interindividual differences in the 3-demthylation of caffeine alias CYP1A2 is determined by both genetic and environmental factors. *Pharmacogenetics* 2002; **12**:473–478.
15. Ingelman-Sundberg M, et al. Influence of cytochrome P450 polymorphisms on drug therapies: pharmacogenetic, pharmacoepigenetic and clinical aspects. *Pharmacol Ther* 2007; **116**:496–526.
16. Stanford University. PharmGKB. 2024 (last accessed August 2024); https://www.pharmgkb.org.
17. Zhou SF, et al. Insights into the substrate specificity, inhibitors, regulation, and polymorphisms and the clinical impact of human cytochrome P450 1A2. *AAPS J* 2009; **11**:481–494.
18. Myriad Genetics. Genesight. 2024 (last accessed August 2024); https://www.genesight.com.
19. Enoch MA, et al. Using ancestry-informative markers to define populations and detect population stratification. *J Psychopharmacol* 2006; **20**:19–26.
20. Genetic Lifehacks. 2024 (last accessed August 2024); https://www.geneticlifehacks.com.
21. Guttman Y, et al. Polymorphism in cytochrome P450 3A4 is ethnicity related. *Front Genet* 2019; **10**:224.
22. Darney K, et al. Inter-ethnic differences in CYP3A4 metabolism: a Bayesian meta-analysis for the refinement of uncertainty factors in chemical risk assessment. *Computational Toxicol* 2019; **12**:100092.

Smoking and psychotropic drugs

Tobacco smoke contains polycyclic aromatic hydrocarbons that induce certain hepatic enzymes (CYP1A2 in particular).[1] Other enzymes that may be induced by smoking are CYP2C19 and, possibly, CYP3A4 and some variants of UGT (glycosyltrans-ferases).[2] The extent of enzyme induction is determined by the number and type of cigarettes smoked and by the degree of smoke inhalation.[3] For some drugs used in psychiatry, smoking significantly reduces drug plasma levels and higher doses are required than in non-smokers. Smoking may also affect alcohol metabolism by inducing CYP2E1.[3]

When people stop smoking, enzyme activity halves roughly every 2 days.[4] It is very important to appreciate that nicotine replacement and vaping have no effect on this process (they do not contain polycyclic aromatic hydrocarbons). Plasma levels of affected drugs will then rise, sometimes substantially. Dose reduction will usually be necessary. If smoking is restarted, enzyme activity increases, plasma levels fall and dose increases are then required. The process is complicated, and effects are difficult to predict. Of course, few people manage to give up smoking completely, so additional complexity is introduced by intermittent smoking and repeated attempts at stopping completely. Close monitoring of plasma levels (where useful), clinical progress and adverse effect severity are essential.

Table 11.7 gives details of psychotropic drugs known to be affected by smoking status.

Table 11.7 Effect of smoking on psychotropic drugs.

Drug	Effect of smoking	Action to be taken on stopping smoking	Action to be taken on restarting smoking
Agomelatine[5]	Plasma levels reduced	Monitor closely. Dose may need to be reduced.	Consider reintroducing previous smoking dose.
Benzodiazepines[3,6]	Plasma levels reduced by 0–50% (depends on drug and smoking status)	Monitor closely. Consider reducing dose by up to 25% over 1 week.	Monitor closely. Consider restarting 'normal' smoking dose.
Carbamazepine[3]	Unclear, but smoking may reduce carbamazepine plasma levels to a small extent.	Monitor for changes in severity of adverse effects.	Monitor plasma levels.
Chlorpromazine[3,6,7]	Plasma levels reduced. Varied estimates of exact effect.	Monitor closely. Consider dose reduction.	Monitor closely. Consider restarting previous smoking dose.
Clozapine[8–10]	Reduces plasma levels by up to 50%. Effect may be maximal at as few as 2–5 cigarettes a day.[11] Plasma level reduction and risk of relapse may be greater in those receiving valproate.[12] Effect is reversed by co-administered fluvoxamine.[13]	Take plasma level before stopping. On stopping, reduce dose gradually (over a week) until around 75% of original dose is reached (i.e. reduce by 25%). Repeat plasma level 1 week after stopping. Anticipate further dose reductions.	Take plasma level before restarting. Increase dose to previous smoking dose over 1 week. Repeat plasma level. Deterioration is common if dose increases allow a fall in blood levels.[14]
Duloxetine[15,16]	Plasma levels may be reduced by up to 50%.	Monitor closely. Dose may need to be reduced.	Consider reintroducing previous smoking dose.

Table 11.7 *(Continued)*

Drug	Effect of smoking	Action to be taken on stopping smoking	Action to be taken on restarting smoking
Escitalopram[17]	In practice, smokers have lower blood levels despite being given higher doses. Reduction in levels may be up to 50% (possibly via induction of CYP2C19).	Monitor closely. Consider 25% dose reduction.	Monitor closely. Reinstate smoking dose.
Fluphenazine[18]	Reduces plasma levels by up to 50%	On stopping, reduce dose by 25%. Monitor carefully over following 4–8 weeks. Consider further dose reductions.	On restarting, increase dose to previous smoking dose.
Fluvoxamine[19]	Plasma levels decreased by around a third	Monitor closely. Dose may need to be reduced.	Dose may need to be increased to previous level.
Haloperidol[20,21]	Reduces plasma levels by around 25–50%	Reduce dose by around 25%. Monitor carefully. Consider further dose reductions.	On restarting, increase dose to previous smoking dose.
Loxapine[22] (inhaled)	Half-life reduced from 15.7 to 13.6 hours	Monitor	Monitor
Mirtazapine[23]	Unclear, but effect probably minimal	Monitor	Monitor
Olanzapine[10,24–26]	Reduces plasma levels by up to 50%. Effect increases with number of cigarettes smoked.[26]	Take plasma level before stopping. On stopping, reduce dose by 25%. After 1 week, repeat plasma level. Consider further dose reductions.	Take plasma level before restarting. Increase dose to previous smoking dose over 1 week. Repeat plasma level.
Risperidone[2,27]	Active moiety concentrations probably lower in smokers. Minor effect (possibly via induction of CYP3A4). Smoking may not affect paliperidone concentrations.[28]	Monitor closely	Monitor closely
Trazodone[29]	Around 25% reduction	Monitor for increased sedation. Consider dose reduction.	Monitor closely. Consider increasing dose.
Tricyclic antidepressants[3,6,30]	Plasma levels reduced by 25–50%. Some studies suggest more limited effect.[2,31]	Monitor closely. Consider reducing dose by 10–25% over 1 week. Consider further dose reductions.	Monitor closely. Consider restarting previous smoking dose.
Zuclopenthixol[32,33]	Unclear, but effect probably minimal	Monitor	Monitor

Note (again: it bears repeating): only tobacco smoking induces hepatic enzymes in the manner described above. This includes cigarettes and cannabis/tobacco 'joints'. Nicotine replacement, vaping devices and electronic cigarettes (which do not contain polycyclic aromatic compounds) have no effect on enzyme activity.[34,35]

CHAPTER 11

References

1. Kroon LA. Drug interactions with smoking. *Am J Health Syst Pharm* 2007; **64**:1917–1921.
2. Scherf-Clavel M, et al. Analysis of smoking behavior on the pharmacokinetics of antidepressants and antipsychotics: evidence for the role of alternative pathways apart from CYP1A2. *Int Clin Psychopharmacol* 2019; **34**:93–100.
3. Desai HD, et al. Smoking in patients receiving psychotropic medications: a pharmacokinetic perspective. *CNS Drugs* 2001; **15**:469–494.
4. Faber MS, et al. Time response of cytochrome P450 1A2 activity on cessation of heavy smoking. *Clin Pharmacol Ther* 2004; **76**:178–184.
5. Servier Laboratories Limited. Summary of product characteristics. Valdoxan (agomelatine). 2021; https://www.medicines.org.uk/emc/medicine/21830.
6. Miller LG. Recent developments in the study of the effects of cigarette smoking on clinical pharmacokinetics and clinical pharmacodynamics. *Clin Pharmacokinet* 1989; **17**:90–108.
7. Goff DC, et al. Cigarette smoking in schizophrenia: relationship to psychopathology and medication side effects. *Am J Psychiatry* 1992; **149**:1189–1194.
8. Haring C, et al. Influence of patient-related variables on clozapine plasma levels. *Am J Psychiatry* 1990; **147**:1471–1475.
9. Diaz FJ, et al. Estimating the size of the effects of co-medications on plasma clozapine concentrations using a model that controls for clozapine doses and confounding variables. *Pharmacopsychiatry* 2008; **41**:81–91.
10. Tsuda Y, et al. Meta-analysis: the effects of smoking on the disposition of two commonly used antipsychotic agents, olanzapine and clozapine. *BMJ Open* 2014; **4**:e004216.
11. Flanagan RJ, et al. Effect of cigarette smoking on clozapine dose and on plasma clozapine and N-desmethylclozapine (norclozapine) concentrations in clinical practice. *J Clin Psychopharmacol* 2023; **43**:514–519.
12. Tsukahara M, et al. Effect of smoking habits and concomitant valproic acid use on relapse in patients with treatment-resistant schizophrenia receiving clozapine: a 1-year retrospective cohort study. *Acta Psychiatr Scand* 2023; **148**:437–446.
13. Augustin M, et al. Effect of fluvoxamine augmentation and smoking on clozapine serum concentrations. *Schizophr Res* 2019; **210**:143–148.
14. Qurashi I, et al. Changes in smoking status, mental state and plasma clozapine concentration: retrospective cohort evaluation. *BJPsych Bull* 2019; **43**:271–274.
15. Fric M, et al. The influence of smoking on the serum level of duloxetine. *Pharmacopsychiatry* 2008; **41**:151–155.
16. Augustin M, et al. Differences in duloxetine dosing strategies in smoking and nonsmoking patients: therapeutic drug monitoring uncovers the impact on drug metabolism. *J Clin Psychiatry* 2018; **79**:17m12086.
17. Scherf-Clavel M, et al. Smoking is associated with lower dose-corrected serum concentrations of escitalopram. *J Clin Psychopharmacol* 2019; **39**:485–488.
18. Ereshefsky L, et al. Effects of smoking on fluphenazine clearance in psychiatric inpatients. *Biol Psychiatry* 1985; **20**:329–332.
19. Spigset O, et al. Effect of cigarette smoking on fluvoxamine pharmacokinetics in humans. *Clin Pharmacol Ther* 1995; **58**:399–403.
20. Jann MW, et al. Effects of smoking on haloperidol and reduced haloperidol plasma concentrations and haloperidol clearance. *Psychopharmacology (Berl)* 1986; **90**:468–470.
21. Shimoda K, et al. Lower plasma levels of haloperidol in smoking than in nonsmoking schizophrenic patients. *Ther Drug Monit* 1999; **21**:293–296.
22. Takahashi LH, et al. Effect of smoking on the pharmacokinetics of inhaled loxapine. *Ther Drug Monit* 2014; **36**:618–623.
23. Grasmader K, et al. Population pharmacokinetic analysis of mirtazapine. *Eur J Clin Pharmacol* 2004; **60**:473–480.
24. Carrillo JA, et al. Role of the smoking-induced cytochrome P450 (CYP)1A2 and polymorphic CYP2D6 in steady-state concentration of olanzapine. *J Clin Psychopharmacol* 2003; **23**:119–127.
25. Lowe EJ, et al. Impact of tobacco smoking cessation on stable clozapine or olanzapine treatment. *Ann Pharmacother* 2010; **44**:727–732.
26. Horvat M, et al. Association of smoking cigarettes, age, and sex with serum concentrations of olanzapine in patients with schizophrenia. *Biochem Med (Zagreb)* 2023; **33**:030702.
27. Schoretsanitis G, et al. Effect of smoking on risperidone pharmacokinetics – a multifactorial approach to better predict the influence on drug metabolism. *Schizophr Res* 2017; **185**:51–57.
28. Schoretsanitis G, et al. Lack of smoking effects on pharmacokinetics of oral paliperidone—analysis of a naturalistic therapeutic drug monitoring sample. *Pharmacopsychiatry* 2021; **54**:31–35.
29. Ishida M, et al. Effects of various factors on steady state plasma concentrations of trazodone and its active metabolite m-chlorophenylpiperazine. *Int Clin Psychopharmacol* 1995; **10**:143–146.
30. Ereshefsky L, et al. Pharmacokinetic factors affecting antidepressant drug clearance and clinical effect: evaluation of doxepin and imipramine – new data and review. *Clin Chem* 1988; **34**:863–880.
31. Lundstrøm NH, et al. The effect of smoking on the plasma concentration of tricyclic antidepressants: a systematic review. *Acta Neuropsychiatr* 2022; **34**:1–9.
32. Jann MW, et al. Clinical pharmacokinetics of the depot antipsychotics. *Clin Pharmacokinet* 1985; **10**:315–333.
33. Jorgensen A, et al. Zuclopenthixol decanoate in schizophrenia: serum levels and clinical state. *Psychopharmacology (Berl)* 1985; **87**:364–367.
34. Blacker CJ. Clinical issues to consider for clozapine patients who vape: a case illustration. *Focus (Am Psychiatr Publ)* 2020; **18**:55–57.
35. Montville DJ, et al. Fluctuation between cigarette smoking and use of electronic nicotine delivery systems: impact on clozapine concentrations and clinical effect. *Ment Health Clin* 2021; **11**:365–368.

Drug interactions with alcohol

Drug interactions with alcohol are complex. Many patient-related and drug-related factors need to be considered. It can be difficult to predict outcomes accurately because a number of processes may occur simultaneously or consecutively.

Pharmacokinetic interactions[1-4]

Alcohol (ethanol) is absorbed from the gastrointestinal tract and distributed in body water. The volume of distribution is smaller in women and the elderly where plasma levels of alcohol will be higher than in young males for a given intake of alcohol. Ingested alcohol is subject to metabolism by alcohol dehydrogenase (ADH). A small proportion of alcohol is metabolised by ADH in the stomach. The remainder is metabolised in the liver by ADH, and by CYP2E1. At low alcohol concentrations only ADH is active; CYP2E1 only begins to contribute when concentrations approach the legal driving limit of many countries (0.08%).[5] CYP2E1 plays a minor role in occasional drinkers but is an important and inducible metabolic route in chronic, heavy drinkers. The induction of CYP2E1 accounts for the apparent tolerance of alcohol in heavy drinkers.[6] CYP1A2, CYP3A4 and many other CYP enzymes also play a minor role in the metabolism of ethanol.[7,8]

  CYP2E1 and ADH convert alcohol to acetaldehyde. This is both the toxic substance responsible for the unpleasant symptoms of the 'Antabuse reaction' (e.g. flushing, headache, nausea, malaise) and the compound implicated in hepatic damage. It may have psychotropic effects – ethanol is metabolised to acetaldehyde by CYP2E1 in the brain.[9] The enzyme catalase is also known to metabolise alcohol to acetaldehyde in the brain and elsewhere.[10] Acetaldehyde is further metabolised by aldehyde dehydrogenase to acetic acid and then to carbon dioxide and water (Figure 11.1).

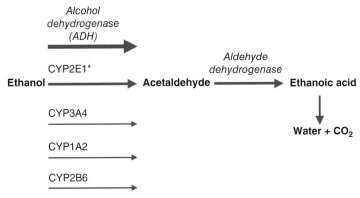

* This is a minor route in occasional drinkers, and a major route in heavy drinkers and at higher blood alcohol concentration. The ubiquitous enzyme catalase is also able to metabolise ethanol but its overall contribution is not known.

Figure 11.1 Metabolism of alcohol.

All of the enzymes involved in the metabolism of alcohol exhibit genetic polymorphism. For example, the majority of people of north Asian origin are poor metabolisers via aldehyde dehydrogenase.[11] Enzyme function can change in response to alcohol. Chronic consumption of alcohol induces CYP2E1 and CYP3A4. The effects of alcohol on other hepatic metabolising enzymes have been poorly studied.

Table 11.8 lists drugs that inhibit ADH and aldehyde dehydrogenase.

Table 11.8 Drugs that inhibit alcohol dehydrogenase and aldehyde dehydrogenase.

Enzyme	Inhibited by	Potential consequences
Alcohol dehydrogenase	Aspirin H$_2$ antagonists	Reduced metabolism of alcohol resulting in higher plasma levels for longer periods of time
Aldehyde dehydrogenase	Chlorpropamide Disulfiram Griseofulvin Isoniazid Isosorbide dinitrate Metronidazole* Nitrofurantoin Sulphamethoxazole Tolbutamide	Reduced ability to metabolise acetaldehyde leading to 'Antabuse' type reaction: facial flushing, headache, tachycardia, nausea and vomiting, arrhythmias and hypotension

*Evidence that metronidazole has any effect on aldehyde dehydrogenase is surprisingly weak.[12–14]

Interactions are difficult to predict in alcohol misusers because two opposing processes may be at work: competition for enzymatic sites during periods of consumption/intoxication (increasing drug plasma levels) and enzyme induction prevailing during periods of sobriety (reducing drug plasma levels[10]). In chronic drinkers, particularly those who binge-drink, blood levels of prescribed drugs may reach toxic levels during periods of intoxication with alcohol and then be sub-therapeutic when the patient is sober. Even in non-intoxicated individuals there is some evidence that co-administered alcohol confers competitive inhibition of CYP3A4, leading to increased exposure to drugs metabolised by this enzyme (Table 11.9).[15] This makes it very difficult to optimise treatment of physical or mental illness.

Table 11.9 Co-administration of alcohol and substrates for CYP2E1 and CYP3A4.[5,6,16]

	Substrates for enzyme (note: this is not an exhaustive list)	Effects in an intoxicated patient	Effects in a chronic, sober drinker
CYP2E1	Isoniazid Paracetamol Phenobarbitone Warfarin Zopiclone	Competition between alcohol and drug leading to reduced rates of metabolism of both compounds. Increased plasma levels may lead to toxicity	Activity of CYP2E1 is increased up 10-fold Increased metabolism of drugs potentially leading to therapeutic failure

Table 11.9 (*Continued*)

	Substrates for enzyme (note: this is not an exhaustive list)	Effects in an intoxicated patient	Effects in a chronic, sober drinker
CYP3A4	Alprazolam Aripiprazole Benzodiazepines Carbamazepine Clozapine Donepezil Galantamine Haloperidol Methadone Mirtazapine Quetiapine Risperidone Sildenafil Tricyclics Valproate Venlafaxine Z-hypnotics	Competition between alcohol and drug leading to reduced rates of metabolism of both compounds. Increased plasma levels may lead to toxicity	Increased rate of drug metabolism potentially leading to therapeutic failure Enzyme induction can last for several weeks after alcohol consumption ceases

Interactions of uncertain aetiology include increased blood alcohol concentrations in people who take verapamil and decreased metabolism of methylphenidate in people who consume alcohol. Alcohol may also, via various routes, impair the function of slow-release tablet mechanisms causing dose-dumping.[17]

Pharmacodynamic interactions[2–4]

Alcohol enhances inhibitory neurotransmission at gamma-aminobutyric acid A (GABA-A) receptors and reduces excitatory neurotransmission at glutamate N-methyl-D-aspartate (NMDA) receptors. It also increases dopamine release in the mesolimbic pathway and may have some effects on serotonin and opiate pathways. Given these actions, alcohol would be expected to cause sedation, amnesia and ataxia (Table 11.10) and give rise to feelings of pleasure (and/or worsen psychotic symptoms in vulnerable individuals).

Table 11.10 Pharmacodynamic interactions with alcohol.

Effect of alcohol	Effect exacerbated by	Potential consequences
Sedation	Other sedative drugs, e.g.: Antihistamines Antipsychotics Baclofen Benzodiazepines Lofexidine Opiates Tizanidine Tricyclics Z-hypnotics	Increased CNS depression ranging from increased propensity to be involved in accidents through to respiratory depression and death

CHAPTER 11

Table 11.10 (*Continued*)

Effect of alcohol	Effect exacerbated by	Potential consequences
Amnesia	Other amnesic drugs, e.g.: Barbiturates Benzodiazepines Z-hypnotics	Increased amnesic effects ranging from mild memory loss to total amnesia. Usually anterograde amnesia: loss of memory of events after the effects of alcohol begin
Ataxia	ACE inhibitors Beta-blockers Calcium channel blockers Nitrates Adrenergic alpha receptor antagonists, e.g.: Clozapine Risperidone Tricyclics	Increased unsteadiness and falls

ACE, angiotensin-converting enzyme; CNS, central nervous system.

Alcohol can cause or worsen psychotic symptoms by increasing dopamine release in mesolimbic pathways. The effect of antipsychotic drugs may be competitively antagonised, rendering them less effective.

Electrolyte disturbances secondary to alcohol-related dehydration can be exacerbated by other drugs that cause electrolyte disturbances (e.g. diuretics). Heavy alcohol consumption can lead to hypoglycaemia in people with diabetes who take insulin or oral hypoglycaemics. Theoretically there is an increased risk of lactic acidosis in patients who take metformin with alcohol. Alcohol can also increase blood pressure.

Chronic alcohol drinkers are particularly susceptible to the gastrointestinal irritant effects of aspirin and non-steroidal anti-inflammatory drugs.

In the presence of pharmacokinetic interactions, pharmacodynamic interactions may be more marked. For example, in a chronic heavy drinker who is sober, enzyme induction will increase the metabolism of diazepam, which may lead to increased levels of anxiety (treatment failure). If the same patient becomes intoxicated with alcohol, the metabolism of diazepam will be greatly reduced as it will have to compete with alcohol for the metabolic capacity of CYP3A4. Plasma levels of alcohol and diazepam will rise (toxicity). As both alcohol and diazepam are sedative (via GABA-A affinity), loss of consciousness and respiratory depression may occur.

Table 11.11 lists drugs that are safe and those that should be avoided in patients who continue drinking.

Table 11.11 Psychotropic drugs: choice in patients who continue to drink.

	Safest choice	Best avoided
Antipsychotics	**Sulpiride and amisulpride Paliperidone,** if depot required (non-sedative and renally excreted)	**Very sedative antipsychotics** such as chlorpromazine and clozapine
Antidepressants	**SSRIs – citalopram, sertraline** Potent inhibitors of CYP3A4 (fluoxetine, paroxetine) may decrease alcohol metabolism in chronic drinkers	**TCAs,** because impairment of metabolism by alcohol (while intoxicated) can lead to increased plasma levels and consequent signs and symptoms of overdose (profound hypotension, seizures, arrhythmias and coma) Cardiac effects can be exacerbated by electrolyte disturbances Combinations of TCAs and alcohol profoundly impair psychomotor skills **Mirtazapine** – often very sedative **MAOIs,** as can cause profound hypotension. Also potential interaction with tyramine-containing drinks which can lead to hypertensive crisis
Mood stabilisers	**Valproate** (where regulations allow) **Carbamazepine** Higher plasma levels achieved during periods of alcohol intoxication may be poorly tolerated	**Lithium,** because it has a narrow therapeutic index and alcohol-related dehydration and electrolyte disturbance can precipitate lithium toxicity

Note: be aware of the possibility of hepatic failure or reduced hepatic function in chronic alcohol misusers. See 'Hepatic impairment' in Chapter 8. Also note the risk of hepatic toxicity with some recommended drugs (e.g. valproate).
MAOIs, monoamine oxidase inhibitors; TCAs, tricyclic antidepressants.

References

1. Zakhari S. Overview: how is alcohol metabolized by the body? *Alcohol Res Health* 2006; **29**:245–254.
2. Tanaka E. Toxicological interactions involving psychiatric drugs and alcohol: an update. *J Clin Pharm Ther* 2003; **28**:81–95.
3. Wan-Chih T. Alcohol-related drug interactions. *Pharmacist's Letter/Prescriber's Letter* 2008; **24**:240106.
4. Smith RG. An appraisal of potential drug interactions in cigarette smokers and alcohol drinkers. *J Am Podiatr Med Assoc* 2009; **99**:81–88.
5. Chan LN, et al. Pharmacokinetic and pharmacodynamic drug interactions with ethanol (alcohol). *Clin Pharmacokinet* 2014; 53:1115–1136.
6. Jiang Y, et al. Alcohol metabolizing enzymes, microsomal ethanol oxidizing system, cytochrome P450 2E1, catalase, and aldehyde dehydrogenase in alcohol-associated liver disease. *Biomedicines* 2020; **8**:50.
7. Salmela KS, et al. Respective roles of human cytochrome P-4502E1, 1A2, and 3A4 in the hepatic microsomal ethanol oxidizing system. *Alcohol Clin Exp Res* 1998; **22**:2125–2132.
8. Hamitouche S, et al. Ethanol oxidation into acetaldehyde by 16 recombinant human cytochrome P450 isoforms: role of CYP2C isoforms in human liver microsomes. *Toxicol Lett* 2006; **167**:221–230.
9. Koster M, et al. Seizures during antidepressant treatment in psychiatric inpatients – results from the transnational pharmacovigilance project 'Arzneimittelsicherheit in der Psychiatrie' (AMSP) 1993–2008. *Psychopharmacology (Berl)* 2013; **230**:191–201.
10. Cederbaum AI. Alcohol metabolism. *Clin Liver Dis* 2012; **16**:667–685.
11. Wall TL, et al. Biology, genetics, and environment: underlying factors influencing alcohol metabolism. *Alcohol Res* 2016; **38**:59–68.
12. Williams CS, et al. Do ethanol and metronidazole interact to produce a disulfiram-like reaction? *Ann Pharmacother* 2000; **34**:255–257.
13. Visapää JP, et al. Lack of disulfiram-like reaction with metronidazole and ethanol. *Ann Pharmacother* 2002; **36**:971–974.
14. Mergenhagen KA, et al. Fact versus fiction: a review of the evidence behind alcohol and antibiotic interactions. *Antimicrob Agents Chemother* 2020; **64**:e02167–02119.
15. Huang Z, et al. Influence of ethanol on the metabolism of alprazolam. *Expert Opin Drug Metab Toxicol* 2018; **14**:551–559.
16. Traccis F, et al. Alcohol-medication interactions: a systematic review and meta-analysis of placebo-controlled trials. *Neurosci Biobehav Rev* 2022; **132**:519–541.
17. Lennernäs H. Ethanol-drug absorption interaction: potential for a significant effect on the plasma pharmacokinetics of ethanol vulnerable formulations. *Mol Pharm* 2009; **6**:1429–1440.

CHAPTER 11

Chapter 12

Other substances

Caffeine

Caffeine is probably the most used psychoactive substance in the world. Mean daily consumption in the UK is 350–620mg.[1] A quarter of the general population and half of those with psychiatric illness regularly consume over 500mg caffeine per day.[2] Consumption of caffeine should be routinely discussed with an individual to assess its effect on their symptoms and presentation.[3] Both caffeine intake and caffeine withdrawal can have a marked effect on mental and physical health.

Most caffeine intake is in the form of coffee and tea but increasingly in the form of energy drinks (Table 12.1). Caffeine is also a constituent of chocolate and hundreds of over-the-counter medicines where it is often included as a co-analgesic.

Table 12.1 Typical caffeine content of drinks.

Drink	Caffeine content
Brewed coffee[4]	100mg/cup (around 100mg per espresso shot)
Red Bull	80mg/can (other energy drinks may contain substantially more; volume of cans varies substantially)
Instant coffee	60mg/cup
Black tea	45mg/cup
Soft drinks (sodas)	25–50mg/can
Green tea	20–30mg/cup
Decaffeinated coffee	3–16mg[5]

The Maudsley® Prescribing Guidelines in Psychiatry, Fifteenth Edition. David M. Taylor, Thomas R. E. Barnes and Allan H. Young.
© 2025 David M. Taylor. Published 2025 by John Wiley & Sons Ltd.

Table 12.2 Dose and psychotropic effects of caffeine.

Dose	Psychotropic effect
Generally	Central nervous system stimulation Increase catecholamine release, particularly dopamine[6]
Low to moderate dose[2,7]	Elation Impulsivity Peacefulness
Large doses >600mg/day[8] (sensitive [non-tolerant] individuals may experience effects at lower doses; tolerance develops in long-term users)	Anxiety Insomnia Psychomotor agitation Excitement Rambling speech Delirium Psychosis

General effects of caffeine

- Acute use can increase systolic and diastolic blood pressure (BP) by up to 10mmHg for up to 4 hours.[3] Chronic moderate use probably has little effect on BP.[9]
- May enhance reinforcing effects of nicotine and possibly other drugs of misuse.[10,11]
- Caffeine has important psychotropic effects (Table 12.2), may worsen existing psychiatric illness and may interact with psychotropic drugs.
- Caffeine is an antagonist at adenosine A1 and A2A receptors, thus stimulating dopamine pathways.

Psychotropic effects of caffeine

Withdrawal

An established withdrawal syndrome exists; symptoms include headache, depressed mood, anxiety, fatigue, irritability, nausea, dysphoria and craving.[12]

Pharmacokinetics

- **Absorption:**
Rapid after oral administration, especially in liquid form.
- **Metabolism:**
  - Half-life of 2.5–4.5 hours.
  - Metabolised by CYP1A2, a hepatic cytochrome enzyme that exhibits genetic polymorphism. This may account for the large interindividual differences that are seen in the ability to tolerate caffeine.[13] Note that CYP1A2 is induced by smoking and inhibited by a number of drugs such as fluvoxamine.
  - This metabolic pathway may become saturated at higher doses.[14]
- **Interactions** (Table 12.3):
  - Caffeine competitively inhibits CYP1A2. Chronic caffeine use may increase plasma levels of drugs metabolised by CYP1A2. Plasma levels of some drugs may be reduced if caffeine is withdrawn.

CHAPTER 12

- The potential effects of caffeine on the metabolism of other drugs, as well as the potential to induce a caffeine withdrawal syndrome, should always be considered before substituting caffeine-free drinks.

Table 12.3 Interactions with caffeine.

Interacting substance	Effect	Comments
CYP1A2 inhibitors: Oestrogens Cimetidine Fluvoxamine (may decrease caffeine clearance by 80%)[15] Disulfiram	Reduce caffeine clearance	Effects of caffeine may be prolonged or increased
		Adverse effects may be increased
		May precipitate caffeine toxicity
Cigarette smoke*	CYP1A2 inducer – increased caffeine metabolism[6]	Smokers may require higher doses of caffeine to gain desired effects[6]
Lithium	High doses of caffeine may reduce lithium levels	Caffeine withdrawal may cause a lithium level rise[16]
MAOIs	May enhance stimulant CNS effects	
Clozapine	Caffeine may increase clozapine plasma concentrations by up to 60%[17]	Thought to be via competitive inhibition of CYP1A2. Other drugs affected by caffeine-induced inhibition of the enzyme include olanzapine, imipramine and clomipramine.
SSRIs	Large doses of caffeine may increase risk of serotonin syndrome[18]	
Benzodiazepines	Caffeine may act as an antagonist	Caffeine reduces the efficacy of benzodiazepines[8]

* Vaping has no effect on CYP1A2 function.
CNS, central nervous system; MAOIs, monoamine oxidase inhibitors.

Caffeine intoxication

The DSM-5[19] defines caffeine intoxication as the recent consumption of caffeine, usually in excess of 250mg, accompanied by five or more of the symptoms in Box 12.1.

In caffeine intoxication, these symptoms cause significant distress or impairment in social, occupational or other important areas of functioning and are not due to a general medical condition or better accounted for by another mental disorder (e.g. an anxiety disorder).

Caffeine abuse or dependence as a clinical syndrome has been reported[3] and caffeine use disorder and caffeine withdrawal are both DSM-5 diagnoses.

Box 12.1 Symptoms of caffeine intoxication

- Restlessness
- Nervousness
- Excitement
- Insomnia
- Flushed face
- Diuresis

- Gastrointestinal disturbance
- Muscle twitching
- Rambling flow of thought and speech
- Tachycardia or cardiac arrhythmia
- Periods of inexhaustibility
- Psychomotor agitation

Energy drinks

So-called energy drinks contain large amounts of caffeine along with sugar, vitamins and a number of other ingredients such as guarana and taurine. There is some evidence that these drinks can improve attention and short-term memory.[20] Marketing is targeted at adolescents and young adults, some of whom consume large volumes of these drinks and seem to be particularly vulnerable to developing signs and symptoms of caffeine intoxication. Symptoms of anxiety and depression, frank suicidal behaviour and seizures have been associated with use of these products by young people.[21–23] When combined with alcohol, aggressive behaviour may result.[24] Excessive intake may lead to acute psychosis[25,26] or mania.[27]

Effects of caffeine on different disorders

Schizophrenia

- Patients with schizophrenia often consume large amounts of caffeine-containing drinks[1] and they are twice as likely as controls to consume >200mg caffeine/day.[6]
- Caffeine-containing drinks may be used to relieve dry mouth (as an adverse effect of some antipsychotic drugs), for the stimulant effects of caffeine (to relieve dysphoria/sedation/negative symptoms)[6] or simply because coffee/tea drinking structures the day or relieves boredom.
- Schizophrenia may increase sensitivity to drug-related cues.[6]
- Moderate caffeine intake may improve cognitive and negative symptoms in schizophrenia.[28,29]
- Large doses of caffeine can worsen psychotic symptoms[6,30] (in particular elation and conceptual disorganisation) and result in the prescription of larger doses of antipsychotic drugs.
- The removal of caffeine from the diets of chronically disturbed (challenging behaviour) patients may ultimately lead to decreased levels of hostility, irritability and suspiciousness[31] although this may not hold true in less disturbed populations.[32]
- Caffeine cessation may be of benefit in clozapine-resistant schizophrenia.[33]

Mood disorders

- Caffeine may elevate mood through increasing noradrenaline release[34] and modest caffeine consumption may protect against depression in those who do not have a pre-existing mood disorder.[35]
- People with mood disorders are more likely to consume caffeine, particularly when depressed.[16,36]
- Depressed patients may be more sensitive to the anxiogenic effects of caffeine.[37,38]
- Excessive consumption of caffeine may precipitate mania.[38,39]
- Caffeine can increase cortisol secretion (gives a false positive in the dexamethasone-suppression test),[40] increase seizure length during electroconvulsive therapy[41] and increase the clearance of lithium by promoting diuresis.[42]

Anxiety disorders

- Caffeine increases vigilance, decreases reaction times, increases sleep latency and worsens sleep quality; effects that may be more marked in poor metabolisers.
- May precipitate or worsen generalised anxiety and panic attacks;[43] vulnerability to these effects may be genetically determined.[11]
- Effects are so marked that caffeine intoxication should always be considered when patients complain of anxiety symptoms or insomnia.
- Symptoms may diminish considerably or even abate completely if caffeine is avoided.[44]
- Patients with panic disorder consume much more caffeine than controls[45] but the reasons for this are not clear. Greater consumption triggers panic attacks in those with panic disorder but not in other populations.[46]

Other disorders

Weak evidence supports the benefit of caffeine in attention deficit hyperactivity disorder (ADHD)[47] and that high caffeine consumption may protect against late-life cognitive decline.[48]

Summary

- Caffeine is present in high quantities in coffee and some soft drinks, particularly energy drinks.
- The intake of caffeine may worsen psychosis and anxiety. Young people may be particularly vulnerable.
- Caffeine inhibits clozapine metabolism.
- Caffeine intoxication is characterised by psychomotor agitation and rambling speech.
- Caffeine may be associated with toxicity when co-administered with CYP1A2 inhibitors such as fluvoxamine.
- Caffeine can enhance the reinforcing effects of nicotine and possibly other drugs of misuse.

References

1. Rihs M, et al. Caffeine consumption in hospitalized psychiatric patients. *Eur Arch Psychiatry Clin Neurosci* 1996; **246**:83–92.
2. Clementz GL, et al. Psychotropic effects of caffeine. *Am Fam Physician* 1988; **37**:167–172.
3. Ogawa N, et al. Clinical importance of caffeine dependence and abuse. *Psychiatry Clin Neurosci* 2007; **61**:263–268.
4. Desbrow B, et al. An examination of consumer exposure to caffeine from retail coffee outlets. *Food Chem Toxicol* 2007; **45**:1588–1592.
5. McCusker RR, et al. Caffeine content of decaffeinated coffee. *J Anal Toxicol* 2006; **30**:611–613.
6. Adolfo AB, et al. Effects of smoking cues on caffeine urges in heavy smokers and caffeine consumers with and without schizophrenia. *Schizophr Res* 2009; **107**:192–197.
7. Grant JE, et al. Caffeine's influence on gambling behavior and other types of impulsivity. *Addict Behav* 2018; **76**:156–160.
8. Sawynok J. Pharmacological rationale for the clinical use of caffeine. *Drugs* 1995; **49**:37–50.
9. O'Keefe JH, et al. Effects of habitual coffee consumption on cardiometabolic disease, cardiovascular health, and all-cause mortality. *J Am Coll Cardiol* 2013; **62**:1043–1051.
10. Pharmaceutical Press. *Martindale: The Complete Drug Reference.* 2024; www.medicinescomplete.com.
11. Bergin JE, et al. Common psychiatric disorders and caffeine use, tolerance, and withdrawal: an examination of shared genetic and environmental effects. *Twin Res Hum Genet* 2012; **15**:473–482.
12. Silverman K, et al. Withdrawal syndrome after the double-blind cessation of caffeine consumption. *N Engl J Med* 1992; **327**:1109–1114.
13. Butler MA, et al. Determination of CYP1A2 and NAT2 phenotypes in human populations by analysis of caffeine urinary metabolites. *Pharmacogenetics* 1992; **2**:116–127.
14. Kaplan GB, et al. Dose-dependent pharmacokinetics and psychomotor effects of caffeine in humans. *J Clin Pharmacol* 1997; **37**:693–703.
15. Pharmaceutical Press. *Medicines Complete: Stockley's Drug Interactions.* 2024; www.medicinescomplete.com.
16. Baethge C, et al. Coffee and cigarette use: association with suicidal acts in 352 Sardinian bipolar disorder patients. *Bipolar Disord* 2009; **11**:494–503.
17. Carrillo JA, et al. Effects of caffeine withdrawal from the diet on the metabolism of clozapine in schizophrenic patients. *J Clin Psychopharmacol* 1998; **18**:311–316.
18. Ohta R, et al. Serotonin syndrome triggered by overuse of caffeine and complicated with neuroleptic malignant syndrome: a case report. *Cureus* 2022; **14**:e22468.
19. American Psychiatric Association. *Diagnostic and Statistical Manual of Mental Disorders,* 5th edn (DSM-5). Arlington, VA: American Psychiatric Association; 2013.
20. Wesnes KA, et al. An evaluation of the cognitive and mood effects of an energy shot over a 6h period in volunteers: a randomized, double-blind, placebo controlled, cross-over study. *Appetite* 2013; **67**:105–113.
21. Szpak A, et al. A case of acute suicidality following excessive caffeine intake. *J Psychopharmacol* 2012; **26**:1502–1510.
22. Trapp GS, et al. Energy drink consumption among young Australian adults: associations with alcohol and illicit drug use. *Drug Alcohol Depend* 2014; **134**:30–37.
23. Pennington N, et al. Energy drinks: a new health hazard for adolescents. *J Sch Nurs* 2010; **26**:352–359.
24. Sheehan BE, et al. Caffeinated and non-caffeinated alcohol use and indirect aggression: the impact of self-regulation. *Addict Behav* 2016; **58**:53–59.
25. Görgülü Y, et al. A case of acute psychosis following energy drink consumption. *Noro Psikiyatri Arsivi* 2014; **51**:79–81.
26. Kelsey D, et al. A case of psychosis and renal failure associated with excessive energy drink consumption. *Case Rep Psychiatry* 2019; **2019**:3954161.
27. Rodrigues Cordeiro C, et al. Triggers for acute mood episodes in bipolar disorder: a systematic review. *J Psychiatr Res* 2023; **161**:237–260.
28. Szoke A, et al. Clinical and pharmacological correlates of caffeine consumption in subjects with schizophrenia – data from the FACE-SZ cohort. *J Psychiatr Res* 2023; **161**:206–212.
29. Han Almis B, et al. Is there a relationship between caffeine intake and smoking and positive and negative symptom severity in schizophrenia? *Psychiatr Danub* 2023; **35**:56–61.
30. Wang HR, et al. Caffeine-induced psychiatric manifestations: a review. *Int Clin Psychopharmacol* 2015; **30**:179–182.
31. De Freitas B, et al. Effects of caffeine in chronic psychiatric patients. *Am J Psychiatry* 1979; **136**:1337–1338.
32. Koczapski A, et al. Effects of caffeine on behavior of schizophrenic inpatients. *Schizophr Bull* 1989; **15**:339–344.
33. Dratcu L, et al. Clozapine-resistant psychosis, smoking, and caffeine: managing the neglected effects of substances that our patients consume every day. *Am J Ther* 2007; **14**:314–318.
34. Achor MB, et al. Diet aids, mania, and affective illness. *Am J Psychiatry* 1981; **138**:392.
35. Wang L, et al. Coffee and caffeine consumption and depression: a meta-analysis of observational studies. *Aust NZ J Psychiatry* 2016; **50**:228–242.
36. Maremmani I, et al. Are "social drugs" (tobacco, coffee and chocolate) related to the bipolar spectrum? *J Affect Disord* 2011; **133**:227–233.
37. Lee MA, et al. Anxiogenic effects of caffeine on panic and depressed patients. *Am J Psychiatry* 1988; **145**:632–635.
38. Rizkallah E, et al. Could the use of energy drinks induce manic or depressive relapse among abstinent substance use disorder patients with comorbid bipolar spectrum disorder? *Bipolar Disord* 2011; **13**:578–580.
39. Machado-Vieira R, et al. Mania associated with an energy drink: the possible role of caffeine, taurine, and inositol. *Can J Psychiatry* 2001; **46**:454–455.
40. Uhde TW, et al. Caffeine-induced escape from dexamethasone suppression. *Arch Gen Psychiatry* 1985; **42**:737–738.
41. Cantu TG, et al. Caffeine in electroconvulsive therapy. *Ann Pharmacother* 1991; **25**:1079–1080.

42. Mester R, et al. Caffeine withdrawal increases lithium blood levels. *Biol Psychiatry* 1995; **37**:348–350.

43. Bruce MS. The anxiogenic effects of caffeine. *Postgrad Med J* 1990; **66** Suppl 2:S18–S24.

44. Bruce MS, et al. Caffeine abstention in the management of anxiety disorders. *Psychol Med* 1989; **19**:211–214.

45. Santos VA, et al. Panic disorder and chronic caffeine use: a case-control study. *Clin Pract Epidemiol Ment Health* 2019; **15**:120–125.

46. Klevebrant L, et al. Effects of caffeine on anxiety and panic attacks in patients with panic disorder: a systematic review and meta-analysis. *Gen Hosp Psychiatry* 2022; **74**:22–31.

47. Ioannidis K, et al. Ostracising caffeine from the pharmacological arsenal for attention-deficit hyperactivity disorder – was this a correct decision? A literature review. *J Psychopharmacol* 2014; **28**:830–836.

48. Panza F, et al. Coffee, tea, and caffeine consumption and prevention of late-life cognitive decline and dementia: a systematic review. *J Nutr Health Aging* 2015; **19**:313–328.

CHAPTER 12

Nicotine

Nicotine is consumed by vaping or tobacco smoking and causes peripheral vasoconstriction, tachycardia and increased blood pressure.[1] People with schizophrenia who smoke are more likely to develop the metabolic syndrome compared with those who do not smoke.[2] Alongside nicotine, cigarettes also contain tar (a complex mixture of organic molecules, many carcinogenic), a cause of cancers of the respiratory tract, chronic bronchitis and emphysema.[3] Electronic cigarettes and vaping devices contain only nicotine (along with some necessary excipients), which has very limited toxicity and is not thought to be carcinogenic. Vaping is thus preferred for all smokers, albeit with some reservations in regard to quality control of content and the so-called re-normalisation of smoking. Vaping is not without risk but this is a complex area beyond the scope of this book.

Nicotine is highly addictive and vulnerability to nicotine addiction may be genetically determined.[4] People with mental illness are 2–3 times more likely than the general population to develop and maintain a nicotine addiction.[5] Chronic smoking contributes to the increased morbidity and mortality from respiratory and cardiovascular disease that is seen in this patient group. Nicotine also has psychotropic effects. Smoking can affect the metabolism (and therefore the efficacy and toxicity) of drugs prescribed to treat psychiatric illness[6] (see 'Smoking and psychotropic drugs' in Chapter 11). Nicotine use may be a gateway drug to experimenting with other psychoactive substances.

Psychotropic effects

Nicotine is highly lipid-soluble and rapidly enters the brain after inhalation. Nicotine receptors are found on dopaminergic cell bodies and stimulation of these receptors leads to dopamine release.[5] Nicotine may be used by people with mental health problems as a form of 'self-medication' (e.g. to alleviate the negative symptoms of schizophrenia or antipsychotic-induced dysphoria or for its anxiolytic effect[7]). Drugs that increase the release of dopamine reduce craving for nicotine. They may also, of course, worsen psychotic illness.

Nicotine improves concentration and vigilance,[5] probably by enhancing the effects of glutamate, acetylcholine and serotonin.[7]

Effects of nicotine on different disorders

Schizophrenia

Before the introduction of vaping, 70–80% of people with schizophrenia regularly smoked cigarettes.[8] Now both tobacco use and vaping are more common among people with psychosis.[9,10] A 2024 study in the USA[11] found that 28% of people with a first episode of psychosis used nicotine in one form or another – roughly double the rate of age-matched controls. In people with longer-standing psychosis in 2023, tobacco use was seen in just over 40% but use of any nicotine product was reported in around 70–80% (i.e. a prevalence no different from before the availability of vaping devices).[12]

This increased tendency to use nicotine predates the onset of psychiatric symptoms[13] and smoking might actually be a causal factor in schizophrenia.[14] Possible explanations are as follows:[15] (i) smoking causes dopamine release, leading to feelings of well-being and a reduction in negative symptoms;[7] (ii) smoking alleviates some of the adverse effects of antipsychotics such as drowsiness and extrapyramidal side effects (EPSEs)[5] and cognitive slowing;[16,17] (iii) smoking serves as a means of structuring the day (a behavioural filler); (iv) smoking arises as a result of a familial vulnerability;[18] or (v) smoking may be used as a means of alleviating the deficit in auditory gaiting that is found in schizophrenia.[19] Nicotine may also improve working memory and attentional deficits.[20–22]

Nicotinic receptor agonists may have beneficial effects on neurocognition,[23,24] although none is licensed for this purpose. Note though that cholinergic agonists may exacerbate nicotine dependence.[25] Interestingly, the greater the occupancy of striatal D_2 receptors by antipsychotic drugs, the more likely the patient is to smoke.[26] This may partly explain the clinical observation that smoking cessation may be more achievable when clozapine (a weak dopamine antagonist) is prescribed in place of a conventional antipsychotic. It has been suggested that people with schizophrenia find it particularly difficult to tolerate nicotine withdrawal symptoms[6] (although some certainly can stop[27]). Switching to nicotine replacement therapy or vaping may thus be the preferred option.[28,29] A switch from tobacco smoking to vaping has been shown to be well tolerated even in severe mental illness.[30]

Depression and anxiety

Moderate consumption of nicotine is associated with pleasure and a decrease in anxiety and feelings of anger.[31] The mechanism of this anxiolytic effect is not understood. People who suffer from anxiety and/or depression are more likely to smoke[32] and find it more difficult to stop.[31,33] Nicotine itself might have antidepressant activity.[34] Nicotine withdrawal can precipitate or exacerbate depression in those with a history of the illness,[31] but cigarette smoking may directly increase the risk of depression.[35] A 2020 study suggested nicotine addiction and depression are independently linked.[36] Some studies suggest that stopping smoking ultimately improves depression and anxiety.[37,38] A 2020 Cochrane review[39] suggests smoking cessation is achievable in depressed smokers, but a later twin study found that depression made smoking cessation much less likely.[40]

Patients with depression are at increased risk of cardiovascular disease. By directly causing tachycardia and hypertension,[1] nicotine may, in theory, exacerbate this problem. More importantly, smoking tobacco is a well-known independent risk factor for cardiovascular disease, probably because it hastens atherosclerosis. Vaping, while not carcinogenic, increases risk of cardiovascular disease.[41]

Attention deficit hyperactivity disorder (ADHD)

People with ADHD are relatively more likely to use nicotine products.[42] Tobacco smoke contains monoamine oxidase inhibitors which may benefit ADHD symptoms.[43] There is ample evidence of complex pharmacodynamic interactions between nicotine and stimulant drugs.[44]

CHAPTER 12

Movement disorders and Parkinson's disease

By increasing dopaminergic neurotransmission, nicotine is thought to provide a protective effect against both drug-induced EPSEs and idiopathic Parkinson's disease. Smokers are less likely to suffer from antipsychotic-induced movement disorders than non-smokers[5] and use anticholinergic drugs less often.[6] Parkinson's disease occurs less frequently in smokers than in non-smokers and the onset of clinical symptoms is delayed.[5,45] This may reflect the inverse association between Parkinson's disease and sensation-seeking behavioural traits, rather than a direct effect of nicotine.[46] The protective effect may not be related to nicotine at all but rather to other compounds in tobacco smoke.[47]

Drug interactions

Polycyclic hydrocarbons in tobacco smoke are known to stimulate the hepatic microsomal enzyme system, particularly CYP1A2,[7] the enzyme responsible for the metabolism of many psychotropic drugs. Smoking can lower the blood levels of some drugs by more than 50%.[7] This can both affect efficacy and influence adverse effects and needs to be taken into account when making clinical decisions. The drugs most likely to be affected are clozapine,[48] fluphenazine, haloperidol, chlorpromazine, olanzapine, many tricyclic antidepressants, mirtazapine, fluvoxamine and propranolol. Vaping has no effect on hepatic enzyme function. See 'Smoking and psychotropic drugs' in Chapter 11.

Smoking cessation and withdrawal symptoms

Withdrawal symptoms occur within 6–12 hours of stopping smoking and include intense craving, depressed mood, insomnia, anxiety, restlessness, irritability, difficulty in concentrating and increased appetite. Nicotine withdrawal can be misdiagnosed as depression, anxiety, sleep disorders and mania.[49] Withdrawal can also exacerbate the symptoms of schizophrenia.[6]

See also 'Nicotine and smoking cessation' in Chapter 4.

References

1. Benowitz NL, et al. Cardiovascular effects of nasal and transdermal nicotine and cigarette smoking. *Hypertension* 2002; **39**:1107–1112.
2. Yevtushenko OO, et al. Influence of 5-HT2C receptor and leptin gene polymorphisms, smoking and drug treatment on metabolic disturbances in patients with schizophrenia. *Br J Psychiatry* 2008; **192**:424–428.
3. Anderson JE, et al. Treating tobacco use and dependence: an evidence-based clinical practice guideline for tobacco cessation. *Chest* 2002; **121**:932–941.
4. Berrettini W. Nicotine addiction. *Am J Psychiatry* 2008; **165**:1089–1092.
5. Goff DC, et al. Cigarette smoking in schizophrenia: relationship to psychopathology and medication side effects. *Am J Psychiatry* 1992; **149**:1189–1194.
6. Ziedonis DM, et al. Schizophrenia and nicotine use: report of a pilot smoking cessation program and review of neurobiological and clinical issues. *Schizophr Bull* 1997; **23**:247–254.
7. Lyon ER. A review of the effects of nicotine on schizophrenia and antipsychotic medications. *Psychiatr Serv* 1999; **50**:1346–1350.
8. Winterer G. Why do patients with schizophrenia smoke? *Curr OpinPsychiatry* 2010; **23**:112–119.
9. Sharma R, et al. Motivations and limitations associated with vaping among people with mental illness: a qualitative analysis of Reddit discussions. *Int J Environ Res Public Health* 2016; **14**:7.
10. Bianco CL. Rates of electronic cigarette use among adults with a chronic mental illness. *Addict Behav* 2019; **89**:1–4.
11. Bennett ME, et al. Tobacco smoking and nicotine vaping in persons with first episode psychosis. *Schizophr Res* 2024; **267**:141–149.
12. Han B, et al. Tobacco use, nicotine dependence, and cessation methods in US adults with psychosis. *JAMA Network Open* 2023; **6**:e234995.
13. Weiser M, et al. Higher rates of cigarette smoking in male adolescents before the onset of schizophrenia: a historical-prospective cohort study. *Am J Psychiatry* 2004; **161**:1219–1223.
14. Hunter A, et al. The effects of tobacco smoking, and prenatal tobacco smoke exposure, on risk of schizophrenia: a systematic review and meta-analysis. *Nicotine Tob Res* 2020; **22**:3–10.

15. Caponnetto P, et al. Tobacco smoking, related harm and motivation to quit smoking in people with schizophrenia spectrum disorders. *Health Psychol Res* 2020; 8:9042.

16. Harris JG, et al. Effects of nicotine on cognitive deficits in schizophrenia. *Neuropsychopharmacology* 2004; 29:1378–1385.

17. Gupta T, et al. Nicotine usage is associated with elevated processing speed, spatial working memory, and visual learning performance in youth at ultra high-risk for psychosis. *Psychiatry Res* 2014; 220:687–690.

18. Ferchiou A, et al. Exploring the relationships between tobacco smoking and schizophrenia in first-degree relatives. *Psychiatry Res* 2012; 200:674–678.

19. McEvoy JP, et al. Smoking and therapeutic response to clozapine in patients with schizophrenia. *Biol Psychiatry* 1999; 46:125–129.

20. Jacobsen LK, et al. Nicotine effects on brain function and functional connectivity in schizophrenia. *Biol Psychiatry* 2004; 55:850–858.

21. Sacco KA, et al. Effects of cigarette smoking on spatial working memory and attentional deficits in schizophrenia: involvement of nicotinic receptor mechanisms. *Arch Gen Psychiatry* 2005; 62:649–659.

22. Smith RC, et al. Effects of nicotine nasal spray on cognitive function in schizophrenia. *Neuropsychopharmacology* 2006; 31:637–643.

23. Olincy A, et al. Proof-of-concept trial of an alpha7 nicotinic agonist in schizophrenia. *Arch Gen Psychiatry* 2006; 63:630–638.

24. Lieberman JA, et al. Cholinergic agonists as novel treatments for schizophrenia: the promise of rational drug development for psychiatry. *Am J Psychiatry* 2008; 165:931–936.

25. Kelly DL, et al. Lack of beneficial galantamine effect for smoking behavior: a double-blind randomized trial in people with schizophrenia. *Schizophr Res* 2008; 103:161–168.

26. De Haan L, et al. Occupancy of dopamine D2 receptors by antipsychotic drugs is related to nicotine addiction in young patients with schizophrenia. *Psychopharmacology (Berl)* 2006; 183:500–505.

27. Gilbody S, et al. Smoking cessation for people with severe mental illness (SCIMITAR+): a pragmatic randomised controlled trial. *Lancet Psychiatry* 2019; 6:379–390.

28. Caponnetto P, et al. Impact of an electronic cigarette on smoking reduction and cessation in schizophrenic smokers: a prospective 12-month pilot study. *Int J Environ Res Public Health* 2013; 10:446–461.

29. Kozak K, et al. Pharmacotherapy for smoking cessation in schizophrenia: a systematic review. *Expert Opin Pharmacother* 2020; 21:581–590.

30. Hickling LM, et al. A pre-post pilot study of electronic cigarettes to reduce smoking in people with severe mental illness. *Psychol Med* 2019; 49:1033–1040.

31. Glassman AH. Cigarette smoking: implications for psychiatric illness. *Am J Psychiatry* 1993; 150:546–553.

32. Cai J, et al. E-cigarette use or dual use of E-cigarette and combustible cigarette and mental health and cognitive impairment: findings from the National Health Interview Survey, 2020–2021. *J Affect Disord* 2024; 351:878–887.

33. Wilhelm K, et al. Clinical aspects of nicotine dependence and depression. *Med Today* 2004; 5:40–47.

34. Gandelman JA, et al. Transdermal nicotine for the treatment of mood and cognitive symptoms in nonsmokers with late-life depression. *J Clin Psychiatry* 2018; 79:18m12137.

35. Boden JM, et al. Cigarette smoking and depression: tests of causal linkages using a longitudinal birth cohort. *Br J Psychiatry* 2010; 196:440–446.

36. Bainter T, et al. A key indicator of nicotine dependence is associated with greater depression symptoms, after accounting for smoking behavior. *PLoS One* 2020; 15:e0233656.

37. Taylor G, et al. Change in mental health after smoking cessation: systematic review and meta-analysis. *BMJ* 2014; 348:g1151.

38. Cather C, et al. Improved depressive symptoms in adults with schizophrenia during a smoking cessation attempt with varenicline and behavioral therapy. *J Dual Diagn* 2017; 13:168–178.

39. Van der Meer RM, et al. Smoking cessation interventions for smokers with current or past depression. *Cochrane Database Syst Rev* 2013; 8:CD006102.

40. Ranjit A, et al. Depressive symptoms predict smoking cessation in a 20-year longitudinal study of adult twins. *Addict Behav* 2020; 108:106427.

41. Zong H, et al. Electronic cigarettes and cardiovascular disease: epidemiological and biological links. *Pflugers Arch* 2024; 476:875–888.

42. Xu G, et al. Association of attention-deficit/hyperactivity disorder with E-cigarette use. *Am J Prev Med* 2021; 60:488–496.

43. Taylor MR, et al. Tobacco and ADHD: a role of MAO-inhibition in nicotine dependence and alleviation of ADHD symptoms. *Front Neurosci* 2022; 16:845646.

44. McNealy KR, et al. The co-use of nicotine and prescription psychostimulants: a review of their behavioral and neuropharmacological interactions. *Drug Alcohol Depend* 2023; 248:109906.

45. Scott WK, et al. Family-based case-control study of cigarette smoking and Parkinson disease. *Neurology* 2005; 64:442–447.

46. Evans AH, et al. Relationship between impulsive sensation seeking traits, smoking, alcohol and caffeine intake, and Parkinson's disease. *J Neurol Neurosurg Psychiatry* 2006; 77:317–321.

47. Rose KN, et al. Clearing the smoke: what protects smokers from Parkinson's disease? *Mov Disord* 2024; 39:267–272.

48. Derenne JL, et al. Clozapine toxicity associated with smoking cessation: case report. *Am J Ther* 2005; 12:469–471.

49. Conti AA, et al. Severity of negative mood and anxiety symptoms occurring during acute abstinence from tobacco: a systematic review and meta-analysis. *Neurosci Biobehav Rev* 2020; 115:48–63.

CHAPTER 12

Chapter 13

Psychotropic drugs in special conditions

Psychotropics in overdose

Suicide attempts and suicidal gestures are frequently encountered in psychiatric and general practice, and psychotropic drugs are often taken in overdose (Table 13.1). This section gives brief details of the toxicity in overdose of commonly used psychotropics. It is intended to help guide drug choice in those thought to be at risk of suicide, to give some indication of safe quantities to prescribe and to help identify symptoms of overdose. This section gives no information on the treatment of psychotropic overdose and readers are directed to specialist poisons centres. In all cases of suspected overdose, urgent referral to acute medical facilities is, of course, strongly advised.

Table 13.1 Psychotropic drugs in overdose.

Drug or drug group	Toxicity in overdose*	Smallest dose likely to cause death	Signs and symptoms of overdose
Antidepressants			
Agomelatine[1,2]	Low	No deaths reported. In early trials, 800mg was maximum tolerated dose. EU SPC reports no serious effects from 2.45g overdose. A mixed overdose of 7.5g caused only drowsiness and mild tachycardia.	Sedation, agitation, stomach pains, dizziness
Brexanolone[3]	Not known	No deaths reported. Two cases of accidental overdose due to pump malfunction.	Sudden loss of consciousness

(Continued)

The Maudsley® Prescribing Guidelines in Psychiatry, Fifteenth Edition. David M. Taylor, Thomas R. E. Barnes and Allan H. Young.
© 2025 David M. Taylor. Published 2025 by John Wiley & Sons Ltd.

Table 13.1 (*Continued*)

Drug or drug group	Toxicity in overdose*	Smallest dose likely to cause death	Signs and symptoms of overdose
Bupropion[4–7]	Moderate	Around 4.5g, although largest overdose of 15g was not fatal.[3,8]	Tachycardia, seizures, QRS prolongation, QT prolongation, arrhythmia. Agitation and toxic psychosis also reported. Fatal serotonin syndrome may occur if taken with venlafaxine.[9]
Dextromethorphan and bupropion[3]	Probably moderate	Unclear. Bupropion inhibits metabolism of the dextromethorphan which may result in more severe/persistent overdose.	Bupropion: as above Dextromethorphan: nausea, vomiting, stupor, coma, respiratory depression, seizures, tachycardia, hyperexcitability, toxic psychosis
Duloxetine[10–13]	Low	Unclear – no deaths from single overdose reported but involved in numerous mixed overdose deaths.	Drowsiness, bradycardia, hypotension May be asymptomatic
Esketamine[14]	Not known	Unclear. No deaths reported.	Predicted to mirror ketamine overdose including sedation, hypertension, tachycardia, respiratory depression.[15]
Ketamine[16]	Moderate	Iatrogenic overdoses of up to 50mg/kg IV are not usually fatal if prompt treatment is given. Mechanical ventilation may be required. Illicit overdose is rarely fatal unless other drugs present.[15]	Sedation, respiratory depression, hypertension, tachycardia
Lofepramine[17,18]	Low	Unclear. Fatality unlikely if lofepramine taken alone.	Sedation, coma, tachycardia, hypotension
MAOIs[17,19–21] (not moclobemide)	High	Phenelzine – 400mg Tranylcypromine – 200mg	Tremor, weakness, confusion, sweating, tachycardia, hypertension
Mianserin[22–24]	Low	Unclear but probably more than 1000mg. Fatality unlikely if mianserin taken alone.	Sedation, coma, hypotension, hypertension, tachycardia, possible QT prolongation
Mirtazapine[4,25–28]	Low	Fatality unlikely in overdose of mirtazapine alone. One death reported following overdose with 990mg.[29]	Sedation. Even large overdose may be asymptomatic. Tachycardia/ hypertension sometimes seen. Agitation.
Moclobemide[30,31]	Low	Unclear, but probably more than 8g. Fatality unlikely if moclobemide taken alone.	Vomiting, sedation, disorientation
Reboxetine[4,32]	Low	Not known. Fatality unlikely in overdose of reboxetine alone.	Sweating, tachycardia, changes in blood pressure
SSRIs[18,33–36]	Low	Unclear. Probably above 1–2g. Fatality unlikely if SSRI taken alone.	Vomiting, tremor, drowsiness, tachycardia, ST depression. Seizures and QT prolongation possible. Citalopram most toxic of SSRIs in overdose[28,37] (coma, seizures, arrhythmia); escitalopram is less toxic.[38,39]

Table 13.1 (*Continued*)

Drug or drug group	Toxicity in overdose*	Smallest dose likely to cause death	Signs and symptoms of overdose
Trazodone[11,40–43]	Low	Unclear but probably more than 10g. Fatality unlikely in overdose of trazodone alone. Mortality rate about 1 in 10,000 overdose exposures.[28]	Drowsiness, nausea, hypotension, dizziness. Rarely QT prolongation, arrhythmia.
Tricyclics[17,19,20,44] (not lofepramine)	High	Around 500mg. Doses over 50mg/kg usually fatal.	Sedation, coma, tachycardia, arrhythmia (QRS, QT prolongation), hypotension, seizures
Venlafaxine[4,45–48] (desvenlafaxine causes similar effects but may be less toxic[49])	Moderate	Probably above 5g, but seizures may occur after ingestion of 1g	Vomiting, sedation, tachycardia, hypertension, seizures, acidosis, hypoglycaemia. Rarely QT prolongation, arrhythmia, rhabdomyolysis. Very rarely cardiac arrest/MI, heart failure.
Vilazodone[50,51]	Low	Doses below 300mg are not fatal. No fatalities recorded in 714 overdose exposures.[28]	Drowsiness, agitation, vomiting, seizures
Vortioxetine[52]	Low	Unclear. An overdose of 250mg caused no symptoms.	Nausea, somnolence, diarrhoea, pruritis

Antipsychotics

Drug or drug group	Toxicity in overdose*	Smallest dose likely to cause death	Signs and symptoms of overdose
Amisulpride[53–55]	Moderate	Around 16g	QT prolongation, arrhythmia, cardiac arrest
Aripiprazole[56–58]	Low	Unclear. Fatality unlikely when taken alone.	Sedation, lethargy, GI disturbance, drooling
Asenapine[59]	Probably low	Unclear. No deaths from overdose reported. Oral absorption very limited.	Sedation, confusion, facial dystonia, benign ECG changes
Brexpiprazole[3]	Probably low	No information available	Presumably agitation and nausea
Butyrophenones[60–62] (e.g. haloperidol)	Moderate	Haloperidol – probably above 500mg. Arrhythmia may occur at 300mg.	Sedation, coma, dystonia, NMS, QT prolongation, arrhythmia
Cariprazine[63]	Low	EU SPC reports one (non-fatal) overdose of 48mg	Sedation, low blood pressure
Clozapine[64,65]	Moderate	Around 2g, but very much lower in those not tolerant to its effects[66]	Lethargy, coma, tachycardia, hypotension, hypersalivation, pneumonia, seizures
Iloperidone[67–69]	Probably moderate	Unclear but probably more than 500mg.	Potent effect on QT interval. Sedation, tachycardia, respiratory depression, hypotension likely
Lumateperone[70]	Probably low	No overdoses reported	Presumably sedation and dizziness

(*Continued*)

Table 13.1 (*Continued*)

Drug or drug group	Toxicity in overdose*	Smallest dose likely to cause death	Signs and symptoms of overdose
Lurasidone[71]	Low	Unclear. An overdose of 1360mg was not fatal.[72] One study reported no deaths in 821 overdose exposures.[28]	Very limited information. Minimal effect on QT interval.
Olanzapine[64,73–76]	Moderate	Unclear. Fatal outcomes have been reported for acute overdoses as low as 450mg.	Lethargy, confusion, myoclonus, myopathy, hypotension, tachycardia, delirium. Possibly QT prolongation.
Olanzapine and samidorphan[3]	Moderate	Unclear. An overdose of 110mg/110mg was not fatal. Possible altered risk of fatality in opioid overdose due to opioid blockade.	As for olanzapine
Phenothiazines[60,77–79] (e.g. chlorpromazine, fluphenazine)	Moderate	Chlorpromazine 5–10g	Sedation, coma, tachycardia, arrhythmia, pulmonary oedema, hypotension, QT prolongation, seizures, dystonia, NMS
Pimavanserin[80]	Not known	No overdoses reported but pimavanserin prolongs QT interval in clinical doses.	Probably QT prolongation and arrhythmia. ?Nausea, vomiting, confusion.[81]
Quetiapine[28,64,82,83]	Moderate	Unclear. Probably more than 5g. Fatalities can occur in single substance overdose.	Lethargy, delirium, tachycardia, QT prolongation, respiratory depression, hypotension, rhabdomyolysis, NMS
Risperidone[64,84,85] (assume the same for paliperidone)	Low	Unclear. Fatality rare in those taking risperidone or paliperidone alone.	Lethargy, dystonia, tachycardia, changes in blood pressure, QT prolongation. Renal failure with paliperidone.
Ziprasidone[86–91]	Low	Around 10g. Fatality unlikely when taken alone.	Drowsiness, lethargy, QT prolongation, Torsades de pointes

Mood stabilisers

Drug or drug group	Toxicity in overdose*	Smallest dose likely to cause death	Signs and symptoms of overdose
Carbamazepine[92–94]	Moderate	Around 20g, but seizures may occur at around 5g; an overdose of 44g was not fatal.	Somnolence, coma, respiratory depression, ataxia, seizures, tachycardia, arrhythmia, electrolyte disturbance
Lamotrigine[95,96]	Low	At least 4g. Two deaths reported – one after 4g, the other after 7.5g, but overdoses of >40g have not proved fatal.	Drowsiness, vomiting, ataxia, seizures, tachycardia, dyskinesia, QT prolongation
Lithium[97–99]	Moderate	Chronic toxicity probably more dangerous but single overdose is occasionally fatal. Six acute overdose deaths recorded in UK 2005–2012.[100]	Nausea, diarrhoea, tremor, confusion, weakness, lethargy, seizures, coma, cardiovascular collapse, bradycardia, arrhythmia, heart block, renal failure
Valproate[101–105]	Moderate	Unclear but probably more than 20g. Doses over 400mg/kg cause severe toxicity.	Somnolence, coma, cerebral oedema, respiratory depression, blood dyscrasia, hypotension, hypothermia, seizures, electrolyte disturbance (hyperammonaemia)

Table 13.1 *(Continued)*

Drug or drug group	Toxicity in overdose*	Smallest dose likely to cause death	Signs and symptoms of overdose
Others			
Benzodiazepines[106–108]	Low	Probably more than 100mg diazepam equivalents. Often involved in fatal mixed overdose but can be fatal when taken alone. Alprazolam is most toxic.	Drowsiness, ataxia, nystagmus, respiratory dysarthria, depression, coma
Buspirone[28]	Low	Limited data. Deaths not reported.	Not known
Daridorexant[3]	Not known	No overdoses reported. In trials, 200mg was maximum dose.	Not known. Likely increased somnolence, muscle weakness, cataplexy-like symptoms, headache.
Lemborexant[3]	Not known	No overdoses reported. In trials, 75mg was maximum dose.	Not known. Likely increased somnolence.
Methadone[109–111]	High	20–50mg may be fatal in non-users. Co-ingestion of benzodiazepines increases toxicity.	Drowsiness, nausea, hypotension, respiratory depression, coma, pulmonary oedema, constricted pupils, rhabdomyolysis
Modafinil[112–114]	Low	Unclear, but no fatalities reported. Overdoses of >6g have not caused death.	Tachycardia, insomnia, agitation, anxiety, nausea, hypertension, dystonia
Pitolisant[115]	Not known	No overdoses reported. In trials, 216mg was maximum dose.	Probably QT prolongation, headache, insomnia, irritability, nausea, abdominal pain
Pregabalin[116–118]	Low	Often involved in fatal mixed overdose (e.g. with opiates) but can be fatal when taken alone. One overdose of 8.4g caused unconsciousness and coma.	May be asymptomatic. Sedation and coma may occur
Solriamfetol[3]	Not known	No overdoses reported. In trials, 1200mg was maximum dose.	Probably hypertension, tachycardia, QT prolongation
Suvorexant[114,119]	Low	Unclear. No deaths reported. An overdose of 100mg caused enhanced sedation.	Sedation, vomiting
Zolpidem[120–122]	Low	Unclear. Probably >200mg, but an overdose of 9g was not fatal. Fatality rare in those taking zolpidem alone.	Drowsiness, agitation, respiratory depression, tachycardia, coma, absent brainstem reflexes
Zopiclone[106,123,124]	Low	Unclear. Probably >100mg. Fatality rare in those taking zopiclone alone.	Ataxia, nausea, diplopia, drowsiness, coma

* High = less than 1 week's supply likely to cause serious toxicity or death.
Moderate = 1–4 weeks' supply likely to cause serious toxicity or death.
Low = death or serious toxicity unlikely even if more than 1 month's supply taken.
GI, gastrointestinal; IV, intravenous; MAOIs, monoamine oxidase inhibitors; MI, myocardial infarction; NMS, neuroleptic malignant syndrome; SPC, summary of product characteristics.

CHAPTER 13

References

1. Howland RH. Critical appraisal and update on the clinical utility of agomelatine, a melatonergic agonist, for the treatment of major depressive disease in adults. *Neuropsychiatr Dis Treat* 2009; 5:563–576.
2. Wong A, et al. Agomelatine overdose and related toxicity. *Toxicol Commun* 2018; 2:62–65.
3. US Food and Drug Administration. Drugs@FDA: FDA-approved drugs. 2023; https://www.accessdata.fda.gov/scripts/cder/daf.
4. Buckley NA, et al. 'Atypical' antidepressants in overdose: clinical considerations with respect to safety. *Drug Saf* 2003; 26:539–551.
5. Mercerolle M, et al. A fatal case of bupropion (Zyban) overdose. *J Anal Toxicol* 2008; 32:192–196.
6. Murray B, et al. Single-agent bupropion exposures: clinical characteristics and an atypical cause of serotonin toxicity. *J Med Toxicol* 2020; 16:12–16.
7. Overberg A, et al. Toxicity of bupropion overdose compared with selective serotonin reuptake inhibitors. *Pediatrics* 2019; 144:e20183295.
8. Robinson S. Treatment of status epilepticus and prolonged QT after massive intentional bupropion overdose with lidocaine. *Am J Emerg Med* 2022; 55:232.e3–232.e4.
9. Alibegović A, et al. Fatal overdose with a combination of SNRIs venlafaxine and duloxetine. *Forensic Sci Med Pathol* 2019; 15:258–261.
10. Menchetti M, et al. Non-fatal overdose of duloxetine in combination with other antidepressants and benzodiazepines. *World J Biol Psychiatry* 2009; 10:385–389.
11. White N, et al. Suicidal antidepressant overdoses: a comparative analysis by antidepressant type. *J Med Toxicol* 2008; 4:238–250.
12. Darracq MA, et al. A retrospective review of isolated duloxetine-exposure cases. *Clin Toxicol (Phila)* 2013; 51:106–110.
13. Scanlon KA, et al. Comprehensive duloxetine analysis in a fatal overdose. *J Anal Toxicol* 2016; 40:167–170.
14. Janssen-Cilag Ltd. Summary of product characteristics. Spravato 28 mg nasal spray, solution. 2023; https://www.medicines.org.uk/emc/product/10977/smpc.
15. Corkery JM, et al. Recreational ketamine-related deaths notified to the National Programme on Substance Abuse Deaths, England, 1997–2019. *J Psychopharmacol* 2021; 35:1324–1348.
16. Green SM, et al. Inadvertent ketamine overdose in children: clinical manifestations and outcome. *Ann Emerg Med* 1999; 34:492–497.
17. Cassidy S, et al. Fatal toxicity of antidepressant drugs in overdose. *BMJ* 1987; 295:1021–1024.
18. Henry JA, et al. Relative mortality from overdose of antidepressants. *BMJ* 1995; 310:221–224.
19. Crome P. Antidepressant overdosage. *Drugs* 1982; 23:431–461.
20. Henry JA. Epidemiology and relative toxicity of antidepressant drugs in overdose. *Drug Saf* 1997; 16:374–390.
21. Waring WS, et al. Acute myocarditis after massive phenelzine overdose. *Eur J Clin Pharmacol* 2007; 63:1007–1009.
22. Chand S, et al. One hundred cases of acute intoxication with mianserin hydrochloride. *Pharmacopsychiatry* 1981; 14:15–17.
23. Scherer D, et al. Inhibition of cardiac hERG potassium channels by tetracyclic antidepressant mianserin. *Naunyn Schmiedebergs Arch Pharmacol* 2008; 378:73–83.
24. Koseoglu Z, et al. Bradycardia and hypotension in mianserin intoxication. *Hum Exp Toxicol* 2010; 29:887–888.
25. Bremner JD, et al. Safety of mirtazapine in overdose. *J Clin Psychiatry* 1998; 59:233–235.
26. LoVecchio F, et al. Outcomes after isolated mirtazapine (Remeron) supratherapeutic ingestions. *J Emerg Med* 2008; 34:77–78.
27. Berling I, et al. Mirtazapine overdose is unlikely to cause major toxicity. *Clin Toxicol (Phila)* 2014; 52:20–24.
28. Nelson JC, et al. Morbidity and mortality associated with medications used in the treatment of depression: an analysis of cases reported to U.S. Poison Control Centers, 2000–2014. *Am J Psychiatry* 2017; 174:438–450.
29. Vignali C, et al. Mirtazapine fatal poisoning. *Forensic Sci Int* 2017; 276:e8–e12.
30. Hetzel W. Safety of moclobemide taken in overdose for attempted suicide. *Psychopharmacology (Berl)* 1992; 106 Suppl:S127–S129.
31. Myrenfors PG, et al. Moclobemide overdose. *J Intern Med* 1993; 233:113–115.
32. Baldwin DS, et al. Tolerability and safety of reboxetine. *Rev Contemp Pharmacother* 2000; 11:321–330.
33. Cheeta S, et al. Antidepressant-related deaths and antidepressant prescriptions in England and Wales, 1998–2000. *Br J Psychiatry* 2004; 184:41–47.
34. Barbey JT, et al. SSRI safety in overdose. *J Clin Psychiatry* 1998; 59 Suppl 15:42–48.
35. Jimmink A, et al. Clinical toxicology of citalopram after acute intoxication with the sole drug or in combination with other drugs: overview of 26 cases. *Ther Drug Monit* 2008; 30:365–371.
36. Tarabar AF, et al. Citalopram overdose: late presentation of torsades de pointes (TdP) with cardiac arrest. *J Med Toxicol* 2008; 4:101–105.
37. Kraai EP, et al. Citalopram overdose: a fatal case. *J Med Toxicol* 2015; 11:232–236.
38. Yilmaz Z, et al. Escitalopram causes fewer seizures in human overdose than citalopram. *Clin Toxicol (Phila)* 2010; 48:207–212.
39. van Gorp F, et al. Clinical and ECG effects of escitalopram overdose. *Ann Emerg Med* 2009; 54:404–408.
40. Gamble DE, et al. Trazodone overdose: four years of experience from voluntary reports. *J Clin Psychiatry* 1986; 47:544–546.
41. Martinez MA, et al. Investigation of a fatality due to trazodone poisoning: case report and literature review. *J Anal Toxicol* 2005; 29:262–268.
42. Dattilo PB, et al. Prolonged QT associated with an overdose of trazodone. *J Clin Psychiatry* 2007; 68:1309–1310.
43. Service JA, et al. QT prolongation and delayed atrioventricular conduction caused by acute ingestion of trazodone. *Clin Toxicol (Phila)* 2008; 46:71–73.
44. Caksen H, et al. Acute amitriptyline intoxication: an analysis of 44 children. *Hum Exp Toxicol* 2006; 25:107–110.
45. Howell C, et al. Cardiovascular toxicity due to venlafaxine poisoning in adults: a review of 235 consecutive cases. *Br J Clin Pharmacol* 2007; 64:192–197.
46. Hojer J, et al. Fatal cardiotoxicity induced by venlafaxine overdosage. *Clin Toxicol (Phila)* 2008; 46:336–337.
47. Taylor D. Venlafaxine and cardiovascular toxicity. *BMJ* 2010; 340:327.

48. Bekka E, et al. Dose-related hypoglycemia in venlafaxine poisoning: a retrospective cohort study. *Clin Toxicol (Phila)* 2022; **60**:1336–1344.

49. Cooper JM, et al. Desvenlafaxine overdose and the occurrence of serotonin toxicity, seizures and cardiovascular effects. *Clin Toxicol (Phila)* 2017; **55**:18–24.

50. Russell JL, et al. Pediatric ingestion of vilazodone compared to other selective serotonin reuptake inhibitor medications. *Clin Toxicol (Phila)* 2017; **55**:352–356.

51. Allergan USA Inc. Highlights of prescribing information: VIIBRYD (vilazodone hydrochloride) tablets for oral use. 2023; https://www.allergan.com/assets/pdf/viibryd_pi.

52. Mazza MG, et al. Vortioxetine overdose in a suicidal attempt: a case report. *Medicine (Baltimore)* 2018; **97**:e10788.

53. Isbister GK, et al. Amisulpride deliberate self-poisoning causing severe cardiac toxicity including QT prolongation and torsades de pointes. *Med J Aust* 2006; **184**:354–356.

54. Ward DI. Two cases of amisulpride overdose: a cause for prolonged QT syndrome. *Emerg Med Australas* 2005; **17**:274–276.

55. Isbister GK, et al. Amisulpride overdose is frequently associated with QT prolongation and torsades de pointes. *J Clin Psychopharmacol* 2010; **30**:391–395.

56. Lofton AL, et al. Atypical experience: a case series of pediatric aripiprazole exposures. *Clin Toxicol (Phila)* 2005; **43**:151–153.

57. Carstairs SD, et al. Overdose of aripiprazole, a new type of antipsychotic. *J Emerg Med* 2005; **28**:311–313.

58. Forrester MB. Aripiprazole exposures reported to Texas poison control centers during 2002–2004. *J Toxicol Environ Health A* 2006; **69**:1719–1726.

59. Taylor JE, et al. A case of intentional asenapine overdose. *Prim Care Companion CNS Disord* 2013; **15**:PCC.13l01547.

60. Haddad PM, et al. Antipsychotic-related QTc prolongation, torsade de pointes and sudden death. *Drugs* 2002; **62**:1649–1671.

61. Levine BS, et al. Two fatalities involving haloperidol. *J Anal Toxicol* 1991; **15**:282–284.

62. Henderson RA, et al. Life-threatening ventricular arrhythmia (torsades de pointes) after haloperidol overdose. *Hum Exp Toxicol* 1991; **10**:59–62.

63. Recordati Pharmaceuticals Limited. Summary of product characteristics. Reagila (cariprazine) 1.5mg, 3mg, 4.5mg and 6mg hard capsules. 2024 (last accessed August 2024); https://www.medicines.org.uk/emc/product/9401/smpc.

64. Trenton A, et al. Fatalities associated with therapeutic use and overdose of atypical antipsychotics. *CNS Drugs* 2003; **17**:307–324.

65. Flanagan RJ, et al. Suspected clozapine poisoning in the UK/Eire, 1992–2003. *Forensic Sci Int* 2005; **155**:91–99.

66. Shigeev SV, et al. [Clozapine intoxication: theoretical aspects and forensic-medical examination]. *Sud Med Ekspert* 2013; **56**:41–46.

67. Vigneault P, et al. Iloperidone (Fanapt®), a novel atypical antipsychotic, is a potent HERG blocker and delays cardiac ventricular repolarization at clinically relevant concentration. *Pharmacol Res* 2012; **66**:60–65.

68. Vanda Pharmaceuticals Inc. Highlights of prescribing information: FANAPT® (iloperidone) tablets. 2021; https://www.fanapt.com/product/pi/pdf/fanapt.pdf.

69. Amon J, et al. A case of iloperidone overdose in a 27-year-old man with cocaine abuse. *SAGE Open Med Case Rep* 2016; **4**:2050313x16660485.

70. Vyas P, et al. An evaluation of lumateperone tosylate for the treatment of schizophrenia. *Expert Opin Pharmacother* 2020; **21**:139–145.

71. CNX Therapeutics Ltd (formerly Sunovion Pharmaceuticals Europe). Summary of product characteristics. Latuda 18.5mg, 37mg and 74mg film-coated tablets. 2022 (last accessed December 2023); https://www.medicines.org.uk/emc/product/3299/smpc.

72. Molnar GP, et al. Acute lurasidone overdose. *J Clin Psychopharmacol* 2014; **34**:768–770.

73. Chue P, et al. A review of olanzapine-associated toxicity and fatality in overdose. *J Psychiatry Neurosci* 2003; **28**:253–261.

74. Waring WS, et al. Olanzapine overdose is associated with acute muscle toxicity. *Hum Exp Toxicol* 2006; **25**:735–740.

75. Morissette P, et al. Olanzapine prolongs cardiac repolarization by blocking the rapid component of the delayed rectifier potassium current. *J Psychopharmacol* 2007; **21**:735–741.

76. Krka US Ltd. Summary of product characteristics. Olanzapine 2.5mg, 5mg, 7.5mg, 10mg, 20mg tablets. 2023 (last accessed August 2024); https://www.medicines.org.uk/emc/product/14727/smpc.

77. Buckley NA, et al. Cardiotoxicity more common in thioridazine overdose than with other neuroleptics. *J Toxicol Clin Toxicol* 1995; **33**:199–204.

78. Li C, et al. Acute pulmonary edema induced by overdosage of phenothiazines. *Chest* 1992; **101**:102–104.

79. Flanagan RJ. Fatal toxicity of drugs used in psychiatry. *Hum Psychopharmacol* 2008; **23** Suppl 1:43–51.

80. Sahli ZT, et al. Pimavanserin: novel pharmacotherapy for Parkinson's disease psychosis. *Exp Opin Drug Discov* 2018; **13**:103–110.

81. Vanover KE, et al. Pharmacokinetics, tolerability, and safety of ACP-103 following single or multiple oral dose administration in healthy volunteers. *J Clin Pharmacol* 2007; **47**:704–714.

82. Ngo A, et al. Acute quetiapine overdose in adults: a 5-year retrospective case series. *Ann Emerg Med* 2008; **52**:541–547.

83. Bertol E, et al. Overdose of quetiapine – a case report with QT prolongation. *Toxics* 2021; **9**:339.

84. Liang CS, et al. Acute renal failure after paliperidone overdose: a case report. *J Clin Psychopharmacol* 2012; **32**:128.

85. Lapid MI, et al. Acute dystonia associated with paliperidone overdose. *Psychosomatics* 2011; **52**:291–294.

86. Gomez-Criado MS, et al. Ziprasidone overdose: cases recorded in the database of Pfizer-Spain and literature review. *Pharmacotherapy* 2005; **25**:1660–1665.

87. Arbuck DM. 12,800-mg ziprasidone overdose without significant ECG changes. *Gen Hosp Psychiatry* 2005; **27**:222–223.

88. Insa Gomez FJ, et al. Ziprasidone overdose: cardiac safety. *Actas Esp Psiquiatr* 2005; **33**:398–400.

89. Klein-Schwartz W, et al. Prospective observational multi-poison center study of ziprasidone exposures. *Clin Toxicol (Phila)* 2007; **45**:782–786.

90. Tan HH, et al. A systematic review of cardiovascular effects after atypical antipsychotic medication overdose. *Am J Emerg Med* 2009; **27**:607–616.

91. Alipour A, et al. Torsade de pointes after ziprasidone overdose with coingestants. *J Clin Psychopharmacol* 2010; **30**:76–77.

92. Spiller HA. Management of carbamazepine overdose. *Pediatr Emerg Care* 2001; **17**:452–456.

93. Schmidt S, et al. Signs and symptoms of carbamazepine overdose. *J Neurol* 1995; **242**:169–173.

94. Pap C, et al. Severe carbamazepine overdose associated with shock, repeated seizures and extreme high serum concentrations treated by extended intermittent hemodiafiltration. 42nd International Congress of the European Association of Poisons Centres and Clinical Toxicologists (EAPCCT) 24–27 May 2022, Tallinn, Estonia. *Clin Toxicol* 2022; **60**:abstract 145.

95. Alabi A, et al. Safety profile of lamotrigine in overdose. *Ther Adv Psychopharmacol* 2016; **6**:369–381.

96. Alyahya B, et al. Acute lamotrigine overdose: a systematic review of published adult and pediatric cases. *Clin Toxicol (Phila)* 2018; **56**:81–89.

97. Tuohy K, et al. Acute lithium intoxication. *Dial Transplant* 2003; **32**:478–481.

98. Chen KP, et al. Implication of serum concentration monitoring in patients with lithium intoxication. *Psychiatry Clin Neurosci* 2004; **58**:25–29.

99. Offerman SR, et al. Hospitalized lithium overdose cases reported to the California Poison Control System. *Clin Toxicol (Phila)* 2010; **48**:443–448.

100. Ferrey AE, et al. Relative toxicity of mood stabilisers and antipsychotics: case fatality and fatal toxicity associated with self-poisoning. *BMC Psychiatry* 2018; **18**:399.

101. Isbister GK, et al. Valproate overdose: a comparative cohort study of self poisonings. *Br J Clin Pharmacol* 2003; **55**:398–404.

102. Spiller HA, et al. Multicenter case series of valproic acid ingestion: serum concentrations and toxicity. *J Toxicol Clin Toxicol* 2000; **38**:755–760.

103. Sztajnkrycer MD. Valproic acid toxicity: overview and management. *J Toxicol Clin Toxicol* 2002; **40**:789–801.

104. Eyer F, et al. Acute valproate poisoning: pharmacokinetics, alteration in fatty acid metabolism, and changes during therapy. *J Clin Psychopharmacol* 2005; **25**:376–380.

105. Robinson P, et al. Severe hypothermia in association with sodium valproate overdose. *NZ Med J* 2005; **118**:U1681.

106. Reith DM, et al. Comparison of the fatal toxicity index of zopiclone with benzodiazepines. *J Toxicol Clin Toxicol* 2003; **41**:975–980.

107. Isbister GK, et al. Alprazolam is relatively more toxic than other benzodiazepines in overdose. *Br J Clin Pharmacol* 2004; **58**:88–95.

108. Kleinman RA, et al. Benzodiazepine-involved overdose deaths in the USA: 2000–2019. *J Gen Intern Med* 2022; **37**:2103–2109.

109. Gable RS. Comparison of acute lethal toxicity of commonly abused psychoactive substances. *Addiction* 2004; **99**:686–696.

110. Caplehorn JR, et al. Fatal methadone toxicity: signs and circumstances, and the role of benzodiazepines. *Aust NZ J Public Health* 2002; **26**:358–362.

111. Martindale Pharma an Ethypharm Group Company. Summary of product characteristics. Methadone 5mg tablets. 2023; (last accessed August 2024) https://www.medicines.org.uk/emc/product/11838/smpc.

112. Spiller HA, et al. Toxicity from modafinil ingestion. *Clin Toxicol (Phila)* 2009; **47**:153–156.

113. Carstairs SD, et al. A retrospective review of supratherapeutic modafinil exposures. *J Med Toxicol* 2010; **6**:307–310.

114. Russell J, et al. Retrospective assessment of toxicity following exposure to Orexin pathway modulators modafinil and suvorexant. *Toxicol Commun* 2019; **3**:33–36.

115. Bioprojet UK Limited. Summary of product characteristics. Wakix 18 mg film-coated tablets (pitolisant). 2023; https://www.medicines.org.uk/emc/product/14454/smpc.

116. Miljevic C, et al. A case of pregabalin intoxication. *Psychiatriki* 2012; **23**:162–165.

117. Wood DM, et al. Significant pregabalin toxicity managed with supportive care alone. *J Med Toxicol* 2010; **6**:435–437.

118. Kriikku P, et al. Pregabalin and gabapentin in non-opioid poisoning deaths. *Forensic Sci Int* 2021; **324**:110830.

119. Trautman W, et al. Orexin antagonist overdose should not keep you up at night: mild toxicity in a large suvorexant overdose. *Clinical Toxicology* 2023; **61** Suppl 2: abstract 205. http://doi.org/10.1080/15563650.2023.2233835.

120. Gock SB, et al. Acute zolpidem overdose – report of two cases. *J Anal Toxicol* 1999; **23**:559–562.

121. Garnier R, et al. Acute zolpidem poisoning – analysis of 344 cases. *J Toxicol Clin Toxicol* 1994; **32**:391–404.

122. De Donatis D, et al. Extremely high-dosage zolpidem poisoning with favorable outcome. *J Clin Psychopharmacol* 2021; **41**:222–223.

123. Pounder D, et al. Zopiclone poisoning. *J Anal Toxicol* 1996; **20**:273–274.

124. Bramness JG, et al. Fatal overdose of zopiclone in an elderly woman with bronchogenic carcinoma. *J Forensic Sci* 2001; **46**:1247–1249.

Driving and psychotropic medicines

Everyone has a legal duty to drive safely and in almost all countries drivers are legally responsible for accidents they cause, whether or not they are under the influence of drugs or alcohol.[1]

Many factors have been shown to affect driving performance. These include age, gender, personality, physical and mental state and being under the influence of alcohol, prescribed medicines, street drugs or over-the-counter medicines.[2,3] Studying the effects of any of these individual factors in isolation is extremely difficult. Some studies have attempted to categorise medicinal drugs according to how they affect driving performance,[4] and some have assessed the effect of medication on tests such as response time and attention,[5] but these tests do not directly measure ability to drive.

As many as 10% of people killed or injured in road traffic accidents (RTAs) are taking psychotropic medication (Table 13.2).[5] Patients with personality disorders and alcoholism have the highest rates of motoring offences and are more likely to be involved in accidents.[5] In most countries, people whose driving ability may be impaired through their illness or prescribed medication are required to inform their motor insurer. Failure to do so is considered to be 'withholding a material fact' and may render the insurance policy void.

Effects of mental illness

In the UK, severe mental disorder is a so-called 'prescribed disability' for the purposes of the Road Traffic Act 1988.[6] Regulations define mental disorder as including mental illness, arrested or incomplete development of the mind, psychopathic disorder or severe impairment of intelligence or social functioning. There is an assessing fitness to drive guide.[7] Among physical conditions commonly seen in mental illness, licence restrictions may also apply to people with diabetes, particularly if treated with insulin or if there are established micro- or macrovascular complications. In the USA, regulations related to driving and mental health disorders vary somewhat from state to state (see US Department of Motor Vehicles website [www.dmvusa.com] for each state).

Many people with early dementia are capable of driving safely.[8,9] In the UK, all drivers with new diagnoses of Alzheimer's disease and other dementias must notify the Driver and Vehicle Licensing Agency (DVLA).[8] The doctor may need to make an immediate decision on safety to drive and ensure that the DVLA is notified.[10] There are no data to support ongoing driving assessments as a way of maintaining driving ability or improving road safety of drivers with dementia.[11,12] In the USA, some states mandate that doctors report a diagnosis of dementia but in others the issue may only arise on licence renewal. Interestingly, states in which reporting is mandatory have a relatively lower rate of dementia diagnosis.[13]

Psychiatric medicines, driving and UK law

Most countries prohibit the use of a range of illicit substances when driving. In the UK drug–driving law gives threshold blood concentration for eight drugs associated with illicit use (with a zero tolerance approach – the threshold is set to reveal any recent use) and eight medicinal drugs.[14] For the latter group, Table 13.3 gives the legal limit and expected plasma concentrations in clinical use.

CHAPTER 13

Table 13.2 Psychotropics and driving.

Drug group	Effect
Alcohol	Alcohol causes sedation and impaired co-ordination, vision, attention and information processing. Alcohol-dependent drivers are twice as likely to be involved in RTAs and offences than licensed drivers as a whole,[5] and a third of all fatal RTAs involve alcohol-dependent drivers.[5] Young drivers who use alcohol in combination with illicit drugs are particularly high risk.[15,16]
Antiseizure medications	Initial, dose-related adverse effects may affect driving ability (e.g. diplopia, ataxia and sedation). In most countries there are strict rules regarding epilepsy and driving that over-ride considerations of medication effects. Carbamazepine has minor adverse effects on driving.[17,18] Lamotrigine may have limited effects on driving ability.[19] Valproate may not increase the risk of RTAs.[20]
Antidepressants	People who are prescribed an antidepressant have an increased risk of being involved in an RTA.[21] SSRIs may have some advantages over TCAs but driving ability is still diminished compared with healthy individuals,[22] suggesting that depression itself may make a major contribution.[23,24] SSRIs tend not to impair driving in healthy volunteers.[25–27] In remitted patients on SSRIs, driving performance may likewise not be impaired.[28] Initiation effects caused by mirtazapine diminish to an extent when it is given as a single dose at night but many people experience substantial hangover which can impair driving.[29] Effects may disappear in chronic treatment.[30] Trazodone also appears to impair driving ability[31] – a review of 27 studies suggested that only trazodone among antidepressants afforded an increased risk of RTAs.[32] Agomelatine and venlafaxine may actually improve driving performance.[33] Vortioxetine has no effect.[30] Intranasal esketamine seems to have no effect on driving ability 8 hours post-dose[34] or the day after.[35]
Antipsychotics	Sedation and EPSEs can impair co-ordination and response time.[2] A high proportion of patients treated with antipsychotics may have an impaired ability to drive.[36,37] One study found patients with schizophrenia taking atypical antipsychotics or clozapine performed better in tests of skills related to car driving ability than patients with schizophrenia taking FGAs,[38] but 25% of all patients were severely impaired with respect to driving skills. SGAs seem to cause less impairment than FGAs[39] and are preferred.
Hypnotics and anxiolytics	Benzodiazepines cause sedation and impairment of attention, information processing, memory and motor co-ordination, and along with opiates are the medicines most frequently implicated in RTAs.[32,40] When used as anxiolytics and hypnotics, benzodiazepines, zopiclone and zolpidem are associated with an increased risk of RTAs.[40] There is some gender variation in the pharmacokinetics of zolpidem with females having higher drug plasma concentrations than males for any given dose; the driving ability of females may therefore be particularly impaired.[3] Zolpidem may additionally be associated with automatism and 'sleep driving'.[41] Zaleplon and the newer hypnotics acting at melatonin or serotonin receptors have not been found to have any negative residual effects on driving ability.[42,43] Orexin receptor antagonists (suvorexant and lemborexant), available in some countries, appear not to impair driving the day after being taken.[44,45] There is some evidence that daridorexant impairs driving ability during the first few days of use.[46]
Lithium	Lithium may impair visual adaptation to the dark[2] but the implications for driving safety are unknown. Many patients treated with lithium can be shown to be unfit to drive[19] although the exact contribution of lithium is difficult to determine. Elderly people who take lithium may be at increased risk of being involved in an injurious RTA.[47] Lithium causes a greater degree of driving impairment than lamotrigine.[39]
Methylphenidate	Some studies have demonstrated that reaction time is longer in patients with ADHD, which may in turn be associated with increased driving risks.[48] Other studies have found that methylphenidate improved driving performance in adults with ADHD,[49] again suggesting that illness may make a bigger contribution to fitness to drive than the specific pharmacology of the treatment.[49]
Opioids	Opioids have major adverse effect on the risk of RTAs.[50] Buprenorphine and methadone reduce driving ability at low doses in non-addicts.[51]

EPSEs, extrapyramidal side effects; RTAs, road traffic accidents; TCAs, tricyclic antidepressants.

Table 13.3 Benzodiazepines concentration in normal dosing and the UK legal limit.

Drug/daily dose	Range of concentrations reported	Legal limit
Clonazepam 0.5–6.0mg[52,53]	5–80mcg/L	50mcg/L
Diazepam 5–30mg[54]	50–1000mcg/L	550mcg/L
Flunitrazepam 0.5–2.0mg[55,56]	10–20mcg/L	300mcg/L
Lorazepam 1–4mg[57,58]	10–70mcg/L	100mcg/L
Oxazepam 15–30mg[59]	250–600mcg/L	300mcg/L
Temazepam 10–20mg[60]	200–900mcg/L	1000mcg/L

In regards to methadone, doses of up to 80mg a day generally give plasma levels below the UK legal limit.[61] The legal limits listed here apply only to those who are lawfully prescribed the drug in question – the driver may be subject to prosecution if it can be proved the drugs were taken illicitly.

Other medicines

Many psychotropics can impair alertness, concentration and driving performance. Medicines that block H_1, α_1-adrenergic or cholinergic receptors may be particularly problematic. Sedative antihistamines used in mental health conditions (promethazine, diphenhydramine) very probably impair driving ability.[62] Effects are particularly marked at the start of treatment and after increasing the dose. Drivers must be made aware of any potential for impairment and are advised to evaluate their driving performance at these times. They must stop driving if adversely affected.[63] The use of alcohol will further increase any impairment.

Some antipsychotics and antidepressants lower the seizure threshold. In the UK, the DVLA advises this is taken into consideration when prescribing for a driver.

Medication-induced sedation

Many psychotropics are sedating. The more sedating a medicine is, the more likely it is to impair driving ability. Other medicines, either prescribed or bought over the counter, may also be sedative and/or affect driving ability (e.g. antihistamines[5]). One study found that 89% of patients taking other psychotropics in addition to antidepressants failed a battery of 'fitness to drive' tests.[64] Since the degree of sedation any individual will experience is very difficult to predict, patients prescribed sedating medicines should be advised not to drive if they feel sedated. In the UK it is the responsibility of the driver to ensure they are fit to drive.

UK DVLA

Duty of the driver

In the UK it is the legal responsibility of the licence holder or applicant to notify the DVLA of any medical condition that may affect safe driving. A list of relevant medical conditions can be found in the DVLA assessing fitness to drive guide.[65]

Duty of the prescriber

Make sure the patient understands that their condition may impair their ability to drive. If the patient is incapable of understanding, notify the DVLA immediately. Explain to the patient that they have a legal duty to inform the DVLA.

Note that the DVLA guidance specifies that patients under Section 17 of the 1983 Mental Health Act must be able to satisfy the standards of fitness for their respective conditions and be free from any effects of medication that would affect driving adversely, before resuming driving. Very few patients will fulfil these criteria.

UK General Medical Council guidelines for prescribers[66]

- Patients who disagree with the diagnosis or the effect of the condition on their ability to drive should seek a second opinion and refrain from driving until this has been obtained.
- If the patient continues to drive while unfit, you should make every reasonable effort to persuade them to stop. This may include telling their next of kin if they agree you may do so.
- If they continue to drive, inform the DVLA. Tell the patient you are going to do this and write to the patient to confirm you have done so. Document the advice given clearly in the patient's notes.

References

1. Annas GJ. Doctors, drugs, and driving – tort liability for patient-caused accidents. *N Engl J Med* 2008; **359**:521–525.
2. Metzner JL, et al. Impairment in driving and psychiatric illness. *J Neuropsychiatry Clin Neurosci* 1993; **5**:211–220.
3. Farkas RH, et al. Zolpidem and driving impairment – identifying persons at risk. *N Engl J Med* 2013; **369**:689–691.
4. Ravera S, et al. A European approach to categorizing medicines for fitness to drive: outcomes of the DRUID project. *Br J Clin Pharmacol* 2012; **74**:920–931.
5. Noyes R, Jr. Motor vehicle accidents related to psychiatric impairment. *Psychosomatics* 1985; **26**:569–580.
6. The National Archives. Road Traffic Act 1991. 1991; http://www.legislation.gov.uk/ukpga/1991/40/contents.
7. Driver and Vehicle Licensing Agency. Guidance: assessing fitness to drive: a guide for medical professionals. 2016 (last updated February 2024, last checked May 2024); https://www.gov.uk/government/publications/assessing-fitness-to-drive-a-guide-for-medical-professionals.
8. Driver and Vehicle Licensing Agency. Assessing fitness to drive – a guide for medical professionals. 2016 (last updated 2018, last accessed May 2024). https://www.gov.uk/dvla/fitnesstodrive.
9. Piersma D, et al. Prediction of fitness to drive in patients with Alzheimer's dementia. *PLoS One* 2016; **11**:e0149566.
10. Breen DA, et al. Driving and dementia. *BMJ* 2007; **334**:1365–1369.
11. Martin AJ, et al. Driving assessment for maintaining mobility and safety in drivers with dementia. *Cochrane Database Syst Rev* 2013; **8**:CD006222.
12. Toups R, et al. Driving performance in older adults: current measures, findings, and implications for roadway safety. *Innov Aging* 2022; **6**:igab051.
13. Jun H, et al. State Department of Motor Vehicles reporting mandates of dementia diagnoses and dementia underdiagnosis. *JAMA Network Open* 2024; **7**:e248889.
14. Department for Transport. Changes to drug driving law. 2013 (last updated August 2017, last accessed May 2024); https://www.gov.uk/government/collections/drug-driving.
15. Biecheler MB, et al. SAM survey on 'drugs and fatal accidents': search of substances consumed and comparison between drivers involved under the influence of alcohol or cannabis. *Traffic Inj Prev* 2008; **9**:11–21.
16. Oyefeso A, et al. Fatal injuries while under the influence of psychoactive drugs: a cross-sectional exploratory study in England. *BMC Public Health* 2006; **6**:148.
17. Kaussner Y, et al. Effects of oxcarbazepine and carbamazepine on driving ability: a double-blind, randomized crossover trial with healthy volunteers. *Psychopharmacology (Berl)* 2010; **210**:53–63.
18. Ramaekers G, et al. A comparative study of the effects of carbamazepine and the NMDA receptor antagonist remacemide on road tracking and car-following performance in actual traffic. *Psychopharmacology (Berl)* 2002; **159**:203–210.
19. Segmiller FM, et al. Driving ability according to German guidelines in stabilized bipolar I and II outpatients receiving lithium or lamotrigine. *J Clin Pharmacol* 2013; **53**:459–462.

20. Bramness JG, et al. An increased risk of road traffic accidents after prescriptions of lithium or valproate? *Pharmacoepidemiol Drug Saf* 2009; **18**:492–496.

21. Olesen AV, et al. Use of psychotropic medication and risk of road traffic crashes: a registry-based case–control study in Denmark, 1996–2018. *Psychopharmacology (Berl)* 2022; **239**:2537–2546.

22. Brunnauer A, et al. The effects of most commonly prescribed second generation antidepressants on driving ability: a systematic review: 70th birthday Prof. Riederer. *J Neural Transm* 2013; **120**:225–232.

23. Bramness JG, et al. Minor increase in risk of road traffic accidents after prescriptions of antidepressants: a study of population registry data in Norway. *J Clin Psychiatry* 2008; **69**:1099–1103.

24. Verster JC, et al. Psychoactive medication and traffic safety. *Int J Environ Res Public Health* 2009; **6**:1041–1054.

25. Iwamoto K, et al. The effects of acute treatment with paroxetine, amitriptyline, and placebo on driving performance and cognitive function in healthy Japanese subjects: a double-blind crossover trial. *Hum Psychopharmacol* 2008; **23**:399–407.

26. Ridout F, et al. A placebo controlled investigation into the effects of paroxetine and mirtazapine on measures related to car driving performance. *Hum Psychopharmacol* 2003; **18**:261–269.

27. Wingen M, et al. Actual driving performance and psychomotor function in healthy subjects after acute and subchronic treatment with escitalopram, mirtazapine, and placebo: a crossover trial. *J Clin Psychiatry* 2005; **66**:436–443.

28. Miyata A, et al. Driving performance of stable outpatients with depression undergoing real-world treatment. *Psychiatry Clin Neurosci* 2018; **72**:399–408.

29. Verster JC, et al. Mirtazapine as positive control drug in studies examining the effects of antidepressants on driving ability. *Eur J Pharmacol* 2015; **753**:252–256.

30. Theunissen EL, et al. A randomized trial on the acute and steady-state effects of a new antidepressant, vortioxetine (Lu AA21004), on actual driving and cognition. *Clin Pharmacol Ther* 2013; **93**:493–501.

31. Ip EJ, et al. The effect of trazodone on standardized field sobriety tests. *Pharmacotherapy* 2013; **33**:369–374.

32. Rudisill TM, et al. Medication use and the risk of motor vehicle collisions among licensed drivers: a systematic review. *Accid Anal Prev* 2016; **96**:255–270.

33. Brunnauer A, et al. Driving performance and psychomotor function in depressed patients treated with agomelatine or venlafaxine. *Pharmacopsychiatry* 2015; **48**:65–71.

34. Van de Loo A, et al. The effects of intranasal esketamine (84 mg) and oral mirtazapine (30 mg) on on-road driving performance: a double-blind, placebo-controlled study. *Psychopharmacology (Berl)* 2017; **234**:3175–3183.

35. Dijkstra FM, et al. The effects of intranasal esketamine on on-road driving performance in patients with major depressive disorder or persistent depressive disorder. *J Psychopharmacol* 2022; **36**:614–625.

36. Grabe HJ, et al. The influence of clozapine and typical neuroleptics on information processing of the central nervous system under clinical conditions in schizophrenic disorders: implications for fitness to drive. *Neuropsychobiology* 1999; **40**:196–201.

37. Wylie KR, et al. Effects of depot neuroleptics on driving performance in chronic schizophrenic patients. *J Neurol Neurosurg Psychiatry* 1993; **56**:910–913.

38. Brunnauer A, et al. The impact of antipsychotics on psychomotor performance with regards to car driving skills. *J Clin Psychopharmacol* 2004; **24**:155–160.

39. Brunnauer A, et al. Driving performance under treatment of most frequently prescribed drugs for mental disorders: a systematic review of patient studies. *Int J Neuropsychopharmacol* 2021; **24**:679–693.

40. Dassanayake T, et al. Effects of benzodiazepines, antidepressants and opioids on driving: a systematic review and meta-analysis of epidemiological and experimental evidence. *Drug Saf* 2011; **34**:125–156.

41. Poceta JS. Zolpidem ingestion, automatisms, and sleep driving: a clinical and legal case series. *J Clin Sleep Med* 2011; **7**:632–638.

42. Verster JC, et al. Hypnotics and driving safety: meta-analyses of randomized controlled trials applying the on-the-road driving test. *Curr Drug Saf* 2006; **1**:63–71.

43. Torres R, et al. Simulated driving performance in healthy adults after night-time administration of 20 mg tasimelteon. *J Sleep Res* 2022; **31**:e13430.

44. Vermeeren A, et al. On-the-road driving performance the morning after bedtime administration of lemborexant in healthy adult and elderly volunteers. *Sleep* 2019; **42**:zsy260.

45. Vermeeren A, et al. On-the-road driving performance the morning after bedtime use of suvorexant 15 and 30 mg in healthy elderly. *Psychopharmacology (Berl)* 2016; **233**:3341–3351.

46. Muehlan C, et al. Driving performance after bedtime administration of daridorexant, assessed in a sensitive simulator. *Clin Pharmacol Ther* 2022; **111**:1334–1342.

47. Etminan M, et al. Use of lithium and the risk of injurious motor vehicle crash in elderly adults: case-control study nested within a cohort. *BMJ* 2004; **328**:558–559.

48. Hashemian F, et al. A comparison of the effects of reboxetine and placebo on reaction time in adults with attention deficit-hyperactivity disorder (ADHD). *Daru* 2011; **19**:231–235.

49. Classen S, et al. Evidence-based review on interventions and determinants of driving performance in teens with attention deficit hyperactivity disorder or autism spectrum disorder. *Traffic Inj Prev* 2013; **14**:188–193.

50. Hetland A, et al. Medications and impaired driving. *Ann Pharmacother* 2014; **48**:494–506.

51. Strand MC, et al. Pharmacokinetics of single doses of methadone and buprenorphine in blood and oral fluid in healthy volunteers and correlation with effects on psychomotor and cognitive functions. *J Clin Psychopharmacol* 2019; **39**:489–493.

52. Sjo O, et al. Pharmacokinetics and side-effects of clonazepam and its 7-amino-metabolite in man. *Eur J Clin Pharmacol* 1975; **8**:249–254.

CHAPTER 13

53. Berlin A, et al. Pharmacokinetics of the anticonvulsant drug clonazepam evaluated from single oral and intravenous doses and by repeated oral administration. *Eur J Clin Pharmacol* 1975; **9**:155–159.

54. Rutherford DM, et al. Plasma concentrations of diazepam and desmethyldiazepam during chronic diazepam therapy. *Br J Clin Pharmacol* 1978; **6**:69–73.

55. Wickstrom E, et al. Pharmacokinetic and clinical observations on prolonged administration of flunitrazepam. *Eur J Clin Pharmacol* 1980; **17**:189–196.

56. Mattila MA, et al. Flunitrazepam: a review of its pharmacological properties and therapeutic use. *Drugs* 1980; **20**:353–374.

57. Greenblatt DJ, et al. Single- and multiple-dose kinetics of oral lorazepam in humans: the predictability of accumulation. *J Pharmacokinet Biopharm* 1979; **7**:159–179.

58. Greenblatt DJ, et al. Pharmacokinetic comparison of sublingual lorazepam with intravenous, intramuscular, and oral lorazepam. *J Pharm Sci* 1982; **71**:248–252.

59. Smink BE, et al. The concentration of oxazepam and oxazepam glucuronide in oral fluid, blood and serum after controlled administration of 15 and 30 mg oxazepam. *Br J Clin Pharmacol* 2008; **66**:556–560.

60. Greenblatt DJ, et al. Clinical pharmacokinetics of the newer benzodiazepines. *Clin Pharmacokinet* 1983; **8**:233–252.

61. Ferrari A, et al. Methadone – metabolism, pharmacokinetics and interactions. *Pharmacol Res* 2004; **50**:551–559.

62. European Monitoring Centre for Drugs and Drug Addiction. Drug use, impaired driving and traffic accidents. 2014 (last accessed May 2024); http://bookshop.europa.eu/uri?target=EUB:NOTICE:TDXD14016:EN:HTML.

63. Department of Transport. Medication and road safety: a scoping study. Road Safety Research Report No. 116. 2010 (last accessed May 2024); https://webarchive.nationalarchives.gov.uk/20101007211118/http://www.dft.gov.uk/pgr/roadsafety/research/rsrr/theme3/report16findings.pdf.

64. Grabe HJ, et al. The influence of polypharmacological antidepressive treatment on central nervous information processing of depressed patients: implications for fitness to drive. *Neuropsychobiology* 1998; **37**:200–204.

65. Driver and Vehicle Licensing Agency. At a glance guide to the current medical standards of fitness to drive. 2013 (last updated February 2024, last checked May 2024); https://www.gov.uk/government/publications/at-a-glance.

66. General Medical Council. Good practice in prescribing and managing medicines and devices. 2021 (last accessed May 2024); https://www.gmc-uk.org/guidance/ethical_guidance/14316.asp.

CHAPTER 13

Chapter 14

Prescribing psychotropics

Working towards adherence

What is adherence?

The first clear statement about adherence comes from Hippocrates (460–377 BC), who vividly described non-adherence and linked it with poor outcomes. The World Health Organization (WHO) has described adherence as 'the extent to which a person's behaviour – taking medication, following a diet, and/or executing lifestyle changes – corresponds with agreed recommendations from a healthcare provider'.[1] In the UK, the National Institute for Health and Care Excellence (NICE) has, more succinctly, defined adherence as 'the extent to which the patient's action matches the agreed recommendations'.[2]

The more traditional notion of the patient 'complying' with the doctor's orders seems patronising and to deny the agency of the patient.[3] 'Concordance' is another term that has been used, which seems to refer to an agreement between the patient and the doctor. This is part of the notion of informed consent and is essential for a 'prescribing partnership' with patients.[4] But, as we know, agreement about a course of action does not necessarily guarantee that the action will happen. Thus 'adherence' will be used in this section to refer to the development of behaviours that will, it is hoped, result in better outcomes for our patients.

How common is non-adherence?

Large numbers of people, in most areas of medicine, do not seem to take their tablets very regularly – and so can be said to be partly or fully non-adherent. This is a phenomenon that arises in other clinical areas as well, such as psychological therapies. For people referred to psychotherapy services in the north of England, 34% did not attend for their first assessment session and, of those who did, only 57% subsequently attended the first treatment session.[5]

The Maudsley® Prescribing Guidelines in Psychiatry, Fifteenth Edition. David M. Taylor, Thomas R. E. Barnes and Allan H. Young.
© 2025 David M. Taylor. Published 2025 by John Wiley & Sons Ltd.

For chronic physical and mental disorders, the picture is not much better. Although 76% of patients with several conditions reported adhering to medication, electronic monitoring suggested that, in fact, only 44% did so.[6] Consistent with previous findings, a 2020 meta-analysis suggested that, overall, about 50% of people with mental health problems do not take their medication as prescribed.[7] This, however, may be an over-simplification. It is probable that a small proportion of patients are fully adherent, the majority are partially adherent to varying degrees, and a few never take any medication at all (of their own volition).[8] These findings are not only characteristic of western medical culture, they are reflected in other parts of the world.[9]

Adherence rates also vary both over time and across settings. For example, 10 days after discharge from hospital, up to 25% of patients with schizophrenia are partially or completely non-adherent with oral treatment and this figure rises to 50% at 1 year and to 75% by 2 years.[10] Other studies have reported 25.8% complete discontinuation of medication within 1 year of discharge from hospital.[11] In some mental healthcare settings, the rate of non-adherence may be as high as 90%.[12] Diagnosis may also be significant. An Austrian study found that significantly more patients with schizophrenia (66%) did not take their medication as prescribed, compared with patients with affective disorders (47%) or those with other psychiatric diagnoses (41%).[13]

A major issue is that poor adherence almost always occurs without the knowledge of the prescriber. In one study, prescribers identified only half of those who were non-adherent.[14] In another, 35% of patients referred for treatment of (apparently) refractory schizophrenia had sub-therapeutic plasma concentrations and many of them had plasma levels of zero.[15]

Impact of non-adherence

Medicines are only effective if taken at a therapeutic dose. And they are effective. A 20-year follow-up study of 62 250 patients with schizophrenia reported a significantly lower suicide mortality during antipsychotic use compared with non-use.[16] Antipsychotic use also decreased overall mortality.

Poor adherence to medication is a major risk factor for worse outcomes including relapse in people with schizophrenia,[17–19] bipolar disorder[20] and depression.[21] Wider health benefits are also lost. Depressed patients who do not take an antidepressant have a 20% increased risk of an incident myocardial infarction compared with those who do.[22]

The serious consequences of non-adherence with medication may be mitigated by implementing routine monitoring. Data were collected as part of the National Confidential Inquiry into Suicide and Homicide by People with Mental Illness.[23] This revealed that healthcare providers who had a policy regarding how to manage patients who are not taking their medication as prescribed had 20% fewer suicides than providers who did not have such a policy.[23] Another reason that poorly adherent individuals do worse is that they may stop their medication abruptly and without monitoring (and without telling anyone). Abrupt cessation of almost all psychotropic drugs tends to worsen prognosis (see *The Maudsley Deprescribing Guidelines*).

One of the findings that clearly illustrate the benefits of adherence is the example of depot antipsychotic medications. They do not differ pharmacologically from their oral equivalents but have consistently been shown to result in lower rates of readmission to hospital. The only difference is that with the depot preparations, adherence is, for a while at least, assured (and known about) – something which cannot be said for oral medications.

Improving adherence offers substantial possibilities for improving the outcomes from treatments. WHO comments that 'increasing the effectiveness of adherence interventions may have far greater impact on the health of the population than any improvements in specific medical treatments'.[1] We must also remember that medication is not the only effective treatment for psychosis. Although a meta-analysis[24] and systematic review[25] of such psychodynamic interventions (which included studies in unmedicated patients) confirmed the superiority of treatment with antipsychotics, the most recent systematic review of psychosocial interventions for psychotic patients (with no or low-dose antipsychotics) found the effect of such interventions to be equal to treatment with antipsychotics.[26] Cognitive behavioural therapy (CBT) for psychosis has been demonstrated to reduce certain symptoms, although its effect on quality of life does not seem to be significant.[27] So – we certainly need better drugs, but we need also to improve adherence.

Factors affecting adherence[7,28]

Table 14.1 lists many of the factors that might affect adherence.

Clearly, not all of these factors necessarily fit into a single category. For example, poor understanding by the patient can either be due to poor health literacy and/or numeracy or can be due to deficiencies in communication by the doctor.

Assessing adherence[29,30]

Table 14.2 outlines methods of assessing medication adherence.

For some antipsychotics such as clozapine, olanzapine, aripiprazole and risperidone, blood tests can be used to directly assess plasma levels. However, the plasma levels of these drugs attained with a fixed dose do vary, as do the therapeutic effects in individuals. It is therefore not possible to accurately determine partial non-adherence. That is to say, total non-adherence will be readily revealed (plasma level = zero) but partial and full adherence may be difficult to tell apart.

Table 14.1 Factors affecting adherence.

Illness-related	Treatment-related	Clinician-related	Patient-related	Environmental
Lack of motivation	Adverse effects	Poor therapeutic alliance	Denial	Disorganised environment
Poor insight	Dysfunctional beliefs	Lack of follow-up	Poor insight	Family's beliefs
Grandiose delusions	Inappropriate medication preparation or packaging	Limited consultation time	Comorbidities	Religious beliefs
Cognitive deficit	Dosing schedules[31,32]	Poor provision of information and explanation	Physical impairments	Health beliefs
Thought disorder			Poor literacy	
Forgetfulness			Poor health literacy[33]	
Disorganisation			Poor understanding of treatment options	

Table 14.2 Assessing adherence.

Method	Variables measured	Advantages	Disadvantages
Direct			
Blood test	Drug/metabolite plasma levels	Accurate	Invasive
			Costly
			Inter-individual variations (e.g. fast and slow metabolisers)
			Not reliable for all drugs (see text)
			Only a result of zero can be definitively interpreted
			Information only relevant for a very limited timeframe
			No information about the patterns of medication-taking behaviour, levels of adherence or factors that may change adherence
Indirect			
Pill count	Number of missing tablets/ missed prescriptions	Simple to use (useful in clinical trials)	Labour-intensive in clinical practice Substantial evidence that pill counts underestimate levels of non-adherence
Electronic database: clinical/pharmacy records	History of non-adherence (but generally with very little detail or formal assessment) Pharmacy dispensing and collection records (e.g. medication possession ratio – MPR)	Readily accessible Easy to identify non-adherent patients Inexpensive Non-invasive	Not reliable – only provides evidence for collection and possession of medication
Self-report	Validated assessment scales (questionnaires) (e.g. Medication Adherence Rating Scale – MARS)	Easy to use Inexpensive	Subject to reporting bias Tendency to please clinicians Massively overestimates adherence Subjective
Electronic monitoring devices (e.g. Medication Event Monitoring System – MEMS)	Number of times medication container has been opened and (assumed) percentage of doses removed	Among the most accurate methods Objective Provides additional information on medication-taking behaviour	Expensive Bulky containers Not evidence for ingestion of medication – only of container opening Patient feels under surveillance

Monitoring adherence and assessing attitudes to medication

Psychiatrists generally prefer to use direct questioning over the use of more intrusive/objective and elaborate methods of assessing adherence. Partly as a result non-adherence may go undetected.[34] NICE recommends that the patient should be asked in a non-judgemental way if they have missed any doses over a specific time period such as the previous week.[35] Issues of forgetfulness aside, whether the patient takes medication or not will be, to a significant extent, determined by their views about medication and its perceived effect on their life and condition.

Rating scales and checklists can help the clinician to guide and structure a discussion of what the patient thinks and feels about medication. The most widely used is the Drug Attitude Inventory (DAI),[36] which consists of a mix of positive and negative statements about medication; 30 statements in its full form and 10 in its short form. The patient completes it by simply agreeing or disagreeing with each statement. The total score is an indicator of the patient's overall perception of the balance between the benefits and harms associated with taking medication, and therefore likely adherence. Attitudes to medication as measured in this way have been shown to be a useful predictor of adherence over time.[37] Other checklists include the Rating of Medication Influences (ROMI) scale,[38] the Beliefs about Medicines Questionnaire[39] and the Medication Adherence Rating Scale (MARS).[19]

Enhancing medication adherence

Adherence to medication requires collaboration between the patient and the prescriber. NICE recommends that, as long as the patient has capacity to consent, their right not to take medication should be respected. If the prescriber considers that this decision may lead to harm, the reasons for the patient's decision and the prescriber's concerns should be recorded.

Adherence is a complex behaviour that is influenced by malleable underlying factors. Consequently, determinants of non-adherence can be modified through patient-specific and factor-focused interventions (Table 14.3). However, most adherence-enhancing interventions are not based on a sound theoretical framework and lack methodological rigour.[40] Low-quality studies and their outcomes are often not duplicated in different settings. This phenomenon was also highlighted by the most recent Cochrane review of adherence interventions when they reported that only 11 studies out of 182 included papers had the lowest risk of bias.[41]

Strategies for improving adherence

Systematic reviews suggest that patient-specific interventions are more likely to enhance adherence in patients with serious mental disorders.[42] NICE has reviewed the evidence for adherence over a range of health conditions and concluded that no specific intervention can be recommended for all patients.

Note that few studies in this area specifically recruited non-adherent patients (the refusal rate in such patients is likely to be high) and the specific barriers to adherence are rarely identified. The small effect size seen in many studies may simply be a consequence of this unfocused approach. An intervention mapping framework[43] provides a way to connect determinants of non-adherence to evidence-based interventions.

CHAPTER 14

Table 14.3 Interventions for non-adherence.[44]

Intentional non-adherence	Unintentional non-adherence
Psychoeducation is the foundation for all adherence interventions, but without behaviour-changing components it is not overwhelmingly effective. Provides both verbal and written information. Motivational interviewing for goal-setting Adherence therapy for exploring dysfunctional beliefs about medication or the illness, providing information and goal setting. It requires more time and multiple sessions. Cognitive behavioural therapy to eradicate or control the residual symptoms that prevent adherence. To address dysfunctional beliefs about treatment. Cognitive remediation to help with cognitive deficit in psychotic patients and thought disorder Mindfulness to help with symptoms Monitor adverse effects regularly and periodically Therapeutic alliance – a non-judgemental clinician allows patients to honestly disclose their thoughts and beliefs about medication Family intervention – psychoeducation and family therapy	Simplify dose regimen – reduce number of medications and/or frequency of administration Dispensing interventions – medication-taking aids EAM (electronic adherence monitoring) – evidence for this is weak[45] Pairing-up medication – taking with a daily activity (e.g. having breakfast, brushing teeth or before bedtime) Use technology – messaging service, email and telephone reminders Pharmacy interventions for those with physical impairment (e.g. opening bottles)

Medication-taking aids

'Compliance aids' are boxes that contain compartments that can accommodate up to four doses of multiple medicines each day. These may be helpful in patients who are clearly motivated to take medication but who are disorganised or who have cognitive deficits. But only 10% of non-adherent patients say that they simply forgot to take medication, so medication-taking aids are not a substitute for lack of insight or lack of motivation. Moreover, some medicines are unstable when removed from blister packaging and placed in a compliance aid. These include oro-dispersible formulations which are often prescribed for non-adherent patients. In addition, medication-taking aids are labour-intensive (expensive) to fill, it can be difficult to change prescriptions at short notice and the process of filling of these devices is particularly error-prone.[46] More sophisticated programmes of practical support, both electronic and in-person, have been shown to be effective.[47]

Depot/long-acting antipsychotics

Meta-analyses of clinical trials have shown that the relative and absolute risks of relapse with depot maintenance treatment were 30% and 10% lower, respectively, than with oral treatment.[48,49] NICE recommends that depots are an option in patients who are known to be non-adherent to oral treatment and/or those who prefer this method of administration. However, it is worth remembering that switching a non-adherent patient from oral antipsychotics to a long-acting injectable formulation does not address the underlying reasons driving that non-adherence. This has been highlighted by a recent systematic review that reported a rate of discontinuation of above 50% in those who had been prescribed second-generation depots.[50] So long-acting antipsychotics do not stop non-adherence but they do prevent sudden cessation of medication and its consequences (all depots provide a slow decline in plasma levels).

Their use can also provide certainty about the level of adherence (the injection is either given or it is not). Depots are probably underused, for example a US study found that depot preparations were prescribed for fewer than one in five patients with a recent episode of non-adherence.[51]

An alternative to depots is the use of long-acting oral antipsychotics such as penfluridol, which can be given weekly.[52] Supervised administration obviates the need for injections but does not provide the same level of certainty over compliance given the facility that patients have demonstrated for disguising the taking of oral medication.

In the USA, Abilify MyCite is approved for use.[53] This is a version of aripiprazole with a transmitting sensor embedded in the formulation which is able to confirm that a tablet has been taken. Evidence for its effectiveness is slim.[54]

Financial incentives

Controlled trials in a number of disease areas support the offer of financial incentives to enhance medication adherence. Paying people to take their medication is extremely controversial, though some clinicians have found this strategy to be effective. The effect could not be maintained in a randomised controlled trial (RCT) at 6- and 24-month follow-up after payments were stopped, and complete adherence was achieved in only 28% of patients receiving the incentives.[55] Other RCTs also have demonstrated a significant increase in adherence during the trial and a decline at follow-up when payments had stopped.[56] Offering financial incentives did not reduce patients' motivation for treatment.[57] A systematic review of acceptability of financial incentives for health-related behaviours has raised concerns about the validity and reliability of these interventions given their methodological limitations.[58]

Psychological interventions

In physical medicine, medication adherence has been found to be associated with health beliefs and psychological variables, such as self-efficacy and locus of control.[59] Family support is also positively related to medication adherence.

It is likely to be the same in psychiatry – but what can be done? One such intervention – called, at the time, 'compliance therapy' – was evaluated at the Maudsley Hospital.[60] This was a pilot of a mixed intervention, consisting of active listening, cognitive behavioural techniques, motivational interviewing and the provision of information and explanation. This showed promising results in terms of increased adherence and reduced admission rates over the next 6 months. However, training for staff and supervision render it time-consuming. A subsequent replication did not show the same improvements,[61] but also did not appear to have incorporated a training or supervisory element for those delivering the therapy. However, a trial of training in compliance therapy did seem to have an effect on the junior doctors involved, who felt that they were more aware of the drivers of non-adherence and of the importance of empathic listening and more able to understand why a patient might not take medication.[62]

One prerequisite for successful adherence to a treatment regimen should be that the patient understands the objectives of treatment, the options on offer and the rationale behind them. However, many – perhaps most – doctors have had no specific training in how to convey information and understanding to patients. Difficulties have been noted

CHAPTER 14

to arise in cancer medicine regarding the benefits and risks of anti-cancer medications.[63] One must assume that we are likely to meet the same difficulties in psychiatry. We also need to consider that our patients may have a very different explanatory model for what is happening to them. For example, not so long ago, only just over a third of white English patients viewed schizophrenia as having a substantially biological origin.[64] So our explanations for a person's psychosis may not be as convincing to them – and their families – as we might imagine. One simple step that might help is to encourage patients with a serious medical illness to read their own notes; one study reported that this helped such patients to better understand why they were prescribed medications.[65] However, this begs the question of why they did not understand in the first place.

The range of practical interventions described in Table 14.3 – and, to a great extent, the psychological interventions contained in the original model of compliance therapy – will need to be tailored to the needs of the individual patient. But this assumes that clinicians have an awareness of the issue, the requisite skills and the time available to use them. The current RCPsych curricula, although they refer to some of the psychological skills modalities mentioned, do not include the management of adherence as an issue in either the core curriculum or the general psychiatry curriculum.[66]

Conclusion

Establishing and maintaining adherence is a quintessentially biopsychosocial activity. It is central to the practice of medicine and, hence, to psychiatry. It demands both an awareness of the problem, a knowledge of practical strategies for its improvement and a repertoire of psychological skills. The neglect of this area of therapeutics in training should not deter prescribers from recognising non-adherence and taking active steps to manage it. An initial gambit might be, at the end of any first prescription, to ask ourselves 'What have I done to help this patient take this medication?' and to record this answer as part of the care plan, as a reminder to ourselves and our colleagues that this issue needs our conscious, structured and regular attention.

References

1. World Health Organization. Adherence to long-term therapies: evidence for action. 2003; https://apps.who.int/iris/bitstream/handle/10665/42682/9241545992.pdf.
2. National Institute for Health and Care Excellence. Medicines adherence: involving patients in decisions about prescribed medicines and supporting adherence. Clinical guideline [CG76]. 2009 (last checked August 2023); https://www.nice.org.uk/guidance/cg76.
3. Piatkowska O, et al. Medication — compliance or alliance? A client-centred approach to increasing adherence. In: Kavanagh DJ, ed. *Schizophrenia: An Overview and Practical Handbook.* Boston, MA: Springer US; 1992:339–355.
4. Bond C, et al. Prescribing and partnership with patients. *Br J Clin Pharmacol* 2012; 74:581–588.
5. Sweetman J, et al. Risk factors for initial appointment non-attendance at Improving Access to Psychological Therapy (IAPT) services: a retrospective analysis. *Psychother Res* 2023; 33:535–550.
6. Foley L, et al. Prevalence and predictors of medication non-adherence among people living with multimorbidity: a systematic review and meta-analysis. *BMJ Open* 2021; 11:e0987.
7. Semahegn A, et al. Psychotropic medication non-adherence and its associated factors among patients with major psychiatric disorders: a systematic review and meta-analysis. *Syst Rev* 2020; 9:17.
8. Masand PS, et al. Partial adherence to antipsychotic medication impacts the course of illness in patients with schizophrenia: a review. *Prim Care Companion J Clin Psychiatry* 2009; 11:147–154.
9. Alosaimi K, et al. Medication adherence among patients with chronic diseases in Saudi Arabia. *Int J Environ Res Public Health* 2022; 19:10053.
10. Leucht S, et al. Epidemiology, clinical consequences, and psychosocial treatment of nonadherence in schizophrenia. *J Clin Psychiatry* 2006; 67 Suppl 5:3–8.

11. Zhou Y, et al. Factors associated with complete discontinuation of medication among patients with schizophrenia in the year after hospital discharge. *Psychiatry Res* 2017; **250**:129–135.

12. Cramer JA, et al. Compliance with medication regimens for mental and physical disorders. *Psychiatr Serv* 1998; **49**:196–201.

13. Geretsegger C, et al. Non-adherence to psychotropic medication assessed by plasma level in newly admitted psychiatric patients: prevalence before acute admission. *Psychiatry Clin Neurosci* 2019; **73**:175–178.

14. Remington G, et al. The use of electronic monitoring (MEMS) to evaluate antipsychotic compliance in outpatients with schizophrenia. *Schizophr Res* 2007; **90**:229–237.

15. McCutcheon R, et al. Antipsychotic plasma levels in the assessment of poor treatment response in schizophrenia. *Acta Psychiatr Scand* 2018; **137**:39–46.

16. Taipale H, et al. 20-year follow-up study of physical morbidity and mortality in relationship to antipsychotic treatment in a nationwide cohort of 62,250 patients with schizophrenia (FIN20). *World Psychiatry* 2020; **19**:61–68.

17. Morken G, et al. Non-adherence to antipsychotic medication, relapse and rehospitalisation in recent-onset schizophrenia. *BMC Psychiatry* 2008; **8**:32.

18. Knapp M, et al. Non-adherence to antipsychotic medication regimens: associations with resource use and costs. *Br J Psychiatry* 2004; **184**:509–516.

19. Jaeger S, et al. Adherence styles of schizophrenia patients identified by a latent class analysis of the Medication Adherence Rating Scale (MARS): a six-month follow-up study. *Psychiatry Res* 2012; **200**:83–88.

20. Lang K, et al. Predictors of medication nonadherence and hospitalization in Medicaid patients with bipolar I disorder given long-acting or oral antipsychotics. *J Med Econ* 2011; **14**:217–226.

21. Mitchell AJ, et al. Why don't patients take their medicine? Reasons and solutions in psychiatry. *Adv Psychiatric Treat* 2007; **13**:336–346.

22. Scherrer JF, et al. Antidepressant drug compliance: reduced risk of MI and mortality in depressed patients. *Am J Med* 2011; **124**:318–324.

23. Appleby L, et al. National Confidential Inquiry into Suicide and Homicide by People with Mental Illness. 2013; http://www.bbmh.manchester.ac.uk/cmhr/research/centreforsuicideprevention/nci/.

24. Malmberg L, et al. Individual psychodynamic psychotherapy and psychoanalysis for schizophrenia and severe mental illness. *Cochrane Database Syst Rev* 2001; **3**:CD001360.

25. Mueser KT, et al. Psychodynamic treatment of schizophrenia: is there a future? *Psychol Med* 1990; **20**:253–262.

26. Cooper RE, et al. Psychosocial interventions for people with schizophrenia or psychosis on minimal or no antipsychotic medication: a systematic review. *Schizophr Res* 2019; **225**:15–30.

27. Health Quality Ontario. Cognitive behavioural therapy for psychosis: a health technology assessment. *Ont Health Technol Assess Ser* 2018; **18**:1–141.

28. Pedley R, et al. Qualitative systematic review of barriers and facilitators to patient-involved antipsychotic prescribing. *BJPsych Open* 2018; **4**:5–14.

29. Forbes CA, et al. A systematic literature review comparing methods for the measurement of patient persistence and adherence. *Curr Med Res Opin* 2018; **34**:1613–1625.

30. Anghel LA, et al. An overview of the common methods used to measure treatment adherence. *Med Pharmacy Rep* 2019; **92**:117–122.

31. Greenberg RN. Overview of patient compliance with medication dosing: a literature review. *Clin Ther* 1984; **6**:592–599.

32. Saini SD, et al. Effect of medication dosing frequency on adherence in chronic diseases. *Am J Manag Care* 2009; **15**:e22–33.

33. Miller TA. Health literacy and adherence to medical treatment in chronic and acute illness: a meta-analysis. *Patient Educ Couns* 2016; **99**:1079–1086.

34. Vieta E, et al. Psychiatrists' perceptions of potential reasons for non- and partial adherence to medication: results of a survey in bipolar disorder from eight European countries. *J Affect Disord* 2012; **143**:125–130.

35. National Institute for Health and Care Excellence. Psychosis and schizophrenia in adults: prevention and management. Clinical guideline [CG178]. 2014 (last checked August 2023); https://www.nice.org.uk/guidance/cg178.

36. Hogan TP, et al. A self-report scale predictive of drug compliance in schizophrenics: reliability and discriminative validity. *Psychol Med* 1983; **13**:177–183.

37. Perkins DO. Predictors of noncompliance in patients with schizophrenia. *J Clin Psychiatry* 2002; **63**:1121–1128.

38. Weiden P, et al. Rating of medication influences (ROMI) scale in schizophrenia. *Schizophr Bull* 1994; **20**:297–310.

39. Horne R, et al. The beliefs about medicines questionnaire: the development and evaluation of a new method for assessing the cognitive representation of medication. *Psychol Health* 1999; **14**:1–24.

40. Zullig LL, et al. Moving from the trial to the real world: improving medication adherence using insights of implementation science. *Annu Rev Pharmacol Toxicol* 2019; **59**:423–445.

41. Nieuwlaat R, et al. Interventions for enhancing medication adherence. *Cochrane Database Syst Rev* 2014; **11**:CD000011.

42. Nosè M, et al. [Systemic review of clinical interventions for reducing treatment non-adherence in psychosis]. *Epidemiol Psichiatr Soc* 2003; **12**:272–286.

43. Kok G, et al. A taxonomy of behaviour change methods: an intervention mapping approach. *Health Psychol Rev* 2016; **10**:297–312.

44. Hartung D, et al. Interventions to improve pharmacological adherence among adults with psychotic spectrum disorders and bipolar disorder: a systematic review. *Psychosomatics* 2017; **58**:101–112.

45. Chan AHY, et al. Effect of electronic adherence monitoring on adherence and outcomes in chronic conditions: a systematic review and meta-analysis. *PLoS One* 2022; **17**:e0265715.

46. Barber ND, et al. Care homes' use of medicines study: prevalence, causes and potential harm of medication errors in care homes for older people. *Qual Safety Health Care* 2009; **18**:341–346.

CHAPTER 14

47. Velligan D, et al. A randomized trial comparing in person and electronic interventions for improving adherence to oral medications in schizophrenia. *SchizophrBull* 2013; **39**:999–1007.

48. Leucht C, et al. Oral versus depot antipsychotic drugs for schizophrenia – a critical systematic review and meta-analysis of randomised long-term trials. *Schizophr Res* 2011; **127**:83–92.

49. Leucht S, et al. Antipsychotic drugs versus placebo for relapse prevention in schizophrenia: a systematic review and meta-analysis. *Lancet* 2012; **379**:2063–2071.

50. Gentile S. Discontinuation rates during long-term, second-generation antipsychotic long-acting injection treatment: a systematic review. *Psychiatry Clin Neurosci* 2019; **73**:216–230.

51. West JC, et al. Use of depot antipsychotic medications for medication nonadherence in schizophrenia. *Schizophr Bull* 2008; **34**:995–1001.

52. Soares BG, et al. Penfluridol for schizophrenia. *Cochrane Database Syst Rev* 2006; **2**:CD002923.

53. Otsuka Pharmaceutical Co. Ltd. Highlights of prescribing information. Abilify Mycite (aripiprazole with sensor) for oral use 2017. https://www.accessdata.fda.gov/drugsatfda_docs/label/2017/207202lbl.pdf.

54. Cosgrove L, et al. Digital aripiprazole or digital evergreening? A systematic review of the evidence and its dissemination in the scientific literature and in the media. *BMJ Evid Based Med* 2019; **24**:231–238.

55. Priebe S, et al. Financial incentives to improve adherence to antipsychotic maintenance medication in non-adherent patients: a cluster randomised controlled trial. *Health Technol Assess* 2016; **20**:1–122.

56. Noordraven EL, et al. Financial incentives for improving adherence to maintenance treatment in patients with psychotic disorders (Money for Medication): a multicentre, open-label, randomised controlled trial. *Lancet Psychiatry* 2017; **4**:199–207.

57. Noordraven EL, et al. The effect of financial incentives on patients' motivation for treatment: results of 'Money for Medication,' a randomised controlled trial. *BMC Psychiatry* 2018; **18**:144.

58. Hoskins K, et al. Acceptability of financial incentives for health-related behavior change: an updated systematic review. *Prev Med* 2019; **126**:105762.

59. Marrero RJ, et al. Psychological factors involved in psychopharmacological medication adherence in mental health patients: a systematic review. *Patient Educ Couns* 2020; **103**:2116–2131.

60. Kemp R, et al. Compliance therapy in psychotic patients: randomised controlled trial. *BMJ* 1996; **312**:345–349.

61. O'Donnell C, et al. Compliance therapy: a randomised controlled trial in schizophrenia. *BMJ* 2003; **327**:834.

62. Surguladze S, et al. Teaching psychiatric trainees 'compliance therapy'. *Psychiatric Bull* 2002; **26**:12–15.

63. Davis C, et al. Communication of anticancer drug benefits and related uncertainties to patients and clinicians: document analysis of regulated information on prescription drugs in Europe. *BMJ* 2023; **380**:e073711.

64. McCabe R, et al. Explanatory models of illness in schizophrenia: comparison of four ethnic groups. *Br J Psychiatry* 2004; **185**:25–30.

65. Blease C, et al. Association of patients reading clinical notes with perception of medication adherence among persons with serious mental illness. *JAMA Netw Open* 2021; **4**:e212823.

66. Royal College of Psychiatrists. Curricula documents and resources. 2022; https://www.rcpsych.ac.uk/training/curricula-and-guidance/curricula-implementation/curricula-documents-and-resources.

Restarting psychotropic medications after a period of non-compliance

When a patient is admitted to hospital it is often because they have been non-compliant with their medications for some time before admission. The clinical question of whether to restart the medication and at which dose is a complex one. The risk of withdrawal symptoms and relapse must be balanced against the risk of adverse drug reactions when medications are reintroduced too quickly. There is little published evidence on this area, with most guidance (often of undeclared provenance) coming from manufacturers. The guidance below should be followed with caution.

Summaries of product characteristics (SPCs) and other formal, regulatory documents tend not to deal with the issue of restarting medication. Official patient information leaflets sometimes give detailed advice. These leaflets are unanimous in advising that on no account should a double dose be given to make up for a missed dose. However, the vast majority of leaflets advise only on what to do if a single dose has been missed. Some leaflets advise taking the missed dose later (providing it is not too close to the next dose), whereas others recommend skipping the missed dose altogether and starting again with the next dose.

In the event that more than one dose has been missed, the first question to ask is whether or not this is the appropriate drug for a patient to be taking. Poor compliance often indicates some dissatisfaction on the part of the patient. If it is a drug with a short half-life or one that requires lengthy re-titration, it may not be appropriate to restart prescribing for a patient who is frequently non-compliant. Similarly, if a patient is intoxicated with alcohol or drugs, it may not be sensible to restart medication at that time. Efforts should be made to find out if there are any particular reasons for non-compliance. Where poor adherence is a result of factors other than tolerability, consider the use of a long-acting injection (although these are only used, officially at least, in schizophrenia and schizoaffective disorder).

When considering whether to restart the drug at the same dose as before or to re-titrate from a lower dose, the time since the last dose is vitally important. If more than a week or two has passed, then all drugs will probably need to be restarted as if it is new treatment (although for many drugs that do not require titration this might mean starting back on the same dose as before). Exceptions include long-acting depot formulations and oral drugs with long half-lives such as aripiprazole, cariprazine and penfluridol. With these, there is a need to reload if the gap in treatment is very long, although shorter gaps (<2 weeks) might be managed by giving the usual dose and then reverting to the original dosing schedule.

Lamotrigine must be considered separately from all other psychotropics because it has been associated with life-threatening cutaneous reactions, especially with high initial doses. The manufacturer's product information advises that if five half-lives have elapsed since the last lamotrigine dose was given, lamotrigine should be titrated as if for the first time. The half-life in healthy subjects on no other medication is around 33 hours. This is affected by other medications and is approximately 14 hours when given with glucuronidation-inducing drugs such as carbamazepine or phenytoin. The half-life is increased to approximately 70 hours when given with valproate. This means that the time before complete re-titration is necessary varies between 3 and 7 days, depending on other drugs co-prescribed.[1]

Table 14.4 summarises some very general recommendations. The drugs in the first column have specific safety issues that mean they require re-titration after the specified

Table 14.4 Restarting medication up to 2 weeks after stopping oral treatment.

Drugs that require re-titration

Drug	Time after which re-titration must be performed	Further guidance	Drugs that are usually safe for restarting at the previous dose	Drugs that are possibly safe for restarting at the previous dose
Clozapine	48 hours	See section in Chapter 1	Acamprosate	Antipsychotics (exceptions in column 1)
Lamotrigine	3–7 days	See text	Asenapine	Carbamazepine (beware
Methadone, buprenorphine	3 days	See section in Chapter 4	Fluoxetine Haloperidol Isocarboxazid	loss on enzyme induction) Cholinesterase inhibitors
Paliperidone long-acting injection	Depends on formulation	See section in Chapter 1	Lofepramine Methylphenidate	CNS stimulants Disulfiram
Aripiprazole long-acting injection	Depends on formulation	See section in Chapter 1	Phenelzine Sulpiride Tranylcypromine	Lithium (titration advised if renal function has changed)
Quetiapine	Suggest 1 week	Tolerance to sedative and hypotensive effects may be lost	Valproate	MAOIs Memantine Naltrexone Pregabalin SSRIs
Risperidone	Suggest 1 week	Tolerance to hypotensive effects may be lost		
Tricyclics	Suggest 1 week	Tolerance to sedative and hypotensive effects may be lost		

MAOIs, monoamine oxidase inhibitors.

length of time. The drugs in the middle column are thought to be safe because the maximum dose is usually no higher than the highest recommended starting dose. The drugs in the right-hand column are thought to be safe to restart at the prior dose because a similar drug appears in the middle column, because clinical experience suggests they are safe or because the risks associated with giving untitrated high doses are thought to be low. Some suggestions are obtained from EU regulatory documents (SPCs),[2] while others are mere suggestions based on clinical experience. If the gap in oral treatment is longer than 2 weeks, start as if it is new treatment (noting the exceptions listed earlier).

References

1. Aurobindo Pharma-Milpharm Ltd. Summary of product characteristics. Lamotrigine 25mg tablets. 2024 (last accessed September 2024); https://www.medicines.org.uk/emc/product/4736/smpc.
2. EMC. *Summaries of Product Characteristics*. 2024 (last accessed September 2024); https://www.medicines.org.uk/emc/.

Relational aspects of prescribing practice

This section provides clinicians with practically useful advice in the relational aspects of prescribing. Evidence exists for the importance of the doctor–patient relationship in improving treatment outcomes.[1-3] The key factors that help develop, maintain and deepen the relationship include instilling trust and regard.[4] Three concepts are important here: object relations, memory and the treatment framework.

Object relations

This means how the individual views themselves and others around them. This view then influences how they process incoming data (e.g. what is happening in an interaction). This view of themselves has been determined from early experience. In essence it means that the present interaction may be experienced inaccurately through the prism of the past (another way to think of this experience is that this is the *transference*). This has implications for both the patient and the clinician. For example, if the patient has had early experience of uncaring parents, they will have greater difficulty in trusting the clinician. In turn, if the clinician's early experience is of demanding parents who expected them to always get it right, a treatment-resistant patient may be a particular challenge for them. This object relations approach allows one to be aware of factors regarding the patient, the clinician and the clinician–patient relationship.

Memory

Up to 95% of our goal-directed activities are executed unconsciously.[5] Thus, the clinician's prescribing may be more influenced by procedural memory than their subjective view that they are using working memory (i.e. there is an illusion of the application of active thinking to solve the specificity of the present problem). By definition, procedural memory and the action flowing from this may not be best suited for a particular clinical situation. Acknowledging the unconscious influence on the present may help bring the conscious mind into play.

Treatment framework

This is using knowledge of the clinician's usual way of working (e.g. following this edition of *The Maudsley Prescribing Guidelines*), and a knowledge of how they tend to personally apply these guidelines. Straying from the guidelines may be based on good clinical judgement but also it may indicate that there is some psychological factor influencing decision-making. Given this psychological factor may be unconscious, the ability to review 'what one usually does' is then a useful check on what may be happening in prescribing. For example, if the prescriber is able to think 'I do not usually prescribe such a high dose of antipsychotic as a starting dose' they may then be able to pose the question 'Am I feeling very anxious to satisfy the demands of this patient?' In effect they may then be able to catch themselves acting out (i.e. replacing thinking with behaviour) in the *countertransference* (in this case their great anxiety to satisfy the patient).

Factors that may influence the patient's use of and adherence to medication

How the individual views themselves, and others, will influence many aspects of a person's behaviour. These issues include their personal and cultural beliefs, readiness to change, ambivalence, expectations of treatment, attachment style and treatment preference. In addition, patients might use medication in countertherapeutic ways. We address each of these in turn in terms of their practical implications.[6,7]

Personal and cultural beliefs

The religious, cultural and socioeconomic contexts shape our beliefs around concepts of illness, health and disability.[8] Adherence to treatments is affected by the patient's subjective beliefs and averages roughly 50% in almost all conditions.[9]

Recommendation: When it comes to prescribing within a culturally diverse population, prescribers need to reflect on their own cultural biases, enquire about the patient's cultural beliefs, and work collaboratively with communities and families.[10]

Readiness to change

Patients' motivation and readiness to change can affect treatment outcomes. Beitman et al.[11] examined stages of change and response to medication in patients with panic disorder and found that readiness to change was associated with better outcomes. The transtheoretical model[12] proposes that people move through different stages of change and that interventions must match the stage of readiness. This model can also be useful for the treatment of other mental health conditions including personality disorder.[13]

Recommendation: The clinician's appreciation of the stages of change, and the work involved in lasting change, can increase compassion and avoid wrongly timed interventions (including wrongly timed prescribing). A recovery-focused and patient-centred approach may help patients to understand entrenched patterns of behaviour, and to actively participate in behavioural change.

Ambivalence

Patients may worry about the safety of psychotropics, and mistrust clinicians. Further, symptoms may have an adaptive and protective function thus making them harder for the patient to relinquish. For example, a patient who has elicited care might be ambivalent about getting better and losing this care. Recovery might portend, for example, confronting a difficult relationship or working through an intolerable loss.[14]

Recent advances in the field of neuropsychoanalysis suggest that unpleasurable feelings at a biological level indicate that the patient's underlying emotional needs are not being satisfied, serving as homeostatic 'error signals'. It is not a surprise then that symptoms (associated with feelings states) can be stubbornly resistant to symptom-focused treatments when the patient's basic emotional needs continue to be unmet.[15]

Recommendation: Exploring patients' ambivalence towards medication and healthcare professionals, and their previous experiences of care, can deepen the therapeutic relationship and is crucial in understanding patients' concerns. Understanding the patient's (often unconscious) underlying conflicts and motivations can explain symptom perseverance despite pharmacological endeavours. Acknowledgement of the patient's ambivalence during the recovery process may help validate their experience, facilitate rapport and enable conversations that the patient might otherwise be reluctant to approach.

Expectations of treatment: placebo and nocebo effect

Expectations of improvement or harm when taking medication exert a significant impact on treatment responses. The powerful 'placebo' response has been well described in medicine as a genuine psychobiological event.[16] Conversely, expectations of harm are associated with negative treatment outcomes known as the 'nocebo' effect. Patients often expect harm from taking antidepressants, fearing dependence and loss of control of their emotions.[17] Interestingly, patients who discussed adverse effects of antidepressants with their doctors were reported less likely to discontinue therapy than patients who did not discuss them.[18]

Recommendation: These findings emphasise the need to use all the elements of the therapeutic relationship in the care of patients.[19] Clinical management of the nocebo effect includes awareness and recognition, focusing on the treatment alliance, carefully naming and working through mistrust, and careful disclosure of potential drug-related adverse effects, while remaining honest and clear.[20]

Attachment style

Healthcare staff often represent attachment figures[21] as they treat patients in times of need and distress. The attachment is particularly important when it comes to the management of long-term conditions. In one study, diabetic patients with dismissive attachment had significantly worse glucose control than patients with preoccupied or secure attachment style, but the effect was mitigated by improved communication between doctors and patients.[22,23]

Concerns about rejection, abandonment, control and intimacy[24] are likely to affect patients' use of their medication. Patients with a dismissive attachment style may fear dependence on medication and services and not adhere to the prescribed interventions. Patients with a fearful-anxious attachment might need regular reassurance, while patients with a disorganised attachment might evoke disorganised and chaotic responses from healthcare staff.

Recommendation: Consider attachment patterns when prescribing. Particular attention and consistency are needed to deliver coherent and reliable care alongside pharmacological interventions.

Treatment preference

The chronic illness model encourages consideration of the patient's treatment preferences. Research suggests that matching treatment to preference might improve outcomes for patients with depression.[25] An RCT matching patients to treatment preference for major depressive disorder concluded that patients had better outcomes on their preferred treatment.[26] These observations might apply to other conditions.

CHAPTER 14

Recommendation: Consider treatment preference as one of the decision factors when prescribing.

Countertherapeutic use of medication

Medication (including overdose) may be used as a way of signalling submission, anger or helplessness. This is especially true in people who lack an emotional vocabulary and secure internal representations of benign care. Medication may become a way of self-management, replacing more developmental coping strategies and relationships.

Recommendation: The clinician should consider the meaning of the emotional communication and be curious about alliance ruptures and system failures (and therefore reflect on the clinician's possible contributions to the rupture).

Summary – a checklist when prescribing

When faced with complex prescribing decisions, a checklist considering the discussed issues from the perspective of the patient, the clinician and the clinician–patient relationship may be helpful.

The patient factor

Q: *'What is my patient's story? What is my patient trying to communicate using words or, as important, through their actions in the here and now?'*

Recommendation: A formulation of the patient's underlying psychological difficulties may help. This may include:

- Predominant relational pattern(s) – attachment style and relationship to care/authority.
- Ambivalence about symptoms – underlying psychological investment in status quo.
- Meaning attached to medication and overall use of medication (including countertherapeutic use of medication).

The clinician factor

Q: *'How do I feel in response to my patient and how does that influence the action I am considering taking (e.g. do I feel helpless, frustrated, incompetent, guilty in the face of the patient's symptoms)? Am I prescribing to avoid unwanted feelings in my relationship with my patient?'*

Recommendation:

1 The first step in identifying countertransference pressure is to recognise and accept it, without always resorting to immediate action.
2 Self-review of practice. The clinician may ask:
   - Am I working within relevant guidelines?
   - Am I doing what I normally do (if not, am I being overly influenced by my countertransference)?
   - Do I have strong feelings about this patient? Do I have *no* feelings about this patient? (Which would be also worth considering.)

- Are any circumstances different, for example do I have managers or other colleagues or the patient's family scrutinising me with this particular patient?
3 Seek support. Use supervision with colleagues and ask support from other members of the multidisciplinary team. It is important to work closely with colleagues (including pharmacists) to triangulate decisions when in complex prescribing dilemmas. Choosing to discuss a problem in supervision and outside of the heat of the consulting room can clarify thinking.

The clinician–patient relationship

Q: '*What might prescribing a medication – or not prescribing – come to represent in my relationship with my patient?*'

Limited consultation time and cancelled clinics might reinforce feelings of rejection and abandonment. Non-adherence to medication or overdose of prescribed medication might be a sign of a rupture in the clinician–patient relationship and further exploration can promote useful insights for patient and clinician.

Recommendation: Consider the meaning of medication in the context of the patient, the clinician and the clinician–patient relationship. Cultivate a pharmacotherapeutic partnership and set limits:[24]

- Reframe prescribing as a partnership, rather than a one-directional activity of the doctor.
- Provide, as much as possible, a stable and consistent consultation setting.
- Set therapeutic limits, confronting unrealistic expectations of care. (This includes maintaining a realistic humility around the limitations of psychopharmacology, and psychoeducating patients regarding what medications can and cannot achieve and their place in the overall journey to recovery and development.)
- Endorse a stance that can promote the pharmacotherapeutic alliance, characterised by emotional presence and warmth, good and honest communication, and support of the patient's autonomy and agency. This includes shared decision-making and respect for the patient's treatment preferences, when clinically indicated.
- Openly discuss overall recovery goals, target symptoms, duration of treatment and potential adverse effects, and address any associated anxieties.
- A clear agreement on treatment objectives, consistent with the overall care plan, and the respective responsibilities of doctor and patient can promote agency and strengthen the pharmacotherapeutic partnership.
- Collaborative crisis planning should be part of this, especially when there are risk concerns.

CHAPTER 14

References

1. Olaisen RH, et al. Assessing the longitudinal impact of physician-patient relationship on functional health. *Ann Fam Med* 2020; 18:422–429.
2. McKay KM, et al. Psychiatrist effects in the psychopharmacological treatment of depression. *J Affect Disord* 2006; 92:287–290.
3. Kelley JM, et al. The influence of the patient-clinician relationship on healthcare outcomes: a systematic review and meta-analysis of randomized controlled trials. *PLoS One* 2014; 9:e94207.
4. Ridd M, et al. The patient-doctor relationship: a synthesis of the qualitative literature on patients' perspectives. *Br J Gen Pract* 2009; 59:e116–e133.
5. Bargh JA, et al. The unbearable automaticity of being. *Am Psychol* 1999; 54:462.
6. Mintz DL, et al. How (not what) to prescribe: nonpharmacologic aspects of psychopharmacology. *Psychiatr Clin North Am* 2012; 35:143–163.
7. Konstantinidou H, et al. Will this tablet make me happy again? The contribution of relational prescribing in providing a pragmatic and psychodynamic framework for prescribers. *BJPsych Advances* 2023; 29:265–273.
8. Ravindran N, et al. Cultural influences on perceptions of health, illness, and disability: a review and focus on autism. *J Child Fam Studies* 2012; 21:311–319.
9. Lam WY, et al. Medication adherence measures: an overview. *BioMed Res Int* 2015; 2015:217047.
10. Brooks LA, et al. Culturally sensitive communication in healthcare: a concept analysis. *Collegian* 2019; 26:383–391.
11. Beitman BD, et al. Patient stage of change predicts outcome in a panic disorder medication trial. *Anxiety* 1994; 1:64–69.
12. Prochaska JO, et al. Stages and processes of self-change of smoking: toward an integrative model of change. *J Consult Clin Psychol* 1983; 51:390–395.
13. Roughley M, et al. Referral of patients with emotionally unstable personality disorder for specialist psychological therapy: why, when and how? *BJPsych Bull* 2021; 45:52–58.
14. Gibbons R. The mourning process and its importance in mental illness: a psychoanalytic understanding of psychiatric diagnosis and classification. *BJPsych Advances* 2024; 30:80–88.
15. Lee T, et al. Managing the clinical encounter with patients with personality disorder in a general psychiatry setting: key contributions from neuropsychoanalysis. *BJPsych Advances* 2023; doi:10.1192/bja.2023.43.
16. Finniss DG, et al. Biological, clinical, and ethical advances of placebo effects. *Lancet* 2010; 375:686–695.
17. Piguet V, et al. Patients' representations of antidepressants: a clue to nonadherence? *Clin J Pain* 2007; 23:669–675.
18. Bull SA, et al. Discontinuation of use and switching of antidepressants: influence of patient-physician communication. *JAMA* 2002; 288:1403–1409.
19. Benedetti F. Placebo and the new physiology of the doctor-patient relationship. *Physiol Rev* 2013; 93:1207–1246.
20. Data-Franco J, et al. The nocebo effect: a clinicians guide. *Aust NZ J Psychiatry* 2013; 47:617–623.
21. Adshead G. Psychiatric staff as attachment figures. Understanding management problems in psychiatric services in the light of attachment theory. *Br J Psychiatry* 1998; 172:64–69.
22. Ciechanowski PS, et al. The patient-provider relationship: attachment theory and adherence to treatment in diabetes. *Am J Psychiatry* 2001; 158:29–35.
23. Ciechanowski PS, et al. The association of patient relationship style and outcomes in collaborative care treatment for depression in patients with diabetes. *Med Care* 2006; 44:283–291.
24. Mintz D. *Psychodynamic Psychopharmacology: Caring for the Treatment-Resistant Patient.* Washington, DC: American Psychiatric Association Publishing; 2022.
25. Lin P, et al. The influence of patient preference on depression treatment in primary care. *Ann Behav Med* 2005; 30:164–173.
26. Kocsis JH, et al. Patient preference as a moderator of outcome for chronic forms of major depressive disorder treated with nefazodone, cognitive behavioral analysis system of psychotherapy, or their combination. *J Clin Psychiatry* 2009; 70:354–361.

Prescribing drugs outside their licensed indications ('off-label' prescribing)

A Product Licence is granted when regulatory authorities are satisfied that the drug in question has proven efficacy in the treatment of a specified disorder, along with an acceptable adverse effect profile, relative to the severity of the disorder being treated and other available treatments. Licensed indications are preparation-specific, outlined in the SPCs, and may be different for branded and generic formulations of the same drug.[1] In the USA, product 'labelling' has a similar legal status to EU licensing.

The decision of a manufacturer to seek a Product Licence for a given indication is essentially a commercial one. Potential sales are balanced against the cost of conducting the necessary clinical trials. Drugs may be effective outside their licensed indications for different disease states, age ranges, doses and durations. The absence of a formal Product Licence or labelling may reflect the absence of controlled trials supporting the drug's efficacy in these areas. In some cases (e.g. sertraline or quetiapine in generalised anxiety disorder [GAD]) there is sufficient evidence but a licence has not been sought by the manufacturer. Importantly, however, it is also possible that trials have been conducted but have given negative or equivocal results.

Clinicians often assume that drugs with a similar mode of action will be similarly effective for a given indication. This may encourage the assumption that the official labelling for one drug indicates efficacy and safety of another, similar drug. However, apparently similar drugs may differ in respect to active metabolites and in regard to receptor affinity.

Prescribing a drug within its licence or labelling does not guarantee that the patient will come to no harm. Likewise, prescribing outside a licence does not mean that the risk–benefit ratio is automatically adverse. For example, sertraline and fluoxetine are no less effective for GAD than alternative, licensed drugs.[2] Prescribing outside a licence, usually called 'off-label', does confer extra responsibilities on prescribers, who will be expected to be able to show that they acted in accordance with a respected body of medical opinion (the Bolam test)[3] and that their action was capable of withstanding logical analysis (the Bolitho test).[4] In the UK, both have effectively been superseded, or at least clarified, by the Montgomery vs Lanarkshire Health Board appeal case decision[5] which stated:

> An adult person of sound mind is entitled to decide which, if any, of the available forms of treatment to undergo, and her consent must be obtained before treatment interfering with her bodily integrity is undertaken. The doctor is therefore under a duty to take reasonable care to ensure that the patient is aware of any material risks involved in any recommended treatment, and of any reasonable alternative or variant treatments. The test of materiality is whether, in the circumstances of the particular case, a reasonable person in the patient's position would be likely to attach significance to the risk, or the doctor is or should reasonably be aware that the particular patient would be likely to attach significance to it.

Thus, in the UK at least, the prescriber has a duty to make a patient aware of any material risks associated with the prescribing of any medicines and to outline alternatives.

CHAPTER 14

The General Medical Council allows doctors to prescribe off-label but only where the prescriber is satisfied that there is enough evidence or experience to support efficacy and safety.[6]

In the USA, it is lawful to prescribe off-label 'within a legitimate health care practitioner–patient relationship'.[7] Marketing of off-label use is forbidden but information may be provided following an unsolicited request.[8] Off-label prescribing represents a significant proportion of prescribing in mental health conditions in the USA.[9,10] A similar degree of off-label prescriptions is seen in other countries.[11–13]

Off-label prescribing in psychiatry is less likely to be supported by a strong evidence base than off-label prescribing in other areas of medicine.[14] In psychiatry, small (underpowered) studies (with wide confidence intervals) often influence practice, particularly with respect to treatment-resistant illness (a great many examples can be found in this book). When these small studies are combined in the form of a meta-analysis, considerable heterogeneity is often found, suggesting publication bias (i.e. that some negative studies are not published). Treatments may therefore become incorporated into 'routine custom and practice' in the absence of robust evidence supporting efficacy and/or tolerability, and these treatments may sometimes continue to be used despite the findings of later, larger and more definitive negative studies and meta-analyses. An example of widespread off-label prescribing of a psychotropic in non-mental health conditions is amitriptyline – 93% of UK primary care prescriptions are off-label.[15]

The psychopharmacology special interest group at the Royal College of Psychiatrists published a consensus statement on the use of licensed medicines for unlicensed uses.[16] They noted that unlicensed use is common in general adult psychiatry, with cross-sectional studies showing that up to 50% of patients are prescribed at least one drug outside the terms of its licence. They also note that the prevalence of this type of prescribing is likely to be higher in patients under the age of 18 or over 65, in those with a learning disability, in women who are pregnant or lactating and in those patients who are cared for in forensic psychiatry settings. The main recommendations in the consensus statement are summarised in Box 14.1.

Box 14.1 Recommendations before prescribing 'off-label'

- Exclude licensed alternatives (e.g. they have proved ineffective or poorly tolerated).
- Ensure familiarity with the evidence base for the intended unlicensed use. If unsure, seek advice from another clinician (and possibly a specialist pharmacist).
- Consider and document the potential risks and benefits of the proposed treatment. Share this risk assessment with the patient, and carers if applicable. Document the discussion and the patient's consent or lack of capacity to consent.
- If prescribing responsibility is to be shared with primary care, ensure that the risk assessment and consent issues are shared with the GP.
- Monitor for efficacy and adverse effects; start a low dose and increase slowly.
- Consider publishing the case to add to the body of knowledge.
- Withdraw any treatment that is ineffective or where emergent risks outweigh the benefits.

The more experimental the unlicensed use is, the more important it is to adhere to the above guidance.

The advice is largely echoed by more recent publications from the American Psychiatric Association[17] (who note that off-label prescribing should be reimbursed) and the Royal Australian and New Zealand College of Psychiatrists[18] who emphasise shared decision-making and the presumption of capacity.

Examples of acceptable use of drugs outside their licences/labels

Table 14.5 gives examples of common unlicensed uses of drugs in psychiatric practice. These examples would all fulfil the Bolam and Bolitho criteria in principle. An exhaustive list of unlicensed uses is impossible to prepare as the evidence base is constantly changing and because the expertise and experience of prescribers vary. A particular strategy may be justified in the hands of a specialist in psychopharmacology based in a tertiary referral centre but be much more difficult to justify if initiated by someone with a special interest in psychotherapy who rarely prescribes.

Note that some drugs do not have a UK licence for any indication. Two commonly prescribed examples in psychiatric practice are immediate-release formulations of melatonin (used to treat insomnia in children and adolescents) and pirenzepine (used to treat clozapine-induced hypersalivation). Awareness of the evidence base and documentation of potential benefits, adverse effects and patient consent are especially important here.

Table 14.5 Examples of common unlicensed uses of drugs in psychiatric practice.

Drug/drug group	Unlicensed use(s)	Further information
Second-generation antipsychotics	Psychotic illness other than schizophrenia	Licensed indications vary markedly, and in most cases are unlikely to reflect real differences in efficacy between drugs.
Clozapine	Bipolar disorder	Substantial evidence to support efficacy when standard treatments have failed to control symptoms
Cyproheptadine	Akathisia	Some evidence to support efficacy in this distressing and difficult to treat adverse effect of antipsychotics
Fluoxetine/sertraline	Generalised anxiety disorder	Substantial supporting evidence
Ketamine (racemate)	Refractory depression	Substantial evidence with both racemate and S-isomer
Melatonin (circadin)	Insomnia in children	Licence covers adults >55 years only. Probably preferable to unlicensed formulations of melatonin.
Naltrexone	Self-injurious behaviour in people with learning disabilities	Limited evidence base Acceptable in specialist hands
Sodium valproate	Treatment and prophylaxis of bipolar disorder	Established clinical practice Evidence from other valproate preparations

References

1. EMC. *Summary of Product Characteristics*. 2024; http://www.medicines.org.uk/emc/.
2. Baldwin D, et al. Efficacy of drug treatments for generalised anxiety disorder: systematic review and meta-analysis. *BMJ* 2011; **342**:d1199.
3. Bolam v Friern Barnet Hospital Management Committee [1957] 1 WLR582.
4. Bolitho v City and Hackney Health Authority [1997] 3 WLR1151.
5. British and Irish Legal Information Institute. Montgomery (Appellant) v Lanarkshire Health Board (Respondent) (Scotland). 2015; http://www.bailii.org/uk/cases/UKSC/2015/11.html.
6. General Medical Council. Good practice in prescribing and managing medicines and devices. 2021 (last checked September 2024); https://www.gmc-uk.org/guidance/ethical_guidance/14316.asp.
7. Buckman Co. v. Plaintiffs' Legal Comm. 531 U.S. 341. 2001; https://www.law.cornell.edu/supct/html/98-1768.ZO.html.
8. FindLaw. Off-label use promotion is protected free speech. 2019 (last accessed September 2024); https://www.findlaw.com/legalblogs/second-circuit/off-label-use-promotion-is-protected-free-speech/.
9. Vijay A, et al. Patterns and predictors of off-label prescription of psychiatric drugs. *PLoS One* 2018; **13**:e0198363.
10. Leslie DL, et al. Off-label use of antipsychotic medications in Medicaid. *Am J Manag Care* 2012; **18**:e109–117.
11. Ishtiak-Ahmed K, et al. Treatment indications and potential off-label use of antidepressants among older adults: a population-based descriptive study in Denmark. *Int J Geriatr Psychiatry* 2022; **37**:10.1002/gps.5841.
12. Martínez CE, et al. Antidepressant use and off-label prescribing in primary care in Spain (2013-2018). *An Pediatr (Engl Ed)* 2022; **97**:237–246.
13. Hefner G, et al. Off-label use of antidepressants, antipsychotics, and mood-stabilizers in psychiatry. *J Neural Transm (Vienna)* 2022; **129**:1353–1365.
14. Epstein RS, et al. The many sides of off-label prescribing. *Clin Pharmacol Ther* 2012; **91**:755–758.
15. Wong J, et al. Off-label indications for antidepressants in primary care: descriptive study of prescriptions from an indication based electronic prescribing system. *BMJ* 2017; **356**:j603.
16. Royal College of Psychiatrists. Use of licensed medicines for unlicensed applications in psychiatric practice (2nd edition) (CR210 Dec 2017). 2017 (last accessed September 2024); https://www.rcpsych.ac.uk/improving-care/campaigning-for-better-mental-health-policy/college-reports/2017-college-reports/use-of-licensed-medicines-for-unlicensed-applications-in-psychiatric-practice-2nd-edition-cr210-dec-2017.
17. American Psychiatric Association. APA official actions: position statement on off-label treatments. 2021 (last accessed September 2024); https://www.psychiatry.org/getattachment/053eae03-9e23-422f-ab75-2ea052eb6c81/Position-Off-Label-Treatments.pdf.
18. Royal Australian New Zealand College of Psychiatrists (RANZCP). 'Off-label' prescribing in psychiatry. Professional Practice Guideline 4. 2023 (last accessed September 2024); https://www.ranzcp.org/getmedia/edc66b1d-005b-411d-b277-5c7fddc71ba2/ppg-4-off-label-prescribing-december-2023.pdf.

The Mental Health Act in England and Wales

The 1983 Mental Health Act (MHA) as amended by the 2007 MHA is the legislation within England and Wales that provides the framework for detaining and treating people with mental disorder in hospital. It also allows for the supervision of people in the community. Mental health law as it pertains to other countries is not covered in this book. The guidance here provides a quick summary of the sections that prescribers are likely to come across in their day-to-day work (Box 14.2). It is not an exhaustive list. The Act has a statutory Code of Practice for practitioners and Chapter 25 of the Code provides detailed guidance on the treatment rules of the Act.[1] The MHA can be accessed at www.legislation.gov.uk.

The power to treat under S58 is only for treatment of mental disorder. Physical treatment (generally) is governed by the normal rules of consent or, if the person lacks capacity, the authority of the Mental Capacity Act.

The Responsible Clinician (RC) is usually the patient's consultant.

For the first 3 months of detention, the RC may give medication with or without consent to a person under one of the detention sections named for the treatment of their mental disorder. Thereafter, the patient's consent or a second opinion must be sought. The 3 months' countdown starts when medication for mental disorder is first administered while the patient is detained. This includes a patient detained under S2 who is then, without a break, detained under S3. For practical purposes the 3-month rule is usually calculated from the date of first detention.

CHAPTER 14

Box 14.2 Civil and forensic detention sections	
Section 2	Admission for assessment which lasts for up to 28 days
Section 3	Admission for treatment which may last up to 6 months and is renewable
Section 36	Remand to hospital for treatment
Section 37	Hospital Order made by the courts (runs like an S3)
Notional 37	Treat as if subject to S37. This term is used informally under a number of different circumstances. One example is where a patient was previously detained under S47/49 and their restriction order expires.
Section 38	Interim Hospital Order
Section 41	Restriction order: an order made by the Crown Court restricting discharge. Accompanies S37 and is written as S37/41.
Section 47	Transfer to hospital of prisoners
Section 49	A restriction order which usually accompanies S47 (written as S47/49)
Section 48	Applies to unsentenced prisoners in need of urgent treatment and is accompanied by S49 (written as S48/49)
Section 58	**Treatment requiring consent or a second opinion** Please note **in law it is the Responsible Clinician (RC) who is accountable for the operation of S58**

If a patient consents to treatment, the RC completes a form **T2**. If a patient has not given consent or has not got the capacity to consent, a Second Opinion Appointed Doctor (SOAD) is called. The SOAD then completes a form **T3**.

A copy of the forms T2 and T3 should be kept with the patient's medication chart as recommended in paragraph 25.75 of the Code of Practice.[1]

Completion of forms T2 and T3

The following should be stated on the forms:

- The name of the drug **or** the class of drug.
- If the class of drug is stated, the number of drugs allowed at any one time.
- The route of administration.
- The maximum dosage with reference to BNF guidance.

For example: Antipsychotic, second generation × 1 (oral) within BNF maximum dose limits.

For a patient who has capacity and is consenting to treatment and is only willing to take a particular drug, it is appropriate for the RC to write the name of the drug instead of the name of the class of drug on the T2.

For example: Olanzapine tablets only(oral) within BNF maximum dose limits.

Psychotropics not found in the BNF may be written on a T2 or T3 with their indication.

For example: Melperone tablets (oral) up to a maximum of 25mg daily for the treatment of schizophrenia.

Non-psychotropics used for the treatment of mental disorder should be included on the T2 and T3, for example omega-3 fatty acids (fish oils) in schizophrenia. Antimuscarinics used to treat hypersalivation and the extrapyramidal side effects of antipsychotics should be included too.

Arranging and preparing for SOAD visits

The Code of Practice 25.51 states: 'Clinicians should consider seeking a review by a specialist mental health pharmacist before seeking a SOAD certificate, particularly if the patient's medication regime is complex or unusual.'

Statutory consultees

The SOAD should consult with two people before issuing a T3. One must be a nurse. The other must not be a nurse or a doctor. Both must have been involved with the patient's treatment. These two people are known as statutory consultees. Mental health pharmacists can perform this role where they have been involved in any recent review of a patient's medication.

The Code of Practice 25.56 states:

Statutory consultees may expect to have a private discussion with the SOAD and to be listened to with consideration. Issues that the consultees may be asked about include, but are not limited to:

- the proposed treatment and the patient's ability to consent to it;
- their understanding of the past and present views and wishes of the patient;
- other treatment options and the way in which the decision on the treatment proposal was arrived at;
- the patient's progress and the views of the patient's carers; and
- where relevant, the implications of imposing treatment on a patient who does not want it and the reasons why the patient is refusing treatment.

What is consent?

The Code of Practice 24.34 defines consent as:

… the voluntary and continuing permission of a patient to be given a particular treatment, based on a sufficient knowledge of the purpose, nature, likely effects and risks of that treatment, including the likelihood of its success and any alternatives to it. Permission given under any unfair or undue pressure is not consent.

For a patient to consent formally they must have the 'capacity' to make a decision.

What is capacity?

The Mental Capacity Act 2005 states that:

- People must be assumed to have capacity unless it is established that they lack capacity.
- People are not to be treated as unable to make a decision unless all practicable steps to help them do so have been taken without success.
- People are not to be treated as unable to make a decision merely because they make an unwise decision.

A patient is deemed to lack capacity if they cannot:

- Understand relevant information about the decision to be made; or
- Retain that information in their mind; or
- Use or weigh that information as part of the decision-making process; or
- Communicate their decision (by talking, using sign language or any other means).

The patient needs to fail on only one of the four points above to be deemed not to have capacity. Capacity may change over time so reassessment is important. A person may lack capacity about one decision but not about another.

CHAPTER 14

Section 62 urgent treatment

If after 3 months medication is needed urgently to treat a patient's mental disorder and it is not covered by a T2 or T3, S62 may be applied.

The Code of Practice 25.38 states:

This applies only if the treatment in question is immediately necessary to:

- save the patient's life;
- prevent a serious deterioration of the patient's condition, and the treatment does not have unfavourable physical or psychological consequences which cannot be reversed;
- alleviate serious suffering by the patient, and the treatment does not have unfavourable physical or psychological consequences which cannot be reversed and does not entail significant physical hazard; or
- prevent patients behaving violently or being a danger to themselves or others, and the treatment represents the minimum interference necessary for that purpose, does not have unfavourable physical or psychological consequences which cannot be reversed and does not entail significant physical hazard.

Each Trust should design a form for the clinician in charge of treatment (usually the consultant) to state what the treatment is, why it is immediately necessary and the length of treatment.

Section 132 duty of managers of hospitals to give information to detained patients

With regard to S132 and consent to treatment the Code of Practice 4.20 states:

Patients must be told what the Act says about treatment for their mental disorder. In particular they must be told:

- the circumstances (if any) in which they can be treated without their consent – and the circumstances in which they have the right to refuse treatment;
- the role of second opinion appointed doctors (SOADs) and the circumstances in which they may be involved; and
- (where relevant) the rules on electroconvulsive therapy (ECT) and medication administered as part of ECT.

Electroconvulsive therapy (ECT)

Section 58a deals with ECT. Treatment for ECT is authorised on forms:

T4	For consenting adults 18 and over, may be written by the RC or SOAD
T5	For consenting patients under 18, to be written by SOAD only
T6	For patients who lack capacity, to be written by SOAD only

All patients under the age of 18 who are to receive ECT, whether or not they are detained under the MHA, must have treatment authorised on a T5 or T6.

Patients who have the capacity to consent must not receive ECT unless they do consent (in emergencies this can, however, be over-ridden under S62 of the Act). There is no 3-month rule with regard to ECT and this also applies to medication given as part of ECT. Hence a form for ECT must always be in place regardless of the first date of detention. The forms should indicate the maximum number of treatments the patient is to receive (Code of Practice paragraph 25.23).

Community patients

Patients on a Community Treatment Order (CTO) should have treatment authorised on one of the following forms:

CTO11	Written by SOAD, after 1 month on a CTO, when the patient lacks capacity
CTO12	Written by the RC when the patient has capacity and is consenting to treatment, after 1 month on a CTO

There is no legal authority to give patients medication in the community if they refuse it.

Reference

1. Gov.UK. Code of practice: Mental Health Act 1983. 2017 (last accessed August 2024); https://www.gov.uk/government/publications/code-of-practice-mental-health-act-1983#history.

Site of administration of intramuscular injections

Table 14.6 gives the sites of administration formally permitted in the individual product's EU licence. Other routes and sites may be possible but pharmacokinetic analysis of administration via these sites is generally not available.

Table 14.6 Sites of administration of intramuscular injections.

Antipsychotic generic name and formulation	Licensed site(s) of administration
Typical antipsychotic (FGA) depots	
Bromperidol decanoate in sesame oil (available in Belgium, Germany, Italy, Luxembourg and the Netherlands[1,2])	Deep intramuscular injection into the **gluteal muscle**. SPCs in some countries recommend to alternate injections into the left and right sides to prevent pain at the injection site.[3]
Flupentixol decanoate in thin vegetable oil derived from coconuts	Deep intramuscular injection into the **upper outer buttock** (dorsogluteal) or **lateral thigh** (vastus lateralis).[4] As with all oil-based injections it is important to ensure, by aspiration before injection, that inadvertent intravascular entry does not occur.[5] This probably applies to dorsogluteal injections only; for all other sites where there are no major blood vessels close to the injection site, this is unnecessary.[4]
Fluphenazine decanoate in sesame oil	Deep intramuscular injection into the **gluteal region**.[4] Has also been administered into the **lateral surface of the thigh muscle** but this is unlicensed. Administration into the deltoid is not recommended by manufacturer.[6] In the USA, licensed to be used 'intramuscularly or subcutaneously'. The site of administration is not specified. Drug leakage appears to be lower after SC injection than after intramuscular administration.[7]
Fluspirilene in vegetable oil[8] (available in some EU countries, Canada, Argentina and Israel[9])	Deep intramuscular injection into the **gluteal muscle** (intragluteal). Because of its microcrystalline form, irritation and inflammation symptoms may occur at the injection site. Manufacturer recommends to alternate between left and right gluteal muscles.[3,10]
Haloperidol decanoate in sesame oil	Deep intramuscular injection into the **gluteal region**.[4] It is recommended to alternate between the two gluteal muscles.[11] As the administration of volumes greater than 3mL is uncomfortable for the patient, such large volumes are not recommended.[11,12] Can also be administered into the **deltoid muscle** according to the manufacturer.[13] Although this is an **unlicensed use**, one trial suggests it is safe and effective.[14]
Perphenazine decanoate in sesame oil (used in the Nordic countries, Belgium, Portugal and the Netherlands[15])	Deep intramuscular injection.[15,16] No other information available.

Table 14.6 *(Continued)*

Antipsychotic generic name and formulation	Licensed site(s) of administration
Perphenazine enanthate in sesame oil (in clinical use in the Nordic countries, Belgium, Portugal and the Netherlands[15])	Deep intramuscular injection into the **gluteal region**.[15,17]
Pipotiazine palmitate in sesame oil[4] (variable availability)	Administration should be by deep intramuscular injection into the **gluteal region**.[18]
Zuclopenthixol decanoate in thin vegetable oil derived from coconuts	Deep intramuscular injection into the **upper outer buttock** (dorsogluteal) or **lateral thigh** (vastus lateralis).[4] As with all oil-based injections it is important to ensure, by aspiration before injection, that inadvertent intravascular entry does not occur.[19]
Atypical antipsychotic (SGA) depots	
Aripiprazole Prefilled syringe for prolonged-release suspension	***Gluteal muscle*** *administration*[4] Gluteal injections should be alternated between the two gluteal muscles. ***Deltoid muscle*** *administration*[4,20] Deltoid injections should be alternated between the two deltoid muscles.[20] The powder and vehicle vials and the prefilled syringe are for single use only.[4]
Aripiprazole lauroxil Prefilled syringe for extended-release suspension	Intramuscular administration into the **deltoid** or **gluteal** (441mg dose only) muscle.[4,21]
Aripiprazole lauroxil nanocrystal dispersion Prefilled syringe for extended-release suspension	Intramuscular injection into the **deltoid** or **gluteal** muscle.[22] Not intended for repeat dosing. Given as a single dose to initiate treatment with aripiprazole lauroxil.[22]
Olanzapine pamoate monohydrate Powder and vehicle for prolonged-release suspension	Olanzapine pamoate monohydrate should **only** be administered by deep intramuscular **gluteal** injection by a healthcare professional trained in the appropriate injection technique and in locations where post-injection observation and access to appropriate medical care in the case of overdose can be assured.[23]
Paliperidone palmitate 1-monthly Prolonged-release suspension for injection every month	Injected slowly, deep into the **deltoid or dorsogluteal muscle** (the two initial loading doses should be administered in the deltoid muscle so as to attain therapeutic concentrations rapidly).[4,24] Following the second initiation dose, monthly maintenance doses can be administered in either the deltoid or gluteal muscle. Administration should be in a single injection. The dose should not be given in divided injections.[24]

(Continued)

CHAPTER 14

Table 14.6 (*Continued*)

Antipsychotic generic name and formulation	Licensed site(s) of administration
Paliperidone palmitate 3-monthly Prolonged-release suspension for injection every 3 months	***Deltoid muscle** administration*[25] The specified needle for administration of Trevicta into the deltoid muscle is determined by the patient's weight (see manufacturer's advice). It should be administered into the centre of the deltoid muscle. Deltoid injections should be alternated between the two deltoid muscles. ***Gluteal muscle** administration*[25] To be administered into the upper outer quadrant of the gluteal muscle. Gluteal injections should be alternated between the two gluteal muscles.
Paliperidone palmitate 6-monthly Prolonged-release suspension for injection every 6 months	Byannli is for **gluteal intramuscular use only. It must not be administered by any other route.** Each injection must be administered only by a healthcare professional giving the full dose in a single injection. It should be injected slowly, deep into the upper outer quadrant of the gluteal muscle. A switch between the two gluteal muscles should be considered for future injections in the event of injection site discomfort. Needles from the 3-monthly or 1-monthly paliperidone palmitate injectable pack or other commercially available needles **must not** be used when administering Byannli.[26]
Risperidone microspheres (Consta) Powder and vehicle for prolonged-release suspension	Following reconstitution, administer via deep intramuscular **deltoid** or **gluteal** injection.[27]
Risperidone ISM (Okedi) Powder and solvent for extended-release suspension	After reconstitution, administer by deep intramuscular **deltoid** or **gluteal** injection.[28]
Risperidone 2-weekly injection (Rykindo) Prefilled syringe and powder vial for prolonged-release suspension	After reconstitution, administer via intramuscular injection into the **gluteal muscle**.[29]
Risperidone subcutaneous long-acting injections (Perseris [RBP-7000], Uzedy [TV-46000]) Extended-release suspension	Subcutaneous administration in the **abdomen** or **upper arm**.[30,31] Prior to administration of Perseris (RBP-7000), the liquid and powder syringes need to be mixed by passing the contents back and forth between the syringes.
Intramuscular injections for rapid tranquilisation	
Aripiprazole Solution for injection	To enhance absorption and minimise variability, injection into the **deltoid or deep within the gluteus maximus muscle**, avoiding adipose regions, is recommended.[32]
Haloperidol Solution for injection	Intramuscular administration.[33] Preferably, the **gluteal muscle** is selected when the dosage volume is high. The **deltoid muscle** is preferred for low doses of the injection. However, there is no information on the dosage limit for these specific muscle groups. Choice of site is at the discretion of the prescriber according to the manufacturer.[34]

Table 14.6 (*Continued*)

Antipsychotic generic name and formulation	Licensed site(s) of administration
Lorazepam Solution for injection	Intramuscular administration. Can be administered into the **gluteal, deltoid or frontal thigh area** according to the manufacturer.[35] A 1:1 dilution of Ativan injection with normal saline or Sterile Water for Injection BP is recommended in order to facilitate intramuscular administration and absorption.[18]
Olanzapine Powder for solution for injection	Inject slowly, deep into the muscle mass. The exact site of administration is not specified and choice of muscle site should be a clinical decision according to the manufacturer.[36] Not to be used intravenously* or subcutaneously. Use the solution immediately within 1 hour of reconstitution.[37] *Intravenous use has been reported[38,39] but is off-licence/label.
Promethazine hydrochloride Solution for injection	By deep intramuscular injection into a large muscle.[40] Can be administered into the **thigh, upper arm or gluteal region**. Ensure muscle mass is sufficient for the volume being injected.[6]
Other intramuscular injections	
Clotiapine 40mg/4mL injection (available in Argentina, Belgium, Israel, Italy, Luxembourg, South Africa, Spain, Switzerland and Taiwan[41])	By intramuscular injection.[41] No other information available.
Clozapine intramuscular injection 25mg/mL (unlicensed)[42,43]	Only for deep intramuscular administration into the **gluteal muscle**. 25mg IM clozapine = 50mg oral. The maximum volume that can be injected into each site is 4mL (100mg). For doses greater than 100mg daily, the dose may be divided and administered into two sites. (Injection sites should be rotated as per usual IM practice.) Administration into the lateral thigh and deltoid muscles has been used in one case series.[42]

FGA, first-generation antipsychotic; ISM, in situ microparticles; SC, subcutaneous; SGA, second-generation antipsychotic; SPC, summary of product characteristics.

CHAPTER 14

References

1. Purgato M, et al. Bromperidol decanoate (depot) for schizophrenia. *Cochrane Database Syst Rev* 2012; **11**:CD001719.
2. Riboldi I, et al. Practical guidance for the use of long-acting injectable antipsychotics in the treatment of schizophrenia. *Psychol Res Behav Manag* 2022; **15**:3915–3929.
3. Eumedica. Medical Information Department – written communication, 2020.
4. Janssen UK. *Guidance on the Administration to Adults of Oil-Based Depot and Other Long-Acting Intramuscular Antipsychotic Injections*, 7th edn. 2022 (last accessed August 2024); https://www.hpft.nhs.uk/media/6180/guidance-on-im-administration-of-oil-based-depots-and-other-long-acting-antipsychotic-injections-7th-edition.pdf.
5. Lundbeck Ltd. Summary of product characteristics. Depixol 20mg/ml solution for injection (flupentixol decanoate). 2021 (last accessed August 2024); https://www.medicines.org.uk/emc/product/995/smpc.
6. Sanofi. Medical Information Department – verbal and written communication, 2017.
7. Glazer WM, et al. Injection site leakage of depot neuroleptics: intramuscular versus subcutaneous injection. *J Clin Psychiatry* 1987; **48**:237–239.
8. Spanarello S, et al. The pharmacokinetics of long-acting antipsychotic medications. *Curr Clin Pharmacol* 2014; **9**:310–317.
9. Abhijnhan A, et al. Depot fluspirilene for schizophrenia. *Cochrane Database Syst Rev* 2007; **2007**:CD001718.
10. iMedikament.de. IMAP. 2024 (last accessed August 2024); https://imedikament.de/imap.

11. Essential Pharma Ltd. Medical Information Department – written communication, 2024.

12. Essential Pharma Ltd (Malta). Summary of product characteristics. HALDOL Decanoate (haloperidol decanoate) 100mg/ml solution for injection. 2023 (last checked August 2024); https://www.medicines.org.uk/emc/product/15246/smpc#gref.

13. Janssen. Medical Information Department – verbal and written communication, 2024.

14. McEvoy JP, et al. Effectiveness of paliperidone palmitate vs haloperidol decanoate for maintenance treatment of schizophrenia: a randomized clinical trial. *JAMA* 2014; **311**:1978–1987.

15. Quraishi S, et al. Depot perphenazine decanoate and enanthate for schizophrenia. *Cochrane Database Syst Rev* 2000; **2**:CD001717.

16. Laakeinfo.fi. PERATSIN DECANOATE solution for injection 108mg/ml (perphenazine decanoate). 2023 (last accessed August 2024); https://laakeinfo.fi/Medicine.aspx?m=2333.

17. Starmark JE, et al. Abscesses following prolonged intramuscular administration of perphenazine enantate. *Acta Psychiatr Scand* 1980; **62**:154–157.

18. myHealthbox 2012-2024. *Summary of Product Characteristics*. 2024 (last accessed August 2024); https://myhealthbox.eu/en/.

19. Lundbeck Ltd. Summary of product characteristics. Clopixol 200mg/ml solution for injection (zuclopenthixol decanoate). 2022 (last accessed August 2024); https://www.medicines.org.uk/emc/product/6414/smpc.

20. Otsuka Pharmaceuticals (UK) Ltd. Summary of product characteristics. Abilify Maintena 300mg powder and solvent for prolonged-release suspension for injection in pre-filled syringe (aripiprazole). 2024 (last accessed August 2024); https://www.medicines.org.uk/emc/product/12955/smpc%202022.

21. Alkermes Inc. Highlights of prescribing information. ARISTADA® (aripiprazole lauroxil) extended-release injectable suspension for intramuscular use. 2018 (last accessed August 2024); https://www.accessdata.fda.gov/drugsatfda_docs/label/2018/207533s013lbl.pdf.

22. Alkermes Inc. Highlights of prescribing information. ARISTADA INITIO® (aripiprazole lauroxil) extended-release injectable suspension, for intramuscular use. 2023; https://www.aristada.com/downloadables/ARISTADA-INITIO-PI.pdf.

23. Eli Lily and Company Ltd. Summary of product characteristics. Zypadhera (olanzapine pamoate monohydrate) 210mg powder and solvent for prolonged release suspension for injection. 2023 (last assessed August 2024); https://www.medicines.org.uk/emc/product/6429/smpc.

24. Janssen-Cilag Ltd. Summary of product characteristics. Xeplion (paliperidone) 25mg, 50mg, 75mg, 100mg, and 150mg prolonged-release suspension for injection. 2023 (last accessed May 2024); https://www.medicines.org.uk/emc/product/7652/smpc.

25. Janssen-Cilag Ltd. Summary of product characteristics. TREVICTA 175mg, 263mg, 350mg, 525mg prolonged release suspension for injection. 2023 (last accessed August 2024); https://www.medicines.org.uk/emc/medicine/32050.

26. Janssen-Cilag Ltd. Summary of product characteristics. Byannli 700mg prolonged-release suspension for injection in pre-filled syringe (paliperidone). 2023 (last accessed August 2024); https://www.medicines.org.uk/emc/product/13307/smpc.

27. Janssen-Cilag Ltd. Summary of product characteristics. RISPERDAL CONSTA 25mg powder and solvent for prolonged-release suspension for intramuscular injection (risperidone). 2022 (last assessed August 2024); https://www.medicines.org.uk/emc/medicine/9939.

28. ROVI Biotech Ltd. Summary of product characteristics. Okedi (risperidone) 100mg powder and solvent for prolonged-release suspension for injection pre-filled syringes. 2023 (last accessed August 2024); https://www.medicines.org.uk/emc/product/13778/smpc.

29. Shandong Luye Pharmaceutical Co Ltd. Highlights of prescribing information. RYKINDO® (risperidone) for extended-release injectable suspension for intramuscular use. 2023 (last checked June 2024); https://www.accessdata.fda.gov/drugsatfda_docs/label/2023/212849s000lbl.pdf.

30. Indivior UK Ltd. Highlights of prescribing information. PERSERIS (risperidone) for extended-release injectable suspension, for subcutaneous use. 2018 (last accessed September 2024); https://www.accessdata.fda.gov/drugsatfda_docs/label/2018/210655s000lbl.pdf.

31. Teva Neuroscience Inc. Highlights of prescribing information. UZEDY (risperidone) extended-release injectable suspension for subcutaneous use. 2024 (last checked June 2024); https://www.uzedy.com/globalassets/uzedy/prescribing-information.pdf.

32. Otsuka Pharmaceutical (UK) Ltd. Summary of product characteristics. Abilify 7.5mg/ml solution for injection (intramuscular) (aripiprazole). 2023 (last accessed August 2024); https://www.medicines.org.uk/emc/product/6239/smpc.

33. ADVANZ Pharma. Summary of product characteristics. Haloperidol injection BP 5mg/ml. 2024 (last accessed August 2024); https://www.medicines.org.uk/emc/product/514.

34. Concordia International. Medical Information Department – verbal and written communication, 2017.

35. Macure Pharma UK Ltd. Medical Information Department – written communication, 2024.

36. Lilly UK. Medical Information Department – verbal and written communication, 2017.

37. Eramol (UK) Ltd. Summary of product characteristics. Xyquila 10mg powder for solution for injection (olanzapine). 2023 (last accessed August 2024); https://www.medicines.org.uk/emc/product/15138/smpc.

38. Wang M, et al. A retrospective comparison of the effectiveness and safety of intravenous olanzapine versus intravenous haloperidol for agitation in adult intensive care unit patients. *J Intensive Care Med* 2022; **37**:222–230.

39. Khorassani F, et al. Intravenous olanzapine for the management of agitation: review of the literature. *Ann Pharmacother* 2019; **53**:853–859.

40. Sanofi. Medical Information Department – written communication, 2024.

41. Carpenter S, et al. Clotiapine for acute psychotic illnesses. *Cochrane Database Syst Rev* 2004; **4**:CD002304.

42. Henry R, et al. Evaluation of the effectiveness and acceptability of intramuscular clozapine injection: illustrative case series. *BJPsych Bull* 2020; **44**:239–243.

43. Casetta C, et al. A retrospective study of intramuscular clozapine prescription for treatment initiation and maintenance in treatment-resistant psychosis. *Br J Psychiatry* 2020; **217**:506–513.

Chapter 15

Miscellany

Biochemical and haematological effects of psychotropics

Almost all psychotropics have haematology- or biochemistry-related adverse effects that may be detected using routine blood tests. While many of these changes are idiosyncratic and not clinically significant, others, such as the agranulocytosis associated with agents such as clozapine, will require regular monitoring of the full blood count. In general, where an agent has a high incidence of biochemical/haematological adverse effects or a rare but potentially fatal effect, regular monitoring is required as discussed in other sections.

For other agents, laboratory-related adverse effects are comparatively rare (prevalence usually less than 1%), are often reversible upon cessation of the putative offending agent and are not always clinically significant. It should further be noted that medical comorbidity, polypharmacy and the effects of non-prescribed agents including substances of abuse and alcohol may also influence biochemical and haematological parameters. In some cases, where a clear temporal association between starting the agent and the onset of laboratory changes is unclear, then withdrawal and rechallenge with the agent in question may be considered. Where there is doubt as to the aetiology and significance of the effect, the appropriate source of expert advice should always be consulted.

Tables 15.1 and 15.2 summarise those agents with identified biochemical and haematological effects from information compiled from various sources.[1–9] In many cases the evidence for these various effects is limited, with information obtained mostly from case reports, case series and information supplied by manufacturers. For further details about each individual agent, the reader is encouraged to consult the appropriate section of this book as well as other specialist sources, particularly product literature relating to individual drugs.

The Maudsley® Prescribing Guidelines in Psychiatry, Fifteenth Edition. David M. Taylor, Thomas R. E. Barnes and Allan H. Young.
© 2025 David M. Taylor. Published 2025 by John Wiley & Sons Ltd.

Table 15.1 Summary of biochemical changes associated with psychotropics.

Parameter	Reference range[10]	Agents reported to raise levels	Agents reported to lower levels
Alanine aminotransferase (ALT)	F: ≤34U/L M: ≤45U/L (may be higher in obesity)	**Antipsychotics:** asenapine, benperidol, cariprazine, clozapine, haloperidol, loxapine, lumateperone tosylate, olanzapine, phenothiazines, quetiapine, risperidone/paliperidone **Antidepressants:** agomelatine, bupropion, MAOIs, mianserin, mirtazapine, SNRIs, SSRIs (especially paroxetine and sertraline), TCAs, trazodone, vortioxetine **Anxiolytics/hypnotics:** barbiturates, benzodiazepines, buspirone, clomethiazole, promethazine, suvorexant, tasimelteon, zolpidem **Mood stabilisers:** carbamazepine, lamotrigine, valproate **Other:** alcohol, atomoxetine, beta-blockers, caffeine, cocaine, disulfiram, naltrexone, opioids, stimulants (abused)	Vigabatrin
Albumin	35–50g/L (gradually decreases after age 40)	Microalbuminuria may be a feature of metabolic syndrome secondary to psychotropic use (especially phenothiazines, clozapine, olanzapine and possibly quetiapine)	Chronic use of amfetamine or cocaine
Alkaline phosphatase	50–120U/L	Baclofen, beta-blockers, benzodiazepines, caffeine (excess/chronic use), carbamazepine, citalopram, clozapine, disulfiram, duloxetine, galantamine, haloperidol, loxapine, memantine, modafinil, nortriptyline, olanzapine, phenytoin, sertraline, topiramate, trazodone, valbenazine, valproate; also associated with agents causing NMS	Buprenorphine, fluoxetine (in children), zolpidem (rarely)
Ammonia	11–32µmol/L (increased following meals and exercise)	Barbiturates, carbamazepine, tobacco smoking, topiramate, valproate (may present with signs of encephalopathy)	None known

Table 15.1 (*Continued*)

Parameter	Reference range[10]	Agents reported to raise levels	Agents reported to lower levels
Amylase	28–100U/L	Alcohol (acute), donepezil, opioids, pregabalin, rivastigmine, SSRIs (rarely) **Agents associated with pancreatitis:** alcohol, carbamazepine, clozapine, olanzapine, valproate	None known
Aspartate aminotransferase (AST)	F: ≤34U/L M: ≤45U/L	As for ALT; baclofen. Note: ALT is preferred as an indicator of liver damage	Trifluoperazine, vigabatrin
Bicarbonate	22–29mmol/L	Laxative abuse	Agents associated with SIADH: all antidepressants, antipsychotics (clozapine, haloperidol, olanzapine, phenothiazines, pimozide, risperidone/paliperidone, quetiapine); carbamazepine; also associated with agents causing metabolic acidosis (alcohol, cocaine, topiramate, zonisamide)
Bilirubin	≤21µmol/L (total)	Amitriptyline, atomoxetine, benzodiazepines, carbamazepine, chlordiazepoxide, chlorpromazine, citalopram, clomethiazole, clozapine, disulfiram, fluphenazine, imipramine, lamotrigine, meprobamate, milnacipran, olanzapine, phenothiazines, phenytoin, promethazine, sertraline, valbenazine, valproate; also associated with agents causing cholestasis/ hepatic damage	Barbiturates
C-reactive protein	<10mg/L	Buprenorphine (rare); also associated with agents causing myocarditis (clozapine)	None known
Calcium	2.20–2.60mmol/L (total, adjusted) 1.15–1.34mmol/L (ionised)	Lithium (rare)	Barbiturates, carbamazepine, haloperidol, valproate
Carbohydrate-deficient transferrin (CDT)	≤1.5%	Alcohol (CDT levels of 1.6–1.9% suggest high intake; levels ≥2% suggest excessive intake)	None known

(*Continued*)

Table 15.1 (Continued)

Parameter	Reference range[10]	Agents reported to raise levels	Agents reported to lower levels
Chloride	95–108mmol/L	Agents causing hyperchloraemic metabolic acidosis: topiramate, zonisamide	Medications associated with SIADH: all antidepressants, antipsychotics (clozapine, haloperidol, olanzapine, phenothiazines, pimozide, risperidone/paliperidone, quetiapine); carbamazepine, laxative abuse
Cholesterol (total)	≤5.2mmol/L (usually compared with recommended action limits rather than reference ranges)	Antipsychotics, especially those implicated in the metabolic syndrome (clozapine, olanzapine, phenothiazines, quetiapine). Rarely: aripiprazole, beta-blockers (additive effects with clozapine), carbamazepine, disulfiram, duloxetine, memantine, mirtazapine, modafinil, phenytoin, rivastigmine, sertraline, venlafaxine	Prazosin, thyroid agents
Creatine kinase	F: 25–200U/L M: 40–320U/L (range for people of European descent; may be higher in other ethnic groups)	Bremelanotide, brexpiprazole, cariprazine, clonidine, clozapine (when associated with seizures), cocaine, dexamfetamine, donepezil, lumateperone, olanzapine, pregabalin; also associated with agents causing NMS and SIADH; agents administered intramuscularly	None known
Creatinine	F: 55–100µmol/L M: 60–120µmol/L	Clozapine, lithium, lurasidone, thioridazine, valproate; medications associated with rhabdomyolysis (benzodiazepines, dexamfetamine, pregabalin, thioridazine); also associated with agents causing renal impairment, NMS and SIADH	None known
Ferritin	F: 15–150mcg/L M: 30–400mcg/L (increases with age)	Alcohol (acutely and in alcoholic liver disease)	None known

CHAPTER 15

Table 15.1 (*Continued*)

Parameter	Reference range[10]	Agents reported to raise levels	Agents reported to lower levels
Gamma-glutamyl transferase (GGT)	F: ≤38U/L M: ≤55U/L (limits twofold higher in persons of African ancestry)	**Antidepressants:** mirtazapine, SSRIs (paroxetine and sertraline implicated), TCAs, trazodone, venlafaxine **Anticonvulsants/mood stabilisers:** carbamazepine, lamotrigine, phenobarbitone, phenytoin, valproate **Antipsychotics:** benperidol, chlorpromazine, clozapine, fluphenazine, haloperidol, olanzapine, quetiapine **Other:** alcohol, barbiturates, clomethiazole, dexamfetamine, modafinil, tobacco smoking	None known
Glucose	Fasting: 2.8–6.1mmol/L Random: <11.1mmol/L	**Antidepressants:** MAOIs, SSRIs/SNRIs,* TCAs* **Antipsychotics:** chlorpromazine, clozapine, haloperidol,* olanzapine,* quetiapine and others **Substances of abuse:** amfetamine, methadone, opioids **Other:** baclofen, beta-blockers,* bupropion,* caffeine* (in diabetics), clonidine, dexmedetomidine,* donepezil, gabapentin, galantamine, lithium,* nicotine, sympathomimetics, thyroid agents, valbenazine	Alcohol; rarely with duloxetine, haloperidol, pregabalin, TCAs. Medications associated with metabolic syndrome may result in raised or decreased glucose levels
HbA$_{1c}$	20–39mmol/mol		Lithium, MAOIs, SSRIs
Lactate dehydrogenase	90–200U/L (levels rise gradually with age)	Benzodiazepines, clozapine, methadone, TCAs (especially imipramine), valproate; also associated with agents causing NMS	None known
Lipoproteins: HDL	>1.2mmol/L	Carbamazepine, nicotine, phenobarbital, phenytoin	Beta-blockers, olanzapine, phenothiazines, valproate
Lipoproteins: LDL	<3.5mmol/L	Beta-blockers, caffeine (controversial), carbamazepine, chlorpromazine, clozapine, iloperidone, memantine, mirtazapine, modafinil, olanzapine, phenothiazines, quetiapine, risperidone/paliperidone, rivastigmine, venlafaxine	Prazosin

Table 15.1 (*Continued*)

Parameter	Reference range[10]	Agents reported to raise levels	Agents reported to lower levels
Phosphate	0.8–1.5mmol/L	Dexamfetamine; also associated with agents causing NMS	Carbamazepine, lithium, mianserin, topiramate
Potassium	3.5–5.3mmol/L	Beta-blockers, lithium	Alcohol, disulfiram, caffeine, cocaine, haloperidol, lithium, mianserin, pregabalin, reboxetine, rivastigmine, sodium oxybate, sympathomimetics, topiramate, zonisamide; may also be a feature of delirium tremens
Prolactin	Normal: <350mU/L Abnormal: >600mU/L	**Antidepressants:** especially amoxapine, MAOIs and TCAs; SSRIs and venlafaxine also implicated **Antipsychotics:** amisulpride, haloperidol, pimozide, risperidone/paliperidone, sulpiride and others (aripiprazole,[†] asenapine, brexpiprazole, cariprazine, clozapine, lurasidone, olanzapine, quetiapine and ziprasidone have minimal effects on prolactin levels) **Other:** benzodiazepines, buspirone, deutetrabenazine, opioids, ramelteon, tetrabenazine, valbenazine	Aripiprazole, dopamine agonists, pirenzepine
Protein (total)	60–80g/L	None known	Olanzapine (rarely)
Sodium	133–146mmol/L	Lithium (in overdose)	**Antidepressants:** especially SSRIs/SNRIs; others also implicated – see section on hyponatraemia in Chapter 3 **Antipsychotics:** all (via SIADH) **Mood stabilisers:** carbamazepine, lithium, valproate **Other:** benzodiazepines, clonidine, donepezil, memantine, rivastigmine
Testosterone	F: 0.22–2.9nmol/L M: 9.9–27.8nmol/L	Diazepam	Opioids, ramelteon
Thyroid-stimulating hormone	0.3–4.0mU/L	Aripiprazole, carbamazepine, lithium, quetiapine, rivastigmine, sertraline, valproate (slightly)	Moclobemide, thyroid agents
Thyroxine	Free: 9–26pmol/L Total: 60–150nmol/L	Rarely; amfetamine (heavy abuse), moclobemide, propranolol	Barbiturates, carbamazepine, liothyronine, lithium (causes decreased T4 secretion), opioids, phenytoin, valproate. Rarely implicated: aripiprazole, clozapine, quetiapine, rivastigmine, sertraline

Table 15.1 (*Continued*)

Parameter	Reference range[10]	Agents reported to raise levels	Agents reported to lower levels
Triglycerides			None known
Triiodothyronine	Free: 3.0–6.8pmol/L Total: 1.2–2.9nmol/L	Heroin, methadone	Free T3: valproate Total T3: carbamazepine, lithium, propranolol
Urate (uric acid)	F: 0.16–0.36mmol/L M: 0.21–0.43mmol/L (increases with age)	Alcohol (acute), caffeine (false positive), clozapine, levodopa, olanzapine, pindolol, prazosin, topiramate, zonisamide	Sertraline (slightly)
Urea	2.5–7.8 mmol/L (increases with age)	Carbamazepine, levodopa; rarely with agents associated with anticonvulsant hypersensitivity syndrome and rhabdomyolysis	None known

*May also be associated with hypoglycaemia.
†May also be associated with subnormal prolactin levels.
F, female; HbA$_{1c}$, haemoglobin A1c; HDL, high-density lipoprotein; LDL, low-density lipoprotein; M, male; MAOIs, monoamine oxidase inhibitors; NMS, neuroleptic malignant syndrome; SIADH, syndrome of inappropriate antidiuretic hormone; TCAs, tricyclic antidepressants.

Table 15.2 Summary of haematological changes associated with psychotropics.

Parameter	Reference range	Agents reported to raise counts/levels	Agents reported to lower counts/levels
Activated partial thromboplastin time	23–33 seconds	Phenothiazines (especially chlorpromazine)	Modafinil (rare)
Basophils	0.0–0.1×10⁹/L	Clozapine, TCAs (especially desipramine)	None known
Eosinophils	0.04–0.40×10⁹/L	Amoxapine, beta-blockers, bupropion, buspirone, carbamazepine, chloral hydrate, chlorpromazine, clonazepam, clozapine, donepezil, fluphenazine, haloperidol, loxapine, meprobamate, maprotiline, methylphenidate (IV abuse only), modafinil, naltrexone (parenterally administered), olanzapine, promethazine, quetiapine, risperidone/paliperidone, SSRIs, TCAs, tetrazepam, tryptophan,* valproate, venlafaxine; may also be a feature of agents causing a hypersensitivity syndrome	None known

CHAPTER 15

Table 15.2 (*Continued*)

Parameter	Reference range	Agents reported to raise counts/levels	Agents reported to lower counts/levels
Erythrocyte sedimentation rate	F: 1–12mm/h M: 1–10mm/h (increases with age)	Clozapine, dexamfetamine, levomepromazine, maprotiline, SSRIs	Buprenorphine
Haemoglobin	F: 115–165g/L M: 130–180g/L	Clozapine, testosterone, tobacco smoking	Aripiprazole, barbiturates, buprenorphine, bupropion, carbamazepine, chlordiazepoxide, chlorpromazine, donepezil, duloxetine, galantamine, MAOIs, memantine, meprobamate, mianserin, phenytoin, promethazine, rivastigmine, tramadol, trifluoperazine, vigabatrin
Lymphocytes	1.5–4.5×10^9/L	Naltrexone, opioids, tobacco smoking, valproate; may also be a feature of drugs causing hypersensitivity syndrome	Alcohol (chronic), chloral hydrate, clozapine, lithium, mirtazapine (rarely)
Mean cell haemoglobin	27–32pg	Medications associated with megaloblastic anaemia, e.g. all anticonvulsants, nitrous oxide	None known
Mean cell haemoglobin concentration	320–360g/L		
Mean cell volume	80–100fL	Alcohol	
Monocytes	0.2–0.8×10^9/L	Haloperidol	None known
Neutrophils	2.0–7.5×10^9/L (may be lower in people of African descent owing to benign ethnic neutropenia)	Bupropion, carbamazepine,[†] citalopram, chlorpromazine, clozapine,[†] duloxetine, fluoxetine, fluphenazine, haloperidol, lamotrigine, lithium, maprotiline, olanzapine, quetiapine, risperidone/paliperidone, rivastigmine, tiotixene, trazodone, venlafaxine	**Agents associated with agranulocytosis:** amoxapine, aripiprazole, barbiturates, carbamazepine, chlordiazepoxide, chlorpromazine, clozapine,[‡] cocaine (adulterated), diazepam, fluphenazine, haloperidol, meprobamate, mianserin, mirtazapine, olanzapine, pirenzepine, promethazine, risperidone/paliperidone, TCAs (especially imipramine), tranylcypromine, valproate **Agents associated with leucopenia:** amitriptyline, amoxapine, asenapine, bupropion, carbamazepine, cariprazine, chlorpromazine, citalopram, clomipramine, clonazepam, clozapine, duloxetine, fluoxetine, fluphenazine, galantamine, haloperidol, lamotrigine, lorazepam, lumateperone, lurasidone, memantine, meprobamate, mianserin, mirtazapine, modafinil, nitrous oxide, olanzapine, oxazepam, phenelzine, pregabalin, promethazine, quetiapine, tranylcypromine, valproate, venlafaxine, ziprasidone **Agents associated with neutropenia:** clozapine, sertraline, trazodone, valproate
Packed cell volume	F: 0.37–0.47L/L M: 0.40–0.52L/L	Clozapine (rare), testosterone	Benzodiazepines (rare), buprenorphine, naltrexone, vigabatrin

Table 15.2 (*Continued*)

Parameter	Reference range	Agents reported to raise counts/levels	Agents reported to lower counts/levels
Platelets	150–450×10⁹/L	Lamotrigine, lithium†	Alcohol, barbiturates, beta-blockers, benzodiazepines, bupropion, buspirone, carbamazepine, chlordiazepoxide, chlorpromazine, clonazepam, clonidine, clozapine,† cocaine, diazepam, donepezil, duloxetine, fluoxetine, fluphenazine, lamotrigine, meprobamate, methadone, methylphenidate, mirtazapine, naltrexone, nitrous oxide, olanzapine, pirenzepine, promethazine, quetiapine, risperidone/paliperidone, rivastigmine, sertraline, TCAs, tranylcypromine, trazodone, trifluoperazine, valproate, venlafaxine, ziprasidone; may also be a feature of drugs causing hypersensitivity syndrome **Agents associated with impaired platelet aggregation:** chlordiazepoxide, citalopram, diazepam, fluoxetine, fluvoxamine, paroxetine, piracetam, sertraline, valproate
Prothrombin time (PT)/international normalised ratio (INR)	PT: 10–13 seconds INR: 0.8–1.2	Chloral hydrate, disulfiram, fluoxetine, fluvoxamine, mirtazapine, valproate; also agents interacting with warfarin	Barbiturates, carbamazepine, phenytoin, tiotixene
Red blood count	F: 3.8–5.8×10¹²/L M: 4.5–6.5×10¹²/L	Lithium, testosterone	Buprenorphine, carbamazepine, chlordiazepoxide, chlorpromazine, donepezil, haloperidol, meprobamate, phenytoin, quetiapine, trifluoperazine
Red cell distribution width	11.5–14.5%	Agents associated with anaemia, e.g. carbamazepine, chlordiazepoxide, citalopram, clonazepam, diazepam, lamotrigine, memantine, mirtazapine, sertraline, tranylcypromine, trazodone, valproate, venlafaxine	None known
Reticulocyte count	0.5–2.5% (or 50–100×10⁹/L)	None known	Carbamazepine, chlordiazepoxide, chlorpromazine, meprobamate, phenytoin, trifluoperazine **Agents associated with pure red cell aplasia:** carbamazepine, clozapine, valproate

*Previous reports of eosinophilia-myalgia syndrome may have been due to a contaminant from a single manufacturer.

†May raise or lower levels.

‡Note that in rare cases clozapine has been associated with a 'morning pseudo-neutropenia' with lower levels of circulating neutrophil levels. As neutrophil counts may follow circadian rhythms, repeating the FBC at a later time of day may be instructive.

F, female; M, male; MAOIs, monoamine oxidase inhibitors; TCAs, tricyclic antidepressants.

References

1. Joint Formulary Committee. *British National Formulary (online)*. London: BMJ and Pharmaceutical Press; https://www.medicinescomplete.com/.

2. Aronson J. *Meyler's Side Effects of Drugs: The International Encyclopedia of Adverse Drug Reactions and Interactions*. Amsterdam: Elsevier Science; 2015.

3. Foster R. *Clinical Laboratory Investigation and Psychiatry. A Practical Handbook*. New York: Informa; 2008.

4. Oyesanmi O, et al. Hematologic side effects of psychotropics. *Psychosomatics* 1999; 40:414–421.

5. Stubner S, et al. Blood dyscrasias induced by psychotropic drugs. Pharmacopsychiatry 2004; 37 Suppl 1:S70–S78.

6. Pharmaceutical Press. *Martindale: The Complete Drug Reference*. 2024; https://www.medicinescomplete.com/.

7. National Institute of Diabetes and Digestive and Kidney Diseases. *LiverTox: Clinical and Research Information on Drug-Induced Liver Injury*. 2012; https://www.ncbi.nlm.nih.gov/books/NBK547852/.

8. Medicines Complete. *AHFS Drug Information*. 2024; https://www.medicinescomplete.com/mc/ahfs/current/.

9. US Food and Drug Administration. *Drugs@FDA: FDA-Approved Drugs*. 2024; https://www.accessdata.fda.gov/scripts/cder/daf/.

10. Association for Laboratory Medicine. *Analyte Monographs Alongside the National Library of Medicine Catalogue*. 2024; https://labmed.org.uk/our-resources/science-knowledge-hub/analyte-monographs.html.

Summary of psychiatric adverse effects of non-psychotropics

It is increasingly recognised that non-psychotropic medications can induce a wide range of psychiatric symptoms.[1] Up to two-thirds of all drugs have potential psychiatric adverse effects listed in their product labelling,[2] although in most cases the evidence supporting a causal link is limited. Psychiatric adverse effects are poorly characterised in drug clinical trials, often only becoming apparent during post-marketing surveillance.[3] Given this level of uncertainty, suspected psychiatric adverse effects should be diagnosed and managed on a case-by-case basis. As a general guide, the psychiatric adverse effects of non-psychotropics are shown in Table 15.3. For individual drugs and agents not listed in this table, additional sources of information and the product literature should be consulted. Note that psychiatric adverse effects of drugs used in psychiatry and drugs for human immunodeficiency virus (HIV) and epilepsy are summarised elsewhere in this book.

Table 15.3 Summary of psychiatric adverse drug reactions (ADRs) with non-psychotropics.[4–7]

Drug	Psychiatric adverse effect	Comment
Analgesics		
Opioids	Sedation, dysphoria, confusion, mood changes including euphoria, sleep disturbances, hallucinations, psychosis, delirium, dependence	Psychiatric ADRs are relatively common with opioids. Psychosis during opioid withdrawal has also been reported rarely.[8]
5HT$_1$ agonists (e.g. sumatriptan)	Fatigue, anxiety, panic attacks	
Antibiotics		
Cephalosporins, penicillins, quinolones (including fluoroquinolones), tetracyclines	Sleep disturbances (insomnia and somnolence, abnormal dreams, nightmares), anxiety, delirium and confusional states, depression and agitation, psychotic symptoms (e.g. hallucinations, suicidal ideation)	All antibiotics can cause delirium. Patients with underlying medical conditions can be at higher risk of developing psychiatric ADRs. Of the quinolones, ciprofloxacin causes the most psychiatric ADRs, including mood disturbances, agitation and confusion. Onset of psychiatric ADRs can be fast, e.g. after one dose.
Isoniazid[9]	Mania, psychosis	Mood-elevating properties have long been noted. In rare cases has been associated with the emergence of manic/psychotic symptoms.
Antimalarials		
Chloroquine, mefloquine	Psychosis including hallucinations, panic attacks, suicidal ideation and attempts, anxiety, depression, restlessness, confusion. Abnormal dreams/nightmares are common with mefloquine.	Symptoms begin early in treatment. Patients should be advised to stop treatment if these develop and seek medical advice. Psychiatric ADRs are more common with mefloquine than chloroquine. Reactions can even occur after discontinuation of the drug. Mefloquine should not be prescribed for patients with an active or a history of a psychiatric diagnosis.

(Continued)

CHAPTER 15

Table 15.3 *(Continued)*

Drug	Psychiatric adverse effect	Comment
Antiparkinsonian treatments		
Levodopa	Visual hallucinations, depression, hypomania, sleep disturbances, abnormal dreams, cognitive impairment, agitation, psychosis, delirium	
Dopamine agonists	Sedation, psychomotor agitation, anxiety, akathisia, sleep disturbances, psychosis, cognitive impairment, delirium, visual hallucinations	These are associated with more psychiatric adverse effects than levodopa
Amantadine	Decreased concentration, sleep disturbances, visual hallucinations, irritability, anxiety, depression, euphoria, fatigue, psychosis, delirium	
Selegiline (MAO-B inhibitor)	Sleep disturbances, agitation, psychosis	Primary metabolites include levamfetamines
Entacapone (COMT inhibitor)	Sleep disturbances, hallucinations, delirium	
Cardiovascular agents		
ACE inhibitors (e.g. captopril, lisinopril)	Fatigue, hallucinations, delirium, mood disturbances	Captopril most strongly associated with mood effects. Overall limited psychiatric ADRs.
Beta-blockers	Fatigue, sedation, sleep disturbances and nightmares, cognitive impairment, depression, hallucinations, psychosis, delirium	Disturbances more common with lipophilic beta-blockers (e.g. propranolol, metoprolol) than with hydrophilic beta-blockers (e.g. atenolol, sotalol, nadolol). Propranolol most commonly associated with depressive symptoms, but even with this drug causality has not clearly been established. Reports of psychiatric ADRs from numerous clinical trials are equivocal.
Calcium channel blockers (e.g. diltiazem, amlodipine)	Mood changes, lethargy, dysphoria, mania, psychosis, delirium, akathisia	Causal association not clearly demonstrated
Statins[10–12] (e.g. simvastatin, atorvastatin)	Cognitive impairment, memory impairment, depression, emotional lability, irritability, sleep disturbance	Causal associations between statins and changes in mood, sleep and cognition have not been established in systematic reviews of RCTs. Statins penetrate the blood–brain barrier; simvastatin has the highest permeability. Switching to hydrophilic statins (e.g. pravastatin, rosuvastatin) has been suggested in suspected cases of moderate to severe psychiatric ADRs.

Table 15.3 (*Continued*)

Drug	Psychiatric adverse effect	Comment
Corticosteroids		
Glucocorticoids (e.g. betamethasone, prednisolone, prednisone)	Mood disorders, mania/hypomania (particularly with higher doses),[13] suicidal ideation, euphoria, agitation, sleep disturbances, psychosis and delirium, dementia, cognitive impairment	Clear causal association. Most substantial associations are with depression and mania.[14] Onset of psychiatric ADRs is often very sudden, and within the first 1–2 weeks of starting treatment. Symptoms generally respond to dose decreases and have been reported in association with several routes of administration (including oral, parenteral and inhaled), although are probably less common with inhalation. Symptoms usually resolve on gradual discontinuation, although duration of symptoms varies considerably.
Other agents		
5α-reductase inhibitors (e.g. finasteride)[15]	Depression, anxiety, suicidality	A pharmacovigilance database study of finasteride found associations with suicidality and other psychological adverse events in younger patients receiving treatment for alopecia but not older patients receiving treatment for BPH.[16]
Chemotherapeutic agents (e.g. 5-fluorouracil, asparaginase, bortezomib, ifosfamide, vincristine)	More commonly: cognitive impairment, delirium, psychosis. Less commonly: depression, anxiety, suicidal ideation	Almost all chemotherapeutic agents are associated with significant psychiatric ADRs, which may be multifactorial in origin (i.e. secondary to the disease process, ADRs and psychological distress). Cancer therapy-associated cognitive changes include difficulty in executive functions, multitasking, short-term memory recall and attention. Cognitive changes seem to be dose-dependent, and certain drugs (methotrexate, fludarabine, cytarabine, 5-fluorouracil, cisplatin) are associated with worse cognitive effects.
Cimetidine	Cognitive impairment, delirium	
Interferons-α and -β	Depression, loss of efficacy of previously effective antidepressants, suicidal ideation, delirium, non-specific psychiatric symptoms. Rare case reports of psychosis and mania with interferon-α.	Psychiatric ADRs are relatively unlikely with interferon-β but much more widely reported with interferon-α. Interferon-α-associated depression responds to antidepressants, use of which can be preventative. Novel diagnostic biomarkers have been investigated to predict which patients are likely to develop interferon-α-associated psychiatric ADRs.

(*Continued*)

CHAPTER 15

Table 15.3 (*Continued*)

Drug	Psychiatric adverse effect	Comment
Isotretinoin[17]	Depression, suicidal ideation, psychosis	Sporadic reports of psychiatric ADRs but a causal link between isotretinoin therapy and depression, anxiety, mood changes or suicidal ideation/suicide has not been established. A recent meta-analysis found no epidemiological evidence to suggest an increased risk of suicide and psychiatric conditions with isotretinoin.[18] Moreover, isotretinoin may be associated with a lower risk of suicide attempt following treatment.[18] Rare, idiosyncratic reactions cannot be ruled out; if they occur the drug should be discontinued. Risk is no higher in those with prior suicide attempts and is not dose- or treatment-duration-related.
Montelukast[19]	Sleep disorders, hallucinations, anxiety, depression, obsessive compulsive symptoms	The UK MHRA has issued warnings about neuropsychiatric reactions associated with montelukast. Reactions have been reported in adults, adolescents and children. Evidence is conflicting, with one systematic review identifying associations with anxiety and sleeping disorders but not suicide and depression-related events.[20]

ACE, angiotensin-converting enzyme; BPH, benign prostatic hyperplasia; COMT, catechol-O-methyltransferase; 5HT, 5-hydroxytryptamine; MAO-B, monoamine oxidase B; MHRA, Medicines and Healthcare products Regulatory Agency; RCTs, randomised controlled trials.

Differential diagnosis of psychiatric adverse effects

A wide range of confounding factors complicate the diagnosis (and perhaps also the recognition) of psychiatric adverse effects. For example, physical illness, co-prescribed medication, non-prescribed agents and pre-existing mental illness may all influence the clinical presentation and outcome. Factors determining the probability of a causal relationship between drugs and psychiatric adverse effects are shown in Box 15.1. To further support clinical decision-making, the Naranjo scale can be used to assess the likelihood of any adverse reaction being drug-related (Table 15.4). Although cessation of the implicated non-psychotropic might be indicated in some cases, such decisions require individual considerations beyond the scope of this book.

Box 15.1 Factors determining the probability of a causal relationship between drugs and psychiatric adverse effects[4,21]

- Temporal relationship between the drug exposure and the psychiatric adverse effect
- Evidence of the specific psychiatric adverse effect occurring with the suspected drug
- Plausible pharmacological mechanism for the psychiatric adverse effect (e.g. dopamine agonists and psychosis)
- Presence of alternative explanations for symptoms (e.g. pre-existing mental illness, de novo psychiatric illness, other drugs)
- Response of symptoms to the withdrawal of the drug
- Effect of rechallenge with the same drug

Table 15.4 Adapted Naranjo adverse drug reaction (ADR) probability scale criteria.[22]

Questions	Yes	No	NA/unknown
1. Are there previous *conclusive* reports on this reaction?	+1	0	0
2. Did the ADR appear after the suspected drug was administered?	+2	−1	0
3. Did the ADR improve when the drug was discontinued?	+1	0	0
4. Did the ADR appear with rechallenge?	+2	−1	0
5. Are there alternative causes for the ADR?	−1	+2	0
6. Did the reaction appear when placebo was given?	−1	+1	0
7. Was the drug detected in the blood at toxic levels?	+1	0	0
8. Was the ADR more severe when the dose was increased, or less severe when the dose was decreased?	+1	0	0
9. Did the patient have a similar reaction to the same or similar drugs in *any* previous exposure?	+1	0	0
10. Was the ADR confirmed by any objective evidence?	+1	0	0

Probability score: ≥9 = definite; 5–8 = probable; 1–4 = possible; ≤0 = doubtful.

CHAPTER 15

References

1. Rudorfer MV, et al. Assessing psychiatric adverse effects during clinical drug development. *Pharmaceut Med* 2012; **26**:363–394.
2. Smith DA. Psychiatric side effects of non-psychiatric drugs. *S D J Med* 1991; **44**:291–292.
3. Holvey C, et al. Psychiatric side effects of non-psychiatric drugs. *Br J Hosp Med (Lond)* 2010; **71**:432–436.
4. Gupta A, et al. Adverse psychiatric effects of non-psychotropic medications. *BJPsych Advances* 2016; **22**:325–334.
5. Huffman JC, et al. Neuropsychiatric consequences of cardiovascular medications. *Dialogues Clin Neurosci* 2007; **9**:29–45.
6. Munjampalli SK, et al. Medicinal-induced behavior disorders. *Neurol Clin* 2016; **34**:133–169.
7. Parker C. Psychiatric effects of drugs for other disorders. *Medicine* 2016; **44**:768–774.
8. Maremmani AG, et al. Substance abuse and psychosis. The strange case of opioids. *Eur Rev Med Pharmacol Sci* 2014; **18**:287–302.
9. Samouco A, et al. Isoniazid-induced mania and the history of antidepressant drugs: case report and literature review. *Bipolar Disord* 2023; **25**:84–87.
10. Ott BR, et al. Do statins impair cognition? A systematic review and meta-analysis of randomized controlled trials. *J Gen Intern Med* 2015; **30**:348–358.
11. Swiger KJ, et al. Statins, mood, sleep, and physical function: a systematic review. *Eur J Clin Pharmacol* 2014; **70**:1413–1422.
12. Tuccori M, et al. Neuropsychiatric adverse events associated with statins: epidemiology, pathophysiology, prevention and management. *CNS Drugs* 2014; **28**:249–272.
13. De Bock M, et al. Corticosteroids and mania: a systematic review. *World J Biol Psychiatry* 2024; **25**:161–174.
14. Koning A, et al. Neuropsychiatric adverse effects of synthetic glucocorticoids: a systematic review and meta-analysis. *J Clin Endocrinol Metab* 2024; **109**:e1442–e1451.
15. Garcia-Argibay M, et al. Association of 5α-reductase inhibitors with dementia, depression, and suicide. *JAMA Netw Open* 2022; **5**:e2248135.
16. Nguyen DD, et al. Investigation of suicidality and psychological adverse events in patients treated with finasteride. *JAMA Dermatol* 2021; **157**:35–42.
17. Liu M, et al. Neurological and neuropsychiatric adverse effects of dermatologic medications. *CNS Drugs* 2016; **30**:1149–1168.
18. Tan NKW, et al. Risk of suicide and psychiatric disorders among isotretinoin users: a meta-analysis. *JAMA Dermatol* 2024; **160**:54–62.
19. Joint Formulary Committee. *British National Formulary (online)*. London: BMJ and Pharmaceutical Press; http://www.medicinescomplete.com.
20. Lo CWH, et al. Neuropsychiatric events associated with montelukast in patients with asthma: a systematic review. *Eur Respir Rev* 2023; **32**:230079.
21. World Health Organization and Uppsala Monitoring Centre. The use of the WHO-UMC system for standardised case causality assessment. 2004; https://www.who.int/docs/default-source/medicines/pharmacovigilance/whocausality-assessment.pdf.
22. Naranjo CA, et al. A method for estimating the probability of adverse drug reactions. *Clin Pharmacol Ther* 1981; **30**:239–245.

Index

Note: Page numbers in **bold** indicate tables and in *italics* indicate figures, where they fall outside the text range.

The Maudsley® Prescribing Guidelines in Psychiatry, Fifteenth Edition. David M. Taylor, Thomas R. E. Barnes and Allan H. Young.
© 2025 David M. Taylor. Published 2025 by John Wiley & Sons Ltd.